Normal and Therapeutic Nutrition

15th edition

Corinne H. Robinson

M.S., D.Sc.(Hon.), R.D.
Professor of Nutrition Emeritus. Formerly, Head, Department of Nutrition and Food, Drexel University, Philadelphia

and

Marilyn R. Lawler, M.S., R.D. Formerly, Associate Director for Patient Services and Teaching, Yale–New Haven Medical Center; Chief Therapeutic Dietitian, Yale–New Haven Medical Center; Instructor, Division of Nursing Education, Southern Connecticut State College, New Haven

Macmillan Publishing Co., Inc.
New York

Collier Macmillan Publishers
London

Earlier editions: *Dietetics for Nurses* by Fairfax T. Proudfit copyright 1918, 1922, 1924, 1927 by Macmillan Publishing Co., Inc., copyright renewed 1946, 1950, 1952, 1955 by Fairfax T. Proudfit; *Nutrition and Diet Therapy* by Fairfax T. Proudfit copyright 1930, 1934, 1938, 1942 by Macmillan Publishing Co., Inc., copyright renewed 1958 by Fairfax T. Proudfit, 1962, 1966 by The First National Bank of Memphis; *Nutrition and Diet Therapy* by Fairfax T. Proudfit and Corinne H. Robinson copyright 1946, 1950, 1955 by Macmillan Publishing Co., Inc., copyright renewed 1974 by Corinne H. Robinson; *Normal and Therapeutic Nutrition* by Fairfax T. Proudfit and Corinne H. Robinson © 1961 by Macmillan Publishing Co., Inc.; *Proudfit-Robinson's Normal and Therapeutic Nutrition* by Corinne H. Robinson © copyright 1967 by Macmillan Publishing Co., Inc.; *Normal and Therapeutic Nutrition* by Corinne H. Robinson copyright © 1972 by Macmillan Publishing Co., Inc.

Macmillan Publishing Co., Inc.
866 Third Avenue, New York, New York 10022

Collier Macmillan Canada, Ltd.

Library of Congress Cataloging in Publication Data

Robinson, Corinne Hogden.
  Normal and therapeutic nutrition.

  Includes bibliographies and index.
  1. Diet in disease. 2. Nutrition.
3. Food—Composition. I. Lawler, Marilyn R.,
joint author. II. Title. [DNLM: 1. Diet
therapy. 2. Nutrition. WB400 R655n]
RM216.R6523 1976   613.2   76-10656
ISBN 0-02-402300-0

The photographs appearing on the verso of title pages for each part were supplied by the following organizations and are used by permission:
Part One: *Aging* Magazine (Oct. 1975), Office of Human Development, Administration on Aging, Department of Health, Education, and Welfare, Washington, D.C.
Part Two: Yale–New Haven Medical Center, New Haven

Printing: 1 2 3 4 5 6 7 8   Year: 7 8 9 0 1 2 3

Preface to the 15th Edition

This revision of *Normal and Therapeutic Nutrition* is published at a time when there is tremendous interest in food, diet, and nutritional science. Students and adults of all ages share such diverse concerns as rapidly rising food costs, world food shortages, vegetarianism, meat from grain-fed animals, food additives, affluence and the effects of excessive intakes, poverty and undernutrition, and need for nutrition education. The authors of this volume have dealt with these and many other concerns of present-day significance.

Normal and Therapeutic Nutrition is intended especially for students of nursing and dietetics. It is a useful reference for the practicing nutritionist, dietitian, physician, nurse, and home economist. As in previous editions, the text is directed toward three objectives: (1) to provide a background in the science of nutrition that individuals can use as the basis for making decisions in dietary planning for themselves or for others in any age group in health and in illness; (2) to show how the principles of nutrition may be integrated with the psychologic, cultural, and economic factors in the daily selection of meals; and (3) to furnish guidelines for education, dietary counseling, and community services.

The concept of dietary balance to maintain or restore the best possible level of health is empha-sized: on the one hand, the diet must furnish sufficient energy and nutrients to meet metabolic needs at all stages of the life cycle; on the other hand, the dangers of excesses that are believed to be etiologic factors in chronic disorders, ranging from dental caries and obesity to cardiovascular and gastrointestinal diseases, are to be avoided. The literature has been extensively reviewed, and the revisions together with the bibliographies are as up-to-date as the time span for book publication permits. Over fifty new illustrations and diagrams are included. Metric measures are used throughout, with English measures given in parentheses.

The text is again divided into two parts. "Normal Nutrition," Part One, includes the following changes and additions: greater clarity for sections on nutrient metabolism (Chapters 4 through 7); emphasis upon trace elements such as zinc (Chapter 8); revision of electrolyte and fluid balance and the inclusion of new line drawings (Chapter 9); mechanisms for vitamin D action (Chapter 10); "health" and "natural" food movements (Chapters 14 and 23); vegetarian diets and diets used by black Americans (Chapter 15); 1974 master food plans and fabricated foods (Chapter 16); food toxicants (Chapter 17); regulations on enrichment and labeling (Chapter 18); overfeeding in infancy and proprietary foods

(Chapter 20); world crisis in food supply (Chapter 23); national nutrition policy, as well as community nutrition programs for women, infants, children, and older Americans, and for heart disease control (Chapter 24).

"Therapeutic Nutrition," Part Two, follows the same organization as in the preceding edition. Much emphasis is given to dietary counseling of the patient in Chapter 25 and for specific conditions in the chapters that follow. Many instructional materials for patient counseling have been listed. Among the additions to Part Two are a table summarizing the effects of drug therapy on nutritive processes (Chapter 25), with further delineation of these effects as specific conditions are discussed; classification of obesity and use of behavior modification in its treatment (Chapter 29); nutritional considerations following jejunoileal bypass surgery for obesity (Chapters 29 and 36), and in esophageal reflux (Chapter 32), anorexia nervosa (Chapter 39), and sickle cell anemia (Chapter 43); high-fiber diet for diverticulosis and related disorders (Chapter 33), diet for type 2a hyperlipoproteinemia (Chapter 40), and food lists for corn-free and soy-free diets (Chapter 44). Several diets have been revised: diet for diabetes mellitus (Chapter 37), ketogenic diet (Chapter 39), diets for chronic renal failure and dialysis (Chapter 42), and elimination diets used in

diagnosis of food allergy (Chapter 44). Information on lactose tolerance (Chapter 34), proprietary tube feedings, and total parenteral nutrition (Chapter 36) has been expanded.

Tabular additions to the Appendix include zinc values in foods (A-2); weight and height tables in metric and English measures (A-8 to A-10); conversions to and from metric measures (A-13); and recommended daily nutrient intakes, 1974, Canada (A-14). The 1976 revised exchange lists for meal planning are included in Table A-4. The table on cholesterol content of foods has been expanded (A-6); also, the table on normal constituents of human blood (A-11) has been revised and enlarged to include examples of situations in which deviations from the normal may be expected. An important addition to the Appendix is a listing of over 100 films and filmstrips, together with brief commentary and correlation with chapters of the text.

Case Studies in Clinical Nutrition: A Workbook and Study Guide for Students of Nursing and Dietetics by Corinne H. Robinson, Marilyn R. Lawler, and Ann E. Garwick has been written to accompany this text.

Corinne H. Robinson
Marilyn R. Lawler

Acknowledgments

Many individuals and organizations have contributed generously to the development of this book. We especially wish to recognize the cooperation of the staff of the Consumer and Research Division, U.S. Department of Agriculture, for data and charts on food composition and food consumption; the comments and suggestions of the many instructors who completed a questionnaire on nutrition and diet therapy; and the editors of journals who gave permission to use their materials.

For photographs and charts new to this edition we thank Ms. Mary Anne Irwin, Ms. Mary Hamil, Mr. Richard Stewart, and Mr. John Brennan, University of Delaware; Dr. Betty Alford, Mrs. Margaret Bogle, Dr. Claire Zane, and Dr. Ralph Pyke, Texas Woman's University; Mrs. Vera Lee Rao and Mrs. Anne Aigner, Delaware County Nutrition Program for the Elderly and Community Nursing Service, Chester, Pa.; Dr. Reva T. Frankle, Weight Watchers International, Inc.; Sister Mary Jamesine and Mrs. Elizabeth Murphy, Marywood College, Scranton, Pa.; Mr. Philip C. Ahn, University of Minnesota; Mrs. Margaret Matheson, St. Paul–Ramsey Hospital and Medical Center; Miss Lorrayne Anderson and Mrs. Nancy Nellgren, University of Minnesota Health Sciences Center; and Mrs. Jean Robb, Diabetes Education Center, Minneapolis. We also appreciate the photographs provided by news and journal editors, governmental agencies, and several food industry organizations.

One of us (M. R. L.) is especially indebted to Mrs. Dorothy Verstraete, Department of Food Science and Nutrition, University of Minnesota. The assistance of Miss Deborah Parant, Consulting Nutritionist, New Haven, in searching the current literature for Part Two is also gratefully acknowledged.

We appreciate the skillful direction given by the staff of the Macmillan Publishing Co., Inc. For several editions it has been a joy to work with Miss Joan C. Zulch, Medical Editor, who is a discerning critic, a gentle taskmaster, and a warm friend.

Contents

PART ONE Normal Nutrition

1. Food and Its Relation to Health   3
2. Introduction to the Study of the Nutritive Processes: Digestion, Absorption, and Metabolism   16
3. Dietary Guides and Their Uses   29
4. Proteins and Amino Acids   41
5. Carbohydrates   61
6. Lipids   76
7. Energy Metabolism   91
8. Mineral Elements   102
9. Fluid and Electrolyte Balance   125
10. The Fat-Soluble Vitamins   148
11. The Water-Soluble Vitamins: Ascorbic Acid   166
12. The Water-Soluble Vitamins: The Vitamin-B Complex   172
13. Food Selection and Meal Planning for Healthy Persons   196
14. Factors Influencing Food Habits and Their Modification   215
15. Cultural Food Patterns in the United States   224
16. Food Selection for Quality and Economy   237
17. Safeguarding the Food Supply   253
18. Controls for the Safety and Nutritive Value of the Food Supply   271
19. Nutrition During Pregnancy and Lactation   284
20. Nutrition During Infancy   298
21. Nutrition for Children and Teen-agers   313
22. Nutrition in Later Maturity   328
23. National and International Problems in Nutrition   337
24. Nutrition Education and Services Through Community Action   351

PART TWO Therapeutic Nutrition

25. Therapeutic Nutrition: Factors in Patient Care   369
26. Counseling and Coordinated Nutritional Services for Patients   380
27. Adaptations of the Normal Diet for Texture: *Normal, Soft, and Fluid Diets*   389
28. Dietary Calculation Using the Food Exchange Lists   399
29. Overweight and Underweight: *Low-Calorie and High-Calorie Diets*   404
30. Protein Deficiency: *High-Protein Diets*   419
31. Diet in Fevers and Infections   426

32. Diet in Diseases of the Esophagus, Stomach, and Duodenum: *Bland Fiber-Restricted Diet in Three Stages* 431

33. Diet in Disturbances of the Small Intestine and Colon: *Very Low-Residue Diet; High-Fiber Diet* 443

34. Malabsorption Syndrome: *Medium-Chain-Triglyceride Diet; Lactose-Restricted Diet; Sucrose-Restricted Diet; Gluten-Restricted Diet* 452

35. Diet in Disturbances of the Liver, Gallbladder, and Pancreas: *High-Protein, High-Carbohydrate, Moderate-Fat Diet; Fat-Restricted Diet* 467

36. Nutrition in Surgical Conditions: *Tube Feedings; High-Protein, High-Fat, Low-Carbohydrate Diet* 479

37. Diabetes Mellitus 491

38. Various Metabolic Disorders: *Purine-Restricted Diet* 507

39. Nutrition in Neurologic Disturbances: *Ketogenic Diet* 518

40. Hyperlipidemia and Atherosclerosis: *Fat-Controlled Diets; Diets for Hyperlipoproteinemia* 526

41. Dietary Management of Acute and Chronic Diseases of the Heart: *Sodium-Restricted Diet* 541

42. Diet in Diseases of the Kidney: *Controlled Protein, Potassium, and Sodium Diet; Calcium- and Phosphorus-Restricted Diet* 552

43. Anemias 570

44. Diet in Allergic and Skin Disturbances: *Elimination Diets* 577

45. Nutrition in Children's Diseases 585

46. Inborn Errors of Metabolism: *Phenylalanine-Restricted Diet; Galactose-Free Diet* 600

Appendixes

Tabular Materials

Foreword 616

Tables

A-1 Nutritive Values of the Edible Part of Foods 617

A-2 Mineral and Vitamin Content of Foods: Sodium, Potassium, Phosphorus, Magnesium, and Zinc; Folacin, Pantothenic Acid, Vitamin B_6, Vitamin B_{12}, and Vitamin E 642

A-3 Nutritive Values of Baby Foods 658

A-4 Exchange Lists for Meal Planning 660

A-5 Amino Acid Content of Selected Foods 665

A-6 Cholesterol Content of the Edible Portion of Food 670

A-7 Composition of Some Alcoholic Beverages 674

A-8 Growth Standards for Boys from Birth to Age 18 675

A-9 Growth Standards for Girls from Birth to Age 18 676

A-10 Suggested Weights for Heights for Men and Women 677

A-11 Normal Constituents of Human Blood 678

A-12 Normal Constituents of the Urine of the Adult 682

A-13 Conversions to and from Metric Measures 683

A-14 Recommended Daily Nutrient Intakes—Canada, Revised 1974 684

List of Audiovisual Materials 686

Common Abbreviations 694

Glossary 695

Index 707

Part One
Normal Nutrition

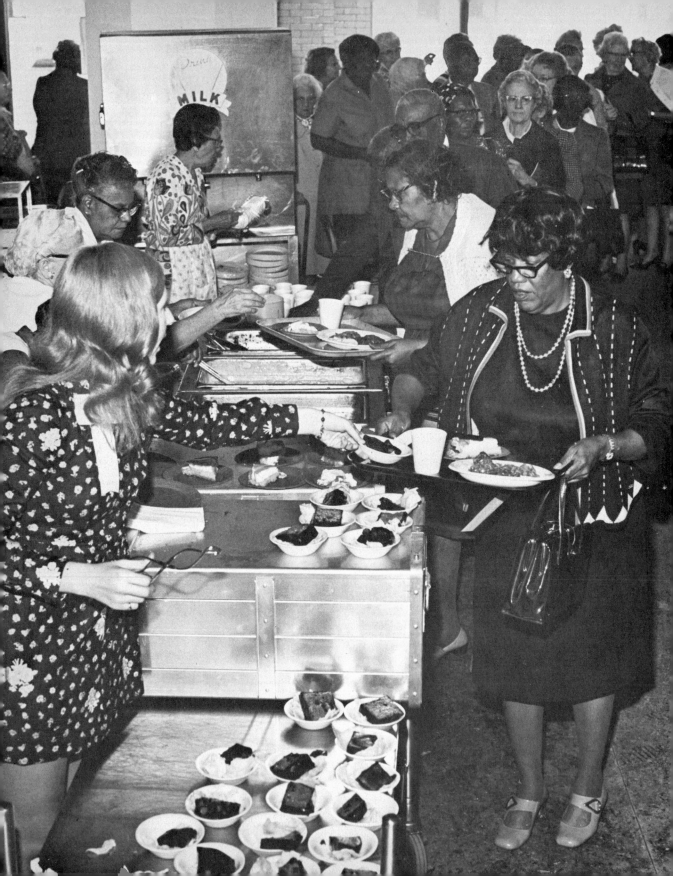

1 Food and Its Relation to Health

The Meanings of Food, Nutrition, and Nutritional Care

What does food mean to you? Food—menu—diet—hunger—nutrition—malnutrition. What images do these words bring to your mind? Are they oriented to your senses? To your social enjoyment? To your concerns about your own well-being? To your emotions? Do they raise questions about the quality of life for your fellow human beings?

When you sit down to your next meal you will have definite ideas—positive or negative—about that meal and the specific foods that are served to you. By your eyes you will delight in the texture variations and color combinations of the food, the artistic touch of a garnish, and the beautiful table appointments; or perhaps your interest will be diminished because the food lacks color and is carelessly served. By your nose you will enjoy the tantalizing odors of meat or of freshly baked rolls, or the fragrance of fully ripened fruit; or possibly you will be repelled because of the odor of grease which has been too hot or of vegetables which have been cooked too long. By your sense of taste you will experience countless flavors—the salty, sweet, bitter, and sour and their variations; you will feel the textures of smooth or fibrous, crisp or soft, creamy or oily, moist or dry foods.

But your senses alone do not describe what your next meal, or any meal, means to you. Is the meal merely a way of staying alive and keeping in health; an opportunity for fellowship with your family and friends; a way to celebrate an event; an occasion for stimulating conversation; a means of satisfying your feelings when you are hurt and depressed; a display of prestige by which you show that you can afford certain foods others cannot; a token of security and love; a means of asserting your independence; a cause of concern because some foods might make you ill; an occasion of self-denial; something you enjoy leisurely; taken for granted as your right; a precious gift from God for which you are thankful? What other feelings are evoked by the food you eat?

Next to the air you breathe and the water you drink, food has been basic to your existence. In fact, food has been the primary concern of man in his physical environment throughout all recorded history. By food, or its lack, the destinies of men are greatly influenced. Man must eat to live, and what he eats will affect in a high degree his ability to keep well, to work, to be happy, and to live long. (See Figures 1–1 and 1–2.)

This chapter will present an overview of the scope of nutrition study, including national and international problems of nutrition, and some suggestions for study objectives. You bring to the study of nutrition your lifetime experience with food which may serve you well in further improving your nutrition and the nutrition of your fellowmen. But it may also be that you have many incorrect ideas and such strong feelings about food that it will take much patience and perseverance on your part to change your attitudes and motivations. As you enter upon this study it is well for you to examine carefully your present feelings about food, as well as your current knowledge of nutrition, so that you can build upon what is good in your dietary pattern and correct that which is undesirable.

Definitions. HEALTH as defined by the World Health Organization of the United Nations is the "state of complete physical, mental and social well-being and not merely the absence of disease or infirmity."[*]

NUTRITION is "the science of foods, the nutrients and other substances therein; their action, interaction, and balance in relationship to health and dis-

[*] *World Health Organization—What It Is, What It Does, How It Works.* Leaflet, Geneva, Switzerland, 1956.

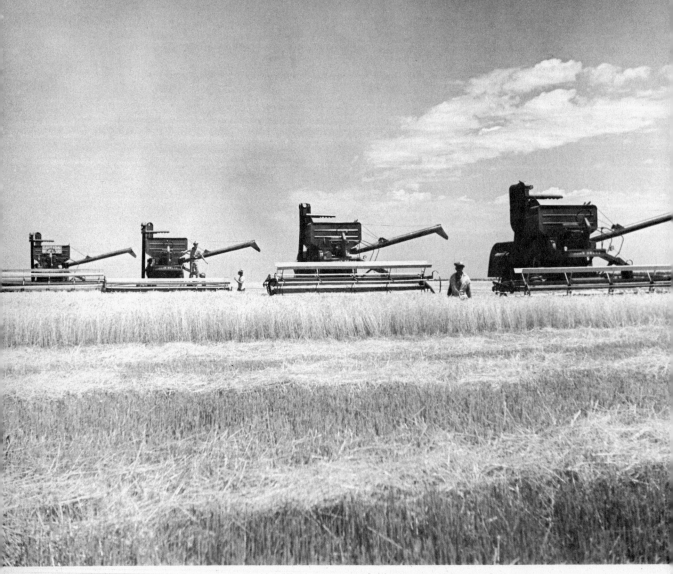

Figure 1-1. Farmers in North America produce an abundance of food that meets the needs not only of the American population but supplies much food for export to food-deficient nations. (Courtesy, Kansas Wheat Commission.)

ease; the processes by which the organism ingests, digests, absorbs, transports, and utilizes nutrients and disposes of their end products. In addition, nutrition must be concerned with social, economic, cultural, and psychological implications of food and eating."[*]

NUTRIENTS are the constituents in food that must

[*] Robinson, W. D.: "Nutrition in Medical Education," in *Proceedings Western Hemisphere Nutrition Congress—1965*, American Medical Association, Chicago, 1966, p. 206.

be supplied to the body in suitable amounts. These include water, proteins and the amino acids of which they are composed, fats and fatty acids, carbohydrates, minerals, and vitamins.

NUTRITIONAL STATUS is the condition of health of the individual as influenced by the utilization of the nutrients. It can be determined only by the correlation of information obtained through a careful medical and dietary history, a thorough physical examination, and appropriate laboratory investigations.

Nutritional care is "the application of the science and art of human nutrition in helping people select and obtain food for the primary purpose of nourishing their bodies in health or in disease throughout the life cycle. This participation may be in single or combined functions: in feeding groups involving food selection and management; in extending knowledge of food and nutrition principles; in teaching these principles for application according to particular situations; and in dietary counseling."[*]

Malnutrition is an impairment of health resulting from a deficiency, excess, or imbalance of

[*]Committee on Goals of Education for Dietetics, Dietetic Internship Council: "Goals of the Lifetime Education of the Dietitian," *J. Am. Diet. Assoc.,* **54:**92, 1969.

nutrients. It includes undernutrition, which refers to a deficiency of calories and/or one or more essential nutrients, and overnutrition, which is an excess of one or more nutrients and usually of calories.

Good nutrition: a multidisciplinary effort. Although each farm worker in the United States produces enough food for 45 persons, millions of people are engaged in the many aspects of meeting human needs for food. The achievement of good nutrition requires (1) application of agricultural science and technology to produce sufficient amounts of plant and animal foods of high nutritive value; (2) processing of foods for maximum retention of nutritive values; (3) adequate storage, transportation, and marketing facilities to make foods available at times and places where needed; (4) appropriate govern-

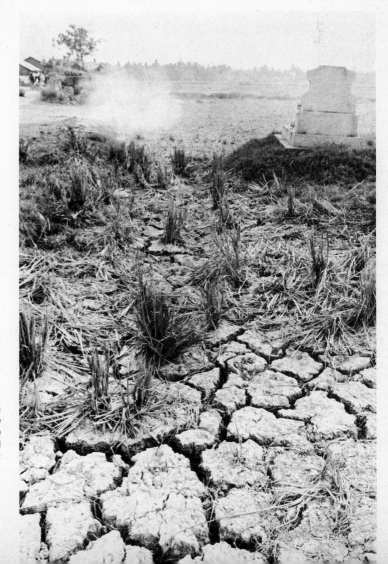

Figure 1–2. Drought, poor thin soil, and pest infestations reduce the amount of food that can be produced in some underdeveloped countries. (Courtesy, UNICEF; photo by Jacques Danois.)

mental controls to ensure wholesomeness and nutritive quality of the food supply; (5) economic conditions that make it possible to procure the necessary foods at a cost within the reach of all; (6) educational programs in nutrition within the schools and at the community level; and (7) efficient use of food within the home, public eating place, and institution.

The perspectives of nutrition held by each of the specialists who help to assure an adequate food supply obviously would be quite different. Thus, the disciplines of the life sciences, human behavior, economics, government, and communications are intertwined in nutrition study. The benefits of good nutrition—health, happiness, efficiency, and longevity—are sought by people all over the world. The achievement of these benefits is like a utopian dream to most of the world's people. (See Figure 1–3.)

DIETARY TRENDS IN THE UNITED STATES

Changes in patterns of living. Since the beginning of this century the population of the United States has shifted from rural to urban areas. Most people must purchase all of their foods, and even on the farm most families purchase a substantial proportion of the foods that they consume. Americans have the benefit of many labor-saving devices in their occupations and in their homes. They work fewer hours in a week, so that the way in which they spend their leisure may be decisive in determining their food needs. Leisure, to many people, means little activity—riding rather than walking, watching television rather than leading an active outdoor life, and so on.

Greater numbers of married women are working away from home than ever before, which means that there is less time for food preparation, more

Figure 1–3. Human nutrition encompasses the study and application of many disciplines.

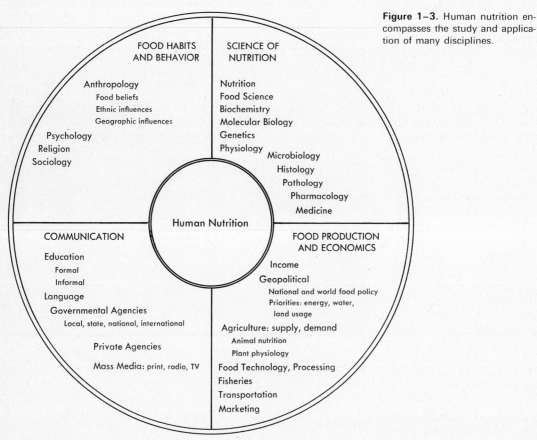

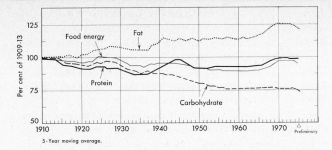

Per cent of 1909-13

125

Food energy   Fat

100

Protein

75

Carbohydrate

50

1910   1920   1930   1940   1950   1960   1970   △ Preliminary

5-Year moving average.

Figure 1–4. Since the beginning of the century there has been a decrease in the consumption of carbohydrate by about one fourth, an increase in fat consumption by about one fifth, and a relatively constant protein intake. (Courtesy, U.S. Department of Agriculture.)

expensive ready-prepared foods are used, and shopping is less frequent. Husbands, as well as wives, are shopping for and preparing foods; sometimes children, especially teen-agers, are given too much freedom in their food choices. Marriages occur at an earlier age with pregnancy often presenting an additional stress on the young woman who has not fully matured.

The average American family of today has a higher income and is spending more of it for food. With this higher income, more meals are eaten in restaurants. More workers are eating in cafeterias at their place of work rather than carrying lunches, and more children are participating in school breakfast and lunch programs. The family eats fewer meals together, and in far too many families some meals may be skipped by one or more persons. Breakfast is an often neglected meal, although some families have found that this is the one time of the day when they can plan to be together.

The scientific and technologic advances reach into every aspect of daily life, including the quantity, quality, variety, and attractiveness of the foods we eat. Frozen foods including complete meals, baked foods of all kinds, mixes, and snacks are commonplace items in the supermarkets. An increasing number of fabricated foods are replacing conventional foods. The number of brands and the variety are so great that the shopper finds it difficult indeed to make wise selections.

Some social changes often have an adverse effect on nutrition: the large number of persons living alone; the increasing proportion of older people; long periods of unemployment; the breakup of families by divorce or death with the attendant emotional turmoil and also the dual role that must be assumed in maintenance of the home and the supply of the income; and the high incidence of alcoholism and drug addiction.

The changing American diet. Major changes have taken place in the American diet during the present century. One way to review these changes is to look at the nutrient values of the food supply available for consumption each year. The U.S. Department of Agriculture keeps such records annually. (See Figure 1–4.)

Protein in the available food supply has ranged from 88 gm in 1935 to 103 gm in 1945–1946. It is now at 99 gm per capita.[1] In 1909 animal foods supplied about half of the total available protein; today they furnish about two thirds of the total protein. There has been a marked increase in beef consumption and some increase in the use of poultry. A marked decline has taken place in the consumption of grain foods. With increasing affluence, Americans and people of other countries consume more animal protein foods and less plant protein foods.

In 1909 carbohydrate represented 56 per cent of the total available calories and now accounts for 46 per cent of the food energy.[2] The consumption of grain foods is about half as high as it was in the beginning of the century, and sugar consumption has increased about one third—from 155 gm to almost 210 gm per capita daily. Of the latter, sucrose alone accounted for 126 gm, or approximately 500 kcal. This is equivalent to about 15 per cent of the total available calories.

The amount of fat available in the national food supply has increased from 127 gm in 1909 to 147 gm at present.[2] During the last five years up to 60 gm of fat has been derived from shortenings and oils.[1-3] This is equivalent to 540 kcal, or about 16 per cent of the total available energy.

Thus, sugars and fats (excluding butter) supply about 30 per cent of the total energy in the diet. Since they do not furnish minerals, vitamins (except vitamin E in vegetable oils), and proteins, the food sources that make up 70 per cent of the available energy must be significant sources of these nutrients. As we shall see, the restriction of fats and sugars becomes more important as the energy requirements of people are reduced with inactivity.

Dietary adequacy. Since 1936 the U.S. Department of Agriculture has conducted five comprehensive surveys of food consumption in the United States. The most recent survey, covering the four seasons from spring 1965 through winter 1966, was a representative sample of the urban and rural regions throughout the United States.[4] Although a more recent survey has not been accomplished, the direction that food consumption has taken based upon available food supplies in the past decade indicates that the 1965 findings are still applicable.[1-3]

The adequacy of the diets was evaluated according to the Recommended Dietary Allowances (RDA) described fully in Chapter 3. This standard describes the desirable levels of nutrient intakes for various age categories and provides a margin of safety for most individuals. In the U.S. Department of Agriculture survey a *good* diet was one that provided the nutrients at levels equal to or in excess of the RDA. A diet was rated *poor* if it provided less than two thirds of the RDA for one or more nutrients. When diets provide less than two thirds of the RDA for a prolonged period of time, it is expected that some individuals may show some signs of deficiency.

From 1955 to 1965 the following changes in the food selection had occurred: (1) less milk and milk products, flour, and cereal foods, vegetables, and fruits; and (2) more meat, fish, poultry, baked foods,

and snack foods such as soft drinks, pretzels, and doughnuts. These changes resulted in a decline in the quality of diets from 1955 to 1965. Only 50 per cent of the diets were rated good in 1965 whereas in 1955 the rating was given to 60 per cent of all diets. Poor diets accounted for 20 per cent of all diets in 1965 and 15 per cent in 1955.

From Figure 1–5 it may be seen that the average intakes of calcium and iron by the various age categories were most seriously below recommended allowances. Females of all ages had diets that were more deficient than did males. Average intakes of iron failed to meet recommended allowances for infants and children. These changes in food consumption and their adverse effect on the nutritive value of diets suggest important points to be emphasized in nutrition education.

NUTRITIONAL PROBLEMS IN THE UNITED STATES

Public concerns about nutrition. In recent years the American public has shown increasing interest and concern about food supplies and nutritional needs. This has come about through dramatic, often exaggerated presentations of newscasts, documentaries, and advertising on radio and television and in the print media. Nutritional terms such as protein, saturated and polyunsaturated fats, the many minerals, and vitamins are familiar, although there are many misconceptions concerning them. This interest provides an excellent opportunity for nutrition education. It also places a responsibility on the professional person in nutrition to provide a sound informational basis for judging the safety of the food supply and for meeting community and world food needs.

What are some of these concerns? Young people especially look upon disruptions in the ecologic balance. Some believe that there is excessive use of pesticides that may harm plant and animal life, and of additives in food processing. They express this concern by selecting foods grown on soils fertilized by manures and without the use of pesticides or chemical fertilizers; they also avoid foods to which additives have been included in food processing. These concerns are exaggerated, as later discussions in the text will show. (See Chapter 17.)

NUTRIENT INTAKE BELOW RECOMMENDED ALLOWANCE
Average Intake of Group Below Recommended Dietary Allowance, NAS-NCR, 1968
U.S. Diets of Men, Women, and Children, One Day in Spring 1965

Sex-Age Group	Protein	Calcium	Iron	Vitamin A value	Thiamin	Riboflavin	Ascorbic acid
Male and Female							
Under 1 year			••••				Below by:
1-2 years			••••				1-10% •
3-5 years			••				11-20% ••
6-8 years							21-29% •••
							30% or more ••••
Male:							
9-11 years		•					
12-14 years		••	•••	•			
15-17 years		•	•				
18-19 years							
20-34 years							
35-54 years		•					
55-64 years		••					
65-74 years		••					
75 years and over		•••		•		••	•
Female:							
9-11 years		•••	••••		•		
12-14 years		•••	•••••	•	•		
15-17 years		••••	•••••		••		
18-19 years		•••	•••••	•	•		
20-34 years		•••	•••••		•	•	
35-54 years		••••	••••		•	••	
55-64 years		••••			•	•	
65-74 years		••••	•	•	••	••	
75 years and over		••••	•	••	••	•••	

Figure 1-5. Females of all ages have average nutrient intakes below recommended allowances, but average intakes by males usually meet allowances. Average calcium and iron intakes for all age groups of females failed to equal recommended levels. (Courtesy, U.S. Department of Agriculture.)

In developing countries people consume an average of 400 pounds of grains per capita annually. In the United States, Canada, and western Europe about 1500 to 2000 pounds of grains are consumed per capita, but most of this is fed to animals that are in turn used for food. Most of the world's people consume diets that contain very little animal protein and manage to maintain health when the plant food supply is varied and abundant. Various forms of vegetarianism have been adopted by significant numbers of Americans in the belief that such diets are more healthful and that they represent a more efficient use of world resources since the food is eaten directly rather than consumed by animals. Some forms of vegetarianism are nutritionally satisfactory; others are not. (See Chapter 15.)

As people approach middle age they are more likely to question whether there are health risks in the present American diet. They are constantly reminded through advertising that some products may reduce one's blood cholesterol and thus lower the risk of cardiovascular disease. More recently the inadequacy of fiber intake is being emphasized through the communications media.

Nutritional deficiencies. In 1967 the first comprehensive National Nutrition Survey was initiated by the Nutrition Program of the Public Health Service.[5] The survey was made on about 70,000 people living in low-income areas of 10 states, including Massachusetts, New York, West Virginia, South Carolina, Michigan, Louisiana, Kentucky, Texas, Washington, and California. The information developed during the survey included socioeconomic data, dietary evaluation, physical examinations, dental examinations, and laboratory analyses of blood and urine. Among the findings were these:

1. Anemia: there was frequent occurrence in all age categories; one third of all children under six years had unacceptable hemoglobin levels.

2. Dental problems: for each 100 persons 90 needed fillings or extractions; 45 had some degree of periodontal disease and 20 had severe periodontal disease; 18 of every 100 persons over 10 years of age had trouble or pain in biting and chewing.

3. Retarded growth: height was considerably below average in children from one to three years: bone development was retarded.

4. Vitamin A deficiency: low serum vitamin A levels were seen in about one third of all children under six years. Eight cases of Bitot's spots on the conjunctiva were reported.

5. Vitamin C deficiency: low serum vitamin C levels were found in 12 to 16 per cent of the various age groups; scorbutic gums were present in 1 person of every 25.

6. Vitamin D deficiency: this was observed in 4 per cent of children under six years; 18 cases of rickets were diagnosed.

7. Protein malnutrition: low serum proteins were found in one of every six persons of all ages. Four to five per cent of children had winged scapula and pot belly indicating protein malnutrition. Seven cases of severe protein-calorie malnutrition (kwashiorkor and marasmus) were diagnosed in preschool children.

Although the initial survey was confined to low-income areas, there is no reason to believe that the conditions described above would be absent in people of ample income. In fact, anemia and dental problems are known to be widely prevalent, and the other deficiencies probably exist to a varying degree.

Problems of nutrient excesses. Many Americans consume diets that are excessively high in calories, saturated fat, cholesterol, and sugars, and that are also excessively refined. All of these excesses are believed to increase the risk of chronic diseases. It must be remembered, however, that there are also other factors that relate to the incidence of chronic diseases.

1. Excessive caloric intake leads to obesity, which is highly prevalent in the American population, and which is associated with chronic diseases such as diabetes mellitus, gallbladder disease, gout, cardiovascular diseases, and others.

2. Excessive intake of fats and sugars that are practically devoid of minerals, vitamins, and proteins may result in suboptimal intakes of these essential nutrients. This imbalance may lead to some of the deficiencies described above.

3. Excessive intakes of saturated fats and cholesterol are believed by many clinicians to be among the important risk factors in the incidence of cardiovascular and cerebrovascular diseases.[6] (See Chapter 40.)

4. Excessive intake of salt has been associated with hypertension.[7]

5. Excessive use of refined foods, on the basis of epidemiologic studies, is believed to increase the incidence of gastrointestinal disorders such as diverticulosis, irritable colon, and possibly colon cancer.[8] (See Chapter 33.)

6. Excessive intakes of vitamins A and D are known to be toxic. (See Chapter 10.)

Nutritional balance. From the preceding discussion it becomes evident that the concept of nutritional balance is important. A good diet must fulfill these criteria: (1) it must furnish the appropriate levels of all nutrients to meet the physiologic and biochemical needs of the body at all stages of the life cycle; and (2) it must avoid excesses of any nutrients that increase the risk of diet-related diseases. PRIMARY PREVENTION implies that the necessary steps are taken to ensure nutritional balance before any detrimental biochemical or physical changes can occur. This positive approach involves careful consideration of nutritional factors throughout the development of the fetus and the years of infancy and childhood. If the factors involved in nutritional balance are maintained, there could be a reduction for the need of correction in later life.

GLOBAL PROBLEMS IN NUTRITION

Scope of malnutrition. Most of the world's people today, as always, are engaged in a struggle for food. In relatively few countries, such as the United

States, Canada, and western European countries, is food abundant and of great variety. More than half the world's people are caught in a relentless sequence of ignorance, poverty, malnutrition, disease, and early death. There are no completely reliable statistics on either morbidity or mortality from malnutrition, but one estimate places the daily death toll from malnutrition at 10,000.[9]

The world's population increases by approximately 180 to 200 thousand persons each day, so that the expansion of food production to keep pace with, and to move ahead of, this population growth must assume staggering proportions. The world production of food increases about 2.5 per cent annually, just keeping ahead of the population increase of 2 per cent annually.[10] Moreover, much of the increase in food production occurs in the developed countries and not in the areas of greatest need.

The energy crisis experienced throughout the world directly affects the food supply. Energy is required for the production of fertilizers, to run farm machinery, to transport foods, and to process foods. Short supplies of energy together with high costs of energy have affected the poor countries most severely.

The first need is for sufficient food to meet the caloric requirements of the population. Qualitatively, the next need is for sufficient protein to supply the amino acids that are used to build and maintain body structures.

Protein-calorie malnutrition is the single greatest world problem in nutrition. In its severe forms, kwashiorkor and marasmus, it affects millions of preschool children. In fact, in some countries, three children may be dead before the first one gets to school. Those children who do survive are physically and mentally retarded—perhaps irreversibly so.

Anemia (especially in mothers and young children), blindness resulting from vitamin A deficiency, and riboflavin deficiency are especially frequent. Rickets, scurvy, pellagra, beriberi, and endemic goiter occur in severe forms in some parts of the world. The characteristics of these deficiencies will be described in the chapters related to the specific nutrients involved.

Responsibility for world nutrition. No thinking man or woman can afford to avoid the fact that so many of the world's people simply do not have enough to eat, nor can he, even in his own self-interest, evade the responsibility for alleviating hunger. In chronic starvation lie the frustration, tension, and envy of masses of people who will ultimately resort to violence.

World peace cannot be guaranteed by supplying adequate food alone, but one road to world peace is surely through a better-fed world population. Beyond this, charity and brotherhood are at the root of the Judeo-Christian religions and indeed of all ethical systems, and to practice them should be on the conscience of mankind.

A number of groups under the United Nations are directly concerned with global problems of nutrition, namely the Food and Agriculture Organization (FAO); World Health Organization (WHO); United Nations Children's Fund (UNICEF); United Nations Educational, Scientific and Cultural Organization (UNESCO). (See Chapter 24.)

SOME OBJECTIVES IN THE STUDY OF NUTRITION

At the beginning of any study it is well for the student to set some specific objectives for himself. These will not be the same for all individuals because students begin the study with quite differing backgrounds of knowledge and experience, and because their professional interests are likely to vary widely. Moreover, it must be anticipated that these will, in fact, change as the study progresses and the student becomes more aware of the field. Worthwhile goals are not fully achieved within the space of a few months but should provide the basis for an ongoing lifetime program of education. The discussion that follows will give the student some background for setting up his own objectives with reference to personal and family nutrition, and toward a professional career in the health sciences.

Personal and family nutrition. Regardless of one's future professional career, the study of nutrition should first be directed to oneself. Physical and mental health are essential assets to meet the exciting, and sometimes arduous, requirements of one's life work. Those who expect to help other people achieve better health through nutrition must be enthusiastic and living examples of the benefits of the application of nutrition knowledge.

Nutrition education applied to the individual also reaches the family. This is especially important for young men and women as they establish their own families. Within the family the wife and mother is the principal decision maker for the family's food. She plans the menus, selects the foods, and prepares them. Although she makes every effort to please her husband, her influence also molds many of his habits. The food habits of children are formed by the prevailing attitudes and practices within the home.

Professional opportunities in nutrition. Professional people in any discipline related to health are engaged in activities related to education, prevention, and therapy.

Nutrition education in schools. Education of the population holds promise of long-range benefits to the greatest numbers. Teachers, nurses, nutritionists, dietitians, home economists, and physicians assume varying responsibilities for individual and group education. The elementary and secondary schools afford the single best opportunity for helping the child to establish attitudes and practices concerning food selection that will lead him to a more healthful, productive life. Nutrition education must begin in the kindergarten and continue through the twelfth grade if it is to achieve maximum effectiveness. It is the responsibility of the elementary teacher as well as teachers of home economics, health, and physical education.

The school nurse, physician, and dentist have many opportunities to note defects in health that suggest the need for improved nutrition; they can influence children in changing their food habits, provide experiences in the classroom, and lend their support to school food service and nutrition education programs.

The school breakfasts and lunches demonstrate that good nutrition and good food are, in fact, partners. School dietitians serve as teachers and also as consultants to teachers.

Nutrition programs for the public. Voluntary and governmental agencies together with industry are accepting responsibility for nutrition programs. The researcher in nutrition and food sciences is equally at home in the laboratories of a food company, a university, a hospital, or in the public health field. Nutritionists, dietitians, and home economists, de-

pending upon their education and particular interests, are the experts who interpret a product for a company; develop new uses for a food; advise mothers and children concerning their diets in a clinic; serve as consultants to a public health team; supervise food service in a college dormitory, industrial cafeteria, or hospital; assist individuals and groups in dietary selection; and teach in nursing schools, colleges, and universities.

Nutrition and health care. The concern of today's health worker is for the maintenance as well as the restoration of health. Traditionally, health care has been directed to the patient—that is, the horizontal individual. Today, health care includes the concept of continuity of care. The health worker soon learns that there must be concern for the patient who makes the transition from the hospital to his home. To implement continuity of care with respect to nutritional needs, the patient may require counseling in the proper choice of foods in the market, assistance in planning for the best use of his food money, and practical suggestions for food preparation with meager facilities, or in the face of physical handicaps. Some of the assistance required by the patient may be provided by the nurse, but more often a team effort—nurse, dietitian, social worker—is needed. (See also Chapters 25 and 26.)

In the community the nurse is often the coordinator of services. The public health nurse encounters a legion of problems and needs related to nutrition: perhaps she needs to show one mother how to prepare an infant formula; another person needs to know how to budget her limited income so that she can buy enough milk; another needs actual instruction in food preparation for an ill member of the family; another has been given a diet that does not fit in with the religious practices of the family; or a pregnant woman may need to know what foods she must eat and how to provide for them in her budget.

Objectives for the student. To achieve the personal and professional objectives the student should strive toward the following behavioral changes.

1. Shows the proper attitude and convictions relative to the importance of nutrition in regulating one's own health, that of the family, and that of individuals of the community.

2. Knows the kinds of health problems arising from poor nutrition that exist in his own community, the nation, and throughout the world.

3. Demonstrates knowledge concerning the science of nutrition:

  a. Functions, digestion, absorption, and metabolism of proteins, fats, carbohydrates, minerals, and vitamins.

  b. The interrelationship of nutrients.

  c. The nutritive requirements of individuals and the variations that may be imposed by activity, climate, stage of life cycle, and disease.

4. Appreciates and understands the meanings that food has for people and how these are related to economic, psychologic, and cultural factors.

5. Interprets the principles of nutrition in the selection of an adequate diet:

  a. By knowing the food sources of the nutrients.

  b. By applying consumer information to the planning of meals and the selection of food for quality and economy.

6. Uses opportunities for improving nutrition through the education of individuals.

7. Counsels people on an individual or group basis by adapting nutrition information to specific health, socioeconomic, and cultural needs.

8. Knows where to look for reliable sources of information and how to evaluate publications on food and nutrition and the claims made through product advertising.

9. Becomes familiar with agencies concerned with nutrition and health in order to utilize their services and contribute to their functioning.

Some guidelines for nutrition study. It is often said that one can judge a workman by the way in which he uses his tools. This is also true of the use a student makes of the study tools available to him. First, one must become acquainted with a tool and gain some practice in using it before it becomes comfortable to use. With your text, for example, look through the table of contents to learn something of the topics that are covered and the sequence of their presentation. Then browse through the book to become aware of the kinds of study aids that are provided.

Terminology in any study is basic to understanding, and the time used in developing the ability to use nutrition terms with accuracy and ease is well spent. Terms with which you should be familiar are set in small capital letters and are defined at the point of their first use. Terms that are used frequently throughout the text have also been listed in the Glossary in the Appendix.

Many tables, diagrams, charts, and photographs emphasize and summarize important points made in the discussion. If you study these, you will find that they reinforce the reading of the text itself. The tables of food composition in the Appendix contain a gold mine of information. Perhaps half of all the questions people will pose to you are concerned with nutritive values, and in these tables you can find the answers. But to use them with confidence means that you must consult them often.

Review questions at the end of each chapter will help you to focus on the important points that have been made. The suggested problems are examples of situations that may be encountered in making applications of the principles of nutrition. You will soon learn to find answers to problems that come within your own daily experiences.

Any student of nutrition should be aware of the current issues before the public. You will find that your interest will be deeper if you try to relate your course of study to some of the reporting in newspapers and magazines, for example. Try to evaluate what you read in the popular publications with what you learn in your study.

Additional references have been included for each chapter to enable you to read more extensively on selected topics, to familiarize you with reliable publications in nutrition, to foster the habit of consulting the literature, and perhaps even to provide the starting point for a paper you may wish to develop. The references included are at a reading level comparable to this text.

PROBLEMS AND REVIEW

1. What is your understanding of the following terms: nutrition, malnutrition, foodstuff, nutrient, health, food, nutritional care, primary prevention?

2. Industrial and economic developments have been a powerful factor in the changing of our food habits. List several of these which have had an influence on our dietary habits within your lifetime.

3. Within your experience give an example of a situation in which the community has fostered better nutrition.

4. Select an article related to food from the daily newspaper or a popular magazine and discuss its merits.

5. In what ways is a knowledge of the following sciences helpful in the study of nutrition: bacteriology, chemistry, sociology, psychology, anthropology?

6. What is the difference between a dietary survey and a nutritional status study?

7. *Problem.* Start a list of resources for the study of nutrition and dietetics. Add to this list as you continue in your study. Include only those books and journals which you have examined. Include the names of official and voluntary agencies in your own community and at state, federal, and international levels as you become familiar with the work they do in the area of nutrition.

8. *Problem.* Compile a list of characteristics which describe a person who is in good nutritional status. How do you measure up with this?

9. *Problem.* Review the suggested objectives for study in this chapter. Then prepare a statement in your own words which best describes the goals you think are most important. Limit your statement to 300 words; be concise but specific.

CITED REFERENCES

1. Friend, B., and Marston, R.: "Nutritional Review," *National Food Situation*, U.S. Department of Agriculture, Nov. 1975, pp. 26–32.
2. Friend, B., and Marston, R.: "Nutritional Review," *National Food Situation*, Nov. 1974, pp. 26–32.
3. Friend, B.: "Nutritional Review," *National Food Situation*, Nov. 1973, pp. 23–28.
4. *Dietary Levels of Households in the United States*, Spring 1965. ARS 62-17, U.S. Department of Agriculture, Washington, D.C., 1968.
5. Schaefer, A. E., and Johnson, O. C.: "Are We Well Fed? The Search for the Answer," *Nutr. Today*, **4** (No. 1):2–11, 1969.
6. Christakis, G.: "The Case for Balanced Moderation, or How to Design a New American Nutritional Pattern Without Really Trying," *Prev. Med.*, **2**:329–36, 1973.
7. Dahl, L. K.: "Salt and Hypertension," *Am. J. Clin. Nutr.*, **25**:231–44, 1972.
8. Burkitt, D. P., and Painter, N. S.: "Dietary Fiber and Disease," *J.A.M.A.*, **229**:1068–74, 1974.
9. "Fortified Foods: the Next Revolution," *Chem. Eng. News*, **48**:36–43, Aug. 10, 1970.
10. Mayer, J.: "Time for Reappraisal. Commentary," *J. Nutr. Educ.*, **7**:8–12, 1975.

ADDITIONAL REFERENCES

Berg, A.: "Priority of Nutrition in National Development," *Nutr. Rev.*, **28**:199–204, 1970.

Brown, L. R.: "Death at an Early Age," *UNICEF News*, Issue 85, 1975, pp. 3–9.

Cobos, L. F., *et al.:* "Will Improved Nutrition Help to Prevent Mental Retardation?" *Prev. Med.*, **1**:185–94, 1973.

Frankle, R. T., and Heussenstam, F. K.: "Food Zealotry and Youth: New Dimensions for Professionals," *Am. J. Public Health*, **64**:11–18, 1974.

Goldsmith, G. E.: "Nutrition and World Health," *J. Am. Diet. Assoc.*, **63**:513–18, 1973.

Harrar, J. G.: "Nutrition and Numbers in the Third World," *Nutr. Rev.*, **32**:97–104, 1974.

Todhunter, E. N.: "The Evolution of Nutrition Concepts—Perspectives and New Horizons," *J. Am. Diet. Assoc.*, **46**:120–28, 1965.

Wade, N.: "World Food Situation: Pessimism Comes Back into Vogue," *Science*, **181**:634–38, 1973.

"White House Conference on Food, Nutrition and Health. Recommendations of Panels on Nutrition Teaching and Education," *J. Nutr. Educ.*, **1**:24–39, Winter 1970.

Books

Anderson, J., Dibble, M. V., Mitchell, H. S., and Rynbergen, H. J.: *Nutrition in Nursing*. J. B. Lippincott Company, Philadelphia, 1972.

Arlin, M. T.: *The Science of Nutrition*, 2nd ed. Macmillan Publishing Co., Inc., New York, 1977.

Bogert, L. J., Briggs, G. M., and Calloway, D. H.: *Nutrition and Physical Fitness*, 9th ed. W. B. Saunders Company, Philadelphia, 1973.

Chaney, M. S., and Ross, M. L.: *Nutrition*, 8th ed. Houghton Mifflin Company, Boston, 1971.

Fleck, H.: *Introduction to Nutrition*, 3rd ed. Macmillan Publishing Co., Inc., New York, 1976.

Goodhart, R. S., and Shils, M. E., eds.: *Modern Nutrition in Health and Disease*, 5th ed. Lea & Febiger, Philadelphia, 1973.

Guthrie, H. A.: *Introductory Nutrition*, 3rd ed. The C. V. Mosby Company, St. Louis, 1975.

Krause, M. V., and Hunscher, M. A.: *Food, Nutrition and Diet Therapy*, 5th ed. W. B. Saunders Company, Philadelphia, 1972.

Lowenberg, M. E., Todhunter, E. N., Wilson, E. D., Savage, J. R., and Lubawski, J. L.: *Food and Man*, 2nd ed. John Wiley & Sons, Inc., New York, 1974.

Mitchell, H. S., Rynbergen, H. J., Anderson, L., and Dibble, M. V.: *Nutrition in Health and Disease*, 16th ed. J. B. Lippincott Company, Philadelphia, 1976.

Stare, F. J., and McWilliams, M.: *Living Nutrition.* John Wiley & Sons, Inc., New York, 1973.

Williams, S. R.: *Nutrition and Diet Therapy*, 2nd ed. The C. V. Mosby Company, St. Louis, 1973.

Wilson, E. D., Fisher, K. H., and Fuqua, M. E.: *Principles of Nutrition*, 3rd ed. John Wiley & Sons, Inc., New York, 1975.

2 Introduction to the Study of the Nutritive Processes: Digestion, Absorption, and Metabolism

Some understanding of the metabolic processes that take place in the body is important to the study of nutrition. The purposes of this chapter are to present an overview of the nutritive processes that will be discussed in somewhat more detail in the chapters pertaining to the nutrients, and to review briefly some aspects of digestion, absorption, and metabolism as a framework for the study of nutrition. Many details have intentionally been omitted, for it is assumed that students who are using this text have already completed courses in physiology and chemistry. The student who desires further review or greater depth of study may consult one of the standard texts of physiology and chemistry, some of which have been listed at the end of this chapter.

The processes of metabolism are so complex that it is impossible to tell the story exactly as it happens. For the sake of simplicity, single aspects are usually described in more or less detail; for example, one can trace the digestion, absorption, and intermediary metabolism of a given carbohydrate, or of any other nutrient, more or less independently of any other. This can give a misleading impression inasmuch as the metabolism of a given nutrient never occurs in isolation but is always interlinked with a multitude of metabolic events. Each metabolic event is affected by other events that preceded it or occurred at the same moment in time. The story of metabolism is an unending one that invites interest and continuing research by physiologists, histologists, cytologists, microbiologists, biochemists, nutritionists, and others.

Composition of the body. Water accounts for roughly two thirds of the body weight and is distributed in all tissues. About three fourths of the water is in the INTRACELLULAR compartment (fluid within the cells), and one fourth is in the EXTRACELLULAR compartment, which includes the blood circulation, the lymph, and the interstitial fluids which bathe all cells. Tissues vary considerably in their water content, with bones, teeth, and adipose tissue, for example, containing appreciably less than muscle and nervous tissue.

Proteins and fats each account for about 18 per cent of body weight, with considerable variations depending upon the amount of fat deposition. The percentage of fat in the newborn infant is relatively low, but in the obese adult the percentage of fat may exceed that of protein by a wide margin.

Only about 300 gm of carbohydrate is present in the body. This is chiefly in the form of fuel storage, with only a small amount being involved in the structure of the tissues.

The predominating chemical elements in the body are oxygen, 65 per cent; carbon, 18 per cent; hydrogen, 10 per cent; and nitrogen, 3 per cent. Together they represent about 96 per cent of body weight and account for the principal elements in water, protein, fat, and glycogen in the body. The remaining 4 per cent is made up of the mineral elements, of which calcium and phosphorus account for three fourths.

Many of the most important body constituents are organic compounds present in such small amounts that they have no significant effect on the total body weight. Among these are the vitamins, hormones, and enzymes.

Cells as functioning units. The human body may be studied at various levels of organization: the organism as a whole; organs and tissues; cells that make up the organs and tissues; and structural components within cells. Nutritional processes of the organism as a whole are the sum total of the physical and chemical activities that take place within the cell and the relationships that exist between the cells and the surrounding environment.

The simplest living organism consists of a single cell such as a bacterium or yeast cell that is capable of respiration, ingestion, digestion, absorption, circulation, synthesis of new materials, breakdown of materials for energy, response to the environment, excretion, and reproduction. Survival of the cell is dependent upon a favorable external environment. The cells of complex organisms such as those in the human being carry out these multiple activities but cannot exist independently; they function through intricate coordination with other cells. Cells are so tiny that they can be seen only with a light microscope. Many structures within cells have been identified by means of the electron microscope that permits magnification of 100,000 times or more. Cells are of infinite variety in size, shape, and specialized functions. They also possess some structures and functions in common so that it is possible to diagram and describe a so-called typical cell. (See Figure 2–1.)

The CELL MEMBRANE surrounds the protoplasm, maintains the constancy of the internal environment, and establishes dynamic equilibrium with the external environment by its highly selective ability to regulate the kinds and amounts of materials that enter and leave the cell.

The NUCLEUS of the cell is the storehouse for deoxyribonucleic acid (DNA), the genetic plan for the construction of proteins that enable new cells to have the characteristics of the parent cell.

The CYTOPLASMIC MATRIX is the continuous phase extending from the cell membrane throughout the cell and surrounding the ORGANELLES, or living structures, as well as certain lifeless materials known as INCLUSIONS. The organelles include the mitochondria, lysosomes, and endoplasmic reticulum.

MITOCHONDRIA are rod-shaped or round structures that vary in size and shape depending upon their activity. Within the mitochondria are hundreds to thousands of oxidative enzymes that are responsible for carrying on the reactions that yield the high-energy compound adenosine triphosphate (ATP). ATP supplies the energy needed by the cell to carry on its activities.

LYSOSOMES are membranes, or bags, that contain

Figure 2–1. Diagram of a cell as it would appear under an electron microscope.

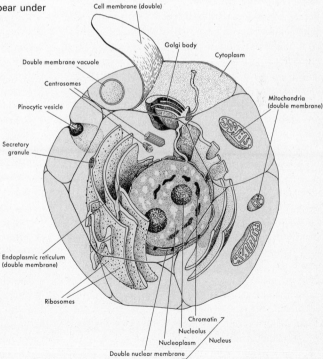

digestive enzymes. When the membrane bursts, the cell itself is digested, this being normal as worn-out cells are replaced by new. Lysosomes also release amino acids from proteins and are able to engulf bacteria and other substances. The phagocytic activity is a special property of the white blood cells.

The ENDOPLASMIC RETICULUM is the system of channels that allows flow of materials to and from the various parts of the cell as well as to the extracellular environment. The endoplasmic reticulum is associated with several special structures that vary considerably according to the type of cell. RIBOSOMES are the site of protein synthesis according to the genetic information supplied by the nucleus. They are abundant in cells where protein synthesis is great, but are lacking in some cells, such as red blood cells, where protein synthesis does not take place. The GOLGI COMPLEX appears as flattened bags and is well developed in secretory cells. It stores and concentrates enzymes and secretes them on demand.

The nature of enzymes. All living tissues, plant and animal, produce thousands of enzymes without which the myriad chemical reactions could not take place. ENZYMES are organic catalysts of a protein nature which remarkably increase the rate of reactions without becoming a part of the reaction products. When protein is denatured (as by heating), the enzyme activity is lost. A small amount of enzyme will accomplish a chemical change on a great deal of substance, sometimes as much as 4,000,000 times its own weight. Enzymes, like all organic materials, are gradually used up, and therefore they must be continuously synthesized by the living cell.

Some enzymes are simple proteins, whereas others consist of a protein and another grouping which is loosely or firmly bound to the protein molecule. In an enzyme system the protein molecule is called the APOENZYME; its attached grouping is called the PROSTHETIC GROUP. For many enzyme systems the prosthetic group is comprised of COENZYMES, which are organic compounds, including several of the vitamins. The same coenzyme, it should be noted, may be used in different enzyme systems; it is the protein molecule that gives an enzyme its particular specificity. Some enzymes may require the presence of a COFACTOR (e.g., a mineral element) for their proper functioning.

Some enzymes are produced in an inactive form known as PROENZYME or ZYMOGEN and require some other substance to activate them. For example:

Trypsinogen $\xrightarrow[\text{(activator)}]{\text{enterokinase}}$ Trypsin
(proenzyme or zymogen) (active enzyme)

Protein + water $\xrightarrow{\text{trypsin}}$ Proteoses, peptones, polypeptides
(substrate)

Most enzymes participate in only one chemical reaction on a single substance, although some act on a class of compounds. They are named for the substances upon which they act, for example, *proteases* for proteins, *lipases* for fats, and so on. Thus, a single cell contains hundreds to thousands of enzymes that are responsible for as many different actions. An enzyme, such as *lactase*, will split only the sugar lactose; it has no action on the sugar sucrose, or on any other sugar, protein, or fat.

Enzymes are classified broadly by the functions they perform. Among the many important functions are hydrolysis, oxidation, dehydrogenation, and transfer of chemical groupings; thus, hydrolases, oxidases, dehydrogenases, and transferases.

Each enzyme has optimum activity at a specific pH. Pepsin, which digests proteins in the stomach, is one of the few enzymes active in the very acid reaction of the stomach, whereas the enzymes found in the small intestine are active at a slightly alkaline pH.

Enzyme activity depends on the amount of exposed surface. For example, much more activity by oxidases occurs if a potato is cut up into small pieces than if it is left whole. Likewise, in digestion, enzyme activity is great because the muscular movements of the tract have reduced the food mass to minute particles with thousands of exposed surfaces.

Enzymes are inactivated but not destroyed at freezing temperatures. When a frozen food or other substance is thawed, the enzyme activity proceeds normally. On the other hand, enzymes are destroyed at temperatures that coagulate proteins.

Metabolism. The series of processes necessary for the building of cells and tissues and their continuous functioning is known as METABOLISM. This broad term implies the coordination of a number of processes:

1. Ingestion, or the intake of food.

2. Digestion, which prepares foods for their use by the body.

3. Absorption of nutrients from the gastrointestinal tract into the circulation.

4. Transportation of nutrients by the circulatory system to the sites for their use, and of wastes to the points of excretion.

5. Respiration, which supplies oxygen to the tissues for the oxidation of food, and which removes waste carbon dioxide. The circulatory system is again responsible for transportation of these gases.

6. Use of materials: oxidation to create heat and energy; incorporation into new cells and tissues.

7. Excretion of wastes: undigested food wastes and certain body wastes from the bowel; carbon dioxide by the lungs; nitrogenous, mineral salt, and other wastes from metabolism by the kidneys and by the skin.

Numerous physical and chemical methods have been developed for measuring the metabolic changes that occur with variations in nutrition. Analyses of blood, of urine, and, somewhat less frequently, of feces for various constituents are utilized in nutrition research. Part of the study of nutrition is concerned with a knowledge of such changes and an interpretation of their significance in assessing the quality of nutrition.

Functions of food. "You are what you eat" is, in a sense, true inasmuch as food supplies the nutrients needed as a source of *energy* for activity of the body, and as *structural materials* for every cell of the body. In the latter capacity, not only do the nutrients furnish the materials that give the body its structure and proportions, but they are used for the synthesis of the numerous *regulatory substances* that are essential to life.

The nutrients that supply energy include carbohydrates, fats, and proteins. In forming body structures, water, proteins, fats, carbohydrates, and minerals all participate. All nutrients—water, amino acids, fatty acids, sugars, mineral elements, and vitamins—are involved in the innumerable regulatory activities.

DIGESTION

Purposes. Only a few substances contained in foods are suitable for use by the body without change, namely, water, simple sugars, and some mineral salts and vitamins. DIGESTION includes the mechanical and chemical processes whereby complex food materials are hydrolyzed to forms that are suitable in size and composition for absorption into the mucosal wall and for utilization by the body. The nutrients that are absorbed include amino acids, fatty acids, glycerol, simple sugars, minerals, and vitamins.

In addition to its hydrolytic activities the gastrointestinal tract controls the amounts of certain substances that will be absorbed, for example, calcium and iron; prevents the absorption of unwanted molecules; synthesizes enzymes and hormones that are required for the digestive process; eliminates the wastes remaining from the digestion of food as well as certain endogenous wastes; and renews its own structure every 24 to 48 hours.

The digestive organs. The gastrointestinal tract is a tube about 7.5 to 9 meters (25 to 30 feet) long in the adult and includes the mouth, esophagus, stomach, small intestine (duodenum, jejunum, and ileum), and large intestine (cecum, colon, rectum, and anal canal). The liver and pancreas, although situated apart from the tract itself, are important for the secretions that they contribute to the digestive process. (See Figure 2–2.)

The structure of the walls of the gastrointestinal tract is grossly similar throughout but is adapted in its detail for the particular functions of a given organ. The wall consists of four layers: a mucosal lining; circular muscle fibers; longitudinal muscle fibers; and an outer covering known as the serosa. (See Figure 2–3.)

Muscular controls are in effect at several points along the tract to permit the influx of food to the next site for digestion and, under normal conditions, to prevent the backward flow of food (regurgitation). These are the cardiac opening from the esophagus to the stomach; the pyloric sphincter at the gastric-duodenal juncture; and the ileocecal valve, which regulates the passage of material from the ileum into the large intestine.

Controls for activity of the digestive tract. The secretion of digestive juices and the motor activity of the tract, and hence the speed and completeness of digestion, are regulated by nervous, chemical, and physical factors.

Everyone is familiar with the fact that the

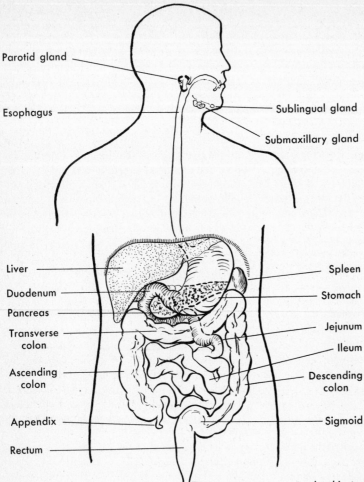

Parotid gland

Esophagus

Sublingual gland

Submaxillary gland

Liver

Duodenum

Pancreas

Transverse
colon

Ascending
colon

Appendix

Rectum

Spleen

Stomach

Jejunum

Ileum

Descending
colon

Sigmoid

Anal sphincter   **Figure 2-2.** The digestive tract.

thought, sight, or smell of foods creates the desire for food and increases the flow of saliva and gastric juices. On the other hand, an unpleasant environment or worry and fear are likely to depress the secretion of digestive juices and thus delay digestion. Strong emotions such as anger often increase gastric secretion, but sometimes depress it.

Of the many digestive processes, the only activities under voluntary control are mastication and defecation. The autonomic nervous system exercises continuous control of the secretory and motor activity throughout the entire tract. The pressure of food against the mucosal surfaces and specific characteristics of foods serve as stimuli to the nerves.

Hormones are the chemical messengers produced at a given site as a result of stimulation by specific foods. Table 2-1 presents a summary of the hormones that affect secretory and motor activity.

Mechanical digestion. Rhythmic coordinated muscle activity causes foods to be reduced to minute particles and intimately mixed with digestive juices so as to facilitate movement throughout the tract, and to provide for maximum exposure to the hydrolyzing enzymes and contact with the absorbing surfaces of the mucosal wall.

By mastication solid foods are cut, ground, mixed with saliva, and prepared for swallowing. Within seconds rhythmic contractions of the muscles of the

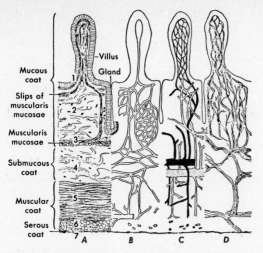

Mucous coat
Villus
Gland
Slips of muscularis mucosae
Muscularis mucosae
Submucous coat
Muscular coat
Serous coat

A   B   C   D

Figure 2–3. Diagram of a cross section of small intestine. *A* shows coats of intestinal wall and tissues of coats: (*1*) columnar epithelium, (*2*) areolar connective tissue, (*3*) muscularis mucosae, (*4*) areolar connective tissue, (*5*) circular layer of smooth muscle, (*6*) longitudinal layer of smooth muscle, (*7*) areolar connective tissue and endothelium. *B* shows arrangement of central lacteal, lymph nodes, and lymph tubes. *C* shows blood supply; arteries and capillaries *black,* veins *stippled. D* shows nerve fibers, the submucous plexus lying in the submucosa, the myenteric plexus lying between the circular and longitudinal layers of the muscular coat. (Courtesy, Miller, M. A., and Leavell, L. C.: *Kimber-Gray-Stackpole's Anatomy and Physiology,* 16th ed. Macmillan Publishing Co., Inc., New York, 1972.)

esophagus force the food particles into the fundus of the stomach, which serves as a reservoir. Each addition of food expands the stomach walls just enough to hold the contents and pushes the mass preceding it forward toward the central part of the organ. Because there is little motor or secretory activity in the fundus, food may remain there for an hour or more, thus allowing salivary digestion of carbohydrates to continue for awhile. Small, regular contractions in the middle region of the stomach gradually increase in rate and intensity. The food is mixed with gastric juice, broken up further, and

Table 2–1. Hormones That Regulate Secretory and Motor Activity of the Digestive Tract

Hormone	Where Produced	Stimulus to Secretion	Action
Gastrin	Pyloric and duodenal mucosa	Food in the stomach, especially proteins, caffeine, spices, alcohol	Stimulates flow of gastric juice
Enterogastrone	Duodenum	Acid chyme, fats	Inhibits secretion of gastric juice; reduced motility
Cholecystokinin	Duodenum	Fat in duodenum	Contraction of gallbladder and flow of bile to duodenum
Secretin	Duodenum	Acid chyme; polypeptides	Secretion of thin, alkaline, enzyme-poor pancreatic juice
Pancreozymin	Duodenum; jejunum	Acid chyme; polypeptides	Secretion of thick, enzyme-rich pancreatic juice
Enterocrinin	Upper small intestine	Chyme	Secretion by glands of intestinal mucosa

finally reduced to a thin, souplike consistency called CHYME.

The principal digestive activity is in the small intestine. Because the stomach has considerable storage capacity and because of the controls exerted by the pyloric valve, only small amounts of chyme enter the duodenum at a given time. The rhythmic movements of the intestine are known as PERISTALSIS. In the small intestine the circular muscle fibers have a constricting and squeezing action so that the chyme is constantly mixed with the digestive enzymes and given maximum exposure to the absorbing surfaces. This motion of the circular muscles is referred to as segmentation. As the longitudinal muscle fibers contract, a wavelike motion is produced that gradually moves the food mass forward. The muscular activity of the tract also serves as a stimulus to the secretion of the digestive juices and increases the blood supply to the digestive organs.

Motility through the tract. The rate at which foods move through the digestive tract depends upon the consistency, composition, and amount of food eaten. Liquids begin to leave the stomach from 15 minutes to $\frac{1}{2}$ hour after ingestion, a fact that explains why liquid diets do not have great satiety value. Carbohydrates, when eaten alone, leave the stomach more rapidly than do proteins. Fats check the secretion of gastric juices and retard peristaltic activity so that their presence in the diet delays the emptying of the stomach. Normally, the stomach empties in two to six hours.

The unabsorbed food residue from the small intestine begins to pass through the ileocecal valve into the large intestine in from 2 to $5\frac{1}{2}$ hours, but 9 hours or more from the time of eating may be required for the last of a large meal to pass this point. The length of time required to eliminate food residues as feces varies widely; a range of 20 to 36 hours after the consumption of the meal is typical.

Chemical digestion. A complex mixture of substances is presented to the various sites of the tract for hydrolysis. Depending upon the location, these include food materials in various stages of hydrolysis, secretions of digestive fluids containing enzymes and hormones, cellular materials from the desquamating mucosa, bile, bacteria, and various products of metabolism within the body that have entered the tract.

About 8 to 9 liters of digestive juices are produced daily by the secretory cells of the digestive tract and by the pancreas and liver. These juices are 98 to 99 per cent water and contain varying proportions of inorganic and organic compounds. One of the organic compounds of importance is MUCIN, a glycoprotein that lends the slippery quality to mucus and thus facilitates the smooth movement of food throughout the tract. Mucus also furnishes a protective coating to the gastric and duodenal mucosa against the corrosive action of hydrochloric acid. Except for bile, the digestive juices contain enzymes that are appropriate for a particular stage of hydrolysis. The final stages of hydrolysis for some nutrients, for example, the disaccharides, occurs within the mucosal cell itself and not in the lumen. Table 2–2 presents a summary of the digestive juices, their components, and the results of enzyme activity. See Chapters 4 to 6 for details of digestion of proteins, fats, and carbohydrates.

Functions of the large intestine. By the time chyme reaches the large intestine practically all of the nutrients and water have been absorbed and the volume has been reduced to about 500 ml. The cecum fills slowly, and the peristaltic waves forcing the residues forward together with antiperistaltic waves forcing them back enable additional amounts of water to be absorbed. The large intestine secretes alkaline juices with a large amount of mucus but no hydrolytic enzymes so that there is practically no hydrolysis or absorption of nutrients at this point. The activity of the large intestine is greatest after meals and after exercise.

The daily excretion of feces is about 100 to 200 gm. The fecal material consists of small amounts of food residues, especially indigestible fiber, billions of bacteria, yeasts, and fungi, wastes from desquamated cells, bile pigments, cholesterol, and unabsorbed minerals such as calcium and iron.

The predominant bacteria in the large intestine are *Escherichia coli.* Bacteria that are fermentative are favored by a high carbohydrate intake, and those that are putrefactive by a high protein intake. Bacterial action in the large intestine releases (1) gases including ammonia, methane, carbon dioxide, and hydrogen, (2) lactic and acetic acids, and (3) certain substances such as indole and phenol that may have toxic properties.

Physicians and clinicians are reemphasizing the importance of ample amounts of fiber in the diet in order to reduce the time fecal residues remain in the large intestine.[1] The reasons for this emphasis are (1) diverticula, present in large proportions of the population by middle age, are less likely to form if the transit time through the colon is shortened, and (2) a more rapid elimination reduces the length of time a potentially toxic substance has contact with the mucosa.

ABSORPTION

The nature of absorption. The process whereby nutrients are moved from the intestinal lumen into the blood or lymph circulation is known as ABSORPTION and results in a net gain of nutrients to the body. It is an *active process* in that substances are moved into the body against forces that would normally cause a flow in the opposite direction. It is also a *selective process* by which some materials, such as glucose, are transported in their entirety across the cell; others, for example, calcium and iron, are absorbed only according to body need; and still others, such as intact proteins, are held back.

Absorption requires that the nutrient penetrate the cell wall, cross the cell, exit from the cell into the lamina propria, and cross the epithelium of the blood or lymph vessels. In some instances absorption includes a metabolic change within the cell before it is transferred to the circulation. The absorption of specific nutrients will be discussed in Chapters 4 to 12.

Sites and rates of absorption. Absorption appears to take place primarily from the duodenum and jejunum.[2] A notable exception is vitamin B_{12}, which has a specific absorption site in the lower ileum. Bile is reabsorbed from the distal part of the intestine. Most, if not all, substances that are proximally absorbed can also be absorbed by the ileum; thus, those substances that escaped absorption proximally are absorbed distally.

Normally, 98 per cent of the carbohydrate, 95 per cent of the fat, and 92 per cent of the protein in the diet is hydrolyzed and the end products are absorbed. These percentages are sometimes referred to as COEFFICIENTS OF DIGESTIBILITY.

Malabsorption can occur under a variety of circumstances: a reduction in the number of functioning villi; an increase in motility so that the time of exposure to absorptive surfaces is inadequate; a lack of specific enzymes or of bile; an interference by insoluble compounds; and removal of part of the intestine by surgery.

The absorptive surface. The small intestine provides an absorbing surface that is probably 600 times as great as its external surface area.[3] This is possible because of the arrangement of the mucosal wall in numerous folds, the 4 to 5 million villi that constitute the mucosal lining, and the 500 to 600 MICROVILLI that form the "brush border" of each epithelial cell of the villus.

VILLI are visible by a light microscope. They are tiny finger-like projections of the mucosa and consist of a single layer of epithelial cells resting on the lamina propria, which is a bed of supporting connective tissue supplied by arterial and venous blood vessels and lacteals or lymph channels.

At the base of each villus is the *crypt of Lieberkühn.* This is where the epithelial cells are formed. As new cells are formed they migrate up the sides of the villus. When they reach the tip of the villus, about one to three days later, they are extruded into the intestinal lumen and are constantly replaced by newly functioning cells.

Microvilli can be seen only by means of an electron microscope. They elaborate some of the hydrolytic enzymes, and the final stages for hydrolysis of some substances such as disaccharides are completed here and not in the lumen of the intestine.

Mechanisms for absorption. Four mechanisms have been postulated to explain absorption, although it must be emphasized that the pores, carriers, and pumps that are hypothesized have not been seen.[3]

1. SIMPLE DIFFUSION THROUGH PORES OR CHANNELS. Substances of very low molecular weight (probably 100 or less), such as water and some electrolytes, appear to move freely across the membrane from the side of higher concentration to the side of lower concentration. This mechanism would operate in the direction of the circulation after meals when the concentration of these small molecules in the intestinal lumen is higher than that in the blood and lymph. Being a two-way channel, this mechanism is effective in maintaining osmotic equilibrium. The molecular size of most nutrients is too great for diffusion by pores.

2. CARRIER-FACILITATED PASSIVE DIFFUSION.

Table 2-2. Digestive Juices and Their Actions

Site of Secretion	Stimuli to Secretion	Daily Volume and pH	Important Constituents	Action
Mouth: saliva Salivary glands Submaxillary Sublingual Parotid	Psychic: thought, sight, smell, taste Mechanical: presence of food in mouth Chemical: contact of sugar, salt, spices, etc., on taste buds	1000–1500 ml pH 5.9–6.8	Mucin Amylase* (ptyalin)	Lubrication Cooked starch → dextrins, maltose Enzyme activity in the mouth is not important
Stomach: gastric juice Parietal cells	Psychic: as above Mechanical: contact with mucosa; distension Hormonal: gastrin increases flow; enterogastrone inhibits	1500–2500 ml pH 2.0–2.5	HCl	Pepsinogen → pepsin Bactericidal Reduces ferric iron to ferrous iron
Chief cells			*Pepsinogen* Pepsin	Inactive form of pepsin Proteins → proteoses, peptones, polypeptides
Columnar epithelium			Mucin ?*Lipase* ?*Rennin* (infants only) Intrinsic factor	Lubrication; protects gastric and duodenal lining Emulsified fats → fatty acids + glycerol (action is negligible) Casein → paracasein Enables absorption of vitamin B_{12}
Liver: bile	Cholecystokinin contracts gallbladder and releases bile to duodenum	500–1100 ml pH 6.9–8.6	Bile salts Bile acids Bile pigments Cholesterol Mucin	Neutralizes acid chyme Emulsifies fats for action of lipase Facilitates absorption of fats and fat-soluble vitamins Path of cholesterol excretion

24

Source	Stimulus/Hormone	Amount, pH	Constituent	Action
Pancreas: pancreatic juice	Secretin	600–800 ml pH 7–8	Thin, watery, alkaline, enzyme-poor juice	Neutralizes acid chyme
	Pancreozymin		*Amylase*	Starch → dextrins, maltose
			Chymotrypsinogen	Inactive form of enzyme
			Chymotrypsin	Proteins → proteoses, peptones, polypeptides
			Trypsinogen	Inactive enzyme
			Trypsin	Proteins → proteoses, peptones, polypeptides
			Lipase	Fats → monoglycerides, fatty acids, glycerol
			Carboxypeptidase	Splits off amino acid with free COOH group
Small intestine: Intestinal juice (succus entericus)	Enterocrinin	2000–3000 ml pH 7–8	*Enterokinase*	Trypsinogen → trypsin
	Presence of food in small intestine		*Aminopeptidase*	Splits off amino acid having free amino group
			Dipeptidase	Dipeptides → amino acids
			Nucleinase	Nucleic acid → nucleotides
			Nucleotidase	Nucleotides → nucleosides + phosphoric acid
			Nucleosidase	Nucleosides → purine or pyrimidine base + pentose
			Lecithinase	Lecithin → diglycerides + choline phosphate
Within mucosal cells			*Sucrase* (invertase)	Sucrose → glucose + fructose
			Maltase	Maltose → glucose + glucose
			Lactase	Lactose → glucose + galactose

*Constituents in italics are enzymes.

Water-soluble nutrients cannot penetrate the lipid-rich membrane of the cell. Therefore, they are attached to "carriers" or "ferries" that facilitate crossing the cell membrane. This is known as *facilitated diffusion*. In passive diffusion the nutrients move downhill, that is, from an area of higher concentration to one of lower concentration; no energy is required for this mechanism. When the concentration of nutrients in the circulation is equal to or exceeds that in the lumen, nutrients can no longer passively diffuse. They would remain in the intestinal tract until excreted in the feces, representing a large wastage of essential nutrients.

3. ACTIVE TRANSPORT. The absorption of most nutrients is probably accounted for by active transport. As in passive diffusion, carriers are necessary for the penetration of the cell membrane. Active transport involves the uphill pumping of nutrients from the lumen into the circulation; that is, the nutrient is moved from a site of lower concentration to one of higher concentration. Energy is required for active transport and is supplied by ATP from the metabolism of glucose within the cell. Sodium plays an essential role in the active transport of water, sugars, and amino acids.[4] The metabolic energy required for the operation of the sodium pump also serves for the transport of these other nutrients, thus serving as an energy-saving device.

4. PINOCYTOSIS. In some instances the cell appears to "drink up" or surround a substance and to extrude it into the interior of the cell. Some fats appear to be absorbed by this process. Occasionally, intact proteins may be absorbed in this fashion, helping to explain the incidence of allergy.

INTERMEDIARY METABOLISM

INTERMEDIARY METABOLISM refers to the physical and chemical changes that take place in the internal environment. As pointed out earlier, these changes are the sum total of the activities occurring within each and every cell. The nutrients diffuse from arterial capillary blood into the interstitial fluids surrounding the cells and thence are absorbed by processes such as those described in the preceding section. Likewise, the cells dispose of waste materials to the interstitial fluid and in turn to the venous circulation.

ANABOLISM refers to those processes by which new substances are synthesized from simpler compounds: for example, enzymes, hormones, and tissue proteins from amino acids, glycogen from glucose, and fats from fatty acids. CATABOLISM refers to the breakdown of complex substances to simpler compounds: for example, the oxidation of glucose to yield energy, carbon dioxide, and water, and the breakdown of fats to glycerol and fatty acids.

The enzyme systems of a given cell determine the specific functioning of that cell. A compound—for example, glucose—that is to be utilized by the cell is attacked by one enzyme after another in assembly-line fashion until the desired end product has been achieved. If a single enzyme in the cell is missing, there is a breakdown in the assembly line and all sorts of problems arise. During the last 25 years a better understanding of enzyme activities has led to the identification, and in some cases effective treatment, of the so-called inborn errors of metabolism seen in far too many infants. The condition *galactosemia* results from the lack of a specific enzyme needed for using galactose; *phenylketonuria*, likewise, results from an enzyme defect that leads to failure to utilize the amino acid phenylalanine.

The metabolic pool. The term METABOLIC POOL is often used to refer to the total supply of a given nutrient that is momentarily available for metabolic purposes. For example, the metabolic pool of amino acids at any given moment would include all the amino acids available from dietary sources plus those available from cellular breakdown. From this mixture of amino acids the cells have available the appropriate ones for synthesizing a new protein. The metabolic pool should not be thought of as having specific physical boundaries from which materials may be drawn, but rather as constituting the environment for the cells and the tissues.

Dynamic equilibrium. Cellular materials are constantly being broken down and equally rapidly synthesized. The rate of cellular turnover is exceedingly high, being especially so in the most active organs such as the intestinal wall and the liver. In spite of the remarkable rate of turnover, the body tends to maintain a state of equilibrium, often referred to as DYNAMIC EQUILIBRIUM, or HOMEOSTASIS; that is, the removal of nutrients and their replenishment are equal. This also implies that any cellular

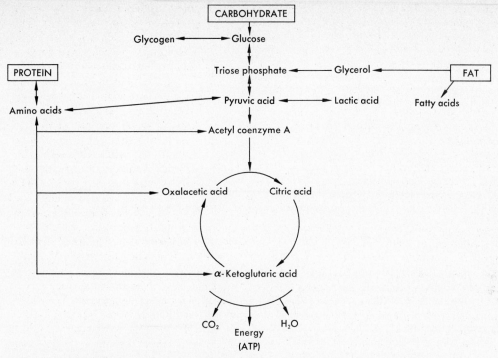

Figure 2–4. Carbohydrates, fats, and proteins are interrelated in anabolic and catabolic reactions. Details of these pathways are shown in Figures 4–4, 4–6, 5–3, and 5–5.

wastes are removed at a rate that does not change the equilibrium. The maintenance of equilibrium is governed by an adequate supply of nutrients, a normal complement of enzyme systems, and the secretion of hormones that regulate metabolic rates.

Common pathways. Carbohydrate, fat, and protein are metabolized in an interdependent fashion. Glucose, fatty acids, and amino acids can enter the common pathway that yields energy. Glucose can be metabolized to fatty acids and cholesterol, and some oxidative products of glucose can combine with amino groups to form amino acids. Amino acids are potential sources of both glucose and fatty acids; and so on. Not only are these major nutrients intertwined in their utilization, but they are dependent upon the correct concentrations of electrolytes and vitamins for making these changes take place. Figure 2–4 is a simplified diagram showing how the metabolism of protein, fat, and carbohydrate is interrelated. Further details of the metabolic pathways are presented in Chapters 4, 5, and 6.

PROBLEMS AND REVIEW

1. What is meant by the following terms: digestion; coefficient of digestibility; peristalsis; segmentation?
2. An enzyme is a catalyst produced by living cells. Name five characteristics of enzymes.
3. In what way does the chewing of food aid digestion in the stomach?
4. It is important that foods be attractively served. How does this facilitate good digestion?
5. Pepsin is a proteolytic enzyme which is secreted by the gastric mucosa as a proenzyme, pepsinogen. How is the pepsinogen activated? What is the substrate on which pepsin acts?
6. Many pediatricians permit children to have foods such as fruit and bread or crackers between meals but

advise against the use of milk for such feedings. Why would milk be more likely to interfere with the appetite for the following meal?

7. In what ways would a deficient secretion of hydrochloric acid interfere with digestion?

8. *Problem.* A meal consisted of 25 gm protein, 35 gm fat, and 50 gm carbohydrate. Using coefficients of digestibility of typical American diets, calculate the amounts that would be actually absorbed.

9. What conditions are necessary so that the tissues can maintain homeostasis?

10. Explain what is meant by passive diffusion; active transport; carrier-mediated transport; pinocytosis.

11. What is the rationale for increasing the fiber content of the diet?

CITED REFERENCES

1. Burkitt, D. P., and Walker, A. R. P.: "Dietary Fiber and Disease," *J.A.M.A.*, **229**:1068–74, 1974.
2. Booth, C. C.: "Sites of Absorption in the Small Intestine," *Fed. Proc.*, **26**:1583–88, 1967.
3. Ingelfinger, F. J.: "Gastrointestinal Absorption," *Nutr. Today*, **2**:2–10, March 1967.
4. Curran, P. F.: "Ion Transport in Intestine and Its Coupling to Other Transport Processes," *Fed. Proc.*, **24**:993–99, 1965.

ADDITIONAL REFERENCES

Asimov, I.: *The Chemicals of Life.* The New American Library of World Literature, New York, 1962.
Bayless, T. M., ed.: "Symposium: Structure and Function of the Gut," *Am. J. Clin. Nutr.*, **24**:44–167, 1971.
Crane, R. K.: "A Perspective of Digestive-Absorptive Function," *Am. J. Clin. Nutr.*, **22**:242–49, 1969.
Floch, M. H., ed.: "Symposium: Current Concepts in Intestinal Absorption and Malabsorption," *Am. J. Clin. Nutr.*, **22**:239–351, 1969.
Guyton, A. C.: *Textbook of Medical Physiology*, 4th ed. W. B. Saunders Company, Philadelphia, 1971.
Mason, M., *et al.: Nutrition and the Cell. The Inside Story.* Year Book Medical Publishers, Chicago, 1973.
Miller, M. A., and Leavell, L. C.: *Kimber-Gray-Stackpole's Anatomy and Physiology*, 16th ed. Macmillan Publishing Co., Inc., New York, 1972.
Nasset, E. S.: "Role of Digestive System in Protein Metabolism," *Fed. Proc.*, **24**:953–58, 1965.
Pansky, B.: *Dynamic Anatomy and Physiology.* Macmillan Publishing Co., Inc., New York, 1975.
Review: "Fat Absorption Physiology and Biochemistry," *Nutr. Rev.*, **26**:168–70, 1968.
———: "Time Response of Jejunal Sucrase and Maltase Activity in Man," *Nutr. Rev.*, **27**:259–61, 1969.
Rosensweig, N. S.: "Dietary Sugars and Intestinal Enzymes," *J. Am. Diet. Assoc.*, **60**:483–86, 1972.
Spencer, R. P.: "Intestinal Absorption of Amino Acids. Current Concepts," *Am. J. Clin. Nutr.*, **22**:292–99, 1969.

3 Dietary Guides and Their Uses

size. Additional modifications are often required for changes in activity and climate.

The bulletin published by the Food and Nutrition Board gives a full description of the bases used to establish the recommended levels of nutrients. Water, carbohydrate, fat, essential fatty acids, vitamin K, pantothenic acid, biotin, and many trace elements are not listed in the table, but a full discussion of these nutrients is included in the bulletin.[1] The allowances for specific nutrients and factors that modify their needs are discussed in more detail in Chapters 4 to 12 inclusive.

Uses of the Recommended Dietary Allowances. The allowances serve as a guide

for planning and procuring food supplies for population groups; for interpreting food consumption records; for establishing standards for public assistance programs; for evaluating the adequacy of food supplies in meeting national nutritional needs; for developing nutrition education programs; for the development of new products by industry; and for establishing guidelines for nutritional labeling of foods.°

Interpretation. It is important to recognize the bases that have been used in the development of the dietary allowances. The stated levels of nutrients have been derived from analyses of the available data on the requirements of different individuals. For each age-sex category the allowances are value judgments of nutritional scientists who are members of the Food and Nutrition Board. It is recognized that much more research is desirable, and to that end the recommended allowances are revised at approximately five-year intervals to incorporate newer knowledge.

The use of the word "allowance" should not be confused with the word "requirement." Because of variations in body build, genetic makeup, and so on, individuals often vary widely from one another in their nutrient requirements. The allowances were set high enough to take care of "practically all of the healthy people in the United States." This means that for most persons the allowances are higher than the actual requirements; that is, a "margin of safety" is included.

° Committee on Dietary Allowances, Food and Nutrition Board: *Recommended Dietary Allowances*, 8th ed. National Research Council—National Academy of Sciences, Washington, D.C., 1974, pp. 1–2.

RECOMMENDED DIETARY ALLOWANCES

Development of dietary allowances. Man has always been concerned about the kinds and amounts of foods that would keep him physically fit. Nevertheless, significant progress in identifying the nutrients needed by the body and the amounts required under varying circumstances has come about principally in this century as a result of thousands of investigations in research laboratories. (See Figure 3–1.) Periodically, summaries of such research have been made in order to recommend the levels of intake desirable for various categories of the population. The first national effort in the United States came about late in 1940 when the Food and Nutrition Board of the National Research Council was organized to guide the government in its wartime nutrition program. One of the first activities of this Board was the careful review of research on human requirements for the various nutrients. This led to the publication of the Recommended Dietary Allowances in 1943. Since that time the Board has evaluated new research and has published revisions of the standards every four to six years.

The 1974 Recommended Dietary Allowances are listed in Table 3–1. They assume a "reference" man and woman weighing 70 and 58 kg, respectively, 23 to 50 years of age, and living in a temperate climate. Adjustments are made in the table for age and body

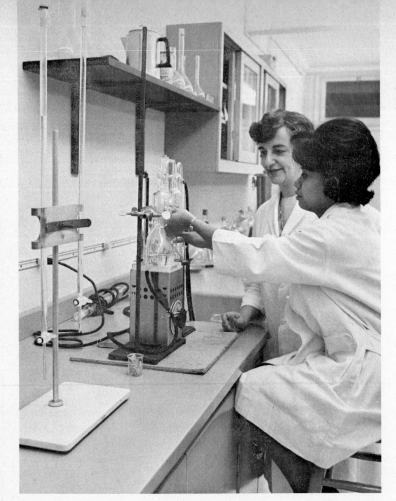

Figure 3–1. Many investigators in research laboratories have contributed to knowledge concerning nutritional needs. (Courtesy, Nesbitt College, Drexel University, Philadelphia.)

Some persons may habitually consume less than the recommended allowances and yet have an adequate diet, simply because their requirements are below the allowances. Nevertheless, there is no practical way to determine which persons have low requirements, which are average in their needs, and which have higher-than-average requirements. For example, suppose that calcium balance studies in a research laboratory had shown that 10 individuals needed the following calcium intakes to maintain satisfactory balance: 425, 540, 570, 590, 600, 610, 630, 710, 770, and 795 mg. The average requirement for this group is 624 mg calcium; five persons are well below the average, two are within 15 mg of the average; and three are well above the average requirement. In this example the allowance of 800 mg calcium provides a generous margin of safety for eight persons and is just sufficient for the two with the highest requirements.

The allowances are the amounts of nutrients to be actually consumed. The food supply brought into the kitchen for a given group must be sufficient to allow for waste in preparation, losses of nutrients in cooking, and plate waste.

In the practice of dietetics the allowances are frequently used to determine the adequacy of the food intake of an individual. When the nutrient intake of a healthy individual is equal to, or exceeds, the recommended allowances, it is highly likely that the diet is meeting the needs of that person in terms of his full potential for growth or productivity. On the other hand, suppose that a particular nutrient or several nutrients are in short supply on a given day. The body has sufficient adaptability that this need be of no concern provided that the average intake over a five-to-eight-day period meets the allowances. An intake below the recommended allowances for a prolonged period of time increases the possibility of nutritional deficiency.

The state of nutritional health cannot be deter-

Table 3–1. Food and Nutrition Board, National Academy of Sciences–National Research Council Recommended Daily Dietary Allowances,[1] Revised 1974

Designed for the maintenance of good nutrition of practically all healthy people in the U.S.A.

	Age (years) From Up to	Weight (kg)	Weight (lb)	Height (cm)	Height (in)	Energy (kcal)[2]	Protein (gm)	Fat-Soluble Vitamins					Water-Soluble Vitamins							Minerals					
								Vitamin A Activity (RE)[3]	Vitamin A Activity (IU)	Vitamin D (IU)	Vitamin E Activity[5] (IU)	Ascorbic Acid (mg)	Folacin[6] (μg)	Niacin[7] (mg)	Riboflavin (mg)	Thiamin (mg)	Vitamin B_6 (mg)	Vitamin B_{12} (μg)	Calcium (mg)	Phosphorus (mg)	Iodine (μg)	Iron (mg)	Magnesium (mg)	Zinc (mg)
Infants	0.0–0.5	6	14	60	24	kg × 117	kg × 2.2	420[4]	1400	400	4	35	50	5	0.4	0.3	0.3	0.3	360	240	35	10	60	3
	0.5–1.0	9	20	71	28	kg × 108	kg × 2.0	400	2000	400	5	35	50	8	0.6	0.5	0.4	0.3	540	400	45	15	70	5
Children	1–3	13	28	86	34	1300	23	400	2000	400	7	40	100	9	0.8	0.7	0.6	1.0	800	800	60	15	150	10
	4–6	20	44	110	44	1800	30	500	2500	400	9	40	200	12	1.1	0.9	0.9	1.5	800	800	80	10	200	10
	7–10	30	66	135	54	2400	36	700	3300	400	10	40	300	16	1.2	1.2	1.2	2.0	800	800	110	10	250	10
Males	11–14	44	97	158	63	2800	44	1000	5000	400	12	45	400	18	1.5	1.4	1.6	3.0	1200	1200	130	18	350	15
	15–18	61	134	172	69	3000	54	1000	5000	400	15	45	400	20	1.8	1.5	2.0	3.0	1200	1200	150	18	400	15
	19–22	67	147	172	69	3000	54	1000	5000	400	15	45	400	20	1.8	1.5	2.0	3.0	800	800	140	10	350	15
	23–50	70	154	172	69	2700	56	1000	5000		15	45	400	18	1.6	1.4	2.0	3.0	800	800	130	10	350	15
	51+	70	154	172	69	2400	56	1000	5000		15	45	400	16	1.5	1.2	2.0	3.0	800	800	110	10	350	15
Females	11–14	44	97	155	62	2400	44	800	4000	400	12	45	400	16	1.3	1.2	1.6	3.0	1200	1200	115	18	300	15
	15–18	54	119	162	65	2100	48	800	4000	400	12	45	400	14	1.4	1.1	2.0	3.0	1200	1200	115	18	300	15
	19–22	58	128	162	65	2100	46	800	4000	400	12	45	400	14	1.4	1.1	2.0	3.0	800	800	100	18	300	15
	23–50	58	128	162	65	2000	46	800	4000		12	45	400	13	1.2	1.0	2.0	3.0	800	800	100	18	300	15
	51+	58	128	162	65	1800	46	800	4000		12	45	400	12	1.1	1.0	2.0	3.0	800	800	80	10	300	15
Pregnant						+300	+30	1000	5000	400	15	60	800	+2	+0.3	+0.3	2.5	4.0	1200	1200	125	18+[8]	450	20
Lactating						+500	+20	1200	6000	400	15	80	600	+4	+0.5	+0.3	2.5	4.0	1200	1200	150	18	450	25

[1] The allowances are intended to provide for individual variations among most normal persons as they live in the United States under usual environmental stresses. Diets should be based on a variety of common foods in order to provide other nutrients for which human requirements have been less well defined. See text for more-detailed discussion of allowances and of nutrients not tabulated.

[2] Kilojoules (KJ) = 4.2 × kcal.

[3] Retinol equivalents.

[4] Assumed to be all as retinol in milk during the first six months of life. All subsequent intakes are assumed to be one-half as retinol and one-half as β-carotene when calculated from international units. As retinol equivalents, three-fourths are as retinol and one-fourth as β-carotene.

[5] Total vitamin E activity, estimated to be 80 per cent as α-tocopherol and 20 per cent other tocopherols. See text for variation in allowances.

[6] The folacin allowances refer to dietary sources as determined by *Lactobacillus casei* assay. Pure forms of folacin may be effective in doses less than one-fourth of the Recommended Dietary Allowances.

[7] Although allowances are expressed as niacin, it is recognized that on the average 1 mg of niacin is derived from each 60 mg of dietary tryptophan.

[8] This increased requirement cannot be met by ordinary diets, therefore, the use of supplemental iron is recommended.

mined by comparing the diet of an individual with the recommended allowances. A diet that fails to meet the allowances could, in fact, be adequate for that particular individual. The determination of nutritional status can be made only by observation of physical signs, and determination of pertinent biochemical indicators. Such data can then be correlated with the pattern of dietary intake, and appropriate recommendations made for correction. (See Figure 3–2.)

The dietary allowances are established for healthy individuals. They are not applicable to persons who have an infection or injury that modifies their requirements or to those individuals who have undergone long periods of stress and depletion. The nutritional needs of these persons must be individually assessed.

The table of allowances lists the recommendations for about one third of the nutrients needed by man. When emphasis is placed upon a wide variety of conventional foods, it is assumed that the needs for the other nutrients will be met. On the other hand, if fabricated foods that supply only the nutrients listed in the table were consumed in significant amounts, deficiency of the unlisted nutrients could result.

Canadian dietary standard. Since 1938 the Canadian Council on Nutrition has published recommendations for nutrient levels for age and sex categories. The most recent revision was published in 1975.[2,3] (See Table A–14 in the Appendix.)

The philosophy for the Canadian standard is essentially the same as that of the Food and Nutrition Board, namely, to recommend nutrient intakes at levels adequate for good health for most Canadians. The standards are above minimum levels and take individual variations into account. The data are derived from essentially the same base lines. The standards are to be used for "planning of diets and food supplies for individuals"[2] and are not to be used as a measure of nutritional status.

An examination of the two tables shows that there are some differences in the recommended levels for nutrients, for example, iron, zinc, and ascorbic acid among others. These differences emphasize that there still exists a good deal of ignorance regarding the criteria for optimum health, the desirable margin of safety, and so on. The assigned levels for each nutrient represent the best judgment of the committees that set up each table.

Dietary guides in other countries. Dietary allowances have been established for populations of many countries. In addition, the Food and Agriculture Organization and the World Health Organization have adopted recommendations for allowances for many nutrients. The aim of the various standards is

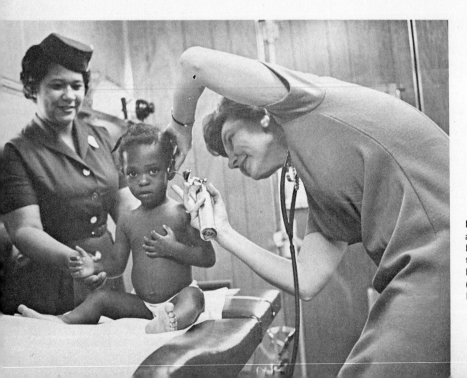

Figure 3–2. The nutritional status and health are determined in part by a physical examination. Laboratory studies and a dietary history help to confirm the findings. (Courtesy, Larry Rana and U.S. Department of Agriculture.)

essentially to provide a level of nutrition that maintains good health for substantially all of the population.[4] The allowances are not minimum requirements, nor are they average needs.

The allowances in various countries differ because they are intended for the population of a given environment—for example, climate, occupation and activity, dietary practices—and therefore they are not interchangeable. For example, more calories would be allowed for men and women in a country where considerable physical activity is involved in daily work than in a country where work is mechanized and activity is sedentary. The increased calorie allowances in turn necessitate increased allowances for some of the B-complex vitamins such as thiamin. The allowances in the various countries also differ because of varying interpretations of data by committees who set up the allowances.[4] As research becomes more extensive these differences are narrowing somewhat. A comparison of allowances set up for men and women for several groups is shown in Table 3-2.

Labeling. The Food and Drug Administration has recently published extensive regulations for food labeling, including nutritional information. The labels for many processed foods now include the caloric, protein, fat, and carbohydrate values per serving and also list the percentages of the U.S. Recommended Daily Allowances (U.S. RDA). Although the latter standard is based upon the Recommended Dietary Allowances, it is a single listing applicable to adults and children over four years of age. It replaces the Minimum Daily Requirements (MDR) used in labeling for many years. The requirements for labeling are fully discussed in Chapter 18.

A DAILY FOOD GUIDE

Foods as sources of nutrients. All foods provide for the energy needs of the body. In addition, most foods furnish nutrients needed for tissue structure and for regulatory functions. No single food meets all these needs. Even a food like milk, which is generally considered to be the most nearly perfect food, does not contain all the food constituents in optimum amounts. Milk is an excellent source of protein for tissue building, it provides more calcium than any other food for bone and tooth formation, and it gives the most abundant supply of riboflavin. In other minerals and vitamins, too, milk is relatively rich. However, its ascorbic acid content is low, so that the need for citrus fruits or other vita-

Table 3-2. Dietary Allowances for Adults by Four Standards

	United States 1974*	Canada 1974*	Food and Agriculture Organization*†	United Kingdom*
Body weight, kg	70–58	70–56	65	65–56
Kilocalories	2700–2000	3000–2100	3200–2300	3000–2500
Protein, gm	56–46	56–41	46–39	87–73
Calcium, mg	800	800–700	400–500‡	800
Iron, mg	10–18	10–14		12
Vitamin A, I.U.:	5000–4000		750 mcg retinol	5000
R.E.	1000–800	1000–800		
Thiamin, mg	1.4–1.0	1.5–1.1	1.3–0.9	1.2–1.0
Riboflavin, mg	1.6–1.2	1.8–1.3	1.8–1.3	1.8–1.5
Niacin, mg	18–13	20–14	21.1–15.2	12–10
Ascorbic acid, mg	45	30		20

*The first figure in each column refers to men, and the second to women. Where the allowance for men and women is the same, only one figure is given.

† Food and Nutrition Board: *Recommended Dietary Allowances,* 7th ed. National Research Council–National Academy of Sciences, Washington, D.C., 1968, pp. 68–69.

‡ This allowance for calcium represents a range for men and women.

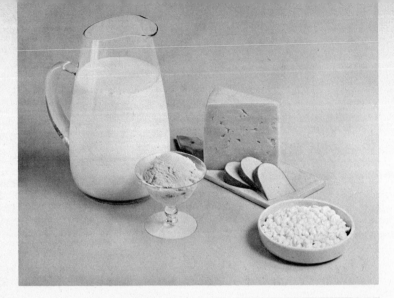

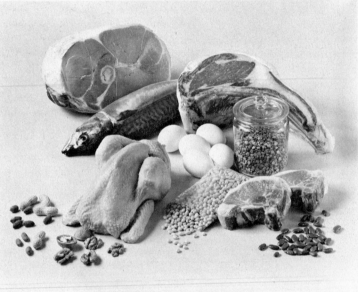

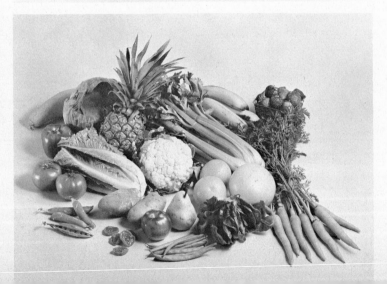

Figure 3–3. A Guide to Good Eating: the Four Food Groups. (Courtesy, National Dairy Council.)

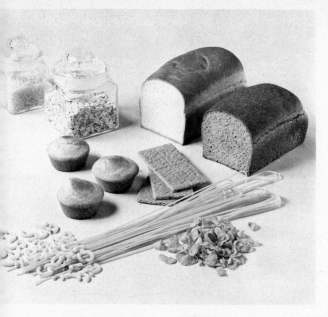

min-C-rich food becomes readily apparent. Milk is also deficient in iron; thus, the place of egg, meats, green leafy vegetables, and fruits becomes evident. One could continue in this manner to evaluate each food. A variety of foods becomes one of the best guarantees that a diet will be adequate.

Four food groups. A standard such as the Recommended Dietary Allowances is of practical value only when it is interpreted into a selection of foods to meet the recommended levels. This may be accomplished through dietary calculations as described in the next section of this chapter. However, simple guides for the general public are essential, and these have been developed by nutrition committees of government agencies and others.

One of these guides, "A Daily Food Guide" (Table 3–3 and Figure 3–3), provides a foundation for a day's meals and includes food choices which permit flexibility for seasonal, regional, and budgetary considerations. The specific nutrient contributions made by foods in each of the Four Food

Table 3–3. A Daily Food Guide*

Milk Group (*8-ounce cups*)
   2 to 3 cups for children under 9 years
   3 or more cups for children 9 to 12 years
   4 cups or more for teen-agers
   2 cups or more for adults
   3 cups or more for pregnant women
   4 cups or more for nursing mothers

Meat Group
   2 or more servings. Count as one serving:
     2 to 3 ounces lean, cooked beef, veal, pork, lamb, poultry, fish—without bone
     2 eggs
     1 cup cooked dry beans, dry peas, lentils
     4 tablespoons peanut butter

Vegetable-Fruit Group (½ *cup serving, or* 1 *piece fruit, etc.*)
   4 or more servings per day, including:
     1 serving of citrus fruit, or other fruit or vegetable as a good source of vitamin C, or 2 servings of a fair source
     1 serving, at least every other day, of a dark-green or deep-yellow vegetable for vitamin A
     2 or more servings of other vegetables and fruits, including potatoes

Bread-Cereals Group
   4 or more servings daily (whole grain, enriched, or restored). Count as one serving:
     1 slice bread
     1 ounce ready-to-eat cereal
     ½ to ¾ cup cooked cereal, cornmeal, grits, macaroni, noodles, rice, or spaghetti

*"A Daily Food Guide" in *Consumers All*. Yearbook of Agriculture, 1965, U.S. Department of Agriculture, Washington, D.C., 1965, p. 394.

Groups will be discussed in the chapters on the nutrients. See also Table 13–2, page 206, for calculation of the nutritive contributions of the Four Food Groups.

The basic diet. The minimum number of servings for the adult of each of the Four Food Groups will be used as a basis for dietary planning throughout this text. The protein, mineral, except for iron, and vitamin needs are substantially met by this plan (see Table 13–2), and the caloric levels are approximately sufficient for basal energy requirements. The size of each portion will obviously need to be modified for preschool and school children and for teenagers to provide the correct amounts of the various nutrients.

To fully meet the energy needs, additional foods may be selected from the fats and sweets or from one or more of the four groups. The nutrient intake will remain essentially at the level calculated for the basic diet if additional energy is provided chiefly from fats and sweets, but the further selection of foods from one or more of the four groups will substantially increase the nutritive value of the diet.

COMPOSITION OF FOODS

Factors affecting food composition. The nutritive values of foods are determined, for the most part, by chemical methods. In some instances, such as the evaluation of protein quality or of digestibility, or the determination of vitamin D, animal feeding (BIOASSAY) is used. Certain of the B vitamins and some of the amino acids are best determined by observing the reproduction, or selected metabolic processes, of microorganisms (MICROBIOLOGIC ASSAY).

The values for nutrients in tables of food composition are customarily expressed as averages of analyses of food samples. For some nutrients numerous analyses have been made, but for other nutrients the number of determinations has been much more limited. Obviously, the actual nutritive value of a food may be expected to vary more or less widely from the average. Some of the more important factors which account for variation in food composition are discussed briefly below.

The nature of the soil might be expected to produce variations in the composition of foods. At the present time, the only correlation that has been fully established is that a low-iodine content of the soil is reflected in a low-iodine content of foods. The quantity of vitamins, or of other nutrients, has been found to be largely independent of the soil composition. Contrary to certain cultists who criticize the use of chemical fertilizers and who emphasize so-called organic farming, Maynard[5] presented evidence that soils that are chemically fertilized are highly productive of foods of good nutritive value.

The variety of plants and the climate are important determinants of nutritive value. The latter cannot be controlled, but much progress has been made in developing plant varieties that have superior nutritive qualities. For example, strains of corn and wheat are helping to improve the food supply in many of the developing countries.

The conditions of storage—length of time, temperature, light—are known to modify the nutritive value of foods. Some nutrients such as ascorbic acid are rapidly lost when the temperature is high or when foods are bruised. Other nutrients may be lost to a varying degree but not quite so readily as ascorbic acid.

Divergent procedures in food preparation are major factors that affect the nutritive value of a food as it is consumed. Losses in food preparation may be brought about through solubility of the nutrient in water, or through destruction of the nutrient. The latter is increased with high temperature and is also dependent upon the pH of the medium in which it is cooked. The amount of peelings removed, the size of pieces subjected to cooking, the temperature used, the length of time for cooking, the amount of water used, the length of time food is held after cooking—as on a steam table—are but a few of the many variables which may result in wide differences between two foods that were identical at the start of the cooking procedure.

Processing techniques enhance or interfere with the nutritive value of foods. Dehydration, canning, and freezing yield foods of high nutritive value, but each, in certain ways, modifies somewhat the nutrient contribution of a given food. No doubt this list could be lengthened, but it should suffice to emphasize to the student that a given value for a nutrient in a table of food composition represents an approximation and not a precise value.

Tables of food composition. In view of the foregoing discussion, one might be tempted to ask what useful purposes can be served by referring to a table of nutritive values. First, tables of food composition serve as a basis for comparing one food with another; for example, an examination of the calcium content of many foods leads one to the conclusion that milk is clearly the best source. Although every medium-sized orange could not be expected to yield exactly the same number of milligrams of ascorbic acid, the tables do give information on the relative magnitude of ascorbic acid in orange as compared with apple, for example. Second, tables of food composition make it possible to calculate the nutritive values of any diet and to compare these values with a given standard. Third, with the information on nutritive values, one can plan diets that meet requirements for specific needs—for example, a high protein diet or a sodium-restricted diet. Finally, the tables provide a ready reference to answer numerous questions concerning the nutritive value of foods; they are useful in counteracting misinformation about nutritive values.

The several tables of food values in the Appendix have been derived from compilations made from time to time, chiefly by investigators in the U.S. Department of Agriculture. Just as the purchase of food involves certain units of measure such as ounces, pounds, pints, quarts, so the amount of nutrients in a food is expressed in certain units—grams (gm), milligrams (mg), sometimes micrograms (mcg), and international units (I.U.). In Table A–1 of the Appendix the nutritive values are expressed for the edible part of household portions of food, thus making it simple to determine the contribution of full or fractional portions of food. Other tables give the nutritive values for 100-gm edible portion of food.

DIETARY EVALUATION

Purposes of dietary evaluation. A dietary evaluation may be qualitative—that is, through questioning of the subject it may be established that certain foods are, or are not, being included; recommendations for dietary improvement can often be made on such a basis without the necessity for detailed calculations. Nurses and dietitians make such evalua-

tions prior to counseling patients regarding a dietary modification. Such qualitative evaluations are also useful as a starting point for nutrition education for the lay public.

The discussion that follows is concerned with dietary calculations since the student and professional person must be able to use tables of food composition with facility. Most tools that are useful in carrying out one's work entail the development of skill on the part of the user. At first a tool may seem cumbersome and awkward; in fact, it may seem to impede progress rather than help to move things forward. So it is with a table of food composition—one of the most valuable of tools in the application of nutritional science. The beginning student often looks upon dietary calculations as being both time consuming and tedious. However, if long-range goals are kept in mind, the time spent in learning to use tables with confidence will be rewarding. Among the outcomes from experience in dietary calculations are the following:

1. A greater consciousness of food habits and their relation to nutrition and health.

2. Familiarity with tables of food composition and the kinds of information they provide.

3. Facility in using food tables whether to calculate a complete dietary or to seek specific answers concerning nutritive values of a single food.

4. Knowledge concerning the important sources of each of the nutrients.

5. Ability to make recommendations for the improvement of dietaries based upon the calculation of dietary intakes.

6. Appreciation of the importance of keeping orderly and accurate records of dietary intake so that any calculations may be as reliable as possible.

7. The habits of preparing neat and concise reports which have been carefully checked for their accuracy so that coworkers may use the information with complete confidence.

Calculation of the nutritive value of a diet. The method described below may be applied to the diet for a day, for one meal, or for a recipe. It may be used for the calculation of a single nutrient such as protein or for all nutrients listed in a given table. Study these steps carefully before you begin your calculations. See sample calculation of a breakfast, Table 3–4.

Table 3–4. Nutritive Value of a Breakfast

Food	Household Measure	Weight gm	Energy calories	Protein gm	Fat gm	Carbohydrate gm	Minerals		Vitamins				
							Ca mg	Fe mg	A I.U.	Thiamin mg	Riboflavin mg	Niacin mg	Ascorbic Acid mg
Prunes, cooked	3	45	49	tr	tr	13	10	0.8	310	0.01	0.03	0.4	tr
Scrambled eggs	2	128	220	14	16	2	102	2.2	1380	0.10	0.36	tr	0
Bacon, cooked	2 strips	15	90	5	8	1	2	0.5	0	0.08	0.05	0.8	—
Toast, enriched	1½ slices	33	105	3	2	20	31	0.9	tr	0.09	0.08	0.9	tr
Butter	2 pats	14	100	tr	12	tr	3	0	470	—	—	—	0
Coffee													
Cream, light	1 tablespoon	15	30	1	3	1	15	tr	130	tr	0.02	tr	tr
Total			594	23	41	37	163	4.4	2290	0.28	0.54	2.1	tr
Recommended Dietary Allowances													
Woman, 23–50 years			2000	46				800	18	4000	1.0	1.2	13	45
Per cent of RDA			30	50				20	24	57	28	45	15	0

1. Study the arrangement of Table A–1, noting especially the units of measure for each nutrient.

2. Keep an accurate record, in household measures, of the foods eaten at each meal. Record the information directly after each meal if at all possible; do not rely on memory. Include any foods or beverages taken between meals. Specify the exact kinds of foods eaten. Note these descriptive terms: *scrambled* eggs; *cooked* prunes; *light* cream; *enriched* toast; *fried* beef liver. These descriptions enable anyone who is making the evaluation to select the correct items from the table of food composition.

3. If the evaluation is for an entire day, list the total amount, in household measures, for the same foods eaten at different meals. For example: one slice enriched bread at breakfast, ¾ slice at lunch, and ½ slice at dinner would be recorded on the calculation sheet as 2¼ slices.

4. Calculate the nutritive values for each food of the diet or recipe by multiplying the values for the stated portion in Table A–1 by the amounts actually eaten. For example, if three cooked prunes are eaten, all nutritive values shown in the table would be multiplied by ⅙, since the values are given for 17 to 18 prunes.

5. When recording the results of your calculations, use only as many decimal places as appear in the original table. For example, 11.3 gm fat is recorded as 11 gm fat; but 11.5 gm fat would be recorded as 12 gm. A calculated value for thiamin of 0.074 mg would be recorded as 0.07 mg since the table lists only two decimal places for thiamin.

6. Check each of your calculations to be sure it is correct before entering the result on the final calculation sheet.

7. Record all data so that numbers are legible and digits and decimal points are aligned.

8. Total the amount of each nutrient contained in the entire diet or recipe.

9. Compare the actual totals of the diet with the Recommended Dietary Allowances of the individual for whom the evaluation was made. If there are wide deviations between the two, it is especially important to look for possible errors in calculations, misplacement of decimal points, or mistakes in additions.

10. Calculate for each of the nutrients the percentage of the Recommended Dietary Allowances provided by the diet.

11. Summarize the study by listing ways in which the diet can be improved.

PROBLEMS AND REVIEW

1. List the Recommended Allowances for yourself. If a dietary calculation indicated that you were getting less than these allowances in one or more respects, how should you interpret this?
2. State the characteristics of the reference woman. How do you differ?
3. List five reasons why two oranges may differ in ascorbic acid content.
4. Two students had hamburger for lunch, each raw hamburger weighing 4 ounces. One student received more calories in her hamburger than did the other. Explain.
5. Examine the tables in the Appendix to become familiar with the information they provide.
6. *Problem.* Using Table A–1, list five fresh fruits that are the most outstanding sources of vitamin A. In your community, which of these, if any, are not practical for dietary planning?
7. *Problem.* Use Table A–1 to find answers to the following questions:
   a. A woman asks whether whole-wheat bread is more nutritious than enriched white bread.
   b. A teen-ager wants to know if potatoes are more fattening than ice cream.
   c. A mother asks if she can substitute tomato juice for orange juice in her child's diet.
   d. A man asks if beefsteak is richer in protein than Swiss cheese.
8. *Problem.* Keep a careful record of your own food intake for three days. See above for directions.
   a. Score your diet according to the Daily Food Guide. What food group, if any, requires more emphasis in order to improve your diet?
   b. Select one of the three days that is most typical of your usual practice. Calculate the nutritive values using Table A–1. Compare your intake with your recommended allowances.
   c. Keep this evaluation for reference as you study the nutrients in chapters that follow.

CITED REFERENCES

1. Food and Nutrition Board: *Recommended Dietary Allowances,* 8th ed., National Research Council—National Academy of Sciences, Washington, D.C., 1974.
2. Campbell, J. A.: "Approaches in Revising Dietary Standards," *J. Am. Diet. Assoc.,* **64:**175–78, 1974.
3. Nutrition Bureau, Health and Welfare: *The Canadian Dietary Standard, Revised 1975.* Canada Health Protection Branch, Ottawa, Canada.
4. Patwardhan, V. A.: "Dietary Allowances—An International Point of View," *J. Am. Diet. Assoc.,* **56:**191–94, 1970.
5. Maynard, L. A.: "Effect of Fertilizers on the Nutritional Value of Foods," *J.A.M.A.,* **161:**1478, 1961.

ADDITIONAL REFERENCES

Goldsmith, G. A.: "Interest and Activities of the Food and Nutrition Board," *J. Am. Diet. Assoc.,* **52:**37–42, 1968.
Gormican, A.: "Inorganic Elements in Foods Used in Hospital Menus," *J. Am. Diet. Assoc.,* **56:**397–403, 1970.
Harper, A. E.: "Recommended Dietary Allowances (Revised 1973)," *Nutr. Rev.,* **31:**393–95, 1973.
Harper, A. E.: "Recommended Dietary Allowances: Are They What We Think They Are?" *J. Am. Diet. Assoc.,* **64:**151–56, 1974.
Harper, A. E.: "Those Pesky RDAs," *Nutr. Today,* **9:**15, March/April 1974.
Hegsted, D. M.: "Dietary Standards," *J. Am. Diet. Assoc.,* **66:**13–21, 1975.
Hertzler, A. A., and Anderson, H. L.: "Food Guides in the United States," *J. Am. Diet. Assoc.,* **64:**19–28, 1974.
Hollingsworth, D. F.: "Recommended Intakes of Nutrients for the United Kingdom," *J. Am. Diet. Assoc.,* **56:**200–202, 1970.
Hopkins, H. T., *et al.:* "Soil Factors and Food Composition," *Am. J. Clin. Nutr.,* **18:**390–95, 1966.
Leverton, R.: "The RDAs Are Not for Amateurs. Commentary," *J. Am. Diet. Assoc.,* **66:**9–11, 1975.
Miller, D. F., and Voris, L.: "Chronologic Changes in the Recommended Dietary Allowances," *J. Am. Diet. Assoc.,* **54:**109–17, 1969.
Todhunter, E. N.: "Food Composition Tables in the U.S.A.," *J. Am. Diet. Assoc.,* **37:**209–14, 1960.
Watt, B. K.: "Concepts in Developing a Food Composition Table," *J. Am. Diet. Assoc.,* **40:**297–300, 1962.

4 Proteins and Amino Acids

Importance of protein. In 1838 a Dutch chemist, Mulder, described certain organic material which is "unquestionably the most important of all known substances in the organic kingdom. Without it no life appears possible on our planet. Through its means the chief phenomena of life are produced."° Berzelius, a contemporary of Mulder, suggested that this complex nitrogen-bearing substance be called *protein* from the Greek word meaning to "take the first place."[1]

PROTEINS is now retained as a group name to designate the principal nitrogenous constituents of the protoplasm of all plant and animal tissues; they are necessary for tissue synthesis and in the regulation of certain body functions. To say that proteins are more important than are other nutrients is not appropriate, however, for we shall see in the study of nutrition that an inadequate dietary supply or an interference with the utilization of any nutrient can have serious consequences.

The shortage of protein is second in importance only to the shortage of calories in the world's food supply. Protein-calorie malnutrition, a broad term that encompasses kwashiorkor and marasmus together with milder stages of these diseases, is the major nutritional problem of the developing coun-

° Mulder, G. J.: *The Chemistry of Animal and Vegetable Physiology.* Quoted in Mendel, L. B.: *Nutrition: The Chemistry of Life.* Yale University Press, New Haven, Conn., 1923, p. 16.

tries of the world. Literally millions of infants and young children are victims of these diseases in Asia, Africa, Central America, the West Indies, and South America. Many of the children who survive are unable to achieve their full physical growth and development. Even more serious is the threat that the most severely malnourished may be retarded in their mental development and that this retardation may be irreversible.

In the United States there is an abundance of protein of good quality but even so some people do not get enough, either because of ignorance concerning the selection of a good diet or because of lack of money to purchase protein foods, which are generally the most expensive items of the diet. Occasionally, an infant is seen with severe protein-calorie malnutrition. This is usually the result of gross ignorance of the infant's food needs, or even of child neglect.

A full understanding of the role of proteins in body functions, of daily requirements, and of food sources to meet these needs is essential for the planning of adequate diets for the healthy in all stages of the life cycle and also for therapeutic modifications for the ill. Moderate to severe protein deficiencies are often encountered during illness because of inadequate intake or faulty absorption or metabolism.

COMPOSITION, STRUCTURE, AND CLASSIFICATION

Composition. Proteins are extremely complex nitrogenous organic compounds in which amino acids are the units of structure. They contain the elements carbon, hydrogen, oxygen, nitrogen, and, with few exceptions, sulfur. Most proteins also contain phosphorus, and some specialized proteins contain very small amounts of iron, copper, and other inorganic elements.

The presence of nitrogen distinguishes protein from carbohydrate and fat. Proteins contain an average of 16 per cent nitrogen and have a molecular weight that varies from 13,000 or less to many millions. Thus, the protein molecule is much larger than those of carbohydrates and lipids. The large protein molecules form colloidal solutions that do not readily diffuse through membranes.

Structure. AMINO ACIDS are organic compounds possessing an amino (NH_2) group and an acid or carboxyl (COOH) group. All the amino acids obtained by hydrolysis from native proteins are α-amino acids; that is, the amino group is attached to the carbon adjacent to the acid group. The structure of an amino acid may be represented thus:

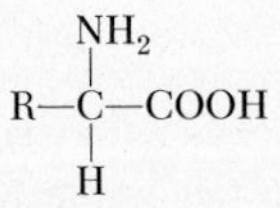

$$\begin{array}{c} NH_2 \\ | \\ R\!-\!C\!-\!COOH \\ | \\ H \end{array}$$

By varying the grouping (R) that is attached to the carbon containing the amino group, many different amino acids are possible. Examples of variations in the R grouping are shown in Figure 4–1. The amino acids, except glycine, are optically active and are of the L-configuration; not all amino acids of the D-configuration are utilized in the body.

Twenty-two amino acids are widely distributed in proteins, and small amounts of four or five additional amino acids have been isolated from one or more proteins. Some amino acids—ornithine and citrulline—are important intermediates in metabolism but are not constituents of intact proteins. See page 52.

Proteins consist of chains of amino acids joined to each other by the peptide linkage; that is, the amino group of one amino acid is linked to the carboxyl group of another amino acid by the removal of water. (See Figure 4–2.) Thus, two amino acids form a dipeptide, three amino acids form a tripeptide, and so on. Proteins consist of hundreds of such linkages.

Specificity of protein. The nature of a protein is first determined by the sequence in which the amino acids are linked and also by the amounts of each amino acid present. For example, tripeptides containing these sequences would differ from each other:

Glycine—Tryptophan—Methionine
Tryptophan—Glycine—Methionine
Glycine—Tryptophan—Valine

Some polypeptide chains might be relatively short; some might be open chains, whereas others might be closed or cyclic chains. Moreover, the nature of the protein is determined by the manner in which the polypeptide chains are bound together to form the protein molecule. *Fibrous* proteins consist of long polypeptide chains bound together in more or less parallel fashion; these are characteristic of proteins of muscle fibers, hair, and collagen. *Globular* proteins are round to ellipsoidal; these include hemoglobin, insulin, and albumins and globulins.

In view of the number of amino acids and the innumerable ways and proportions by which they may be combined, it should not be surprising that proteins are so numerous and so highly specific. Each species synthesizes protein that is characteristic. Moreover, each species also synthesizes for its manifold functions proteins that are tailored to these specific needs. Thus, serum albumin, insulin, hemoglobin, keratin, collagen, and myosin have specific structures and functions; they are not interchangeable.

Classification. Proteins may be classified on the basis of their physical and chemical properties or their nutritional qualities.

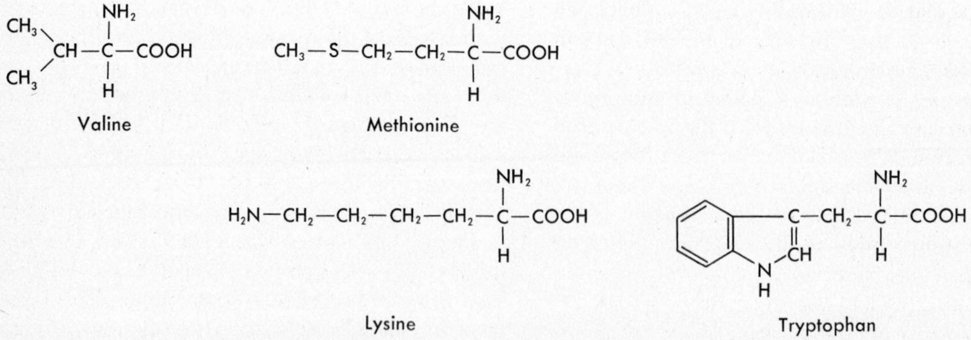

Figure 4–1. Amino acids with different groupings attached to the carbon that holds the amino group.

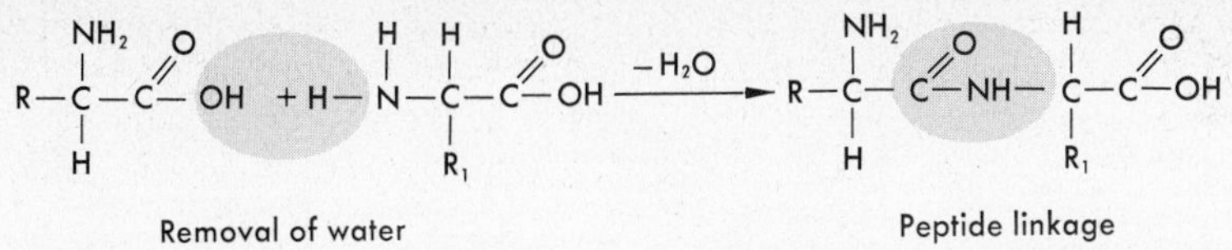

Removal of water   Peptide linkage

Figure 4–2. Peptide linkage (CONH). The carboxyl group of one amino acid is linked to the amino group of another amino acid by removal of water. Proteins consist of long chains of amino acids thus linked. The peptide linkage is broken by hydrolysis as in digestion.

Physical-chemical properties. Each of the three groups within this classification may be subdivided into a number of classes according to solubility.

1. Simple proteins upon hydrolysis by acids, alkalies, or enzymes yield only amino acids or their derivatives. Examples of this group are albumins and globulins found within all body cells and in the blood serum; keratin, collagen, and elastin in supportive tissues of the body and in hair and nails; globin in hemoglobin and myoglobin; and zein in corn, gliadin and glutenin in wheat, legumin in peas, and lactalbumin and lactoglobulin in milk.

2. Conjugated proteins are composed of simple proteins combined with a nonprotein substance. This group includes *lipoproteins,* the vehicles for the transport of fats in the blood; *nucleoproteins,* the proteins of the cell nuclei; *phosphoproteins,* such as casein in milk and ovovitellin in eggs; *metalloproteins,* such as the enzymes that contain mineral elements; *mucoproteins,* found in connective tissues, mucin, and gonadotropic hormones; *chromoproteins,* such as hemoglobin and visual purple; and *flavoproteins,* which are enzymes that contain the vitamin riboflavin.

3. Derived proteins are substances resulting from the decomposition of simple and conjugated proteins. These include rearrangements within the molecule without breaking the peptide bond, such as that occurring with coagulation, and also substances formed by hydrolysis of the protein to smaller fragments.

Essential and dispensable amino acids. In 1915 Osborne and Mendel observed that rats failed to grow or even survive if some amino acids were omitted from the diet, but that the elimination of other amino acids had no such harmful effects. (See Figure 4–3.) Later work by others, especially Dr. William C. Rose,[2] established that this was also true for human beings. Thus, amino acids came to be classified as *essential or indispensable* and *nonessential or dispensable.*

Essential amino acids are those that cannot be synthesized in the body and must be provided in the diet. The human adult requires nine essential amino acids. Histidine, for which the requirement by adults has long been uncertain, has now been found to be essential.[3] Methionine, an essential amino acid, can be converted to cystine, but cystine cannot be converted to methionine. Likewise, phenylalanine can be converted to tyrosine, but tyrosine cannot be converted to phenylalanine. Since the requirements for methionine and phenylalanine are reduced when cystine and tyrosine, respectively, are present in the diet, the latter amino acids are considered to be *semiessential.*

The nonessential or dispensable amino acids are those that the body can synthesize provided that there is an available source of nitrogen. If the full requirement for the essential amino acids is met by the diet, the body can synthesize any nonessential amino acid that is not present in the diet in sufficient amounts to meet metabolic needs.

Complete and incomplete proteins. A complete protein contains enough of the essential amino acids to maintain body tissues and to promote a normal rate of growth and is sometimes referred to as having a high-biologic value. Egg, milk, and meat (including poultry and fish) proteins are all complete but not necessarily identical in quality. Wheat germ and dried yeast have a biologic value approaching that of animal sources.

Partially complete proteins will maintain life, but they lack sufficient amounts of some of the amino acids necessary for growth. Gliadin, which is one of a number of proteins found in wheat, is a notable example of proteins of this class. Adults under no physiologic stress can maintain satisfac-

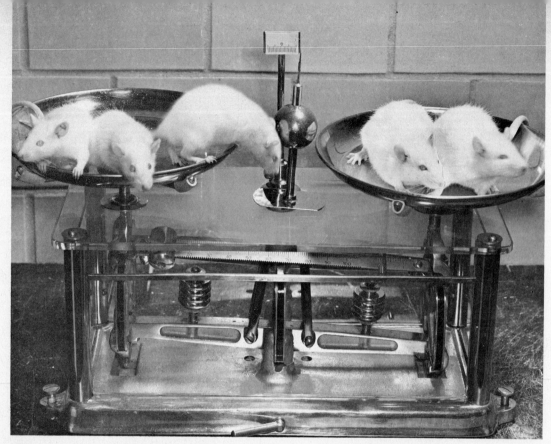

Figure 4–3. Effect of protein quality. These rats of the same age were fed a bread diet. The lysine content of wheat is too low to promote optimum growth. The two rats on the right received bread to which lysine had been added. This improvement of the protein quality led to greater gain. (Courtesy, E. I. DuPont de Nemours and Company, Inc.)

Table 4–1. Classification of Amino Acids

Classification	Essential Amino Acids	Nonessential Amino Acids
Neutral—one amino and one carboxyl group		
Aliphatic	Threonine	Glycine
	Valine	Alanine
	Leucine	Serine
	Isoleucine	
Aromatic—contains benzene ring	Phenylalanine	Tyrosine*
Heterocyclic	Tryptophan	Proline
		Hydroxyproline
	Histidine	
Sulfur containing	Methionine	Cystine*
		Cysteine
Basic—two amino and one carboxyl group	Lysine	Arginine
		Hydroxylysine
Acid—one amino and two carboxyl groups		Aspartic acid
		Glutamic acid

*These amino acids are classed as semiessential. See text (page 43).

tory nutrition for indefinite periods when consuming sufficient amounts of protein from certain cereals or legumes.

Totally INCOMPLETE PROTEINS are incapable of replacing or building new tissue, and hence cannot support life, let alone promote growth. Zein, one of the proteins found in corn, and gelatin are classic examples of proteins that are incapable of even permitting life to continue.

FUNCTIONS

Maintenance and growth. Proteins constitute the chief solid matter of muscles, organs, and endocrine glands. They are major constituents of the matrix of bones and teeth; skin, nails, and hair; and blood cells and serum. In fact, every living cell and all body fluids, except bile and urine, contain protein. The first need for amino acids, then, is to supply the materials for the building and the continuous replacement of the cell proteins throughout life.

Regulation of body processes. Body proteins have highly specialized functions in the regulation of body processes. For example, hemoglobin, an iron-bearing protein that is the chief constituent of the red blood cells, performs a vital role in carrying oxygen to the tissues. The plasma proteins are of fundamental importance in the regulation of osmotic pressure and in the maintenance of water balance. The blood proteins have a role in the maintenance of the normal slightly alkaline reaction of the blood. The body's resistance to disease is maintained in part by antibodies which are protein in nature.

Enzymes that are specific catalysts for metabolic processes are protein in nature. Governing the metabolic reactions are hormones, many of which are protein in nature—insulin, epinephrine, and thyroid hormone, to name but a few.

Amino acids also have specific functions in metabolism. Tryptophan serves as a precursor for niacin, one of the B-complex vitamins; methionine supplies labile methyl groups for the synthesis of choline, a compound that helps to prevent storage of fat in the liver; glycine contributes to the formation of the porphyrin ring in the hemoglobin molecule and is also an important constituent of the purines and pyrimidines in nucleic acid.

Energy. Proteins are a potential source of energy, each gram of protein yielding on the average 4 kilocalories. The energy needs of the body take priority over other needs, and if the diet does not furnish sufficient calories from carbohydrate and fat, the protein of the diet as well as tissue proteins will be catabolized for energy. When amino acids are used for energy, they are then lost for synthetic purposes. Conversely, when amino acids are incorporated into the protein molecule, they are not furnishing energy until such time as the tissue proteins are again being catabolized.

DIGESTION AND ABSORPTION

Digestion. The purposes of digestion are to hydrolyze proteins to amino acids so that they can be absorbed and to destroy the biologic specificity of the proteins by such hydrolysis. (See also Chapter 2.) In addition to the foods ingested, the mixture to be digested includes a sizable amount of protein that is constantly being released from the worn-out cells of the mucosa and of the digestive enzymes themselves.[4] The endogenous and exogenous sources of the amino acids are indistinguishable and present a mixture for absorption that differs from that provided by the diet alone.

Saliva contains no proteolytic enzyme, and thus the only action in the mouth is an increase in the surface area of the food mass as a result of the chewing of food. Digestion of protein involves the splitting of the peptide linkages. (See Figure 4–2.) Most of the hydrolysis of protein occurs in the stomach, duodenum, and jejunum. The protein molecule is split to smaller fragments by the proteases with final cleavage by the peptidases. The enzymes are secreted in their inactive form and are activated when they are needed for protein hydrolysis. Each enzyme is highly specific and is capable of splitting only one type of peptide linkage.[5] For example, pepsin attacks only those peptide linkages where phenylalanine or tyrosine provides the amino group. The rate of hydrolysis appears to be regulated to the rate of absorption so that there is never a large excess of amino acids in the intestinal lumen. Table 4–2 summarizes the important enzymes in protein digestion and the linkages with which they react.

Effect of protein denaturation. Proteolytic en-

Table 4–2. Enzyme Activity in Protein Digestion

Enzyme and Its Location	Action
Stomach	
Pepsinogen	Activated to pepsin by hydrochloric acid
Pepsin	Splits peptide chain where phenylalanine or tyrosine furnishes amino group
Small intestine	
Trypsinogen*	Activated to trypsin by enterokinase
Trypsin	Splits peptide chain where lysine or arginine furnishes carboxyl group
Chymotrypsinogen*	Activated to chymotrypsin by trypsin
Chymotrypsin	Splits peptide chain where carboxyl group is furnished by tryptophan, methionine, tyrosine, or phenylalanine
Intestinal mucosa	
Aminopeptidase	Splits peptide linkage next to a terminal amino group
Carboxypeptidase*	Splits peptide linkage next to a terminal carboxyl group

*These enzymes are secreted by the pancreas.

zymes not only bring about the splitting of the peptide linkages but they also split the crosslinks that connect the peptide chains. During moderate heating of proteins some of the cross-linkages are split, thereby facilitating digestion. On the other hand, excessive heating results in the formation of linkages that are resistant to the digestive enzymes. As a consequence the amino acids so linked may not be available at a rate that is necessary for incorporation into new proteins.

One resistant linkage is that of lysine with carbohydrate as a result of high heat, usually prolonged. The brown crust of bread contains less available lysine than does the white crumb; toasting of bread results in small losses. If breakfast cereals are processed at high temperatures, they are also subject to such losses. These changes may be important when relatively low-protein diets of poor quality are consumed.

Effect of enzyme inhibitors. Some foods such as navy beans and soybeans contain substances that inhibit activity of enzymes such as trypsin. Heating inactivates these inhibitors, thereby improving the digestibility of the protein.

Absorption. Amino acids are absorbed from the proximal intestine into the portal circulation. The rates of absorption are regulated by complex mechanisms not fully understood. These rates are dependent upon (1) the total load of amino acids released through digestion, (2) the proportions of the various amino acids present in the mixture to be absorbed, (3) the availability of carriers to ferry the amino acids into the mucosal cells, and (4) the uptake of amino acids by tissues. Because the liberation of amino acids through digestion is coordinated with the rate of absorption, there is a minimal loss of amino acids in the feces. The rate of absorption also appears to be controlled by the levels existing in the blood. Amino acids are rapidly removed from the circulation, and the concentration in the blood at any given time is relatively low.

Active transport and specific carriers. Amino acids are absorbed by active transport, but some diffusion of amino acids also occurs. The amino acids are in competition for the carriers, some amino acids being absorbed much more rapidly than others. In one study an essential amino acid mixture in amounts usually present in a protein meal was administered into the jejunum of normal adults, and the rates of absorption were measured.[6] Methionine, leucine, isoleucine, and valine had the highest rates of absorption, and these were two to three times as rapid as that for threonine, which was the lowest. Whether these same rates would apply to a protein meal fed intact is not known. If they do, as is strongly suspected, a protein that might contain an excess of a rapidly absorbed amino acid such as leucine would be less effective than a more balanced protein inasmuch as carriers would be less available for the amino acids with the lower rates of absorption.

On the average, 92 per cent of the amino acids present in the typical American diet are released through digestion and absorbed. Proteins that are well balanced in their amino acid composition, as in milk, eggs, and meat, show even higher rates of absorption. Most plant proteins have excesses of some amino acids and deficiencies of others, and the percentage of amino acids absorbed is somewhat less. In part this results from the competition of amino acids for carriers to transport them across the mucosal cells, and in part it may be explained by linkages resistant to digestion as explained above. A point of practical importance in dietary planning is that some protein of good quality should be present in each meal so that the available mixture of amino acids at any given time is optimum in quality as well as quantity.

METABOLISM

Strictly speaking, the metabolism of proteins is the metabolism of the amino acids. Each cell within the body utilizes the available amino acids to synthesize all the numerous proteins required for its own functions and also makes use of amino acids to furnish energy. In addition, some specialized cells, such as those of the liver, also synthesize proteins and nonprotein nitrogenous substances that are required for the functioning of the body as a whole. Whether the fate of an amino acid, at any given moment, is that of anabolism or catabolism is determined by a number of interrelated factors. (See Figure 4–4.)

Methods for study of protein metabolism. Many techniques are available to the biochemist and nutritionist for the study of protein metabolism. Hundreds of investigators since the nineteenth century have assayed the quality of proteins from single foods and food mixtures and have measured the requirements for proteins or amino acids under varying dietary and physiologic conditions by means of *nitrogen balance* studies. These studies on infants, children, and adults as well as on experimental animals—especially rats—have included measurements of the dietary intake of protein or amino acids and of the excretion of nitrogen in the urine and feces. The nitrogen balance technique requires continuous supervision of subjects for weeks so that precise controls of dietary intake and 24-hour quantitative collections of urine and feces are assured. The method is time consuming, tedious, and expensive. By nitrogen balance only the total nitrogen metabolism of the body is measured, without information on what is happening in specific tissues.

Other methods that supplement or take the place of nitrogen balance studies include the determination of the concentration in the blood of the protein fractions, amino acids, and nonprotein nitrogenous

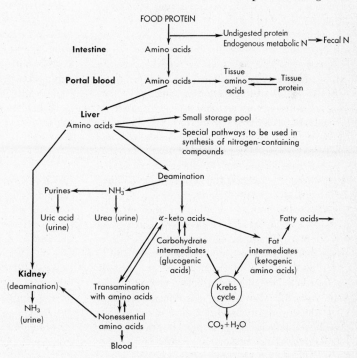

Figure 4–4. The metabolism of protein.

constituents—total nonprotein nitrogen, urea nitrogen, creatinine, and uric acid. Tracers are often used to study the fate of an amino acid including its absorption, its incorporation into tissues, its pathway through intermediate substances, or its excretion in the urine.

Through a study of the nitrogenous constituents in the urine it is possible to determine the level of nitrogen catabolism that is taking place, to detect abnormalities in amino acid metabolism (as in phenylketonuria) or in nonprotein nitrogenous compounds (as in gout), and to evaluate the ability of the kidney to excrete nitrogenous products. (See Tables A–11 and A–12.)

Nitrogen balance. Nitrogen balance studies are based on the fact that protein, on the average, contains 16 per cent nitrogen; thus, 1 gm nitrogen is equivalent to 6.25 gm protein. The balance may be expressed thus:

$$\text{Nitrogen balance} = \text{Nitrogen intake} - \text{nitrogen excretion (urine + feces + skin)}$$

Nitrogen excretion. The fecal nitrogen includes that from undigested dietary protein and also nitrogen from undigested endogenous sources. The latter are composed of the undigested protein fractions of desquamated cells of the intestinal mucosa, the used-up enzymes from the digestive juices, and bacterial cells. The daily fecal excretion of nitrogen by the adult is approximately 1 gm, but this varies with the quality of the protein fed, the gastrointestinal motility, and so on. The difference between the amount of nitrogen in the diet and the fecal nitrogen is the amount of nitrogen absorbed and available for tissue use.

More than 90 per cent of the urinary nitrogen results from the deamination of the amino acids in the body and is excreted chiefly as urea with small amounts of ammonia. Nonprotein nitrogenous end products include creatinine, uric acid, and a number of others. When the calorie intake is fully adequate and the protein intake is just sufficient to cover the repletion of body tissues, the urinary nitrogen is at its lowest level. As the protein intake increases above the tissue maintenance requirement, the excess amino acids are not stored but are deaminized and used for energy or stored as fat, thereby increasing the amount of urinary nitrogen.

Therefore, in studies of the minimum protein requirement by the nitrogen balance technique it is always necessary to determine the balance at gradually decreasing levels of intake until the point of negative balance is reached. That level just above negative balance that is just sufficient for tissue replacement represents the *minimum* protein requirement under the conditions of the experiment.

Nitrogen is also lost through perspiration and from the desquamated cells of the skin surfaces, the hair, and the nails. Such losses are extremely difficult to measure. A few studies have shown that the average daily losses by the adult male are about 1.4 gm nitrogen. When people live and work at high environmental temperatures so that sweating is profuse, the losses from the skin have been found to be as high as 3.75 gm nitrogen (equivalent to 23 gm protein) in 24 hours.[7]

States of balance. NITROGEN EQUILIBRIUM is that state of balance when the intake of nitrogen is equal to that which is excreted. A state of equilibrium is normal for the healthy adult. It is established at any level of protein intake that exceeds the minimum requirement, provided that the calorie intake is also adequate.

POSITIVE NITROGEN BALANCE is that state in which the intake of nitrogen exceeds the excretion. It indicates that new protein tissues are being synthesized, as in growing children or during pregnancy. Positive nitrogen balance also occurs when tissues depleted of protein during illness or injury are being replenished, or when muscles are being developed, as in athletic training. Positive nitrogen balance should not be interpreted as storage in the usual sense. There is no further addition of protein to already well-nourished cells.

NEGATIVE NITROGEN BALANCE is that condition in which the excretion of nitrogen exceeds the intake. An individual with a negative nitrogen balance is losing nitrogen from tissues more rapidly than it is being replaced—an undesirable state of affairs. It may occur because (1) the calorie content of the diet is inadequate and therefore tissues are being broken down to supply energy; (2) the quality of the protein is poor and the needs for tissue replacement are not being met; or (3) injury, immobilization, and disease are causing excessive breakdown of tissues.

Dynamic equilibrium. The liver is the key organ in the metabolism of protein. It selectively removes amino acids from the portal circulation for the synthesis of its own proteins and for many of the specialized proteins such as lipoproteins, plasma albumins, globulins, and fibrinogen as well as nonprotein nitrogenous substances such as creatine. The liver is also the principal organ for the synthesis of urea.

Amino acids are transported throughout the body by the systemic circulation and are rapidly removed from the circulation by the various tissue cells. Likewise, amino acids and products of amino acid metabolism are constantly added to the circulation by the tissues. The AMINO ACID POOL available to any given tissue at any given moment thus includes dietary sources (exogenous) and tissue breakdown (endogenous sources). These sources are indistinguishable. Body proteins are not static structures, but there is a continuous taking up and release of amino acids. In the adult the gains and losses are about equal, and the state is known as *dynamic equilibrium.*

The rate of turnover varies widely in body tissues. The intestinal mucosa, for example, renews itself every one to three days—a fantastic rate of repletion! The liver also has a high rate of turnover. Muscle proteins have a much slower rate of turnover, but the size of the muscle mass in the body is so great that the net daily release of amino acids is considerable. The turnover rate of collagen is very slow and that of the brain cells is negligible.

Protein reserves. Although the body does not store protein in the sense that it stores fat, or glycogen, or vitamin A, certain "reserves" are available from practically all body tissues for use in an emergency. Based upon animal studies, about one fourth of the body protein can be depleted and repleted.[8] Thus, the vital functions of the organism may be protected for 30 to 50 days of total starvation or for much longer periods of partial starvation. It should be apparent that the use of these reserves eventually requires restoration of tissue to their normal protein composition.

Anabolism or catabolism? Whether an amino acid is utilized for the synthesis of new proteins or is deaminized and used for energy depends upon a number of factors.

1. The "all-or-none" law. All the amino acids needed for the synthesis of a given protein must be simultaneously present in sufficient amounts. If a single amino acid is missing, the protein cannot be constructed. If a given amino acid is present only to a limited extent, the protein can be formed only as long as the supply of that amino acid lasts. The amino acid in short supply is known as the LIMITING AMINO ACID. If one or more amino acids are missing from the pool, the remaining amino acids are unavailable for later synthesis and will be catabolized for energy.

2. Adequacy of calorie intake. For protein synthesis to proceed at an optimum rate, the calorie intake must be sufficient to supply the energy needs. A deficiency of calories necessitates the use of some dietary and tissue proteins for energy.

3. The nutritional and physiologic state of the individual. The rate of synthesis is high during growth and in tissue repletion following illness or injury. In the adult synthesis just balances tissue depletion when the calorie intake is adequate.

Protein catabolism is greatly increased immediately following an injury, burns, and immobilization because of illness. It is also increased as a result of fear, anxiety, or anger. For example, unmarried pregnant girls who are worried about their future often have a negative nitrogen balance in spite of diets that appear to be adequate.

4. Development of specific tissues. Some tissues may be synthesized even though the overall nitrogen balance might be negative. Thus, the fetus and maternal tissues may be developed at the expense of the mother when her diet is inadequate. Another example of specific tissue development is that of rapidly growing tumors that use amino acids at the expense of normal tissues.

5. Hormonal controls. The pituitary growth hormone has an anabolic effect during infancy and childhood, and the estrogens and androgens exert an anabolic effect during preadolescent and adolescent years. By bringing about normal carbohydrate metabolism insulin has an indirect anabolic effect by reducing the breakdown of proteins to supply glucose. Insulin probably facilitates the transport of amino acids into the cell. In normal amounts thyroid hormone also stimulates growth.

Among the hormones that increase the catabolism of body tissues are adrenocortical hormones, which stimulate the breakdown of tissue proteins to yield glucose. An excessive production of thyroxine also increases the breakdown of proteins.

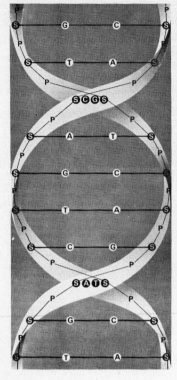

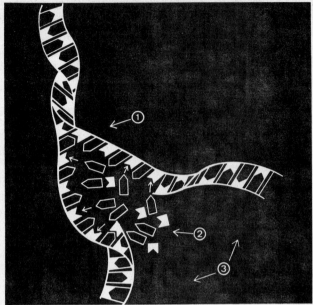

Figure 4–5. (*Left*) The Watson-Crick DNA model. Shown here are only a few of the thousands of turns in the double-helix structure of the molecule. The two outer ribbons are the backbone of the molecule, consisting of the sugar (*S*) deoxyribose and phosphate (*P*). Cross-links between the two ribbons are pairs of bases: adenine (*A*), guanine (*G*), cytosine (*C*), and thymine (*T*). (Courtesy, World Health Organization.)

   (*Right*) Shows replication of the molecule. The two chains of the DNA molecule are "unzipped" at (*1*); sugars, phosphates, and bases move about in the nucleus (*2*) and attach to form two new double-helix arrangements (*3*). (Courtesy, World Health Organization.)

Synthesis of proteins. Each cell is capable of synthesizing all the proteins for its own functions but not those of a different type of cell. The specific protein that will be synthesized is governed by the GENETIC CODE, or amino acid program, that exists within the nucleus of each cell. The synthesis of protein takes place in the cytoplasm of the cell. The model for protein synthesis was established by Watson and Crick in 1962. (See Figure 4–5.)

Within the nucleus of the cell are giant molecules of a substance known as deoxyribonucleic acid (DNA). These molecules consist of two intertwining chains containing 5-carbon sugar (deoxyribose) and phosphate groupings that form a long double-helix molecule. These chains are the backbone of the molecule. Four nitrogenous bases (adenine, guanine, cytosine, and thymine) are joined in pairs and at-

tached by hydrogen bonds to the sugar-phosphate chain to give a firm sturcture that resembles a spiral staircase. The arrangement of the bases within the molecule designates the specific amino acids that will be used and the sequence of their attachment to one another.

Since the synthesis of the protein takes place in the cytoplasm, the plan must be carried from the DNA molecules in the nucleus. This is the function of MESSENGER RIBONUCLEIC ACID (mRNA). Ribonucleic acid is a compound that resembles DNA except that the 5-carbon sugar is ribose and uracil is substituted for thymine. The information in DNA is copied within the nucleus to mRNA, which then moves to the ribosomes, which are the site of synthesis in the cytoplasm.

Amino acids enter the cell by active transport

from the metabolic pool. Some of the nonessential amino acids may be synthesized within the cell itself. The amino acids are activated in a reaction that requires the energy-rich compound ATP. Then they form a complex with another type of RNA, known as TRANSFER RNA; the transfer RNA is specific for each amino acid. The RNA-amino acid complex is then moved to the messenger RNA where the peptide linkage is formed according to the pattern carried from DNA. When the synthesis has been completed, the protein is set free from the ribosomes to perform its function in the cell, and the transfer RNA is also released to pick up amino acids for another sequence of synthesis.

The daily synthesis of protein in the adult has been estimated to be about 1.3 gm per kilogram, or about 91 gm for the 70-kg man.[9] Almost all the amino acids for this daily replacement are supplied by tissue proteins that have been broken down, supplemented with amino acids from dietary sources.

Synthesis of nonessential amino acids. The materials for the formation of the nonessential amino acids are keto acids such as pyruvic and α-ketoglutaric acid formed in the metabolism of carbohydrates (see Fig. 5–5) and ammonia that is released through deamination of amino acids. The synthesis involves a process known as TRANSAMINATION in which an amino group is transferred to a keto acid. Enzymes known as *transaminases* and pyridoxal phosphate, a coenzyme containing vitamin B_6, are involved. By this mechanism a new amino acid is formed without the appearance of ammonia in the free state. Glutamic acid often serves as a donor of nitrogen in this reaction. The general reaction is as follows:

$$R_1CHNH_2COOH + R_2COCOOH \rightleftharpoons$$
Amino acid$_1$ Keto acid$_2$

$$R_2CHNH_2COOH + R_1COCOOH$$
Amino acid$_2$ Keto acid$_1$

Catabolism. When amino acids are used for energy, the amino group is removed and a keto acid remains. Most of the deamination of amino acids occurs in the liver, but some also occurs in the kidney. Ammonia is liberated from the amino acids by oxidative enzymes according to the following general reaction:

$$RCHNH_2COOH + \tfrac{1}{2} O_2 \rightarrow RCOCOOH + NH_3$$
Amino acid   Keto acid   Ammonia

The two fractions resulting from the deamination of the amino acids are disposed of in the following ways.

Keto acids. The keto acids enter the common pathway for energy metabolism at various points of the cycle depending upon the amino acids from which they were derived. There they may be completely oxidized to yield energy, carbon dioxide, and water. The common pathway for the release of energy is described in Chapter 5 (page 68). (See also Figure 4–6.)

Some of the amino acids, accounting for about 58 per cent of the molecule, are said to be GLUCOGENIC; that is, after deamination they can be synthesized to glycogen. Other amino acids, slightly less than half of the protein molecule, are potentially KETO-GENIC; that is, they can be synthesized to fat. These distinctions are not fully valid. For example, from Figure 4–6 it may be noted that a number of amino acids are converted to pyruvic acid, which, in turn, can form glucose or can combine with coenzyme A and proceed to form fatty acids.

Disposal of ammonia. Most of the ammonia released through deamination is synthesized to urea. A small amount of ammonia may be used in the formation of new amino acids or purines, pyrimidines, creatine, and other important nonprotein nitrogenous substances. The transfer of amino groups by transamination has been described in the left column.

The liver is the primary organ for the synthesis of urea. This is an essential mechanism for the disposal of ammonia, which is highly toxic if it enters the systemic circulation. When the function of the liver is seriously impaired, ammonia enters the circulation and produces harmful effects on the central nervous system.

The KREBS-HENSELEIT CYCLE is a mechanism that explains the formation of urea. (See Figure 4–7.) This is an energy-requiring process. The ammonia combines with carbon dioxide (available from oxidation in the Krebs cycle) and ATP to form a carbamyl phosphate. This compound combines with ornithine—an amino acid—to initiate the urea cycle. A second molecule of ammonia is contributed to the cycle from aspartic acid. In the presence of argi-

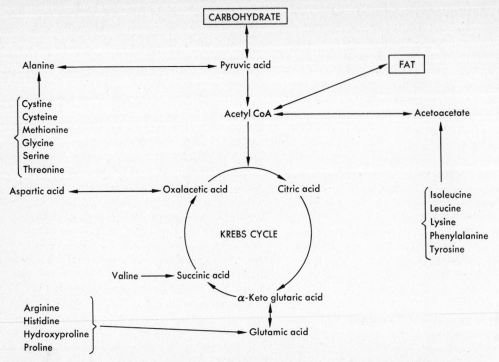

Figure 4–6. Amino acids enter the pathways common to carbohydrate and fat metabolism. Most amino acids are glucogenic; some are ketogenic; and a few may be either glucogenic or ketogenic.

nase, an enzyme, and magnesium, arginine yields one molecule of urea and of ornithine. Thus, one turn of the cycle has effected the release of ammonia in the form of urea and is able to recycle again.

The excretion of urea and other nitrogenous products in the urine entails an obligatory excretion of fluid as well. In the absence of sufficient fluid the work of the kidney will be increased.

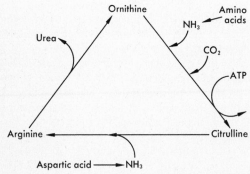

Figure 4–7. The Krebs-Henseleit cycle. A mechanism for disposing of ammonia by urea synthesis.

Dietary Protein Allowances

Factors affecting requirement. From the preceding discussion of metabolism it should be evident that the amount of protein required by any given individual depends on many factors. These are summarized as follows:

1. Daily nitrogen losses. Sufficient protein for adults is needed to cover daily nitrogen losses in the urine, feces, desquamated skin, hair, nails, perspiration, and other secretions.

2. Quality of protein. Indispensable amino acids must be present in sufficient amounts for tissue regeneration.

3. Calorie adequacy. Sufficient carbohydrates and fat to spare protein for tissue maintenance.

4. Needs for growth, including development of fetus and maternal tissues, as well as growth of infants and children.

5. Needs for lactation.

6. Prior state of nutrition. If poor, additional protein is needed to replete tissues.

7. Stress factors, such as fever, injury, immobilization, which increase the protein requirement.

Recommended allowances. The Food and Nutrition Board has set the protein allowance at 56 gm for the 70-kg man and 46 gm for the 58-kg woman.[10] These allowances are equivalent to 0.8 gm protein per kilogram, or 0.4 gm per pound. The allowances include individual variability and an increment for efficiency of various proteins. They have been derived as follows:

	gm per kg
Protein requirement based on nitrogen balance studies	0.47
Allowance for individual variability (+30 per cent)	0.14
	0.61
Adjustment for efficiency of protein in typical American diets of 75 per cent 0.61 ÷ 0.75 =	0.8

Allowances for growth. The allowances for infants are based upon human milk as the source of protein. The allowance decreases from 2.2 gm per kilogram during the first six months to 2.0 gm per kilogram for the second half year. For children from 1 to 10 years the daily allowances range from 23 to 36 gm. On the basis of body weight, these are equivalent to 1.8 to 1.2 gm per kilogram, the higher level being given during the second and third years and gradually decreasing with age.

An additional 30 gm protein per day during pregnancy will take care of the growth of the fetus and of the maternal tissues. During lactation, an increase in the protein allowance of 20 gm is satisfactory for the production of an upper limit of 1200 ml milk.

Essential amino acid requirements. Dr. Rose[11,12] has determined the quantitative requirements of the essential amino acids for healthy young men by feeding a controlled diet which included a mixture of pure amino acids flavored with lemon juice and sugar, and wafers made of cornstarch, sucrose, centrifuged butterfat, corn oil, and vitamins. Similar studies have been reported for young women and for infants.[13,14] The requirements on the basis of these studies are summarized in Table 4–3; they suffice only when the diet provides enough nitrogen for the synthesis of the nonessential amino acids so that the essential amino acids will not be used for this purpose. On a weight basis, it will be noted that the infant requirements are several times as high—a

Table 4–3. Estimated Amino Acid Requirements of Man*

Amino Acid	Requirement (per kg of body weight) mg per day			Amino Acid Pattern for High-Quality Proteins mg/gm of Protein
	Infants§ (3–6 mo)	Child (10–12 yr)	Adult	
Histidine	33	?	?	17
Isoleucine	80	28	12	42
Leucine	128	42	16	70
Lysine	97	44	12	51
Total S-containing amino acids†	45	22	10	26
Total aromatic amino acids‡	132	22	16	73
Threonine	63	28	8	35
Tryptophan	19	4	3	11
Valine	89	25	14	48

*Food and Nutrition Board: *Recommended Dietary Allowances,* 8th ed. National Academy of Sciences–National Research Council, Washington, D.C., 1974, p. 44.

† Methionine plus cystine.

‡ Phenylalanine plus tyrosine.

§ Two grams of protein per kilogram of body weight per day of the quality listed in column 4 would meet the amino acid needs of the infant.

fact that one would expect in view of the high rate of tissue synthesis during infancy.

Food Sources

Protein content of foods and American diets. The average protein composition of common foods is shown in Table 4–4. The protein concentration is high in dry milk, meat, fish, poultry, cheese, and nuts; intermediate in eggs, legumes, flours and cereals, and liquid milk; and low in most fruits and vegetables. One pint of liquid milk furnishes one fourth to one third of the recommended allowance for most age categories. Breads and cereals supply an appreciable amount of protein by virtue of the amounts that are consumed in a day.

The protein contribution made by the recommended number of servings from the Four Food Groups is shown in Figure 4–8. Inasmuch as some of the foods added to this basic diet for calories usually would contain some protein, the daily intake would be more than sufficient to meet the needs of healthy people of all ages.

In the United States the food supply available for consumption furnishes 99 gm protein per capita daily. The percentages supplied by each food group are: meat, fish, and poultry, 42; eggs, 5; legumes and nuts, 6; milk and milk products, 22; fruits and vegetables, 7; and flour and cereal products, 18.[15] (See Figure 4–9.)

The Basic Diet pattern and typical American diets furnish substantially more protein than is recommended by the Food and Nutrition Board. A protein-rich diet is also likely to supply much of the requirement for some minerals such as iron and other trace minerals as well as the B-complex vitamins. Indeed, if the protein intake were to be kept at recommended levels, good dietary planning would become difficult.[16] Nonetheless, it may well be questioned whether so large a proportion of protein should come from animal sources in view of eco-

Table 4–4. Average Protein Content of Foods in Four Food Groups*

Food	Average Serving	Protein gm	Protein Quality Limiting Amino Acids
Milk Group			
Milk, whole or skim	1 cup	9	Complete
Nonfat dry milk	⅞ ounce (3–5 tablespoons)	9	Complete
Cottage cheese	2 ounces	10	Complete
American cheese	1 ounce	7	Complete
Ice cream	⅛ quart	3	Complete
Meat Group			
Meat, fish, poultry	3 ounces, cooked	15–25	Complete; higher protein for lean cuts
Egg	1 whole	6	Complete
Dried beans or peas	½ cup cooked	7–8	Incomplete; methionine
Peanut butter	1 tablespoon	4	Incomplete; several amino acids borderline
Vegetable-Fruit Group			
Vegetables	½ cup	1–3	Incomplete
Fruits	½ cup	1–2	Incomplete
Bread-Cereals Group			
Breakfast cereals, wheat	½ cup cooked ¾ cup dry	2–3	Incomplete; lysine
Bread, wheat	1 slice	2–3	Incomplete; lysine
Macaroni, noodles, spaghetti	½ cup cooked	2	Incomplete; lysine
Rice	½ cup cooked	2	Incomplete; lysine and threonine
Cornmeal and cereals	½ cup cooked	2	Incomplete, lysine and tryptophan

*These values represent approximate group averages. For specific food items, consult Table A–1, in the Appendix.

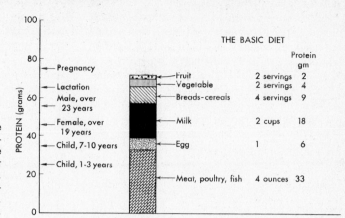

Figure 4-8. The Four Food Groups of the Basic Diet meet the recommended allowances for protein for most categories of the population. The addition of 1 cup of milk or 1 ounce of meat will fulfill increased needs. Note the high proportion of complete protein furnished by the milk and meat groups. See Table 13-2 for complete calculation.

Figure 4-9. Animal sources of protein account for over three fifths of the present total protein consumption in the United States. Note the marked reduction in protein from flour and cereal products since 1909. (Courtesy, Agricultural Research Service, U.S. Department of Agriculture.)

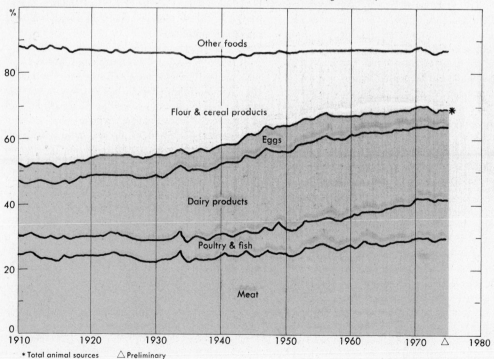

logic, economic, and health concerns as well as the urgent needs for food in the developing countries.

Protein quality of foods. Not only the quantity of protein but also the quality of protein is important in dietary planning. It has been pointed out that typical American diets with their high proportion of protein from animal foods are of high biologic value. The biologic value of a protein is a measure of its ability to meet the body's needs. It is measured by determining the nitrogen content of the diet, the urine, and the feces. The following calculation is made from these data:

$$BV = \frac{\text{Dietary N} - (\text{Urinary N} + \text{Fecal N})}{\text{Dietary N} - \text{Fecal N}} \times 100$$

A protein that has a biologic value of 70 or more is capable of supporting growth provided that sufficient calories are also ingested. The biologic values of proteins in foods are as follows: egg, 100; milk, 93; rice, 86; casein, fish, and beef, 75; corn, 72; peanut flour, 56; and wheat gluten, 44.

Limiting amino acids. The biologic value of a protein depends, in the final analysis, upon the quantity and proportions of the amino acids present in a food. The amino acid composition of foods may be calculated from values listed in Table A–5. Plant foods usually contain insufficient quantities of one or more of these four amino acids: lysine, methionine, tryptophan, and threonine. Plant foods often contain poor balances of other amino acids so that excesses of some interfere with the absorption and utilization of those that are more limiting.

Supplementary value of proteins. Foods are said to have SUPPLEMENTARY VALUE when they supply the essential amino acids that are missing in another food. For example, most cereals are deficient in lysine and threonine, and most legumes are low in methionine. When the foods are eaten together, however, the deficiencies in one are corrected by the adequacy of the amino acids in the other.

Plant food mixtures. One of the tremendously important areas of nutrition research is directed toward the development of mixtures of plant proteins whereby the limiting amino acid of one food is provided by another. *Incaparina* was the first such mixture used successfully in child feeding.[17] Many other mixtures have been developed and used successfully in the developing countries of the world.

Amino acid supplementation. Some essential amino acids such as lysine and methionine can be produced at costs sufficiently low to make it practical to add them to foods that are deficient. The lysine supplementation of bread, for example, has been tested and found to improve the biologic value of the bread. (See Figure 4–3.) The addition of amino acids to food products must be used with caution since the possibility exists that an imbalance of amino acids could be created in low-protein diets, thereby depressing growth.[18]

Vegetarian diets. Most of the world's people consume diets in which the protein is derived principally or solely from plant foods. In the United States many people have adopted vegetarian diets for religious, ecologic, or economic reasons. Some of these diets are satisfactory but others are not.

Lactovegetarian diets. Lactovegetarians consume milk and cheese along with a variety of plant foods. *Lacto-ovo-vegetarians* eat eggs as well as milk and cheese. When an appreciable amount of plant proteins is fed with a small amount of animal proteins, the quality of the mixture is as effective as if only animal proteins had been fed. For example, small amounts of milk, egg, or cheese will supply the lysine that is limiting in cereal foods. Thus, macaroni and cheese, cereal and milk, and bread and milk are supplementary.

Pure vegetarians. A variety of food combinations is used by persons who consume no animal foods whatsoever. The adequacy of the diets depends upon the combinations of foods that are used and their supply of the essential amino acids. Legumes and grains are the principal sources of proteins in vegetarian diets. The legumes include peas, chickpeas, navy beans, Lima beans, pinto beans, black-eyed peas, kidney beans, lentils, and soybeans. When corn and beans are eaten together, as in the countries of Central America, the biologic value is satisfactory. Hardinge and his associates found that legumes, whole grains, nuts, and vegetables provide a satisfactory combination of amino acids for a group of pure vegetarians.[19] Many resources are available for the planning of diets for vegetarian groups.[20,21]

Vegetarian diets that offer little variety can be extremely dangerous. One example is the Zen macrobiotic diet in which the final stage of diet consists principally of brown rice.[22] It is true that rice can meet the protein needs of the healthy adult when sufficient amounts of rice are consumed to also meet the caloric requirements. But rice alone cannot meet the protein needs of infants, children, pregnant women, and protein-depleted persons. Moreover, a diet consisting principally of rice fails to supply essential minerals and vitamins, and serious metabolic derangements occur, including interference with protein metabolism.

PROTEIN DEFICIENCY

Because the protein intake in the United States is high, and because the quality is exceptionally good, one would not expect to see many individuals exhibiting the clinical symptoms of severe deficiency. A reduced protein intake over an extended period of time leads eventually to depletion of the tissue reserves and then to lowering of blood protein levels. The speed with which the deficiency develops depends upon the quality and quantity of the protein intake, the caloric intake, the age of the individual, and other factors. Nutritional edema is an early clinical sign; it becomes more marked in the legs at the end of the day. With increasing severity the edema becomes more generalized.

Protein deficiency is sometimes seen among pregnant women from low-economic groups ignorant of the essentials of a good diet. Miscarriage, premature birth, and anemia are frequent in these women. Other vulnerable groups are the elderly who have too little income to secure food, insufficient understanding of the importance of diet, lack of incentive to eat, or poor health; and the chronically ill who have poor appetites and disorders of absorption together with increased protein requirements. Although symptoms of protein deficiency may not be detectable, the stress of an infection or surgery on such an individual may result in delayed convalescence or poor wound healing.

Protein-calorie malnutrition. KWASHIORKOR (meaning "the displaced child") occurs in children shortly after weaning, usually between ages one and four years, and is characterized by growth failure, edema, skin lesions, and changes in hair color. The liver is extensively infiltrated with fat. The principal dietary defect is a lack of protein in the foods available to the child when he is weaned. (See Figure 4–10.)

MARASMUS (from a Greek word meaning "withering") is usually seen at a somewhat earlier age than

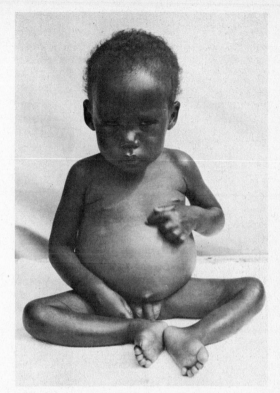

Figure 4–10. Child suffering from kwashiorkor—Africa. (Courtesy, M. Autret and the Food and Agriculture Organization.)

kwashiorkor and is caused by a deficiency of both protein and calories. Growth failure is even more severe than in kwashiorkor, but edema is usually absent.

One of the most serious problems associated with protein-calorie malnutrition is the possibility that mental development may be permanently impaired. The protein-calorie deficiencies constitute the major nutritional problem in the world today and will be discussed more extensively in Chapter 24.

SOME POINTS FOR EMPHASIS IN NUTRITION EDUCATION

1. Proteins are made up of building units called amino acids. They are required by people of all ages to replace tissues that are constantly

being broken down. Children and pregnant and lactating women need additional protein for synthesis of new proteins.

2. Proteins, like carbohydrates and fats, contribute calories to the diet. If too few calories are included in the diet, protein will be used for energy. Then it cannot also be used for building tissues.

3. Muscular work does not increase the requirement for protein.

4. Nine amino acids, called essential, must be supplied in the diet because the body cannot make them.

5. Animal protein foods, except gelatin, are complete because they contain balanced proportions of the essential amino acids. Include some good-quality protein at each meal.

6. About one sixth of the day's allowance for protein for the adult will be supplied by 1 ounce meat, fish, or poultry, or 1 cup milk, or 1 egg, or 1 ounce cheese.

7. Proteins from plant foods are incomplete but they are useful in reducing the amount of expensive animal protein that is needed. Breads, cereals, dry beans and peas, and peanut butter when combined with small amounts of eggs, cheese, meat, fish, and poultry give just as good an assortment of amino acids as a large amount of animal foods.

8. In vegetarian diets a variety of plant proteins can provide the amounts and kinds of essential amino acids required. Thus, cereal grains and legumes when consumed together provide satisfactory biologic value. Since the protein concentration in plant foods is lower than that in flesh foods, the bulk of the diet is greater.

PROBLEMS AND REVIEW

1. Describe the synthesis of tissue proteins. Under what circumstances would synthesis be accelerated?
2. Name four ways in which proteins are used in the regulation of body functions.
3. Explain why proteins are considered to be a wasteful source of energy.
4. *Problem.* Prepare an outline or diagram which shows the steps in the digestion of protein.
5. What is meant by an essential amino acid; complete protein; high biologic value; limiting amino acid; supplementary value of protein?
6. What is meant by positive nitrogen balance; negative nitrogen balance; nitrogen equilibrium? When does each condition occur?
7. How can you explain the fact that a person on a low-protein, high-calorie diet is less likely to go into negative nitrogen balance than one who is on a low-calorie diet of the same protein level?
8. How can you explain the fact that some vegetarians maintain good protein nutrition while others do not?
9. *Problem.* Plan a diet for a woman that provides 46 gm of protein, of which not more than one third is in the form of animal protein. What foods are especially important in such a diet plan?
10. What happens to protein that is eaten in excess of body requirements? Why is it important to provide a margin of safety in planning for the daily protein allowance?
11. What foods would you include in your own diet to ensure an adequate protein intake? How would you modify this plan for a growing child?
12. *Problem.* A diet contains 3000 kcal and 150 gm of protein. What percentage of the calories is supplied by protein?
13. *Problem.* One pint of milk supplies 18 gm of protein. What amounts of these foods would be required to replace the protein of the milk: nonfat dry milk; ice cream; Cheddar cheese; eggs; halibut; beef liver; sirloin steak; peanut butter; dry navy beans; oatmeal? How does the quality of protein in the various foods listed above compare?
14. *Problem.* On the basis of current market prices, calculate the cost for the amounts of foods which were needed to replace the protein of 1 pint milk (problem 13). What conclusions can you draw from this calculation?

15. A friend asks you whether she should buy lysine-enriched bread in preference to the usual enriched loaf of bread. How would you reply?
16. What are the effects of insufficient protein in the diet?

CITED REFERENCES

1. Vickery, H. B.: "The Origin of the Word Protein," *Yale J. Biol. Med.,* **22:**387–93, 1950.
2. Rose, W. C., *et al.:* "Further Experiments on the Role of Amino Acids in Human Nutrition," *J. Biol. Chem.,* **148:**457–58, 1943.
3. Kopple, J. D., and Swendseid, M. E.: "Evidence That Histidine Is an Essential Amino Acid in Normal and Chronically Uremic Man," *J. Clin. Invest.,* **55:**881–91, 1975.
4. Nasset, E. S.: "Role of the Digestive Tract in the Utilization of Protein and Amino Acids," *J.A.M.A.,* **164:**172–77, 1957.
5. Albanese, A. A., and Orto, L. A.: "The Proteins and Amino Acids," in Goodhart, R. E., and Shils, M. E., eds.: *Modern Nutrition in Health and Disease,* 5th ed. Lea & Febiger, Philadelphia, 1973, p. 32.
6. Adibi, S. A., and Gray, S. J.: "Intestinal Absorption of Essential Amino Acids in Man," *Gastroenterology,* **52:**837–45, 1967.
7. Consolazio, C. F.: "Comparisons of Nitrogen, Calcium, and Iodine Excretion in Arm and Total Body Sweat," *Am. J. Clin. Nutr.,* **18:**443–48, 1966.
8. Allison, J. B., and Wannamacher, R. N., Jr.: "The Concept and Significance of Labile and Over-all Protein Reserves of the Body," *Am. J. Clin. Nutr.,* **16:**445–52, 1965.
9. Sprinson, D. B., and Rittenberg, D.: "The Rate of Interaction of the Amino Acids of the Diet with Tissue Proteins," *J. Biol. Chem.,* **180:**715–26, 1949.
10. Food and Nutrition Board: *Recommended Dietary Allowances,* 8th ed. National Academy of Sciences—National Research Council, Washington, D.C., 1974, pp. 37–48.
11. Staff Report: "Rose Reports Human Amino Acid Requirements," *Chem. Eng. News,* **27:**1364, 1949.
12. Rose, W. C., *et al.:* "The Amino Acid Requirements of Man. XV. The Valine Requirements: Summary and Final Observations," *J. Biol. Chem.,* **217:**987–95, 1955.
13. Leverton, R. M., *et al.:* "The Quantitative Amino Acid Requirements of Young Women," *J. Nutr.,* **58:**59, 83, 219, 341, 355, 1956.
14. Holt, L. E., and Snyderman, S. E.: "The Amino Acid Requirements of Children," in Cole, W. H., ed.: *Some Aspects of Amino Acid Supplementation.* Rutgers University Press, New Brunswick, N.J., 1956, pp. 60–68.
15. Friend, B., and Marston, R.: "Nutritional Review," *National Food Situation,* U.S. Department of Agriculture, November 1975, pp. 26–32.
16. Calloway, D. H.: "Recommended Dietary Allowances for Protein and Energy," *J. Am. Diet. Assoc.,* **64:**157–62, 1974.
17. Scrimshaw, N. S.: "Progress in Solving World Nutrition Problems," *J. Am. Diet. Assoc.,* **35:**441–48, 1959.
18. Elvehjem, C. A.: "Amino Acid Balance in Nutrition," *J. Am. Diet. Assoc.,* **32:**305–308, 1956.
19. Hardinge, M. G., *et al.:* "Nutritional Studies of Vegetarians. V. Proteins and Essential Amino Acids," *J. Am. Diet. Assoc.,* **48:**25–28, 1966.
20. *Diet Manual,* 4th ed. Seventh-Day Adventist Dietetic Association, Box 75, Loma Linda, California, 1975.
21. Register, U. D., and Sonnenberg, L. M.: "The Vegetarian Diet. Scientific and Practical Considerations," *J. Am. Diet. Assoc.,* **62:**253–61, 1973.
22. Council on Foods and Nutrition: "Zen Macrobiotic Diets," *J.A.M.A.,* **218:**397, 1971.

ADDITIONAL REFERENCES

Asimov, I.: *The New Intelligent Man's Guide to Science.* Basic Books, Inc. New York, 1965, pp. 487–530; 561–76.
Brown, W.: "Present Knowledge of Protein Nutrition," *Postgrad. Med.,* **41:**A109–16, Feb. 1967; A107–12, March 1967; A119–26, April 1967.

Clark, H. E., *et al.:* "Nitrogen Balances of Adult Human Subjects Fed Combinations of Wheat, Beans, Corn, Milk, and Rice," *Am. J. Clin. Nutr.,* **26:**702–706, 1973.

Consolazio, C. F., *et al.:* "Protein Metabolism During Intensive Physical Training in the Young Adult," *Am. J. Clin. Nutr.,* **28:**29–35, 1975.

Fisher, H., *et al.:* "Reassessment of Amino Acid Requirements of Young Women on Low Nitrogen Diets. III. Isoleucine, Threonine, Phenylalanine and Summation," *Am. J. Clin. Nutr.,* **27:**130–34, 1974.

Food and Agriculture Organization: *Amino Acid Content of Foods and Biological Data on Proteins.* Nutr. Studies 24, FAO, Rome, 1970.

Hegsted, D. M.: "Minimum Protein Requirements of Adults," *Am. J. Clin. Nutr.,* **21:**352–57, 1968.

Joint Committee, FAO/WHO: *Energy and Protein Requirements.* WHO Tech. Rep. 522, World Health Organization, Geneva, 1973.

Review: "Tissue Protein Turnover Rates," *Nutr. Rev.,* **27:**181–82, 1969.

Scrimshaw, N. S., *et al.:* "Lysine Supplementation of Wheat Gluten at Adequate and Restricted Energy Intakes in Young Men," *Am. J. Clin. Nutr.,* **26:**965–72, 1973.

Scrimshaw, N. S.: "Nature of Protein Requirements. Way They Can Be Met in Tomorrow's World," *J. Am. Diet. Assoc.,* **54:**94–102, 1969.

"Soy Protein Products: Technology and Nutritive Value," *J. Am. Diet. Assoc.,* **64:**398–401, 1974.

Turk, R. E., *et al.:* "Adequacy of Spun-soy Protein Containing Egg Albumin for Human Nutrition," *J. Am. Diet. Assoc.,* **63:**519–24, 1973.

Williams, C. D.: "The Story of Kwashiorkor," *Nutr. Rev.,* **31:**334–40, 1973.

5 Carbohydrates

Photosynthesis. Carbohydrates are the most abundant organic compounds in the universe. They include the structural parts of plants in the form of cellulose as well as stores of starches and sugars. The sun is the ultimate source of energy for living organisms. By an exceedingly complex process known as PHOTOSYNTHESIS the energy of the sun is utilized by chlorophyll, the green coloring matter in leaves, to synthesize carbohydrate from carbon dioxide of the air and water of the soil.

$$6\ CO_2 + 6\ H_2O + \text{light energy} \rightarrow C_6H_{12}O_6 + 6\ O_2$$
$$\text{chemical energy}$$

The ability of plants to harness solar energy in usable form is basic to the continuance of life by all species. The energy stored in the leaves, stems, roots, and seeds is used in turn by animal species.

Dietary significance. Starches and sugars account for about half of the caloric intake in the United States and up to four fifths of the calories in diets of the people of Africa and the Orient. In addition, carbohydrate-rich foods are the principal sources of protein for most people of the world.

Try to imagine meals that exclude all foods containing starches and sugars such as breads, cakes, cookies, pastries, and puddings; breakfast cereals, macaroni, rice, spaghetti, noodles; fruits and vegetables; jellies, jams, candies, and sweetened beverages. As you think of such a limitation you soon realize how important carbohydrate-rich foods are for the energy, satiety, variety, and palatability they afford the diet.

A liberal use of carbohydrate has a number of distinct advantages. The yield of energy per acre of land is far greater from plant foods than from animal foods because the animal must first convert the energy of the plants it consumes into protein and fat. Cereal grains, legumes, and roots are somewhat less subject to deterioration than are animal foods. For these reasons, carbohydrate-rich foods are less expensive. Generally, as the income decreases, the consumption of carbohydrate foods increases, and that of protein-rich foods decreases.

Carbohydrates are sparing of the body economy, for they are easily digested, and also help to conserve tissue proteins. When the dietary selection is made from whole-grain or enriched cereals and breads, rather than refined foods, a bonus of B-complex vitamins and iron is added.

Composition. CARBOHYDRATES are simple sugars or polymers such as starch that can be hydrolyzed to simple sugars by the action of digestive enzymes or by heating with dilute acids. Like thousands of organic compounds, they contain carbon, hydrogen, and oxygen. Generally, but not always, the hydrogen and oxygen are present in the proportion to form water; hence the term *carbohydrate*. However, many compounds such as acetic acid ($C_2H_4O_2$) and lactic acid ($C_3H_6O_3$) that are not carbohydrate also contain hydrogen and oxygen in the same proportions as water.

CLASSIFICATION, DISTRIBUTION, AND CHARACTERISTICS

Carbohydrates are classified as monosaccharides, or simple sugars, disaccharides, or double sugars, and polysaccharides, which include many molecules of simple sugars.

MONOSACCHARIDES are compounds that cannot be hydrolyzed to simpler compounds. Although naturally occurring simple sugars may contain three to seven carbon atoms, only the hexoses (6-carbon atoms) are of dietary importance.

Glucose, galactose, fructose, and mannose have the same empiric formula, $C_6H_{12}O_6$. They differ in the arrangement of the groupings about the carbon

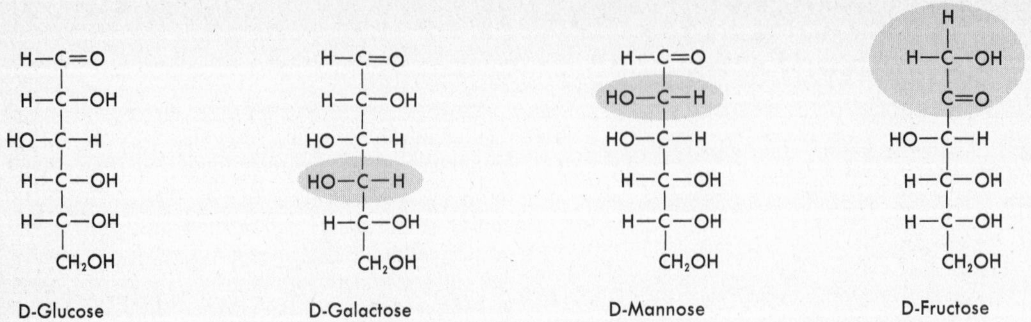

Figure 5–1. These hexoses differ in the arrangement of the groupings about the carbon atoms. The encircled grouping shows how the sugar differs from glucose in its structure. Fructose is a ketose; the others are aldoses.

atoms (see Figure 5–1) and are distinctive in their physical properties, such as solubility and sweetness. Glucose, galactose, and mannose possess an aldehyde grouping (CHO) and are known as aldohexoses. Fructose possesses a ketone grouping (CO) and is known as a ketohexose.

Solutions of glucose, galactose, and mannose rotate the plane of polarized light to the right (dextrorotatory), whereas fructose rotates the plane to the left (levorotatory). These natural sugars are designated as D-sugars, not because of their plane of rotation, but because the asymmetric carbon atom next to the primary alcohol group has the same orientation as in the triose D-glycerose (CHO·CHOH·CH$_2$OH).

Glucose, also known as dextrose, grape sugar, or corn sugar, is somewhat less sweet than cane sugar and is soluble in hot or cold water. It is found in sweet fruits such as grapes, berries, and oranges and in some vegetables such as sweet corn and carrots. It is prepared commercially as corn syrup or in its crystalline form by the hydrolysis of starch with acids. Glucose is the chief end product of the digestion of the di- and polysaccharides, is the form of carbohydrate circulating in the blood, and is the carbohydrate utilized by the cell for energy.

Fructose (levulose or fruit sugar) is a highly soluble sugar that does not readily crystallize. It is much sweeter than cane sugar and is found in honey, ripe fruits, and some vegetables. It is also a product of the hydrolysis of sucrose.

Galactose is not found free in nature, its only source being from the hydrolysis of lactose. *Mannose* is of limited distribution in foods, is poorly absorbed, and is of little consequence in nutrition.

Ribose, xylose, and *arabinose* are three pentoses (5-carbon sugars) that do not occur free in nature but are constituents of pentosans in fruits and the nucleic acids of meats. Ribose is of great physiologic importance as a constituent of riboflavin, a B-complex vitamin, and of ribonucleic acid (RNA) and deoxyribonucleic acid (DNA). It is rapidly synthesized by the body and is not a dietary essential.

DISACCHARIDES, or double sugars, result when two hexoses are combined with the loss of one molecule of water, the empiric formula being C$_{12}$H$_{22}$O$_{11}$. They are water soluble, diffusible, and crystallizable and vary widely in their sweetness. They are split to simple sugars by acid hydrolysis or by digestive enzymes.

Sucrose is the table sugar with which we are familiar and is found in cane or beet sugar, brown sugar, sorghum, molasses, and maple sugar. Many fruits and some vegetables contain small amounts of sucrose.

Lactose, or milk sugar, is produced by mammals and is the only carbohydrate of animal origin of significance in the diet. It is about one sixth as sweet as sucrose and dissolves poorly in cold water. The concentration of lactose in milk varies from 2 to 8 per cent, depending upon the species of animal.

Maltose, or malt sugar, does not occur to any appreciable extent in foods. It is an intermediate product in the hydrolysis of starch. Maltose is produced in the malting and fermentation of grains and is present in beer and malted breakfast cereals. It is also used with dextrins as the source of carbohydrate for some infant formulas.

POLYSACCHARIDES, (C$_6$H$_{10}$O$_5$)$_n$, are complex compounds with a relatively high molecular weight.

They are amorphous rather than crystalline, are not sweet, are insoluble in water, and are digested with varying degrees of completeness. Starches, dextrins, glycogen, and several indigestible carbohydrates are of nutritional interest.

Starch is the storage form of carbohydrate in the plant and a valuable contributor to the energy content of the diet. The starch granules are encased in a cellulose-type wall and are distinctive in size and shape for each source. The characteristics of the starch molecule depend upon the way in which the 2000 or so glucose units that make up the molecule are linked. Two types of glucose chains are present: (1) *amylose,* consisting of long straight chains of glucose, accounts for 10 to 20 per cent of the molecule; and (2) *amylopectin,* consisting of short branched chains of glucose units, accounts for the major part of the molecule. (See Figure 5–2.)

When starch is cooked in moist heat, the granules absorb water and swell, and the walls of the cell are ruptured, thus permitting more ready access to the digestive enzymes. Amylopectin has colloidal properties so that thickening of a starch-water mixture occurs when heat is applied.

Dextrins are intermediate products in the hydrolysis of starch and consist of shorter chains of glucose units. Some dextrins are produced when flour is browned or bread is toasted.

Glycogen, the so-called "animal starch," is similar

G–G–G–G–G–G–G–G–G–G–G–

Amylose

Amylopectin

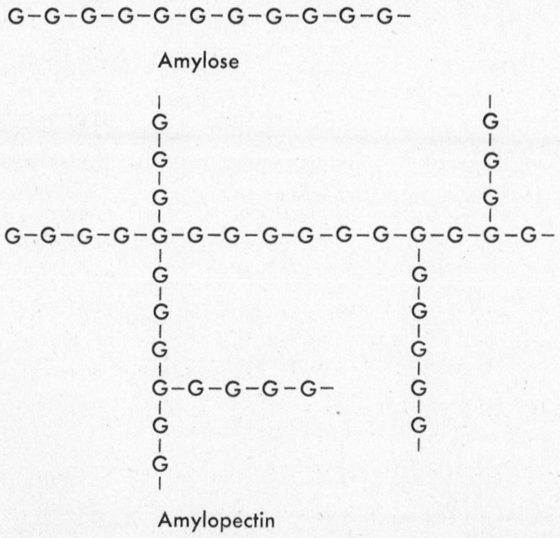

Figure 5–2. The starch molecule is composed of (1) amylose, with straight chains of glucose units, and (2) amylopectin, with branched chains of glucose units.

in structure to the amylopectin of starch, but contains many more branched chains of glucose. It is rapidly synthesized from glucose in the liver and muscle.

Indigestible polysaccharides. Cellulose is the most abundant organic compound in the world, comprising at least 50 per cent of the carbon in vegetation. Wood and cotton are chiefly cellulose, but the skins of fruits, the coverings of seeds, and the structural parts of edible plants are the only forms of cellulose and hemicellulose with which we are concerned in the study of nutrition. Ruminants are able to utilize cellulose for energy because of the presence of specific enzymes in the rumen, but for man cellulose is an indigestible dietary constituent.

Several indigestible polysaccharides have useful properties in food processing. *Pectins,* found in ripe fruits, have the ability to absorb water and to form gels, a property utilized in making fruit jellies. *Agar* is obtained from seaweed and is useful for its gelling properties. *Carrageen* (Irish moss) and *alginates* from seaweed are often used to enhance the smoothness of foods such as ice cream and evaporated milk.

Carbohydrate derivatives. Sugars react chemically to form sugar alcohols, amino sugars, glycosides, uronic acids, and many complex compounds with lipids and proteins. *Glycerol* is the 3-carbon alcohol that is a component of glycerides. *Sorbitol,* a sugar alcohol, is sweet, is water soluble, and is found in cherries, plums, and berries. *Inositol* is an alcohol related to the hexoses. It occurs in the bran of cereal grains. When combined with phosphate it forms phytic acid, a compound that interferes with the absorption of minerals such as calcium, iron, and zinc.

Ascorbic acid, one of the water-soluble vitamins, is a hexose derivative that can be synthesized by plants and by some animals but not by the human being. Numerous carbohydrate derivatives are constituents of connective, nervous, and other tissues and are involved in many metabolic functions.

FUNCTIONS

Body distribution. The amount of carbohydrate in the adult body is about 300 to 350 gm. Of this, 100 gm is stored as glycogen in the liver, another 200 to 250 gm is present as glycogen in cardiac, smooth, and skeletal muscles, and about 15 gm makes up the glucose in the blood and extracellular fluid. Very small amounts of carbohydrate are constituents of numerous essential body compounds.

Energy. Each gram of carbohydrate when oxidized yields, on the average, 4 kcal. Following absorption from the intestinal tract, the carbohydrate meets these principal fates: (1) immediate use to meet energy needs of tissue cells; (2) conversion to glycogen and storage in the liver or muscle for later release to meet energy needs; and (3) conversion to fat as a larger reserve for energy. The total glycogen reserves in the body would meet about half of one day's energy needs of the adult. Glycogen stored in the liver can be converted to glucose to maintain the sugar level of the blood. Glycogen in muscle can be used to supply energy needs of muscle cells but is not available for regulation of the blood sugar level. The amount of energy stored as fat can be large and is a ready and continuing supply to meet energy needs when glycogen stores are depleted.

Protein-sparing action. The body will use carbohydrate preferentially as a source of energy when it is adequately supplied in the diet, thus sparing protein for tissue building. Since meeting energy needs of the body takes priority over other functions, any deficiency of calories in the diet will be made up by using adipose and protein tissues.

Regulation of fat metabolism. Some carbohydrate is necessary in the diet so that the oxidation of fats can proceed normally. When carbohydrate is severely restricted in the diet, fats will be metabolized faster than the body can take care of the intermediate products. The accumulation of these incompletely oxidized products leads to ketosis. As little as 50 gm carbohydrate in the diet will prevent ketosis under normal conditions. In uncontrolled diabetes mellitus ketosis is often present.

Role in gastrointestinal function. Several regulatory functions have been attributed to lactose. One of these is the promotion of the growth of desirable bacteria in the small intestine. Some of these bacteria are useful in the synthesis of certain B-complex vitamins. Lactose also enhances the absorption of calcium. It is undoubtedly no accident of nature that milk, which is the outstanding source of calcium, is also the only dietary source of lactose.

Cellulose, hemicellulose, and pectins yield no nutrients to the body. These indigestible substances aid in the stimulation of the peristaltic movements of the gastrointestinal tract, by absorbing water give bulk to the intestinal contents, and reduce the length of time food wastes remain in the colon.

Carbohydrate in body compounds. Structurally, carbohydrate accounts for a very small part of the weight of the body. Nevertheless, monosaccharides are vitally important constituents of numerous compounds that regulate metabolism. Among these are:

Glucuronic acid, which occurs in the liver and is also a constituent of a number of mucopolysaccharides. Glucuronic acid in the liver combines with toxic chemicals and bacterial by-products and is thus a detoxifying agent.

Hyaluronic acid, a viscous substance that forms the matrix of connective tissue.

Heparin, a mucopolysaccharide, a substance that prevents the clotting of blood.

Chondroitin sulfates found in skin, tendons, cartilage, bone, and heart valves.

Immunopolysaccharides as part of the body's mechanism to resist infections.

Deoxyribonucleic acid (DNA) and ribonucleic acid (RNA), the compounds that possess and transfer the genetic characteristics of the cell.

Galactolipins as constituents of nervous tissue.

Glycosides as components of steroid and adrenal hormones.

DIGESTION AND ABSORPTION

Digestion. The purpose of carbohydrate digestion is to hydrolyze the di- and polysaccharides of the diet to their constituent simple sugars. This is accomplished by enzymes of the digestive juices and yields these end products:

$$\text{Starch} \xrightarrow{\text{amylase}} \text{Glucose}$$

$$\text{Sucrose} \xrightarrow{\text{sucrase}} \text{Glucose} + \text{fructose}$$

$$\text{Maltose} \xrightarrow{\text{maltase}} \text{Glucose} + \text{glucose}$$

$$\text{Lactose} \xrightarrow{\text{lactase}} \text{Glucose} + \text{galactose}$$

Although some hydrolysis of starch to maltose occurs in the mouth by the action of salivary amylase and continues in the stomach until the food mass is acidified, the principal site of digestion of carbohydrate is in the small intestine. Salivary amylase does not act upon raw starch but pancreatic amylase hydrolyzes both raw and cooked starch to dextrins and, in turn, to maltose. Cooked starch is more rapidly hydrolyzed because the cell walls have been ruptured and the enzymes have more ready access to the starch granules.

Disaccharidases are produced within the mucosal cell and are not secreted into the lumen of the intestine.[1] Sucrose, lactose, and maltose are hydrolyzed within the brush border of the epithelial cell.

Fiber. Cellulose and hemicellulose cannot be hydrolyzed by enzymes of the human digestive tract, therefore yield no energy, and are excreted in the feces. Tough fibers including seeds, skins, and structural parts of plant foods are broken into smaller particles, whereas the more tender fibers of young plants are partially disintegrated by bacterial action within the large intestine. The cooking of foods also softens fibers and partially disintegrates them.

Available carbohydrate. The total carbohydrate values reported in tables of food composition include not only the fully digestible starches and sugars but also nondigestible components such as cellulose, hemicellulose, and pectins. Thus, the amount of carbohydrate actually available to the body is the difference between the total carbohydrate and the amount of fiber that is present. The carbohydrate of refined flours and cereals, sugars, and sweets is completely, or almost completely, digested, whereas that from fibrous vegetables, fruits with seeds, and whole-grain cereals and flours is somewhat less completely digested.

Absorption. The process by which the monosaccharides are absorbed is by no means simple. As indicated above, the disaccharides have been hydrolyzed to their component single sugars at the brush border of the epithelial cells lining the tract and are ready for absorption to the internal environment. The single sugars must enter the epithelial cell, be transported across the cell, enter the interstitial fluid, and then pass through the walls of the blood capillaries for transport to the portal circulation and then to locations of use within the body.

Glucose and galactose can be absorbed by passive diffusion with a carrier as an intermediary as long as the concentration at the luminal surface is greater than that in the circulation. Passive diffusion accounts for only a small amount of the total glucose that is absorbed. When the concentration in the circulation exceeds that at the luminal surfaces, active transport is required. This is effected by the sodium pump and a mobile carrier system.[1] The same energy that is required to pump sodium out of the cell also serves to transport glucose and galactose. The energy to operate the sodium pump is provided by ATP that has been generated from a supply of glucose within the cell. Active transport undoubtedly accounts for the principal means whereby glucose and galactose are absorbed. Fructose apparently is absorbed only by passive diffusion.

Most absorption occurs from the jejunum. When the concentration of sugar in the intestine is great, the need for carriers to ferry sugars across the epithelial cells may exceed the numbers present; hence, some sugars will move along the tract to carrier sites in the ileum.

The rate of absorption is about equal for galactose and glucose, whereas fructose is absorbed about half as rapidly. Mannose and xylose are poorly absorbed, indicating a high level of selectivity at the absorption sites.

About 97 to 98 per cent of the carbohydrate in diversified American diets is digested and absorbed. The fuel factor of 4 kcal per gram is based upon this level of absorption. In countries where plant foods comprise most of the diet so that the unavailable carbohydrate is correspondingly higher, the percentage of carbohydrate absorbed is lower, and the energy value per gram of dietary carbohydrate is somewhat lower.

INTERMEDIARY METABOLISM

Glucose is quantitatively the most important carbohydrate available to the body whether it be by absorption from the diet or by synthesis within the body. Galactose and fructose from the diet or from endogenous sources are rapidly synthesized to glucose in the liver. Therefore, any discussion of carbohydrate metabolism is essentially that of glucose. (See Figure 5–3.)

Interrelation with other nutrients. Glucose metabolism consists of an interrelated series of biochemical reactions that are facilitated by enzymatic

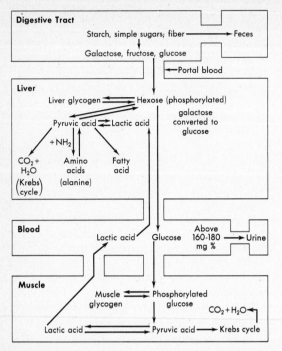

Figure 5-3. Pathways of carbohydrate metabolism.

activity. Glucose metabolism cannot be completely separated from the metabolism of fats and proteins. On the one hand, proteins and fats are potential sources of glucose, and on the other, glucose can be converted to fatty acids, glycerol, and certain amino acids. A number of points in the sequence of glucose metabolism are also the crossroads for amino acid and fatty acid metabolism, and in some respects one nutrient can substitute for another. For example, a decrease in carbohydrate metabolism is accompanied by an increase in fatty acid oxidation. Trace amounts of magnesium, iron, and other mineral elements and several of the B-complex vitamins are essential for enzyme activity. Thus, the metabolism of the nutrients is interdependent, and the lack of any one of them affects the total metabolism of the organism. For example, when there is a deficiency of any one of the vitamins, the result is a failure of the reaction to take place at the point where that vitamin is essential. Any reactions subsequent to this point, therefore, cannot occur.

The details of these elegant metabolic mechanisms are beyond the scope of this text, but they are well described in a number of texts on biochemistry. Nevertheless, the nurse and nutritionist frequently encounter patients with some defect in carbohydrate metabolism. The following paragraphs will furnish a general understanding of the mechanisms for the regulation of the blood glucose and a broad outline of the anaerobic and aerobic phases of glucose metabolism.

The liver in carbohydrate metabolism. Following absorption from the small intestine, the monosaccharides are carried by the portal vein to the liver. Just as the control tower in an airport regulates the flow of traffic in the air, so the liver exercises the principal control of the pathways that glucose (and other nutrients) shall take. The purposes of the transformations that take place in the liver are to serve as the chief storage house for glycogen, to regulate the level of glucose in the blood (not too much and not too little), and to synthesize certain essential compounds from glucose.

The chemical changes are facilitated by enzymes that are specific for each reaction. The liver is under the influence of hormones secreted by the pancreas and the adrenal, pituitary, and thyroid glands. Inasmuch as the liver is the chief organ for the regulation of glucose metabolism, it is understandable that any disturbance in liver function can have more or less profound effects on carbohydrate metabolism. The paragraphs that follow will help to explain how the liver maintains the regulation of the blood glucose.

The blood glucose. By means of the blood circulation glucose is made continuously available to each and every cell of the body as a source of energy and for the synthesis of a variety of substances. The glucose taken from the circulation by the cells is constantly replaced so that the blood glucose level is maintained within relatively narrow limits. (See Figure 5-4.)

In the fasting state the blood glucose concentration is normally 60 to 85 mg per 100 ml. Shortly after a meal it rises to about 140 to 150 mg per 100 ml, but within a few hours the concentration will have returned to the fasting level. Should the blood sugar level reach 160 to 180 mg per 100 ml some glucose will be excreted in the urine (GLUCOSURIA). This level, varying somewhat from one individual to another, is known as the RENAL THRESHOLD FOR GLUCOSE. The regulation of the blood sugar

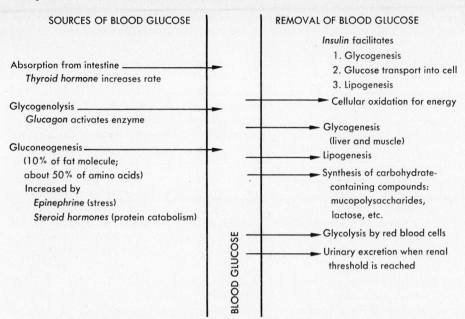

SOURCES OF BLOOD GLUCOSE | REMOVAL OF BLOOD GLUCOSE

Insulin facilitates
1. Glycogenesis
2. Glucose transport into cell
3. Lipogenesis

Absorption from intestine
   Thyroid hormone increases rate

→ Cellular oxidation for energy

Glycogenolysis
   Glucagon activates enzyme

→ Glycogenesis
   (liver and muscle)

Gluconeogenesis
   (10% of fat molecule;
   about 50% of amino acids)
   Increased by
      Epinephrine (stress)
      Steroid hormones (protein catabolism)

→ Lipogenesis

→ Synthesis of carbohydrate-
   containing compounds:
   mucopolysaccharides,
   lactose, etc.

→ Glycolysis by red blood cells

→ Urinary excretion when renal
   threshold is reached

BLOOD GLUCOSE

Figure 5–4. The blood glucose is maintained within physiologic limits by replacement as rapidly as it is removed to meet metabolic needs. Glycogenesis, lipogenesis, and excretion at the renal threshold are mechanisms that prevent hyperglycemia in the normal individual.

level by the liver is so efficient that glucosuria does not normally occur. Occasionally, an individual who has a lower renal threshold for glucose but who has no other abnormalities will excrete some glucose following meals that are especially rich in carbohydrate.

A blood sugar concentration in excess of normal levels is known as HYPERGLYCEMIA; this is characteristic of diabetes mellitus. A glucose concentration below normal levels is known as HYPOGLYCEMIA and may occur in certain abnormalities of liver function, or when insulin is produced in excessive amounts by the pancreas.

Sources of blood glucose. Glucose is available to the circulation (1) from absorbed sugars from the diet; (2) by breakdown of liver glycogen (GLYCOGEN-OLYSIS); (3) by conversion from glucogenic amino acids and the glycerol of fats (GLUCONEOGENESIS); and to a lesser extent (4) by the reconversion of pyruvic and lactic acids formed in the glycolytic pathway. Fatty acids and ketogenic acids do not contribute to the blood glucose nor does muscle glycogen.

Since absorbed sugars are only intermittently available, the liver maintains a constant supply of sugar to the blood by the release of glucose from glycogen. If the glycogen reserves are depleted, protein and fat from body reserves or from dietary sources are used to replenish the glucose of the blood. Amino acids must be deaminized before the remainder of the molecule can enter the pathway of carbohydrate metabolism. Approximately half the amino acids are glucogenic. Only the glycerol fraction of fats, representing about 10 per cent of the total fat molecule, can be converted to glucose.

Hormones. Several mechanisms under the influence of hormones increase the supply of glucose to the blood. *Thyroid hormone* increases the rate of absorption from the gastrointestinal tract. *Glucagon*, a hormone secreted by the cells of the pancreas, is believed to activate phosphorylase, thus initiating glycogenolysis. *Epinephrine*, produced by the adrenal gland under conditions of stress, increases the rate of glycogen breakdown. *Steroid hormones* accelerate the catabolism of proteins, thus bringing about gluconeogenesis. *Adrenocorticotropic hormone* is antagonistic to the action of insulin and thus prevents the blood sugar level from dropping.

Figure 5-5. Glucose is oxidized anaerobically to pyruvic and lactic acids—the Embden-Meyerhof pathway. Glucose may also be oxidized through the pentose shunt. Pyruvic acid is decarboxylated to form acetate. Active acetate condenses with oxalacetic acid, and each turn of the Krebs cycle releases 2 molecules of CO_2 and 8 hydrogen ions and uses up 2 molecules of water.

Removal of glucose from the blood. Six pathways are available for the removal of glucose from the blood: (1) the continuous uptake of glucose by every cell in the body and its oxidation for energy; (2) the conversion of glucose to glycogen by the liver (GLYCOGENESIS); (3) the synthesis of fats from glucose (LIPOGENESIS); (4) the synthesis of numerous carbohydrate derivatives (see page 64); (5) glycolysis in the red blood cells; and (6) elimination of glucose in the urine when the renal threshold is exceeded.[2]

The amount of glycogen that can be formed is limited, but there is no limit to the amount of fat that is formed. Glycogen reserves are maintained at their maximum level by diets high in carbohydrate. A diet high in protein and relatively low in carbohydrate will result in moderate glycogen reserves, but a diet high in fat and low in carbohydrate and protein will result in poor glycogen reserves.

Insulin. Only one hormone is known to lower the blood sugar. An increase in the concentration of blood glucose stimulates the release of INSULIN, the hormone produced by the beta cells of the islands of Langerhans. Insulin lowers the blood glucose by several actions: (1) facilitating the synthesis of glycogen in the liver; (2) the active transport of glucose across cell membranes; and (3) the conversion of glucose to fatty acids.

Oxidation of glucose. The oxidation of glucose takes place within each of the billions of cells that make up the body. This is not a single explosive reaction, but the glucose molecule is taken through a complex series of steps whereby the rate of energy release is so controlled that the maximum efficiency is achieved. Each of the numerous reactions is catalyzed by a specific enzyme. (See Figure 5-5.)

The catabolism of glucose includes (1) GLYCOLYSIS, principally an anaerobic phase that breaks glucose down to pyruvic acid and lactic acid, and (2) the CITRIC ACID CYCLE, an aerobic phase in which energy, carbon dioxide, and water are released. A number of the intermediate products formed in these pathways are the crossroads for carbohydrate, fat, and protein metabolism.

High-energy phosphate compounds. Certain phosphate compounds trap large amounts of energy and are known as high-energy phosphate compounds, designated thus $\sim$. ADENOSINE TRIPHOSPHATE (ATP) is one such compound. It contains three phosphate groupings, two of which are held to the rest of the molecule by high-energy bonds. On demand ATP gives up one of its phosphate groupings to yield a burst of energy for the work of the cell. The energy required to reconvert ADP to ATP is supplied by the metabolism of glucose. In the glycolytic pathway the net yield of energy is only

$$A - P \sim P \sim P = ATP \qquad A - P \sim P = ADP$$

2 moles of ATP, whereas in the citric acid cycle it is about 15 times as great.

Glycolysis. The chemical reactions that constitute glycolysis, also known as the *Embden-Meyerhof pathway* for the men who first described them, take place in the cytoplasmic matrix of the cell. These reactions degrade glucose to pyruvic acid in preparation for entrance into the mitochondria. They are catalyzed by a specific enzyme in each case, some of which require the presence of inorganic phosphate, inorganic ions, NAD (nicotinamide adenine dinucleotide), and NADP (nicotinamide adenine dinucleotide phosphate). The reactions do not require oxygen. Almost all of the glucose catabolized in the body undergoes breakdown through these steps.

Phosphorylation. The entrance of glucose into the cell is facilitated by insulin. Within the cell the first step in glycolysis is the combination of glucose with ATP in the presence of glucokinase and magnesium to form glucose-6-phosphate and ADP. The phosphorylated glucose then proceeds through the glycolytic pathway to pyruvic acid and lactic acid, or to the synthesis of glycogen, or, to a lesser extent, through an alternate oxidative pathway known as the *pentose shunt.*

Conversion to trioses. The hexose molecule is split to trioses, which undergo a series of changes until pyruvic acid ($CH_3COCOOH$) is formed. One of the trioses—dihydroxyacetone phosphate—instead of proceeding to pyruvic acid may be sidetracked to

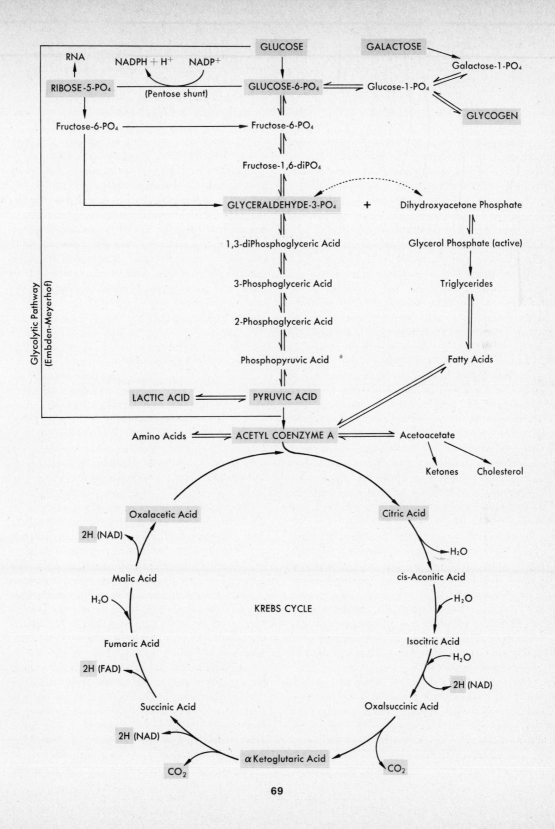

form α-glycerophosphate, which furnishes the glycerol molecule for the synthesis of neutral fats. (See page 85.)

Lactic acid. Pyruvic acid can proceed anaerobically to form lactic acid, which is utilized for muscle contraction under conditions when the energy need exceeds the supply of oxygen. Under normal conditions only a small amount of lactic acid is formed. About one fifth of the lactic acid produced in the muscle is further oxidized through the citric acid cycle; the rest reenters the blood circulation and is synthesized to glycogen by the liver.

The pentose shunt. An aerobic bypass for glycolysis may be utilized especially by the liver and adipose tissue. This is also known as the *hexose monophosphate shunt* or the *oxidative shunt.* Through the reactions occurring in this pathway, ribose, which is a constituent of RNA, is synthesized. Also, NADPH is produced, which is essential for the synthesis of fatty acids and for the utilization of lactic acid in muscular work.

Aerobic metabolism. Most of the pyruvic acid formed in the glycolytic pathway enters the mitochondria of the cells and is there oxidized. By a complex series of steps pyruvic acid is decarboxylated to a 2-carbon fragment (acetate), which reacts with coenzyme A to form ACETYL COENZYME A also known as ACTIVE ACETATE. These reactions require NAD, thiamin, pyrophosphate, lipoic acid, magnesium, coenzyme A, and a series of enzymes. In this conversion 3 moles of ATP are formed, or 6 moles for each glucose molecule.

COENZYME A is a complex molecule of which pantothenic acid, a B-complex vitamin, is a constituent. Acetyl coenzyme A is derived not only from pyruvic acid but also from the oxidation of fatty acids (see page 85) and from certain amino acids (see page 51). Acetyl coenzyme A is something like the hub of a wheel in that it can proceed in a number of directions, namely, through the citric acid cycle to yield energy or to form a number of new compounds.

Citric acid cycle. This is also known as the *tricarboxylic acid cycle* (because the acids involved contain three carboxyl groups) or the *Krebs cycle* (for the man who first formulated the sequence). Through this cycle about 90 per cent of the energy of the body is produced.

The citric acid cycle is initiated by the condensation of acetyl coenzyme A with oxalacetic acid to form citric acid. In one turn of the cycle the two carbon atoms from acetyl coenzyme A are oxidized to form carbon dioxide and water. The overall reaction is:

$$CH_3COOH + 2\ O_2 \rightarrow 2\ CO_2 + 2\ H_2O$$

One molecule of carbon dioxide is released in the formation of ketoglutaric acid and one in the formation of succinyl coenzyme A. (See Figure 5–5.) A full turn of the cycle yields one molecule of oxalacetic acid, which combines with a new molecule of acetyl coenzyme A for another cycle. Through the citric acid cycle the energy from glucose, fatty acids, and some amino acids is converted to the form the body can use, namely ATP. (See oxidative phosphorylation, page 68.)

CARBOHYDRATE IN THE DIET

Dietary allowances. The low-carbohydrate diet of the Eskimos and the high-carbohydrate diet of many people in Far Eastern countries indicate that man can be healthy with wide variations in carbohydrate intake. This wide variation is compatible with health because of the interrelations with fatty acids and amino acids in meeting energy needs of the body.

The minimum requirement for carbohydrate is not known, but at least 50 to 100 gm carbohydrate daily is deemed desirable by the Food and Nutrition Board to maintain metabolic processes and to prevent ketosis.[3] Most Americans consume diets that include between 200 and 300 gm carbohydrate.

Many years ago Cowgill[4] recommended a fiber intake of 100 mg per kilogram, or about 5 to 6 gm per day for the adult. There has been little research to verify this level or to suggest another. Vegetarians who had four times as much fiber in the diet as nonvegetarians did not experience any adverse effects on the digestive tract.[5] The fiber content of typical American diets has declined in the last half century because of the increasing refinement of foods. Some clinicians believe that a low fiber intake is responsible for several gastrointestinal disorders including diverticulosis and cancer of the bowel.[6]

Dietary sources. Flour and cereal products furnish about 35 per cent and sugars and sweets about 38 per cent of the carbohydrate in the food supply in the United States. The remainder of the carbohydrate is provided by fruits, vegetables, and dairy products.

The carbohydrate composition of typical foods is shown in Table 5-1. Pure sugars are 100 per cent carbohydrate, and syrups, jellies, and jams contain 65 to 80 per cent. Cereal foods, flours, and crackers contain 65 to 85 per cent carbohydrate on a dry weight basis, chiefly in the form of starch.

Fruits and vegetables vary widely in their carbo-

hydrate concentration. Those with a high water content such as spinach, cabbage, other leafy vegetables, and melons contain 6 per cent or less of carbohydrate and are correspondingly low in calories. Potatoes, sweet potatoes, Lima beans, corn, and bananas are somewhat lower in water content and furnish approximately 20 per cent carbohydrate or more. Dried beans and peas and dried fruits have a carbohydrate content in excess of 60 per cent. For convenience in dietary planning, fruits and vegetables have been grouped according to their carbohydrate content. (See Table A-4.)

Table 5-1. Carbohydrate Content of Some Typical Foods

Food	Per 100 gm of Food gm	Per Serving Portion Measure	Weight gm	Carbohydrate gm
*Complex Carbohydrates**				
Bread, all kinds	50–56	1 slice	25	13
Cereals, breakfast, dry	68–84	1 cup wheat flakes	30	24
Crackers, all kinds	67–73	4 saltines	11	8
Flour, all kinds	71–80	2 tablespoons	14	11
Legumes, dry	60–63	½ cup navy beans, cooked	95	20
Macaroni, spaghetti, dry	75	½ cup cooked	70	16
Nuts	15–20	¼ cup peanuts	36	7
Pie crust, baked	44	⅙ shell	30	13
Potatoes, white, raw	17	1 boiled	122	18
Rice, dry	80	½ cup cooked	105	25
Complex and Simple Carbohydrates (½ and ½)				
Cake, plain and iced	52–68	1 piece layer, iced	75	45
Cookies	51–80	1 chocolate chip	10	6
Simple Carbohydrates				
Beverages, carbonated	8–12	8 ounces cola	246	24
Candy (without nuts)	75–95	1 ounce milk chocolate	28	16
Fruit, dried	59–69	4 prunes	32	18
Fruit, fresh	6–22	1 apple	150	18
		1 orange	180	16
Fruit, sweetened, canned or frozen	16–28	½ cup peaches	128	26
		3 ounces frozen strawberries	85	24
Ice cream	18–21	½ cup	67	14
Milk	5	1 cup	244	12
Pudding	16–26	½ cup vanilla	128	21
Sugar, all kinds	96–100	1 tablespoon white	11	11
Syrups, molasses, honey	65–82	1 tablespoon molasses	20	13
Vegetables	4–18	½ cup green beans	63	4
		½ cup peas	80	10

*Foods are grouped according to the predominating type of carbohydrate present.

The degree of ripeness determines the relative proportions of sugars and starches in fruits and vegetables. Green bananas are high in starch and low in sugar, whereas ripe bananas have little starch and consist primarily of sugars. Freshly picked and immature vegetables, on the other hand, for example, sweet corn, tender peas, and young carrots, contain more sugar and less starch than mature vegetables.

Milk is the only animal food contributing to the daily carbohydrate intake. Freshly opened oysters and scallops contain some glycogen, but the amount is of no practical significance. The glycogen in liver is rapidly converted to lactic and pyruvic acids when the animal is slaughtered.

The principal sources of fiber are whole-grain breads and cereals, raw fruits, especially those with skins and seeds, and vegetables such as celery, corn, and Lima beans.

Problems related to carbohydrate consumption. The daily per capita consumption of carbohydrate has decreased about 100 gm since the beginning of the century. (See Figure 5-6.) This has resulted from a sharp decline in the use of flours and cereals. On the other hand, the per capita consumption of sugar has increased from 155 to about 210 gm daily.[7] In 1909–1913 sugars accounted for only one third of the total carbohydrate consumed, but today they account for more than half of the total carbohydrate. About 23 per cent of the sugar consumed is used for the manufacture of soft drinks. In 1960 the annual consumption of soft drinks per person was 192 8-ounce units, and in 1974 this had risen to 430 8-ounce units.[8] These shifts in the sources of carbohydrate can have an adverse effect on health.

Nutritional adequacy. An excessive intake of sugars, pastries, cakes, cookies, and candies crowds out essential foods, thus resulting in nutrient deficiencies as well as problems of overweight. For example, the increasing use of soft drinks tends to reduce the intake of milk. The establishment of food habits early in life with respect to judicious consumption of sweets can scarcely be overemphasized.

Some individuals consume normal levels of carbohydrate but their choices are restricted to the refined sugars and sweets. Others, believing that breads and cereals contribute to overweight, omit the bread-cereal group from their diets. In either instance the intake of B-complex vitamins and iron is correspondingly reduced. Four servings of whole-grain or enriched breads and cereals should be included daily before nutritionally inferior carbohydrate foods are added.

Dental caries. The causes of tooth decay are many and complex. Nevertheless, if the consumption of sweets by a child leads to reduced intake of other foods, some defects in tooth structure may be expected if some of the essential nutrients are missing. Any carbohydrates in contact with the tooth surfaces for a period of time provide a favorable medium for the rapid growth of bacteria; sticky candies and other sweets are especially harmful. Brushing the teeth after eating sweets or, at the very least, rinsing the mouth with water is

Figure 5–6. Sugars account for over half of the carbohydrate in today's diets. Early in the century starchy foods accounted for about two thirds of the carbohydrate intake. (Data from "Nutritional Review," by B. Friend and R. Marston, *National Food Situation*, U.S. Department of Agriculture, November 1974, p. 29.)

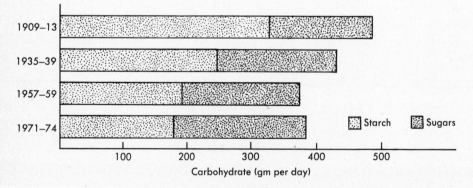

helpful in removing the carbohydrate residues from the teeth.

Gastrointestinal irritation. An excessive intake of concentrated sweets sometimes leads to irritation of the gastrointestinal mucosa and, in certain disorders, favor[9] increased fermentation and gas production. Some individuals experience distention, flatulence, and diarrhea after drinking milk because of a deficiency of the enzyme lactase in the intestinal mucosa.

Serum lipids. The shift from the complex carbohydrates to the simpler forms brings about an elevation in the serum triglycerides in some susceptible individuals.[9-11] This increase in serum triglycerides is believed to increase the incidence of cardiovascular disease. Other research workers have pointed out that these changes are not of the same order of magnitude as those seen with alterations in the amount and nature of fat. (See also Chapter 6.)

SOME POINTS FOR EMPHASIS IN NUTRITION EDUCATION

1. Carbohydrates include sugars, starches, and fiber from plant foods. Milk, which contains lactose, or milk sugar, is the only important animal source of carbohydrate.

2. The principal function of carbohydrate is to furnish energy for the body. In the United States about half of the energy value of the diet is provided by carbohydrate.

3. Equally good nutrition can be maintained on diets that are low in carbohydrate and those that are high in carbohydrate. In certain disease conditions carbohydrates may need to be moderately or severely restricted, whereas in other conditions a high carbohydrate intake is necessary.

4. Only a small amount of carbohydrate is stored in the body in the form of glycogen. If there is an excess of carbohydrate beyond the body's immediate need, it is stored as fat.

5. Wheat, corn, rice, potatoes, sweet potatoes, sugars, and sweets are the important sources of carbohydrate and calories in the American diet because they are used so frequently and appear in so many forms.

6. Weight for weight, fresh fruits and vegetables contain much less carbohydrate than breads and cereals. The fiber of fruits and vegetables is important for helping to maintain normal elimination.

7. Enriched and whole-grain breads and cereals are best buys for low-cost diets. They contribute not only energy but substantial amounts of protein, B-complex vitamins, and iron. Whole grains are good sources of fiber.

8. Sugars and sweets are concentrated sources of energy and are valued for the palatability they give to the diet.

9. Sugars and sweets should not replace essential foods needed for proteins, minerals, and vitamins. Unless used with discretion they may contribute to dental caries, especially in children.

10. Dark-brown sugar and molasses contain some minerals, especially iron. The contribution made to the daily intake of minerals is, however, likely to be small.

PROBLEMS AND REVIEW

1. What are the important differences between the three classes of carbohydrates?
2. In the United States about half of the calories are furnished by carbohydrate. Under what circumstances would you expect this proportion to increase?
3. Drinking a glass of fruit juice removes feelings of hunger quickly but for a relatively short period of time. Explain this on the basis of the physiologic and biochemical reactions that have taken place.
4. Even though you eat a diet that is high in carbohydrate the blood glucose will not usually reach the renal threshold. Explain the mechanisms whereby the blood sugar is maintained within such narrow limits.
5. If an individual is not eating, what mechanisms provide for the maintenance of a normal blood sugar?
6. If carbohydrate is eaten in excess of the body's need for energy, what happens to it?

7. Of what practical importance is cellulose in the diet?
8. *Problem.* Calculate the carbohydrate content of 60 gm bread; 120 gm potato; 150 gm orange.
9. *Problem.* Calculate the carbohydrate and caloric content of your diet for one day. What percentage of the calories were derived from carbohydrate? What percentage of your calories were derived from cereal foods and breadstuffs; cakes, pies, and other baked sweets; sugars, candy, carbonated beverages? What improvements could you suggest for the selection of carbohydrates in your diet?
10. *Problem.* Plan a midafternoon and bedtime snack that will furnish 100 gm carbohydrate. What points should you consider in planning for these snacks?
11. What reasons can you give for reducing the intake of sugars and sweets? What legitimate role do they have in the diet?

CITED REFERENCES

1. Levine, R.: "Carbohydrates," in Goodhart, R. S., and Shils, M. E., eds.: *Modern Nutrition in Health and Disease*, 5th ed. Lea & Febiger, Philadelphia, 1973, p. 102.
2. West, E. S., *et al.: Textbook of Biochemistry*, 4th ed. Macmillan Publishing Co., Inc., New York, 1966, p. 1039.
3. Food and Nutrition Board: *Recommended Dietary Allowances*, 8th ed. National Academy of Sciences—National Research Council, Washington, D.C., 1974, p. 34.
4. Cowgill, G. R., and Anderson, W. E.: "Laxative Effects of Wheat Bran and 'Washed' Bran in Healthy Men. A Comparative Study," *J.A.M.A.*, **98:**1866–75, 1932.
5. Hardinge, M. G., *et al.:* "Nutritional Studies of Vegetarians. III. Dietary Levels of Fiber," *Am. J. Clin. Nutr.*, **6:**523–25, 1958.
6. Burkitt, D. P., *et al.:* "Dietary Fiber and Disease," *J.A.M.A.*, **229:**1068–74, 1974.
7. Friend, B. and Marston, R.: "Nutritional Review," *National Food Situation*, Economic Research Service, U.S. Department of Agriculture, November 1974, pp. 26–32.
8. "Sugar and Tropical Products—Situation and Outlook," *National Food Situation*, Economic Research Service, U.S. Department of Agriculture, Washington, D.C., August 1974, pp. 20–23.
9. Yudkin, J.: "Dietary Fat and Dietary Sugar in Relation to Ischaemic Heart Disease and Diabetes," *Lancet*, **2:**4–5, July 4, 1964.
10. Grande, F., *et al.:* "Effects of Carbohydrates of Leguminous Seeds, Wheat, and Potatoes on Serum Cholesterol Concentrations in Man," *J. Nutr.*, **86:**313–17, 1965.
11. Antar, M. A., *et al.:* "Changes in Retail Market Food Supplies in the United States in the Last Seventy Years in Relation to the Incidence of Coronary Heart Disease, with Special Reference to Dietary Carbohydrate and Essential Fatty Acids," *Am. J. Clin. Nutr.*, **14:**169–78, 1964.

ADDITIONAL REFERENCES

Ahrens, R. A.: "Sucrose, Hypertension, and Heart Disease. An Historical Perspective." *Am. J. Clin. Nutr.*, **27:**403–22, 1974.
Anderson, J. T.: "Dietary Carbohydrate and Serum Triglycerides," *Am. J. Clin. Nutr.*, **20:**168–75, 1967.
Bibby, B. G.: "Cariogenicity of Foods," *J.A.M.A.*, **177:**316–21, 1961.
Glass, R. L., and Fleisch, S.: "Diet and Dental Caries: Dental Caries Incidence and the Consumption of Ready-to-Eat Cereals," *J. Am. Dent. Assoc.*, **88:**807–13, 1974.
Groen, J. J.: "Effect of Bread in the Diet on Serum Cholesterol," *Am. J. Clin. Nutr.*, **20:**191–97, 1967.
Hardinge, M. G., *et al.:* "Carbohydrate in Foods," *J. Am. Diet. Assoc.*, **46:**197–204, 1965.
"Idea Exchange: Fiber in the Diet," *J. Am. Diet. Assoc.*, **66:**50–53, 1975.
Mendeloff, A. I.: "Dietary Fiber," *Nutr. Rev.*, **33:**321–26, 1975.
Paige, D. M., *et al.:* "Lactose Hydrolyzed Milk," *Am. J. Clin. Nutr.*, **28:**818–22, 1975.
Review: "Frequency of Eating and Dental Caries Prevalence," *Nutr. Rev.*, **32:**139–41, 1974.
Review: "Glucose Ingestion and the Control of Lipogenesis," *Nutr. Rev.*, **31:**287–89, 1973.

Review: "Mechanisms of Carbohydrate-induced Hypertriglyceridemia," *Nutr. Rev.*, **32:**74–75, 1974.

Review: "The Role of Sugars in Hyperlipidemia," *Nutr. Rev.*, **32:**40–42, 1974.

Stevens, H. A., and Ohlson, M. A.: "Estimated Intake of Simple and Complex Carbohydrates," *J. Am. Diet. Assoc.*, **48:**294–96, 1966.

Yudkin, J.: "Evolutionary and Historical Changes in Dietary Carbohydrates," *Am. J. Clin. Nutr.*, **20:**108–15, 1967.

6 Lipids

vantages to such changes? The informed nurse, dietitian, and physician are people who can look at specific questions with an overall perspective and provide sound guidance to the public.

COMPOSITION, CLASSIFICATION, AND CHARACTERISTICS

Composition. LIPIDS include fats, oils, and fatlike substances that have a greasy feel and that are insoluble in water but soluble in certain organic solvents such as ether, alcohol, and benzene. Like carbohydrates, fats are organic compounds of carbon, hydrogen, and oxygen, but the resemblance ends there. Fats have a much smaller proportion of oxygen than do carbohydrates and differ importantly in their structure and properties. Some lipids also contain carbohydrates, phosphates, or nitrogenous compounds.

Classification. Lipids are usually classified in three groups:

1. *Simple lipids* are esters of glycerol and fatty acids. GLYCEROL is a 3-carbon alcohol with three hydroxyl groups, each of which can combine with a fatty acid. A MONOGLYCERIDE is formed by combining a fatty acid with one of the hydroxyl groups of the glycerol molecule; DIGLYCERIDES contain two fatty acids; TRIGLYCERIDES, also referred to as *neutral fats*, contain three fatty acids.

A *simple triglyceride* is one in which the three fatty acids are the same. A *mixed triglyceride* is one in which at least two fatty acids are different. (See Figure 6–1.) Mixed triglycerides account for 98 per

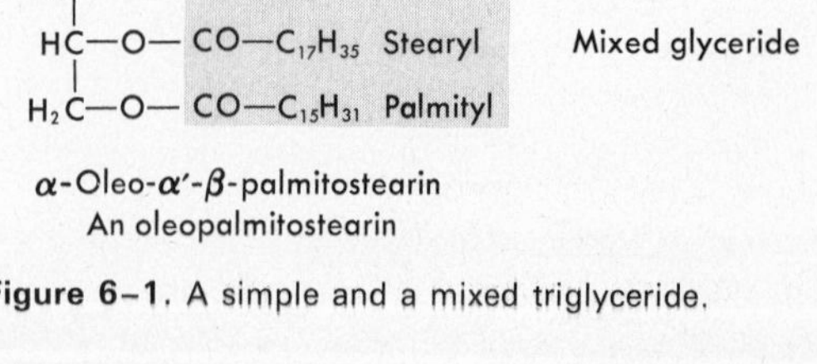

Dietary significance. Fats are prominent constituents of the American diet, supplying as much as two fifths of the total calorie intake. Anyone who has been forced to drastically restrict his intake of fats appreciates how much they contribute to the palatability of the diet whether it be the butter or margarine on bread, sauces for meats and vegetables, dressings on salads, or cakes, cookies, pastries, and other desserts.

Because fats are a concentrated source of energy it is possible to ingest the needed calories without excessively bulky diets. Meals that are moderate in fat content also have greater satiety than those that are low in fat. This results from the longer time that a food mixture containing fat remains in the stomach, thus delaying hunger.

The fat in many foods is also a carrier of fat-soluble vitamins. For example, the elimination of butter or margarine, whole milk, whole-milk cheeses, and egg yolk means that the diet must be planned with especial care to include sufficient vitamin A from other sources.

Many Americans today, on the basis of research reports as well as food advertising, are raising important questions about the fat content of their diets. They ask: Should we reduce the fat in our diets? Should we omit whole milk and eggs because they are high in saturated fats and in cholesterol? What are the possible benefits of substituting special margarines and cooking oils for regular margarines, butter, and solid fats? Are there any disad-

$$H_2C\text{—}O\text{—}CO\text{—}C_{17}H_{35}$$
$$HC\text{—}O\text{—}CO\text{—}C_{17}H_{35}$$
$$H_2C\text{—}O\text{—}CO\text{—}C_{17}H_{35}$$

Simple glyceride

Glyceryl tristearate
Tristearin

$$H_2C\text{—}O\text{—}CO\text{—}C_{17}H_{33}\ \ Oleyl$$
$$HC\text{—}O\text{—}CO\text{—}C_{17}H_{35}\ \ Stearyl$$
$$H_2C\text{—}O\text{—}CO\text{—}C_{15}H_{31}\ \ Palmityl$$

Mixed glyceride

α-Oleo-α'-β-palmitostearin
An oleopalmitostearin

Figure 6–1. A simple and a mixed triglyceride.

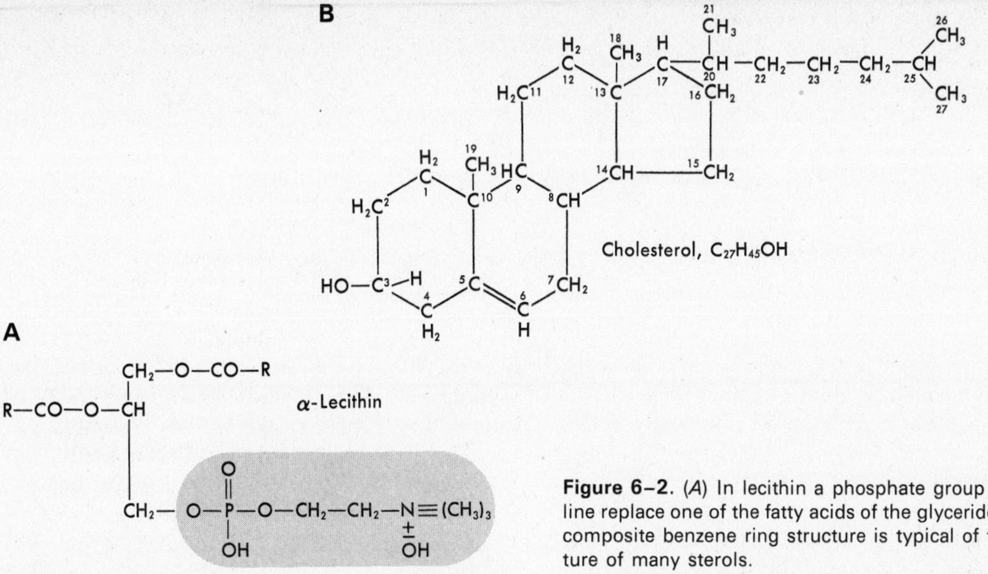

B

Cholesterol, $C_{27}H_{45}OH$

A

α-Lecithin

Figure 6-2. (A) In lecithin a phosphate group and choline replace one of the fatty acids of the glyceride. (B) The composite benzene ring structure is typical of the structure of many sterols.

cent of fats in foods and over 90 per cent of fat in the body.

Waxes are esters of fatty acids and long-chain or cyclic alcohols. This group includes the esters of cholesterol, vitamin A, and vitamin D.

2. *Compound lipids.* These are esters of glycerol and fatty acids, with substitution of other components such as carbohydrate, phosphate, and/or nitrogenous groupings. Phospholipids such as lecithin and cephalin contain a phosphate and nitrogen grouping replacing one of the fatty acids in the molecule. (See Figure 6-2.) Glycolipids such as the cerebrosides contain a molecule of glucose or galactose. Lipoproteins include a variety of lipid molecules bound to protein molecules in order to facilitate transport in the aqueous medium of the blood.

3. *Derived lipids.* These include fatty acids; alcohols (glycerol and sterols); carotenoids; and the fat-soluble vitamins, A, D, E, and K.

Fatty acids. Most fatty acids in foods and in the body are straight, even-numbered carbon chains, containing as few as 4 or as many as 24 carbon atoms. Short-chain fatty acids contain four and six carbon atoms, medium-chain fatty acids contain 8 to 12 carbon atoms, and long-chain fatty acids contain more than 12 carbon atoms.

Fatty acids are "saturated" or "unsaturated." A fatty acid in which each of the carbon atoms in the chain has two hydrogen atoms attached to it is

saturated:
$$-\underset{\underset{H}{|}}{\overset{\overset{H}{|}}{C}}-\underset{\underset{H}{|}}{\overset{\overset{H}{|}}{C}}-.$$
An unsaturated fatty acid is one in which a hydrogen atom is missing from each of two adjoining carbon atoms, thus necessitating a double bond between the two carbon atoms:
$$-\overset{\overset{H}{|}}{C}=\overset{\overset{H}{|}}{C}-.$$
A monounsaturated fatty acid has one double bond; oleic acid is widely distributed in food and body fats. A polyunsaturated fatty acid (PUFA) contains two or more double bonds; linoleic, linolenic, and arachidonic acids are nutritionally important examples of this group. The formulas for four fatty acids that contain 18 carbon atoms but that differ in their saturation are shown in Figure 6-3.

Unsaturated fatty acids can exist as geometric isomers. In the *cis* form the molecule folds back upon itself at each double bond. In the *trans* form the molecule extends to its maximum length.

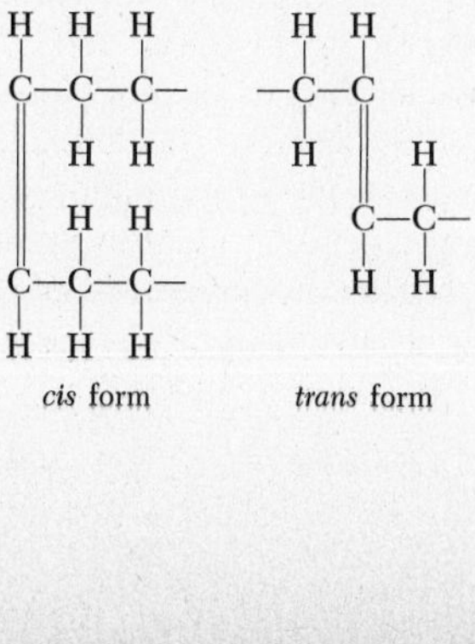

cis form   *trans* form

$CH_3(CH_2)_{16}COOH$ Stearic acid (saturated)

$CH_3(CH_2)_7$ $CH{=}CH$ $(CH_2)_7COOH$ Oleic acid (monounsaturated)

$CH_3(CH_2)_4$ $CH{=}CH$ CH_2 $CH{=}CH$ $(CH_2)_7COOH$ Linoleic acid (2 double bonds; polyunsaturated)

CH_3CH_2 $CH{=}CH$ CH_2 $CH{=}CH$ CH_2 $CH{=}CH$ $(CH_2)_7COOH$ Linolenic acid (3 double bonds; polyunsaturated)

Figure 6–3. These fatty acids contain 18 carbon atoms but differ in the level of saturation.

The form in which a fatty acid occurs markedly influences the melting point and other properties of the fat. Food and body fats exist principally in the *cis* form.

Characteristics of fats. The nature of fats—their hardness, melting point, and flavor—is determined by the length of the carbon chain and the level of saturation of the fatty acids as well as the order in which the fatty acids are attached to the glycerol molecule. Although pure triglycerides are practically tasteless, they have the ability to hold flavors and aromas. A tremendous number of fats exist in nature. Each food fat—beef, lamb, chicken, olive oil, for example—has its distinctive flavor and hardness.

Hardness. Fatty acids containing 12 carbon atoms or less and unsaturated fatty acids are liquid at room temperature. Saturated fatty acids containing 14 carbon atoms or more are solid at room temperature. Food and body fats contain mixtures of short- and long-chain fatty acids and of saturated and unsaturated fatty acids. No natural fat is made up completely of either saturated or unsaturated fatty acids.

The distribution of fatty acids in a number of fats is shown in Table 6–1. Only about 5 per cent of fatty acids in food and body fats contain less than 14 carbon atoms, coconut oil being an exception. Oleic, palmitic, and stearic acids predominate in animal fats. These fats are solid at room temperature and are often referred to as "saturated." In general, herbivora have harder fats than carnivora, and land animals have harder fats than aquatic animals. Lamb and beef fat, with their high content of palmitic and stearic acids, are much harder than pork and chicken fat, which contain somewhat more of the unsaturated fatty acids. Fats from fish have a high proportion of polyunsaturated fatty acids containing 20 to 24 carbon atoms. The proportion of saturated fatty acids is high in milk fat, but this fat is soft because of the presence of many short-chain fatty acids.

Oleic and linoleic acids predominate in vegetable fats, except for coconut oil. Corn, cottonseed, and soybean oils are very rich in linoleic acid, whereas peanut and olive oils are rich in oleic acid and correspondingly lower in linoleic acid. Of the vegetable fats, coconut oil is unique in that it is composed largely of the 12-carbon lauric acid, which is liquid at room temperature. Coconut oil is classed as a "saturated" fat, and other vegetable fats as "unsaturated." Those fats that have a high proportion of fatty acids with two or more double bonds are referred to as "polyunsaturated."

Hydrogenation. In the presence of a catalyst such as nickel, liquid fats can be changed to solid fats by HYDROGENATION; this consists of the addition of hydrogen at the double bonds of the carbon chain. In the manufacture of vegetable shortenings and margarines, some, but not all, of the double bonds in the oils are hydrogenated, thereby giving fats that are somewhat soft and plastic. During hydrogenation some of the fatty acids are changed from the *cis* to the *trans* form, but both forms are utilized by the body. Hydrogenation reduces the linoleic acid content of the fat.

Emulsification. Fats are capable of forming emulsions with liquids, a property that is essential for their digestion and absorption. Emulsification of fats is also utilized in the homogenization of milk and in the preparation of mayonnaise.

Saponification. The combination of a fatty acid with a cation to form a soap is known as SAPONIFICATION. In the alkaline medium of the intestine, for

Table 6-1. Typical Major Fatty Acid Analyses of Some Fats of Animal and Plant Origin*†

| | Saturated | | | | | | | Unsaturated | | | | | |
	4-8	Capric 10.0	Lauric 12.0	Myristic 14.0	Palmitic 16.0	Stearic 18.0	Arachidic 20.0	Behenic 22.0	Palmitoleic 16.1	Oleic 18.1	Linoleic 18.2	Linolenic 18.3	Arachidonic 20.4	Other Polyenoic Acids
Animal														
Lard				1.5	27.0	13.5			3.0	43.5	10.5	0.5		
Chicken			2.0	7.0	25.0	6.0			8.0	36.0	14.0			
Egg					25.0	10.0				50.0	10.0	2.0	3.0	
Beef				3.0	29.0	21.0	0.5		3.0	41.0	2.0	0.5	0.5	
Butter	5.5	3.0	3.5	12.0	28.0	13.0			3.0	28.5	1.0			
Human milk		1.5	7.0	8.5	21.0	7.0	1.0		2.5	36.0	7.0	1.0	0.5	
Menhaden				9.0	19.0	5.5			16.0					48.5
Human adipose‡			0.1-2	2-6	21-25	2-8			3-7	39-47	4-25			2-8
Vegetable														
Corn					12.5	2.5	0.5			29.0	55.0	0.5		
Peanut					11.5	3.0	1.5	2.5		53.0	26.0			
Cottonseed				1.0	26.0	3.0			1.0	17.5	51.5			
Soybean					11.5	4.0				24.5	53.0	7.0		
Olive					13.0	2.5			1.0	74.0	9.0	0.5		
Coconut	7.0	6.0	49.5	19.5	8.5	2.0				6.0	1.5			

* Food and Nutrition Board: *Dietary Fat and Human Health.* Pub. 1147, National Academy of Sciences—National Research Council, Washington, D.C., 1966, p. 6.

† Composition is given in weight percentages of the component fatty acids (rounded to nearest 0.5) as determined by gas chromatography. The number of carbon atoms and the number of double bonds is indicated under the common name of the fatty acid. These data were derived from a variety of sources. They are representative determinations rather than averages, and considerable variation is to be expected in individual samples from other sources.

‡ Adapted from West, E. S., *et al.: Textbook of Biochemistry,* 4th ed. Macmillan Publishing Co., Inc., New York, 1966, p. 134.

example, free fatty acid may combine with calcium to form an insoluble compound that is excreted in the feces. In certain diseases characterized by poor fat absorption—sprue, for example—the loss of calcium in this manner could be significant.

Rancidity. Air at room temperature can induce oxidation of fats, resulting in the changes in odor and flavor commonly known as rancidity. These changes are accelerated upon exposure to light and in the presence of traces of certain minerals. They occur more readily in fats that have a high proportion of unsaturated fatty acids. Some fats are naturally protected from rapid oxidation by the presence of antioxidants, one of which is vitamin E. Commercially processed fats and oils are usually protected by the addition of small amounts of antioxidants.

Effect of heat. Excessive heating of fats leads to the breakdown of glycerol, producing a pungent compound (acrolein) which is especially irritating to the gastrointestinal mucosa. Fatty acids are also oxidized by prolonged heating at high temperatures. Under ordinary conditions of home or commercial frying no adverse effects on nutritional properties have been found.

FUNCTIONS

Important source of energy. The primary function of fat is to supply energy, each gram of fat yielding approximately 9 kcal when oxidized. This energy is continuously available from the stores in adipose tissue. The high density and low solubility of fats make them an ideal form in which to store energy. In fact, not only fats as such are stored in adipose tissue, but any glucose and amino acids not promptly utilized are also synthesized into fats and stored.

Adipose tissue, which consists principally of triglycerides, is stored in the subcutaneous tissues and in the abdominal cavity. It also surrounds the organs and is laced throughout muscle tissue. Many examples could be cited of individuals who have survived total starvation for 30 or 40 days, or partial starvation for much longer periods of time. Their survival was possible only because of the energy available from the adipose tissues.

Insulation and padding. The subcutaneous layer of fat is an effective insulator and reduces losses of body heat in cold weather. Excessive layers of sub-cutaneous fat, as in obesity, interfere with heat loss during warm weather, thus increasing discomfort. The vital organs such as the kidney are protected against physical injury by a padding of fat. Fats and oils also have some value as a lubricant for the gastrointestinal tract.

Essential fatty acids. LINOLEIC ACID, the 18-carbon acid with two double bonds, is an essential fatty acid; that is, it cannot be synthesized in the body and must be present in the diet. In the body linoleic acid is rapidly converted to ARACHIDONIC ACID, the physiologically functioning polyunsaturated fatty acid. Young animals that are fed a diet deficient in polyunsaturated fatty acids fail to grow and are afflicted with an eczemalike dermatitis. These conditions are corrected when linoleic acid is added to the diet. Similarly, Hansen[1] found that the inclusion of essential fatty acids in the diet of infants who had eczema led to improvement of the skin and to greater gains in weight. (See Figure 6–4.)

The essential fatty acids are constituents of phospholipids that form cellular membranes and thus appear to have a role in regulating cell permeability. They also are involved in the transport of lipids and have a lowering effect on the blood cholesterol. Arachidonic acid is a precursor of PROSTAGLANDINS, a group of hormonelike compounds. They play a role in smooth muscle contraction, gastric secretion, pancreatic function, and control of blood pressure.[2]

Linolenic acid, another of the polyunsaturated fatty acids, promotes normal growth in animals but it does not cure the dermatitis that occurs from fatty acid deficiency. It is, therefore, not an essential fatty acid and is not a substitute for linoleic acid.

Phospholipids. All cells contain phospholipids, but brain, nervous tissue, and liver are especially rich in them. The phospholipid level in the body is not reduced even in starvation, suggesting the vital role that they must play in metabolism. Phospholipids are powerful emulsifying agents and have an affinity for water. Hence, they are essential to the digestion and absorption of fats and they facilitate the uptake of fatty acids by the cells.

Phospholipids comprise a significant proportion of the blood lipoproteins but their function in lipid transport is not clearly understood. They are manufactured and removed by the liver and apparently do not enter the tissue cells, which readily synthesize their own supply of phospholipid.

Cholesterol. The concentration of cholesterol is

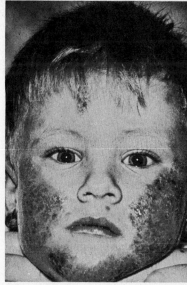 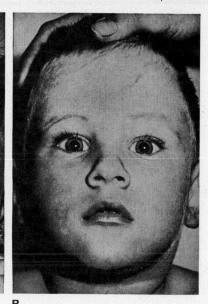

Figure 6–4. Child, 2½ years old, showing (*A*) eczema present since two months of age; (*B*) condition one month after fresh lard was added to the diet. (Courtesy, Dr. A. E. Hansen, Galveston, Texas.)

A

B

high in the liver, the adrenal, the white and gray matter of the brain, and the peripheral nerves. It is present in small amounts in almost all body tissues and constitutes an important fraction of the blood lipoproteins. It is synthesized by the liver to meet body needs regardless of dietary intake. Cholesterol furnishes the nucleus for the synthesis of provitamin D, adrenocortical hormones, steroid sex hormones, and bile salts.

DIGESTION AND ABSORPTION

Digestion. Almost all the fats presented to the digestive tract for hydrolysis are triglycerides. Only a small fraction of dietary fat consists of cholesterol esters and phospholipids. Fats are hydrolyzed primarily in the small intestine. Although gastric lipase brings about some hydrolysis of finely divided fats from foods such as egg yolk and cream, the action is not important.

As the chyme enters the duodenum, the presence of fat stimulates the intestinal wall to secrete CHOLECYSTOKININ, a hormone that is carried to the gallbladder by the bloodstream. Cholecystokinin stimulates the contraction of the gallbladder, thereby forcing bile into the common duct and thence into the small intestine.

Bile has several important functions in fat diges-

tion and absorption: (1) it stimulates peristalsis; (2) it neutralizes the acid chyme so as to provide the optimum hydrogen ion concentration for enzyme activity; (3) it emulsifies fats, thereby increasing the surface area exposed to enzyme action; and (4) it lowers the surface tension so that intimate contact between the fat droplets and the enzymes is possible.

The triglycerides are hydrolyzed stepwise by lipase; that is, one of the end fatty acids is removed at the time yielding in turn a diglyceride and then a monoglyceride. Only about one fourth to one half of the triglycerides are completely hydrolyzed to glycerol and fatty acids. Phospholipids are hydrolyzed by a number of phospholipases that can attack the several linkages of the molecule. The end products of lipid hydrolysis that are presented for absorption include fatty acids, glycerol, monoglycerides, and probably some diglycerides and triglycerides. (See Figure 6–5.)

Speed of digestion. Fats reduce the motility of the gastrointestinal tract, and hence any diet containing fat remains in the stomach longer than one that is low in fat. Fats that are liquid at body temperature are hydrolyzed more rapidly than those that are solid at body temperature. Typical mixed diets contain complex mixtures of fats including short- and long-chain as well as saturated and unsaturated fatty acids. Adults normally expe-

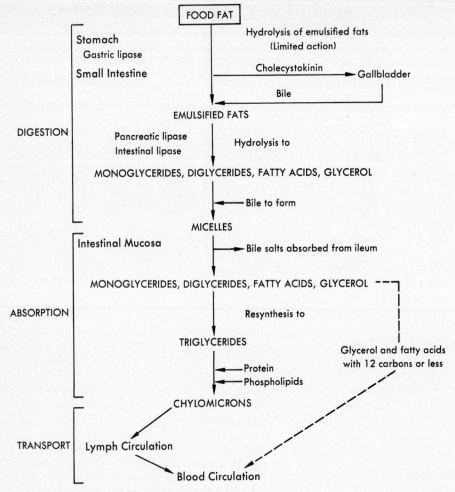

Figure 6–5. Digestion, absorption, and transport of fat.

rience no difficulty in digesting fats from any source. Infants and young children, as well as some elderly persons, seem to have somewhat better tolerance for the softer, more highly emulsified fats such as those in dairy products. They also may experience some discomfort following meals that are high in fat.

Fried foods are digested somewhat more slowly than foods prepared by other methods of cookery because the food particles coated with fat must be broken up before they can be acted upon by enzymes. Properly fried foods do not normally cause digestive difficulties, even for persons who require therapeutic diets. When the frying temperature is too low, foods absorb excessive amounts of fat, thus lengthening the time required for digestion. On the other hand, if foods are fried at too high a temperature the resulting decomposition products may be irritating to the intestinal mucosa.

Absorption. The free fatty acids, monoglycerides, some diglycerides and triglycerides, and cholesterol are complexed with bile salts to form MICELLES, which are water-soluble microscopic particles that can penetrate the mucosal membrane. At the point of contact of the micelle with the brush border of the epithelial cell, the lipids are apparently released from the complex and enter the cell by mechanisms not fully understood. *Pinocytosis*, that is, engulfing the fat and subsequently releasing it to the interior of the cell, is believed to be one of the operative mechanisms. When the lipids are released from the micelle, new products of hydrolysis of fats can again combine with the bile salts. Most of the absorption of fats occurs from the jejunum.

Fatty acids that contain 12 carbon atoms or less are absorbed into the portal circulation without reesterification in the mucosal cell. They are attached to albumin for their transportation, and they may be used within the liver or released to other tissues in the body. The glycerol resulting from fat hydrolysis is also carried by the portal circulation.

Fatty acids that contain 14 carbon atoms or more are resynthesized to new triglycerides within the epithelial cell of the mucosa before they are extruded into the lymph circulation. The new fats are formed by the addition of two fatty acids to a monoglyceride molecule or by esterification of glycerol with three fatty acids. See page 85 for a further description of fat synthesis. Cholesterol is also reesterified within the epithelial cell.

Enterohepatic circulation. Bile salts are utilized over and over again through the cycle known as the ENTEROHEPATIC CIRCULATION. This consists of (1) the secretion of bile into the duodenum, (2) the reabsorption of bile salts by active transport from the ileum, (3) the entrance of the salts into the hepatic circulation, and (4) the secretion of bile once again into the duodenum. The total body pool of bile salts is estimated to be about 3 gm, but this pool can be recirculated as much as 10 times in a day. This results in the effectiveness of 30 gm bile salts daily. The liver normally synthesizes about 0.5 gm bile salts daily, an amount that just about covers the excretion in the feces.

Chylomicrons. In order to penetrate the lipoprotein membrane of the epithelial cell for entrance to the lymph circulation, the newly formed fats are made soluble by surrounding them with a lipoprotein envelope consisting chiefly of phospholipids and a very small amount of protein. These particles are known as CHYLOMICRONS, having first been identified in chyle (lymph). They are of very low density and give to the lymph a milky appearance.

Completeness of digestion and absorption. Normally about 95 per cent of dietary fats and 80 per cent of dietary cholesterol are absorbed. Mineral oil, which is not a true fat, is not absorbed from the intestine. This fact is mentioned in order to empha-

size that mineral oil should never be used in food preparation inasmuch as it seriously interferes with the absorption of fat-soluble vitamins. When mineral oil is used as a laxative, it should not be taken at mealtime.

A number of factors reduce the amount of fat that is digested and absorbed. Among these are increased motility so that food is moved along the tract too rapidly for complete enzyme action; disease of the biliary tract so that the secretion of bile is deficient or does not reach the small intestine; disease of the pancreas so that lipase is not secreted; and reduction in the absorbing surfaces as in celiac disease or following surgery on the small intestine. When fat absorption is decreased, large amounts of fat are excreted in the feces (steatorrhea) with a consequent serious loss of calories. (See Chapter 34.)

METABOLISM

The blood is the means of transportation of lipids from one site to another, and the liver and adipose tissues are the specialized organs that control lipid metabolism. The synthesis of new lipids (LIPOGENESIS) and the catabolism of lipids (LIPOLYSIS) are continuously taking place. These reactions are catalyzed by specific enzymes under the control of nervous and hormonal mechanisms. (See Figure 6-6.)

Blood lipids. Since fats are insoluble in water, proteins provide the mechanism for their transport in the aqueous medium of the blood. These protein-lipid complexes are known as lipoproteins. The chylomicrons synthesized in the intestinal mucosa (see above) are large particles consisting principally of triglycerides. They give a milky appearance to blood serum shortly after a fat-rich meal, but they are rapidly hydrolyzed by lipoprotein lipase and the released fats are used by the tissues. The blood serum is thus "cleared."

Alpha- and beta-lipoproteins. The greatest concentration of lipids in the blood consists of two classes of lipoproteins. *High-density* or *α-lipoproteins* contain a large proportion of protein, phospholipid, and cholesterol. This class is little affected by changes in diet or by age. *Low-density* or *β-lipoproteins* include a number of groups that vary widely in density and in their proportions of tri-

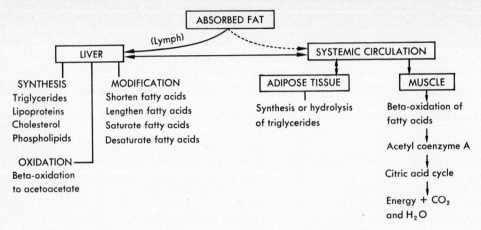

Figure 6–6. The liver and adipose tissue are principal organs of fat metabolism.

glycerides, cholesterol, phospholipids, and protein. Those that approach the particle size of chylomicrons consist principally of triglycerides and only small amounts of protein and other lipids. This class is especially elevated in carbohydrate-induced hyperglyceridemia.

Another group of β-lipoproteins contains a large proportion of cholesterol and is elevated with increasing age and when diets are rich in saturated fatty acids, and to a lesser extent when diets contain substantial amounts of cholesterol. Patients who have had a myocardial infarction, those who have angina pectoris, and those individuals who are considered to be high risks for cardiovascular disease usually show increased concentrations of the β-lipoprotein group (HYPERLIPOPROTEINEMIA). Other pathologic conditions in which this group is often elevated include diabetes mellitus, nephrosis, hypothyroidism, and xanthomatosis.[3]

Free fatty acids (FFA), also designated as nonesterified fatty acids (NEFA), are the principal source of fatty acids made available to the cells for energy. They enter the circulation as the result of the hydrolysis of triglycerides, chiefly by adipose tissue. The fatty acids are attached rather tightly to plasma albumin and do not circulate in their free state. At the cell surfaces the fatty acid is released with ease from its carrier. The concentration of FFA in the blood at any given time is quite low, but the rate of turnover is so rapid that several thousand calories are transported daily in the circulation in this way. The concentration of free fatty acids is somewhat higher in the circulation during fasting, indicating more rapid release from adipose tissue. It is somewhat lower when carbohydrate is being absorbed, indicating that carbohydrate is being used for energy as well as synthesized to fat.

Adipose tissue and fat metabolism. Like other tissues, adipose tissue is constantly being remolded. It synthesizes, stores, and releases fat. It consists chiefly of triglycerides and is supplied with the enzymes that are required for lipogenesis and lipolysis. Fat synthesis and breakdown take place continuously, but they are in equilibrium when the energy needs of the body are exactly met.

If the energy supplied to the body is in excess of the body's needs, lipogenesis exceeds the rate of lipolysis and adipose tissue is stored (weight is gained) regardless of whether calories are derived from fat, carbohydrate, or protein. Insulin is required for the synthesis of fats. The number of adipose cells is determined early in life. Overfeeding of the infant and young child results in a great increase in the number of adipose cells. Later in life, as these numerous cells become saturated with fat through overeating, obesity results.[4]

When a calorie deficit exists, the adipose tissue will be catabolized more rapidly than it is being synthesized (weight is lost). The release of fatty acids from adipose tissue is accelerated by the same hormones that increase glucose breakdown: epinephrine, norepinephrine, glucagon, growth hormone, adrenocorticotropic hormone, and thyrotropic hormone.

The liver and fat metabolism. The liver is the key organ in the regulation of fat metabolism. It is able to accomplish the shortening or lengthening of the carbon chain of the fatty acids and to introduce double bonds into fatty acids. For example, a double bond can be introduced into stearic acid to yield oleic acid. On the other hand, a second double bond cannot be introduced into oleic acid to yield linoleic acid. With a dietary supply of linoleic acid, this essential fatty acid can be converted to arachidonic acid by adding a 2-carbon unit and by introducing two additional double bonds.

The liver hydrolyzes the triglycerides brought to it, re-forms new triglycerides, and again releases them to the circulation. It converts FFA to triglycerides and phospholipids and synthesizes lipoproteins. It releases them to the circulation and also removes them from the circulation, thus maintaining control over the blood levels.

The liver is probably the chief regulator of the total body content of cholesterol and of the circulating blood cholesterol. It governs the endogenous synthesis of cholesterol, the removal of cholesterol from the circulation, the production of bile acids from cholesterol, and the excretion of cholesterol and bile acids by way of the bile into the intestine.

Certain LIPOTROPIC SUBSTANCES must be present to prevent the accumulation of fat in the liver. They include choline, vitamin B_{12}, betaine, and possibly inositol. Methionine, one of the essential amino acids, donates methyl groups for the synthesis of choline and is therefore a lipotropic substance.

Synthesis of fats. Triglycerides are synthesized by the epithelial cells of the intestinal mucosa, by the adipose tissue, and by the liver. In order to synthesize triglycerides, a source of α-glycerophosphate is essential. This is furnished by the normal oxidation of glucose that occurs in each of these tissues through the Embden-Meyerhof pathway (see page 68). A second source of α-glycerophosphate is available from the glycerol released from fat hydrolysis in the intestinal mucosa and in the liver.[5] The glycerol so released combines with ATP in the presence of glycerokinase to form α-glycerophosphate. Adipose tissue does not contain glycerokinase and cannot convert glycerol to the active form.

The fatty acids for the triglyceride molecule are available from the hydrolysis of fats and also through synthesis from acetyl coenzyme A derived through the oxidation of fats, glucose, and some amino acids. The synthesis of unsaturated fatty acids and the elongation of existing fatty acid chains are accomplished by the mitochondria.

The synthesis of fats from acetyl coenzyme A is accomplished essentially by building up the carbon chain by successive additions of 2-carbon fragments. NADPH, a niacin-containing coenzyme, is required for this synthesis. It is made available through the pentose shunt of the glycolytic pathway (see page 70). The synthesis of fatty acids from acetyl coenzyme A is thus seen to be dependent upon normal carbohydrate metabolism and to require insulin. Free fatty acids are not esterified directly with glycerophosphate but must first be converted to fatty acyl coenzyme A. They are then attached stepwise to glycerophosphate to form the triglyceride.

Oxidation of fatty acids. All cells of the body except those of the central nervous system and red blood cells can oxidize fatty acids to yield energy. Although glucose is the source of energy for the central nervous system, the brain cells after a period of total starvation can adapt to the utilization of ketone bodies derived from fat and amino acids.[6]

The oxidation of fatty acids takes place in the cell mitochondria. BETA OXIDATION is the major pathway for oxidation. By this process oxidation occurs at the carbon that is beta from the carboxyl group. To prime the reaction ATP is required. The oxidation is accomplished in five steps, the end result of which is a fatty acid that is two carbons shorter plus a molecule of acetyl coenzyme A. Thus, the complete breakdown of an 18-carbon fatty acid requires 45 reactions.

$$CH_3(CH_2)_{16}COOH + \text{Coenzyme A} \rightarrow$$
$$\text{Stearic acid}$$

$$CH_3(CH_2)_{14}COOCoA + CH_3COOCoA$$
$$\text{Palmityl coenzyme A} \quad \text{Acetyl coenzyme A}$$

Each molecule of acetyl coenzyme A can (1) enter the Krebs cycle for oxidation to energy, carbon dioxide, and water, or (2) be used for the synthesis of new fatty acids, cholesterol, and other compounds.

The glycerol made available from the hydrolysis of fatty acids enters the glycolytic pathway by combining with ATP to form glycerophosphate. Thus, it is a potential source of glucose, glycogen, and energy or may be the backbone for the new glyceride molecule.

Ketogenesis. Within the liver two molecules of acetyl coenzyme A can condense to form acetoacetyl coenzyme A, which in turn yields acetoacetic acid, beta-hydroxybutyric acid, and acetone. These compounds are known as KETONE BODIES and the process as KETOGENESIS. The ketone bodies are normally produced in small amounts by the liver. Although the liver cells do not possess the enzymes necessary for their further oxidation, muscle and other cells can utilize them to yield energy.

In certain circumstances, such as uncontrolled diabetes mellitus and starvation, carbohydrate metabolism is greatly reduced, and the production of acetyl coenzyme A from fat oxidation is greatly increased. The reduction in carbohydrate metabolism means that the amount of oxalacetate available to combine with acetyl coenzyme A in the Krebs cycle is also reduced. The liver synthesizes vastly increased amounts of the ketones—far beyond the ability of the tissues to oxidize them. The principal effect of the increased production is a disturbance of the acid-base balance. Acetoacetic acid and β-hydroxybutyric acid are fairly strong acids and combine with the available base. They are excreted (KETONURIA) and the alkali reserve is reduced. Acetone, being volatile, is excreted by the lungs.

Cholesterol metabolism. The liver and intestine are the chief sites of cholesterol synthesis, but all cells are able to produce some cholesterol. The endogenous production of cholesterol has been variously estimated at 1000 to 2000 mg daily and is apparently independent of the dietary supply. Acetyl coenzyme A is the direct precursor of cholesterol, and thus any donor of acetyl coenzyme A—fatty acids, glucose, and some amino acids—is a potential source of cholesterol.

The body is unable to break down the cholesterol nucleus, but the liver converts it by enzyme action to bile acids. This is apparently rate limited,[7] and therefore any excess supply poses problems of disposal. Cholesterol as such and bile acids are constituents of bile, and excretion occurs from the intestine.

As stated in a preceding section, cholesterol is transported in the blood in the lipoproteins. The determination of the cholesterol concentration in blood serum is conveniently made in the laboratory, and any increase in blood levels correlates well with the increase in the concentration of the class of β-lipoproteins that occur in certain pathologic conditions. The serum cholesterol concentration in apparently normal adults ranges from 150 to 250 mg per 100 ml, although a level above 200 mg per 100 ml is now considered by many investigators to be undesirable. About three fourths of the serum cholesterol is esterified. The concentration of cholesterol varies considerably and is increased during periods of emotional stress, physical inactivity, and overeating. A single determination is probably of limited significance.

FAT IN THE DIET

Dietary allowances. People of the Orient consume diets that provide around 10 per cent or less of the calories from fat, whereas Americans derive 40 per cent or more of their calories from fat. These extremes of intake cannot be described categorically as being damaging to health or as affording promise of good health.

The Food and Nutrition Board has not set precise recommendations for either the quantity or type of fat that should be included in the diet. Since the energy value of the diet is derived mainly from fat and carbohydrate, any drastic restriction in the one means that the other must be increased in order to maintain caloric equilibrium. In normal individuals it is debatable whether it is desirable to markedly increase the carbohydrate intake in order to restrict the fat intake, let us say, to 20 to 25 per cent of the calories.

The American Heart Association[8] recommends a fat intake not to exceed 35 per cent of calories. It is further suggested that not more than 10 per cent of calories be derived from saturated fat and up to 10 per cent of calories be furnished by polyunsaturated fatty acids. Such a proportion of fat intake would give a polyunsaturated to saturated ratio (P/S RATIO) of 1.0. In general, American diets are high in saturated fats so that the P/S ratio ranges between 0.2 and 0.5. Such a ratio is considered to be incompatible with desirable blood lipid levels.

A moderate reduction of cholesterol intake, 400

to 500 mg daily, is probably desirable for all persons. This is readily achieved by restricting the intake of eggs to four per week.

As little as 1 to 2 per cent of the calories from linoleic acid is sufficient to prevent symptoms of fatty acid deficiency.[9] Essential fatty acid deficiency has not been demonstrated in adults, and the exact requirement for linoleic acid is not known. The average mixed diet supplies more than adequate amounts. When a diet is modified to provide greatly increased amounts of linoleic acid, the need for vitamin E is also increased.

Food sources. In the United States the fat available for consumption in 1975 was 147 gm.[10] The percentages contributed by each food group were: fats and oils including butter, 42.4; meat, poultry, and fish, 34.1; dairy products excluding butter, 13.2; legumes, 3.7; eggs, 3; flour and cereals, 1.4; and fruits and vegetables, 1.0. The so-called "visible" fats include oils, lard, hydrogenated shortening, butter, margarine, fat back of pork, bacon, and salad dressings, and are concentrated sources of fat. A small amount of them contribute importantly to the caloric level of the diet.

"Invisible" fats include meat, poultry, fish, eggs, whole milk, cream, cheese, and baked products. Meats, poultry, and fish vary widely in their fat content. The amount of fat ingested from meat will depend upon the cut that was used, whether fat was carefully trimmed, whether fat drippings were used, and upon the method of preparation. Lean cuts of beef, pork, lamb, and veal differ little in their fat content. Fish is somewhat lower in fat than is meat. Fish that have a colored flesh are somewhat higher in fat than those with white flesh.

All of the fat in the egg is in the yolk, about one third of this being in the form of phospholipid. Whole milk, cream, ice cream, and whole-milk cheeses furnish appreciable amounts of fat. Fruits, vegetables, legumes, cereals, and flours are low in fat. On the other hand, nuts contain an appreciable amount of fat.

Linoleic acid. Corn, cottonseed, and soy oils are good sources of linoleic acid. Some special margarines now available in food markets are processed by adding hydrogenated fat to oils, thereby retaining a greater proportion of linoleic acid. These margarines are much softer than regular margarines. In the labeling of such margarines the words *liquid oil* appear first, followed by a listing of hydrogenated oil and other ingredients. Fish and poultry furnish small amounts of linoleic acid.

Cholesterol. Only animal foods furnish cholesterol. Liver, egg yolk, kidney, brains, sweetbreads, and fish roe are rich sources. Much smaller concentrations are found in whole milk, cream, butter, cheese, and meat. (See Table A–6.)

An individual who eats no eggs or organ meats probably ingests not more than 200 mg cholesterol daily; if, in addition, he uses skim milk and substitutes vegetable margarine for butter, the intake will be further reduced to 100 to 150 mg daily. Each egg yolk adds about 250 mg cholesterol.

Fat in the American diet. The fat content of the basic diet pattern is shown in Table 6–2. Note that the basic list of foods supplies approximately equal amounts of saturated and oleic acids, a proportion that is quite characteristic of American diets. The choice of additional foods to supply the needed energy requirements affords a wide range of possibilities for modifying the kind as well as the amount of fat that is included. In the example given, the use of salad dressing and corn oil increases the linoleic acid content considerably.

Some important changes have taken place in the consumption of fat in the United States since the beginning of this century. The total amount of fat available for consumption at the present time is 147 gm daily.[10] This represents about 42 per cent of the total calories available. Socioeconomic changes have resulted in a steady decline in the intake of cereal foods, breadstuffs, and potatoes, which are low in fat, and an increase in the intake of meats and fat-rich foods including ice cream, table spreads, and other fats. The use of butter has sharply declined, but this has been replaced by margarine. Hydrogenated shortenings have replaced, to a large extent, shortenings of animal origin. Vegetable oils are used much more widely so that the average intake of linoleic acid is greater than that in earlier decades.

Problems related to fat in the diet. Because fats are so concentrated a source of energy, small quantities rapidly increase the calorie intake. It should be self-evident that the individual who does not exercise moderation in the use of fats can rapidly

Table 6–2. Fat Content of Basic Diet

| | Measure | Total Fat gm | Fatty Acids | | | Cholesterol |
			Saturated gm	Oleic gm	Linoleic gm	mg
Milk, whole	2 cups	18	10	6	tr	68
Egg	1	6	2	3	tr	252
Meat, fish, poultry, lean	4 ounces	10	4	5	1	104
Vegetables-fruit	4 servings	tr	tr	tr	tr	—
Bread	3 slices	3	tr	1	tr	—
Total fat in basic diet		37	16	15	1	424
Typical Additions of Fat to Basic Diet						
Butter	3 teaspoons	12	6	4	tr	35
French dressing	1 tablespoon	6	1	1	3	—
Corn oil in cooked foods	1 tablespoon	14	1	4	7	—
Cherry pie	1 piece	15	4	7	3	—
Total fat		84	28	31	14	459

increase his caloric intake beyond his needs and thus become overweight.

There is considerable evidence that a high intake of saturated fats and of cholesterol increases the concentration of blood cholesterol and certain lipoprotein fractions. These elevated levels of blood lipids appear to be highly correlated with the incidence of cardiovascular diseases. Persons who are considered to be at high risk include especially males over 40 years who have hypertension, who are overweight, and who smoke. Physicians often recommend that such persons restrict the intake of saturated fats and cholesterol and increase the intake of polyunsaturated fats. (See also Chapter 40.)

SOME POINTS FOR EMPHASIS IN NUTRITION EDUCATION

1. Fats are essential constituents of the body, being the principal way in which the body stores energy.

2. Fats are the most concentrated source of energy in the diet and furnish more than twice as many calories, gram for gram, as do carbohydrates and proteins. Consequently, a small volume of fatty food will increase the calorie intake considerably.

3. When an individual consumes a diet that provides more calories than he needs, the excess calories will be stored as fat regardless of the composition of the diet. On the other hand, when an individual consumes a diet that supplies fewer calories than he needs, adipose tissue will furnish the additional needs.

4. A diet that provides 35 per cent of the calories from fat allows a wide latitude of food choice that is acceptable to Americans. Some of the foods chosen should be good sources of vitamin A.

5. Foods fried at the proper temperature may be used in moderation by most people. Preferably they should not be given to very young children.

6. Cholesterol is an essential constituent of body tissues and is required for the regulation of important body functions. It does not need to be in the diet because the liver readily synthesizes it.

7. Linoleic acid is an essential fatty acid abundantly supplied by corn, cottonseed, soy, and safflower oils.

8. Lecithin and other phospholipids are es-

sential constituents of nervous tissue and important for the transport of fats. The liver readily synthesizes the phospholipids so that their presence in the diet is not essential. An additional intake of lecithin does not convey unique benefits to health and is not necessary.

9. A diet that contains a high proportion of saturated fatty acids and of cholesterol is one of many factors that is believed to contribute to cardiovascular disease.

10. In advising Americans about ways to modify their diets without resorting to distorted dietary patterns or faddism, the following guidelines seem appropriate: (a) Include first those basic foods that are essential for protein, minerals, and vitamins. (b) Select fats for food preparation from oils rich in linoleic acid as well as from solid fats. (c) Trim visible fats from meats; use more poultry and fish. (d) Substitute fruits and low-calorie desserts more frequently for high-fat desserts. (e) In choosing foods for additional calories, place emphasis on the maintenance of normal weight.

Problems and Review

1. Prepare an outline that shows the digestion, absorption, and metabolic fate of triglycerides supplied by the diet.
2. Give several reasons why fat is a useful constituent of the diet.
3. What is a hydrogenated fat? Give several examples. How does it compare in nutritional value with the fat from which it was made?
4. What effect will the inclusion of fatty foods such as fried potatoes and pork chops have on the digestion of the meal as a whole?
5. *Problem.* Compare the fat and calorie values of ½ cup ice cream; 1 tablespoon mayonnaise; 1 ounce cream cheese; 2 teaspoons butter; 1 cup milk.
6. *Problem.* Calculate your own fat intake for one day. Which of the foods you ate are good sources of linoleic acid? What percentage of the total calories in your diet was derived from fat?
7. A margarine may be manufactured from 100 per cent vegetable oil but may still be a poor source of linoleic acid. Explain why this might be true.
8. *Problem.* Examine the labels of three or four brands of special types of margarine. What information do they give you about their value as sources of linoleic acid? How do these margarines compare with regular margarines in cost?
9. What is the nutritional significance of linoleic acid? Of cholesterol? Of phospholipids?
10. A patient tells you that he has not been eating butter, eggs, or whole milk because he read in a magazine that cholesterol causes heart disease. How would you respond to this?

Cited References

1. Hansen, A. F.: "Essential Fatty Acids in Infant Feeding," *J. Am. Diet. Assoc.*, **34**:239–41, 1958.
2. Pickles, V. R.: "Prostaglandins," *Nature*, **224**:221–25, 1969.
3. Fredrickson, D. S., *et al.: The Dietary Management of Hyperlipoproteinemia. A Handbook for Physicians.* National Institutes of Health, U.S. Department of Health, Education and Welfare, Washington, D.C., 1970.
4. Stern, J. S., and Greenwood, M. R. C.: "A Review of Development of Adipose Cellularity in Man and Animals," *Fed. Proc.*, **33**:1952–55, 1974.
5. Isselbacher, K. J.: "Metabolism and Transport of Lipid by Intestinal Mucosa," *Fed. Proc.*, **24**:16–22, 1965.
6. Cahill, G. F., Jr., *et al.*: "Hormone-Fuel Interrelationships During Fasting," *J. Clin. Invest.*, **45**:1751–69, 1966.
7. Connor, W. E., *et al.*: "Cholesterol Balance and Fecal Neutral Steroid and Bile Acid Excretion in Normal Men Fed Dietary Fats of Different Fatty Acid Composition," *J. Clin. Invest.*, **48**:1363–75, 1969.

8. *Diet and Coronary Heart Disease.* Leaflet, American Heart Association, New York, 1973.
9. Alfin-Slater, R. B.: "Fats, Essential Fatty Acids, and Ascorbic Acid," *J. Am. Diet. Assoc.,* **64:**168–70, 1974.
10. Friend, B., and Marston, R.: "Nutritional Review," *National Food Situation,* Economic Research Service, U.S. Department of Agriculture, Washington, D.C., November 1975, pp. 26–32.

ADDITIONAL REFERENCES

Bennion, M., and Park, R. L.: "Changes in Frying Fats with Different Foods," *J. Am. Diet. Assoc.,* **52:**308–12, 1968.
Burr, G. O., and Burr, M. M.: "A New Deficiency Disease Produced by the Rigid Exclusion of Fat from the Diet," (A nutrition classic, 1929) reprinted in *Nutr. Rev.,* **31:**248–49, 1973.
Connor, W. E., and Connor, S. L.: "The Key Role of Nutritional Factors in the Prevention of Coronary Heart Disease," *Preventive Med.,* **1:**49–83, 1972.
Fleischman, A. I., *et al.:* "Studies on Cooking Fats and Oils," *J. Am. Diet. Assoc.,* **42:**394–98, 1963.
Food and Nutrition Board: *Dietary Fat and Human Health.* Pub. 1147. National Academy of Sciences—National Research Council, Washington, D.C., 1966.
Hansen, A. E., *et al.:* "Role of Linoleic Acid in Infant Nutrition," *Pediatrics,* **31** (Pt. II):171–92, 1963.
Hodges, R. E.: "Dietary and Other Factors Which Influence Serum Lipids," *J. Am. Diet. Assoc.,* **52:**198–201, 1968.
Holt, P. R.: "Fats and Bile Salts. 1. Physiologic Considerations," *J. Am. Diet. Assoc.,* **60:**491–95, 1972.
Kilgore, L., and Windham, F.: "Degradation of Linoleic Acid in Deep-fried Potatoes," *J. Am. Diet. Assoc.,* **63:**525–27, 1973.
Paulsrud, J. R., *et al.:* "Essential Fatty Acid Deficiency in Infants Induced by Fat-free Intravenous Feeding," *Am. J. Clin. Nutr.,* **25:**897–904, 1972.
Review: "Acetoacetate Production in Starvation Ketosis," *Nutr. Rev.,* **26:**147–49, 1968.
————: "Fat and Cholesterol in the Diet," *Nutr. Rev.,* **23:**3–6, 1965.
————: "Glyceride Structure and Fat Absorption," *Nutr. Rev.,* **27:**18–20, 1969.
————: "Safety of Used Frying Fats," *Nutr. Rev.,* **26:**210–12, 1968.
Santos, M., *et al.:* "Conversion of Free Fatty Acids to Triglycerides," *Arch. Intern. Med.,* **134:**457–60, 1974.
West, R. O., and Hayes, O. B.: "Diet and Serum Cholesterol Levels. A Comparison Between Vegetarians and Non-vegetarians in a Seventh Day Adventist Group," *Am. J. Clin. Nutr.,* **21:**853–62, 1968.

7 Energy Metabolism

The amount of available energy has become a crucial issue in our times, whether it be the oil, gas, coal, or electrical power to heat, air-condition, or light our homes, drive our automobiles, run our factories, and so on; or whether, in direct human terms, it be the amount of available food to yield the energy required to accomplish the involuntary and voluntary activities of the body. Sufficient food to meet the energy needs is the first nutritional priority. When the supply of calories is moderately reduced, the capacity to work is also reduced, and in children growth is retarded or ceases. As the energy available to the body continues to decrease, the body's own substance will be utilized until eventually no more of the body mass can be sacrificed and death ensues.

ENERGY TRANSFORMATION

ENERGY is the capacity to do work. The sun is the original source of all energy, arising from nuclear reactions. Through the action of chlorophyll with sunlight, by the process known as photosynthesis, plants synthesize carbohydrates from carbon dioxide and water. The carbohydrates stored by the plants are then available as energy to animals and to man. All of man's energy is derived from the plant and animal foods he eats. Carbohydrates, fats, and proteins are the energy-yielding substances. In a typical American diet carbohydrate furnishes 45 to 55 per cent of the calories, fats, 35 to 45 per cent, and proteins about 15 per cent.

Forms of energy. Potential (storage) energy is continuously available in the body from the small amounts of glycogen in muscle and liver, the sizable fat depots, and the cellular mass itself. The potential energy is transformed to other forms to accomplish the work of the body: for example, *mechanical* energy for muscle contraction; *osmotic* energy to maintain the transport of fluids and nutrients; *electrical* energy for the transmission of nerve impulses; *chemical* energy as in the synthesis of new compounds; and *thermal* energy for heat regulation.

Whenever one form of energy is produced, another form is reduced by exactly the same amount. This is known as the law of CONSERVATION OF ENERGY, which states that energy can be neither created nor destroyed. When foods supply more energy than is needed for the work of the body, the excess is stored as fat; it has resulted in weight gain. This store of energy is available at such a time as the food supply might furnish too few calories for the body's activities.

Transformation to ATP. If the potential energy of glucose, fatty acids, and amino acids were released in one step, much of it would be lost and wasted as heat. The cell utilizes energy efficiently by releasing small amounts of it at a time in a series of steps that occur in the mitochondria of the cell. The energy liberated in these steps is trapped in the form of adenosine triphosphate (ATP). This compound has two high-energy phosphate bonds, one of which is released in the innumerable transactions of the body that require energy (ATP → ADP). For example:

$$\text{Glucose} + \text{ATP} \rightarrow \text{Glucose-6-phosphate} + \text{ADP}$$

The reactions that occur in the catabolism of glucose, fatty acids, and amino acids liberate energy, and thereby ATP is again formed (ADP → ATP). ATP is sometimes called the "legal tender" or "currency" for energy of the living organism, for, like the convenience of small coins of money, it is the convenient form for small bursts of energy.

The formation of ATP occurs in the metabolic pathways described in the preceding chapters on carbohydrates, fats, and proteins. Initially these nutrients are oxidized independently to the "common denominators," namely, pyruvic acid, acetyl coenzyme A, and alpha-ketoglutaric acid. In this first phase some of the reactions require ATP for their initiation; other reactions release small amounts of energy so that ATP is regenerated from ADP, but the net yield is not great.

The common denominators enter the tricarboxylic acid (TCA) cycle, which is the common pathway for the oxidation of glucose, fatty acids, and amino acids. About 90 per cent of the energy liberated from food occurs by this pathway.

Oxidative phosphorylation. Each turn of the TCA cycle yields four pairs of hydrogens and electrons. These hydrogens are never in their free state but are accepted by dehydrogenases NAD (nicotinamide adenine dinucleotide) and FAD (flavin adenine dinucleotide). These enzymes can exist in the oxidized or reduced form ($NAD \leftrightarrow NADH_2$ and $FAD \leftrightarrow FADH_2$). The hydrogen is transported to the nearby CYTOCHROME SYSTEM, also known as the *electron transport system* or the *respiratory chain*.

The CYTOCHROMES are a series of iron-containing enzymes. They accept hydrogens from the dehydrogenases and transfer them step by step from one cytochrome to another until they react with oxygen to form water. The acceptance of hydrogen by the dehydrogenases and the transfer along the respiratory chain yields three molecules of ATP for each pair of hydrogens. Thus, each turn of the TCA cycle yields 12 molecules of ATP, and each molecule of glucose results in the formation of 24 molecules of ATP throughout the cycle alone.

Potentially, the total yield of ATP from one molecule of glucose is 38 molecules of ATP. The amount of energy converted to ATP from glucose and fat is, at a maximum, 38 to 40 per cent of the potential energy. The remainder is dissipated as heat. Hegsted[1] has described several ways by which the potential yield of 38 molecules of ATP from glucose is not likely to be realized. First, the coupling in the respiratory chain is not always complete so that three molecules of ATP are not always obtained. Second, the abundance of phosphatases may result in the wasteful removal of high-energy bonds from ATP. Third, the energy cost of producing new tissue is high. These and other variations emphasize how complex the maintenance of energy balance becomes.

MEASUREMENT

Kilocalories. The potential energy value of foods and the energy exchanges of the body are expressed in terms of the calorie, which is a heat unit. By definition, a KILOCALORIE (kcal) is the amount of heat required to raise the temperature of 1 kg water 1° C (from 15° to 16°). Older nutrition literature indicates energy values as Calories, or calories. It should be remembered that such designations always refer to kilocalories, and that this unit is 1000 times as large as the small calorie used in the sciences of chemistry and physics.

The joule. The JOULE (J) is the unit of energy used in the metric system. It is used internationally in the sciences, and it is logical that it also be used for expressing energy values in nutrition, which is so closely related to chemistry and physics. The VIIIth International Congress of Nutrition in Prague in 1969 and the Committee on Nomenclature of the American Institute of Nutrition in 1970 have recommended the adoption of the joule in place of the calorie.

The conversion of tables of food composition and dietary allowances from calories to joules will require a considerable period of time. Also, some adjustment is required by those who are accustomed to thinking in terms of calories.

One calorie is equivalent to 4.184 joules; a kilocalorie is equivalent to 4.184 kilojoules (kJ). Thus, a dietary allowance of 2000 kcal is 8368 kJ.

The bomb calorimeter. The fuel values of foods are readily determined by means of an apparatus known as a BOMB CALORIMETER. (See Figure 7–1.) A weighed sample of food is placed in a heavy steel container called a "bomb." After the bomb is charged with oxygen, the sample is ignited and the heat is dissipated into a known volume of water surrounding the bomb. By noting the change in the temperature of water, one can calculate the energy value of the food by applying the definition for a calorie. The following caloric values are obtained:

1 gm pure carbohydrate yields	4.1 kcal
1 gm pure fat yields	9.45 kcal
1 gm pure protein yields	5.65 kcal
1 gm pure alcohol yields	7.1 kcal

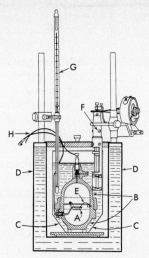

Figure 7–1. Diagram of bomb calorimeter with bomb in position. (Courtesy, the Emerson Apparatus Company.)

(*A*) Platinum dish holding weighed food sample.
(*B*) Bomb filled with pure oxygen enclosing food sample.
(*C*) Can holding water of known weight in which the bomb is submerged.
(*D*) Outer double-walled insulating jacket.
(*E*) Fuse, which is ignited by an electric current.
(*F*) Motor-driven water stirrer.
(*G*) Thermometer calibrated to 1/1000°C.
(*H*) Electric wires to send current through fuse.

Physiologic fuel factors. Certain small losses occur in digestion so that it is necessary to reduce the values obtained in the bomb calorimeter to those that are physiologically available. For the typical American diet the coefficient of digestibility is 98 per cent for carbohydrate 95 per cent for fat, and 92 per cent for protein. In addition, the end products of protein metabolism such as urea and other nitrogenous products are combustible; their loss in the urine is equivalent to about 1.25 kcal per gram protein. The PHYSIOLOGIC FUEL FACTORS, first derived by Atwater, thus become:

0.98×4.1 kcal $\ = 4.02$ kcal (4 kcal per gram pure carbohydrate)

0.95×9.45 kcal $\ = 8.98$ kcal (9 kcal per gram of pure fat)

0.92×5.65 kcal $\ = 5.20$ kcal $- 1.25$ kcal
$\qquad\qquad\qquad = 3.95$ kcal (4 kcal per gram of pure protein)

In terms of joules, these fuel factors are 17 kJ for pure carbohydrate and protein, and 38 kJ for pure fat.

Specific fuel factors. Each food has a specific coefficient of digestibility, and thus the fuel value likewise would be specific for each given good. For example, the coefficient of digestibility for the protein in milk, eggs, and meat is 97 per cent, but for the protein of whole ground cornmeal it is only 60 per cent; the coefficient of digestibility for the carbohydrate of wheat is 98 per cent when white flour (70 to 74 per cent extraction) is used, but is 90 per cent when whole-wheat flour (97 to 100 per cent extraction) is used. The errors introduced by the variations in digestibility are small for the typical mixed American diet, and for any calculations the student is likely to make Atwater's physiologic fuel values are sufficiently reliable.

Whenever the diet differs markedly from the typical diet on which Atwater based his data, considerable error is introduced with the use of average fuel values. For example, the caloric value of a diet which is predominant in cereal foods would be overestimated. This can be a serious problem when it involves suitable allocation of food to populations where the food supply is short. The Nutrition Division of FAO[2] has published a table for estimating calories based on these specific factors rather than on the average values. The energy values listed in tables of food composition developed by the U.S. Department of Agriculture employ specific fuel factors for each food.

MEASUREMENT OF ENERGY EXCHANGE OF THE BODY

Direct and indirect calorimetry. DIRECT CALORIMETRY is the measurement of the amount of heat produced by the body. By this method the individual is placed in a specially constructed chamber called a respiration calorimeter. The chamber is so well insulated that no heat can enter into or escape through the walls. The heat given off by the individual is picked up by water flowing through coils in the chambers. Measurements are made of the temperature of the water at the beginning of the study, at intervals, and at the termination of the study. The volume of water flowing through the coils is also measured, and the calories expended can be calculated from these data. These calorimeters are very expensive to construct and require careful attention to many details of measurement. They are used only in a few research centers.

The respiration calorimeter is so designed that the oxygen consumption and the carbon dioxide excretion can be measured at the same time the heat production is measured. From numerous studies the relationship of oxygen usage to heat production under varying conditions has been established. Therefore, it is possible to determine the level of energy metabolism by the less time-consuming and far less costly procedures of indirect calorimetry.

INDIRECT CALORIMETRY measures the amount of oxygen consumed in a given time period and, in other than basal conditions, the amount of carbon

Figure 7–2. This student's energy expenditure while bicycling is being measured by using a respirometer under controlled conditions. (Courtesy, Department of Nutrition and Food Sciences, Texas Woman's University, Denton.)

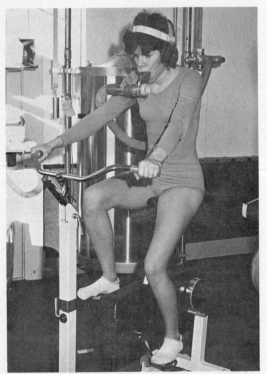

dioxide excreted. The amount of oxygen consumed is proportional to the amount of heat that is being produced. Numerous experiments on people of all ages have shown that 1 liter of oxygen is equal to 4.825 kcal when the conditions for a basal metabolism test, described below, are met.

The energy expenditure at varying levels of activity can be measured by a respirometer under controlled conditions when the subject walks on a treadmill or rides on a stationary bicycle. (See Figure 7–2.) In other situations such as mountain climbing, or typing, or ironing, a portable apparatus is used. This lightweight piece of equipment, weighing 4 kg or less, consists of a meter for measuring the volume of expired air and a bag for collecting the sample of expired air. The air samples are analyzed for their amounts of oxygen and carbon dioxide, and from the data it is possible to determine caloric equivalents.

Basal metabolism test. The amount of energy required to carry on the involuntary work of the body is known as the *basal metabolic rate*. It includes the functional activities of the various organs such as the brain, heart, liver, kidneys, and lungs, the secretory activities of the glands, the peristaltic movements of the gastrointestinal tract, the oxidations occurring in resting tissues, and the maintenance of muscle tone and body temperature. The brain and nervous tissue account for about one fifth of the energy utilized in the basal state, and the liver, kidneys, gastrointestinal tract, and heart for an additional two fifths.

The basal metabolic rate is measured by indirect calorimetry under the following specific conditions.

1. Postabsorptive state: 12 to 16 hours after the last meal; usually performed in the morning.

2. Reclining, but awake: one-half to one hour of rest before the test is necessary if there has been any activity in the morning.

3. Relaxed and free from emotional upsets or fear of the test itself.

4. Normal body temperature.

5. Comfortable room temperature and humidity: about 70° to 75° F.

Under these conditions, normal individuals fall within ± 15 per cent of standards established for their body size, sex, and age. Suppose a young woman consumes 1200 cc oxygen in a six-minute test period; in a 24-hour period her basal heat expenditure is calculated as follows:

$$\frac{10 \times 1200 \times 24}{1000} = 288 \text{ liters oxygen in 24 hours}$$

$$288 \times 4.825 \text{ kcal} = 1390 \text{ kcal}$$

Factors influencing the basal metabolic rate. The adult basal metabolic rate is approximately 1 kcal per kilogram per hour for men and about 0.9 kcal per kilogram per hour for women. Thus, the range of basal metabolism for normal adults is about 1300 to 1700 kcal (5439 to 7113 kJ). This accounts for the largest proportion of the total energy requirement for most people. The rate of basal metabolism is influenced by size, shape, and weight of the individual, sex, age, rate of growth, the activity of the endocrine glands, sleep, body temperature, and state of nutrition.

Surface area. About 80 per cent of the energy from glucose and fat is lost as heat, all but 15 per cent of heat loss being from the skin. The remaining heat loss occurs from the lungs and through the excreta. Since the heat loss is proportional to the skin surface, the basal heat production is directly proportional to the surface area. A tall, thin person has a greater surface area than an individual of the same weight who is short and fat, and the former therefore will have a higher basal metabolism.

Sex. Women have a metabolic rate about 6 to 10 per cent lower than that of men. Formerly this was attributed to the fact that women had relatively higher proportions of adipose tissue, believed to be metabolically inert. However, this explanation is not fully satisfactory inasmuch as adipose tissue is now known to be metabolically active. The influence of the sex hormones may account for some of the difference.

Age. Per unit of surface area the basal metabolic rate is at its highest during the first two years of life. It declines gradually throughout childhood and accelerates slightly in adolescence. Thereafter the decline continues throughout life with somewhat more rapid decrease in the later years. The rapid growth rate explains the high metabolic rate in early childhood. In later years the lessened muscle tone and the reduction in muscle mass account for the lower rate.

Sleep. During the sleeping hours the basal metabolism is about 10 per cent lower than in the waking state. However, this is quite variable depending upon the amount of motion of the individual while asleep.

Body temperature. An elevation of the body temperature for each degree F increases the basal metabolism by 7 per cent.

Endocrine glands. The thyroid gland regulates the rate of energy metabolism, and any change in thyroid activity is reflected in the metabolic rate. If the thyroid is overactive (HYPERTHYROIDISM), the metabolism may be speeded up as much as 75 to 100 per cent; if the activity of the gland is decreased (HYPOTHYROIDISM), the metabolism may be reduced by 30 to 40 per cent.

The measurement of *protein-bound iodine* has now largely replaced the basal metabolism test as a measure of thyroid activity. This test is based upon the fact that the level of protein-bound iodine circulating in the blood is proportional to the degree of thyroid activity. The basal metabolism test is still the method of choice for nutritional studies.

Other endocrine secretions have a more transitory effect on the basal metabolism. An increased excretion of epinephrine during excitement or fear temporarily raises the metabolic rate. Disturbances of the pituitary gland may also modify the metabolic rate. Just prior to the onset of the menstrual period the metabolism is increased slightly, but it is a little lower than normal during the period. These slight changes are of no overall significance in determining the energy requirement.

State of nutrition. In starvation the rate of oxidation by active lean tissue mass is similar to that occurring normally. Some underweight schoolchildren appear to have a higher-than-normal metabolic rate because the proportion of active lean tissue is higher. When undernutrition is severe, the destruction of body tissues lowers the rate.

Pregnancy. During the last trimester of pregnancy the basal metabolism increases from 15 to 25 per cent. This increase can be accounted for almost entirely by the increase in weight of the woman and the high rate of metabolism of the fetus.

TOTAL ENERGY REQUIREMENT

Factors influencing the total energy requirement. Superimposed upon the energy expenditure for maintaining the involuntary activities of the body are such factors as voluntary muscular activity, the effect of food, and the maintenance of the body temperature.

Muscular activity. Next to the basal metabolism, activity accounts for the largest energy expenditure; in fact, for some persons who are vigorously active, the energy needs for activity may exceed those for the basal metabolism. Sedentary work, which includes office work, bookkeeping, typing, teaching, and so forth, calls for less energy than more active and strenuous occupations such as nursing, homemaking, or gardening. A still greater amount of energy is required by those individuals who do hard manual labor such as ditch digging, shifting freight, and lumbering. (See Figure 7–3.)

The energy expenditure for many activities has been measured in adults and children,[3,4] and the data serve as a guide in setting standards for various groups of people. A wide range of activities has been classified in five groups in Table 7–1. The calorie expenditures listed for each category include the basal metabolism and are representative for adults. The lower figure for each category would apply to women, and the higher figure to men. Of course, it must be realized that these would vary from one individual to another not only on the basis of body size but especially because of variations of intensity of effort expended.

If an exact record of activity for a given 24-hour period were kept, it would be possible with data such as those in Table 7–1 to estimate the daily caloric requirement of an adult. However, such calculations are time consuming and give, at best, only rough approximations since individuals vary widely in the efficiency of their work and in their muscle tone.

The figures in Table 7–1 illustrate the value of exercise in weight control, for it is quite evident that the student who sits quietly watching television, for example, is expending only half as many calories as one who is walking leisurely, and only one fourth as many calories as one who swims for an hour.

Not infrequently the question is raised as to the reason for the differing caloric needs of two people of the same build and body weight who are doing the same kind of work. The energy needs will be greater for the person who wastes many motions in the performance of a piece of work, who works under greater muscle tension, or who finds it difficult to relax completely even when at rest.

Mental effort. The nervous system is continuously active, and its energy requirement is a significant part of the basal rate. However, the energy expenditure beyond the basal rate for intense mental effort as in problem solving or writing examinations does not add appreciably to the caloric requirement.

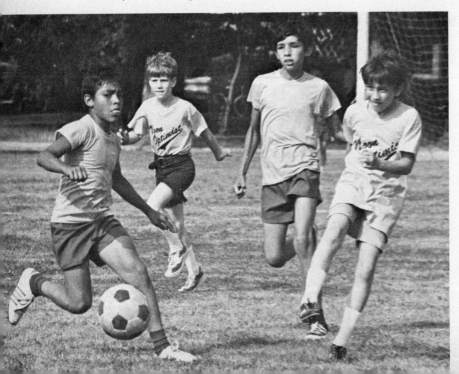

Figure 7–3. A great deal of energy is expended in active sports such as this soccer game. (Courtesy, Department of Nutrition and Food Sciences, Texas Woman's University, Denton.)

Table 7-1. Calorie Expenditure for Various Kinds of Activity*

Type of Activity	Kilocalories per Hour†
Sedentary Reading; writing; eating; watching television or movies; listening to the radio; sewing; playing cards; typing; and miscellaneous office work and other activities done while sitting that require little or no arm movement	80 to 100
Light Preparing and cooking food; doing dishes; dusting; hand washing small articles of clothing; ironing; walking slowly; personal care; miscellaneous office work and other activities done while standing that require some arm movement; and rapid typing and other activities done while sitting that are more strenuous	110 to 160
Moderate Making beds; mopping and scrubbing; sweeping; light polishing and waxing; laundering by machine; light gardening and carpentry work; walking moderately fast; other activities done while standing that require moderate arm movement; and activities done while sitting that require more vigorous arm movement	170 to 240
Vigorous Heavy scrubbing and waxing; hand washing large articles of clothing; hanging out clothes; stripping beds; other heavy work; walking fast; bowling; golfing; and gardening	250 to 350
Strenuous Swimming; playing tennis; running; bicycling; dancing; skiing; and playing football	350 and more

*Adapted from Page, L., and Fincher, L. J.: *Food and Your Weight.* Home and Garden Bulletin No. 74, U.S. Department of Agriculture, 1960, p. 4.

† Lower figures apply to women, higher figures to men. The figures include the metabolism at rest as well as for the activity.

Some students become tense and restless in the solving of problems, but the increased expenditure of energy in such a situation is not primarily that of mental work.

Calorigenic effect of food. The ingestion of food results in increased heat production known as the *calorigenic effect* or SPECIFIC DYNAMIC ACTION OF FOOD. It represents the energy required for digestion and absorption and also the stimulating effect of nutrients upon metabolism. Protein when eaten alone has been shown to increase the metabolic rate by 30 per cent, whereas carbohydrates and fats will produce much smaller increases in metabolism. On the basis of the mixed diets usually eaten, the specific dynamic action is approximately 6 per cent of the energy requirement.[5]

Maintenance of body temperature. Under normal conditions the temperature of the body is controlled by the amount of blood brought to the skin. When the surrounding temperature is low, most of the heat is lost by radiation and conduction, but when the environmental temperature is high, the body heat is lost chiefly through evaporation. It is a well-known fact that more heat is lost by evaporation when the air is dry than when it is humid.

During cold weather, man avoids excessive heat losses from his body by the use of suitable clothing and the heating of his home or place of work. Moreover, body heat is conserved if there is a layer of adipose tissue under the skin. The subcutaneous fat serves to keep heat in the body rather than allowing it to be dissipated through the skin—an advantage in cold weather, but a disadvantage in warm weather. Infants and young children have a relatively large surface area and lose much heat from the body when they are exposed.

When the body is subjected to extreme cold, the body temperature is maintained by an increase in involuntary and often voluntary activity. The blood vessels constrict so that there is less blood reaching the skin surface; the muscles become tense; and shivering follows. These involuntary activities result in a considerable increase in the metabolic rate. As anyone knows who has been exposed to a cold winter day, one is not likely to stand still. In addition, then, to the increased energy expenditure occasioned by the involuntary activities, the individual increases his voluntary activity.

Growth. The building of new tissue represents a storage of energy in one form or another; for example, every gram of protein in body tissue represents about 4 kcal. When growth is rapid, as during the first year of life, the energy allowance must be high. In fact, the caloric need is greater per unit of body weight than at any other time in life. In pregnancy, likewise, the energy needs are increased to cover the building of new tissues. These needs are discussed in more detail in Chapters 19, 20, and 21.

CALORIC ALLOWANCES

Daily allowances. The Recommended Dietary Allowances[6] for calories take into account sex, body size, age, climate, and activity. Unlike the allowances for the various nutrients, the recommended allowances for energy do not afford a margin of safety. They are based on the maintenance of desirable body weight or a suitable rate of growth and must be adjusted upward or downward to meet individual needs. The allowances are a rough guide in dietary planning for groups. A given individual may vary widely from the stated allowances. The bases for the allowances are described in the following paragraphs. (See Table 7–2.)

Reference standard. The allowances for men and women are stated in terms of persons who are in good health, who live in an environment with a mean annual temperature of 20° C (68° F), and who weigh 70 kg (154 lb) and 58 kg (128 lb), respectively. Their physical activity is "light" and they are engaged in occupations that could be described as sedentary. For the man 23 to 50 years the allowance is 2700 kcal and for the woman the allowance is 2000 kcal.

Adjustments for body size. Those activities that involve the whole body in motion will require greater expenditure by individuals who are large and heavy than those who are of smaller size. For example, the person who weighs 180 pounds will use more energy in walking 3 miles than another person who weighs only 120 pounds. On the other hand, there is much less difference in energy expenditure when such persons are engaged in sedentary activities such as reading, typing, and so on. It is customary to adjust calorie allowances to the desirable weight for one's height and health. For example, the following adjustments for a woman 23 to 50 years are typical:

kg	lb	kilocalories
50	110	1800
55	121	1950
58	128	2000
60	132	2050
65	143	2200
70	154	2300

Table 7–2. Recommended Daily Dietary Allowances for Energy*

	Age years	Weight kg	lb	Energy kcal		Age years	Weight kg	lb	Energy kcal
Infants	0.0–0.5	6	14	kg × 117	Males (cont.)	23–50	70	154	2700
	0.5–1.0	9	20	kg × 108		51 +	70	154	2400
Children	1–3	13	28	1300	Females	11–14	44	97	2400
	4–6	20	44	1800		15–18	54	119	2100
	7–10	30	66	2400		19–22	58	128	2100
Males	11–14	44	97	2800		23–50	58	128	2000
	15–18	61	134	3000		51 +	58	128	1800
	19–22	67	147	3000	Pregnancy				+300
					Lactation				+500

*Food and Nutrition Board: *Recommended Dietary Allowances*, National Academy of Sciences—National Research Council, Washington, D.C., 1974.

Adjustments for age. The highest calorie requirement for males occurs between ages 15 and 22, and for females between ages 11 and 14. Beginning in early adulthood there is a gradual decline in basal metabolism and physical activity. The decline in resting metabolism for adults is about 2 per cent for each decade. It is difficult to estimate how much physical activity declines over the years. For persons engaged in light occupations the activity is fairly constant from 20 to 45 years. It is about 200 kcal less between 45 and 75 years, and 500 kcal less after 75 years. Since the desirable weight at 25 years is a goal to maintain throughout life, the calorie intake needs to be correspondingly reduced. The Basic Diet pattern (Table 13–2) furnishes about 1200 kcal. Thus, it becomes apparent that women especially need to choose their additional calories with care so that all the nutrient needs will be met.

Adjustment for climate. In summer and winter most Americans live in an environmental temperature of 20° to 25° C. In winter they wear warm clothing, live and work in well-heated buildings, and travel by heated means of transportation. Likewise, in summer many of them live and work in air-conditioned buildings. Therefore, adjustments for temperature are not usually necessary.

A small increase in calories (2 to 5 per cent) may be necessary in winter for the person carrying a weight of heavy clothing. When a person is inadequately clothed, the calorie expenditure increases considerably.

When men are physically active at high environmental temperatures, an increase in the calorie allowance of 0.5 per cent for each degree above 30° C is indicated. This increase is necessary to cover the slight increase that occurs in the metabolic rate and in the extra energy expenditure to maintain normal body temperature. In warm climates, most individuals tend to reduce their activity and thus their caloric needs.

Adjustments for activity. Today the average work week is 35 to 40 hours; sleep accounts for 50 to 60 hours; eating and travel to and from work consumes 20 hours, more or less; and leisure time amounts to 50 or 60 hours in a given week. The leisure activities may range from reading, watching television, movies, or stamp collecting, on the one hand, to such vigorous activities as tennis, gardening, golf, and swimming, on the other hand. Obviously, to set up a

caloric allowance in terms of one's activity at work alone is to ignore a large part of one's day.

For persons who are moderately active the allowances should be increased by about 300 kcal. Very active individuals such as athletes, military recruits, and construction workers may require 600 to 900 kcal above the recommended allowances.

The best guide to the adequacy of the caloric intake lies in the maintenance of desirable weight by adults and the normal rate of growth by children. When there is weight gain despite adherence to a diet that furnishes the recommended levels of calories, the amount of activity should be increased rather than relying on a low-calorie diet alone. Many Americans are overweight because of a very sedentary way of life. When calories are restricted to lose weight, it is difficult to obtain sufficient levels of some nutrients such as iron and magnesium. The problems of weight control are discussed further in Chapter 29.

FOODS FOR ENERGY

The inclusion of minimum amounts of each of the Four Food Groups provides energy at approximately basal levels for the adult. (See Figure 7–4.) To complete the caloric requirement, preference should be given to additional amounts of foods from the food groups. This is especially important for women and for older persons whose caloric requirements are lower but who have the same nutrient requirements.

Foods that are high in fat, sugar, or starch content but low in water are concentrated sources of calories. By contrast, foods high in water content are low in calories. For example, a teaspoon of margarine contains 35 kcal, a tablespoon of sugar 45 kcal, and $\frac{1}{2}$ cup tomatoes 25 kcal. Thus, the addition of small amounts of concentrated foods to the diet increases the calorie intake rapidly, and vegetables and fruits can be eaten in appreciable amounts without great increases in caloric intake.

Persons who use alcoholic beverages daily may derive 5 to 10 per cent of their caloric intake from this source.[6] It has been reported that some individuals consume up to 1800 kcal from this source on a daily basis. Such consumption has an adverse effect on the nutritive adequacy of the diet since alcohol provides no nutrients.

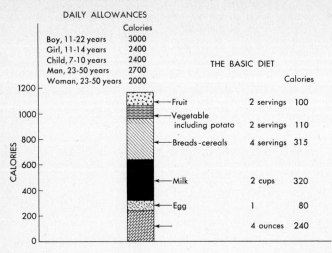

THE BASIC DIET

DAILY ALLOWANCES

	Calories
Boy, 11-22 years	3000
Girl, 11-14 years	2400
Child, 7-10 years	2400
Man, 23-50 years	2700
Woman, 23-50 years	2000

		Calories
Fruit	2 servings	100
Vegetable including potato	2 servings	110
Breads-cereals	4 servings	315
Milk	2 cups	320
Egg	1	80
	4 ounces	240

Figure 7-4. The Basic Diet provides just about half of the energy requirement of the teen-age girl and almost three fifths of that for the woman of 23 years. See Table 13-2 for complete calculations.

SOME POINTS FOR EMPHASIS IN NUTRITION EDUCATION

1. The calorie is a unit of heat. It measures the amount of energy available from foods and the energy exchange taking place in the body.

2. A calorie is the same whether it comes from carbohydrates, fats, or proteins. Carbohydrates and proteins furnish 4 kcal per gram and fats 9 kcal per gram.

3. Weight for weight, foods that are dry or greasy are relatively high in calories: for example, cereals, cookies, cakes, pastries, sweets, butter, fatty meats. Foods that have a high concentration of water are much lower in calories: for example, fruits and vegetables.

4. The basal metabolism is the amount of energy the body uses at rest. It ranges from about 1300 to 1700 kcal for adults and accounts for about half or more of the total calories needed by the average American.

5. The amount of activity is the important factor determining the number of calories needed above the basal metabolism. For the average young woman in America about 2000 kcal are needed daily; the average young man needs about 2700 kcal. Sedentary young adults require less than this, and older persons require considerably fewer calories.

6. In addition to furnishing most of the needed amounts of protein, minerals, and vitamins, the Four Food Groups in the recommended amounts provide almost 1200 kcal. Thus, a young woman can use a reasonable amount of desserts, fats, and sugars without exceeding her energy requirement, but the older woman has very little leeway in using these foods if she is also going to meet her nutritional requirements.

7. The body is in energy balance when the calories supplied by food are exactly equal to the energy needed for all the involuntary and voluntary activities of the body. Weight is neither gained nor lost.

8. If the calorie intake is greater than the body needs, weight is gained, and if the calorie intake is less than the body needs, weight is lost.

PROBLEMS AND REVIEW

1. Define or explain what is meant by calorie; basal metabolism; bomb calorimeter; respiratory calorimeter; physiologic fuel factor; joule.
2. *Problem.* Using data from Table A-1, calculate the number of grams required of each of the following foods to furnish 100 kcal; butter, milk, cheese, egg, potato, apple, banana, orange, sugar, bread, lean beef, cooked rice, chocolate cake.

3. Why are the physiologic fuel factors not suitable for calculating calorie values for the staple foods used in Asia and Africa?

4. What are the standard conditions for performing a basal metabolism test? What factors might make the basal metabolism of two adult individuals of the same age vary? How does age itself affect the basal metabolism?

5. Explain how the following factors affect the total energy requirement: muscular activity; food; climate; clothing; growth; muscle tension; endocrine secretions. Which of these has the greatest effect?

6. *Problem.* Calculate your own calorie intake for one day. What percentage of your calories was derived from each of the Four Food Groups? What percentage from sweets, fats, desserts, and snack foods?

7. Why would you expect the caloric requirement of many poor people to be higher during cold weather than that of people in better economic circumstances?

8. What is the best indication of adequate caloric intake?

CITED REFERENCES

1. Hegsted, D. M.: "Energy Needs and Energy Utilization," *Nutr. Rev.*, **32**:33–38, 1974.
2. Committee on Calorie Conversion Factors and Food Consumption Tables: *Energy Yielding Components of Food and Computation of Calorie Values.* Food and Agriculture Organization, 1947.
3. Taylor, C. M., and MacLeod, G.: *Rose's Laboratory Handbook of Dietetics*, 5th ed. The Macmillan Company, New York, 1949, p. 73.
4. Passmore, R., and Durnin, J. V. G. A.: "Human Energy Expenditure," *Physiol. Rev.*, **34**:801–40, 1955.
5. Swift, R. W., *et al.:* "The Effect of High Versus Low Protein Equicaloric Diets on the Heat Production of Human Subjects," *J. Nutr.*, **65**:89–102, 1958.
6. Food and Nutrition Board: *Recommended Dietary Allowances*, 8th ed. National Academy of Sciences—National Research Council, Washington, D.C., 1974.

ADDITIONAL REFERENCES

Adams, W. C.: "Influence of Age, Sex, and Body Weight on the Energy Expenditure of Bicycle Riding," *J. Appl. Physiol.*, **22**:539–45, 1967.

Ames, S. R.: "The Joule—Unit of Energy," *J. Am. Diet. Assoc.*, **57**:415–16, 1970.

Bray, G. A., *et al.:* "The Acute Effects of Food Intake on Energy during Cycle Ergometry," *Am. J. Clin. Nutr.*, **27**:254–59, 1974.

Buskirk, E. R., and Mendez, J.: "Nutrition, Environment and Work Performance with Special Reference to Altitude," *Fed. Proc.*, **26**:1760–67, 1967.

Calloway, D. H.: "Recommended Dietary Allowances for Protein and Energy," *J. Am. Diet. Assoc.*, **64**:157–62, 1974.

Energy and Protein Requirements, FAO Nutrition Meetings Report Series 52, Geneva, 1973.

Flatt, J.-P., and Blackburn, G. L.: "The Metabolic Fuel Regulatory System. Implications for Protein-sparing Therapies During Caloric Deprivation and Disease," *Am. J. Clin. Nutr.*, **27**:175–87, 1974.

Groen, J. J.: "An Indirect Method for Approximating Caloric Expenditure of Physical Activity. A Recommendation for Dietary Surveys," *J. Am. Diet. Assoc.*, **52**:313–17, 1968.

Havel, R. J.: "Caloric Homeostasis and Disorders of Fuel Transport," *N. Engl. J. Med.*, **287**:1186–92, 1972.

Hawkins, W. W.: "The Calorie, the Joule," *J. Nutr.*, **102**:1553–54, 1972.

Hirst, E.: "Food-related Energy Requirement," *Science*, **184**:134–38, 1974.

Kleiber, M.: "Joules vs Calories in Nutrition," *J. Nutr.*, **102**:309–12, 1972.

Konishi, F.: "Food Energy Equivalents of Various Activities," *J. Am. Diet. Assoc.*, **46**:186–88, 1965.

Lehninger, A. L.: "Energy Transformation in the Cell," *Sci. Am.*, **202**:102–14, 1960.

Review: "Energy Expenditure during Exercise," *Nutr. Rev.*, **31**:11–12, 1973.

Richardson, M., and McCracken, E. C.: *Energy Expenditures of Woman Performing Selected Activities.* Home Econ. Res. Rept. 11, U.S. Department of Agriculture, Washington, D.C., 1960.

Swindells, Y. E.: "The Influence of Activity and Size of Meals on Caloric Response in Women," *Br. J. Nutr.*, **27**:65–73, 1972.

Wilder, R. M.: "Calorimetry, The Basis of the Science of Nutrition," *Arch. Intern. Med.*, **103**:146–54, 1959.

8 Mineral Elements

The story of each mineral element required by the human being is every bit as dramatic as that of proteins, or vitamins, or the energy-yielding components. With new developments in laboratory technology it is now possible to trace minute amounts of mineral elements in living tissues, and many an element formerly considered to be a contaminant in foods has joined the ranks of the essential nutrients.

This chapter is concerned with calcium, phosphorus, sulfur, magnesium, iron, iodine, and zinc. A brief discussion is presented of several trace minerals for which recommended allowances have not been set. Sodium, potassium, and chlorine together with water balance and acid-base balance are discussed in Chapter 9.

Mineral composition of the body. MINERALS are those elements that remain largely as ash when plant or animal tissues are burned. About 4 per cent of the body weight consists of mineral matter. Seven MACRONUTRIENTS—that is, those occurring in appreciable amounts—account for most of the body content of minerals. Calcium and phosphorus account for three fourths of all mineral matter.

Some 15 to 20 elements are present in such minute amounts that they are generally referred to as TRACE ELEMENTS or MICRONUTRIENTS. In recent years some elements such as chromium and selenium, long considered to be contaminants, have been found to be essential. It is altogether possible that functions will be found for lead, mercury, gold, and others; no such evidence presently exists. Certainly the ecologic balance is important. On the one hand, there is a critical need for some trace elements; on the other hand, excesses of these same elements are toxic. Table 8–1 summarizes the mineral composition of the body, including approximate concentrations of some minerals.

General functions. Mineral elements are present in organic compounds such as phosphoproteins, phospholipids, hemoglobin, and thyroxine; as inorganic compounds such as sodium chloride and calcium phosphate; and as free ions. They enter into the structure of every cell of the body. Hard skeletal structures contain the greater proportions of some elements such as calcium, phosphorus, and magnesium, and soft tissues contain relatively higher proportions of potassium.

Mineral elements are constituents of enzymes such as iron in the catalases and cytochromes; of hormones such as iodine in thyroxine; and of vitamins such as cobalt in vitamin B_{12} and sulfur in thiamin. Their presence in body fluids regulates the permeability of cell membranes; the osmotic pressure and water balance between intracellular and extracellular compartments; the response of nerves to stimuli; the contraction of muscles; and the maintenance of acid-base equilibrium.

The amount of an element present gives no clue to its importance in body functions. For example, a few milligrams of an element such as iodine can make a critical difference in the health of an individual.

Dynamic equilibrium. For the normal adult a balance usually exists between the intake of an element and its excretion. On the one hand, absorption and excretion are constantly adjusted to guard against an overload that might produce toxic effects. On the other hand, precise mechanisms carefully conserve needed amounts of mineral elements.

Homeostasis is maintained in spite of the fact that a continuous flow of nutrients into the cell and away from the cell is taking place. For example, bone, often thought of as being inert, is an exceedingly active tissue in its constant uptake and release of mineral constituents. Nevertheless, a state of balance or dynamic equilibrium is maintained provided that the supply of nutrients is adequate.

Foods as sources of mineral elements. When selecting foods for their mineral content, these factors must be considered: (1) the concentration of the

Table 8–1. Mineral Composition of the Body

Know Chart

	Amount in the Body*		Micronutrients (no estimate of amounts)	
	per cent	Per 70 Kilograms gm		
Macronutrients			*Essential for Body Functions*	
Calcium	1.5–2.2	1050–1540	Chromium	Molybdenum
Phosphorus	0.8–1.2	560–840	Cobalt	Selenium
Potassium	0.35	245	Fluoride	Zinc
Sulfur	0.25	175		
			Possibly Essential (needed by animals)	
Sodium	0.15	105	Cadmium	Tin
Chlorine	0.15	105	Nickel	Vanadium
Magnesium	0.05	35	Silicon	
Micronutrients			*No Known Function*	
Iron	0.004	2.8	Aluminum	Bromine
Manganese	0.0003	0.21	Arsenic	Gold
Copper	0.00015	0.105	Barium	Lead
Iodine	0.00004	0.024	Boron	Mercury
				Strontium

*Calculations are on the basis of elementary composition of the body as stated by H. C. Sherman in *Chemistry of Food and Nutrition,* 8th ed. Macmillan Publishing Co., Inc., New York, 1952, p. 227.

mineral in the food; (2) how much of a given food is ordinarily consumed; (3) whether the food has lost some of its minerals through refinement or in cooking processes; and (4) whether the food contains the mineral in available form.

The best assurance that the diet will supply sufficient amounts of the essential mineral elements is to select a wide variety of foods, using the Four Food Groups as the basis. Fats and sugars are practically devoid of mineral elements, and highly refined cereals and flours are poor sources of most of them. Fabricated foods may lack important trace minerals for which no recommended allowances have been set. Many adolescent girls and women are unable to obtain sufficient iron even from a good diet and still keep within their caloric requirement.

CALCIUM

Distribution and functions. Of the approximately 1200 gm of calcium in the adult body, 99 per cent is combined as the salts that give hardness to the bones and teeth. The bones not only provide the rigid framework for the body, but they also furnish the reserves of calcium to the circulation so that the concentration in the plasma can be kept constant at all times.

The remaining 1 per cent of the calcium in the adult—about 10 to 12 gm—is distributed throughout the extracellular and intracellular fluids of the body. It fulfills important functions such as these:

1. Activates a number of enzymes including pancreatic lipase, adenosine triphosphatase, and some proteolytic enzymes.

2. Is required for the synthesis of ACETYLCHOLINE, a substance necessary for transmission of nerve impulses.

3. Increases the permeability of cell membranes, thus aiding in the absorptive processes.

4. Aids in the absorption of vitamin B_{12} from the ileum.

5. Regulates the contraction and relaxation of muscles, including the heartbeat.

6. Catalyzes two steps in the clotting of blood. When tissue cells are injured the following sequence takes place:

Cell injury: blood platelets $\xrightarrow{Ca++}$ thromboplastin

Thromboplastin + prothrombin $\longrightarrow$ thrombin

Thrombin + fibrinogen $\xrightarrow{Ca++}$ fibrin (the clot)

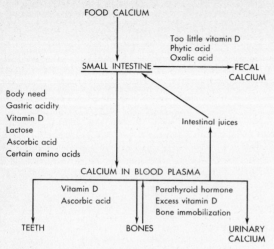

FOOD CALCIUM

Too little vitamin D
Phytic acid
Oxalic acid

SMALL INTESTINE ⟶ FECAL CALCIUM

Body need
Gastric acidity
Vitamin D
Lactose
Ascorbic acid
Certain amino acids

Intestinal juices

CALCIUM IN BLOOD PLASMA

Vitamin D   Parathyroid hormone
Ascorbic acid   Excess vitamin D
                   Bone immobilization

TEETH   BONES   URINARY CALCIUM

Figure 8–1. The utilization of calcium.

Absorption. Calcium is absorbed by active transport, an energy-requiring process, chiefly from the duodenum. Passive diffusion of calcium across the intestinal mucosa also occurs from the jejunum and ileum. (See Figure 8–1.)

Factors favoring absorption. Body need is the major factor governing the amount of calcium that is absorbed. Healthy adults receiving a diet that meets the recommended allowances absorb approximately 40 per cent of their dietary calcium. At higher levels of intake the proportion that is absorbed is lower but the absolute amount that crosses the intestinal membranes depends upon need. In many areas of the world, the diet supplies low amounts of calcium. People in these areas have adapted to these low levels and absorb a high proportion of the intake. During growth the absorption is increased to take care of increase in size and hardness of the skeleton.

Several mechanisms control the amount of calcium that is absorbed. Two of these are the hormone secreted by the parathyroid gland, PARATHORMONE, and vitamin D. Parathormone is secreted when the blood calcium level is lowered. One of its functions appears to be to stimulate the kidney to synthesize vitamin D hormone. One function of the metabolically active vitamin D is believed to be as a catalyst in the synthesis of a specific protein that binds calcium, and thus facilitates its transport across the mucosal membrane.[1] (See Vitamin D, Chapter 10.)

An acid reaction aids in the absorption of calcium since calcium salts are then more soluble. Once bile and pancreatic juice have mixed with the chyme, the reaction becomes strongly alkaline and the solubility of the calcium salts is reduced. The presence of ascorbic acid and some amino acids facilitates absorption by increasing the solubility of the calcium salts.

The ability of lactose to increase absorption has long been recognized. Being slowly absorbed, lactose favors the growth of intestinal microorganisms that increase the acidity of the intestinal contents. It is also believed that lactose chelates with calcium so that the formation of insoluble salts is minimized.

Factors interfering with absorption. The lack of vitamin D seriously impairs the absorption of calcium. Such lack may arise from inadequate exposure to sunlight or failure to ingest vitamin D in some form. A reduction in the amount of acid, sometimes found in elderly persons, reduces the solubility of the calcium salts. A marked increase in gastrointestinal motility reduces the length of time that calcium remains in contact with the intestinal mucosa. Emotional stress also reduces the utilization of calcium.

The presence of oxalic acid or phytic acid in foods and an abnormal calcium-to-phosphorus ratio are known to result in the formation of insoluble calcium complexes and thus interfere with calcium absorption. These effects can be clearly demonstrated on experimental animals when a decidedly abnormal diet is fed. None of these factors are of sufficient magnitude to be of practical importance in typical American diets.

Oxalic acid is found in spinach, Swiss chard, beet tops, cocoa, and rhubarb. Spinach, for example, contains sufficient calcium to bind the oxalic acid, and none of the calcium in other foods eaten at the same meal would be adversely affected.[2] The amount of cocoa that could be ingested at a time is too small to reduce the absorption of calcium significantly; thus, one would expect chocolate-flavored milk to supply about the same amounts of calcium for absorption as plain milk.

PHYTIC ACID is an organic phosphorus compound found in the outer layers of cereal grains. It binds calcium into insoluble complexes, but the effect would be important only when whole-grain cereals comprised a major part of the diet and when the calcium intake was also low, as is true in some vegetarian diets in which unleavened bread is a major part of the caloric intake. Yeast fermentation in a bread sponge destroys much of the phytate present in whole meals, and therefore leavened bread should be recommended.[3]

The effect of fats on absorption is reported variously by different investigators. On the one hand, fats reduce intestinal motility so that there is longer contact with the absorbing surfaces. On the other hand, free fatty acids combine with calcium to form insoluble soaps that are excreted. Foods high in unsaturated fatty acids have little effect, whereas those high in saturated fatty acids are more likely to yield some soaps.

Metabolism. The concentration of calcium in the plasma is kept within the narrow range of 9 to 11 mg per 100 ml (4.5 to 5.5 mEq per liter). About 40 per cent of the calcium is bound to plasma protein and 60 per cent is diffusible. The plasma level is regulated by (1) vitamin D hormone synthesized by the kidney, (2) parathormone, and (3) CAL-CITONIN, a hormone secreted by the thyroid gland.

When the blood calcium level is lowered, parathormone is secreted. The kidney is stimulated to synthesize vitamin D hormone either by the action of parathormone or by the flow of the blood with its lower calcium content through the kidney. The calcium level of the blood is increased by three actions: (1) increased absorption from the intestinal tract; (2) release of calcium from the bone (RESORPTION); and (3) increased reabsorption of calcium by the renal tubules. The excretion of phosphate in the urine is also increased, thereby maintaining a normal calcium-to-phosphorus ratio in the blood.

Calcitonin is antagonistic to parathormone and lowers the blood calcium when it becomes abnormally high. It does this by inhibiting bone resorption.

Bone. Bone consists of organic and inorganic substances. The principal organic substance is the protein COLLAGEN, and the ground substance consists of small amounts of mucoproteins and mucopolysaccharides, especially chondroitin sulfate. The formation of bone is initiated early in fetal life with the development of the cartilagenous matrix. During the latter part of pregnancy some mineralization of the fetal skeleton takes place so that the infant at birth has a body calcium content of about 28 gm.

During growth the addition of mineral to bone exceeds the amounts that are removed. The bone hardness consists of a gradual addition of minerals by the process referred to as MINERALIZATION or OSSIFICATION. During fetal development and the first few months after birth the bones achieve sufficient mineralization so that the skeleton can support the weight of the baby when he walks. Throughout childhood and adolescence the bones increase in length and diameter. This increase in size is dependent upon adequate protein as well as mineral elements. The hardness of bones increases throughout the first 20 years—sometimes longer. About 165 mg calcium are added to the skeleton daily during the early growing years. At adolescence the retention is as high as 300 mg a day, with a yearly increase as high as 90 gm.

The complex mineral substance in bone consists of an amorphous phase and a crystalline phase that is similar to HYDROXYAPATITE—$Ca_{10}(PO_4)_6(OH)_2$. Small amounts of calcium can be replaced by magnesium, sodium, potassium, lead, or strontium. Likewise, the anions sulfate, fluoride, citrate, carbonate, and chloride can enter the structure.

Bone is the principal reserve of calcium and phosphorus in the body. Contrary to popular belief, bones are continuously remodeled and reshaped by OSTEOBLASTS (bone-forming cells) and OSTEOCLASTS (bone-destroying cells). About 700 mg calcium enter and leave the bone each day in the adult.[4] Because of the turnover of calcium within the bone, widely varying intakes of calcium have no direct effect on the blood calcium.

In the well-nourished individual the readily available stores of calcium are in the ends of the long bones, and are known as TRABECULAE. In the absence of trabeculae calcium is withdrawn from the shaft of the long bone.

Teeth. Like bones, teeth are complex structures consisting of a protein matrix (keratin in the enamel, and collagen in the dentin) and mineral salts, principally calcium and phosphorus as hydroxyapatite. In the fetus the development of teeth begins by the fourth month and calcification proceeds during the growth of the fetus. Prenatally and during infancy and childhood tooth development requires adequate supplies of many diet factors including not only calcium and phosphorus, but also vitamins A and D, and protein. The deciduous teeth of the infant are fully mineralized by the end of the first year of life, but the calcification of permanent teeth is completed at various times during childhood and adolescence; for some teeth the mineralization is not completed until early adult years.

The turnover of calcium in teeth is very slow, but, unlike calcium in bone, once the calcium in teeth is lost it cannot be replaced. Thus, any factor that increases the solubility of mineral salts at the tooth surfaces will lead to decay: for example, the activity of microorganisms when sugars stick to the teeth. On the other hand, the presence of fluoride in the salts of tooth enamel increases the hardness, thereby reducing their decay. (See page 119.) Because of the slow rate of turnover of calcium in teeth, the fetus does not take much calcium from the mother's teeth, and the popular notion of the loss of "a tooth for every child" is false.

Excretion. The urinary excretion for a given individual remains relatively constant regardless of calcium intake, but varies widely from one individual to another. The calcium excretion is increased as the protein intake is increased.[5-7] In one investigation adults were fed a diet containing 800 mg calcium and 47, 95, and 142 gm protein.[5] The urinary calcium excretion on the three levels of protein were 217, 303, and 426 mg, respectively. The calcium balances were +12, +1, and −85 mg, respectively. Thus, high protein diets used in osteoporosis, weight reduction, and other clinical situations could lead to negative calcium balances.

Fecal calcium includes endogenous calcium that is not reabsorbed from the digestive juices and dietary calcium. The fecal calcium varies directly with the dietary calcium. Under normal conditions the skin losses are small. When people work strenuously at very high temperatures and perspire profusely, the calcium losses could be considerable.

Daily allowances. The recommended allowance for calcium is 800 mg for adults and for children 1 to 10 years; 1200 mg for boys and girls 11 to 18 years and for pregnant and lactating women; and 360 to 540 mg during the first year of life.[8] The allowance for adults is based upon replacement of daily losses including 175 mg in the urine, 125 mg as endogenous loss from digestive juices in the feces, and 20 mg from the skin. Assuming absorption to be 40 per cent, this daily loss of 320 mg would necessitate an allowance of 800mg.

A great deal of controversy exists concerning the requirement for calcium. The calcium balance technique for determining the calcium requirement has been criticized by many. People who ingest high levels of calcium are in negative balance if they suddenly shift to a lower intake, but in time most of them adjust to the lower level of intake. Adults throughout the world consume diets that often provide 400 mg or less of calcium, yet they do not show any adverse effects.

The FAO/WHO committee has recommended 400 to 500 mg calcium as a "practical allowance" for adults.[9] Such levels can be realized in most countries for the entire population, whereas higher levels would be impractical in terms of available food supplies. The Canadian allowance for men is 800 mg and for women is 700 mg, with an additional 500 mg allowance for pregnancy and lactation.

Food sources of calcium. The calcium content of some typical foods is shown in Table 8–2, and the calcium contribution of the basic diet pattern is charted in Figure 8–2. Milk is the outstanding source of calcium in the diet; without it, a satisfactory intake of calcium is extremely difficult. Whole or skimmed, homogenized or nonhomogenized, plain or chocolate-flavored, sweet or sour milks are equally good. For the adult 2 to 3 cups milk daily and for the child 3 to 4 cups daily will ensure adequate calcium intake. Cheddar cheese is an excellent source of calcium. Cottage cheese and ice cream are good sources but will not adequately substitute for milk. The dairy products, excluding butter, account for three fourths of the calcium in the American dietary.

All of the foods other than dairy products when considered together contribute not more than 200 to 300 mg calcium daily. Certain green leafy vegetables such as mustard greens, turnip greens, kale, and collards are important sources of calcium when they are eaten frequently. Canned salmon with the bones, clams, oysters, and shrimp are likewise good sources, but they are not eaten with frequency. Meats and cereal grains are poor sources. The use of nonfat dry milk, dough conditioners, and mold inhibitors in bread enhances the calcium value of the diet. Calcium is also an optional enrichment ingredient in flours and breads.

Calcium deficiency. The evidence regarding the effect of a low intake of calcium on deficiency symptoms is contradictory. If a low calcium intake alone could cause deficiency, one would expect to

Table 8–2. Calcium Content of Some Typical Foods

	Household Measure	Calcium mg	Per Cent of Adult Daily Allowance*
Milk, fresh	1 cup	288	36
Milk, nonfat dry, low-density	⅓ cup	288	36
Cheese, American process	1 ounce	198	25
Salmon, pink, canned	3 ounces	167†	21
Collards, cooked	½ cup	145	18
Turnip greens, cooked	½ cup	126	16
Clams or oysters	½ cup	113	14
Mustard greens, cooked	½ cup	97	12
Shrimp	3 ounces	98	12
Ice cream	⅛ quart	87	11
Cottage cheese, uncreamed	3 ounces	77	10
Kale, cooked	½ cup	74	9
Soybeans, mature, cooked	½ cup	73	9
Broccoli, cooked	½ cup	66	8
Orange, whole	1 medium	54	7
Sweet potato, boiled	1 medium	47	6
Molasses, light	1 tablespoon	33	4
Egg, whole	1 medium	27	3
Cabbage, raw, shredded	½ cup	22	3
Carrots, cooked	½ cup	24	3
Bread, 4 per cent nonfat dry milk	1 slice	21	3

*Recommended Dietary Allowance of calcium for the adult is 800 mg.
†Includes bones packed with salmon.

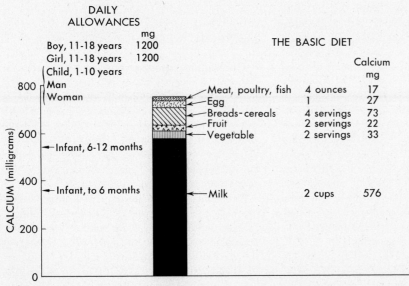

Figure 8–2. The milk group furnishes almost three fourths of the calcium allowance of the adult. The addition of 1 to 2 cups milk ensures sufficient calcium during periods of growth, in pregnancy, and in lactation. See Table 13–2 for complete calculation.

see much more deficiency throughout the world than actually exists. There are, however, a number of disturbances of calcium metabolism that have serious consequences.

Bone resorption is increased during immobilization from illness or injury. The loss of calcium from bone occurs almost immediately, as demonstrated in the space flights by the astronauts.[10] The release of calcium from the bones of those who are bedfast for long periods of time sometimes leads to calcium deposits in soft tissues and the formation of renal calculi.

Failure to provide vitamin D by exposure to sunshine or in the diet reduces the absorption and utilization of calcium. Eventually this leads to rickets in the young or osteomalacia in adults. (See also Chapter 10.) OSTEOMALACIA is a reduction in the mineral content of the bone without reduction in bone size. A recent report describes osteomalacia in a Bedouin woman who had a calcium intake of less than 500 mg daily, but apparently adequate source of vitamin D.[11] More than half of the calories were furnished by whole-grain unleavened bread. The phytate content of the unleavened bread was sufficient to combine with all of the calcium in the diet.

OSTEOPOROSIS is a reduction in the total bone mass. It occurs in millions of American women after age 50 and to a somewhat lesser extent in men. According to Lutwak, a low-calcium diet for 20 to 40 years is an important etiologic factor in periodontal disease and 5 to 10 years later in osteoporosis.[12] The loss of mineral from bone is not detected by radiography until 30 to 40 per cent has disappeared. Lutwak believes that a daily intake of 800 to 1000 mg calcium would reduce the incidence of osteoporosis. Hegsted, on the other hand, has presented evidence that low calcium intakes are not necessarily causative nor are high intakes preventive.[13]

In malabsorption diseases such as sprue large amounts of fat are excreted. The fat combines with calcium in the intestinal lumen to form soaps and the absorption of calcium as well as fat-soluble vitamins is greatly decreased. Hypocalcemia, tetany, and osteoporosis are frequently seen.

Chronic renal disease has long been recognized as contributing to hypocalcemia, osteitis, and osteomalacia. The cause of the metabolic disorder is the failure of the malfunctioning kidney to synthesize the metabolically active vitamin D_3. When the synthetic hormone is given, the calcium absorption and utilization are improved.[1]

TETANY is a condition characterized by a low blood calcium, increased excitability of the nerves, and uncontrolled contractions of the muscles. It is not caused by a dietary lack of calcium, but is the consequence of lowered parathyroid function. Administration of parathormone brings the blood calcium back to normal.

Hypercalcemia. A number of conditions can cause HYPERCALCEMIA, or increase in the blood calcium. It is accompanied by increased deposition of calcium in the soft tissues and increased calcium excretion in the urine. A high intake of calcium is not, in itself, a causative factor.

One of the situations in which hypercalcemia occasionally occurs is the milk-alkali syndrome in which patients with peptic ulcer have used excessive amounts of readily absorbed alkalies together with large amounts of milk over a period of years. The hypercalcemia in these patients was accompanied by vomiting, gastrointestinal bleeding, and increase in blood pressure.

Hypercalcemia occurs in infants who are given an excess of vitamin D. Gastrointestinal upsets are noted and growth is retarded. The condition is corrected by the removal of the excess vitamin from the diet.

PHOSPHORUS

Distribution. Phosphorus accounts for about 1 per cent of body weight or one fourth of the total mineral matter in the body. About 85 per cent of the phosphorus is in inorganic combination with calcium as the insoluble apatite of bones and teeth. In bones the proportion of calcium to phosphorus is about 2 to 1. Soft tissues contain much higher amounts of phosphorus than of calcium. Most of this phosphorus is in organic combinations.

Functions. Perhaps no mineral element has as many widely differing functions as does phosphorus. In fact, reference has been made to phosphorus compounds at many points in preceding chapters of the text, and some of the many roles are listed here for review purposes:

1. Phosphorus is a constituent of the sugar-phosphate linkage in the structures of DNA and RNA, the substances that control heredity (see page 50).

2. Phospholipids are constituents of cell membranes, thus regulating the transport of solutes into and out of the cell. The phosphorus-containing lipoproteins facilitate the transport of fats in the circulation.

3. Phosphorylation is a key reaction in many metabolic processes: for example, the phosphorylation of glucose for absorption from the intestine, the uptake of glucose by the cell, and the reabsorption of glucose by the renal tubules. Likewise, monosaccharides are phosphorylated in the initial stages of metabolism to yield energy (see page 68).

4. Phosphorous compounds are essential for the storage and controlled release of energy—the ADP-ATP system (see page 68); in the niacin-containing coenzymes required for oxidation-reduction reactions—NADP-NADPH (see page 179); and for the active form of thiamin for decarboxylation reactions—TPP (see page 173).

5. Inorganic phosphates in the body fluids constitute an important buffer system in the regulation of body neutrality (see page 140).

Metabolism. Much of the phosphorus in foods is in organic combinations that are split by intestinal phosphatases to free the phosphate. The phosphorus is absorbed as inorganic salts. About 70 per cent of dietary phosphorus is normally absorbed.

The inorganic phosphorus content of blood serum ranges from 2.5 to 4.5 mg per cent and is slightly higher in children. The level is kept constant through regulation by the kidney. All of the plasma inorganic phosphate is filtered through the renal glomeruli but most of it is reabsorbed. Vitamin D increases the rate of reabsorption by the tubules, and parathormone decreases the reabsorption.

Daily allowances. The phosphorus allowances recommended by the Food and Nutrition Board[8] are the same as those for calcium, except for infants. With ordinary diets, the phosphorus intake exceeds the calcium intake, but within a relatively wide range of calcium-to-phosphorus ratios there are no adverse effects in children and adults.

During the first six months of life the phosphorus allowance is 240 mg, and during the remainder of the first year the allowance is 400 mg. By keeping the phosphorus allowance below that of calcium during the first weeks of life, hypocalcemic tetany is avoided.

Food sources. Phosphorus is widely distributed in foods, the milk and meat groups being important contributors. Thus, a diet that furnishes enough protein and calcium will also provide sufficient phosphorus. Whole-grain cereals and flours contain much more phosphorus than refined cereals and flours; however, much of this occurs in phytic acid, which combines with calcium to form an insoluble salt that is not absorbed. Vegetables and fruits contain only small amounts of phosphorus. (See Table A–2.)

MAGNESIUM

Distribution. The amount of magnesium in the body is much smaller than that of calcium and phosphorus. Of the 20 to 35 gm in the adult body, about 60 per cent is present as phosphates and carbonates chiefly at the surfaces of the bones. Most of the remaining magnesium is within the cells where it ranks next to potassium in magnitude.

Extracellular fluids account for about 2 per cent of the body's magnesium. The normal concentration of magnesium in blood serum is 2 to 3 mg per cent, about 80 per cent of this being ionized; the remainder is bound to protein.

Functions. Magnesium is essential for all living cells. In plants magnesium is present in chlorophyll in a chemical structure similar to the iron in hemoglobin. In addition to its function in the skeletal structures, magnesium is a catalyst in numerous metabolic reactions. It is involved in protein synthesis through its action on the aggregation of ribosomes. It is an activator for the enzymes involved in the oxidative phosphorylation of ADP to ATP (see page 92), and also for all enzymes that bring about the transfer of phosphate from ATP to a phosphate acceptor. These reactions are essential whenever energy is expended, as in active transport across cell membranes, and the accomplishment of physical work.

Magnesium, together with calcium, sodium, and potassium, must be in balance in the extracellular fluids so that transmission of nerve impulses and the consequent muscle contraction can be regulated.

Metabolism. Magnesium is absorbed by active transport and competes with calcium for carrier sites. Thus, a high intake of either element interferes with absorption of the other. Many of the factors that enhance calcium absorption such as acidity, or that interfere with calcium absorption such as oxalic and phytic acids, also affect the absorption of magnesium. Neither vitamin D nor parathyroid hormone is believed to influence magnesium absorption. The absorption of magnesium varies inversely with the intake; at low levels of intake it is as high as 75 per cent, and at high levels of intake it may be as low as 25 per cent. The absorption on typical intakes in America is about 45 per cent.[14]

In magnesium deficiency the kidneys and the intestinal mucosa have a marked ability to retain magnesium. Thus, homeostasis can be maintained over a wide range of intake. The urinary excretion of magnesium in adults normally ranges between 100 and 200 mg. Almost all of the magnesium in the feces represents unabsorbed dietary magnesium.

Daily allowances. The Food and Nutrition Board has recommended a daily allowance of magnesium for men at 350 mg and for women at 300 mg.[8] During pregnancy and lactation a daily allowance of 450 mg is recommended. The allowances range from 60 to 70 mg during the first year of life and thereafter gradually increase from 150 mg for the toddler to 250 mg for the child of 7 to 10 years.

Food sources. In the food supply available for consumption in the United States, dairy products excluding butter furnish about 23 per cent of the total magnesium; vegetables, 20 per cent; flours and cereals, 18 per cent; meat, fish, poultry, and eggs, 13 per cent; legumes, 11 per cent; and fruits, 6 per cent.[15] Green leafy vegetables are especially good sources as are also dry beans and peas, soybeans, nuts, and whole grains. High losses of magnesium occur in the refinement of foods, and some losses are sustained when cooking waters are discarded. (See Table A–2 for magnesium content of foods.)

The average mixed American diet supplies about 120 mg magnesium per 1000 kcal.[8] Thus, if girls and women stay within their caloric requirements it would appear that they could not easily meet the recommended allowances. There is no evidence, however, that magnesium deficiency occurs except under conditions described below. The contributions of the Basic Diet pattern are shown in Figure 8–3.

Effects of imbalance. Under normal conditions of health and food intake, magnesium deficiency is not likely to occur. Unlike calcium, magnesium is only slowly mobilized from bone. Therefore, a generally

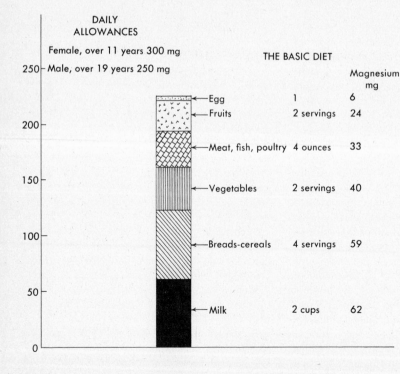

Figure 8–3. The Basic Diet furnishes about three fourths of the daily allowance for magnesium for women. If most of the foods that make up the remaining caloric need are chosen from the Four Food Groups the full daily allowance can be met. See Table 13–3 for calculations.

poor intake of magnesium, if it is also accompanied by increased excretion, leads to rapid lowering of the plasma magnesium. The ionic imbalance thus produced in the extracellular fluid upsets the regulation of nervous irritability and muscle contraction. Characteristic symptoms of magnesium deficiency include muscle tremor, paresthesias, and sometimes convulsive seizures and delirium. Since these symptoms are similar to hypocalcemic tetany, a differentiation can usually be made by determining the blood levels of the two cations.

Among the circumstances under which magnesium deficiency is encountered are these: chronic alcoholism, cirrhosis of the liver, malabsorption syndromes such as sprue, kwashiorkor, severe vomiting, prolonged use of magnesium-free parenteral fluids, diabetic acidosis, and diuretic therapy. In most of these instances the deficiency has occurred because of curtailment of food intake or lowered absorption or both. The loss of magnesium from the body is increased during diuretic therapy, and also in diabetic acidosis.

High blood magnesium levels are sometimes encountered when there is an unusual increase in absorption or a marked reduction in urinary excretion. The symptoms of such excess include extreme thirst, a feeling of excessive warmth, marked drowsiness, a decrease in muscle and nerve irritability, and atrial fibrillation. The early stages of hypermagnesemia are readily corrected by giving calcium gluconate.

SULFUR

Distribution. Sulfur accounts for about 0.25 per cent of body weight, or 175 mg in the adult male. It is present in all body cells, chiefly as the sulfur-containing amino acids methionine, cystine, and cysteine. Sulfur is a constituent of thiamin and biotin, two vitamins that must be present in the diet. Connective tissue, skin, nails, and hair are especially rich in sulfur.

Functions and metabolism. Sulfur is an essential element for all animal species inasmuch as they all require the sulfur-containing amino acid methionine. Almost all of the sulfur absorbed from the intestinal tract is in organic form, principally as the sulfur amino acids. Inorganic sulfates, present in only small amounts in foods, are poorly absorbed.

Sulfur is a structurally important constituent of mucopolysaccharides such as chondroitin sulfate found in cartilage, tendons, bones, skin, and the heart valves. Sulfolipids are abundant in such tissues as liver, kidney, the salivary glands, and the white matter of the brain. Other important sulfur-containing compounds are insulin (page 68) and heparin, an anticoagulant.

Sulfur compounds are essential in many oxidation-reduction reactions. Included among these compounds are a number of coenzymes discussed elsewhere in this text: thiamin (page 173); biotin (page 184); coenzyme A (page 183); and lipoic acid (page 189). Glutathione, an important compound in oxidation-reduction reactions, is a tripeptide of glutamic acid, cysteine, and glycine. The concentration of glutathione is especially high in the red blood cells.

The metabolism of the sulfur amino acids within the cells yields sulfuric acid, which is immediately neutralized and excreted as the inorganic salts. One of the important reactions of sulfuric acid is the conjugation with phenols, cresols, and the steroid sex hormones, thereby detoxifying compounds that would otherwise be harmful.

Excretion. About 85 to 90 per cent of the sulfur excreted in the urine is in the inorganic form, being derived almost entirely from the metabolism of the sulfur amino acids. The ratio of nitrogen to sulfur excreted in the urine is about 13 to 1. The range of excretion by the adult is 1 to 2 gm. On a low-protein diet the excretion would be much less than on a high-protein diet.

From 5 to 10 per cent of the sulfur excreted is in the form of organic esters produced in the detoxification reactions. The fecal excretion of sulfur is about equal to the inorganic sulfur content of the diet.

Cystinuria is a relatively rare hereditary defect in which large amounts of cystine as well as lysine, arginine, and ornithine are excreted because of a failure of renal reabsorption. Being somewhat insoluble, the cystine forms renal calculi.

Requirements and sources. The daily requirement for sulfur has not been determined. A diet that is adequate in methionine and cystine is considered to meet the body's sulfur needs.

The sulfur content of foods depends upon the

concentration of methionine and cystine. Food proteins vary from 0.4 to 1.6 per cent in their sulfur content, with an average of 1 per cent for a typical mixed diet. Thus, meat, milk, eggs, and legumes may be considered to be important sources.

TRACE ELEMENTS OR MICRONUTRIENTS

IRON

Distribution. The amount of iron in the body of the adult male is about 50 mg per kilogram, or a total of 3.5 gm; in the woman it is about 35 mg per kilogram, or a total of 2.3 gm. All body cells contain some iron. Approximately 75 per cent of the iron is in the hemoglobin, 5 per cent is held as myoglobin, 5 per cent is present in cellular constituents including the iron-containing enzymes, and 20 per cent is stored as FERRITIN or HEMOSIDERIN by the liver, spleen, and bone marrow. In healthy men the iron reserve is about 1000 mg, but in menstruating women it is not more than 200 to 400 mg.

Iron circulates in the plasma bound to a β-globulin, TRANSFERRIN—also known as SIDEROPHILIN. The concentration of iron in the serum for men ranges from 80 to 165 mcg per 100 ml, and for women from 65 to 130 mcg per 100 ml. Normally, the saturation of transferrin with iron ranges from 20 to 40 per cent.

Functions. Hemoglobin is the principal component of the red blood cells and accounts for most of the iron in the body. It acts as a carrier of oxygen from the lungs to the tissues and indirectly aids in the return of carbon dioxide to the lungs.

MYOGLOBIN is an iron-protein complex in the muscle which stores some oxygen for immediate use by the cell. Enzymes such as the catalases, the cytochromes in hydrogen ion transport (see page 92), and xanthine oxidase contain iron as an integral part of the molecule. Iron is required as a cofactor for other enzymes.

Metabolism. The amount of iron that will be absorbed from the intestinal tract is governed by (1) the body's need for iron, (2) the conditions existing in the intestinal lumen, and (3) the food mixture that is fed. (See Figure 8–4.) Iron is absorbed into the mucosal cells as (1) nonheme iron from inorganic salts in foods, and (2) as heme iron.[16] In the latter the porphyrin ring is split open in the cell and the iron is released into the blood circulation.

The absorption of iron is meticulously regulated by the intestinal mucosa according to body need. An increase in erythropoiesis leads to withdrawal of iron from the iron-transferrin complex in the circulation, and the lowering of transferrin saturation in turn brings about an increase in the amount of iron that is absorbed. Thus, growing children, pregnant women, and anemic individuals will have a higher rate of absorption than healthy males. The absorptive mechanism is also highly effective in preventing an overload of iron entering the body and causing toxic reactions. Although excess iron can be absorbed, extremely large intakes would be necessary for a long period of time before toxic reactions would result.

In the acid medium of the stomach and upper duodenum ferric iron is reduced to ferrous iron, a more soluble form that is readily absorbed. Achlorhydria, observed in many elderly persons and present in pernicious anemia, reduces the absorption of iron. Likewise, the surgical removal of the portion of the stomach that produces acid will also result in lower absorption of iron. The alkaline reaction of pancreatic juice reduces the solubility of iron so that little absorption takes place from the jejunum and ileum. Absorption of iron is also hindered in malabsorption syndromes, and in the presence of excess phytates.

The absorption of iron from foods varies widely, but in the healthy adult it averages about 5 to 10 per cent. From animal foods the absorption ranges from 10 to 30 per cent, whereas for vegetables it may be as little as 2 to 10 per cent.[7] Absorption from plant sources improves when animal foods are simultaneously fed, probably because the amino acids released from the proteins enhance solubility. The presence of ascorbic-acid-rich foods also increases the absorption of iron in that ferric iron is reduced to ferrous iron.

Transport and utilization. Iron in the plasma is made available from three sources: (1) absorption from the intestinal tract, (2) release from body reserves, and (3) release from the breakdown of hemoglobin that takes place constantly. Within a 24-hour

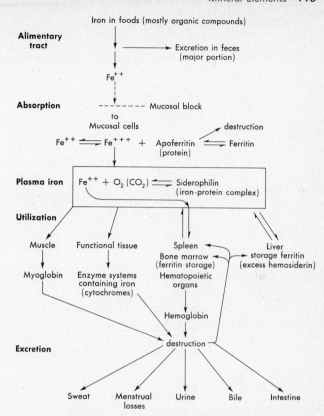

Figure 8–4. The utilization of iron.

period the turnover of iron is about 27 to 28 mg.[18] Only 1 to 1.5 mg of this has been available from absorption.

Iron is withdrawn from the plasma into the bone marrow for the synthesis of HEMOGLOBIN, which is a complex substance composed of a basic protein, GLOBIN, linked to a prosthetic group, HEME. The heme molecule consists of protoporphyrin with reduced iron at its center; four heme molecules together with globin make up the hemoglobin. Copper plays a catalytic role in the incorporation of iron into the protoporphyrin molecule.

The body exercises amazing economy in the use of iron. When the red blood cell has fulfilled its life cycle of about 120 days, more or less, the cell is destroyed within the reticuloendothelial system. The amino acids of the stroma and the globin, and the lipids, are utilized again. Heme is disintegrated to release iron once again to the circulation and the bile pigments are synthesized from the remainder of the molecule.

Excretion. The daily excretion of body iron by adults is about 0.1 mg from the urine and 0.3 to 0.5 mg into the intestinal lumen. Small amounts of iron are also lost in the perspiration and by exfoliation of the skin. The iron losses through menstruation range from 0.3 to 1.0 mg on a daily basis, but about 5 per cent of women have losses in excess of 1.4 mg daily.[8] Thus, the total iron losses by women are 1 to 2 mg daily.

Most of the iron in the feces represents the unabsorbed iron from the diet, or 90 per cent of the intake. A small amount of fecal iron is of endogenous origin, namely, that derived from the sloughing off of mucosal cells, and some is contained in the digestive juices.

Daily allowances. Dietary iron is required for (1) replacement of the daily losses of all individuals; (2) an expanding blood volume and increasing amounts of hemoglobin in growing children; (3) replacement of the varying losses through menstruation; (4) development of the fetus and to avoid anemia in

Table 8–3. Daily Iron Requirements*

	Absorbed Iron Requirement mg/day	Food Iron Requirement† mg/day	Recommended Dietary Allowance mg/day
Normal men and nonmenstruating women	0.5 – 1	5–10	10
Menstruating women	0.7 – 2	7–20	18
Pregnant women	2 – 4.8	20–48‡	18+
Adolescents	1 – 2	10–20	18
Children	0.4 – 1	4–10	10–15
Infants	0.5 – 1.5	1.5 mg/kg§	10–15 mg

*Adapted from: Committee on Iron Deficiency, Council on Foods and Nutrition: "Iron Deficiency in the United States," *J.A.M.A.*, **203**:407–14, Feb. 5, 1968; and Food and Nutrition Board: *Recommended Dietary Allowances*, 8th ed. National Academy of Sciences—National Research Council, Washington, D.C., 1974.

†Assuming an absorption of 10 per cent.

‡This amount of iron cannot be derived from diet and should be met by iron supplementation in the latter half of pregnancy.

§To a maximum of 15 mg.

pregnant and lactating women; and (5) a reserve of iron that is available when blood loss occurs from any cause whatsoever.

Table 8–3 lists the amounts of iron that must be absorbed to replace losses and to meet the synthetic requirements of various age groups. Assuming an average absorption of 10 per cent, the amounts of iron that must be provided in the diet are also listed. These values are compared with the recommended allowances of the Food and Nutrition Board.

Food sources. Of all nutrients, the iron allowance is the most difficult to provide in the diet. The iron content of typical diets adequate in other respects is estimated to be 6 mg per 1000 kcal.[8] (See Figure 8–5.) Thus, men and boys with their caloric requirements can easily meet their iron needs, but girls and women with their lower caloric requirements cannot supply their needs even with a good selection of diet.

Much more research is required to determine the

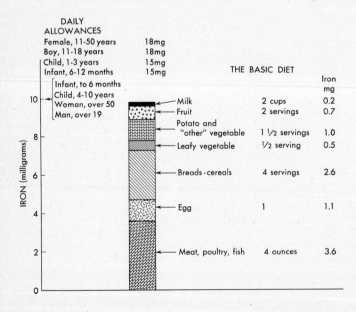

Figure 8–5. The Four Food Groups of the Basic Diet fulfill the iron allowance for the man. For teen-age girls and women it is difficult to meet the iron allowance without exceeding the caloric requirement. The allowances can be met by increased fortification of foods or by the use of iron supplements. See Table 13–2 for calculations.

availability of iron from various food sources and the conditions that enhance or detract from that availability. Lean meats, deep-green leafy vegetables, and whole-grain or enriched cereals and breads are the foods of the daily diet that must be depended upon for their iron. Milk, cheese, and ice cream are poor sources of iron—a fact that explains why infant diets must be fortified with iron-rich foods at an early age. Liver, other organ meats, dried fruits, legumes, shellfish, and molasses are iron-rich foods that deserve frequent use.

Cooking procedures are an important determinant in the amount of iron that is actually ingested. Some mineral salts are leached out when large amounts of water are used and subsequently discarded. Cast-iron cookware was widely used many years ago, and the uptake of iron from such cooking vessels added appreciably to the daily intake. Today, iron skillets are about the only such cookware used frequently. There are substantial differences between the iron content of foods cooked in cast-iron ware and the same foods cooked in glass or aluminum.[19]

Effects of imbalance. The characteristics of iron-deficiency anemia are a low serum level of iron, high iron-binding capacity, low hemoglobin, low red cell volume, and low mean corpuscular hemoglobin. The serum ferritin is a good indicator of iron stores.[20] However, inflammation, liver disease, and increased red cell turnover as in hemolytic anemia raise serum ferritin levels to a degree disproportionate to stores. Iron-deficiency anemia is characterized by reduced red cell and hemoglobin levels in the blood and by small, pale cells (microcytic, hypochromic). It is widely prevalent in the United States and throughout the world, but the exact incidence is not known. Infants, preschool children, adolescent girls, and pregnant women are especially susceptible. See Chapter 43 for discussion of anemias.

HEMOSIDEROSIS is a disorder of iron metabolism in which large deposits of iron are made especially in the liver and in the reticuloendothelial system. The transferrin of the circulation becomes saturated and is unable to bind all of the iron that is absorbed. This disorder affects a high proportion of the adult Bantu population in South Africa and is believed to be caused by an overload of dietary iron.[21] Bantu men commonly ingest 30 mg iron daily and frequently as much as 100 mg per day. The beer that they drink is fermented in iron pots, and likewise the acid-fermented cereal foods and sour porridge are cooked in these pots. The resulting foods have a high iron content.

Hemosiderosis also occurs when there is abnormal destruction of the red blood cells as in hemolytic anemia. It may also occur following prolonged iron therapy when it is not needed. The iron overload leads to deposits of iron in the liver cells, following which typical symptoms of cirrhosis develop. The excess iron may also be deposited in the lungs, pancreas, and heart.

IODINE

Distribution and function. About one third of the iodine in the adult body, variously estimated from 25 to 50 mg, is found in the thyroid gland where it is stored in the form of THYROGLOBULIN. The concentration of iodine in the thyroid gland is about 2500 times as great as that in any other tissues.

The only known function of iodine is as a constituent of the thyroid hormones, THYROXINE and TRIIODOTHYRONINE. Tyrosine, one of the amino acids, incorporates four atoms of iodine to form thyroxine. The thyroid hormones regulate the rate of oxidation within the cells and in so doing influence physical and mental growth, the functioning of the nervous and muscle tissues, circulatory activity, and the metabolism of all nutrients.

Metabolism. Iodine is ingested in foods as inorganic iodides and as organic compounds. In the digestive tract iodine is split from organic compounds and is rapidly absorbed as inorganic iodide. The degree of absorption is dependent upon the level of circulating thyroid hormone.

Iodine is transported by the circulation as free iodide and as PROTEIN-BOUND IODINE. The protein-bound fraction (PBI) is sensitive to changes in the level of thyroid activity; it rises during pregnancy and with hypertrophy of the gland and falls with hypofunction of the gland. The measurement of PBI, therefore, is a specific diagnostic tool for thyroid activity and has largely replaced the basal metabolism test as a study of thyroid function.

Another measure of thyroid activity is the uptake of radioactive iodine 24 hours after a measured dose of ^{131}I has been given. Normally, the thyroid gland takes up about 40 to 50 per cent of the dose given; this is increased in hyperthyroidism, and decreased in hypothyroidism.

Thyroid activity is controlled by the thyroid-stimulating hormone (TSH) secreted by the anterior lobe of the pituitary. When the blood level of the thyroid hormone is low, the activity of the thyroid is increased by TSH. By this action the thyroid gland withdraws iodide from the circulation, concentrates it, oxidizes it to iodine, and incorporates it into tyrosine to form diiodotyrosine, triiodothyronine, and thyroxine. These iodine-containing amino acids then become part of the thyroglobulin complex.

When thyroid hormone is utilized for cellular oxidation, iodine is released into the circulation. About one third of the released iodine is again incorporated into thyroid hormone and the remainder is excreted in the urine.

Daily allowances. The recommended allowance for men 19 to 22 years is 140 mcg; 23 to 50 years, 130 mcg; and 51 years and over, 110 mcg. For women from 19 to 50 years the allowance is 100 mcg, and for those 51 years and over, 80 mcg. Infants should receive 35 to 45 mcg during the first year, and children up to 10 years, 60 to 110 mcg. The allowances in pregnancy and lactation are 125 and 150 mcg, respectively.[8]

Sources. The most important dietary sources of iodine are iodized salt and bread to which iodates have been added as dough conditioners. Samples of continuous-process bread showed that 1 pound of bread furnishes about 4 mg iodine; thus, one slice of this bread would just about meet the recommended allowance.[8] Batch process bread supplies much smaller amounts of iodine.

The concentration of iodine used in salt is 1 part sodium or potassium iodide per 10,000 parts of salt. One gram of salt would furnish about 76 mcg iodine. About half of the table salt sold in the United States is iodized. Salt used in the processing of food and bulk salt for institutional use is rarely iodized.[8]

Seaweed, saltwater fish, and shellfish contain important amounts of iodine for people who consume these foods on a regular basis. The iodine content of eggs, dairy products, and meats depends upon the iodine content of the animal's diet. Vegetables grown on iodine-rich soils near the seacoast are good sources of iodine; those grown on iodine-poor soils, generally inland, contain little iodine.

Effects of deficiency. ENDEMIC GOITER, the iodine-deficiency disease, occurs in those areas where the iodine content of the soil is so low that insufficient iodine is obtained through food and water, and when no provision is made for supplying iodized salt. Among the areas of iodine-poor soils are the Great Lakes region, the Pacific Northwest, Switzerland, Central American countries, mountainous areas of South America, New Zealand, and the Himalayas. The World Health Organization has estimated that up to 200 million people throughout the world may be affected. The iodine intake in the United States is generally adequate, and deficiency is no longer considered to be a problem.

Lack of iodine leads to an increase in the size and number of epithelial cells in the thyroid gland and thus an enlargement of the gland. This condition known as simple or endemic goiter, presents no other abnormal physical findings. The basal metabolism remains normal. The deficiency is more prevalent in females than males and is more frequent during adolescence and pregnancy.

The most urgent reason for stressing iodine as a preventive measure is not the goiter itself but the cretinism which is its ultimate sequel in areas severely deficient in iodine. Cretinism occurs in the infant when the pregnant woman is so severely depleted that she cannot supply iodine for the development of the fetus. CRETINISM is characterized by a low basal metabolism, muscular flabbiness and weakness, dry skin, enlarged tongue, thick lips, arrest of skeletal development, and severe mental retardation. Desiccated thyroid given early enough to the infant results in marked improvement of physical development; mental retardation may be less severe, but any damage which has occurred to the central nervous system cannot be reversed. Endemic cretinism is rare or nonexistent in the United States today.

Goitrogens. Certain substances called GOITROGENS are known to interfere with the use of thyroxine and will produce goiters, at least in experimental animals, even though the iodine intake would normally be adequate. Goitrogens are present in rutabagas,[22] peanuts—especially in the red skin[23]—and seeds of the *Brassica* family (cabbage, Brussels sprouts, cauliflower). The substances are inactivated by cooking, and there is currently no evidence that goiters in endemic regions are caused by them.

ZINC

Distribution in the body. About 2 to 3 gm zinc is present in the adult body. It is widely distributed in all tissues but not evenly so. High concentrations are found in the eye, especially the iris and retina, in the liver, bone, prostate and prostatic secretions, and in the hair. In the blood about 85 per cent of the zinc is in the red blood cells. Each leukocyte contains about 25 times as much zinc as each red blood cell.

Functions. Zinc is essential for all living organisms. Its numerous functions include the following:

1. As an integral part of at least 20 enzymes that belong to a large group known as metalloenzymes. Among these are:

CARBONIC ANHYDRASE, an enzyme isolated and purified in 1940 and found to contain zinc. Carbonic anhydrase is as essential to the transport of carbon dioxide to the lungs as hemoglobin is to the transport of oxygen.

LACTIC DEHYDROGENASE involved in the interconversion of pyruvic and lactic acid in the glycolytic pathway.

ALKALINE PHOSPHATASE required in bone metabolism. The concentration is especially high in white blood cells.

CARBOXYPEPTIDASE and AMINOPEPTIDASE, which bring about removal of the terminal carboxyl and amino groups in the digestion of proteins.

2. As a cofactor in the synthesis of DNA and RNA, and thus proteins. In this role it is especially important in cellular systems that undergo rapid turnover, as in the gastrointestinal tract including the taste buds. Thus, zinc plays a role in the sensory systems that control food intake.[24]

3. The mobilization of vitamin A from the liver to maintain normal concentrations in the blood circulation.

4. Enhancement of the action of follicle-stimulating hormone and luteinizing hormone.

Metabolism. Most of the zinc is absorbed from the duodenum and jejunum. Although absorption ranges widely, the usual uptake by the intestinal mucosa is probably less than 50 per cent. Large intakes of calcium, vitamin D, and phytate interfere with absorption.

Upon absorption zinc combines with a protein for transport. The rate of turnover in the liver, pancreas, kidney, and pituitary is rapid. The normal serum concentration of zinc is about 100 to 140 mcg per 100 ml. There is little day-to-day variation in plasma concentrations and no increase in the blood level after meals. Unlike iron, the body stores of zinc are not readily utilized.

Zinc is excreted primarily by pancreatic and intestinal juices. The normal urinary loss is about 500 mcg daily.

Recommended allowances. Only a limited amount of research has been conducted on the requirements for zinc. The recommended allowances are 15 mg for adults; 3 to 5 mg for infants; 10 mg for children; 20 mg during pregnancy; and 25 mg for the lactating woman.[8]

Food sources. Data on food composition are sparse, and there is little information on the variability from sample to sample. Rich sources include oysters, liver, high-protein foods, and whole-grain cereals. Beef, lamb, and pork contain three to four times as much as fish; and dark meat of chicken furnishes about three times as much as light meat. Legumes, peanuts, and peanut butter are good sources, but fruits and most vegetables are poor sources. The zinc in plant proteins is less available than that in animal proteins. Vegetarian diets and low-protein diets are likely to be deficient in zinc. (See Table A–2.)

Deficiency. The first description of human deficiency of zinc was reported from Iran and Egypt.[25-27] Dwarfs in those countries were observed to consume a diet in which more than half of the calories were furnished by unleavened whole-grain bread. Although the whole-grain cereals are good sources of zinc, practically all of the mineral is tied up by the high concentration of phytate in the unleavened bread. In addition to growth failure, there were hypogonadism, enlarged liver, and severe anemia. Serum zinc levels were about 50 mcg per 100 ml. With the addition of zinc to the diet there was considerable improvement in growth and development of the sexual organs. This type of growth failure is rare in the United States, although it has been observed in children who had grossly inadequate diets.[28]

Impaired taste and odor acuity is a consequence of zinc deficiency. HYPOGEUSIA is a decrease in taste acuity; DYSGEUSIA is an unpleasant, perverted, and obnoxious taste. HYPOSMIA is a decrease in odor acuity; DYSOSMIA is a disagreeable odor. Patients often complain of persistent foul odor in the nasopharynx, metallic taste in the absence of food; or saltiness, sweetness, sourness, or bitterness.[29] Studies by electron microscope have shown the taste buds to be fewer in number, smaller, and with a number of histologic changes.

In some patients, no preceding events can account for the disagreeable symptoms. In many, an upper respiratory infection with fever has been associated with zinc deficiency.[30] Patients with severe burns have serum zinc levels about two thirds of normal, urinary excretions are doubled, and anorexia is severe. Therapy with zinc has improved the appetite so that food intake begins to approximate the high protein and caloric needs for recovery.[31] Hyposmia, dysosmia, and hypogeusia are often severe in acute viral hepatitis, cirrhosis of the liver, hepatic coma, and kwashiorkor.

Toxicity. Zinc salts are relatively nontoxic. About 60 to 120 times the recommended allowance will induce vomiting, cramps, and diarrhea in 3 to 12 hours but the symptoms subside shortly. Intake of excessive zinc has been reported when acid foods or beverages such as lemonade were prepared and stored in galvanized containers. The acidity of the food dissolves enough zinc to produce the toxic symptoms.

COPPER

Distribution. The presence of copper in blood was first recognized in 1875, but the nutritional significance was not established until Hart and Elvehjem at the University of Wisconsin found that traces of copper were essential for the formation of hemoglobin. The body of the human adult contains about 75 to 150 mg of copper. Traces of copper are found in all tissues, but by far the highest concentrations are found in the liver, brain, heart, and kidney. In the fetus and at birth the levels in these organs are several times as high, and they decrease during the first year.

Metabolism and function. Copper is absorbed from the stomach and from the upper gastrointestinal tract. About 95 per cent of the copper in blood plasma is firmly bound to a protein complex, CERULOPLASMIN, and 5 per cent is loosely bound to albumin.

Molybdenum and zinc are antagonistic to copper; thus, an increased intake of these trace elements increases the requirement for copper. Almost all of the excretion of copper is in the feces, chiefly through the excretion of bile.

Copper is required for diverse functions, including taste sensitivity, melanin pigment formation, electron transport, integrity of the myelin sheath, maturation of collagen, elastin formation, phospholipid synthesis, bone development, and hemoglobin formation. Copper has been identified as a constituent of a number of enzymes: butyryl coenzyme A dehydrogenase required for the oxidation of fatty acids; tyrosinase required for melanin pigment formation; uricase in purine metabolism; and in the cytochrome oxidation system for energy production. The functions of several copper-containing proteins such as hepatocuprein and erythrocuprein are not known.

Daily allowances. A daily allowance of 2 mg copper is considered to be satisfactory for the adult. For infants an allowance of 0.08 mg per kilogram daily is sufficient.

Food sources. Typical diets furnish from 2 to 5 mg copper. Even a diet that is poor in other nutrients is likely to furnish enough copper. The copper content of foods is somewhat dependent upon the copper content of soil. Among rich sources are organ meats, shellfish, whole-grain cereals, legumes, and nuts. Milk is a poor source.

Effects of imbalance. Dietary deficiency of copper is not likely in humans. Low blood levels of copper have been observed in kwashiorkor, the nephrotic syndrome, and sprue, and occasionally in patients with iron-deficiency anemia.

In excessive amounts copper is toxic. A rare hereditary disorder known as Wilson's disease is characterized by a marked reduction of blood ceruloplasmin and greatly increased deposits of copper in the liver, brain, and other organs. The excess copper in these tissues leads to hepatitis, lenticular degeneration, renal malfunction, and neurologic disorders.

FLUORINE

Distribution and function. Fluoride occurs normally in the body primarily as a calcium salt in the bones and teeth. Small amounts of fluoride bring about striking reductions in tooth decay, probably because the tooth enamel is made more resistant to the action of acids produced in the mouth by bacteria.

Carefully controlled studies in a number of cities for more than 10 years have established that fluoridation of the water supplies at a level of 1 part fluoride per million (1 ppm) may be expected to reduce the incidence of dental caries in children by approximately 50 to 60 per cent. Several thousand communities in the United States have now initiated water fluoridation as an effective public health measure. Children who have been drinking fluoridated water since infancy show the greatest benefits; those who begin the ingestion of fluoridated water in later school years are helped to a lesser extent.

Fluorides may be involved in some way in the maintenance of bone structure. Some studies have shown that osteoporosis occurs less frequently in elderly persons who live in areas supplied with fluoridated water.[32] The fluoride salts of calcium are less readily lost from bone during immobilization or following the menopause.

Metabolism. Fluorides are absorbed readily from the gastrointestinal tract. They replace the hydroxyl groups in the calcium-phosphorus salts of bones and teeth to form fluoroapatite. The fluoride crystals are less readily resorbed than are crystals of hydroxyapatite. Most of the fluoride ingested is excreted in the urine. An average daily excretion is about 3 mg.

Food sources. Fluoride occurs in all soils, water supplies, plants, and animals, and is a normal constituent of the diet. The amounts present are in direct correlation with the fluoride concentration of water and soils. In low-fluoride areas the daily diet furnishes only 0.3 mg; in high-fluoride areas the daily intake from food is about 3.1 mg.[8] Six glasses of water containing 1 ppm will provide an additional 1.2 mg.

Effects of excess. Chronic dental FLUOROSIS results when the concentration of fluoride in drinking water is in excess of 1.5 ppm. The teeth become MOTTLED; that is, the tooth enamel becomes dull and unglazed with some pitting. At higher concentrations of fluoride some dark-brown stains appear. Although aesthetically undesirable, such teeth are surprisingly free of dental caries.

Large excesses of fluorine—20 to 80 mg daily for several years—lead to bone fluorosis with symptoms resembling arthritis.

OTHER TRACE ELEMENTS

Manganese, molybdenum, selenium, chromium, and cobalt are essential trace elements. Their principal functions are as integral constituents of enzymes or as activators of enzymes.

No recommended allowances have been set for these elements inasmuch as only a few studies have been conducted on the requirements. Data on the distribution and the availability of these elements in foods are also sparse. A diet that is adequate in other nutrients, and that does not contain a high proportion of refined foods, is considered to satisfy the needs for these trace elements. Dietary deficiency is not likely in human beings.

Experimental studies on animals have shown that the mineral elements are closely interrelated. Thus, an excess of one element may increase the need for another. Excessive amounts of trace elements produce symptoms of toxicity in animals.

Manganese. About 2.5 to 7 mg manganese are supplied in the daily diet of the adult.[8] Seeds of plants—nuts, legumes, and whole-grain cereals—are good sources, but animal foods are much lower in their content. Manganese is rather poorly absorbed from the small intestine by a mechanism similar to that for the absorption of iron. It is loosely bound to a protein and transported as TRANSMANGANIN. Tissues that are rich in mitochondria take up manganese readily from the blood. A dynamic equilibrium exists between intracellular and extracellular manganese. Most of the metabolic manganese is excreted into the intestine as a constituent of bile, but much of this is again reabsorbed, indicating an effective body conservation. Very little manganese is excreted in the urine.

Studies on experimental animals have shown that manganese is required for normal bone growth and development, normal lipid metabolism, reproduction, and regulation of nervous irritability. Manganese is an activator for a number of enzymes including arginase, which is required for the formation of urea, and a number of peptidases that bring about the hydrolysis of proteins in the intestine. Manganese can substitute for magnesium in a number of enzymes required for oxidative phosphorylation.

Molybdenum. A precise balance of molybdenum is essential for plant and animal life. Nitrogen-fixing bacteria require this metal for their growth, and thus the synthesis of proteins and ultimately animal life are affected. A deficiency of molybdenum will adversely affect the growth of legumes. Also, in molybdenum deficiency the growth of certain fungi that produce mycotoxins is favored. These mycotoxins have been shown to be carcinogenic in animals. (See also Chapter 17.)

Molybdenum is found especially in legumes, whole-grain cereals, and organ meats. It is absorbed as molybdate and is concentrated especially in the liver, adrenal, and kidney. It is a cofactor for a number of flavoprotein enzymes and is found in XANTHINE OXIDASE, an enzyme that brings about the oxidation of xanthine to uric acid.

Molybdenum competes with copper for the same metabolic sites, and an excess of molybdenum will result in symptoms of copper deficiency. Cattle grazing on lands that have a high molybdenum content develop a condition known as *teart* and characterized by diarrhea, brittle bones, loss of pigmentation, and weight loss. When the sulfate content of the diet is increased, the symptoms of toxicity are avoided inasmuch as the excretion of molybdenum is increased. This affords an interesting example of the interrelationship of sulfur, copper, and molybdenum.

Selenium. Some selenium is present in all tissues, with the highest concentrations in kidney, liver, spleen, pancreas, and testes. In whole blood the average concentration of selenium is about 25 mcg per 100 ml. Values as low as 11 mcg per cent have been found in children with protein-calorie malnutrition, and as high as 81.3 mcg per cent in Venezuelan children living in seleniferous areas.[33]

For many years it has been known that selenium and vitamin E could spare each other. Both factors can behave as antioxidants. Recently selenium has been shown to be a constituent of the enzyme GLUTATHIONE OXIDASE, which is capable of destroying lipid peroxides.[34]

Meats and seafoods are rich sources of selenium. Cereals contribute varying amounts depending upon the soil concentration. Unlike some elements there is relatively little loss in the milling of grains. Vegetables and fruits are poor sources. Frozen foods and some baby foods were found to contain marginal amounts of selenium.[33] The concentration of selenium in foods correlates closely with the protein content.

The effects of selenium deficiency in man are not known. Animals consuming a selenium-deficient diet show a variety of symptoms: faulty development of the vascular system, cataracts, and alopecia in rats; degeneration of the pancreas in chicks. Many attempts have been made to correlate selenium deficiency with specific diseases, but none have been successful.

Excess selenium is toxic. Many cattle grazing in areas where the soil has a high selenium content suffer from "alkali disease" characterized by stiffness, blindness, deformity of the hooves, loss of hair, and sometimes death. An increase in dental caries in Oregon schoolchildren who lived in seleniferous areas has been reported.[35]

Chromium. The adult body contains about 6 mg chromium. There are high concentrations in the hair, spleen, kidney, and testes, and lower concentrations in the heart, pancreas, lungs, and brain. The plasma chromium is about 3 parts per billion.[36] With age there is a decline in body chromium, possibly caused by an accumulated dietary deficit.[33]

The usable form of chromium is the GLUCOSE TOLERANCE FACTOR (GTF), an organic compound containing glycine, glutamic acid, cysteine, and niacin. The absorption of the trivalent chromium in GTF is about 10 to 25 per cent; only 1 per cent of inorganic chromium is absorbed.

Glucose tolerance factor is essential for the efficient use of insulin. It enhances the removal of glucose from the blood. Its action appears to increase the uptake of glucose by the cells, the oxidation of glucose to carbon dioxide, the incorporation of glucose carbon into fat, and the synthesis of proteins. Chromium is also an activator of several enzymes.

Diets in the United States furnish about 52 to 78 mcg chromium,[36] a level that is lower than in Italy, Egypt, South Africa, and India. Yeast, beer, liver, whole-grain cereals and breads, meat, and cheese are good sources. The milling of grains removes up to 83 per cent of chromium.[33] Milk, white flour and bread, chicken breast, fish, and vegetables are low in chromium. Even diets that are considered to be adequate in other respects may be marginal in chromium.

Chromium deficiency is believed to be relatively common in the United States and is manifested by impaired glucose tolerance. It is seen especially in older persons, in maturity-onset diabetes, and in infants with protein-calorie malnutrition. Supplements with chromium have been found to improve the glucose tolerance in diabetic patients and in persons with impaired glucose tolerance.

Cobalt. This element is an essential constituent of vitamin B_{12} and must be ingested in the form of the vitamin molecule inasmuch as humans cannot synthesize the vitamin. No other function of cobalt has been established.

A summary of mineral elements and review questions appear at the end of Chapter 9.

Cited References

1. Haussler, M. R.: "Vitamin D: Mode of Action and Biochemical Applications," *Nutr. Rev.*, **32**:257–66, 1974.
2. Johnston, F. A.: "Calcium Retained by Young Women Before and After Adding Spinach to the Diet," *J. Am. Diet. Assoc.*, **28**:933–38, 1952.
3. Reinhold, J. C.: "Phytate Destruction by Yeast Fermentation in Whole Wheat Meals," *J. Am. Diet. Assoc.*, **66**:38–41, 1975.
4. Whedon, G. D.: "The Combined Use of Balance and Isotopic Studies in the Study of Calcium Metabolism," in Mills, C. F., and Passmore, R., eds. *Proceedings VI International Congress of Nutrition*, E. & S. Livingstone, Ltd., Edinburgh, 1964, pp. 425–38.
5. Walker, R. M., and Linkswiler, H. M.: "Calcium Retention in the Adult Human Male as Affected by Protein Intake," *J, Nutr.*, **102**:1297–1302, 1972.
6. Anand, C. R., and Linkswiler, H. M.: "Effect of Protein Intake on Calcium Balance of Young Men Given 500 mg Calcium Daily," *J. Nutr.*, **104**:695–700, 1974.
7. Margen, S., *et al.*: "Studies in Calcium Metabolism. I. The Calciuretic Effect of Dietary Protein," *Am. J. Clin. Nutr.*, **27**:584–89, 1974.
8. Food and Nutrition Board: *Recommended Dietary Allowances*, 8th ed. National Academy of Sciences, Washington, D.C., 1974.
9. FAO/WHO Expert Committee: *Calcium Requirements*. WHO Tech. Rep. Ser. No. 230, WHO, Geneva, 1962.
10. Mack, P. B., and LaChance, P. A.: "Effects of Recumbency and Space Flight on Bone Density," *Am. J. Clin. Nutr.*, **20**:1194–1205, 1967.
11. Berlyne, G. M., *et al.*: "Bedouin Osteomalacia Due to Calcium Deprivation Caused by High Phytic Acid Content of Unleavened Bread," *Am. J. Clin. Nutr.*, **26**:910–11, 1973.
12. Lutwak, L.: "Continuing Need for Dietary Calcium Throughout Life," *Geriatrics*, **29**:171–78, 1974.
13. Hegsted, D. M.: "Calcium and Phosphorus," in Goodhart, R. S., and Shils, M. E., eds.: *Modern Nutrition in Health and Disease*, 5th ed. Lea & Febiger, Philadelphia, 1973, pp. 268–86.
14. Shils, M. E.: "Magnesium," in Goodhart, R. S., and Shils, M. E., eds.: *Modern Nutrition in Health and Disease*, 5th ed. Lea & Febiger, Philadelphia, 1973, pp. 287–96.
15. Friend, B., and Marston, R.: "Nutritional Review," *National Food Situation*, NFS-150, Washington, D.C., November 1974, pp. 26–32.
16. Review: "The Value of Iron Fortification of Food," *Nutr. Rev.*, **31**:275–77, 1973.
17. Finch, C. A.: "Iron Metabolism," *Nutr. Today*, **4**:2–7, Summer 1969.
18. Gubler, C. J.: "Absorption and Metabolism of Iron," *Science*, **123**:87–90, 1956.
19. White, H. S.: "Current Use and Changes in Use of Cast-Iron Cookware," *J. Home Econ.*, **60**:724–27, 1968.
20. Lipschitz, D. A., *et al.*: "A Clinical Evaluation of Serum Ferritin as an Index of Iron Stores," *N. Engl. J. Med.*, **290**:1213–16, 1974.
21. deBruin E. J. P., *et al.*: "Iron Absorption in the Bantu," *J. Am. Diet. Assoc.*, **57**:129–31, 1970.
22. Greer, M. A.: "Goitrogenic Substances in Food," *Am. J. Clin. Nutr.*, **5**:440–44, 1957.
23. Srinivasin, V., *et al.*: "Studies on Goitrogenic Agents in Food. I. Goitrogenic Action of Groundnut," *J. Nutr.*, **61**:87–95, 1957.

24. McConnell, S. D., and Henkin, R. I.: "Altered Preference for Sodium Chloride, Anorexia, and Changes in Plasma and Urinary Zinc in Rats Fed a Zinc-Deficient Diet," *J. Nutr.*, **104**:1108–14, 1974.

25. Prasad, A. D., *et al.*: "Zinc and Iron Deficiencies in Male Subjects with Dwarfism and Hypogonadism but Without Ancylostomiasis, Schistosomiasis, or Severe Anemia," *Am. J. Clin. Nutr.*, **12**:437–44, 1963.

26. Halsted, J. A., *et al.*: "A Conspectus of Research on Zinc Requirements of Man (Monograph)," *J. Nutr.*, **104**:345–78, 1974.

27. Ronaghy, H. A., *et al.*: "Zinc Supplementation of Malnourished Schoolboys in Iran: Increased Growth and Other Effects," *Am. J. Clin. Nutr.*, **27**:112–21, 1974.

28. Hambidge, K. M., *et al.*: "Low Levels of Zinc in Hair, Anorexia, Poor Growth, and Hypogeusia in Children," *Pediatr. Res.*, **6**:868–74, 1972.

29. Henkin, R. I., *et al.*: "Idiopathic Hypogeusia, Hyposmia and Dysosmia: A New Syndrome," *J.A.M.A.*, **217**:434–40, 1971.

30. Hussey, H. H.: "Taste and Smell Deviations: Importance of Zinc," *J.A.M.A.*, **228**:1669–70, 1974.

31. Cohen, I. K., *et al.*: "Hypogeusia, Anorexia, and Altered Zinc Metabolism Following Thermal Burn," *J.A.M.A.*, **223**:914–16, 1973.

32. Rich, C., and Ensinck, J.: "Effect of Sodium Fluoride on Calcium Metabolism of Human Beings," *Nature*, **191**:184–85, 1961.

33. Levander, O. A.: "Selenium and Chromium in Human Nutrition," *J. Am. Diet. Assoc.*, **66**:338–44, 1975.

34. Rotruck, J. T., *et al.*: "Relationship of Selenium to GSH Peroxidase" (abstract), *Fed. Proc.*, **31**:691, 1972.

35. Tank, G., and Storvick, C. A.: "Effect of Naturally Occurring Selenium and Vanadium on Dental Caries," *J. Dent. Res.*, **39**:473–88, 1960.

36. Hambidge, K. M.: "Chromium Nutrition in Man," *Am. J. Clin. Nutr.*, **27**:505–14, 1974.

ADDITIONAL REFERENCES

Calcium and Phosphorus

Bronner, F., and Harris, R. S.: "Absorption and Metabolism of Calcium in Human Beings Studied with Calcium[45]," *Ann. N.Y. Acad. Sci.*, **64**:314–25, 1956.

Hankin, J. H., *et al.*: "Contribution of Hard Water to Calcium and Magnesium Intakes of Adults," *J. Am. Diet. Assoc.*, **56**:212–24, 1970.

Irwin, M. I., and Kienholz, E. W.: "Monograph: A Conspectus of Research on Calcium Requirements of Man," *J. Nutr.*, **103**:1019–95, 1973.

Lotz, M. E., *et al.*: "Evidence for a Phosphorus-Depletion Syndrome in Man," *N. Engl. J. Med.*, **278**:409–15, 1968.

McBean, L. D., and Speckman, E. W.: "A Recognition of the Interrelationship of Calcium with Various Dietary Components," *Am. J. Clin. Nutr.*, **27**:603–609, 1974.

Moon, Wan-Hee, *et al.*: "Phosphorus Balances of Adults Consuming Several Food Combinations," *J. Am. Diet. Assoc.*, **64**:386–90, 1974.

Review: "Calcium Transport and Mobilization Mediated by 1,25-Dihydroxycholecalciferol," *Nutr. Rev.*, **31**:58–59, 1973.

Review: "Calcium Transport in the Ileum," *Nutr. Rev.*, **33**:84–85, 1975.

Spencer, H. J., *et al.*: "Effect of High Phosphorus Intake on Calcium and Phosphorus Metabolism in Man," *J. Nutr.*, **86**:125–32, 1965.

Tewell, J. T., *et al.*: "Phosphorus Balances of Adults Fed Rice, Milk, and Wheat Flour Mixtures," *J. Am. Diet. Assoc.*, **63**:530–35, 1973.

Chromium

Mayer, J.: "Chromium in Medicine," *Postgrad. Med.*, **49**:235–36, Jan. 1971.

Mertz, W.: "Effects and Metabolism of Glucose Tolerance Factor," *Nutr. Rev.*, **33**:129–35, 1975.

Mertz, W., *et al.*: "Present Knowledge of the Role of Chromium," *Fed. Proc.*, **33**:2275–80, 1974.

Mitman, F. W., *et al.*: "Urinary Chromium Levels of Nine Young Women Eating Freely Chosen Diets," *J. Nutr.*, **105**:64–68, 1975.

Morgan, J. M.: "Hepatic Chromium Content in Diabetic Subjects," *Metabolism*, **21**:313–16, 1972.

Copper

Butler, L. C., and Daniel, J. M.: "Copper Metabolism in Young Women Fed Two Levels of Copper and Two Protein Sources," *Am. J. Clin. Nutr.*, **26:**744–49, 1973.

Dowdy, R. P.: "Copper Metabolism," *Am. J. Clin. Nutr.*, **22:**887–92, 1969.

Frieden, E.: "Ceruloplasmin, a Link Between Copper and Iron Metabolism," *Nutr. Rev.*, **28:**87–91, 1970.

Hill, C. H.: "A Role of Copper in Elastin Formation," *Nutr. Rev.*, **27:**99–102, 1969.

Krishnamachari, K. A. V. R.: "Some Aspects of Copper Metabolism in Pellagra," *Am. J. Clin. Nutr.*, **27:**108–11, 1974.

Review: "Copper and the Aorta," *Nutr. Rev.*, **27:**325–28, 1969.

Review: "Copper and Taste Sensitivity," *Nutr. Rev.*, **26:**175–77, 1968.

Review: "Copper Toxicity, Rats and Wilson's Disease," *Nutr. Rev.*, **33:**51–53, 1975.

Fluoride

American Dietetic Association: "Policy Statement on Fluoridation," *J. Am. Diet. Assoc.*, **64:**68, 1974.

Bernstein, D. S., *et al.:* "Prevalence of Osteoporosis in High- and Low-Fluoride Areas in North Dakota," *J.A.M.A.*, **198:**499–504, 1966.

Kramer, L., *et al.:* "Dietary Fluoride in Different Areas in the United States," *Am. J. Clin. Nutr.*, **27:**590–94, 1974.

Review: "Skeletal Fluorosis and Dietary Calcium, Vitamin C, and Protein," *Nutr. Rev.*, **32:**13–15, 1974.

Smith, E. H.: "Fluoridation of Water Supply," *J.A.M.A.*, **230:**1569, 1974.

Iodine

Fierro-Benitez, R., *et al.:* "Endemic Goiter and Endemic Cretinism in the Andean Region," *N. Engl. J. Med.*, **280:**296–302, 1969.

Food and Nutrition Board: *Iodine Nutriture in the United States.* National Academy of Sciences—National Research Council, Washington, D.C., 1970.

Kidd, P. S., *et al.:* "Sources of Dietary Iodine," *J. Am. Diet. Assoc.*, **65:**420–22, 1974.

Matovinovic, J., *et al.:* "Goiter and Other Thyroid Diseases in Tecumseh, Michigan," *J.A.M.A.*, **192:**234–40, 1965.

Review: "Endemic Goiter and Antithyroid Agents," *Nutr. Rev.*, **33:**171–72, 1975.

Review: "The Etiology of Endemic Cretinism," *Nutr. Rev.*, **29:**227–30, 1971.

Staff Report: "Iodized Salt," *Nutr. Today*, **4:**22–25, Spring 1969.

Trowbridge, F. L., *et al.:* "Findings Relating to Goiter and Iodine in the Ten-State Nutrition Survey," *Am. J. Clin. Nutr.*, **28:**712–16, 1975.

Iron

Amine, E. K., and Hegsted, D. M.: "Biological Assessment of Available Iron in Food Products," *J. Agr. Food Chem.*, **22:**470–76, 1974.

Cook, J. D., *et al.:* "Absorption of Fortification Iron in Bread," *Am. J. Clin. Nutr.*, **26:**861–72, 1973.

Council on Foods and Nutrition: "Fortification of Flour and Bread with Iron," *J.A.M.A.*, **223:**322, 1973.

Crosby, W. H.: "Bureaucratic Clout and a Parable. Commentary," *J.A.M.A.*, **228:**1651–52, 1974.

Gaines, E. G., and Daniel, W. A., Jr.: "Dietary Iron Intakes of Adolescents," *J. Am. Diet. Assoc.*, **65:**275–80, 1974.

Layrisse, M., *et al.:* "Measurement of the Total Daily Dietary Iron Absorption by the Extrinsic Tag Model," *Am. J. Clin. Nutr.*, **27:**152–62, 1974.

Norman, C.: "Iron Enrichment," *Nutr. Today*, **8:**16–17, Nov. 1973.

Review: "Problems in Iron Enrichment and Fortification of Foods," *Nutr. Rev.*, **33:**46–47, 1975.

Rundels, J. C.: "Iron Deficiency in Children," *Nurs. Care*, **6:**16–18, Sept. 1973.

Vaghefi, S. B., *et al.:* "Availability of Iron in an Enrichment Mixture Added to Bread," *J. Am. Diet. Assoc.*, **64:**275–80, 1974.

Waddell, J.: "The Bioavailability of Iron Sources and Their Utilization in Food Enrichment," *Fed. Proc.*, **33:**1779–83, 1974.

Wallack, M. K., and Winkelstein, A.: "Acute Iron Intoxication in an Adult," *J.A.M.A.*, **229**:1333–34, 1974.

Wintrobe, M. W.: "The Proposed Increase in the Iron Fortification of Wheat Products," *Nutr. Today*, **8**:18–20, Nov. 1973.

Magnesium

Flink, E. B.: "Magnesium Deficiency Syndrome in Man," *J.A.M.A.*, **160**:1406–1409, 1956.

Hathaway, M. L.: *Magnesium in Human Nutrition*. Home Econ. Res. Rept. 19, U.S. Department of Agriculture, Washington, D.C., 1962.

Hunt, S. M., and Schofield, F. A.: "Magnesium Balance and Protein Intake Level in Adult Human Female," *Am. J. Clin. Nutr.*, **22**:367–73, 1969.

Jones, J. E., *et al.*: "Magnesium Requirements in Adults," *Am. J. Clin. Nutr.*, **20**:632–35, 1967.

Review: "Hypermagnesemia," *Nutr. Rev.*, **26**:12–15, 1968.

Review: "Hypomagnesemia in Protein-Calorie Malnutrition," *Nutr. Rev.*, **29**:89–90, 1971.

Review: "Magnesium Toxicity in the Newborn," *Nutr. Rev.*, **26**:139–40, 1968.

Shils, M. E.: "Experimental Human Magnesium Depletion. I. Clinical Observations and Blood Chemistry Alterations," *Am. J. Clin. Nutr.*, **15**:133–43, 1964.

Wacker, W. E. C., and Parisi, A. F.: "Magnesium Metabolism," *N. Engl. J. Med.*, **278**:658–63; 712–17; 772–76, 1968.

Zinc

Henkin, R. I.: "Zinc in Wound Healing," *N. Engl. J. Med.*, **291**:675–76, 1974.

Mills, C. F., *et al.*: "Metabolic Role of Zinc," *Am. J. Clin. Nutr.*, **22**:1240–49, 1969.

Murphy, E. W., *et al.*: "Provisional Tables on the Zinc Content of Foods," *J. Am. Diet. Assoc.*, **66**:345–55, 1975.

Prasad, A. S., ed.: *Zinc Metabolism*. Charles C Thomas, Springfield, Ill., 1966.

Review: "Growth and Zinc Deficiency," *Nutr. Rev.*, **31**:145–46, 1973.

Review: "Zinc in Hair as a Measure of the Zinc Nutriture of Human Beings," *Nutr. Rev.*, **28**:209–11, 1970.

Review: "Zinc Availability in Leavened and Unleavened Bread," *Nutr. Rev.*, **33**:18–19, 1975.

Sandstead, H. H.: "Zinc Nutrition in the United States," *Am. J. Clin. Nutr.*, **26**:1251–60, 1973.

Smith, J. C., *et al.*: "Zinc: A Trace Element Essential in Vitamin A Metabolism," *Science*, **181**:954–55, 1973.

Other Trace Elements

Carlisle, E. M.: "Silicon as an Essential Element," *Fed. Proc.*, **33**:1758–66, 1974.

Cohen, N. L., and Briggs, G. M.: "Trace Minerals in Nutrition," *Am. J. Nurs.*, **68**:807–11, 1968.

Hopkins, L. L., Jr., and Mohr, H. E.: "Vanadium as an Essential Nutrient," *Fed. Proc.*, **33**:1773–75, 1974.

Krehl, W. A.: "Mercury, the Slippery Metal," *Nutr. Today*, **7**:4–15, Nov. 1972.

Krehl, W. A.: "Selenium—the Maddening Mineral," *Nutr. Today*, **5**:26–32, Winter 1970.

Margen, S., and King, J. C.: "Effect of Oral Contraceptive Agents on the Metabolism of Some Trace Elements," *Am. J. Clin. Nutr.*, **28**:392–402, 1975.

Mertz, W.: "Recommended Dietary Allowances Up to Date—Trace Minerals," *J. Am. Diet. Assoc.*, **64**:163–67, 1974.

Morris, V. C., and Levander, O. A.: "Selenium Content of Foods," *J. Nutr.*, **100**:1383–88, 1970.

Nielsen, F. H., and Ollerich, D. A.: "Nickel: A New Essential Trace Element," *Fed. Proc.*, **33**:1767–72, 1974.

Nielsen, F. H., and Sandstead, H. H.: "Are Nickel, Vanadium, Silicon, Fluorine, and Tin Essential for Man? A Review," *Am. J. Clin. Nutr.*, **27**:515–20, 1974.

Review: "Does Lead Make Children Hyperactive?" *Nutr. Rev.*, **31**:88–90, 1973.

Schroeder, H. A., *et al.*: "Essential Trace Metals in Man: Manganese. A Study in Homeostasis," *J. Chron. Dis.*, **19**:545–71, 1966.

Schroeder, H. A., *et al.*: "Essential Trace Elements in Man: Molybdenum," *J. Chronic Dis.*, **23**:481–99, 1970.

Schwartz, K.: "Recent Dietary Trace Element Research Exemplified by Tin, Fluorine, and Silicon." *Fed. Proc.*, **33**:1748–57, 1974.

Scott, M. L.: "The Selenium Dilemma," *J. Nutr.*, **103**:803–10, 1973.

Underwood, E. J.: *Trace Elements in Human and Animal Nutrition*, 3rd ed. Academic Press, New York, 1971.

Underwood, E. J.: "Cobalt," *Nutr. Rev.*, **33**:65–69, 1975.

9 Fluid and Electrolyte Balance

The interchange that constantly takes place between the body and its external environment, and within the body between cells, tissues, and organs and their environment, is dependent upon the fluid medium that is precisely regulated in its volume, composition, and concentration. The electrolytes and nonelectrolytes held in solution in this aqueous medium maintain normal osmotic pressure relationships, control nervous irritability and muscle contraction, regulate acid-base balance, and facilitate movement of nutrients into cells and removal of wastes from cells.

This chapter includes a discussion of the role of water; the electrolyte composition of body fluids; three important electrolytes, namely, sodium, potassium, and chloride; the role of the kidney; mechanisms for fluid-electrolyte balance; and acid-base balance.

WATER

The body's need for water is second only to that for oxygen. One can live for weeks without food, but death is likely to follow a deprivation of water for more than a few days. A 10 per cent loss of body water is a serious hazard, and death usually follows a 20 per cent loss.

Distribution. Water makes up 50 to 70 per cent of the weight of the human body. Lean individuals have a higher percentage of body water than do obese individuals. Also, men have a higher propor-

tion of body water than women inasmuch as even women of normal weight have more adipose tissue.

All body tissues contain water, but the variations in tissue contents are wide. For example, the approximate percentage of water in teeth is 5; fat and bone, 25; and striated muscle, 80.

Fluid compartments. Body fluids exist in two so-called compartments that are disseminated throughout the entire body. The INTRACELLULAR FLUID is that which exists within the cells. It accounts for about 45 per cent of body weight. The EXTRACELLULAR FLUID is subdivided as follows: (1) the plasma fluid, accounting for 5 per cent of body weight, which contains protein as well as numerous substances that easily penetrate the capillary membrane; and (2) the interstitial fluid, representing about 15 per cent of body weight, which is similar to plasma fluid except in its much lower concentration of protein. Also included in the extracellular fluids are the lymph circulation and secretions such as those of the lacrimal glands, pancreas, liver, gastrointestinal mucosa, and others. (See Figure 9–1.)

Functions. Most of the many functions of water are self-evident. Water is a structural component and a cushion of all cells. Each gram of protein holds about 4 gm water, and each gram of fat is associated with about 0.2 gm water. In some instances, as in bone, water is tightly bound, but in most tissues a constant interchange between intracellular and extracellular fluid is occurring in order to maintain osmotic pressure relationships.

Water is the medium of all body fluids including the digestive juices, the lymph, the blood, the urine, and the perspiration. All the physiochemical changes that occur in the cells of the body take place in the precisely regulated environment of the body fluids. Water enters into many essential reactions, such as hydrolysis that occurs in digestion. In oxidation-reduction reactions water is often the end product as in the oxidation of glucose.

Water is a solvent for the products of digestion, holding them in solution and permitting them to pass through the absorbing walls of the intestinal tract into the bloodstream. Because nutrients and cellular wastes are soluble in water, it is the means whereby nutrients are carried to the cells and wastes are removed to the lungs, kidney, gut, and skin. The metabolic wastes are diluted by water, thereby preventing cellular injury.

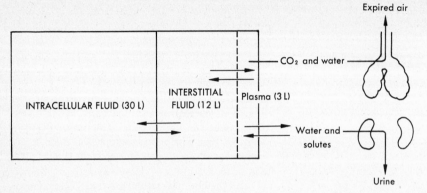

Figure 9–1. Fluid compartments of the body, and interchanges from one compartment to another.

Water regulates body temperature by taking up the heat produced in cellular reactions and distributing it throughout the body. About 25 per cent of the heat lost from the body occurs by evaporation from the lungs and skin. Each liter of water lost in perspiration represents a heat loss of about 600 kcal. When there is an increase in body temperature, centers in the hypothalamus stimulate increased sweating and hence greater evaporation and loss of body heat.

Water is essential as a body lubricant: the saliva that makes possible the swallowing of food; the mucous secretions of the gastrointestinal, respiratory, and genitourinary tracts; the fluids that bathe the joints; and so on.

Sources of water to the body. Water to meet the body's needs is supplied by (1) the ingestion of water and beverages, (2) the preformed water in foods, and (3) the water resulting from the oxidation of foodstuffs.

As may be seen below, water is the principal constituent by weight of almost all foods, pure sugars and fats being the important exceptions.

	Per Cent Water
Milk	87
Eggs	75
Meat, well done	40
Meat, rare	75
Fruits, vegetables	70–95
Cereals, ready to eat	1–5
Cereals, cooked	80–88
Breads	35

The oxidation of glucose, fatty acids, and amino acids yields water; for example:

$$C_6H_{12}O_6 + 6\,O_2 \rightarrow 6\,H_2O + 6\,CO_2$$

The following amounts of water are produced in the oxidation of foodstuffs:

	ml Water
100 gm fat	107
100 gm carbohydrate	56
100 gm protein	41

Using these equivalents, the water of oxidation for a 2100-kcal diet consisting of 80 gm protein, 90 gm fat, and 220 gm carbohydrate is approximately 250 ml.

Daily losses of water. The daily losses of water include:

	ml
Feces	100–200
Urine	1000–1500
Lungs	250–400
Insensible perspiration	400–600
Visible perspiration	None to 10,000

Some losses of water are OBLIGATORY, that is, they are essential for the maintenance of physicochemical equilibrium. The losses in the feces, through the lungs, and in the insensible perspiration occur regardless of intake.

Renal losses. The amount of water loss from the kidney that is obligatory depends upon the amount of wastes that must be dissolved. Under normal circumstances it is about 600 ml. Urea and sodium chloride are the principal solids that are excreted, and thus any reduction in their production will correspondingly reduce the obligatory loss of water in the urine. A diet that is high in carbohydrate to minimize tissue catabolism and low in protein is one that reduces the formation of urea and thus will spare body water. FACULTATIVE WATER EXCRETION by the kidney is in addition to the obligatory losses, and varies according to body needs.

Skin. Insensible perspiration accounts for a relatively constant amount of water loss that is proportional to the surface area of the body. It is so called because the evaporation takes place from the skin immediately and the water loss is not noticeable. This evaporation is an important means by which body temperature is maintained. An infant weighing 10 pounds or so has a surface area that is about one third that of the adult, and thus the infant is much more vulnerable to water losses from the skin and rapid changes in body temperature.

The water losses by visible perspiration are highly variable, ranging from zero in cool weather to several liters during very warm weather under conditions of strenuous activity. Whenever a great deal of water is lost by perspiration, body water is conserved by the elimination of a much more concentrated urine.

Lungs. Air expired from the lungs also contains water. Any condition that would increase the rate of respiration—for example, fever—likewise increases the water loss by this route. The individual engaged in vigorous activity will lose more water by this route than the one who is sedentary.

Requirement. The 24-hour water requirement is that amount that replaces the losses by the kidneys, lungs, skin, and bowel. Ordinarily, thirst is an accurate guide to supplying the necessary amounts of water. Under ideal conditions including a low-solute diet, a minimum of physical activity, and absence of sweating, the water need for the adult is about 1.5 liters from beverages, food, and water of oxidation.

Although conditions are variable, the daily requirement is about 1 ml per kilocalorie for adults and 1.5 ml per kilocalorie for infants.

Table 9–1 illustrates a typical balance between water intake and water losses from the body. The mechanisms for the regulation of fluid balance and some of the problems of imbalance are discussed on pages 136 through 138.

ELECTROLYTES

Definitions and measurement. An ION is an atom or group of atoms that carries an electrical charge. CATIONS (Na^+, K^+, Ca^{++}, Mg^{++}) carry positive electrical charges; they are electron donors. ANIONS (Cl^-, HCO_3^-, HPO_4^{--}, SO_4^{--}) carry negative electrical charges; they are electron acceptors. In any solution the total cations are exactly equal to the total anions.

An ELECTROLYTE is any substance that dissociates into its component ions when dissolved in water. It is so named because an electrical current can be transmitted by a solution containing any one of these substances. The dissociation for a given substance is constant, but the degree of dissociation varies widely from one substance to another. Strong electrolytes are those substances such as inorganic acids or bases that dissociate almost completely.

The concentrations of physiologic solutions are expressed, and most easily compared, in milliequivalents (mEq) rather than in weights per 100 ml or per liter. A MILLIEQUIVALENT is the weight in milligrams of an element that combines with or replaces 1 mg of hydrogen. Snively and Brown[2] used a dance analogy to describe this concept. For a dance one would invite equal numbers of boys and girls—not 1400 pounds of boys and 1400 pounds of girls. It is the number of boys to pair off with girls that is

Table 9–1. Normal Water Balance for an Adult*

Available Water	gm	Excreted Water	gm
Water, coffee, tea, etc.	1200	In urine	1350
Water in foods, including milk	900	In stool	200
Water of oxidation	250	In vapor from lungs	400
Total	2350	From skin	400
		Total	2350

*Assumes light activity and no visible sweating.

important, not their weight. With an equal number of boys and girls, any boy could dance with any girl.

Likewise, with cations and anions; any cation can pair off with any anion. For example, 1 milliequivalent of sodium combines with 1 milliequivalent of chloride. Expressed in weight, 23 mg sodium have combined with 35 mg chloride. But 1 milliequivalent of potassium can also combine with 1 milliequivalent of chloride; in this instance, 39 mg potassium have combined with 35 mg chloride. Another example: calcium, with two positive charges, can pair off with two chloride ions; it can, instead, pair off with one phosphate ion, since phosphate carries two negative charges. Thus, it is the *chemical combining power* rather than the weights of the substances that is most convenient in measuring electrolyte concentrations. The calculation of milliequivalents of an electrolyte, when the concentration in milligrams is known, may be expressed as follows:

$$mEq/liter = \frac{mg\ per\ liter}{Equivalent\ weight}$$

$$Equivalent\ weight = \frac{Atomic\ weight}{Valence\ of\ the\ element}$$

Suppose the concentration of calcium in blood serum is 9.5 mg per 100 ml. Since the atomic weight of calcium is 40 and the valence is 2, the equivalent weight is $40 \div 2 = 20$.

$$mEq/liter = \frac{9.5 \times 10}{20} = 4.75$$

Electrolyte composition of body fluids. The electrolyte balance of the body is studied principally by determining the electrolyte concentrations in blood plasma. The electrolyte compositions of plasma and of cellular fluid are compared in Table 9–2. The electrolyte patterns for plasma and interstitial fluid are almost identical except for the much greater concentration of protein in the plasma. Note that within each fluid compartment the total milliequivalents of cations exactly balance the total milliequivalents of anions. There are remarkable differences in the electrolyte composition of plasma and intracellular fluid, yet the concentrations are such that osmotic balance is maintained. Because of the higher protein within the cell, the total of all electrolytes is higher than that in extracellular fluid. Each protein molecule carries eight negative charges thus combining with eight potassium ions;

Table 9–2. Electrolyte Composition of Body Fluids*

	Blood Plasma		Cellular Fluid
	mg per 100 ml	mEq per liter	mEq per liter
Cations			
Sodium (Na⁺)	327	142	10
Potassium (K⁺)	19	5	148
Calcium (Ca⁺⁺)	10	5	2
Magnesium (Mg⁺⁺)	3.6	3	40
Total cations		155	200
Anions			
Chloride (Cl⁻)	365	103	
Bicarbonate (HCO₃⁻)	165	27	8
Phosphate (HPO₄⁻⁻)	9.6	2	
including other nonprotein ions			136
Sulfate (SO₄⁻⁻)	4.8	1	
Organic acids⁻		6	
Proteinate⁻		16	56
Total anions		155	200

*Adapted from Tables 17–3 and 17–4 in West, E. S., *et al.*: *Textbook of Biochemistry,* 4th ed. Macmillan Publishing Co., Inc., New York, 1966, pp. 689, 690.

the protein molecule and the eight potassium ions would thus yield only nine osmotically active particles.

Extracellular fluid. Sodium accounts for over 90 per cent of the cations in plasma and interstitial fluid; potassium, magnesium, and calcium are found in very small, though physiologically important, concentrations. The principal anion of plasma is chloride; there are smaller concentrations of bicarbonate and proteinate and very small amounts of phosphate, sulfate, and organic acids.

Wide variations in electrolyte concentrations are found in the digestive juices. For example, in the acid gastric juice, the concentration of sodium is low, and that of chloride is high and is balanced by hydrogen ions. Intestinal juice and bile compare with plasma in their principal electrolytes.

Intracellular fluid. By contrast, potassium is the principal cation in intracellular fluid, with magnesium, sodium, and calcium accounting for the remainder. Phosphate as the organic phosphate in adenosine triphosphate, creatine phosphate, and sugar phosphate as well as inorganic phosphate is the principal balancing anion. Proteinate accounts for about one fourth of the anions in intracellular fluid, and the amounts of bicarbonate, chloride, and sulfate are small.

SODIUM

Throughout the history of man salt has occupied a unique position. Mosaic law prescribed the use of salt with offerings made to Jehovah, and there are frequent Biblical references to the purifying and flavoring effects of salt. Greek slaves were bought and sold with salt, and a good slave was said to be "worth his weight in salt." Because salt was scarce and greatly prized, the Via Salaria of Rome was a carefully guarded artery for the transport of salt. Salt served as a medium of exchange; thus the word *salary* from the Latin *salaria.* To own salt was a privilege, and royal banquet halls had imposing salt cellars. Important persons were invited to "sit above the salt" and those of lesser importance were seated "below the salt." Today salt is so commonplace that only those who are denied its free use give more than casual thought to it.

Distribution. About 50 per cent of the body's sodium is present in the extracellular fluid, 40 per cent in bone, and 10 per cent or less in intracellular fluid. Much of the sodium in bone is readily interchangeable with extracellular fluid, but some of it is located deeply in dense long bones. In terms of concentration, the sodium content of blood plasma is about 14 times that of intracellular fluid. (See Table 9–2.)

Functions. Sodium is the principal electrolyte in extracellular fluid for the maintenance of normal osmotic pressure and water balance. It is the largest component of the extracellular total base and supplies the alkalinity of the gastrointestinal secretions. It functions mutually with some and antagonistically with other ions in maintaining the normal irritability of nerve cells and the contraction of muscles, and in regulating the permeability of the cell membrane. The sodium "pump" maintains electrolyte differences between intracellular and extracellular fluid compartments. (See page 135.)

Metabolism. Most of the sodium in the diet is in the form of inorganic salts, principally sodium chloride. The absorption of sodium from the gastrointestinal tract is rapid and practically complete, there being only small amounts of sodium in the feces. The kidneys regulate the sodium level in the body. When the intake of sodium is high, the excretion is likewise high. But if the intake of sodium is low, the excretion of sodium is likewise decreased. An analysis of a 24-hour collection of urine is a good measure of the level of intake in the normal individual. When sodium is drastically restricted in the diet, the excretion of sodium by the normal kidney practically reaches the vanishing point, and sodium is almost completely conserved. The mechanisms for these controls will be discussed further on page 136.

The losses of sodium in perspiration depend upon the concentration and the total volume of sweat. In very warm weather the initial losses may be so high that the sodium depletion syndrome occurs unless compensation is made by increasing salt and fluid intake. With acclimatization there is a gradual reduction in the concentration of sodium in perspiration and hence the amount of sodium that will be lost through the skin. Concentrations of sodium in sweat ranging from 12 to 120 mEq per liter have been reported.[3]

Requirements. The average daily intake of salt is 6 to 15 gm, equivalent to 2500 to 6000 mg sodium.

This is far in excess of physiologic requirements and reflects the desire for salt. Some people desire so much salt that they add salt to food without even tasting it, whereas others prefer only a light salting of food. The exact requirements for sodium are not known, but in the absence of visible perspiration the need is very low. Patients who are consuming diets restricted to 500 mg sodium daily, or even less, have been able to maintain sodium balance.

Food sources. The principal source of sodium in the diet is sodium chloride by virtue of its universal use in food preservation, in cookery, and at the table. One teaspoon of salt contains almost 2000 mg sodium. The Basic Diet pattern (Table 13–2) furnishes about 500 mg sodium if all foods are prepared and cooked without the addition of salt or other sodium-containing compounds. About half of this is obtained from milk. Other naturally occurring sources of sodium are egg white, meat, poultry, fish, and certain salt-loving vegetables such as spinach, beets, celery, and chard. Most vegetables, fruits, cereals, and legumes are naturally low in sodium. Most drinking waters contain less than 20 mg sodium per liter, but in some areas the sodium content is considerably higher. (See also Table A–2).

Numerous sodium compounds other than salt are also used in food preparation and processing, and in many drugs: baking soda and baking powder; sodium alginate, sodium propionate, sodium citrate, sodium sulfite to enhance some quality of a food product.

Sodium imbalance. Epidemiologic studies have shown that hypertension occurs more frequently in populations such as the Japanese who have a high intake of salt throughout a lifetime.[4,5] The critical level at which salt intake becomes a high risk is not known. Any disturbance in the concentration of sodium in extracellular fluids has a serious effect on osmotic pressure and on acid-base balance.

In cardiac or renal failure the excretion of sodium is reduced. Consequently, sodium and fluids are retained in tissues and the condition is known as edema. An excessive excretion of cortical hormones, as by adrenal tumors, leads to increased retention of sodium. Likewise adrenocorticotropic hormone used therapeutically in a variety of conditions also increases the retention of sodium.

Excessive sodium losses during hot weather have already been mentioned. A deficiency of adrenocortical hormone that is characteristic of Addison's disease is characterized by such large losses of sodium that the patient hungers for salt.

In diarrhea and vomiting sodium is continuously drawn into the gastrointestinal tract, and ultimately the extracellular fluid is depleted of its normal sodium content.

POTASSIUM

Distribution. The total potassium content of the adult body is about 250 gm. Of this, about 97 per cent is within the tissue cells with the remainder being distributed in the extracellular fluid compartment. From Table 9–2 it may be seen that the concentration of potassium in cellular fluid is about 30 times that in the plasma.

Functions. Potassium is an obligatory component of all cells and increases in proportion to the increase in the body's cell mass. Because a fixed proportion of potassium is bound to protein, the measurement of body potassium is often used to determine the total lean body mass.

Within the cell potassium is the principal cation for the maintenance of osmotic pressure and fluid balance, just as sodium is the principal cation in extracellular fluid.

Potassium is required for enzymatic reactions taking place within the cell. Some potassium is bound to phosphate and is required for the conversion of glucose to glycogen; this potassium is released during glycogenolysis.

The small concentration of potassium in extracellular fluid is essential, together with other ions, for the transmission of the nerve impulse and for contraction of muscle fibers.

Metabolism. Potassium is readily absorbed from the gastrointestinal tract. Although the digestive juices contain relatively large amounts of potassium, most of this is reabsorbed and the losses in the feces are small.

Under conditions of protein synthesis, glycogen formation, and cellular hydration, potassium is rapidly removed from the circulation. With the removal of sodium from the cell to the extracellular fluid by the sodium pump, potassium ions move in, thus balancing the cations between the fluid compartments. Potassium leaves the cell during protein catabolism, dehydration, or glycogenolysis.

Excess potassium is excreted by the kidney. Aldosterone secretion increases potassium excretion. Although the normal kidney readily excretes excess potassium, the ability to conserve potassium in the face of a deficit is much less rigid than that for sodium. Even in the absence of any potassium intake and with low tissue levels, the urinary losses may be 15 to 30 mEq per day.[6]

Requirements. The exact requirements for potassium are not known, but on the basis of obligatory losses it is estimated that 1 to 3 mEq per kilogram per day will suffice. The daily intake on typical diets far exceeds this level.

Food sources. Because potassium is widely distributed in foods, the daily intake increases as the caloric intake increases. Typical diets furnish 50 to 150 mEq (2 to 6 gm) daily.[1] Meats, poultry, and fish are good sources. Fruits, vegetables, and whole-grain cereals are especially high in potassium. Bananas, potatoes, tomatoes, carrots, celery, oranges, and grapefruit are rich sources. (See Table A–2 for potassium values in foods.)

Potassium deficiency. Potassium deficiency is not primarily of dietary origin but there are numerous circumstances under which it can occur. One of these is defective food intake such as that in severe malnutrition, chronic alcoholism, anorexia nervosa, or some illness that seriously interferes with the appetite. Any condition that reduces the availability of nutrients for absorption can lead to potassium depletion: for example, prolonged vomiting, gastric drainage, and diarrhea. Adrenal tumors that increase aldosterone secretion lead to potassium loss. Losses may exceed replacement in severe tissue injury, following surgery, in burns, and during prolonged fevers. Some therapeutic measures may also initiate potassium deficiency: for example, prolonged parenteral feeding without potassium in the parenteral fluids; excessive adrenocortical steroid therapy; or halogenated thiazide diuretics used in the treatment of hypertension and edema. Rapid infusions of glucose and insulin in diabetic acidosis bring about such rapid shifts of potassium into the cell that the plasma potassium levels may be reduced to levels that could bring about cardiac failure.

Potassium deficiency is characterized by low plasma levels of potassium (hypopotassemia or hypokalemia). The symptoms of deficiency include nausea, vomiting, listlessness, apprehension, muscle weakness, paralytic ileus, hypotension, tachycardia,

arrhythmia, and an altered electrocardiogram. The heart may stop in diastole.

Potassium excess. Hyperpotassemia (hyperkalemia) is a frequent complication in renal failure, in severe dehydration, following too rapid parenteral administration of potassium, and in adrenal insufficiency. Hyperkalemia is characterized by paresthesias of the scalp, face, tongue, and extremities; muscle weakness; poor respiration; cardiac arrhythmia; and changes in the electrocardiogram. Cardiac failure may follow with the heart stopping in systole. Hyperkalemia is corrected by using a low-potassium, low-protein, liberal-carbohydrate diet. Carbohydrate intake results in the formation of glycogen and the movement of potassium into the cells.

CHLORIDE

Distribution. Chlorine exists in the body almost entirely as the chloride ion. Most of the 100 gm or so of chloride in the body is present in the extracellular fluid but it also occurs to some extent in the red blood cells and to a lesser degree in other cells.

Functions. Chloride accounts for two thirds of the total anions of extracellular fluid. It is important in the regulation of osmotic pressure, water balance, and acid-base balance. It is the chief anion of gastric juice and is accompanied by the hydrogen ion rather than the sodium ion, thus providing the acid medium for the activation of the gastric enzymes and the digestion in the stomach. Chloride is one of several activators of salivary amylase.

Metabolism. For the secretion of gastric juice chloride is withdrawn from the blood circulation, and changes in dietary intake do not modify its production. The gastric juice mixes with foods and moves along the intestinal tract. The chloride from foods and that from the gastric juice is readily absorbed into the circulation.

The CHLORIDE SHIFT between the red blood cells and the plasma is a mechanism whereby changes in pH are minimized. When the blood reaches the lungs, the blood CO_2 tension is decreased, the bicarbonate ions in the red blood cells decrease, bicarbonate ions move from the plasma into the cells, and chloride and OH ions move from the cells into the plasma. When the blood returns to the tissues, the partial pressure of CO_2 increases and these ionic shifts are reversed.

Chloride, like other ions, is filtered by the glomerulus and selectively reabsorbed from the renal tubules. Excess chloride is readily excreted. The chloride excretion usually parallels the excretion of sodium, but when it is essential to conserve sodium the kidney will substitute the ammonium ion. Sweat and feces contain variable amounts of chloride accompanied by sodium or potassium.

Dietary intake. The requirement for chloride has not been determined, but the liberal intake of sodium chloride assures more than adequate intake under normal circumstances. Most of the chloride ingested is from the salt used in food processing and preparation.

Chloride imbalance. Severe vomiting, drainage, or diarrhea leads to large losses of chloride and an alkalosis because of the replacement of chloride with bicarbonate.

ROLE OF THE KIDNEY

Structural unit. The NEPHRON, of which there are approximately one million in each kidney, is the functioning unit of the kidney. (See Figure 9–2.) Each nephron consists of the GLOMERULUS, which is a tuft of capillaries surrounded by a capsule (Bowman's capsule), and a TUBULE, including (1) the proximal convoluted tubule, (2) the loop of Henle, and (3) the distal convoluted tubule. The nephrons finally empty into collecting tubules.

Blood flows into the glomerulus through an *afferent arteriole* and leaves through an *efferent arteriole* and then flows through a system of *peritubular capillaries* that surround the tubules.

Functions of the kidney. Every meal we eat would seriously upset metabolic balances were it not for the function of the kidneys. The primary function of the kidneys is to maintain the constant composition and volume of the blood. This includes the regulation of (1) the osmotic pressure, (2) the electrolyte and water balance, and (3) the acid-base balance. By regulation of the composition of the blood, homeostasis in the interstitial and intracellular fluid compartments of the body is achieved.

The production of urine permits the elimination of excess water and solutes such as sodium, chloride,

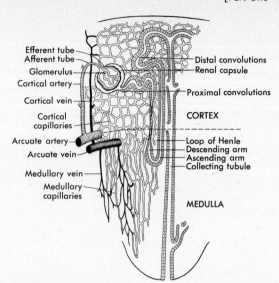

Figure 9–2. The nephron is the functioning unit of the kidney. (Courtesy, Leavell, L. C., and Miller, M. A.: *Anatomy and Physiology,* 15th ed. Macmillan Publishing Co., Inc., New York, 1966.)

and others, the by-products of metabolism such as urea, and ingested substances that may be toxic.

Glomerular filtration. About 1200 ml of blood flow through the kidneys each minute, this being about one fourth of the total cardiac output. The total amount of glomerular filtrate produced is about 125 ml per minute for a 24-hour total of 180 liters. The glomerular filtrate has essentially the same composition as the blood plasma except that it contains no protein or other large colloidal particles.

FILTRATION is the movement of fluid and solutes through a membrane when the pressure on one side is greater than on the other. The blood pressure in the glomerular capillary is 90 mm mercury (Hg). This is opposed by the colloidal osmotic pressure of the plasma proteins equal to 25 mm Hg and the hydrostatic pressure of the tubular fluid equal to 15 mm Hg. Thus, the net pressure in the glomerular capillary of 50 mmg Hg pushes the fluid into the tubule.[7] (See Figure 9–3.)

The many branching capillaries in the glomerulus reduce the rate of renal flow, thus promoting filtration. These capillary branches unite to form the efferent arteriole, which has a much smaller diameter. This further resists flow and increases filtration.

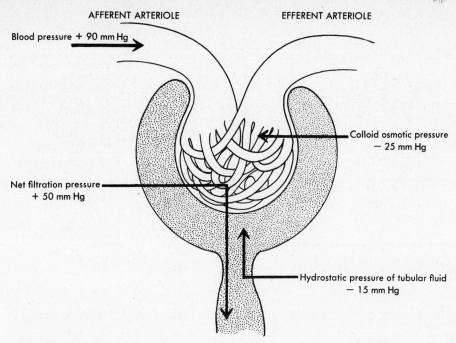

AFFERENT ARTERIOLE   EFFERENT ARTERIOLE

Blood pressure + 90 mm Hg

Colloid osmotic pressure
— 25 mm Hg

Net filtration pressure
+ 50 mm Hg

Hydrostatic pressure of tubular fluid
— 15 mm Hg

Figure 9–3. The blood pressure is opposed by the osmotic pressure and the hydrostatic pressure. The net filtration pressure of 50 mm Hg leads to filtration of fluid and solutes through the membrane into the tubule.

Functions of the tubules. There are two broad functions of the tubules: (1) selective reabsorption, and (2) secretion. If it were not for reabsorption from the tubules the body would lose all of its water, sodium, bicarbonate, glucose, and other filtered substances within half an hour and death would ensue.

As the glomerular filtrate moves through the proximal convoluted tubule, all of the glucose, amino acids, acetoacetic acid, and a number of other substances are reabsorbed if blood levels are within normal limits. For example, when glucose loads in the blood are within normal limits, all the glucose will be reabsorbed. Only when glucose levels in the blood exceed normal limits—as in diabetes mellitus—is some glucose not reabsorbed.

About 80 per cent of the water and electrolytes are reabsorbed from the proximal tubule. Since the tubular epithelium is almost impermeable to waste products such as urea, these substances continue to pass along the tubule.

By the time the filtrate has reached Henle's loop,

marked changes in composition have occurred. Most of the remaining sodium and some of the remaining water are reabsorbed into the circulation from Henle's loop.

About 3 per cent of the electrolytes and 13 per cent of the water still remain in the filtrate that reaches the distal convoluted tubule. At this point the final adjustments in the concentration of water and solutes are made by mechanisms that are described in more detail on page 136. (See Figure 9–4.)

Energy requirements. Only the liver exceeds the kidney in its metabolic activities. Water and urea move across the membranes by passive diffusion, which does not require energy. However, most substances are reabsorbed by active transport, thus entailing considerable energy expenditure. Fatty acids are the principal source of energy in the aerobic oxidations occurring in the cortex, but glucose, fructose, and other substrates can also be oxidized. In the renal medulla oxidation is principally by anaerobic glycolytic pathway, glucose being the chief substrate. (See page 68.)

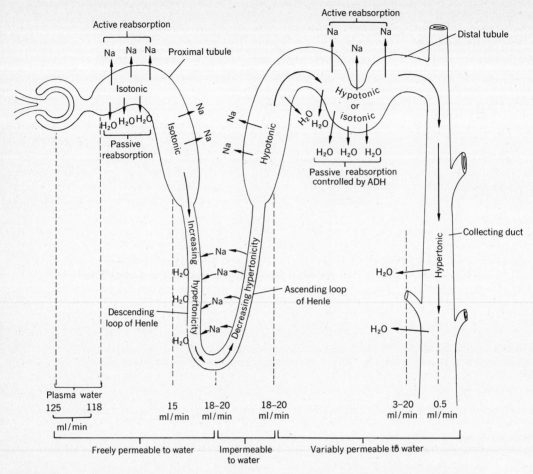

Figure 9-4. Function of the nephron in adjusting the reabsorption of sodium and water, and the formation of urine. (Courtesy, Pansky, B.: *Dynamic Anatomy and Physiology.* Macmillan Publishing Co., Inc., New York, 1975.)

Secretory activities. The final control of acid-base balance is brought about by the distal portion of the tubule. Hydrogen ions are continually released from carbonic acid by the action of carbonic anhydrase into the tubules. The tubules synthesize ammonia (NH_3), which combines with the hydrogen ions to form the ammonium (NH_4^+) ion, thus releasing bicarbonate ions to the blood, thereby replacing the alkaline reserve.

Recently it has been found that the final stage in the conversion of vitamin D to the metabolically active 1,25-dihydroxyvitamin D_3 takes place in the renal tubule. (See page 156.)

Composition of urine. As the glomerular filtrate passes through the tubules, the metabolic wastes—unlike water and electrolytes—are poorly reabsorbed. Their concentration therefore increases as the filtrate moves along the tubules with the resultant formation of urine. Urine consists of about 95 per cent water and 5 per cent solids. The kidney can produce a urine varying in specific gravity from about 1.008 to 1.035 depending upon the proportions of water and solids to be excreted. The average daily excretion of solids is about 50 to 70 gm, with three fifths of this being nitrogenous and two fifths inorganic salts. Urea is the predominating nitrogenous substance in the urine, along with much smaller amounts of uric acid, ammonia, and creatinine. (See Table A–12.)

Inorganic ions in the urine include Na^+, K^+, Ca^{++}, Mg^{++}, Cl^-, SO_4^{--}, and PO_4^{--}. These are not true wastes inasmuch as they are essential to cellular function. They are excreted only when they are in excess of body needs, and the quantity excreted depends upon dietary intake.

With an increase in solid wastes, the fluid required for their excretion would also be increased. Among the situations in which increased solid wastes are produced are the following: (1) protein intake in excess of tissue needs so that large amounts of amino acids are deaminized and the urea production is increased; (2) increased tissue catabolism following any stress such as surgery, injury, burns, or fever; and (3) increased intake of salt. Whenever the kidney is unable to concentrate urine, the fluid requirement for excretion of wastes is greatly increased.

REGULATION OF FLUID AND ELECTROLYTE BALANCE

Fluid exchange. Although the sources of water to the body and the losses from the body are in balance, the fluid exchanges that take place in a 24-hour period are of tremendous magnitude and impressive in the precision of their regulation. For the digestive process alone the estimated daily volume of fluid that enters and leaves the gastrointestinal tract is estimated to be about 10 liters and is made up of the following:[8]

	ml
Water intake as beverage and in food	2,000
Saliva	1,500
Gastric juice	2,500
Bile	500
Intestinal juice	3,000
Pancreatic juice	700
	10,200

The fluid exchanges between the gastrointestinal tract and the blood circulation are variable from hour to hour; yet they are so balanced that normally the volume of the blood and the fluids within the tract are in equilibrium. Inasmuch as the daily losses from the bowel are no more than 100 to 200 ml, it is evident that the outpouring of digestive juices into the intestinal tract is continuously balanced by the reabsorption of water from the gut. That the kidneys are highly efficient conservators of body water has been pointed out on page 133. The magnitude of water exchange that occurs between the blood circulation, the interstitial fluid, the lymph vessels, and the cells is no doubt very great.

Factors influencing fluid and electrolyte balance. The movements of water and solutes from one compartment to another are influenced by many factors: (1) the permeability of membranes to water and other substances; (2) the hydrostatic pressure within the capillaries; (3) the colloid osmotic pressure exerted by large molecules such as proteins; (4) the osmotic effect of electrolytes in the fluids of extracellular and intracellular fluids; (5) the lymph flow; (6) the mechanisms for active transport; (7) the competition of substances for carriers to transport materials across cell membranes; and (8) the hormonal and nervous controls influencing each of these factors.

The transport of most solutes across cell membranes has been described on page 23. Water can move in and out of cells by OSMOSIS, which is the passage of fluid from the less concentrated to the more concentrated side of the membrane. Osmotic pressure is the difference in the force exerted on each side of the membrane. Thus, the solution that is more concentrated exerts a pull on the water in the more dilute solution.

Sodium has little effect on the osmotic pressure between the capillaries and the interstitial fluid because its concentration in the two fluids is about equal. However, sodium is the principal cation in intercellular fluid and potassium in intracellular fluid so that these electrolytes effect important osmotic controls between these fluid compartments. A reduction of extracellular sodium, for example, results in the entrance of fluid into the cell, whereas an increase in extracellular sodium results in the withdrawal of fluid from the cell.

Proteins are large molecules that form colloidal (gluelike) solutions. They cannot pass through membranes and exert COLLOIDAL OSMOTIC PRESSURE within the blood vessels. Plasma albumin is the principal force that maintains fluid equilibrium between the interstitial fluid and the plasma. The plasma albumin exerts a constant pull of fluid from the interstitial fluid to the plasma. Thus, the colloid osmotic pressure opposes and balances the flow of materials out of the capillaries that is exerted by filtration pressure. When the concentration of plasma albumin is reduced, the osmotic pressure is reduced and the fluid remains in the tissue spaces; this is sometimes referred to as "nutritional edema." (See Figure 9-3.)

Mechanisms for the regulation of water balance. The sensation of thirst is one means whereby the body meets its water need. When the ionic concentration of the extracellular fluid is increased, the cells in the *drinking center* of the hypothalamus become dehydrated and the desire to drink water is initiated.

Water reabsorption from the renal tubule is modified according to the extracellular fluid concentration. This depends upon the *osmoreceptor system*, which is effective in two ways. One of these is the change in osmotic pressure that occurs in the interstitial fluid of the renal medulla. The loops of Henle of the renal tubules extend into the medulla. Because rapid, active absorption of sodium and chloride occurs, the interstitial fluid of the medulla has a high concentration of sodium and chloride and hence exerts increased osmotic pressure. As the tubular fluid passes into the collecting ducts located in the medulla, water is rapidly absorbed from the ducts.[9]

Water reabsorption by the tubules is also controlled by the secretion of antidiuretic hormone by the posterior pituitary gland. Osmoreceptors especially in the supraoptic nuclei of the hypothalamus are sensitive to increases in the osmolarity of the extracellular fluid. Under conditions of increased concentration, impulses are initiated that stimulate production of ADH. The hormone enters the circulation and passes to the kidney where it increases the permeability of the distal and collecting tubules so that the amount of water that is reabsorbed is greatly increased. If the concentration of electrolytes is low, no stimulation of the osmoreceptors occurs and hence the hormone is not produced. The cell permeability is then decreased so that more water will be excreted, thereby restoring normal electrolyte concentration. (See Figure 9-5.)

Regulation of ionic balance. The regulation of sodium concentration in the extracellular fluid is better understood than that of other ions, but it is believed that the mechanisms that control the concentrations of other electrolytes are similar. These mechanisms are under nervous and hormonal control.

A low concentration of sodium in the extracellular fluid stimulates the secretion of aldosterone and, to a lesser extent, other mineralocorticoids by the adrenal cortex. The sequence for the stimulation of the adrenal is believed to be as follows: with a drop in blood pressure of the juxtaglomerular cells, the kidney is stimulated to produce RENIN, an enzyme,

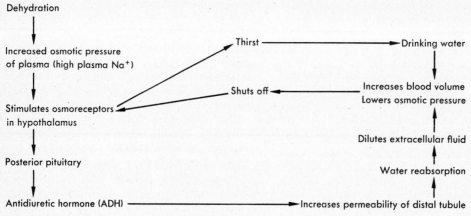

Figure 9-5. The regulation of water balance by thirst and antidiuretic hormone mechanisms.

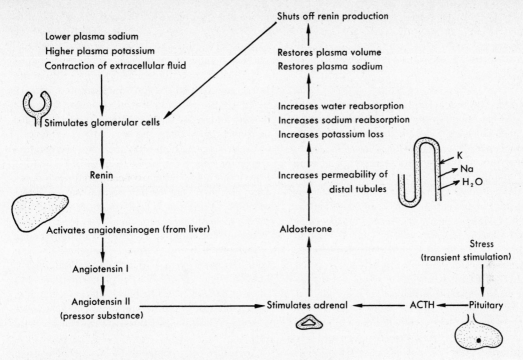

Lower plasma sodium
Higher plasma potassium
Contraction of extracellular fluid

Stimulates glomerular cells

Renin

Activates angiotensinogen (from liver)

Angiotensin I

Angiotensin II
(pressor substance)

Shuts off renin production

Restores plasma volume
Restores plasma sodium

Increases water reabsorption
Increases sodium reabsorption
Increases potassium loss

Increases permeability of
distal tubules

K
Na
H₂O

Aldosterone

Stress
(transient stimulation)

Stimulates adrenal ← ACTH ← Pituitary

Figure 9–6. The regulation of sodium concentration in extracellular fluid.

which in turn acts on a globulin substance in blood, ANGIOTENSINOGEN, to convert it to ANGIOTENSIN I, an inactive substance. An enzyme in the plasma converts angiotensin I to angiotensin II; the latter substance in the blood circulation stimulates the production of aldosterone by the adrenal cortex. Upon reaching the renal circulation, aldosterone increases the permeability of the distal and collecting tubules so that more sodium is reabsorbed into the peritubular capillaries. When the extracellular sodium concentration is high, the adrenal cortex stops secreting aldosterone, and thus greater amounts of sodium will be excreted. When sodium is reabsorbed it carries positive electrical charges which draw negative ions, principally chloride, through the tubular membrane. Thus, the reabsorption of chloride closely parallels that of sodium. (See Figure 9–6.)

Potassium ions are passively secreted into the distal and collecting tubules. This secretion is greater when the potassium content of the extracellular fluid is high. The retention of sodium under the influence of aldosterone is accompanied by an increased loss of potassium.

Fluid imbalance. A deficiency of fluid may occur because of inadequate intake, or abnormal loss, or a combination of the two. Abnormal loss of water occurs from prolonged vomiting, hemorrhage, diarrhea, protracted fevers, burns, excessive perspiration, drainage from wounds, and so on. It leads to decrease in peristaltic action, reduced blood volume, poor absorption of nutrients, impairment of renal function, and circulatory failure. Loss of fluid is accompanied by electrolyte losses as well. Thus, the adjustment of fluid balance requires also the consideration of electrolyte concentration.

In some pathologic conditions the body is in *positive* water balance; that is, the intake of fluids is greater than the excretion, and the patient is said to have an *edema*. The effect of the lowered plasma albumin has been mentioned (see page 135). Congestive heart failure, cirrhosis of the liver, nephritis, and nephrosis are examples of cardiovascular and renal disturbances in which sodium excretion is reduced, thereby contributing to the retention of water.

ACID-BASE BALANCE

Acid-base balance refers to the regulation of the hydrogen ion concentration of body fluids. Normal metabolic processes result in the continuous production of acids that must be eliminated. On a given day, the equivalent of 20 to 40 liters of 1 N acid are eliminated by the lungs and 50 to 150 ml 1 N acid are excreted by the kidney.[10] The mechanisms for maintaining body neutrality are so efficient that the healthy individual does not need to give any thought whatsoever to the nature of his diet insofar as acid-producing or alkali-producing elements are concerned.

Many pathologic conditions, however, are characterized by serious disturbances in acid-base balance: for example, acidosis in uncontrolled diabetes mellitus, following severe dehydration, and in renal failure. Through the study of physiology and biochemistry the student has gained an understanding of electrolyte and fluid balance, the chemistry of respiration, and the regulation of acid-base balance. The scope of this text and the limitations of space permit only a brief summary of this important subject. Several references at the end of the chapter may be consulted by the student who desires a review or more extensive study.

Definitions and measurement. An ACID is a substance that gives off or donates protons (H$^+$ ions); a BASE is a substance that combines with or accepts protons. For example, HCl, a *strong* acid, dissociates almost completely in water to H$^+$ and Cl$^-$; the chloride ion is a very *weak* base because it has practically no capacity for combining with the hydrogen ions in the solution. Carbonic acid (H_2CO_3) is a *weak* acid; it dissociates only slightly in solution to H$^+$ and HCO_3^-. The bicarbonate ion is a relatively *strong* base because it combines readily with hydrogen ions to form a weak acid.

The acidity of a fluid is measured by its concentration of hydrogen ions; the greater the concentration of hydrogen ions, the greater the acidity. The weight of hydrogen ions in a liter of plasma is exceedingly small, and concentrations would be expressed as decimal fractions or as negative exponents, for example, $10^{-7.45}$ mole H$^+$ per liter. In order to avoid this cumbersome designation, the symbol pH is used. The PH is a logarithmic function of the actual hydrogen ion concentration, and a pH difference of one unit represents a tenfold difference in the actual hydrogen ion concentrations. Thus, a pH of 4 represents a hydrogen ion concentration of 0.0001, and a pH of 5 represents a hydrogen ion concentration of 0.00001.

In an aqueous solution at room temperature where the concentration of hydrogen ions and hydroxyl ions is equal, the pH is designated as 7.0 and the solution is said to be "neutral." An alkaline reaction is expressed as a pH above 7.0—for example, 7.1. With increasing acidity, the pH value decreases; for example, a pH of 6.9 is slightly acid.

The pH of blood plasma is maintained within very narrow limits of 7.35 to 7.45—a slightly alkaline reaction. The extremes of pH compatible with life are 6.8 and 7.8; obviously, at these extremes individuals are very ill and prompt therapeutic measures must be instituted if the person is to survive.

Acids formed in metabolism. The principal end products of metabolic activities are acid, chiefly carbonic acid. The oxidation of carbohydrates, fatty acids, and amino acids in the Krebs cycle (see page 70) yields carbon dioxide and water; carbonic acid is the hydrated form of carbon dioxide. Intermediate products in metabolism are also acid, such as lactic and pyruvic acid formed in carbohydrate metabolism, keto acids formed in fatty acid oxidation, and amino acids resulting from the hydrolysis of proteins. Urea synthesis is an acid-producing process, and nucleoproteins give rise to uric acid. Sulfuric acid is formed in the body from the sulfur-containing amino acids and phosphoric acid from the phospholipids and phosphoproteins.

The reaction of foods. If the cations (Na$^+$, K$^+$, Mg^{++}, and Ca^{++}) remaining in the body on the metabolism of a food exceed the anions (PO_4^{--}, SO_4^{--}, and Cl$^-$), the food is said to produce an ALKALINE ASH and the excess cations will allow the body to retain more bicarbonate ions, thus producing an alkaline reaction. Vegetables, fruits, milk, and some nuts yield excess cations.

Meat, fish, poultry, eggs, cheese, cereals, and some nuts when metabolized yield an excess of anions that are not removed from the body immediately. These foods are said to produce an ACID ASH. The excess anions carrying a negative charge must be balanced approximately with some cations. This yields an acid reaction because less bicarbonate, which also carries a negative charge, can exist in the body. The excess bicarbonate ions form carbonic acid, increasing the acidity.

Fats, sugar, and starches contain no mineral elements and are metabolized quickly to carbon dioxide and water which are rapidly removed from the body. These foods, therefore, do not form excess cations or anions which would disturb the neutrality regulation.

Although lemons, oranges, and certain other fruits contain some free organic acids that give them a taste of acid (sour), they yield an alkaline ash because the body quickly oxidizes the anions of the acid to carbon dioxide and water and leave excess cations that are removed more slowly from the body. Plums, cranberries, and prunes contain aromatic organic acids that are not metabolized in the body, and therefore they increase the acidity of the body fluids.

The regulation of body neutrality. The reaction of the body fluids is kept within a narrow range by the following mechanisms:

1. Dilution is an important defense against the effects of the metabolic acids. The total volume of body fluid, representing about two thirds of body weight, is so great that the considerable amounts of carbon dioxide produced result in only a slight increase in the bicarbonate concentration because of the distribution throughout the fluid system.

2. Acid-base buffer systems are an important mechanism for the regulation of acid-base balance. A BUFFER is a substance that will react chemically with either acids or alkalies so that there is not a marked change in the pH of the solution. The buffers consist of weak acids and their sodium or potassium salts. The bicarbonate-carbonic acid (HCO_3^-/H_2CO_3) system is one important buffer of the blood in maintaining neutrality. The ease and speed with which the body can get rid of carbon dioxide obtained from this buffer mixture constitute one of the first lines of defense. The plasma bicarbonate is an indicator of the alkaline reserve of the body. Serious disturbances may occur if the alkaline reserve is depleted to a low level. Other buffer systems include:

$$\frac{Protein}{H.protein} \quad \frac{HPO_4^=}{H_2PO_4^-} \quad \frac{Hb^-}{HHb} \quad \frac{HbO_2^-}{HHbO_2}$$

3. Besides its buffer action hemoglobin aids in the transport of carbon dioxide in two ways which prevent great changes in reaction. The acid strength of hemoglobin is decreased when oxyhemoglobin loses oxygen whereby an extra amount of carbon dioxide can be transported without any change of reaction (isohydric transport). Hemoglobin can also transport a limited amount of carbon dioxide by forming a carbamate, which releases most of the carbon dioxide from the hemoglobin complex at the lung as the hemoglobin takes up oxygen.

4. The respiratory rate regulates the losses of carbon dioxide and the intake of oxygen. In one minute the resting individual will have lost about 200 cc carbon dioxide and absorbed about 250 cc oxygen. Any increase in activity will raise the exchange of gases taking place by a very large amount. This is accomplished by increasing the respiratory rate. If the hydrogen ion concentration is increased, the respiratory center in the brain causes an increase in the rate of pulmonary ventilation. The increased ventilation increases the loss of carbon dioxide, and the hydrogen ion concentration of the body fluids returns to normal. If the hydrogen ion concentration is lowered, the respiratory center is inhibited and the rate of ventilation is reduced; thus, the carbonic acid concentration of the body fluids rises.

5. The kidney makes the final adjustment that keeps the body pH within normal limits. The glomerular filtrate has a pH of 7.4, but the kidney can excrete a urine that is as acid as pH 4.5 or as alkaline as pH 8; normally, the average urine pH is 6.0. Bicarbonate ions are filtered into the tubular fluid and their loss from plasma represents loss of alkali. Hydrogen ions are secreted into the tubules, and their loss from plasma represents a loss of acid. When the hydrogen ions of the plasma are increased, the secretion of the hydrogen ions into the tubular fluid also increases and exceeds the loss of bicarbonate, thus permitting the return of plasma to its normal pH. The urine excreted is then more acid. Conversely, in alkalosis the hydrogen ion secretion into the tubules is decreased, thus allowing greater loss of bicarbonate. The urine then becomes more alkaline.

The kidney cannot excrete strong acids such as HCl and H_2SO_4. The hydrogen ions secreted into the lumen of the tubule are excreted by combining with disodium phosphate to form monosodium acid phosphate. By excreting practically all of the phosphate as acid phosphate ($H_2PO_4^-$, instead of HPO_4^{--}) only one phosphate is lost instead of two, thus reducing by half the number of milliequivalents of fixed anions that are excreted; this permits the return of more fixed anions to the circulation.

The kidney is also able to synthesize ammonia from glutamine and other amino acids. The ammonia combines with hydrogen ions to form the ammonium ion (NH_4^+), which can then replace cations such as sodium or potassium. The latter are exchanged for the hydrogen ions so that they can be returned to the blood to carry more carbon dioxide as the bicarbonate ion.

Acidosis and alkalosis. The acid-base balance of the body can be upset by an increase in hydrogen ions, a loss of hydrogen ions, an increase in base, or a loss of base. In each instance the treatment can be instituted only after evaluation of symptoms that are present, the determination of the carbon dioxide content of the blood plasma and the pH, and the cause of the imbalance. (See Figure 9–7.)

An ACIDOSIS is a condition in which the hydrogen ion concentration is increased or there is an excessive loss of base (mineral cations); the ratio of bicarbonate to carbonic acid is less than 20:1 and the pH is below 7.35. An ALKALOSIS is a condition in which the hydrogen ion concentration is decreased or the base is increased; the ratio of bicarbonate to carbonic acid is greater than 20:1, and the pH is above 7.45.

With changes in concentrations of hydrogen ions and base, the lungs and kidneys attempt to compensate. Ventilation by the lungs is increased when there is an increase in hydrogen ions, and the kidney attempts to adjust by excreting a more acid urine and conserving base with the synthesis of more ammonia. When there is an increase in base, the respiration is depressed, and the hydrogen ions are retained and more base is excreted by the kidneys. If these adjustments succeed in keeping the bicarbonate-carbonic acid ratio at 20:1, the pH remains at 7.35 to 7.45; the acidosis or alkalosis is said to be "compensated." When the pH is outside these limits, the acidosis or alkalosis is "uncompensated."

Respiratory acidosis or alkalosis results from an abnormality of the control of the normal CO_2 tension. Hypoventilation such as that seen in pneumonia, pulmonary edema, suppression of breathing as with morphine, and asphyxia lead to acidosis. The kidneys partially compensate by increasing the excretion of hydrogen ions and the synthesis of ammonia, thereby increasing the return of bicarbonate to the blood.

Respiratory alkalosis occurs when there is overventilation of the lungs so that excessive amounts of carbonic acid are lost. This may result from hysteria, from salicylate poisoning, in fevers and infections, and at high altitudes. By reducing the excretion of hydrogen ions and the synthesis of ammonia and by increasing the excretion of sodium, the kidneys compensate in part.

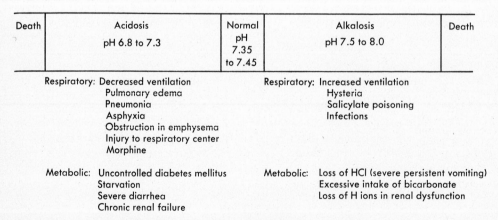

Figure 9–7. Normal and abnormal pH ranges in body fluids.

Metabolic acidosis or alkalosis refers to changes resulting from faulty intake or output of acids or bases other than carbonic acid. Metabolic acidosis occurs in a variety of circumstances: the rapid production of ketones in uncontrolled diabetes mellitus; the inability of the kidney to excrete acid phosphates in chronic renal failure; the ketosis of starvation; or the loss of bicarbonate and sodium that occurs with severe diarrhea. Ventilation of the lungs is greatly increased, and air hunger is characteristic of the patient in diabetic acidosis. The synthesis of ammonia by the kidney may increase tenfold in an effort to conserve base.

Metabolic alkalosis occurs when there is a severe loss of hydrochloric acid as a result of vomiting, or by the ingestion of soluble alkalinizing salts such as sodium bicarbonate.

SOME POINTS FOR EMPHASIS IN NUTRITION EDUCATION

1. Mineral elements perform varied and interrelated functions in the body. Among these functions are:

a. The hardness of bones and teeth especially by calcium and phosphorus.

b. The association with proteins in numerous ways: potassium with protein within cells; iron with hemoglobin; phosphorus with phosphoproteins; and so on.

c. The regulation of the transmission of the nerve impulse and the contraction of muscles; contraction of the heart muscle is one example.

d. The maintenance of the proper environment around and within all cells and tissues of the body—acid-base balance.

2. Mineral elements do not yield energy, as do carbohydrates, fats, and proteins; yet they are essential in the processes whereby the body derives its energy from foods.

3. Only calcium, iron, and iodine require particular attention in the planning of diets for normal individuals. Diets that are adequate in protein and calories and that include normal amounts of fruits and vegetables can be expected to supply all the other mineral elements in satisfactory amounts.

4. For most persons the calcium allowance can be met only when the diet includes 2 to 4 cups of milk, depending upon age. Cheese may be substituted for part of the milk allowance.

5. A deficiency of calcium may not become apparent for a long time because the bones supply the blood with its needs. Eventually, sufficient calcium is withdrawn from bones so that they become brittle and break easily, and osteoporosis may occur later in life.

6. Iron-deficiency anemia is widely prevalent, especially in infants, preschool children, teenage girls, and pregnant women. The only practical way by which these groups can obtain their iron needs is through the use of foods highly fortified with iron or by oral supplements of iron salts.

7. Iodine deficiency leads to endemic goiter. It can be prevented by the use of iodized salt.

8. Variations in the intake of acid-producing or alkali-producing foods do not result in acidosis or alkalosis in healthy individuals.

PROBLEMS AND REVIEW

1. Give several examples of the ways in which minerals function together in the body structure; in regulatory activities.
2. List four functions of calcium; of phosphorus.
3. What anions may combine with calcium in the intestinal tract and thus interfere with absorption? In which foods do these predominate? Of what practical significance is this in American diets?
4. Many adults believe that their needs for calcium are low because their bones are fully developed. Explain why this reasoning is wrong.
5. Iron is essentially a one-way substance. What does this mean? How does this affect the daily requirement?

(Problems continued on page 146.)

Table 9-3. Summary of the Minerals

Minerals	Functions in the Body	Metabolism	Food Sources	Daily Allowances
Calcium	Hardness of bones, teeth Transmission of nerve impulse Muscle contraction Normal heart rhythm Activate enzymes Increase cell permeability Catalyze thrombin formation	*Absorption:* about 15–40 per cent, according to body need; aided by gastric acidity, vitamin D, lactose; excess phosphate, fat, phytate, oxalic acid interfere *Storage:* trabeculae of bones; easily mobilized *Utilization:* needs parathyroid hormone, vitamin D *Excretion:* 60–85 per cent of diet intake in feces; small urinary excretion; high protein intake increases urinary excretion *Deficiency:* retarded bone mineralization; fragile bones; stunted growth; rickets; osteomalacia; osteoporosis	Milk, hard cheese Ice cream, cottage cheese Greens: turnip, collards, kale, mustard, broccoli Oysters, shrimp, salmon, clams	Infants: 360–540 mg Children: 800 mg Teen-agers: 1200 mg Adults: 800 mg Pregnancy: 1200 mg Lactation: 1200 mg
Phosphorus	Structure of bones, teeth Cell permeability Metabolism of fats and carbohydrates: storage and release of ATP Sugar-phosphate linkage in DNA and RNA Phospholipids in transport of fats Buffer salts in acid-base balance	*Absorption:* about 70 per cent; aided by vitamin D *Utilization:* about 85 per cent in bones; controlled by vitamin D, parathormone *Excretion:* about one third of diet in feces; metabolic products chiefly in urine *Deficiency:* poor bone mineralization; poor growth; rickets	Milk, cheese Eggs, meat, fish, poultry Legumes, nuts Whole-grain cereals	Infants: 200 to 400 mg Children: 800 mg Adults: 800 mg Pregnancy: 1200 mg Lactation: 1200 mg
Magnesium	Constituents of bones, teeth Activates enzymes in carbohydrate metabolism Muscle and nerve irritability	*Absorption:* parallels that of calcium; competes with calcium for carriers *Utilization:* slowly mobilized from bone *Excretion:* chiefly by kidney *Deficiency:* seen in alcoholism, severe renal disease; hypomagnesemia, tremor	Whole-grain cereals Nuts; legumes Meat Milk Green leafy vegetables	Infants: 60 to 70 mg Children: 150 to 250 mg Women: 300 mg Men: 350 mg Pregnancy and lactation: 450 mg

Element	Physiological Function	Absorption/Metabolism	Food Sources	Daily Allowances
Sulfur	Constituent of proteins, especially cartilage, hair, nails Constituent of melanin, glutathione, thiamin, biotin, coenzyme A, insulin High-energy sulfur bonds Detoxication reactions	Absorbed chiefly as sulfur-containing amino acids Excreted as inorganic sulfate in urine in proportion to nitrogen loss	Protein foods rich in sulfur-amino acids Eggs Meat Milk, cheese Nuts, legumes	Not established Diet adequate in protein meets need
Sodium	Principal cation of extracellular fluid Osmotic pressure; water balance Acid-base balance Regulate nerve irritability and muscle contraction "Pump" for glucose transport	*Absorption:* rapid and almost complete *Excretion:* chiefly in urine; some by skin and in feces; parallels intake; controlled by aldosterone *Deficiency:* rare; occurs with excessive perspiration and poor diet intake; nausea, diarrhea, abdominal cramps, muscle cramps	Table salt Milk Meat, fish, poultry Egg white	Not established Probably about 500 mg except with excessive perspiration Diets supply substantial excess
Potassium	Principal cation of intracellular fluid Osmotic pressure; water balance; acid-base balance Nerve irritability and muscle contraction, regular heart rhythm Synthesis of protein Glycogenesis	*Absorption:* readily absorbed *Excretion:* chiefly in urine; increased with aldosterone secretion *Deficiency:* following starvation, correction of diabetic acidosis, adrenal tumors; muscle weakness, nausea, tachycardia, glycogen depletion, heart failure	Widely distributed in foods Meat, fish, fowl Cereals Fruits, vegetables	Not established Diet adequate in calories supplies ample amounts
Chlorine	Chief anion of extracellular fluid Constituent of gastric juice Acid-base balance; chloride-bicarbonate shift in red cells	*Absorption:* rapid, almost complete *Excretion:* chiefly in urine; parallels intake *Deficiency:* with prolonged vomiting, drainage from fistula, diarrhea	Table salt	Not established Daily diet contains 3 to 9 gm, far in excess of need
Iodine	Constituent of diiodotyrosine, triiodothyronine, thyroxine; regulate rate of energy metabolism	*Absorption:* controlled by blood level of protein-bound iodine *Storage:* thyroid gland; activity regulated by thyroid-stimulating hormone *Excretion:* in urine *Deficiency:* simple goiter; if severe, cretinism—rarely seen in U.S.	Iodized salt is most reliable source Seafood Foods grown in non-goitrous coastal areas	Infants: 35–45 mcg Children: 60–110 mcg Teen-agers: 115–150 mcg Men: 130 mcg Women: 100 mcg Pregnancy: 125 mcg Lactation: 150 mcg

Table 9–3. (Cont.)

Minerals	Functions in the Body	Metabolism	Food Sources	Daily Allowances
Iron	Constituent of hemoglobin, myoglobin, and oxidative enzymes: catalase, cytochrome, xanthine oxidase	*Absorption:* about 5 to 10 per cent; regulated according to body need; aided by gastric acidity, ascorbic acid *Transport:* bound to protein, transferrin *Storage:* as ferritin in liver, bone marrow, spleen *Utilization:* chiefly in hemoglobin; daily turnover about 27 to 28 mg; iron used over and over again *Excretion:* men, about 1 mg; women, 1 to 2 mg; in urine, perspiration, menstrual flow; fecal excretion is from unabsorbed diet *Deficiency:* anemia; frequent in infants, preschool children, teenage girls, pregnant women	Liver, organ meats Meat, poultry Egg yolk Enriched and whole-grain breads, cereals Dark-green vegetables Legumes Molasses, dark Peaches, apricots, prunes, raisins Diets supply about 6 mg per 1000 kcal	Infants: 10 to 15 mg Children: 10 to 15 mg Teen-agers: 18 mg Men: 10 mg Women: 18 mg Pregnancy: 18+ mg Lactation: 18 mg
Manganese	Activation of many enzymes: oxidation of carbohydrates, urea formation, protein hydrolysis Bone formation	*Absorption:* limited *Excretion:* chiefly in feces *Deficiency:* not known	Legumes, nuts Whole-grain cereals	Not established
Copper	Aids absorption and use of iron in synthesis of hemoglobin Electron transport Melanin formation Myelin sheath of nerves Purine metabolism Metabolism of ascorbic acid	*Transport:* chiefly as protein, ceruloplasmin *Storage:* liver, central nervous system *Excretion:* bile into intestine *Deficiency:* rare; occurs in severe malnutrition Abnormal storage in Wilson's disease	Liver, shellfish Meats Nuts, legumes Whole-grain cereals Typical diet provides 2 to 5 mg	Infants and children: 0.08 mg per kg Adults: 2 mg

144

Mineral	Functions	Metabolism	Food Sources	Requirements
Zinc	Constituent of enzymes: carbonic anhydrase, carboxypeptidase, lactic dehydrogenase	*Absorption:* limited; competes with calcium for absorption sites *Storage:* liver, muscles, bones, organs *Excretion:* chiefly by intestine *Deficiency:* only in severe malnutrition	Seafoods Liver and other organ meats Meats, fish Wheat germ Yeast Plant foods are generally low Usual diet supplies 10 to 15 mg	Infants: 3–5 mg Children: 10 mg Teen-agers: 15 mg Adults: 15 mg Pregnancy: 20 mg Lactation: 25 mg
Fluorine	Increases resistance of teeth to decay; most effective in young children Moderate levels in bone may reduce osteoporosis	*Storage:* bones and teeth *Excretion:* urine Excess leads to mottling of teeth	Fluoridated water: 1 ppm	Not established
Molybdenum	Cofactor for flavoprotein enzymes; present in xanthine oxidase	Absorbed as molybdate Stored in liver, adrenal, kidney Related to metabolism of copper and sulfur	Organ meats Legumes Whole-grain cereals	Not established
Selenium	Antioxidant Constituent of glutathione oxidase	Stored especially in liver, kidney Spares vitamin E	Meat and seafoods Cereal foods	Not established
Chromium	Efficient use of insulin in glucose uptake; conversion of glucose to fat, glucose oxidation, protein synthesis Activation of enzymes	Usable form in organic compound: glucose tolerance factor	Liver, meat Cheese Whole-grain cereals	Not established

6. *Problem.* Calculate your daily intake of calcium and iron for two days. Compare your intake with the recommended allowances. What were the important sources of calcium in your diet? Of iron?

7. *Problem.* Using the basic diet calculation on page 206, show how the iron level can be increased to 18 mg. Include your calculations for iron and for calories.

8. What is the principal function of iodine? What happens if the intake is inadequate?

9. To which groups of individuals is the prophylactic use of iodine especially important?

10. If you consume 10 gm of iodized salt in a day, how much iodine would you ingest if the level of iodization is 0.005 per cent?

11. What is the significance of fluorine in nutrition? What levels of fluorine are recommended in drinking water?

12. What is meant by dental fluorosis? At what levels of intake does it occur?

13. Name the principal mineral elements that contribute to an alkaline ash. Which foods are classed as alkali producing?

14. Name the principal mineral elements that contribute to an acid ash. Which foods are classed as acid producing?

15. What is the metabolic effect of an excess of acid-producing or of alkali-producing foods?

16. Describe the ways in which the lungs function to maintain the normal blood pH. Describe how the kidneys make the final adjustments to maintain acid-base balance.

17. Describe the water compartments of the body in terms of (a) relative size; (b) electrolyte composition.

18. What are the daily sources of water to the body? What are the routes of excretion by the healthy individual?

19. Describe the functioning parts of the kidney in terms of the results achieved by each of these parts.

20. What hormones control the excretion of water? Of sodium and potassium?

21. What is meant by obligatory water loss? If you found yourself in a situation where drinking water was extremely limited in supply, how could you reduce the loss of water from your body?

CITED REFERENCES

1. Food and Nutrition Board: *Recommended Dietary Allowances,* 8th ed. National Academy of Sciences—National Research Council, Washington, D.C., 1974.

2. Statland, H., cited by Snively, W. D., Jr., and Brown, B. J.: "In the Balance," *Am. J. Nurs.,* **58:**55–57, 1958.

3. West, E. S., *et al.: Textbook of Biochemistry,* 4th ed. Macmillan Publishing Co., Inc., New York, 1966, p. 686.

4. Prior, I. A. M.: "The Price of Civilization," *Nutr. Today,* **6:**2–11, July 1971.

5. Dahl, L. K.: "Salt and Hypertension," *Am. J. Clin. Nutr.,* **25:**231–44, 1972.

6. Krehl, W. A.: "The Potassium Depletion Syndrome," *Nutr. Today,* **1:**20, June 1966.

7. Griffiths, M.: *Introduction to Human Physiology.* Macmillan Publishing Co., Inc., New York, 1974, p. 333.

8. Brook, C. E., and Anast, C. S.: "Oral Fluid and Electrolytes," *J.A.M.A.,* **179:**792–97, 1962.

9. Wright, A.: *Rypins' Medical Licensure Examination.* J. B. Lippincott Company, Philadelphia, 1970, p. 98.

10. Frisell, W. R.: *Acid-Base Chemistry in Medicine.* Macmillan Publishing Co., Inc., New York, 1968, p. 51.

ADDITIONAL REFERENCES

Abbey, J. C.: "Nursing Observations of Fluid Imbalance," *Nurs. Clin. North Am.,* **3:**77–86, 1968.

Burgess, R. E.: "Fluids and Electrolytes," *Am. J. Nurs.,* **65:**90–95, 1965.

Camien, M. N., *et al.:* "A Critical Reappraisal of 'Acid-Base' Balance," *Am. J. Clin. Nutr.,* **22:**786–93, 1969.

Earley, L. E., and Daugharty, T. M.: "Sodium Metabolism," *N. Engl. J. Med.,* **281:**72–86, 1969.

Fenton, M.: "What to Do About Thirst," *Am. J. Nurs.,* **69:**1014–17, 1969.

Frazier, H. S.: "Renal Regulation of Sodium Balance," *N. Engl. J. Med.*, **279**:868–75, 1968.

Grant, M. M., and Kubo, W. M.: "Assessing the Patient's Hydration Status," *Am. J. Nurs.*, **75**:1306–11, 1975.

Klahr, S., *et al.:* "Acid-Base Disorders in Health and Disease," *J.A.M.A.*, **222**:567–73, 1972.

Krehl, W. A.: "Sodium: A Most Extraordinary Dietary Essential," *Nutr. Today*, **1**:16, Dec. 1966.

Laragh, J. H.: "Potassium, Angiotensin and the Dual Control of Aldosterone Secretion," *N. Engl. J. Med.*, **289**:745–47, 1973.

Lee, C. A., *et al.:* "Extracellular Volume Imbalance," *Am. J. Nurs.*, **74**:888–91, 1974.

Review: "Sodium Intake and Blood Pressure," *Nutr. Rev.*, **27**:280–82, 1969.

Robinson, J.: "Water the Indispensable Nutrient," *Nutr. Today*, **5**:16, 1970.

Sharer, J. E.: "Reviewing Acid-Base Balance," *Am. J. Nurs.*, **75**:980–83, 1975.

10 The Fat-Soluble Vitamins

INTRODUCTION TO THE STUDY OF THE VITAMINS

The story of the vitamins—their discovery, their positive functions in maintaining health, and their usefulness in healing deficiency diseases—is fascinating and deserving of considerable study. Popular interest was early aroused by the discovery of the role of vitamins in preventing such severe deficiency diseases as scurvy, pellagra, beriberi, and others. It is now known that vitamins function primarily in enzyme systems which facilitate the metabolism of amino acids, fats, and carbohydrates. Those who understand the functions of vitamins do not minimize their importance in relation to the utilization of food. However, it is important that no one be misled into believing that vitamins are "cure-alls" for disease. The properties of vitamins, their functions in metabolism, their distribution in foods, and the effects of deficiency will be discussed in he sections below.

Definition and nomenclature. The term *vitamins* was first coined in 1912 by Funk, a Polish chemist, who believed that the water-soluble antiberiberi substance he was describing was a "vital amine"; that is, an amine with life-giving properties. The final "e" was soon dropped because the substance was found, in reality, to be a group of essential compounds not all of which were amines. VITAMINS is the name given to a group of potent organic compounds other than protein, carbohydrate, and fat that are necessary in minute quantities in foods and are essential for specific body functions of maintenance, growth, and reproduction. Vitamins differ from hormones in that they must be supplied by the diet and are not formed by ductless glands in the body. During the last decade important studies have shown that vitamin D is an exception in that its metabolically active form is a hormone. See page 156.

Early classifications listed two groups of vitamins: fat soluble and water soluble. This classification is still used although it is arbitrary. Within each of the classes the vitamins differ widely in their properties, functions, and distribution. Vitamins were first named for their curative properties and were given a convenient letter name according to the order of their discovery; for example, antiscorbutic vitamin or vitamin C. The nomenclature used today includes chemically descriptive terms, but letter designations are also used.

Measurement. Before the chemical nature of vitamins was discovered, their potency could be measured only by their ability to promote growth or to cure a deficiency when test doses were fed to experimental animals such as rats, guinea pigs, pigeons, and chicks. Such measurement is known as *bioassay* and has been expressed in units. Vitamins A, D, and E are still expressed in international units (I.U.). Other vitamins are measured by their ability to promote the growth of microorganisms; this is known as *microbiologic assay*. Many vitamins formerly measured by bioassay are now measured by *chemical assay* in units of weight. Some vitamins are measured in milligram (mg) amounts; for example, the adult allowance for vitamin C is 45 mg. Other vitamins are measured in microgram (mcg or μg) amounts; the adult allowance for vitamin B_{12} is 3 mcg. Thus, the weight of ascorbic acid needed is 15,000 times that for vitamin B_{12}.

Selection of foods for vitamin content. In selecting the foods to furnish vitamins in the diet it is well to keep in mind the following points: (1) under normal circumstances it is better to use common food sources than concentrates, because foods furnish other essential factors as well; (2) it is important to determine how often any given food will be used in the dietary; (3) the amount of food which would ordinarily be used must be ascertained; (4)

the effects of processing and preparation of foods on the vitamin retention must be clearly understood; and (5) economic factors such as availability and cost must be considered. For example, 100 gm of parsley furnish about 8500 I.U. of vitamin A, whereas 100 gm of milk supply only 140 I.U. of vitamin A. Parsley, as a garnish, will have limited use, whereas 1 pint of milk a day, essential in an adequate diet, furnishes about 670 I.U. or 15 per cent of the day's allowance for men and women.

Vitamin supplementation of the diet. Any diet selected on the basis of the Four Food Groups will provide the necessary amounts of the vitamins. Undoubtedly the sale of supplements far exceeds the need for them. As a matter of fact, the water-soluble vitamins in excess of body needs will be excreted in the urine. Vitamin A, being fat soluble, is stored in appreciable amounts in the liver; other fat-soluble vitamins are stored to a lesser degree. Excessive intakes of vitamins A and D are toxic. In the United States there is probably a greater health hazard through overuse than through deficiency.

Vitamin D supplementation for infants, growing children, and pregnant or lactating women is needed if fortified milk is not available or if exposure to sunlight is inadequate.

Vitamin supplements are needed in some clinical situations, for example, illness characterized by inability to consume a normal diet, following surgery or severe injury such as burns, in diseases of malabsorption, and so on. Sometimes supplements are needed to restore reserves when the diet has been inadequate because of ignorance, poor eating habits, or inability to obtain the necessary foods.

VITAMIN A

Discovery. In 1913 McCollum and Davis of the University of Wisconsin[1] and Osborne and Mendel of Yale University[2] independently discovered that rats consuming purified diets with lard as the only source of fat failed to grow and developed soreness of the eyes. When butterfat or ether extract of egg yolk was added to the diet, growth resumed and the eye condition was corrected. The term *fat-soluble A* was applied by McCollum to the organic complex present in the ether extract that was necessary for normal growth.

A PRECURSOR is a substance that precedes another, or a substance from which an active compound can be synthesized. In 1919 Steenbock at the University of Wisconsin[3] demonstrated that the yellow pigment in plants, the CAROTENES, had vitamin A activity. Thus, the carotenes are precursors of vitamin A, and are also referred to as PROVITAMIN A.

Chemistry and characteristics. Vitamin A is active in many forms, the nomenclature being as follows:[4]

Vitamin A, vitamin A alcohol—RETINOL. (See Figure 10–1.)
Vitamin A aldehyde, retinene, retinal—RETIN-ALDEHYDE
Vitamin A acid—RETINOIC ACID
Vitamin A esters—RETINYL ESTERS

Collectively, these forms may be referred to as vitamin A.

In its pure form vitamin A is a pale-yellow crystalline compound. It occurs naturally in the animal kingdom and has been synthesized so that it is available commercially. It is soluble in fat and fat solvents but insoluble in water, and it is relatively stable to heat and to acids and alkalies. It is easily oxidized; rapid destruction occurs by exposure to high temperatures in the presence of air, by ultraviolet irradiation, or in rancid fats.

The ultimate source of all vitamin A is the carotenes, which are synthesized by plants. Animals in turn, and man as well, convert a considerable proportion of the carotene of the foods they eat into vitamin A. The carotenes are dark-red crystalline compounds that give a deep-yellow coloration to plants such as carrots and sweet potatoes. In deep-green plants, also rich in carotenes, the color is masked by the chlorophyll. Alpha-, beta-, and gamma-carotene and possibly cryptoxanthin are of nutritional significance. Upon hydrolysis each molecule of beta-carotene ($C_{40}H_{56}$) theoretically yields two molecules of vitamin A; the biologic activity, however, is only about half that of vitamin A.

Measurement. Vitamin A is measured in international units. The equivalents are:

1 I.U. = 0.3 mcg retinol

1 I.U. = 0.6 mcg beta-carotene

1 I.U. = 1.2 mcg other carotenoids

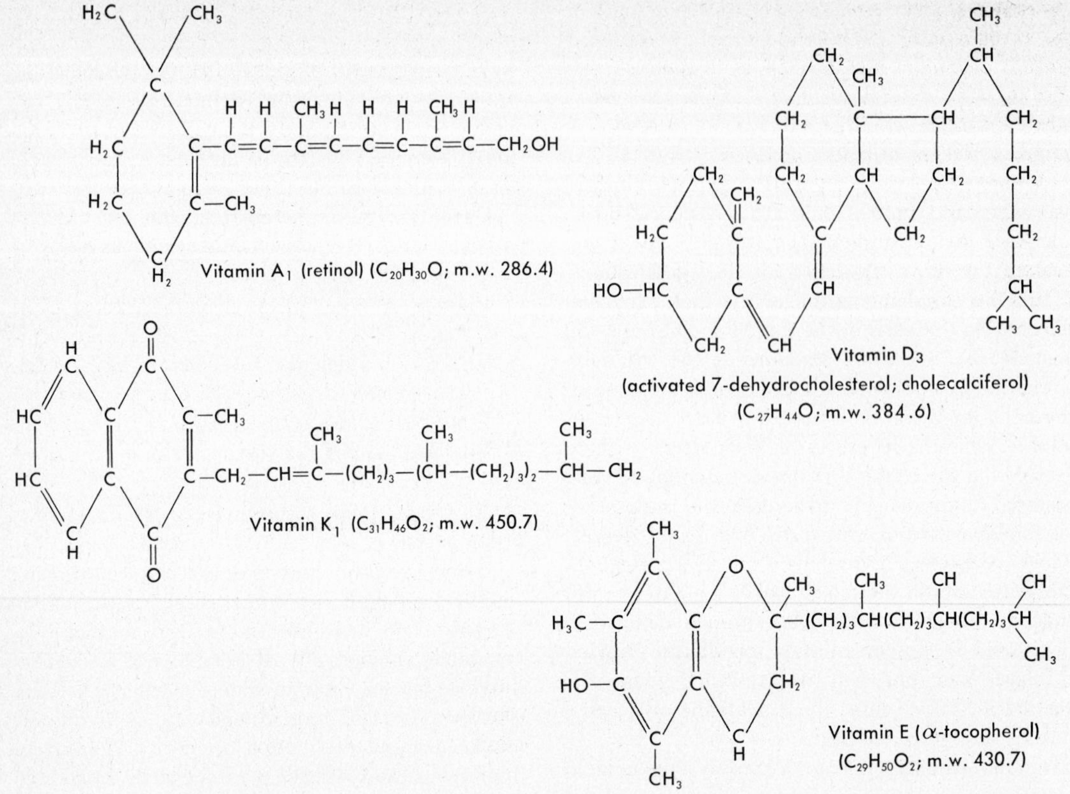

Figure 10–1. Each of the fat-soluble vitamins exists in several forms, only one of which is shown here. Note the similarity of structure of vitamin D to that of cholesterol.

The Food and Nutrition Board has recommended that RETINOL EQUIVALENTS (R.E.) replace the international unit.[5] This system of measurement takes into account the amount of absorption of the carotenes as well as the degree of conversion to vitamin A, and thus is a more precise system of measures. The equivalents are:

1 R.E. = 1 mcg retinol (3.33 I.U.)

1 R.E. = 6 mcg beta-carotene (10 I.U.)

1 R.E. = 12 mcg other carotenoids (10 I.U.)

Values for vitamin A in this chapter will be expressed in R.E. with the corresponding values in I.U. placed in parentheses. Tables of food values at present express the values for vitamin A in international units.

Absorption, storage, and transport. The carotenes are split in the intestinal tract and retinaldehyde is formed, and then reduced to retinol. Most of the retinol is reesterified to retinyl ester in the intestinal mucosa and transported by the lymph circulation.

The absorption of vitamin A and the carotenes, like that of fat, is facilitated by bile. When a diet is very low in fat, or when there is an obstruction of the bile duct, the absorption of vitamin A and the carotenes is seriously impaired.

The simultaneous presence of vitamin E in the intestinal tract prevents the excessive oxidation of vitamin A that would otherwise occur. On the other hand, the presence of mineral oil reduces the absorption. Since mineral oil itself is not absorbed, it carries with it vitamin A and other fat-soluble vitamins. When used as a laxative, mineral oil should not be taken at or near mealtime.

Retinol is completely absorbed from the gastrointestinal tract but the absorption of carotenes is about one third. Since about half of the absorbed beta-carotene is converted to retinol, only one sixth of the intake in food is actually utilized. For other carotenoids only one fourth is converted to retinol; thus, only one twelfth of the intake in foods is available.[6] (See retinol equivalents, page 150.)

The principal conversion of carotenes to vitamin A takes place in the intestinal mucosa, but some conversion also occurs in the liver and kidney. Like other fat-soluble materials, vitamin A is attached to a specific protein for transport in the circulation. The vitamin-A-protein complexes enter the lymph circulation for transport to the liver.

About 90 per cent of body stores of vitamin A are found in the liver, with the remainder being present in the kidney, lungs, adrenal glands, and adipose tissue. The healthy adult has reserves that are adequate for several months to a year. Infants and young children have not built up such reserves and therefore are much more susceptible to the effects of deficiency.

Normal concentrations of vitamin A in blood serum range from 25 to 90 mcg per 100 ml and of carotene from 40 to 125 mcg per 100 ml. The liver maintains the level in the blood as long as there is an adequate reserve. Only when the liver reserves are depleted will the blood concentration be lowered.

Functions. Although the existence of vitamin A has been known for over 60 years, its functions have not been fully explained. Retinyl esters, retinol, and retinaldehyde are readily converted from one form to the other, but retinoic acid cannot be converted to other forms. Retinoic acid fulfills some of the functions of vitamin A but does not function in the visual cycle.

Vision. The best understood function of vitamin A is related to the maintenance of normal vision in dim light. The retina of the eye contains two kinds of light receptors: the rods for vision in dim light and the cones for vision in bright light and color vision. The rods produce a photosensitive pigment, RHODOPSIN or VISUAL PURPLE, and the cones produce IODOPSIN or VISUAL VIOLET. In both these pigments retinaldehyde is the prosthetic group, but the proteins to which the aldehyde is attached are different. When light strikes the pigments, they are split to their component parts, retinaldehyde and protein. In healthy persons the rates of bleaching and regeneration are equal. Some retinaldehyde is lost in each cycle so that a constant supply from the blood must be present. A simplified diagram of the visual cycle is shown in Figure 10–2.

Epithelial tissues. Vitamin A is required for healthy epithelium whether covering the body externally or lining the mucous membranes. It effects the synthesis of constituents of mucus such as the mucoproteins and the mucopolysacccharides. The mucous secretions maintain the integrity of the epithelium, especially the membranes that line the eyes, the mouth, and the gastrointestinal, respiratory, and genitourinary tracts. These membranes maintained in their optimum condition offer resistance to bacterial invasion; to that extent vitamin A gives protection against infection. The designation *anti-infective* is unfortunate insofar as it often leads people, mistakenly, to believe that large intakes of vitamin A will confer additional protective benefits.

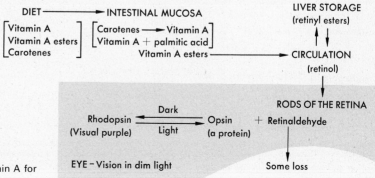

Figure 10–2. Metabolism of vitamin A for vision in dim light.

Growth and other functions. Vitamin A is essential for normal skeletal and tooth development. With a deficiency of vitamin A bones do not grow in length and the normal remodeling process does not take place. Studies on experimental animals have shown that vitamin A is essential for spermatogenesis in the male and normal estrus cycle in the female. If vitamin A is not available to the animal during fetal development, many malformations result. The synthesis of hydrocortisone from cholesterol is facilitated in the adrenal cortex by vitamin A. The stability of biologic membranes appears to be maintained by interaction of vitamins A and E.

Daily allowances. The recommended allowances for vitamin A are stated in retinol equivalents and international units.[5] When international units are calculated to retinol equivalents, it is assumed that one half of the vitamin A is retinol and one half is beta-carotene. Thus, 5000 I.U. = 1000 R.E.:

$$2500 \text{ I.U.} \div 3.33 = 750 \text{ R.E.}$$
$$2500 \text{ I.U.} \div 10 = \underline{250 \text{ R.E.}}$$
$$1000 \text{ R.E.}$$

The vitamin A allowance for males over 11 years is 1000 R.E. or 5000 I.U. and for females over 11 years it is 800 R.E. or 4000 I.U. The allowances for infants over six months and children up to 10 years are 400 to 700 R.E., for pregnancy 1000 R.E., and for lactation 1200 R.E.

Food sources. Only animal foods contain vitamin A as such, fish-liver oils being outstanding. These oils are generally not classed with common foods, but milk, butter, fortified margarines, whole-milk cheese, liver, and egg yolk contain vitamin A.

The principal source of vitamin A in the diet is likely to be from the carotenes, which are widespread in those plant foods that have high green or yellow colorings. There is a direct correlation between the greenness of a leaf and its carotene content. Dark-green leaves are rich in carotene, but the pale leaves, in lettuce and cabbage for example, are insignificant sources. Abundant sources of carotene are found in foods such as:

Green leafy vegetables—spinach, turnip tops, chard, beet greens
Green stem vegetables—asparagus, broccoli
Yellow vegetables—carrots, sweet potatoes, winter squash, pumpkin
Yellow fruits—apricots, peaches, cantaloupe

The vitamin A contribution of the Four Food Groups is indicated in Figure 10–3. The meat group contributes only when liver or an organ meat is

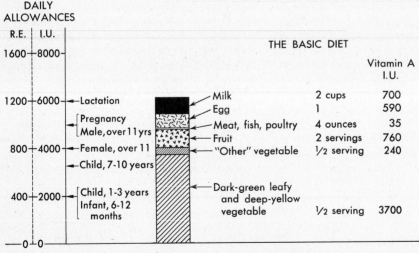

Figure 10–3. The Four Food Groups of the Basic Diet provide a liberal allowance of vitamin A for all age categories. Note the contribution made by dark-green, leafy, and deep-yellow vegetables. Breads, cereals, flours, and white potato do not provide vitamin A. See Table 13–2 for complete calculations.

served once every week to 10 days. One egg provides about one tenth of the daily allowance.

Retention of food values. Since vitamin A is
stable to the usual cooking temperatures, only slight
losses are likely to occur in food preparation. The
wilting of vegetables or dehydration of foods results
in considerable losses. Canned and frozen foods
retain maximal values for nine months or longer.
Vitamin A activity is rapidly lost in rancid fats.

Effects of vitamin A deficiency. In the United
States vitamin A deficiency should be practically
nonexistent inasmuch as there are abundant dietary
sources of vitamin A available. Nevertheless, the
1965 household survey of diets showed that one diet
in every four failed to supply the recommended
allowances and that 1 diet in every 10 supplied less
than two thirds of the recommended allowances.
The National Nutrition Survey conducted on low-
income groups disclosed that serum vitamin A levels
were less than adequate in about 13 per cent of the
population surveyed.[7] The predominance of low
serum levels was in young children. About one
fourth of the children aged 6 to 9 years had low
levels and one third of preschool children had unacceptable serum levels of vitamin A.

Vitamin A deficiency is the most prevalent vitamin deficiency throughout the world and ranks
second only to protein-calorie malnutrition in its
incidence. When the two conditions are present in
the same child, the prognosis is very poor. Severe
forms of vitamin A deficiency are practically nonexistent in the United States, but throughout the
world up to 80,000 persons, chiefly children, become blind each year because of vitamin A lack.[8]
The predominant regions of severe deficiency are
the Middle East, India, Malaysia, Latin America,
and South America.

It is ironic that the most severe forms of vitamin
A deficiency occur in areas where there is an abundance of green plant foods. Through ignorance the
young child is not given these foods. Vitamin A
deficiency has been a major problem in areas of
famine such as occurred in Bangladesh and in Africa. Vitamin A deficiency also results from faulty
absorption in such diseases as sprue, celiac disease,
and other malabsorptive disorders.

Night blindness. One of the earliest signs of vitamin A deficiency is night blindness, or NYCTALOPIA

(see Figure 10–4). This is a condition in which the
individual is unable to see well in dim light, especially on coming into darkness from a bright light as
in entering a darkened theater. Drivers who are
easily blinded (glare blindness) by the headlights of
other automobiles and who consequently see road
markers, pedestrians, etc., with difficulty constitute
a special traffic hazard.

Nyctalopia occurs when there is insufficient vitamin A to bring about prompt and complete regeneration of visual purple. Blood carotene and vitamin
A levels and a substantiating dietary history are
useful in establishing a diagnosis of vitamin A deficiency. Other causes of night blindness must be
ruled out. If a therapeutic dose of vitamin A does
not bring about relief of night blindness after a few
weeks' trial, it may be assumed that the condition is
not a vitamin A deficiency.

Epithelial changes. An inadequate supply of vitamin A may lead to definite changes in the epithelial
tissues throughout the body: KERATINIZATION, or a
noticeable shrinking, hardening, and progressive
degeneration of the cells, occurs, which increases
the susceptibility to severe infections of the eye, the
nasal passages, the sinuses, middle ear, lungs, and
genitourinary tract.

Skin changes in severe vitamin A deficiency
known as FOLLICULAR HYPERKERATOSIS have been
described. The skin becomes rough, dry, and scaly.
The keratinized epithelium plugs the sebaceous
glands so that goose-pimple-like follicles appear first
along the upper forearms and thighs, and then
spread along the shoulders, back, abdomen, and
buttocks.

Xerophthalmia. The term XEROPHTHALMIA
means dryness of the eye. Progressive stages of this
condition have been described by Oomen, who was
a physician in Indonesia and a nutritionist for the
World Health Organization.[9] The first mild symptoms of epithelial changes in the eye are suggested
by night blindness. The young child, most likely to
be affected, is unable to describe this condition, but
the mother, upon questioning, may be aware that
the child does not see well at dusk. Then XEROSIS of
the conjunctiva occurs, characterized by dryness
and dullness. BITOT'S SPOTS, which are grayish
plaques appearing on the conjunctiva, may or may
not be seen. This is followed by xerosis of the

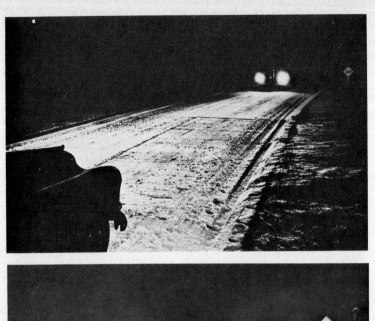

A

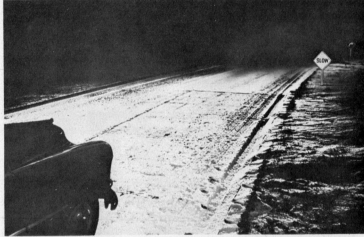

B

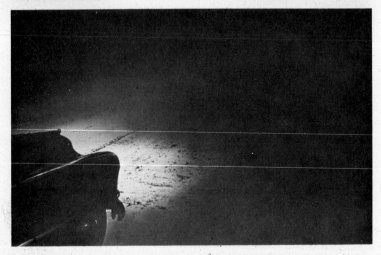

C

Figure 10–4. Night blindness. (*A*) Safe driving at night depends, in part, on the ability of one's eyes to adjust to the glare of lights. (*B*) Properly focused headlights of an approaching automobile do not impede a good view of the road when the eye has an adequate supply of vitamin A. (*C*) The edge of the road and distances far ahead cannot be seen immediately after meeting an automobile when there is insufficient vitamin A available to the eye. (Courtesy, The Upjohn Company.)

cornea, which becomes dry and opaque. At this stage the condition is reversible if promptly treated. The corneal xerosis rapidly progresses to involvement of the deeper layers of the cornea, perforation, keratomalacia, scarring, and loss of sight.

Prevention and treatment. Much vitamin A deficiency could be prevented if carotene-rich foods were included in the diet. A very low fat intake, common in many dietaries, reduces the efficiency of absorption. When skim milk is used for the correction of protein-calorie malnutrition, it is essential that it be fortified with vitamin A; such fortification is now prevalent.

When deficiency occurs, treatment is rapidly effective with large doses of vitamin A provided that the eye conditions have not become irreversible. Massive doses of vitamin A (200,000 I.U.) every three to six months given under medical supervision have been used successfully to prevent the high incidence of blindness.[10] Vitamin E is given simultaneously to bring about effective storage of vitamin A and to reduce the tendency to hypervitaminosis.

Hypervitaminosis A. In the United States the ingestion of large excesses of vitamin A perhaps poses a greater health hazard than does lack of vitamin A. There has been ample documentation of the toxicity of vitamin A when ingested in excess of 50,000 I.U. daily for months or years.[11,12] Infants who received 18,500 to 60,000 I.U. daily showed signs of toxicity in 12 weeks.[13] The common symptoms of toxicity are anorexia, hyperirritability, and drying and desquamation of the skin. Loss of hair, bone and joint pain, bone fragility, headaches, and enlargement of the liver and spleen are quite frequent. When vitamin A is discontinued, recovery takes place.

Vitamin D

Cod-liver oil has been recommended as a remedy for rickets ever since the Middle Ages but does not appear to have been used with any consistency until the present century. During World War I, Hess and Unger noted the effect of cod-liver oil in protecting Negro children in New York City against rickets. Then in 1919 Mellanby found that the skeletal structure of puppies was influenced by some fat-soluble substance in food. McCollum, Steenbock,

and Drummond simultaneously reported that cod-liver oil in which vitamin A had been destroyed still retained its antirachitic properties, and hence it was shown that vitamin A was not the antirachitic factor. Steenbock and Hess in 1924 independently found that foods that had been exposed to ultraviolet rays possessed antirachitic properties. Pure vitamin D was isolated in crystalline form in 1930 and was called calciferol.

Chemistry and characteristics. Vitamin D is a group of chemically distinct sterol compounds possessing antirachitic properties. The vitamin is produced by irradiating a precursor or provitamin D with ultraviolet light; in other words, substances like ergosterol are exposed to ultraviolet light to form calciferol. Of nutritional interest are (1) vitamin D_2 (ERGOCALCIFEROL, CALCIFEROL, or VIOSTEROL—ERGOSTEROL being the chief vitamin D precursor found in plants, and (2) vitamin D_3 (CHOLECALCIFEROL)—the chief form occurring in animal cells and developed in the skin on exposure of 7-DEHYDROCHOLESTEROL to ultraviolet light from sunshine. (See Figure 10–1.) Pure vitamins D are white odorless crystals that are soluble in fats and fat solvents. They are insoluble in water, and they are stable to heat, alkalies, and oxidation.

Measurement. One international unit (I.U.) of vitamin D is the activity of 0.025 mcg pure crystalline vitamin D.

The LINE TEST is used for measuring the potency of vitamin D in materials. Young rats from mothers having a deficient supply of vitamin D are kept on a rachitogenic diet so that no calcification occurs in the ends of the long bones. When a test material is fed, its value as a source of vitamin D is measured by the amount that must be fed for 7 to 10 days to produce a good calcium line (line test) in the ends of the long bones. Standard cod-liver oil is fed to a similar group of animals and is used as a basis of comparison. No satisfactory chemical or microbiologic assay is yet available. (See Figure 10–5.)

Functions. That vitamin D is necessary for calcium and phosphorus metabolism has long been known. Vitamin D improves the absorption of calcium and probably also phosphorus from the intestine, and mobilizes calcium, and consequently phosphorus, from bone. These actions increase the calcium and phosphorus levels of the blood thereby permitting normal mineralization of the cartilage

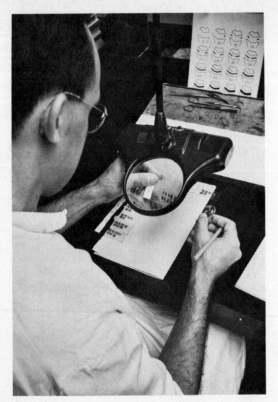

Figure 10–5. The line test is still used for determination of vitamin D. On charts in background, the darker the line, the better the healing. The amount of healing is related to the amount of vitamin D supplied to the test animal by the diet. (Courtesy, Food and Drug Administration.)

and bone matrix, and also maintaining the correct concentration of calcium in extracellular fluids for muscle contraction and nerve irritability.

Metabolism. Although the functions of vitamin D have, in general, been known for decades, the mechanisms of the activity have been poorly understood. Very exciting research by DeLuca and his coworkers at the University of Wisconsin[14] and others [15,16] has resulted in significant progress not only in determining the modes of action but also in making available new therapeutic agents for serious bone diseases.

Vitamin D is absorbed along with food fats from the jejunum and ileum and is transported in the chylomicrons through the lymph circulation. Bile is essential for effective absorption, and anything that interferes with fat absorption, such as pancreatitis,

sprue, and malabsorption disorders, also affects the completeness of vitamin D absorption.

Vitamin D itself is the inert, storage form of the vitamin that is concentrated in the liver and to a lesser extent in the skin, spleen, lungs, brain, and kidney. In the liver vitamin D is rapidly hydroxylated to 25-HYDROXYVITAMIN D_3 (25-OH-D_3), also known as 25-HYDROXYCHOLECALCIFEROL (25HCC). This form of the vitamin is two to five times as active as vitamin D and is the principal form circulating in the blood. In the kidney a second hydroxylation occurs to produce 1,25-DIHYDROXY-VITAMIN D_3 (1,25-$(OH)_2$-D_3), also known as 1,25-DIHYDROXYCHOLECALCIFEROL (1,25 DHCC). This compound is a sterol hormone that regulates the transport of calcium from the intestine and bone. It is the first instance of a vitamin behaving as a hormone. (See Figure 10–6.)

The parathyroid gland is sensitive to the calcium level in the blood. When the serum calcium level falls, the gland produces parathormone, which activates a hydroxylase in the kidney to produce 1,25-$(OH)_2$-D_3. The hormone circulates to the intestine where it stimulates the absorption of calcium, and possibly also phosphorus. Calcium is apparently attached to a specific protein for transport across the intestinal mucosa. In the intestine the vitamin D hormone is effective without the presence of parathormone.

The mobilization of calcium from bone, and consequently phosphorus as well, is increased by the action of 1,25-$(OH)_2$-D_3 and parathormone. With the increased absorption and also the mobilization of calcium from bone, the serum level of calcium is increased thereby facilitating the mineralization of bone matrix and cartilage.

Daily allowances. As little as 100 I.U. vitamin D will promote bone development and prevent rickets. The recommended allowance of 400 I.U. is well documented for full-term and premature infants. Additional amounts do not confer greater benefits and are not required. Vitamin D should be supplied to breast-fed and bottle-fed infants.

The allowances for growing children, adolescents, and pregnant and lactating women are difficult to establish because of the exposure to sunlight, but 400 I.U. are recommended daily. Adults with normal exposure to sunlight do not require a dietary supplement.

Sources. Exposure to sunlight, fortified foods,

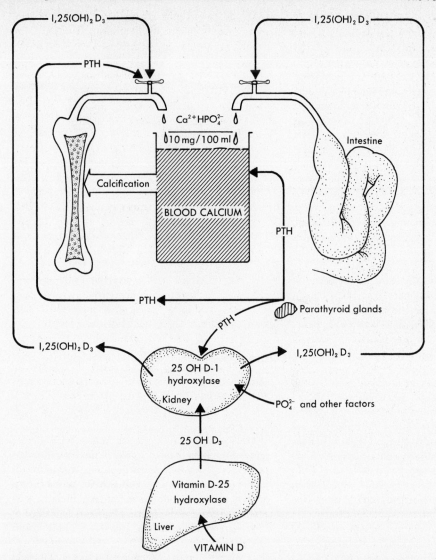

Figure 10–6. Hormonal loop derived from vitamin D. Diagram shows calcium homeostatic system. In the intestine 1,25-(OH)$_2$D$_3$ functions without the presence of parathyroid hormone; in bone the presence of parathyroid hormone is essential. (Reprinted from *Federation Proceedings*, **33**:2215, 1974. Courtesy, Dr. H. F. DeLuca and *Federation Proceedings*.)

fish-liver oils, and commercial vitamin D preparations are the sources of vitamin D. Natural foods are poor sources of vitamin D, although small amounts are present in egg yolk, liver, and fish such as herring, sardines, tuna, and salmon.

About 85 per cent of fresh milk and almost all evaporated milk are fortified with 400 I.U. vitamin D per quart. Milk is especially suitable for fortifica-

tion since it contains the calcium and phosphorus whose absorption it facilitates, and because it is an important food consumed by children. The fortification of foods other than milk is of dubious value since the ingestion of several foods so treated could lead to excessive intake.

Exposure of the skin to sunlight brings about the synthesis of vitamin D from the precursor 7-dehydrocholesterol. Sunlight cannot always be depended upon to supply the body with adequate ultraviolet rays to manufacture vitamin D, because these rays are so easily strained out by dust, smoke, fog, clothing, and ordinary window glass—all of which act as barriers to prevent the rays from reaching the skin.

Hypervitaminosis D. The tolerance for vitamin D varies widely. As little as 1800 I.U. over a long period of time may be mildly toxic to children, whereas massive doses of 100,000 I.U. may be necessary and are tolerated by those rare individuals who have vitamin-D-resistant rickets. The symptoms of toxicity include nausea, vomiting, diarrhea, excessive thirst, weight loss, polyuria, and nocturia. As the toxicity becomes more severe, renal damage and calcification of the soft tissues such as the heart, blood vessels, bronchi, stomach, and tubules of the kidney occur.

Effects of vitamin D deficiency. A deficiency of vitamin D leads to inadequate absorption of calcium and phosphorus from the intestinal tract and to faulty mineralization of bone and tooth structures. The inability of the soft bones to withstand the stress of weight results in skeletal malformations.

Rickets. Infantile rickets is rarely seen in the United States because of the widespread use of fortified milk or of vitamin D preparations in prophylaxis. When such preventive measures are not taken, rickets is more prevalent in northern regions than in warm, sunny climates. It is more likely to develop in dark, overcrowded sections of large cities where the ultraviolet rays of sunshine, especially in the winter months, cannot penetrate through the fog, smoke, and soot. Poverty and ignorance may acccount for failure to obtain enough vitamin D from concentrates, fortified milk, or skin exposure. Dark-skinned children are more susceptible to rickets than those of the white race.

Premature infants are more susceptible to rickets than full-term infants since the growth rate and the calcification of the skeleton impose additional demands for vitamin D.

Fully developed cases of rickets present the following characteristics (see Figure 10–7):

1. Delayed closure of the fontanelles, softening of the skull (craniotabes), and bulging or bossing of the forehead, giving the head a boxlike appearance.

2. Soft, fragile bones leading to widening of the

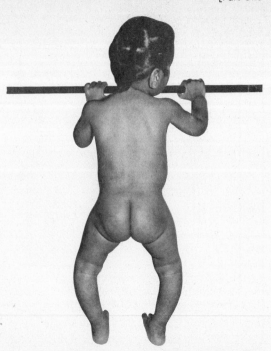

Figure 10–7. Early skeletal deformities of rickets often persist throughout life. Bowlegs that curve laterally, as shown here, indicate that the weakened bones have bent after the second year, as the result of standing. (Courtesy, Dr. Rosa Lee Nemir, Professor of Pediatrics, New York University—Bellevue Medical Center, and *The Vitamin Manual,* published by The Upjohn Company.)

ends of the long bones; bowing of the legs; enlargement of the costochondral junction with rows of knobs or beads forming the RACHITIC ROSARY; projection of the sternum as in "pigeon breast"; narrowing of the pelvis; spinal curvature.

3. Enlargement of wrist, knee (knock-knees), and ankle joints.

4. Poorly developed muscles; lack of muscle tone—pot belly—being the result of weakness of abdominal muscles; weakness, with delayed walking.

5. Restlessness and nervous irritability.

6. High serum phosphatase; lowered inorganic blood phosphorus; lowered serum citrate.

Rickets is treated by giving relatively large amounts of vitamin D concentrates, the dosage being prescribed by the physician.

Tetany. Tetany is characterized by a low serum calcium (7.5 mg per 100 ml or less), muscle twitchings, cramps, and convulsions. It results from insufficient absorption of calcium or vitamin D, or from a disturbance of the parathyroid gland. The physician prescribes calcium salts to control the acute spasms, a diet liberal in calcium, and vitamin D.

Dental health. In rachitic infants and children there may be delayed dentition and malformation of the teeth. Permanent teeth forming in the jaw are more subject to decay.

Osteomalacia. Frequently referred to as "adult rickets," OSTEOMALACIA literally means bone softening. It occurs when there is lack of vitamin D and calcium. In the Orient it is seen in women who have had many pregnancies, who subsist on a meager cereal diet, and who have little exposure to sunshine.

Osteomalacia may occur when there is interference with fat absorption, and hence also vitamin D absorption. The steatorrhea also reduces the absorption of calcium. In chronic renal disease patients often complain of bone pain, and osteodystrophy may be severe. There is little absorption of calcium apparently because the kidney is unable to produce $1,25\text{-}(OH)_2\text{-}D_3$.

The following changes take place in osteomalacia:

1. A softening of the bones, which may be so severe that the bones of the legs, spine, thorax, and pelvis bend into deformities.

2. Pain of the rheumatic type in bones of the legs and lower part of the back.

3. General weakness with difficulty in walking, and especially difficulty in climbing stairs.

4. Spontaneous multiple fractures.

The synthetic forms of $25\text{-}(OH)\text{-}D_3$ and $1,25\text{-}(OH)_2\text{-}D_3$ show considerable promise in the treatment of these bone disorders. The effective dosages are much smaller than those of vitamin D.[17]

Vitamin E

Discovery. Evans and Bishop established the fact that a fat-soluble factor was necessary for reproduction in rats. They showed that absence of vitamin E, or the antisterility factor, as it was designated, led to irreparable damage of the germinal epithelium in male rats, and female rats which had diets deficient in vitamin E were unable to carry their young to term. In severe deficiency the fetus dies and is resorbed completely. In the female the damage is not permanent; that is, normal reproduction could again take place if the diet were once more adequate in this factor.

Chemistry and characteristics. Vitamin E activity is exhibited by a number of compounds of related chemical structure called TOCOPHEROLS. This term is derived from the Greek words *tokos* meaning "birth" and *phero* "to carry." The ending *-ol* indicates that the substance is an alcohol. Alpha-tocopherol is the compound possessing the greatest vitamin E activity. (See Figure 10–1.) Vitamin E and the sex hormones are chemically related.

High temperatures and acids do not affect the stability of vitamin E, but oxidation takes place readily in the presence of rancid fats or lead and iron salts. Decomposition occurs in ultraviolet light. Vitamin E itself acts as an antioxidant.

Measurement. Vitamin E is expressed in international units or in milligrams of α-tocopherol. One international unit of vitamin E is equal to 1 mg synthetic $dl\text{-}\alpha$-tocopherol acetate. The activity of the natural form, d-α-tocopherol acetate, is 1.36 I.U. per milligram; and that of the free alcohol, d-α-tocopherol, is 1.49 I.U. milligram.[5] Dietary evaluations are concerned primarily with alpha-tocopherol. Other tocopherols in foods contribute vitamin E activity equal to about 20 per cent of the alpha-tocopherol content of the diet.

Physiology. Vitamin E requires the presence of fat and of bile salts for absorption into the intestinal wall. The vitamin is carried with the chylomicrons into the lymph circulation and to the liver. Small amounts of vitamin E are present in all body tissues with the highest concentrations in the pituitary, adrenal gland, and testes. The bulk of the body stores of vitamin E is in the muscle and adipose tissue. No toxicity to vitamin E, even in large amounts, has been shown.

The total plasma tocopherol ranges from 0.5 to 1.2 mg per 100 ml. A level below 0.5 mg is undesirable. There is little transfer of vitamin E across the placenta to the fetus. Hence, newborn infants have low tissue stores.

Functions. The metabolic roles of vitamin E are poorly understood. The principal role appears to be as an antioxidant. By accepting oxygen, vitamin E helps to prevent the oxidation of vitamin A and ascorbic acid, thereby sparing these vitamins. In the tissues vitamin E reduces the oxidation of the polyunsaturated fatty acids, thereby helping to maintain the integrity of the cell membranes.

Vitamin E is probably related to some synthetic processes. One of these is the incorporation of pyrimidines into nucleic acid, especially in the formation of red blood cells in the bone marrow. Vitamin E is also required for the synthesis of coenzyme Q, a factor that is essential in the respiratory chain that releases energy from carbohydrates and fats. In some manner small amounts of selenium can partially replace vitamin E in animal diets.

Daily allowances. The Food and Nutrition Board recommends a daily intake of 4 to 5 I.U. during the first year of life, 12 I.U. for women, 15 I.U. during pregnancy and lactation, and 15 I.U. for men. These allowances are based upon metabolic body size.

The need for vitamin E is higher when the intake of polyunsaturated fatty acids is increased. Since the principal source of vitamin E is from vegetable oils and margarines, the increased intake of linoleic acid from these fats is accompanied by a satisfactory intake of vitamin E. At the present time evidence indicates that there is no fixed ratio of vitamin E to polyunsaturated fatty acids that can be recommended.[18]

Sources. The principal sources of vitamin E in the diet are vegetable oils (corn, soy, cottonseed, safflower), hydrogenated fats from these oils, whole grains, and dark-green leafy vegetables, nuts, and legumes. Foods of animal origin are low in vitamin E. Human milk provides adequate vitamin E for the infant, but cow's milk is low. See Table A–2 for vitamin E content of foods.

The content of tocopherols in foods varies widely. In general, the tocopherol level in oils increases as the linoleic acid content increases. There is considerable loss in fried foods that are frozen and also in the heating of oils. The milling of grains removes about 80 per cent of the vitamin E.

Typical diets in the United States provided 4.4 to 12.7 mg alpha-tocopherol, with an average of 9 mg (13.5 I.U.).[19] In addition, the gamma-tocopherol content was estimated to be about two and a half times that of alpha-tocopherol. The biologic activity of this amount of gamma-tocopherol was estimated to be equal to 25 per cent of the alpha-tocopherol,

or 2.25 mg (4.1 I.U.). Thus, the typical diet would furnish 11.25 mg (16.8 I.U.) tocopherol. In view of the absence of signs of dietary deficiency of vitamin E, the diets in the United States are presumed to meet body needs.

Effects of deficiency. Vitamin E deficiency is extremely rare. It has been observed in some infants with severe kwashiorkor. There was increased hemolysis of the red blood cells, macrocytic anemia, and creatinuria.[20] These conditions were corrected by the administration of vitamin E. Premature infants show an extremely low level of tocopherol in the serum and increased capillary fragility.

When men were consuming diets extremely low in tocopherols over a period of several years, there was increased hemolysis of red blood cells. The length of time to bring about the onset of hemolysis was shortened when the intake of polyunsaturated fats was increased.[21]

Exaggerated claims for vitamin E. When animals are placed on diets devoid of vitamin E a wide range of symptoms is observed, with considerable variation from one species to another. Among the changes observed have been reproductive failure, macrocytic anemia, shorter life-span of the red cells, creatinuria, liver necrosis, encephalomalacia, and muscular dystrophy. The results of these studies have been widely misinterpreted and applied to human nutrition. The fact that human diets generally provide ample amounts of vitamin E is ignored.

Vitamin E has been recommended for such widely varying conditions as heart disease, muscular dystrophy, acne, ulcers, habitual abortion, disorders of the menopause, and sexual impotence. However, objective studies do not support any of these exaggerated claims.[22-24] In view of the excessive amounts of the vitamin ingested by many people it is indeed fortunate that the vitamin does not exert toxic effects.

VITAMIN K

The existence of vitamin K was first suggested by Dr. Dam of Copenhagen who in 1935 found that a "Koagulations Vitamin" was necessary to prevent fatal hemorrhages in chicks by promoting normal blood clotting.

Chemistry and characteristics. Vitamin K consists

of a number of related compounds known as *quinones;* vitamin K_1, also known as *phytylmenaquinone,* was first isolated from alfalfa, and vitamin K_2, also termed *menaquinone,* was produced from putrefied fish meal and is also the form synthesized by intestinal bacteria. (See Figure 10–1.) *Menadione* is a synthetic compound that is two to three times as potent as the natural vitamin. Vitamin K is fat soluble, resistant to heat, but easily destroyed by acids, alkalies, light, and oxidizing agents.

Measurement. The activity of test materials is measured in micrograms by its ability to prevent hemorrhage in young chicks. Menadione is used as the standard for measuring vitamin K potency.

Physiology. Vitamin K can be synthesized by bacteria of the lower intestinal tract. Being fat soluble, vitamin K requires the presence of bile for its absorption, most of which occurs in the upper part of the small intestine. Probably only a small amount of the intestinal synthesis is actually utilized. A large amount of vitamin K is excreted in the feces. Limited stores of vitamin K are maintained but the concentration in no tissues is high.

The newborn infant has a very limited supply of vitamin K, and synthesis by the relatively sterile intestinal tract does not take place for several days. Human milk supplies about one fourth as much vitamin K as does cow's milk. Thus, the first few days may be critical for the infant.

Function. Vitamin K is essential for the formation of PROTHROMBIN and other clotting proteins by the liver. (See page 103.) A high prothrombin level of the blood indicates good ability to coagulate blood, whereas low blood levels of prothrombin are associated with a slow rate of coagulation. Vitamin K probably also participates in oxidative phosphorylation in the tissues.

Daily allowances. The variations in intestinal synthesis and in the diet have made it impossible to establish a daily allowance. Dietary deficiency is not believed to be a problem.

Sources. Green leaves of plants such as spinach and kale are excellent sources of vitamin K as are also cabbage, cauliflower, and pork liver. Cereals, fruits, and other vegetables are poor sources.

Effects of deficiency. A low blood level of prothrombin and other clotting factors leads to increased tendency to hemorrhage. Premature infants, anoxic infants, and those whose mothers have been taking anticoagulants are most susceptible to deficiency. The hemorrhagic disease of the newborn can be prevented by a single dose of vitamin K_1 administered to the infant immediately after birth. The practice of giving vitamin K to the mother prior to delivery has been questioned since too much may lead to hemolytic anemia in the infant.

Dietary deficiency of vitamin K is not likely. Deficiency may occur in adults because of a failure in absorption, or interference with the synthesis in the intestine, or inability to form prothrombin by the liver. Oral therapy with sulfa drugs and antibiotics interferes with the synthesis of the vitamin in the intestine. Obstruction of the biliary tract and severe diarrhea as in sprue, celiac disease, and colitis may seriously interfere with absorption. In severe disease of the liver the synthesis of the clotting factors is impaired even though the source of vitamin K is adequate.

If absorption is inadequate, vitamin K may be prescribed orally together with bile salts. Parenteral administration may be required when there is severe intestinal disease. Vitamin K_1 may be used for oral therapy, but menadione taken orally leads to vomiting.

Dicumarol is an anticoagulant often used to treat coronary thrombosis. It is antagonistic to the action of vitamin K and prevents the formation of prothrombin. Anticoagulant therapy carries the risk of hemorrhage. When an excessive amount of anticoagulant is given, vitamin K may be administered to counteract it.

PROBLEMS AND REVIEW

1. What is the relationship of carotene to vitamin A? What are the important sources of carotene?
2. Why are young children more susceptible than adults to deficiency of vitamin A or D? Describe the signs of deficiency that may be seen in children.
3. *Problem.* Calculate the vitamin A content of your own diet for two days. What percentage of your daily allowance is provided by sources rich in vitamin A? By sources rich in the provitamin?

Table 10–1. Summary of the Fat-Soluble Vitamins

Nomenclature	Important Sources	Physiology and Functions	Effect of Deficiency	Daily Allowances*
Vitamin A Retinol Retinal Retinyl ester Retinoic acid Provitamin A Alpha-, beta-, gamma-carotene, cryptoxanthin	*Animal* Fish-liver oils Liver Butter, cream Whole milk Whole-milk cheeses Egg yolk *Plant* Dark-green leafy vegetables Yellow vegetables Yellow fruits Fortified margarines	Bile necessary for absorption Stored in liver Maintains integrity of mucosal epithelium, maintains visual acuity in dim light Large amounts are toxic	Faulty bone and tooth development Night blindness Keratinization of epithelium—mucous membranes and skin *Xerophthalmia*	Children: 400–700 R.E. (2000–3300 I.U.) Men: 1000 R.E. (5000 I.U.) Women: 800 R.E. (4000 I.U.) Pregnancy: 1000 R.E. (5000 I.U.) Lactation: 1200 R.E. (6000 I.U.)
Vitamin D Vitamin D_2 Ergocalciferol Vitamin D_3 Cholecalciferol Antirachitic factor	Fish-liver oils Fortified milk Activated sterols Exposure to sunlight Very small amounts in butter, liver, egg yolk, salmon, sardines	Synthesized in skin by activity of ultraviolet light Liver synthesizes 25-OH-D_3 Kidney synthesizes 1,25-$(OH)_2$-D_3 Functions as steroid hormone to regulate calcium and phosphorus absorption, mobilization and mineralization of bone Large amounts are toxic	*Rickets* in children Soft, fragile bones Enlarged joints Bowed legs Chest, spinal, pelvic, bone deformities Delayed dentition *Tetanic* convulsions in infants *Osteomalacia* in adults	Need is small for adults Children, pregnant or lactating women: 400 I.U.
Vitamin E Alpha-, beta-, gamma-tocopherol Antisterility vitamin	Plant tissues—vegetable oils; wheat germ, rice germ; green leafy vegetables; nuts; legumes Animal foods are poor sources	Not stored in body to any extent Related to action of selenium *Humans:* reduces oxidation of vitamin A, carotenes, and polyunsaturated fatty acids *Animals:* normal reproduction; utilization of sex hormones, cholesterol	*Humans:* hemolysis of red blood cells; mild anemia; deficiency is not likely *Animals:* sterility in male rats; resorption of fetus in female rats; muscular dystrophy; creatinuria; macrocytic anemia	Men: 15 I.U. Women: 12 I.U. Pregnancy: 15 I.U. Infants: 4–5 I.U.
Vitamin K Phytylmenaquinone (K_1) Menaquinone (MK_n) Menadione	Green leaves such as alfalfa, spinach, cabbage Liver Synthesis in intestine	Bile necessary for absorption Formation of prothrombin Sulfa drugs and antibiotics interfere with absorption Large amounts are toxic	Prolonged clotting time Hemorrhagic disease in newborn infants	Not known

*See Recommended Dietary allowances for complete listing, Table 3–1.

162

4. Why is the fortification of milk with vitamin D generally recommended? Why is the fortification of other foods not desirable?

5. Which of the fat-soluble vitamins are toxic? What intakes are likely to lead to toxicity? What are the manifestations of the toxicity?

6. What interrelationship exists between these factors: vitamin A and E; vitamin D and phosphorus; vitamin D and calcium; vitamin E and selenium; vitamin E and polyunsaturated fatty acids?

7. What is the relation of vitamin K to blood clotting? Under what circumstances is a deficiency of vitamin K likely to occur?

8. What is the principal function of vitamin E? What conditions are necessary to produce a deficiency of vitamin E?

9. Which of the fat-soluble vitamins functions as a hormone? How is the hormone formed? What is the role of parathormone?

10. Describe the mechanism by which retinaldehyde participates in night vision.

11. A diet supplies 2000 I.U. retinol and 3000 I.U. beta-carotene. To how many R.E. are these equivalent? Does the diet meet the need of the pregnant woman?

CITED REFERENCES

1. McCollum, E. V., and Davis, M.: "The Necessity of Certain Lipins in the Diet during Growth," *J. Biol. Chem.*, **15**:167–75, 1913. See "Nutrition Classic," *Nutr. Rev.*, **31**:280–81, 1973.

2. Osborne, T. B., and Mendel, L. B.: "The Relation of Growth to the Chemical Constituents of the Diet," *J. Biol. Chem.*, **15**:311–26, 1913.

3. Steenbock, H.: "White Corn versus Yellow Corn and a Probable Relation between the Fat Soluble Vitamin and Yellow Plant Pigments," *Science*, **50**:352–53, 1919.

4. "Nomenclature Policy: Generic Descriptions and Trivial Names for Vitamins and Related Compounds," *J. Nutr.*, **104**:144–50, 1974.

5. Food and Nutrition Board: *Recommended Dietary Allowances*, 8th ed. National Academy of Sciences, Washington, D.C., 1974.

6. FAO/WHO: *Requirements of Vitamin A, Thiamine, Riboflavine, and Niacin.* WHO Tech. Rept. Ser. No. 362, WHO, Geneva, 1967.

7. Schaefer, A. E., and Johnson O. C.: "Are We Well Fed? The Search for the Answer," *Nutr. Today*, **4**:2–11, Spring 1969.

8. McClaren, D. S.: News note in "Medical News Around the World," *Med. World News*, Jan. 26, 1968, p. 11.

9. Oomen, H. A. P. C.: "Vitamin A Deficiency, Xerophthalmia and Blindness," *Nutr. Rev.*, **32**:161–70, 1974.

10. Bauernfeind, J. C., *et al.:* "Vitamin A and E Nutrition via Intramuscular or Oral Route," *Am. J. Clin. Nutr.*, **27**:234–53, 1974.

11. Committee on Drugs and on Nutrition, American Academy of Pediatrics: "The Use and Abuse of Vitamin A," *Nutr. Rev.*, **32**, (Suppl. 1):41–43, 1974.

12. Fisher, G., and Skillern, P. G.: "Hypercalcemia Due to Hypervitaminosis A," *J.A.M.A.*, **227**:1413–14, 1974.

13. Review: "Vitamin A Intoxication in Infancy," *Nutr. Rev.*, **23**:263–65, 1965.

14. DeLuca, H. F.: "A New Look at an Old Vitamin," *Nutr. Rev.*, **29**:179–81, 1971.

15. Haussler, M. R.: "Vitamin D: Mode of Action and Biomedical Applications," *Nutr. Rev.*, **32**:257–66, 1974.

16. Fraser, D. R., and Kodicek, E.: "Unique Biosynthesis by Kidney of a Biologically Active Vitamin D Metabolite," *Nature*, **228**:764–66, 1970.

17. DeLuca, H. F.: "Vitamin D: The Vitamin and the Hormone," *Fed. Proc.*, **33**:2211–19, 1974.

18. Bieri, J. G., and Evarts, R. P.: "Vitamin E Adequacy in Vegetable Oils," *J. Am. Diet. Assoc.*, **66**:134–39, 1975.

19. Bieri, J. G., and Evarts, R. P.: "Tocopherols and Fatty Acids in American Diets," *J. Am. Diet. Assoc.*, **62**:147–51, 1973.

20. Roels, O. A.: "Present Knowledge of Vitamin E," *Nutr. Rev.*, **25**:33–37, 1967.

21. Horwitt, M. K., *et al.*: "Effects of Limited Tocopherol Intake in Man with Relationships to Erythrocyte Hemolysis and Lipid Oxidation," *Am. J. Clin. Nutr.*, **4**:408–18, 1956.
22. "Vitamin E—Miracle or Myth?" *Nutr. Rev.*, **32** (Suppl. 1):35–36, July 1974.
23. Anderson, T. W., and Reed, D. B. W.: "A Double-Blind Trial of Vitamin E in Angina Pectoris," *Am. J. Clin. Nutr.*, **27**:1174–78, 1974.
24. Committee on Nutritional Misinformation, Food and Nutrition Board: "Supplementation of Human Diets with Vitamin E," *Nutr. Rev.*, **31**:327–28, 1973.

ADDITIONAL REFERENCES

Vitamin A

Bloch, C. E.: "Clinical Investigation of Xerophthalmia in Infants and Young Children," *J. Hygiene*, **19**:283–301, 1921; Nutrition Classic reproduced in part in *Nutr. Rev.*, **32**:176–79, 1974.

Furman, K. I.: "Acute Hypervitaminosis A in an Adult," *Am. J. Clin. Nutr.*, **26**:575–77, 1973.

Ganguly, A. J.: "Absorption of Vitamin A," *Am. J. Clin. Nutr.*, **22**:923–33, 1969.

High, E. G.: "Some Aspects of Nutritional Vitamin A Levels in Preschool Children of Beaufort County, South Carolina," *Am. J. Clin. Nutr.*, **22**:1129–32, 1969.

Katz, C. M., and Tzagournis, M.: "Chronic Adult Hypervitaminosis A with Hypercalcemia," *Metabolism*, **21**:1171–76, 1972.

Lala, V. R., and Reddy, V.: "Absorption of β-Carotene from Green Leafy Vegetables in Undernourished Children," *Am. J. Clin. Nutr.*, **23**:110–13, 1970.

Pereira, S. M., *et al.*: "Vitamin A Therapy in Children with Kwashiorkor," *Am. J. Clin. Nutr.*, **20**:297–304, 1967.

Rao, C. N., and Rao, B. S. N.: "Absorption of Dietary Carotenes in Human Subjects," *Am. J. Clin. Nutr.*, **23**:105–109, 1970.

Review: "Interrelationships between Vitamins A and E," *Nutr. Rev.*, **23**:82–84, 1965.

Rodriguez, M. E., and Irwin, M. I.: "A Conspectus of Research on Vitamin A Requirements of Man," *J. Nutr.*, **102**:909–68, 1972.

Russell, R. M., *et al.*: "Hepatic Injury from Chronic Hypervitaminosis A Resulting in Portal Hypertension and Ascites," *N. Engl. J. Med.*, **291**:435–40, 1974.

Sweeney, J. P., and Marsh, A. C.: "Effect of Processing on Provitamin A in Vegetables," *J. Am. Diet. Assoc.*, **59**:238–43, 1971.

Wald, G.: "Molecular Basis of Visual Excitation," *Science*, **162**:230–39, 1968.

Vitamin D

Committee on Nutrition Misinformation, Food and Nutrition Board: "Hazards of Overuse of Vitamin D," *Nutr. Rev.*, **33**:61–62, 1975.

Committee on Nutrition, American Academy of Pediatrics: "The Relation between Infantile Hypercalcemia and Vitamin D—Public Health Implications in North America," *Pediatrics*, **40**:1050–61, 1967.

Dale, A. E., and Lowenberg, M. E.: "Consumption of Vitamin D in Fortified and Natural Foods and in Vitamin Preparations," *J. Pediatr.*, **70**:952–55, 1967.

Editorial: "Vitamin D, Another Frontier," *J.A.M.A.*, **210**:550, 1969.

McCollum, E. V., *et al.*: "Studies on Experimental Rickets. XXI. Experimental Demonstration of a Vitamin Which Promotes Calcium Deposition," *J. Biol. Chem.*, **53**:293–312, 1922; Nutrition Classic reproduced in part in *Nutr. Rev.*, **33**:48–50, 1975.

Omdahl, J. L., and DeLuca, H. F.: "Vitamin D," in Goodhart, R. S., and Shils, M. E., eds.: *Modern Nutrition in Health and Disease*, 5th ed. Lea & Febiger, Philadelphia, 1973, pp. 158–65.

Palmisano, P. A.: "Vitamin D: A Reawakening," *J.A.M.A.*, **224**:1526–27, 1973.

Review: "The Role of 1,25-Dihydroxyvitamin D_3 in Phosphate Metabolism," *Nutr. Rev.*, **32**:247–49, 1974.

Review: "Recent Clinical Correlates of Vitamin D Metabolites and Calcium Metabolism," *Nutr. Rev.*, **33**:209–10, 1975.

Review: "Phytate and Rickets," *Nutr. Rev.*, **31**:238–39, 1973.

Review: "Control of Vitamin D Metabolism," *Nutr. Rev.*, **31**:187–88, 1973.

Stearns, G.: "Early Studies of Vitamin D Requirement during Growth," *Am. J. Public Health,* **58**:2027–35, 1968.

Weick, Sr. M. T.: "A History of Rickets in the United States," *Am. J. Clin. Nutr.,* **20**:1234–41, 1967.

Vitamin E

Dicks-Bushnell, M. W., and Davis, K. C.: "Vitamin E Content of Infant Formulas and Cereals," *Am. J. Clin. Nutr.,* **20**:262–69, 1967.

Draper, H. H., and Csallany, A. S.: "Metabolism and Function of Vitamin E," *Fed. Proc.,* **28**:1690–95, 1969.

Herting, D. C.: "Perspective on Vitamin E," *Am. J. Clin. Nutr.,* **19**:210–18, 1966.

Hodges, R. E.: "Vitamin E and Coronary Heart Disease," *J. Am. Diet. Assoc.,* **62**:638–42, 1973.

Horwitt, M. K.: "Status of Human Requirements for Vitamin E," *Am. J. Clin. Nutr.,* **27**:1182–93, 1974.

Olson, R. E.: "Vitamin E and Its Relation to Heart Disease," *Circulation,* **48**:179–84, 1973.

Oski, F. A., and Barness, L. A.: "Vitamin E Deficiency: A Previously Unrecognized Cause of Hemolytic Anemia in the Premature Infant," *J. Pediatr.,* **70**:211–20, 1967.

Review: "Compounds with Vitamin E Activity," *Nutr. Rev.,* **27**:92–94, 1969.

Review: "Vitamin E Status of Adults on a Vegetable Oil Diet," *Nutr. Rev.,* **24**:41–43, 1966.

Review: "Hypervitaminosis E and Coagulation," *Nutr. Rev.,* **33**:269–70, 1975.

Vitamin K

Campbell, H. A., and Link, K. P.: "Studies on the Hemorrhagic Sweet Clover Disease. IV. The Isolation and Crystallization of the Hemorrhagic Agent," *J. Biol. Chem.,* **138**:21–33, 1941; Nutrition classic reproduced in part in *Nutr. Rev.,* **32**:244–46, 1974.

Dam, H.: "The Antihaemorrhagic Vitamin of the Chick," *Biochem. J.,* **29**:1273–85, 1935; Nutrition classic reproduced in part in *Nutr. Rev.,* **31**:121, 1973.

Filer, L. J., Jr., *et al.:* "Vitamin K Supplementation for Infants Receiving Milk Substitute Infant Formulas and for Those with Fat Malabsorption," *Pediatrics,* **48**:483–87, 1971.

Garrison, W.: "Vitamin K. Savior of Bleeding Babies," *Today's Health,* **47**:42, Sept. 1969.

Goldman, H. I., and Amadio, P.: "Vitamin K Deficiency After the Newborn Period," *Pediatrics,* **44**:745–49, 1969.

Olson, R. E.: "The Mode of Action of Vitamin K," *Nutr. Rev.,* **28**:171–76, 1970.

Review: "Vitamin K Deficiency in Adults," *Nutr. Rev.,* **26**:165–67, 1968.

Review: "Vitamin K and Prothrombin Structure," *Nutr. Rev.,* **32**:279–81, 1974.

Suttie, J. W.: "Vitamin K and Prothrombin Synthesis," *Nutr. Rev.,* **31**:105–109, 1973.

11 The Water-Soluble Vitamins: Ascorbic Acid

incidence of scurvy on his seagoing voyages by stocking up on fresh fruits and vegetables whenever he was in port, and also by including sauerkraut as part of the rations. The sauerkraut kept well and was a good preventive of scurvy.

The scientific era of vitamin C began in 1907 when two Norwegian scientists, Holst and Frölich, produced scurvy in guinea pigs. The isolation and chemical nature of vitamin C, or ascorbic acid, was accomplished by Dr. Charles G. King and his co-workers at the University of Pittsburgh and by Dr. Szent-Györgyi of Hungary in the early 1930s.

Chemistry and characteristics. ASCORBIC ACID is a white crystalline compound of relatively simple structure, and closely related to the monosaccharide sugars. It is synthesized from glucose and other simple sugars by plants and by most animal species. It can be prepared synthetically at low cost from glucose. Vitamin C activity is possessed by two forms: L-ascorbic acid (the reduced form) and L-dehydroascorbic acid (the oxidized form). (See Figure 11–1.) The latter is oxidized further with complete loss of activity.

Of all vitamins, ascorbic acid is the most easily destroyed. It is highly soluble in water. The oxidation of ascorbic acid is accelerated by heat, light, alkalies, oxidative enzymes, and traces of copper and iron. Oxidation is inhibited to a marked degree in an acid reaction, and when the temperature is reduced.

Measurement. Ascorbic acid is determined by chemical assay, and the concentration in tissues and foods is expressed in milligrams.

Metabolism. So far only five species are known to require a dietary source of ascorbic acid: man, monkeys, guinea pigs, Indian fruit bat, and the red-vented bulbul bird, native to India. Ascorbic acid is

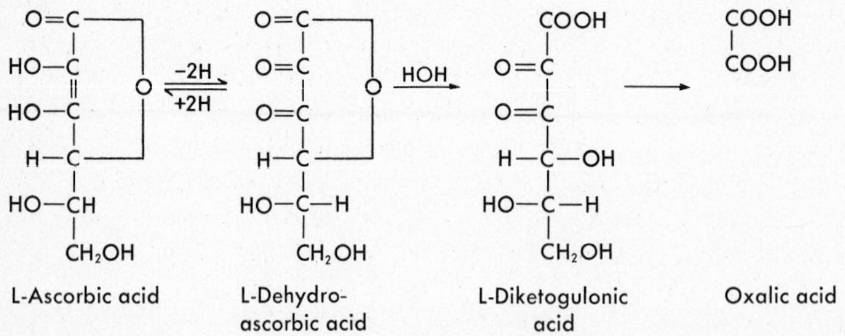

Discovery. Scurvy has been known as a dread disease since ancient times. It was described as early as 1550 B.C. by the Egyptians in the Papyrus Ebers, a treatise on medicine. It particularly plagued the seagoing adventurers of the sixteenth and seventeenth centuries who lost thousands of men to scurvy. Jacques Cartier in his explorations in Canada was slightly more fortunate for the Indians showed how a brew of pine needles and bark could cure scurvy, and many men were thus saved.

In 1747, Dr. James Lind, a British physician, tested six remedies on 12 sailors who had scurvy. He found that oranges and lemons were curative. But it took another 50 years before the British Navy required rations of lemons or limes on the sailing vessels. From that day to the present the British sailor has been known as a "limey." During this same period Captain Cook was able to reduce the

L-Ascorbic acid $\quad$ L-Dehydro-ascorbic acid $\quad$ L-Diketogulonic acid $\quad$ Oxalic acid

Ascorbic acid, $(C_6H_8O_6;$ m.w. 176.1)

Figure 11–1. Ascorbic acid and dehydroascorbic acid are biologically active. These forms are easily converted to diketogulonic acid, which is inactive. Note the similarity of the structure of ascorbic acid to that of glucose.

rapidly absorbed from the gastrointestinal tract and distributed to the various tissues of the body. The adrenal gland and the retina of the eye contain an especially high concentration of vitamin C, but other tissues such as the spleen, intestine, bone marrow, pancreas, thymus, liver, pituitary, and kidney also contain appreciable amounts.

A plasma level of 0.6 mg ascorbic acid per 100 ml indicates tissue saturation, and a body storage equivalent to 1500 mg in the adult. Adequate vitamin C nutrition is indicated when plasma concentrations range between 0.40 and 0.59 mg per 100 ml, representing a body pool of 600 to 1499 mg.[1] Smokers will store less of a given dose of ascorbic acid than nonsmokers.[2]

The kidney exercises some control over the excretion of ascorbic acid. If tissues are saturated, most of a large dose of vitamin C will be excreted. If tissues are depleted, only a small amount of vitamin C will be excreted. Ascorbic acid is excreted as such, or as metabolites including oxalic acid and ascorbic acid sulfate.

The body efficiently utilizes either synthetic L-ascorbic acid or the vitamin in its natural form as in orange juice.[3]

Functions. One of the principal functions of ascorbic acid is the formation of collagen, an abundant protein that forms the intercellular substance in cartilage, bone matrices, dentin, and the vascular epithelium. For the synthesis of collagen ascorbic acid brings about the HYDROXYLATION (introduction of —OH groups) of proline and lysine to hydroxyproline and hydroxylysine. These hydroxy amino acids are important constituents of collagen. This function helps to explain the importance of vitamin C in wound healing and the ability to withstand the stresses of injury and infection.

Another important hydroxylation reaction occurs in the conversion of tryptophan to serotonin, a compound that raises blood pressure through vasoconstrictor action. The conversion of cholesterol to bile acids also requires hydroxylation reactions. By this conversion the cholesterol content of the blood is reduced.[4]

Ascorbic acid is an important antioxidant and thus has a role in the protection of vitamins A and E and the polyunsaturated fatty acids from excessive oxidation. Ascorbic acid reduces ferric iron to ferrous iron in the gastrointestinal tract, thereby increasing the absorption of iron. It also aids in the release of iron from transferrin in the circulation so that it can be incorporated into tissue ferritin. The conversion of folacin, a B-complex vitamin, to its active form folinic acid requires vitamin C.

Based upon animal studies, ascorbic acid together with ATP and magnesium chloride has a role in the deactivation of adipose tissue lipase. The mobilization of fat from adipose tissue requires lipase, but such mobilization ceases when the three controlling agents are present.[5] Other studies have shown that ascorbic acid increases the rate of removal of amide groups from certain amino acids. Still another role appears to be in the sulfation (introduction of sulfur groups) of certain compounds.[6,7] For example, cholesterol sulfate is a water-soluble compound that is more readily excreted. Ascorbic acid may be involved in the synthesis of epinephrine and steroid hormones by the adrenal gland. At the present time there is no evidence that links vitamin C with enzyme activity.

Recommended allowances. As little as 10 mg ascorbic acid will prevent scurvy. This level may be regarded as a minimum requirement but it does not ensure fully satisfactory tissue levels. Each day the adult male removes about 30 mg ascorbic acid from body stores. The recommended allowance has been set at 45 mg for males and females over 11 years, 35 mg for infants, 40 mg for children, and 60 mg for pregnancy and lactation.[8]

During infections such as tuberculosis, rheumatic fever, and pneumonia and severe stress such as burn injuries the ascorbic acid requirement is increased.

Food sources. Almost all of the daily intake of ascorbic acid is obtained from the vegetable-fruit group. (See Figure 11–2.) In the American diet the vitamin C in the available food supply is furnished from food groups in these percentages: citrus fruits, 27.6; other fruits, 11.2; potatoes and sweet potatoes, 17.5; dark-green and deep-yellow vegetables, 8.2; other vegetables including tomatoes, 27.3.[9]

Vitamin C has been called the "fresh-food vitamin" since it is found in highest concentrations just as the food is fresh from the plant. In general, the active parts of the plant contain appreciable amounts, and mature or resting seeds are devoid of the vitamin.

Raw, frozen, or canned citrus fruits such as oranges, grapefruit, and lemons are excellent sources

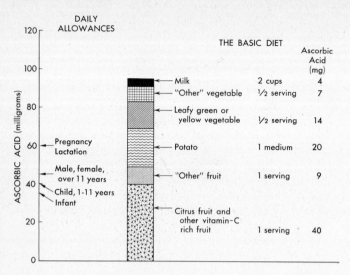

Figure 11–2. The vegetable-fruit group accounts for almost all of the ascorbic acid in the diet. See Table 13–2 for complete calculation of the Basic Diet.

of the vitamin. Orange sections including the thin white peel contain more vitamin C than an equal weight of strained juice.

Fresh strawberries, cantaloupe, pineapple, and guavas are also excellent sources. Other nonacid fresh fruits such as peaches, pears, apples, bananas, and blueberries contribute small amounts of the vitamin; when eaten in large amounts these fruits may be an important dietary source. The concentration of ascorbic acid in the nonacid canned fruits is considerably reduced.

Broccoli, Brussels sprouts, spinach, kale, green peppers, cabbage, and turnips are excellent-to-good sources even when cooked. The use of potatoes and sweet potatoes as staple food items enhances the vitamin C intake considerably provided that preparation methods have been good.

Milk, eggs, meat, fish, and poultry are practically devoid of vitamin C as they are consumed. If the mother's diet has been adequate, human milk contains four to six times as much ascorbic acid as cow's milk and is able to protect the infant from scurvy. Liver contains a small amount of vitamin C, but most of this is lost during cookery.

Retention of food values. A warm environment, exposure to air, solubility in water, heat, alkali, and dehydration are detrimental to the retention of ascorbic acid in foods. The cutting of vegetables releases oxidative enzymes and increases the surfaces exposed to leaching by water. Since the vitamin is so soluble, losses are considerable when large amounts of water are used. Vegetables should be added to a small quantity of boiling water, covered tightly, and cooked until just tender for high retention of ascorbic acid. Retention is also good when a pressure cooker is used, provided that the cookery time is carefully controlled. The practice of adding baking soda to retain green color of vegetables not only reduces the vitamin C level but may also modify the flavor and texture of the vegetable. Leftover vegetables lose a large proportion of the ascorbic acid, although losses are reduced somewhat when the container is tightly covered in the refrigerator. On the other hand, citrus juices and tomatoes retain practically all the vitamin C value for several days.

Effects of deficiency. According to the 1965 dietary survey in the United States, 27 per cent of the diets provided less than the recommended dietary allowances for ascorbic acid; half of these diets furnished less than two thirds of the RDA. The National Nutrition Survey showed that 12 to 16 per cent of people in all age categories had unacceptable serum levels of ascorbic acid.[10] Of all subjects surveyed in this study, 4 per cent had scorbutic gum lesions.

A deficiency of ascorbic acid results in the defective formation of the intercellular cement substance. Fleeting joint pains, irritability, retardation of growth in the infant or child, anemia, shortness of breath, poor wound healing, and increased susceptibility to infection are among the signs of defi-

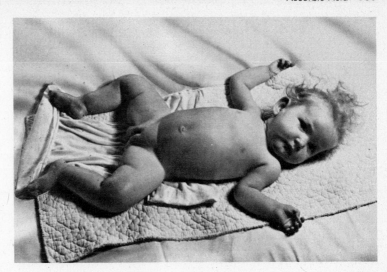

Figure 11–3. Child in scorbutic position. (Courtesy, Dr. Bernard S. Epstein, The Long Island Jewish Hospital, New Hyde Park, New York, and *The Vitamin Manual*, published by The Upjohn Company.)

ciency, but none of these can establish a diagnosis. A dietary history, the concentration of ascorbic acid in the blood plasma and in the white blood cells, and a measure of the excretion of a test dose in the urine help to establish the diagnosis.

Scurvy. The classic picture of scurvy is rarely seen in adults in the United States. The incidence is also uncommon in infants, but a gross deficiency of ascorbic acid results in scurvy during the second six months of life. Infections, fevers, and hyperthyroidism may precipitate the symptoms when the intake has been inadequate. The symptoms are related to the weakening of the collagenous material.

Pain, tenderness, and swelling of the thighs and legs are frequent symptoms of infantile scurvy. The baby shows a disinclination to move and assumes a position with legs flexed for comfort (see Figure 11–3). He is pale and irritable and cries when handled. Loss of weight, fever, diarrhea, and vomiting are frequently present. If the teeth have erupted, the gums are likely to be swollen, tender, and hemorrhagic. Bone calcification is faulty because of degeneration or lack of proper development of the bone matrix. The cartilage supporting the bones is weak, and bone displacement results. The ends of the long bones and of the ribs are enlarged somewhat is in rickets, but tenderness is a distinguishing characteristic in scurvy.

Scurvy in adults results after several months of a diet devoid of ascorbic acid. The symptoms include swelling, infection, and bleeding of the gums—gingivitis; tenderness of the legs; anemia; and petechial hemorrhages. The teeth may become loose and eventually may be lost. As the disease progresses, the slightest injury produces excessive bleeding, and large hemorrhages may be seen underneath the skin. There is degeneration of the muscle structure and of the cartilage generally.

Acute scurvy responds within a few days to the administration of 100 to 200 mg ascorbic acid given in the synthetic form or as orange juice. Chronic changes that have occurred, such as bone deformities and anemia, require much longer periods for their correction.

Megadoses of ascorbic acid. Since the publication of Dr. Linus Pauling's Book,[11] thousands of people take large doses of ascorbic acid—1.0 to 5.0 gm daily for prophylaxis, and up to 15 gm daily to treat colds. Such dosages are 20 to 100 times the recommended allowances, and should be regarded as pharmaceutic agents. A group of investigators in Canada studied the preventive and therapeutic effects of vitamin C on a group of 818 volunteers during the winter months.[12] Half of the volunteers were given 1.0 gm ascorbic acid daily and half were given placebos that could not be distinguished from the vitamin tablets. Only the person holding the code knew which individuals consumed ascorbic acid and which individuals consumed placebos. There was a slight reduction in the incidence of colds and also a lesser length of time confined to the house (1.3 days for the vitamin group and 1.87 days for the placebo group) in persons who took the ascorbic acid tablets. The authors felt that the results did not justify a recommendation for using large doses of vitamin C and that studies were needed to establish the safety of ingesting large amounts.

Although no toxicity has been encountered with large doses of ascorbic acid, this problem has not been sufficiently studied. Hodges and Baker have discussed some potential hazards: increased absorption of iron beyond desirable levels, especially in males; increased mobilization of bone minerals; interference with anticoagulant therapy; formation of uric acid stones by persons who have a tendency to gout; formation of oxalate stones since ascorbic acid is metabolized to oxalic acid; possible dependency upon large doses of vitamin C so that smaller doses no longer meet nutritional needs.[1]

In view of the small response to large doses of vitamin C in preventing colds, and in the absence of studies establishing the safety of large amounts, it would seem that excessive intakes of ascorbic acid serve no useful purpose.

A summary of ascorbic acid appears at the end of Chapter 12.

PROBLEMS AND REVIEW

1. In what way is ascorbic acid related to the functioning of each of these substances: iron, collagen, folacin, cholesterol, lipase, vitamin A, tryptophan?
2. What are the clinical manifestations of a deficiency of ascorbic acid?
3. What is the effect of an intake of ascorbic acid in excess of the body's needs?
4. Why is a formula-fed baby more prone to scurvy than a breast-fed baby?
5. List the instructions you would give for the preparation and service of these foods in order that the maximum ascorbic acid would be retained: tossed green salad, buttered cabbage?
6. *Problem.* Calculate the ascorbic acid content of your own diet for two days. Compare your intake with the recommended allowances.
7. *Problem.* Calculate the amounts of each of the following foods necessary to furnish 25 mg of ascorbic acid: orange juice, tomato juice, sweet potato, cabbage, grapefruit, endive, strawberries, cantaloupe, apple, lettuce.
8. Mashed potatoes served in a restaurant probably should not be relied upon as a source of ascorbic acid. Give several reasons why this is true.

CITED REFERENCES

1. Hodges, R. E., and Baker, E. M.: "Ascorbic Acid," in Goodhart, R. S., and Shils, M. E., eds.: *Modern Nutrition in Health and Disease*, 5th ed. Lea & Febiger, Philadelphia, 1973, pp. 245–55.
2. Pelletier, O.: "Smoking and Vitamin C Levels in Humans," *Am. J. Clin. Nutr.*, **21:**1259–67, 1968.
3. Pelletier, O., and Keith, M. O.: "Bioavailability of Synthetic and Natural Ascorbic Acid," *J. Am. Diet. Assoc.*, **64:**271–75, 1974.
4. Review: "Ascorbic Acid and the Catabolism of Cholesterol," *Nutr. Rev.*, **31:**154–56, 1973.
5. Review: "New Roles for Ascorbic Acid," *Nutr. Rev.*, **32:**53–55, 1974.
6. Baker, E. M., III, *et al.*: "Ascorbate Sulfate: A Urinary Metabolite of Ascorbic Acid in Man," *Science*, **173:**826–27, 1971.
7. Review: "Ascorbic Acid Sulfate (AAS): A Metabolite of Ascorbic Acid with Antiscorbutic Activity," *Nutr. Rev.*, **31:**251–52, 1973.
8. Food and Nutrition Board: *Recommended Dietary Allowances*, 8th ed. National Academy of Sciences—National Research Council, Washington, D.C., 1974.
9. Friend, B., and Marston, R.: "Nutritional Review," in *National Food Situation*, U.S. Department of Agriculture, November, 1975, pp. 26–32.
10. Schaefer, A. E., and Johnson, O. C.: "Are We Well Fed? The Search for the Answer," *Nutr. Today*, **4:**2–9, Spring 1969.
11. Pauling, L.: *Vitamin C and the Common Cold*. W. H. Freeman and Company, San Francisco, 1970.

12. Anderson, T. W., *et al.:* "Vitamin C and the Common Cold: A Double-Blind Trial," *Canad. Med. Assoc. J.,* **107:**503–508, 1972.

ADDITIONAL REFERENCES

Anderson, T. W., *et al.:* "The Effect on Winter Illness of Large Doses of Vitamin C," *Canad. Med. Assoc. J.,* **111:**31–36, 1974.

Beeuwkes, A.: "The Prevalence of Scurvy Among Voyageurs to America 1493–1600," *J. Am. Diet. Assoc.,* **24:**300–303, 1947.

Committee on Drugs, American Academy of Pediatrics: "Vitamin C and the Common Cold, *Nutr. Rev.,* **32** (Suppl. 1); 39–40, July 1974.

Coulehan, J. L., *et al.:* "Vitamin C Prophylaxis in a Boarding School," *N. Engl. J. Med.,* **290:**6–10, 1974.

Hodges, R. E., *et al.:* "Experimental Scurvy in Man," *Am. J. Clin. Nutr.,* **22:**535–48, 1969.

Hodges, R. E., *et al.:* "Clinical Manifestations of Ascorbic Acid Deficiency in Man," *Am. J. Clin. Nutr.,* **24:**432–43, 1971.

Lopez, A., *et al.:* "Influence of Time and Temperature on Ascorbic Acid Stability," *J. Am. Diet. Assoc.,* **50:**308–10, 1967.

Noble, I.: "Ascorbic Acid and Color of Vegetables," *J. Am. Diet. Assoc.,* **50:**304–307, 1967.

Review: "Vitamin C and the Common Cold," *Nutr. Rev.,* **31:**303–305, 1973.

Schwartz, P. L.: "Ascorbic Acid in Wound Healing—a Review," *J. Am. Diet. Assoc.,* **56:**497–503, 1970.

Sherlock, P., and Rothschild, E. O.: "Scurvy Produced by a Zen Macrobiotic Diet," *J.A.M.A.,* **199:**794–98, 1967.

12 The Water-Soluble Vitamins: The Vitamin-B Complex

In areas of the world where polished rice is a staple food, beriberi, a serious disease affecting the nerves, has been known for generations. Takaki, a Japanese medical officer, studied the high incidence of the disease among men of the Japanese navy during the years 1878–1883. Among 276 men serving on one sailing vessel he found 169 cases of beriberi including 25 deaths at the end of nine months, but only 14 cases with no deaths occurred among a similar number of men on a second vessel who had received more meat, milk, and vegetables in their diet. Takaki believed this difference was related to the protein content of the diet.

About 15 years later (1897) Eijkman, a Dutch physician in the East Indies, noted that illness in fowls that ate scraps of hospital food consisting chiefly of polished rice was similar to beriberi seen in humans. He subsequently showed that the addition of rice polishings to the diet would cure the disease. He theorized that the starch of the polished rice was toxic to the nerves, but that the outer layers of the rice kernel were protective. Another Dutch physician, Grijns, interpreted the findings as a deficiency of an essential substance in the diet.

A number of chemists demonstrated the effects of extracts from rice. Funk in 1911 coined the term *vitamine* for the substance which he found to be effective in preventing beriberi. McCollum and Davis applied the term *water-soluble B* to the concentrates which cured beri-beri.

The water-soluble vitamin B described by Funk and others was soon discovered to be not a single substance but a group of compounds which we now designate as the vitamin-B complex. Many of these have been synthesized, and their chemical and physical properties are fairly well understood. Principally these vitamins combine with specific proteins to function as parts of the various oxidative enzyme systems which are concerned with the breakdown of carbohydrate, protein, and fat in the body. Thus, they are interrelated and are intimately involved in the mechanisms which release energy, carbon dioxide, and water as the end products of metabolism.

THIAMIN

Discovery. Crystalline thiamin (vitamin B_1) was isolated from rice bran by Jansen and Donath in Java in 1926. The synthesis and structure were accomplished in 1936 by Dr. R. R. Williams, who had worked for a quarter of a century on studies of beriberi and on the factor in rice polishings which brought about cure of the disease. Because of the presence of sulfur in the molecule, the vitamin was named THIAMIN.

Chemistry and characteristics. Thiamin is available commercially as thiamin hydrochloride in a crystalline white powder. (See Figure 12–1.) It has a faint yeastlike odor and a salty nutlike taste, and is readily soluble in water. The vitamin is stable in its dry form, and heating in solutions at 120° C in an acid medium (pH 5.0 or less) has little destructive effect. On the other hand, cooking foods in neutral or alkaline reaction is very destructive.

Measurement. Thiamin is now measured in milligrams or micrograms. It is determined by chemical or microbiologic methods.

Physiology. The thiamin ingested in food is available in the free form or bound as thiamin pyrophosphate or in a protein-phosphate complex. The bound forms are split in the digestive tract after which absorption takes place principally from the upper part of the duodenum where the reaction is acid. The amount of thiamin stored in the body is not great—probably about 50 mg in all. The liver, kidney, heart, brain, and muscles have somewhat higher concentrations than the blood. The tissues

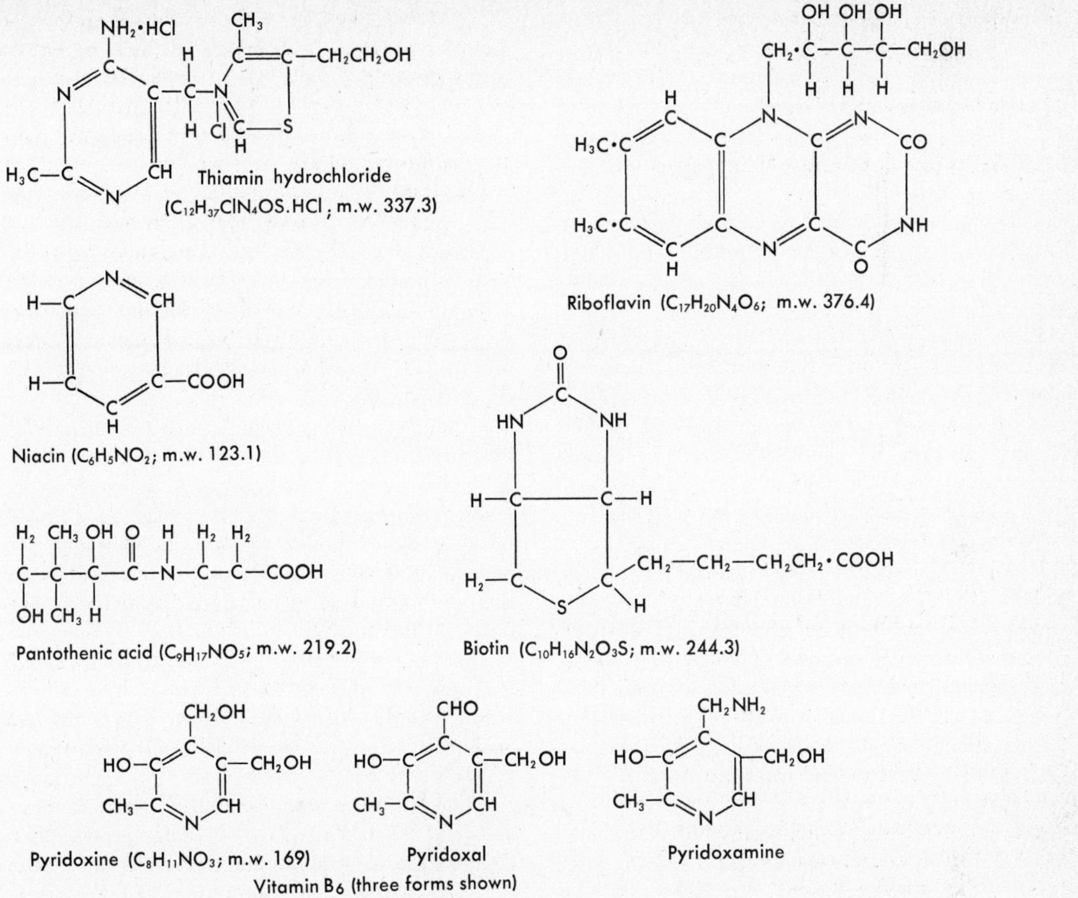

Thiamin hydrochloride
($C_{12}H_{37}ClN_4OS \cdot HCl$; m.w. 337.3)

Riboflavin ($C_{17}H_{20}N_4O_6$; m.w. 376.4)

Niacin ($C_6H_5NO_2$; m.w. 123.1)

Pantothenic acid ($C_9H_{17}NO_5$; m.w. 219.2)

Biotin ($C_{10}H_{16}N_2O_3S$; m.w. 244.3)

Pyridoxine ($C_8H_{11}NO_3$; m.w. 169)   Pyridoxal   Pyridoxamine

Vitamin B₆ (three forms shown)

Figure 12-1. These B-complex vitamins are essential for coenzymes in metabolic reactions involving carbohydrates, fats, and proteins. Note wide variations in structure.

are rapidly depleted during a dietary deficiency.

The functioning form of thiamin is THIAMIN PYROPHOSPHATE (TPP), also known as COCARBOXYLASE. For the phosphorylation of thiamin, ATP is required. Cocarboxylase in the presence of magnesium ions combines with a specific protein to form CARBOXYLASE, the active enzyme. Thiamin pyrophosphate is the coenzyme for a number of enzyme systems.

If thiamin is ingested in excess of tissue needs, it is excreted in the urine. With a low dietary intake, the urinary excretion promptly falls.

THIAMINASE is an enzyme present in uncooked clams, some fishes, and shrimp that splits the thiamin molecule, thereby inactivating it. In most situations this presents no problem since cooking inactivates thiaminase.

Functions. One of the critical points at which cocarboxylase functions in carbohydrate metabolism is in the oxidative decarboxylation of pyruvic acid and the subsequent formation of acetyl coenzyme A, which in turn enters the Krebs cycle. (See Figure 5-5.) This is one of the most complex reactions in carbohydrate metabolism and, in addition to TPP, also requires these cofactors: coenzyme A, which contains pantothenic acid (see page 183); nicotinamide adenine dinucleotide (NAD), which contains niacin (see page 179); magnesium ions; and lipoic acid (see page 189).

Another point in carbohydrate metabolism that

involves oxidative decarboxylation is in the Krebs cycle in the conversion of α-ketoglutaric acid to succinic acid. Because fats and amino acids as well as carbohydrate can contribute to α-ketoglutaric acid, thiamin and the other factors listed above are involved in the metabolism of the three energy-producing nutrients.

Thiamin pyrophosphate is also a cofactor for TRANSKETOLASE, an enzyme required to produce active glyceraldehyde through the pentose shunt. See Figure 5–5.

Daily allowances. The thiamin requirement is proportional to the calorie requirement. The minimum requirement is about 0.33 to 0.35 mg of thiamin per 1000 kcal, and the recommended allowance has been set at 0.5 mg per 1000 kcal.[1] This provides a margin of safety for individual variation and affords some protection during periods of stress.

The daily allowance for men aged 23 to 50 years is 1.4 mg and for women of the same age it is 1.0 mg. Elderly persons utilize thiamin somewhat less efficiently, and therefore an allowance of at least 1.0 mg is recommended even though the calorie requirement may be below 2000. The allowance for pregnant and lactating women is increased by 0.3 mg. Infants should receive 0.3 to 0.5 mg daily, and children up to 10 years are allowed 0.7 to 1.2 mg daily.

Sources. Thiamin is widely distributed in many foods, but most foods do not furnish especially high concentrations. Although brewers' yeast and wheat germ are rich sources, they do not form an important part of most diets. The American food supply provides 1.87 mg per capita.[2] Of this about one third is furnished by whole-grain or enriched cereals, flours, and breads.

The meat group supplies another third of the daily intake of thiamin. Lean pork—fresh and cured—is especially high in its thiamin concentration; its frequent inclusion in the diet thus makes it a highly significant source. Liver, dry beans and peas, soybeans, and peanuts are also excellent sources. The thiamin in egg, a fair source, is concentrated in the yolk.

Although the concentration of thiamin in vegetables and fruits is low, the quantities of these foods eaten may be such that important contributions are made to the daily total. Milk is likewise a fair source because of the amounts taken in the daily diet and because milk is not subjected to treatment other than pasteurization, which does not materially reduce the thiamin level.

The thiamin contribution of the basic diet pattern is shown in Figure 12–2.

Retention of food values. Little loss of thiamin occurs in the preparation of cooked breakfast cereals inasmuch as the water used in preparation is consumed. On the other hand, losses are considerable when rice is washed before cooking and when it is cooked in a large volume of water that is later

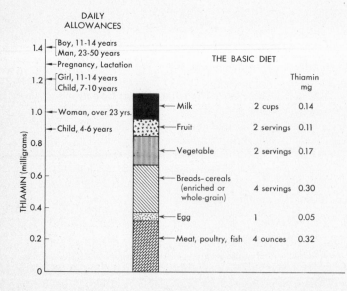

Figure 12–2. The Four Food Groups meet the recommended allowances for thiamin for women and children. The additional allowances for teen-agers and men are easily met by using increased amounts of these food groups. See Table 13–2 for complete calculation.

drained off. Losses are minimized if rice is cooked in just enough water so that all of it is absorbed by the grains. "Converted" rice retains more of the thiamin than does regular rice because in its processing the water-soluble nutrients are distributed throughout the grain. In the baking of bread about 15 to 20 per cent of the thiamin content is lost.

Thiamin losses are 25 per cent or less when meats are broiled or roasted. When meats are cooked in liquid, the losses approach 50 per cent if the liquid is discarded. If the liquid in which meat is cooked is consumed, the loss is about 25 per cent.

Thiamin losses in vegetable cookery are minimal if vegetables are cooked in a small amount of water for a short time without the addition of baking soda. In general, when the principles for retention of ascorbic acid are observed in food preparation, the maximum thiamin content will also be preserved.

Effects of deficiency. Severe thiamin deficiency is rare in the United States. The incidence of mild deficiency is not known. One group that is susceptible is the alcoholic population. Deficiency may also occur following gastrointestinal disturbances accompanied by persistent vomiting or diarrhea, or subsequent to febrile diseases or surgery when the dietary intake has been poor.

Beriberi still occurs in the Orient where high-carbohydrate diets are common and where enrichment of rice and wheat is not practiced. Williams demonstrated the effectiveness of rice enrichment in the Philippines, an area where the incidence of beriberi has been high.[3]

Diagnosis. The symptoms of mild deficiency are so vague that a diagnosis of thiamin lack is difficult. The activity of an enzyme, erythrocyte transketolase, which is found in the red blood cells correlates closely with thiamin nutrition,[4] and is believed to be useful in detecting marginal deficiency before clinical symptoms have become apparent. An elevated level of pyruvic and lactic acids in the blood, especially after exercise and the administration of a standard amount of glucose, together with a low concentration of thiamin in the urine is suggestive of deficiency. If such tests are further substantiated with a dietary history of thiamin lack plus the appearance of peripheral neuritis and disorders of the cardiovascular system, thiamin deficiency is apparent.

Symptoms. The individual who daily receives less than the minimum amount of thiamin builds up an increasing deficiency which affects the gastrointestinal, cardiovascular, and peripheral nervous systems. The early symptoms are nonspecific for thiamin lack and include fatigue, lack of interest in one's affairs, emotional instability, irritability, depression, anger and fear, and loss of appetite, weight, and strength. As the deficiency becomes more marked, the patient may complain of indigestion, constipation, headaches, insomnia, and tachycardia after moderate exercise. There appears a feeling of heaviness and weakness of the legs which may be followed by cramping of the calf muscles and burning and numbness of the feet—an indication of the development of peripheral neuritis.

The neuritic effects are first noted in the foot, then the muscles of the calf, and then the thigh. The muscle degeneration may be so pronounced that coordination is impossible and a characteristic high-stepping gait results.

The heart becomes enlarged, and tachycardia, dyspnea, and palpitation occur on exertion. In the acute type of beriberi, acute cardiac failure may be fatal before the seriousness of the disease has been fully appreciated.

Beriberi is sometimes referred to as "wet" beriberi because the chief manifestation is a severe edema which masks the emaciation that is also present. "Dry" beriberi is characterized primarily be emaciation and multiple neuritic symptoms.

Infantile beriberi. In the Far East infants are especially susceptible to beriberi because the mother has had a deficient intake of thiamin and the milk she supplies to the infant consequently contains a very low level of thiamin. The onset is often sudden and is characterized by pallor, facial edema, irritability, vomiting, abdominal pain, loss of voice, and convulsion. The infant may die within a few hours. With thiamin therapy, recovery is dramatic.

Treatment. Because beriberi is a complex vitamin deficiency disease, patients make the greatest improvement when B-complex vitamins rather than thiamin alone are prescribed. In addition to the B-complex concentrates, it is customary to prescribe a diet that is high in protein and calories.

RIBOFLAVIN

Discovery. As early as 1879 a pigment which possessed a yellow-green fluorescence had been discovered in milk. Other workers later obtained it from such widely varying sources as liver, yeast, heart, and egg white. The pigments which possess these fluorescent properties were designated as "flavins."

In the early 1920s the substance in yeast which prevented polyneuritis was shown to be more than one vitamin. The antineuritic fraction which was destroyed by heat was called vitamin B_1. Another fraction not destroyed by heat did not prevent or cure polyneuritis but it was needed for growth. It was designated as vitamin B_2 or vitamin G; it is now known as RIBOFLAVIN.

In 1932 a yellow enzyme necessary for cell respiration was isolated from yeast by Warburg and Christian, who also discovered that a protein and the pigment component were two factors in the enzyme. It then remained for Kuhn and his coworkers in 1935 to report on the synthesis of riboflavin and to note the relation of its activity to the green fluorescence, thereby establishing that lactoflavin and the vitamin are one and the same thing. This was the first example of a vitamin functioning as a coenzyme.

Chemistry and characteristics. Riboflavin was so named because of the similarity of part of its structure to that of the sugar ribose and because of its relation to the general group of flavins. (See Figure 12–1.) In its pure state, this vitamin is a bitter-tasting, orange-yellow, odorless compound in which the crystals are needle shaped. It dissolves sparingly in water to give a characteristic greenish-yellow fluorescence. In solution it is quickly decomposed by ultraviolet rays and visible light, and is sensitive to strongly alkaline solutions. This vitamin is stable to heat, to oxidizing agents, and to acids.

Measurement. Riboflavin is measured in terms of milligrams or micrograms by chemical and microbiologic methods.

Physiology. Riboflavin is present in the free state in foods, or in combination with phosphate, or with protein and phosphate. Riboflavin is absorbed from the upper part of the small intestine and is phosphorylated in the intestinal wall. It is present in body tissues as the coenzyme or as flavoproteins.

The body guards carefully its stores of riboflavin so that even in severe deficiency as much as one third of the normal amount has been found to be present in the liver, kidney, and heart of experimental animals. Apparently the flavin content of the body tissues cannot be increased beyond a certain point since the urinary excretion increases markedly if intake exceeds 0.75 mg per 1000 kcal.[1] On the other hand, a decided reduction in the supply leads to restriction or even curtailment of the urinary excretion.

Functions. Riboflavin is a constituent of two coenzymes: riboflavin monophosphate or FLAVIN MONONUCLEOTIDE (FMN) and FLAVIN ADENINE DINUCLEOTIDE (FAD). Both these coenzymes are prosthetic groups for aerobic dehydrogenases that act as hydrogen acceptors. The enzymes are required for the completion of several reactions in the energy cycle by which ATP is generated and in which hydrogen is transferred from one compound to another until eventually it reaches oxygen and forms water. Functionally, these enzymes are closely associated with the niacin-containing enzymes.

Riboflavin is also a component of L- and D-amino acid oxidases that oxidize amino acids and hydroxy acids to α-keto acids, and of xanthine oxidase, an enzyme that catalyzes the oxidation of a number of purines.

Daily allowances. At various times the allowances for riboflavin have been based on the calorie intake, the protein allowance, and the metabolic size. Regardless of the base used, the calculated allowance is about the same. The present recommendation of the Food and Nutrition Board is 0.6 mg per 1000 kcal for persons of all ages.[1]

The recommended allowance for males 23 to 50 years is 1.6 mg and for females is 1.2 mg. For pregnancy and lactation, the allowances are increased by 0.3 and 0.5 mg, respectively. The infant's allowance is 0.4 to 0.6 mg, and for children to 10 years 0.8 to 1.2 mg are recommended.

Hyperthyroidism, fevers, the stress of injury or surgery, and malabsorption are among the factors that increase the requirement. Achlorhydria may precipitate deficiency because the vitamin is so quickly destroyed in an alkaline medium.

Food sources. On a per capita basis the American food supply furnishes 2.29 mg riboflavin daily; 40 per cent of this is supplied by milk, 25 per cent by meat, poultry, and fish, and 18 per cent by cereal and flour products.[2] A diet that supplies 2 cups milk and a serving of meat daily is not likely to be deficient in riboflavin.

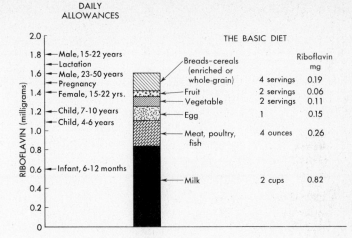

DAILY ALLOWANCES

THE BASIC DIET

RIBOFLAVIN (milligrams)

		Riboflavin mg
Male, 15-22 years		
Lactation		
Male, 23-50 years		
Pregnancy		
Female, 15-22 yrs.	Breads–cereals (enriched or whole-grain) 4 servings	0.19
	Fruit 2 servings	0.06
Child, 7-10 years	Vegetable 2 servings	0.11
Child, 4-6 years	Egg 1	0.15
	Meat, poultry, fish 4 ounces	0.26
Infant, 6-12 months		
	Milk 2 cups	0.82

Figure 12–3. Note the important contribution of milk to the total riboflavin content of the diet. See Table 13–2 for complete calculation of the Basic Diet.

Liver, kidney, and heart contain considerable quantities of riboflavin, and other meats, eggs, and green leafy vegetables supply smaller, but nevertheless important, amounts. Cereals and flours are ordinarily low in riboflavin; their enrichment adds significantly to the riboflavin content of the diet.

Fruits, roots, and tubers are poor sources of riboflavin, and fats and oils are practically devoid of the vitamin. The contribution of the basic diet is shown in Figure 12–3.

Retention of food values. Pasteurization, irradiation for vitamin D, evaporation, or drying of milk accounts for loss of not more than 10 to 20 per cent of the initial riboflavin content of milk. On the other hand, milk that is bottled in clear glass loses up to 75 per cent with $3\frac{1}{2}$ hours exposure in direct sunlight. The distribution of milk in opaque containers prevents this loss.

Meats that have been stewed, roasted, or braised retain more than three fourths of the riboflavin; most of the remainder can be accounted for in the drippings. Because riboflavin is sparingly soluble, the usual cooking procedures for vegetables do not contribute to much loss, but the addition of sodium bicarbonate to preserve green color is destructive.

Effect of deficiency. Ariboflavinosis is believed to be one of the most common of deficiency diseases. It is rare that an individual seeks medical advice for it alone, but it may accompany other deficiencies especially of the B complex.

Symptoms. In 1939 Sebrell and Butler studied a group of women whom they placed upon a diet

extremely low in riboflavin. This diet in the course of 94 to 130 days led to such symptoms as a greasy dermatitis around the folds of the nose, a cracking of the lips at the corners (CHEILOSIS), glossitis, and increased vascularization of the cornea.[5] The lips and tongue assume a purplish-red and shiny appearance in contrast to the scarlet color seen in niacin deficiency. (See Figure 12–4.)

Ocular manifestations are believed to be among the earliest signs of riboflavin deficiency. The eyes become sensitive to light and easily fatigued. There is also blurring of the vision, itching, watering, and soreness of the eyes. An increased number of capillaries develop in the cornea, and the eye becomes bloodshot in appearance. These eye changes were not observed by Horwitt.[6]

Growth failure is characteristic in young animals, and would also apply if children fail to receive minimum requirements for riboflavin. The appetite, attitude, and activity are not adversely affected with riboflavin lack as they are in thiamin deficiency. No human deaths have been reported because of riboflavin deficiency.

NIACIN (NICOTINIC ACID AND NICOTINAMIDE)

Early studies. In 1735 a Spanish physician, Casals, described a disease, *mal de la rosa*, which came to be known as PELLAGRA, a term of Italian origin meaning "rough skin." In the early part of this century it was one of the leading causes of mental

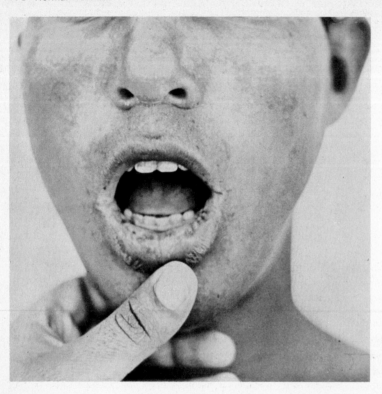

Figure 12-4. Cheilosis—lesions of the lips and fissures at the angles of the mouth. (Courtesy, Nutrition Section, National Institutes of Health.)

illness and of death in this country. Its causes had been variously ascribed to toxic substances present in corn, infections from microorganisms, of toxicity produced by exposure to the sun, lack of tryptophan in the diet, and amino acid imbalance.

Goldberger, of the United States Public Health Service, who was assigned to study the problem of pellagra in the South, early noted that the disease was almost always associated with poverty and ignorance, and that hospital attendants who worked with the patients never contracted the disease. In 1915 he performed a classic experiment on 12 prisoners who were promised release in return for their cooperation in eating a diet representative of the poorer classes in the southern states.[7] The diet consisted of sweet potatoes, corn bread, cabbage, rice, collards, fried mush, brown gravy, corn grits, syrup, sugar, biscuits, and black coffee. After a few weeks the prisoners developed headache, abdominal pain, and general weakness, and in about five months the typical dermatitis of pellagra appeared. Goldberger then suggested the existence of a pellagra-preventing (P-P) factor and related it to the B vitamins.

Identification of the vitamin. Goldberger in 1922 concluded that blacktongue in dogs was similar to pellagra in humans. Nicotinic acid had been known as a chemical substance since 1867, but it remained for Elvehjem and his coworkers in 1937 to discover its effectiveness as a curative agent for blacktongue in dogs.[8] Following this discovery, Smith, Spies, and others were soon making reports of dramatic clinical improvement in pellagrous patients who had been given nicotinic acid. The term *niacin* was suggested by Cowgill to avoid association with the nicotine of tobacco.

Chemistry and characteristics. NIACIN and NIACINAMIDE (see Figure 12-1) are organic compounds of relatively simple structure with equal biologic activity. Niacin is the generic term that includes both forms. The two forms are white, bitter-tasting compounds, moderately soluble in hot water but only slightly soluble in cold water. Niacin is very stable to alkali, acid, heat, light, and oxidation; even boiling and autoclaving do not decrease its potency.

Measurement. Niacin is measured in milligrams by using chemical methods or microbiologic assay.

Physiology. Niacin is readily absorbed from the small intestine. Some reserves are found in the body, but, as with other B-complex vitamins, the amount appears to be limited so that a day-to-day supply is desirable. Any excess of niacin is excreted in the urine as N-methylnicotinamide and N-methyl pyridone. In a deficiency such as pellagra the metabolites in the urine diminish markedly or are absent.

Tryptophan, one of the essential amino acids, is a precursor of niacin so that a diet that contains a liberal amount of tryptophan will provide enough niacin even though the diet is low in preformed niacin. Milk and eggs are excellent sources of tryptophan but poor sources of preformed niacin; their pellagra-preventive characteristics have long been known.

Niacin is not toxic in amounts that considerably exceed recommended allowances. In therapeutic doses it brings about some vasodilation and consequent flushing of the skin and tingling sensations; niacinamide reduces these reactions, and is preferred as a therapeutic agent for pellagra. From 3 to 6 gm niacin have been prescribed to reduce the blood levels of cholesterol, beta-lipoproteins, and triglycerides.[9]

Functions. Like other B-complex vitamins, niacin is a constituent of coenzymes involved in glycolysis, tissue respiration, and fat synthesis. NICOTINAMIDE ADENINE DINUCLEOTIDE (NAD) contains nicotinamide, ribose, two phosphate groups, and adenine; it is also referred to in the literature as diphosphopyridine nucleotide (DPN) or coenzyme I. NICOTINAMIDE ADENINE DINUCLEOTIDE PHOSPHATE (NADP) is similar to NAD except that it contains three phosphate groupings; it was formerly known as triphosphopyridine nucleotide (TPN) or coenzyme II.

NAD and NADP are hydrogen acceptors involved in many reactions. For example, the complex reaction required for the decarboxylation of pyruvic acid and the formation of acetyl coenzyme A requires dehydrogenation by NAD (see also page 70); NAD and NADP are involved in dehydrogenation reactions in the Krebs cycle; hydrogen is transferred from NAD to FAD to cytochrome c in the respiratory chain in which ATP is liberated. (See page 92.)

In the pentose shunt (see page 70) NADP is the hydrogen acceptor for two reactions, thereby forming NADPH. The latter is required for the synthesis of fatty acids and cholesterol, and for the conversion of phenylalanine to tyrosine.

Daily allowances. The symptoms of pellagra are prevented by a daily intake of 4.4 mg niacin per 1000 kcal. The recommended allowances provide about 50 per cent margin of safety, and are based upon 6.6 mg niacin per 1000 kcal. Although these levels are stated as niacin, it is recognized that 1 mg niacin is derived from each 60 mg dietary tryptophan as well as from preformed niacin in the diet.[10-12]

For the reference man, 23 to 50 years, the allowance is 18 mg, and for the reference woman is 13 mg. The allowances for pregnancy and lactation are 15 and 17 mg, respectively. From 5 to 8 mg are recommended during the first year, and 9 to 16 mg for children to 10 years. For boys and girls, 11 to 14 years, allowances are 18 and 16 mg, respectively.

As with the other B-complex vitamins, the niacin requirements are increased whenever metabolism is accelerated as by fever and the stress of injury or surgery.

Sources. A diet that furnishes the recommended allowances for protein also provides enough niacin inasmuch as protein will supply tryptophan for conversion to niacin, and the protein-rich foods are generally, except for milk, rich sources of preformed niacin. Animal proteins contain about 1.4 per cent tryptophan, and plant proteins about 1 per cent tryptophan.[13] If one assumes that a mixed diet provides 1 per cent of the protein as tryptophan, then an intake of 65 gm protein is equivalent to 650 mg tryptophan, or 10.8 mg niacin.

Poultry, meats, and fish constitute the most important single food group insofar as preformed niacin is concerned. (See Figure 12–5.) Organ meats, peanuts, peanut butter, and brewers' yeast are rich sources, but are not ordinarily consumed in sufficient amounts to greatly affect the dietary level.

Whole grains are fair sources of niacin but most of this is in a bound form which may not be completely available.[13] The effect of cooking on the bound form is not known.

Potatoes, legumes, and some green leafy vegetables contain fair amounts of preformed niacin, but most fruits and vegetables are poor sources—as are also milk and cheese.

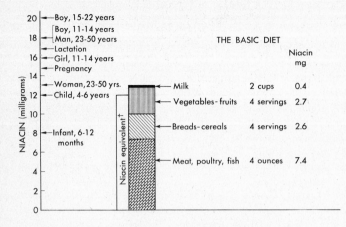

Figure 12–5. The meat group contributes most of the preformed niacin in the Basic Diet. Milk and eggs contain only small amounts of preformed niacin, but they are excellent sources of tryptophan. Note that the tryptophan in this diet contributes almost as much niacin as the preformed content. See Table 13–2 for complete calculation of Basic Diet.

Retention of food values. The cookery of foods does not result in serious losses of niacin, except insofar as part of the soluble vitamin may be discarded in cooking waters which are not used. The application of principles for the retention of ascorbic acid and thiamin which have been discussed earlier will result in maximum retention of niacin as well.

Effect of deficiency. Pellagra appears after months of dietary deprivation. The phenomenal decrease in the incidence of pellagra in the United States may be attributed to several factors including the enrichment program which is mandatory in some states, the concerted efforts in nutrition education, and the improvement in income. Pellagra is still a public health problem in some countries such as Spain, Yugoslavia, and certain areas of Africa.

Symptoms and clinical findings. Pellagra involves the gastrointestinal tract, the skin, and the nervous system. Although no two cases of pellagra are exactly alike, the following symptoms are characteristic.

1. Early signs include fatigue, listlessness, headache, backache, loss of weight, loss of appetite, and general poor health.

2. Sore tongue, mouth, and throat, with glossitis extending throughout the gastrointestinal tract, are present. The tongue and lips become abnormally red in color. The mouth becomes so sore that it is difficult to eat and swallow.

3. A deficiency of hydrochloric acid with a resultant anemia similar to pernicious anemia may be found.

4. Nausea and vomiting are followed by severe diarrhea.

5. A characteristic symmetric dermatitis especially on the exposed surfaces of the body—hands, forearms, elbows, feet, legs, knees, and neck—appears (see Figure 12–6). The dermatitis is sharply separated from the surrounding normal skin. At first the skin becomes red, somewhat swollen, and tender, resembling a mild sunburn; if the condition is untreated, the skin becomes rough, cracked, and scaly and may become ulcerated. Sunshine and exposure to heat aggravate the dermatitis.

6. Neurologic symptoms which include confusion, dizziness, poor memory, and irritability, and leading to hallucinations, delusions of persecution, and dementia, are noted as severity increases.

The classic "D's" are the final stages of the disease—dermatitis, diarrhea, dementia, and death.

Treatment and prophylaxis. Niacinamide is given in therapeutic doses of 50 to 250 mg daily.[14] With such therapy it is possible to progress rapidly from an all-fluid to a soft and then a high-protein regular diet. Obviously, prophylaxis must include careful and persistent education in dietary improvement, emphasis upon enrichment programs, and efforts to improve the economic status of affected populations.

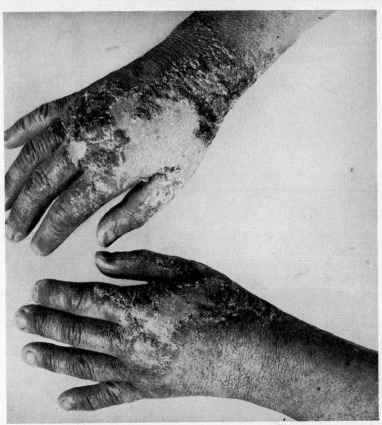

Figure 12–6. Dermatitis of pellagra.

VITAMIN B$_6$

Discovery. Goldberger and Lillie in 1926 provided a description of dermatitis in rats that was recognized several years later to be characteristic of vitamin B$_6$ deficiency. In 1934 György reported that vitamin B$_2$ consisted of two factors—riboflavin, and another factor which he named vitamin B$_6$ that prevented skin lesions (acrodynia) in rats. In 1938 the isolation of a crystalline compound with vitamin B$_6$ activity was reported by several laboratories, followed by identification of the chemical structure by Harris and Folkers and its synthesis by Kuhn and Wendt in 1939.

Chemistry and characteristics. Vitamin B$_6$ consists of a group of related pyridines: PYRIDOXINE, PYRIDOXAL, and PYRIDOXAMINE. (See Figure 12–1.) These may appear in tissues and foodstuffs in the free form, or combined with phosphate, or with phosphate and protein. The preferred terminology is vitamin B$_6$; pyridoxine, being only one of the three active forms, is not entirely synonymous.

Vitamin B$_6$ is soluble in water and relatively stable to heat and to acids. It is destroyed in alkaline solutions and is also sensitive to light. Of the three forms, pyridoxine is more resistant to food processing and storage conditions and probably represents the principal form in food products.

Measurement. Vitamin B$_6$ concentrations are expressed in milligrams or micrograms. The vitamin is determined in tissues and foods by chemical or fluorometric procedures. Because the vitamin occurs in various bound forms, some difficulties have been experienced in providing acceptable tabulations for food values.

Physiology. The active form of vitamin B$_6$ is the

coenzyme pyridoxal phosphate, which can be formed from any of the three compounds. Since vitamin B_6 is water soluble, the body stores are small; about half of it is in the form of glycogen phosphorylase. All forms of the vitamin may be excreted in the urine, but the principal metabolite is pyridoxic acid.

Functions. Pyridoxal phosphate is the coenzyme for a large number of enzyme systems, most of which are involved in amino acid metabolism. A few examples are given below:

Decarboxylation. The removal of the carboxyl group from amino acids requires enzymes that contain pyridoxal phosphate. Each of the amino acids is decarboxylated by a specific enzyme. For example, the decarboxylation of tryptophan produces tryptamine and carbon dioxide. Serotonin is also produced by decarboxylation of tryptophan and is a potent vasoconstrictor as well as an agent in the regulation of brain and other tissues.

Transamination. Each of the many transaminases involves a distinct protein for which pyridoxal phosphate is the coenxyme. One example of transamination is shown on page 51. In the reaction, the amino group is removed from an amino acid and transferred to a keto acid, thus forming a new amino acid. This reaction is important in the formation of the nonessential amino acids.

Transulfuration. This involves the removal and transfer of sulfur groups from the sulfur-containing amino acids such as cysteine by transulfurases.

Tryptophan conversion to niacin. The importance of tryptophan as a source of niacin has been described on page 179. Several steps are required in this conversion, one of which is catalyzed by vitamin B_6.

Pyridoxal phosphate is also required for glycogen phosphorylase, an enzyme by which glycogen is broken down to glucose; for the formation of antibodies; for the synthesis of a precursor of the porphyrin ring which is part of the hemoglobin molecule; and possibly for the conversion of linoleic acid to arachidonic acid.

Daily allowances. The need for vitamin B_6 is proportional to the amount of protein metabolized. The recommended allowance for the reference man and woman is 2.0 mg daily.[1] This provides a reasonable margin of safety and permits a protein intake of 100 gm or more. Those who ingest a low-protein diet (40 to 50 gm) require only 1.2 to 1.5 mg.

The allowance for infants is 0.3 to 0.4 mg; for children from 1 to 10 years, it increases gradually from 0.6 to 1.2 mg; and for adolescents, the range is 1.6 to 2.0 mg. During pregnancy and lactation 2.5 mg is recommended.

Food sources. The vitamin B_6 available in the American food supply per capita is 2.25 mg. The principal source is meat, poultry, and fish, with this group accounting for 45 per cent of the total amount available. Potatoes, sweet potatoes, and vegetables account for about 23 per cent of the total supply; dairy products, 10 per cent; and flour and cereals, 9 per cent.[2] Whole grains are good sources of pyridoxine, but most of this is lost in the milling of the grains.

Effects of deficiency. The TRYPTOPHAN LOAD TEST is the most widely used measure of vitamin B_6 adequacy. In this test a measured dose of tryptophan is given after which the 24-hour urinary excretion of xanthurenic acid is measured. XANTHURENIC ACID is an intermediary metabolite of tryptophan metabolism that is excreted when there is insufficient vitamin B_6 to catalyze the reactions throughout the normal pathway. An excretion of more than 50 mg is indicative of vitamin B_6 deficiency. Reduced levels of serum and red blood cell transaminases and lowered excretion of pyridoxic acid are also found in vitamin B_6 deficiency.

Deficiency in infants. In the 1950s vitamin B_6 deficiency was reported in infants who had received a commercial formula in which the pyridoxine had been inadvertently destroyed in the processing of the milk. The infants showed nervous irritability and convulsive seizures. Other related symptoms included anemia, vomiting, weakness, ataxia, and abdominal pain. The convulsive seizures responded dramatically to the administration of pyridoxine.[15,16]

Deficiency in adults. College students who ingested a vitamin-B_6-deficient diet for seven weeks showed a rapid decrease in the blood level of pyridoxine and increased excretion of xanthurenic acid with the tryptophan load test.[17] Despite the biochemical evidence of deficiency, no clear-cut symptoms have been observed in adults. However, when an antagonist such as deoxypyridoxine is fed together with a diet deficient in vitamin B_6, seborrheic dermatitis around the eyes, eyebrows, and angles of the mouth has been described.[18] Large doses of vitamin B_6 will counteract the effect of the antagonist.

Isonicotinic acid hydrazide (INH) is widely used in the treatment of tuberculosis. It is chemically related to pyridoxine and acts as an antagonist to vitamin B_6 activity. Patients who have been treated with this drug have experienced neuritic symptoms believed to be caused by the imposed vitamin B_6 deficiency, and corrected when additional vitamin supplements were prescribed. Penicillamine, a drug used in the treatment of Wilson's disease and cystinuria, is also an antagonist of vitamin B_6. Vitamin B_6 supplements are usually prescribed when this drug is used.

During pregnancy and in women who are using the steroid contraceptive pill there is increased excretion of xanthurenic acid following the tryptophan load test and lower blood transaminase activity. The biochemical changes are readily corrected by increasing the intake of vitamin B_6 but there is little indication that there is any physiologic advantage.[1]

Vitamin B_6 dependency. An inborn error of metabolism has been described in which convulsive seizures are controlled by up to 200 to 600 mg pyridoxine hydrochloride daily.[19]

The effect of megadoses of pyridoxine was tested on normal individuals by giving 200 mg pyridoxine daily for 33 days. When these large doses were withdrawn, the individuals required greater-than-normal intakes of vitamin B_6 to maintain normal biochemical levels.[1] Because such megadoses can induce vitamin B_6 dependency, their use is contraindicated as a routine measure.

PANTOTHENIC ACID

Discovery. Pantothenic acid was isolated in 1938 by Dr. R. J. Williams and synthesized in 1940 by workers in the laboratories of Merck and Company. Although tests showed its vitamin nature by its ability to prevent certain deficiencies in animals, little interest was shown in this vitamin until about a decade later. In 1946 Lipmann and his associates showed that coenzyme A was essential for acetylation reactions in the body, and in 1950 reports from this same laboratory showed pantothenic acid to be a constituent of coenzyme A. The name for this vitamin is derived from the Greek word *panthos*, meaning "everywhere." The universal distribution of this vitamin in biologic materials suggests the key role that it plays in metabolism.

Characteristics. PANTOTHENIC ACID, as the free acid, is an unstable, viscous yellow oil, soluble in water. (See Figure 12–1.) Commercially, it is available as the sodium or calcium salt, which is slightly sweet, water soluble, and quite stable. There is little loss of the vitamin with ordinary cooking procedures, except in acid and alkaline solutions.

The pantothenic acid content of tissues and foods is determined by microbiologic methods, and values are expressed in milligrams or micrograms.

Functions. Coenzyme A is the form in which pantothenic acid functions in the body. Coenzyme A is a complex molecule consisting of a sulfur-containing compound, adenine, ribose, phosphoric acid, and pantothenic acid. The sulfur linkage is highly reactive.

Coenzyme A functions in reactions that accept or remove the acetyl group ($-CH_3CO$). One of these reactions is the formation of acetylcholine, a substance of importance in the transmission of the nerve impulse. Coenzyme A participates in the oxidation of pyruvate, α-ketoglutarate, and fatty acids. (See Figure 5–5 and page 70.) Coenzyme A reacts with pyruvic acid to form acetyl coenzyme A, which, in turn, combines with oxalacetate to form citrate, thus initiating the tricarboxylic acid cycle for the release of energy. Coenzyme A is also involved in the synthesis of fatty acids, cholesterol and other sterols, and porphyrin in the hemoglobin molecule.

Coenzyme A is synthesized in all cells and apparently does not cross cell membranes. Liver, kidney, brain, adrenal, and heart tissues, being metabolically active, contain high concentrations.

Requirement. The daily requirement is not known, but the Food and Nutrition Board has suggested an allowance of 5 to 10 mg for adults. This level is readily available from diets that are adequate in other nutrients.[1] An intake of 4 to 5 mg by children is believed to be satisfactory.

Food sources. Most of the pantothenic acid in animal tissues is in the form of coenzyme A. As its name indicates, pantothenic acid is widely distributed in animal foods and in whole grains and legumes. Liver, yeast, egg yolk, and meat are particularly good sources. Fruits, vegetables, and milk contain smaller amounts. About 50 per cent of the pantothenic acid of grains is lost in their milling, and dry processing of foods also leads to significant losses.

Effects of deficiency. No clear-cut demonstration of pantothenic acid deficiency has been afforded by experimental diets low in pantothenic acid. When an antagonist, omega methyl panthothenic acid, was fed with deficient diets, the following symptoms were observed: loss of appetite, indigestion, abdominal pain; sullenness, mental depression; peripheral neuritis with cramping pains in the arms and legs; burning sensations in the feet; insomnia; and respiratory infections. In these subjects there was an increased sensitivity to insulin, an increased sedimentation rate for erythrocytes, and marked decrease in antibody formation.[20,21]

The neuropathy observed in alcoholics is possibly related to pantothenic acid deficiency. However, when diets are deficient in pantothenic acid, they are also deficient in many other factors, and therefore the separation of symptoms attributable to various nutrient lacks becomes exceedingly difficult.

BIOTIN

Discovery. In the 1920s a factor essential for the growth of yeast was described and named *bios*. In the 1930s Dr. Helen Parsons and her coworkers and others reported on the symptoms observed in rats that were fed a diet including raw egg white. The animals lost their fur, particularly around the eyes, giving a spectacle-like appearance; there was rapid loss of weight, paralysis of the hind legs, and eventual cyanosis and death. The symptoms did not occur when cooked egg white was used.[22]

Small quantities of the active factor were isolated from egg yolk in 1936 by Kögl and were later established as being identical with the yeast growth factor and the anti-egg-white injury factor.

The substance in raw egg white has been found to be a glycoprotein that binds biotin and thereby prevents its absorption from the intestinal tract. It is called AVIDIN, which means "hungry albumin." Heating of egg white inactivates the binding capacity of avidin.

Characteristics. BIOTIN is a relatively simple compound, a cyclic urea derivative and containing a sulfur grouping. (See Figure 12–1.) In its free form it is a crystalline substance, very stable to heat, light, and acids. It is somewhat labile to alkaline solutions and to oxidizing agents. In tissues and in foods it is usually combined with protein.

Functions and metabolism. Biotin is a coenzyme of a number of enzymes that participate in carboxylation, decarboxylation, and deamination reactions. For example, it is required in the synthesis of fatty acids. Another reaction catalyzed by biotin-containing enzymes is the fixation of CO_2 in the conversion of pyruvate to oxalacetate, an important reaction that generates the tricarboxylic acid cycle (see Figure 5–5). Within the TCA cycle, biotin is also required for the conversion of succinate to fumarate and oxalsuccinate to ketoglutarate.

Biotin is essential for the introduction of CO_2 in the formation of purines, these compounds being essential constituents of DNA and RNA. The deaminases for threonine, serine, and aspartic acid also require biotin as a coenzyme.

Biotin is stored in minute amounts principally in the metabolically active tissues such as the kidney, liver, brain, and adrenal. The biotin content of the feces and likewise of the urinary excretion is considerably greater than the dietary intake. This indicates the intestinal synthesis of biotin and the absorption of the vitamin from this source.

Dietary needs. The requirement for biotin has not been established. The average diet is estimated to contain 100 to 300 mcg daily.

Good dietary sources of biotin include organ meats, egg yolk, legumes, and nuts. Cereal grains, muscle meats, and milk contain only small amounts.

Effects of deficiency. Biotin deficiency has been described in human beings only when large amounts of raw egg whites were fed. Four volunteer subjects were fed an experimental diet containing approximately 3000 kcal, low in biotin, and including 928 of the total calories from egg white (equivalent to about 60 egg whites!) for a period of 10 weeks. Beginning with the third to fourth weeks symptoms appeared approximately in this order: scaly desqua-

Food sources. Most of the pantothenic acid in animal tissues is in the form of coenzyme A. As its name indicates, pantothenic acid is widely distributed in animal foods and in whole grains and legumes. Liver, yeast, egg yolk, and meat are particularly good sources. Fruits, vegetables, and milk contain smaller amounts. About 50 per cent of the pantothenic acid of grains is lost in their milling, and dry processing of foods also leads to significant losses.

Effects of deficiency. No clear-cut demonstration of pantothenic acid deficiency has been afforded by experimental diets low in pantothenic acid. When an antagonist, omega methyl panthothenic acid, was fed with deficient diets, the following symptoms were observed: loss of appetite, indigestion, abdominal pain; sullenness, mental depression; peripheral neuritis with cramping pains in the arms and legs; burning sensations in the feet; insomnia; and respiratory infections. In these subjects there was an increased sensitivity to insulin, an increased sedimentation rate for erythrocytes, and marked decrease in antibody formation.[20,21]

The neuropathy observed in alcoholics is possibly related to pantothenic acid deficiency. However, when diets are deficient in pantothenic acid, they are also deficient in many other factors, and therefore the separation of symptoms attributable to various nutrient lacks becomes exceedingly difficult.

BIOTIN

Discovery. In the 1920s a factor essential for the growth of yeast was described and named *bios*. In the 1930s Dr. Helen Parsons and her coworkers and others reported on the symptoms observed in rats that were fed a diet including raw egg white. The animals lost their fur, particularly around the eyes, giving a spectacle-like appearance; there was rapid loss of weight, paralysis of the hind legs, and eventual cyanosis and death. The symptoms did not occur when cooked egg white was used.[22]

Small quantities of the active factor were isolated from egg yolk in 1936 by Kögl and were later established as being identical with the yeast growth factor and the anti-egg-white injury factor.

The substance in raw egg white has been found to be a glycoprotein that binds biotin and thereby prevents its absorption from the intestinal tract. It is called AVIDIN, which means "hungry albumin." Heating of egg white inactivates the binding capacity of avidin.

Characteristics. BIOTIN is a relatively simple compound, a cyclic urea derivative and containing a sulfur grouping. (See Figure 12–1.) In its free form it is a crystalline substance, very stable to heat, light, and acids. It is somewhat labile to alkaline solutions and to oxidizing agents. In tissues and in foods it is usually combined with protein.

Functions and metabolism. Biotin is a coenzyme of a number of enzymes that participate in carboxylation, decarboxylation, and deamination reactions. For example, it is required in the synthesis of fatty acids. Another reaction catalyzed by biotin-containing enzymes is the fixation of CO_2 in the conversion of pyruvate to oxalacetate, an important reaction that generates the tricarboxylic acid cycle (see Figure 5–5). Within the TCA cycle, biotin is also required for the conversion of succinate to fumarate and oxalsuccinate to ketoglutarate.

Biotin is essential for the introduction of CO_2 in the formation of purines, these compounds being essential constituents of DNA and RNA. The deaminases for threonine, serine, and aspartic acid also require biotin as a coenzyme.

Biotin is stored in minute amounts principally in the metabolically active tissues such as the kidney, liver, brain, and adrenal. The biotin content of the feces and likewise of the urinary excretion is considerably greater than the dietary intake. This indicates the intestinal synthesis of biotin and the absorption of the vitamin from this source.

Dietary needs. The requirement for biotin has not been established. The average diet is estimated to contain 100 to 300 mcg daily.

Good dietary sources of biotin include organ meats, egg yolk, legumes, and nuts. Cereal grains, muscle meats, and milk contain only small amounts.

Effects of deficiency. Biotin deficiency has been described in human beings only when large amounts of raw egg whites were fed. Four volunteer subjects were fed an experimental diet containing approximately 3000 kcal, low in biotin, and including 928 of the total calories from egg white (equivalent to about 60 egg whites!) for a period of 10 weeks. Beginning with the third to fourth weeks symptoms appeared approximately in this order: scaly desqua-

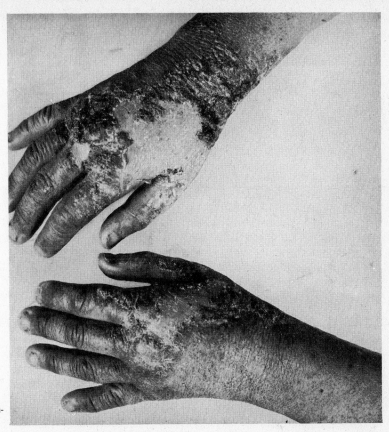

Figure 12–6. Dermatitis of pellagra.

VITAMIN B_6

Discovery. Goldberger and Lillie in 1926 provided a description of dermatitis in rats that was recognized several years later to be characteristic of vitamin B_6 deficiency. In 1934 György reported that vitamin B_2 consisted of two factors—riboflavin, and another factor which he named vitamin B_6 that prevented skin lesions (acrodynia) in rats. In 1938 the isolation of a crystalline compound with vitamin B_6 activity was reported by several laboratories, followed by identification of the chemical structure by Harris and Folkers and its synthesis by Kuhn and Wendt in 1939.

Chemistry and characteristics. Vitamin B_6 consists of a group of related pyridines: PYRIDOXINE, PYRIDOXAL, and PYRIDOXAMINE. (See Figure 12–1.) These may appear in tissues and foodstuffs in the free form, or combined with phosphate, or with phosphate and protein. The preferred terminology is vitamin B_6; pyridoxine, being only one of the three active forms, is not entirely synonymous.

Vitamin B_6 is soluble in water and relatively stable to heat and to acids. It is destroyed in alkaline solutions and is also sensitive to light. Of the three forms, pyridoxine is more resistant to food processing and storage conditions and probably represents the principal form in food products.

Measurement. Vitamin B_6 concentrations are expressed in milligrams or micrograms. The vitamin is determined in tissues and foods by chemical or fluorometric procedures. Because the vitamin occurs in various bound forms, some difficulties have been experienced in providing acceptable tabulations for food values.

Physiology. The active form of vitamin B_6 is the

coenzyme pyridoxal phosphate, which can be formed from any of the three compounds. Since vitamin B_6 is water soluble, the body stores are small; about half of it is in the form of glycogen phosphorylase. All forms of the vitamin may be excreted in the urine, but the principal metabolite is pyridoxic acid.

Functions. Pyridoxal phosphate is the coenzyme for a large number of enzyme systems, most of which are involved in amino acid metabolism. A few examples are given below:

Decarboxylation. The removal of the carboxyl group from amino acids requires enzymes that contain pyridoxal phosphate. Each of the amino acids is decarboxylated by a specific enzyme. For example, the decarboxylation of tryptophan produces tryptamine and carbon dioxide. Serotonin is also produced by decarboxylation of tryptophan and is a potent vasoconstrictor as well as an agent in the regulation of brain and other tissues.

Transamination. Each of the many transaminases involves a distinct protein for which pyridoxal phosphate is the coenzyme. One example of transamination is shown on page 51. In the reaction, the amino group is removed from an amino acid and transferred to a keto acid, thus forming a new amino acid. This reaction is important in the formation of the nonessential amino acids.

Transulfuration. This involves the removal and transfer of sulfur groups from the sulfur-containing amino acids such as cysteine by transulfurases.

Tryptophan conversion to niacin. The importance of tryptophan as a source of niacin has been described on page 179. Several steps are required in this conversion, one of which is catalyzed by vitamin B_6.

Pyridoxal phosphate is also required for glycogen phosphorylase, an enzyme by which glycogen is broken down to glucose; for the formation of antibodies; for the synthesis of a precursor of the porphyrin ring which is part of the hemoglobin molecule; and possibly for the conversion of linoleic acid to arachidonic acid.

Daily allowances. The need for vitamin B_6 is proportional to the amount of protein metabolized. The recommended allowance for the reference man and woman is 2.0 mg daily.[1] This provides a reasonable margin of safety and permits a protein intake of

100 gm or more. Those who ingest a low-protein diet (40 to 50 gm) require only 1.2 to 1.5 mg.

The allowance for infants is 0.3 to 0.4 mg; for children from 1 to 10 years, it increases gradually from 0.6 to 1.2 mg; and for adolescents, the range is 1.6 to 2.0 mg. During pregnancy and lactation 2.5 mg is recommended.

Food sources. The vitamin B_6 available in the American food supply per capita is 2.25 mg. The principal source is meat, poultry, and fish, with this group accounting for 45 per cent of the total amount available. Potatoes, sweet potatoes, and vegetables account for about 23 per cent of the total supply; dairy products, 10 per cent; and flour and cereals, 9 per cent.[2] Whole grains are good sources of pyridoxine, but most of this is lost in the milling of the grains.

Effects of deficiency. The TRYPTOPHAN LOAD TEST is the most widely used measure of vitamin B_6 adequacy. In this test a measured dose of tryptophan is given after which the 24-hour urinary excretion of xanthurenic acid is measured. XANTHURENIC ACID is an intermediary metabolite of tryptophan metabolism that is excreted when there is insufficient vitamin B_6 to catalyze the reactions throughout the normal pathway. An excretion of more than 50 mg is indicative of vitamin B_6 deficiency. Reduced levels of serum and red blood cell transaminases and lowered excretion of pyridoxic acid are also found in vitamin B_6 deficiency.

Deficiency in infants. In the 1950s vitamin B_6 deficiency was reported in infants who had received a commercial formula in which the pyridoxine had been inadvertently destroyed in the processing of the milk. The infants showed nervous irritability and convulsive seizures. Other related symptoms included anemia, vomiting, weakness, ataxia, and abdominal pain. The convulsive seizures responded dramatically to the administration of pyridoxine.[15,16]

Deficiency in adults. College students who ingested a vitamin-B_6-deficient diet for seven weeks showed a rapid decrease in the blood level of pyridoxine and increased excretion of xanthurenic acid with the tryptophan load test.[17] Despite the biochemical evidence of deficiency, no clear-cut symptoms have been observed in adults. However, when an antagonist such as deoxypyridoxine is fed

together with a diet deficient in vitamin B_6, seborrheic dermatitis around the eyes, eyebrows, and angles of the mouth has been described.[18] Large doses of vitamin B_6 will counteract the effect of the antagonist.

Isonicotinic acid hydrazide (INH) is widely used in the treatment of tuberculosis. It is chemically related to pyridoxine and acts as an antagonist to vitamin B_6 activity. Patients who have been treated with this drug have experienced neuritic symptoms believed to be caused by the imposed vitamin B_6 deficiency, and corrected when additional vitamin supplements were prescribed. Penicillamine, a drug used in the treatment of Wilson's disease and cystinuria, is also an antagonist of vitamin B_6. Vitamin B_6 supplements are usually prescribed when this drug is used.

During pregnancy and in women who are using the steroid contraceptive pill there is increased excretion of xanthurenic acid following the tryptophan load test and lower blood transaminase activity. The biochemical changes are readily corrected by increasing the intake of vitamin B_6 but there is little indication that there is any physiologic advantage.[1]

Vitamin B_6 dependency. An inborn error of metabolism has been described in which convulsive seizures are controlled by up to 200 to 600 mg pyridoxine hydrochloride daily.[19]

The effect of megadoses of pyridoxine was tested on normal individuals by giving 200 mg pyridoxine daily for 33 days. When these large doses were withdrawn, the individuals required greater-than-normal intakes of vitamin B_6 to maintain normal biochemical levels.[1] Because such megadoses can induce vitamin B_6 dependency, their use is contraindicated as a routine measure.

PANTOTHENIC ACID

Discovery. Pantothenic acid was isolated in 1938 by Dr. R. J. Williams and synthesized in 1940 by workers in the laboratories of Merck and Company. Although tests showed its vitamin nature by its ability to prevent certain deficiencies in animals, little interest was shown in this vitamin until about a decade later. In 1946 Lipmann and his associates

showed that coenzyme A was essential for acetylation reactions in the body, and in 1950 reports from this same laboratory showed pantothenic acid to be a constituent of coenzyme A. The name for this vitamin is derived from the Greek word *panthos*, meaning "everywhere." The universal distribution of this vitamin in biologic materials suggests the key role that it plays in metabolism.

Characteristics. PANTOTHENIC ACID, as the free acid, is an unstable, viscous yellow oil, soluble in water. (See Figure 12-1.) Commercially, it is available as the sodium or calcium salt, which is slightly sweet, water soluble, and quite stable. There is little loss of the vitamin with ordinary cooking procedures, except in acid and alkaline solutions.

The pantothenic acid content of tissues and foods is determined by microbiologic methods, and values are expressed in milligrams or micrograms.

Functions. Coenzyme A is the form in which pantothenic acid functions in the body. Coenzyme A is a complex molecule consisting of a sulfur-containing compound, adenine, ribose, phosphoric acid, and pantothenic acid. The sulfur linkage is highly reactive.

Coenzyme A functions in reactions that accept or remove the acetyl group ($-CH_3CO$). One of these reactions is the formation of acetylcholine, a substance of importance in the transmission of the nerve impulse. Coenzyme A participates in the oxidation of pyruvate, α-ketoglutarate, and fatty acids. (See Figure 5-5 and page 70.) Coenzyme A reacts with pyruvic acid to form acetyl coenzyme A, which, in turn, combines with oxalacetate to form citrate, thus initiating the tricarboxylic acid cycle for the release of energy. Coenzyme A is also involved in the synthesis of fatty acids, cholesterol and other sterols, and porphyrin in the hemoglobin molecule.

Coenzyme A is synthesized in all cells and apparently does not cross cell membranes. Liver, kidney, brain, adrenal, and heart tissues, being metabolically active, contain high concentrations.

Requirement. The daily requirement is not known, but the Food and Nutrition Board has suggested an allowance of 5 to 10 mg for adults. This level is readily available from diets that are adequate in other nutrients.[1] An intake of 4 to 5 mg by children is believed to be satisfactory.

mation, lassitude, muscle pains, hyperesthesia, pallor of skin and mucous membranes, anorexia, and nausea. The hemoglobin levels were lowered, the blood cholesterol levels were increased, and the urinary excretion of biotin dropped to about one tenth of the normal levels. All of these abnormalities were cured within five days when 150 mcg biotin was given daily.[23]

Recently biotin deficiency was reported in a 62-year-old woman with Laennec's cirrhosis who, on a physician's advice, had ingested six raw eggs daily for 18 months in an effort to regenerate liver tissue. Her symptoms included anorexia, nausea, vomiting, pallor, lassitude, scaly dermatitis, and desquamation of the lips. All these promptly disappeared or significantly improved within a few days following the daily parenteral administration of 200 mcg biotin.[24]

VITAMIN B$_{12}$

Discovery. Until the 1920s pernicious anemia was an invariably fatal disease. Then came the dramatic announcement by Minot and Murphy[25] that large amounts of liver—about a pound a day—would control the anemia and prevent the neurologic changes.

Castle set forth the hypothesis that liver contained a substance which he termed the EXTRINSIC FACTOR (now known to be vitamin B$_{12}$) and that its absorption required another principle in normal gastric secretion which he called the INTRINSIC FACTOR. Patients with pernicious anemia were lacking the intrinsic factor. Nevertheless, when very large amounts of liver were consumed, some absorption of the extrinsic factor took place by simple diffusion.

The active principle in liver was extracted in the 1930s and provided the basis for the treatment of patients by injection. Then in 1948 came the announcement by Rickes and his associates in the United States[26] and Smith and Parker in England[27] of the isolation of a few micrograms of a red crystalline substance that was shown to be dramatically effective in the remission of pernicious anemia. The structure of this complex molecule was elucidated in 1955, and synthesis was accomplished by Woodward and others just 25 years after its isolation.[28]

Characteristics. Vitamin B$_{12}$ is the most complex of all vitamin molecules and contains a single atom of cobalt held in a structure similar to that which holds iron in hemoglobin and magnesium in chlorophyll. (See Figure 12–7.) It occurs in several forms designated as COBALAMINS; cyanocobalamin is one of the most active forms.

The deep-red needle like crystals are slightly soluble in water, stable to heat, but inactivated by light and by strong acid or alkaline solutions. There is little loss of the vitamin by ordinary cooking procedures.

Vitamin B$_{12}$ is assayed microbiologically or by radioassay, and is measured in micrograms or picograms (pg, $\mu\mu$g, micromicrograms).

Metabolism. Vitamin B$_{12}$, being a very large molecule, requires a special mechanism for absorption, including at least five steps: (1) vitamin B$_{12}$ is separated from its polypeptide linkages with food by the gastric acid and enzymes; (2) vitamin B$_{12}$ is bound to intrinsic factor which is secreted by the parietal cells in the cardia and fundus of the stomach; (3) the vitamin B$_{12}$-intrinsic factor complex in the presence of calcium is bound to receptor sites in the ileum; (4) the vitamin is released from the complex and transferred across the mucosal epithelium; (5) vitamin B$_{12}$ is bound to a protein, TRANSCOBALAMIN, for transport in the blood circulation.

Intrinsic factor regulates the amount of absorption to about 2.5 to 3 mcg daily.[29] When the dietary intake is only 1 to 2 mcg daily, 60 to 80 per cent is absorbed. With good diets young men averaged 10 per cent absorption and elderly men about 5 per cent. Absorption is greater if the vitamin is present in three meals than if it is all provided in a single meal.

The liver is the principal site of storage for vitamin B$_{12}$. Storage in the bone marrow is limited, and amounts to only 1 to 2 per cent of that in the liver. The enterohepatic circulation varies from 0.6 to 6 mcg daily of vitamin B$_{12}$ with practically complete reabsorption taking place. Thus, the normal liver store of 2000 to 5000 mcg is sufficient to take care of body needs for three to five years.

The serum concentration of vitamin B$_{12}$ is 200 to 900 pg per milliliter. A level of 80 pg per milliliter represents unequivocal deficiency.

Functions. Vitamin B$_{12}$ functions in all cells, but especially those of the gastrointestinal tract, the nervous system, and the bone marrow. Within the bone marrow a vitamin B$_{12}$ coenzyme participates

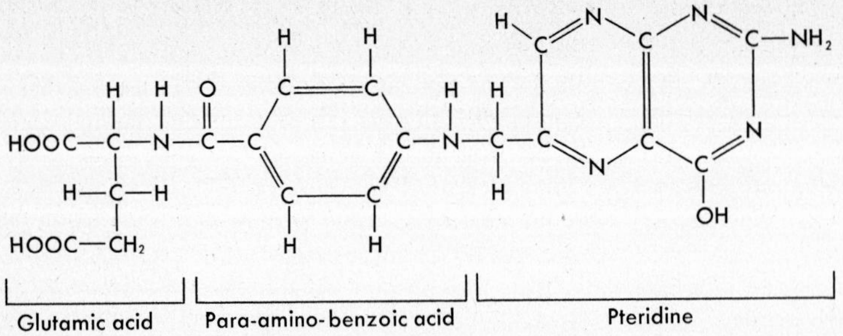

Glutamic acid · Para-amino-benzoic acid · Pteridine

Folic acid ($C_{19}H_{19}N_7O_6$; m.w. 441.4)

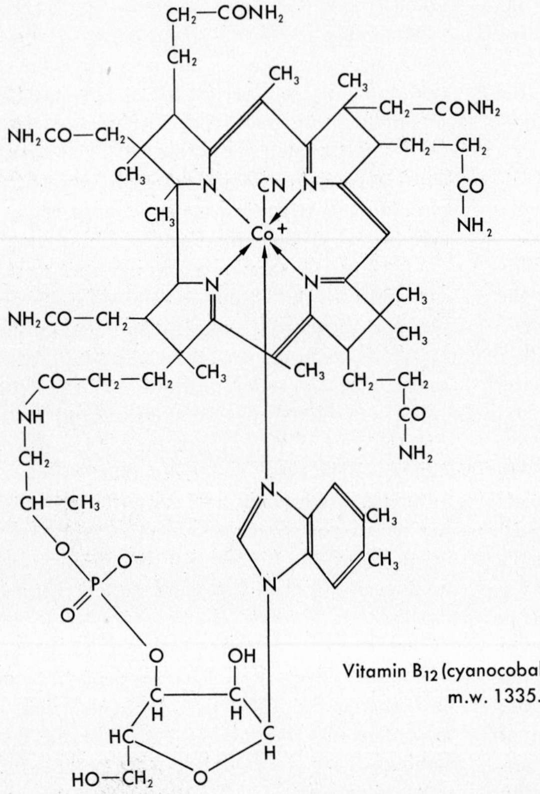

Vitamin B_{12} (cyanocobalamin shown; $C_{63}H_{88}CoN_{14}O_{14}P$; m.w. 1335.4)

Figure 12–7. Folic acid and vitamin B_{12} are essential for the regeneration of red blood cells. Vitamin B_{12} has the most complex structure of any of the vitamins. Note the similarity of the position of cobalt in this structure to the position of iron in hemoglobin, and of magnesium in chlorophyll.

in the synthesis of DNA. When DNA is not being synthesized, the erythroblasts do not divide but increase in size, becoming megaloblasts which are released into the circulation. Whether the influence of vitamin B_{12} is a direct action or a facilitation of the use of folic acid is not understood.

Vitamin B_{12} is also required for enzymes that accomplish the synthesis and transfer of single-carbon units such as the methyl group, for example, the synthesis of methionine and choline, which are important lipotropic factors.

Dietary needs. A minimum intake of 0.6 to

1.2 mcg of vitamin B_{12} daily is sufficient for normal hematopoiesis and good health, but will not replenish liver stores. The recommended allowance for males and females over 11 years is 3 mcg daily, and for pregnancy and lactation is 4 mcg.[1] For infants, 0.3 mcg is recommended daily, and for children the allowance increases from 1.0 mcg at 1 to 3 years to 2.0 mcg at 7 to 10 years.

The vitamin B_{12} available per capita in the American food supply is 9.5 mcg, of which 71 per cent is supplied by meats, poultry, and fish, 20 per cent by dairy foods excluding butter, and 8 per cent from eggs. Plant foods do not supply vitamin B_{12}.

Effects of deficiency. Vitamin B_{12} deficiency is a defect of absorption and rarely of dietary lack. Pernicious anemia is a disease, probably of genetic origin, in which intrinsic factor is not produced, and consequently vitamin B_{12} is not absorbed. The bone marrow is unable to produce mature red blood cells, but releases fewer number of large cells (macrocytes) into the circulation. Thus, the capacity to carry hemoglobin is reduced. The characteristic symptoms include lemon-yellow pallor, anorexia, dyspnea, prolonged bleeding time, abdominal discomfort, loss of weight, glossitis, neurologic disturbances including unsteady gait, and mental depression. Patients respond to as little as 1 mcg given parenterally; usually, initial therapy provides 50 to 100 mcg until the anemia is corrected, after which maintenance therapy is given monthly and averages 1 mcg daily.[30]

Megaloblastic anemia from vitamin B_{12} deficiency also occurs following surgical removal of the part of the stomach that produces intrinsic factor, or the part of the ileum where the absorption sites are located. Such deficiency occurs three to five years following the surgery and can be prevented by injections of vitamin B_{12} at periodic intervals. Malabsorption syndromes such as sprue may also be characterized by megaloblastic anemias resulting from deficient absorption of vitamin B_{12} as well as folic acid.

Dietary deficiency of vitamin B_{12} has been described in vegetarians who consumed no animal foods whatsoever.[31] They showed low serum levels of vitamin B_{12}, glossitis, paresthesias, and some changes in the spinal cord but did not have the characteristic anemia. For strict vegetarians a supplement of vitamin B_{12} is indicated.

A few cases of children with genetic disorders interfering with vitamin B_{12} utilization have been described.[32] In one of these the defect was apparently an inability to bind the vitamin B_{12}-intrinsic factor complex to the ileal receptor sites. In another there was absence of the protein that binds vitamin B_{12} in the circulation. A defect in transport across the mucosal membrane was observed in another. Injections of vitamin B_{12}, sometimes in large doses, were required to maintain normal blood values.

FOLACIN (FOLIC ACID)

Discovery. During the 1930s and 1940s many investigators had described water-soluble factors required by various animal species and microorganisms and given them names such as factor U (unknown factor required for chick growth); vitamin B_c (antianemia factor for chicks); Wills factor for treatment of tropical macrocytic anemia of pregnancy described by Dr. Lucy Wills; vitamin M, essential for monkeys; L-casei factor, citrovorum factor, and SLR factor for growth of various microorganisms. Folic acid was named in 1941 by Mitchell and his associates because of its prevalence in green leaves; *folium* is the Latin word for leaf. In 1945 the identification of the structure and the synthesis of folic acid by Angier and his coworkers at Lederle Laboratories established that these variously named factors were one and the same substance. That same year Dr. Tom Spies showed that folic acid was effective in the treatment of megaloblastic anemia of pregnancy and of tropical sprue.

Characteristics. FOLACIN is the generic term for folic acid, pteroylglutamic acid, and other compounds having the activity of folic acid. It consists of three linked components: a pteridine grouping, para-aminobenzoic acid, and glutamic acid, an amino acid. (See Figure 12–7.) It may consist of one, three, or seven glutamate groupings and is thus designated as mono-, tri-, or hepta-pteroylglutamate. Pure folic acid occurs as a bright-yellow crystalline compound, only slightly soluble in water and quite stable at pH 5 and above even with heating at 100° C. It is easily oxidized in an acid medium and is sensitive to light.

Folic acid is measured in micrograms or nanograms (ng, millimicrograms) and is assayed micro-biologically, or by colorimetric or fluorometric methods.

Metabolism. About 25 per cent of folacin in foods is in the free form and is readily absorbed. The folic acid that is bound must be freed by conjugase, an enzyme, in the mucosal cells of the proximal intestine before it can be absorbed. The amount absorbed is not known.

Folacin is stored principally in the liver. The active form is TETRAHYDROFOLIC ACID. Ascorbic acid prevents the oxidation of this active form and thus maintains an adequate level of the folate for metabolic needs.[33]

Functions. After absorption folacin undergoes a series of reactions to form coenzymes known as tetrahydrofolates. These are linked to single carbon groupings: methyl ($-CH_3$); hydroxymethyl ($-CH_2OH$); formyl ($-OCH$); and formimino ($-CH=NH$). The ability to link up with and to donate these single carbon units leads to the synthesis of methionine from homocysteine; the formation of choline; and the synthesis of serine, a 3-carbon amino acid, from glycine, a 2-carbon amino acid. Folacin is essential to DNA synthesis, and thus, together with vitamin B_{12}, regulates the formation of normal red blood cells in the bone marrow.

Recommended allowances. An allowance of 400 mcg is recommended for adults. For pregnancy the allowance is 800 mcg and for lactation it is 600 mcg; during the first year of life the needs are met with 50 mcg daily.

Food sources. Folic acid is widely distributed in foods in both free and conjugate forms. The availability of the latter to meet body needs is not known. Liver, kidney, yeast, and deep-green leafy vegetables are excellent sources; lean beef, veal, eggs, and whole-grain cereals are good sources; and root vegetables, dairy foods, pork, and light-green vegetables are relatively low in the vitamin.

Effects of deficiency. Folic acid deficiency results from inadequate dietary intake or is secondary to disease. In many instances dietary surveys have shown the intake to be considerably below the recommended allowances, but without accompanying biochemical or subjective signs of deficiency.[34] This suggests that utilization of conjugated forms may be higher than anticipated in setting up the allowances, or that the margin of safety is high.

With a deficiency the serum folate level is reduced and changes take place in the production of red blood cells in the bone marrow. The anemia that results from folic acid deficiency is characterized by a reduction in the number of red blood cells, the release into the blood circulation of large nucleated cells (hence the designation macrocytic, or megaloblastic, anemia), low hemoglobin levels but a high color content of each cell, and lowered leukocyte and platelet levels.

The anemia has been observed in elderly patients who have had poor diets and who have various organic diseases, in pregnant women, in some women using contraceptive pills, and in infants whose formulas may be inadequate in folic acid or ascorbic acid. It frequently accompanies disease conditions in which the requirement for the vitamin is greatly increased, as in Hodgkin's disease and leukemia. Malabsorption syndromes, notably tropical sprue, are characterized by the presence of megaloblastic anemias.

The administration of folic acid to patients with megaloblastic anemia brings about dramatic reversal of the changes in the bone marrow. The red blood cells become normal in size, their number increases, the total hemoglobin increases, and the leukocyte levels return to normal. Many of the patients have a glossitis and diarrhea especially associated with malabsorption; these too are improved.

Folacin will bring about remission of the anemia in pernicious anemia but is not effective in preventing or correcting the neurologic disturbances. Therefore, folacin is not a substitute for vitamin B_{12} in the treatment of this disorder.

OTHER FACTORS

Choline. All living cells contain CHOLINE, $C_5H_{15}NO_2$, principally in phospholipids. Choline is known as a lipotropic factor in that it prevents the deposit of fat in the liver. It is an important constituent of acetylcholine and thus is essential for the transmission of nerve impulses. One of the important functions of choline is the donation of methyl groups that can be utilized in numerous reactions.

Choline has been shown to be essential for various

animal species, but the need for it by human beings has not been clearly established. Probably synthesis of choline within the body is sufficient.

Egg yolk is especially rich in choline, but legumes, organ meats, milk, muscle meats, and whole-grain cereals are also good sources. A typical diet furnishes from 200 to 600 mg daily. These relatively large amounts indicate that choline is probably not a true vitamin.

Inositol. INOSITOL, $C_6H_{12}O_6$, is a water-soluble, sweet-tasting substance distributed in fruits, vegetables, whole grains, meats, and milk. It possesses lipotropic activity but its significance in human nutrition has not been established.

Lipoic acid. LIPOIC ACID is a sulfur-containing, fat-soluble substance also known as *thioctic acid* and *protogen*. Strictly speaking, it is not a vitamin because it is not necessary in the diet of animals. It functions, however, in the same manner as many of the B-complex vitamins. It is a component of the complexes involved in the decarboxylation of keto acids such as pyruvic acid and α-ketoglutaric acid. (See page 70.)

SOME POINTS FOR EMPHASIS IN NUTRITION EDUCATION (A GENERAL SUMMARY)

1. Vitamins are compounds of known chemical nature occurring in minute amounts in foods. They have exact functions in the body for the use of carbohydrates, fats, and proteins for energy and for the synthesis of tissues, enzymes, and other body regulators. Thus, vitamins help to maintain healthy tissues and normal functions of all organs.

2. Each vitamin has specific functions and cannot substitute for another. Many reactions in the body require several vitamins, and a lack of any one can interfere with the function of another.

3. Synthetic vitamins and the vitamins occurring naturally in foods have the same chemical formulas and, weight for weight, are of equal use in the body.

4. A diet that includes recommended amounts of the Four Food Groups will furnish sufficient amounts of all the vitamins (except vitamin D) required by healthy persons of all age categories.

5. Each food group makes a special vitamin contribution to the diet. All the vitamin needs are not easily met if one or more of these food groups are omitted. For example, fruits and vegetables are the principal sources of ascorbic acid; dark-green leafy vegetables and deep-yellow vegetables and fruits are a major source of carotene; milk is a principal source of riboflavin; meats, poultry, and fish are outstanding for niacin, vitamin B_6, vitamin B_{12}, and thiamin; and whole-grain and enriched breads and cereals are especially important for thiamin and niacin.

6. Vitamin D is present in natural foodstuffs in only small amounts. Infants, children, pregnant and lactating women, and people who have little exposure to sunlight should use vitamin D milk or a supplement.

7. All vitamins are susceptible to destruction under certain conditions. However, for practical purposes, if the homemaker observes rules for the preservation of ascorbic acid, thiamin, and riboflavin, all other vitamins are likely to be satisfactorily retained. For riboflavin, the principal destruction comes about when milk in clear-glass bottles is allowed to stand in direct sunlight. The retention of ascorbic acid, thiamin, and other vitamins is assured if (1) some raw foods such as salads are freshly prepared and used daily, (2) cutting and exposure of surfaces are reduced to the shortest possible period of time, (3) cookery takes place in a small volume of liquid, (4) the use of alkali to retain green color is avoided, (5) foods are cooked only to the point of tenderness, and (6) foods are served promptly after preparation.

8. Vitamins A and D are toxic, and high-potency supplements should be used only when prescribed by a physician for specific deficiencies.

9. If taken in greater amounts than the body needs, the water-soluble vitamins are excreted in the urine; hence, supplements in addition to a good diet are probably an economic waste.

10. Vitamin deficiencies can be diagnosed only by means of accurate dietary and medical history, physical examination, and laboratory

Table 12–1. Summary of Water-Soluble Vitamins (see also Points for Emphasis, page 189)

Nomenclature	Important Sources	Physiology and Function	Effects of Deficiency	Recommended Allowances
Ascorbic acid Vitamin C	Citrus fruits; tomatoes; melons; cabbage; broccoli; strawberries; fresh potatoes; green leafy vegetables	Very little storage in body Formation of intercellular cement substance; synthesis of collagen Absorption and use of iron Prevents oxidation of folacin	Weakened cartilages and capillary walls Cutaneous hemorrhage; sore, bleeding gums, anemia Poor wound healing Poor bone and tooth development Scurvy	Men: 45 mg Women: 45 mg Pregnancy: 60 mg Lactation: 60 mg Infants: 35 mg Children under 10: 40 mg Boys and girls: 45 mg
Thiamin Vitamin B$_1$	Whole-grain and enriched breads, cereals, flours; organ meats, pork; other meats, poultry, fish; legumes, nuts; milk; green vegetables	Limited body storage Thiamin pyrophosphate (TPP) is coenzyme for decarboxylation and transketolation; chiefly involved in carbohydrate metabolism	Poor appetite; atony of gastrointestinal tract, constipation Mental depression, apathy, polyneuritis Cachexia, edema Cardiac failure Beriberi	Men: 1.4 mg Women: 1.0 mg Pregnancy: 1.3 mg Lactation: 1.3 mg Infants: 0.3–0.5 mg Children under 10: 0.7–1.2 mg Boys and girls: 1.1–1.5 mg
Riboflavin Vitamin B$_2$	Milk; organ meats; eggs; green leafy vegetables	Limited body stores, but reserves retained carefully Coenzymes for removal and transfer of hydrogen; flavin mononucleotide (FMN) and flavin adenine dinucleotide (FAD)	Cheilosis (cracks at corners of lips) Scaly desquamation around nose, ears Sore tongue and mouth Burning and itching of eyes Photophobia	Men: 1.6 mg Women: 1.2 mg Pregnancy: 1.5 mg Lactation: 1.7 mg Infants: 0.4–0.6 mg Children under 10: 0.8–1.2 mg Boys and girls: 1.3–1.8 mg
Niacin Nicotinic acid Nicotinamide	Meat, poultry, fish; whole-grain and enriched breads, flours, cereals; nuts, legumes Tryptophan as a precursor	Coenzyme for glycolysis, fat synthesis, tissue respiration. Coenzymes NAD and NADP accept hydrogen and transfer it	Anorexia, glossitis, diarrhea Dermatitis Neurologic degeneration Pellagra	Men: 18 mg Women: 13 mg Pregnancy: 15 mg Lactation: 17 mg Infants: 5–8 mg Children under 10: 9–16 mg Boys and girls: 14–20 mg
Vitamin B$_6$ Three active forms: pyridoxine, pyridoxal, pyridoxamine	Meat, poultry, fish; potatoes, sweet potatoes, vegetables	Pyridoxal phosphate is coenzyme for transamination, decarboxylation, transulfuration Conversion of tryptophan to niacin; conversion of glycogen to glucose	Nervous irritability, convulsions Weakness, ataxia, abdominal pain Dermatitis; anemia	Adults: 2.0 mg Pregnancy: 2.5 mg Lactation: 2.5 mg Infants: 0.3–0.4 mg Children under 10: 0.6–1.2 mg Boys and girls: 1.6–2.0 mg

Vitamin	Food Sources	Functions	Deficiency	Requirement
Pantothenic acid	Meat, poultry, fish; whole-grain cereals; legumes Smaller amounts in fruits, vegetables, milk	Constituent of coenzyme A: oxidation of pyruvic acid, α-ketoglutarate, fatty acids; synthesis of fatty acids, sterols, and porphyrin	Deficiency seen only with severe multiple B-complex deficits; then, gastrointestinal disturbances, neuritis, burning sensations of feet	Not known; probably about 5–10 mg
Biotin	Organ meats, egg yolk, nuts, legumes	Avidin, a protein in raw egg white, blocks absorption; large amounts of raw eggs must be eaten Coenzyme for deamination, carboxylation, and decarboxylation	Deficiency only when many raw egg whites are consumed for long periods of time Dermatitis, anorexia, hyperesthesia, anemia	Not known; probably about 150 mcg
Vitamin B$_{12}$ Cyanocobalamin Hydroxycobalamin	In animal foods only: organ meats, muscle meats, fish, poultry; eggs; milk	Requires intrinsic factor for absorption Biosynthesis of methyl groups Synthesis of DNA and RNA Formation of mature red blood cells	Lack of intrinsic factor leads to deficiency: pernicious anemia, following gastrectomy Macrocytic anemia Neurologic degeneration	Adults: 3 mcg Pregnancy: 4 mcg Lactation: 4 mcg Infants: 0.3 mcg Children: 1–2 mcg Boys and girls: 3 mcg
Folacin Folic acid Tetrahydrofolic acid	Organ meats, deep-green leafy vegetables; muscle meats, poultry, fish, eggs; whole-grain cereals	Active form is folinic acid; requires ascorbic acid for conversion Coenzyme for transmethylation; synthesis of nucleoproteins; maturation of red blood cells Interrelated with vitamin B$_{12}$	Megaloblastic anemia of infancy, pregnancy, tropical sprue	Adults: 400 mcg Pregnancy: 800 mcg Lactation: 600 mcg Infants: 50 mcg Children under 10: 100–300 mcg Boys and girls: 400 mcg
Choline	Egg yolk, meat, poultry, fish, milk, whole grains	Probably not a true vitamin Donor of methyl groups: lipotropic action Component of acetylcholine	Has not been observed in humans	Not known; typical diet supplies 200–600 mg
Lipoic acid Thioctic acid Protogen		Probably not a true vitamin Coenzyme for decarboxylation of keto acids		Not known
Inositol	Widely distributed in all foods	Lipotropic agent Vitamin nature not established	Has not been observed in humans	Not known

*See also Table 3–1 for complete listing of allowances.

studies. Self-diagnosis and therapy are wasteful and can be dangerous.

11. Vitamin deficiency diseases can occur (1) if the dietary intake is generally poor, (2) if a food group is consistently omitted without making appropriate compensation for such omission, and (3) when there is too little money to buy an adequate diet.

12. A large proportion of vitamin deficiencies in the United States are secondary to disease, including anorexia and vomiting and failure to eat, malabsorption as in diarrhea, sprue, and other conditions, and increased metabolic requirements because of fever and other stress factors.

13. Specific vitamin deficiencies require therapy with the vitamins that are lacking. Usually, synthetic vitamins are used to correct the deficiency inasmuch as large dosages can bring about rapid improvement.

PROBLEMS AND REVIEW

1. Explain how the following nutrients are interrelated:

riboflavin and niacin	pyridoxine and protein	cobalt and vitamin B_{12}
tryptophan and niacin	tryptophan and vitamin B_6	folic acid and ascorbic acid
glucose and thiamin		choline and fat

2. What is the effect on carbohydrate metabolism of a deficiency of thiamin? What are clinical signs of such deficiency?

3. What is the role of niacin in metabolism? What clinical symptoms are observed in a niacin deficiency?

4. How can you explain the fact that milk is a pellagra-preventive food even though it contains very little niacin?

5. The dietary intake of vitamins may appear to be satisfactory when compared with recommended allowances, but a physician may prescribe a vitamin supplement. Under what circumstances would you expect such a supplement to be necessary?

6. What is the possible significance of each of the following in human nutrition: folacin; choline; biotin; pantothenic acid; pyridoxine; inositol; vitamin B_{12}?

7. *Problem.* Compare the label information on three packages of dry cereal, including whole grain, enriched or restored, and fortified. Which of these would give the highest nutritional value for an expenditure of 10 cents? Show your calculations.

8. *Problem.* Mrs. Smith has asked for your guidance in the selection, storage, and preparation of food so that maximum nutritive value will be retained. On the basis of your information concerning the stability of vitamins, indicate briefly a set of instructions for guiding Mrs. Smith. Show how these rules apply to the preparation of a meal that includes roast beef, potatoes, green beans, cole slaw, milk, and fruit cup. Which vitamin or vitamins are especially concerned in each rule you have laid down?

9. *Problem.* Calculate the thiamin, riboflavin, and niacin content of your own diet for two days. Compare your intake with the recommended allowances. If there are any deficits, show how you could correct them.

10. *Problem.* A dietary calculation showed an intake of 80 gm protein and 12 mg niacin. Calculate the total niacin equivalent of this diet.

11. *Problem.* Calculate the percentage of your own daily requirement for thiamin and riboflavin which 2 cups of milk would supply. For each of these nutrients list two foods which would serve as effective supplements to the milk in supplying your daily needs.

CITED REFERENCES

1. Food and Nutrition Board: *Recommended Dietary Allowances,* 8th ed. National Academy of Sciences—National Research Council, Washington, D.C., 1974.

2. Friend, B., and Marston, R.: "Nutritional Review," *National Food Situation*, U.S. Department of Agriculture, Washington, D.C., Nov. 1975, pp. 26–32.

3. Williams, R. R.: "The World Beriberi Problem," *J. Clin. Nutr.*, **1**:513–16, 1953.

4. Brin, M.: "Erythrocytes as a Biopsy Tissue for Functional Evaluation of Thiamine Adequacy," *J.A.M.A.*, **187**:762–66, 1964.

5. Sebrell, W. H., and Butler, R. E.: "Riboflavin Deficiency in Man," *Public Health Rep.*, **54**:2121–31, 1939.

6. Horwitt, M. K., *et al.*: "Effects of Dietary Depletion of Riboflavin," *J. Nutr.*, **39**:357–73, 1949.

7. Goldberger, J.: "The Prevention of Pellagra. A Test Diet Among Institutional Inmates," *Public Health Rep.*, **30**:3117–31, 1915; Nutrition classic reproduced in part in *Nutr. Rev.*, **31**:152–53, 1973.

8. Elvehjem, C. A., *et al.*: "The Isolation and Identification of the Anti-black Tongue Factor," *J. Biol. Chem.*, **123**:137–49, 1938; Nutrition classic reproduced in part in *Nutr. Rev.*, **32**:48–50, 1974.

9. Miller, O. N., *et al.*: "Investigation of the Mechanism of Action of Nicotinic Acid in Serum Lipid Levels in Man," *Am. J. Clin. Nutr.*, **8**:480–90, 1960.

10. Horwitt, M. K., *et al.*: "Tryptophan-Niacin Relationships in Man," *J. Nutr.*, **60** (Suppl. 1):1–43, 1956.

11. Goldsmith, G. A., *et al.*: "Efficiency of Tryptophan as a Niacin Precursor in Man," *J. Nutr.*, **73**:172–76, 1961.

12. Vivian, V. M.: "Relationship Between Tryptophan-Niacin Metabolism and Changes in Nitrogen Balance," *J. Nutr.*, **82**:395–400, 1964.

13. Mickelson, O.: "Present Knowledge of Niacin," in *Present Knowledge of Nutrition*, The Nutrition Foundation, Inc., New York, pp. 96–100.

14. Horwitt, M. K.: "Niacin," in Goodhart, R. S., and Shils, M. E.: *Modern Nutrition in Health and Disease*, 5th ed., Lea & Febiger, Philadelphia, 1973, pp. 198–202.

15. Snyderman, S.E., *et al.*: "Pyridoxine Deficiency in the Human Infant," *Am. J. Clin. Nutr.*, **1**:200–207, 1953.

16. Coursin, D. B.: "Convulsive Seizures in Infants with Pyridoxine-Deficient Diet," *J.A.M.A.*, **154**:406–408, 1954.

17. Cheslock, K. E., and McCully, M. T.: "Response of Human Beings to a Low-Vitamin B_6 Diet," *J. Nutr.*, **70**:507–13, 1960.

18. Mueller, J. F., and Vilter, R. W.: "Pyridoxine Deficiency in Human Beings Induced with Desoxy-pyridoxine," *J. Clin. Invest.*, **29**:193–201, 1950.

19. Frimpter, G. W., *et al.*: "Vitamin B_6-Dependency Syndromes: New Horizons in Nutrition," *Am. J. Clin. Nutr.*, **22**:794–805, 1969.

20. Glusman, N.: "The Syndrome of 'Burning Feet' (Nutritional Melalgia) as a Manifestation of Nutritional Deficiency," *Am. J. Med.*, **3**:211–23, 1947.

21. Hodges, R. E., *et al.*: "Human Pantothenic Acid Deficiency Produced by Omega-Methyl Pantothenic Acid," *J. Clin. Invest.*, **38**:1421–25, 1959.

22. Parsons, H. T., *et al.*: "Interrelationship Between Dietary Egg White and Requirements for Protective Factor in Cure of Nutritional Disorder Due to Egg White," *Biochem. J.*, **31**:424–32, 1937.

23. Sydenstricker, V. P., *et al.*: "Preliminary Observations on 'Egg White Injury' in Man and Its Cure with a Biotin Concentrate," *Science*, **95**:176–77, 1942.

24. Baugh, C. M., *et al.*: "Human Biotin Deficiency. A Case History of Biotin Deficiency Induced by Raw Egg Consumption in a Cirrhotic Patient," *Am. J. Clin. Nutr.*, **21**:173–82, 1968.

25. Minot, G. R., and Murphy, W. P.: "Treatment of Pernicious Anemia by a Special Diet," *J.A.M.A.*, **87**:470–76, 1926.

26. Rickes, E. L., *et al.*: "Crystalline Vitamin B_{12}," *Science*, **107**:396–97, 1948.

27. Smith, E. L., and Parker, L. F. J.: "Purification of Anti-pernicious Anemia Factors from Liver," *Nature*, **161**:638, 1948.

28. Staff Report: "Discovery and Synthesis of Vitamin B_{12} Celebrated," *Nutr. Today*, **8**:24–27, Jan.–Feb. 1973.

29. Heyssel, R. M., *et al.*: "Vitamin B_{12} Turnover in Man," *Am. J. Clin. Nutr.*, **18**:176–84, 1966.

30. McCurdy, P. R.: "B_{12} Shots," *J.A.M.A.*, **229**:703–704, 1974.

31. Smith, A. D. M.: "Veganism: A Clinical Survey with Observations on Vitamin B_{12} Metabolism," *Br. Med. J.*, **1**:1655–58, 1962.

32. Review: "Rare Forms of Familial Vitamin B_{12} Malabsorption in Children," *Nutr. Rev.*, **31**:149–51, 1973.

33. Stokes, P. L., *et al.:* "Folate Metabolism in Scurvy," *Am. J. Clin. Nutr.,* **28**:126–29, 1975.
34. Daniel, W. A., Jr., *et al.:* "Dietary Intakes and Plasma Concentrations of Folate in Healthy Adolescents," *Am. J. Clin. Nutr.,* **28**:363–70, 1975.

ADDITIONAL REFERENCES

Thiamin, Riboflavin, and Niacin

Ariaey-Nejad, M. R., *et al.:* "Thiamin Metabolism in Man," *Am. J. Clin. Nutr.,* **23**:764–78, 1970.
Goldsmith, G. A.: "Experimental Niacin Deficiency," *J. Am. Diet. Assoc.,* **32**:312–16, 1956.
Gopalan, C.: "Leucine and Pellagra," *Nutr. Rev.,* **26**:323–26, 1968.
Henshaw, J. L., *et al.:* "Method for Evaluating Thiamine Adequacy in College Women," *J. Am. Diet. Assoc.,* **57**:436–41, 1970.
Horwitt, M. K.: "Nutritional Requirements of Man with Special Reference to Riboflavin," *Am. J. Clin. Nutr.,* **18**:458–66, 1966.
Keefer, C. S.: "The Beriberi Heart," *Arch. Intern. Med.,* **45**:1–22, 1930; Nutrition classic reproduced in part in *Nutr. Rev.,* **32**:304–307, 1974.
Noble, I.: "Thiamine and Riboflavin Retention in Cooked Variety Meats," *J. Am. Diet. Assoc.,* **56**:225–28, 1970.
Review: "Conversion of Tryptophan to Niacin in Man," *Nutr. Rev.,* **32**:76–77, 1974.
Sydenstricker, V. P., *et al.:* "The Ocular Manifestations of Ariboflavinosis," *J.A.M.A.,* **114**:2437–45, 1940.
Williams, R. R.: *et al.:* "Observations on Induced Thiamine Deficiency in Man," *Arch. Intern. Med.,* **66**:785–99, 1940.
Williams, R. R.: *Toward the Conquest of Beriberi.* Harvard University Press, Cambridge, Mass., 1961.

Vitamin B₆, Pantothenic Acid, and Biotin

Baker, E. M., *et al.:* "Vitamin B_6 Requirement for Adult Men," *Am. J. Clin. Nutr.,* **15**:59–66, 1964.
Bridgers, W. F.: "Present Knowledge of Biotin," *Nutr. Rev.,* **25**:65–68, 1967.
Brown, R. R., *et al.:* "Urinary 4-pyridoxic Acid, Plasma Pyridoxal Phosphate, and Erythrocyte Aminotransferase Levels in Oral Contraceptive Users Receiving Controlled Intakes of Vitamin B_6," *Am. J. Clin. Nutr.,* **28**:10–19, 1975.
Cohenour, S. H., and Calloway, D. H.: "Blood, Urine, and Dietary Pantothenic Acid Levels of Pregnant Teenagers," *Am. J. Clin. Nutr.,* **25**:512–17, 1972.
Fox, H. M., and Linkswiler, H.: "Pantothenic Acid Excretion on Three Levels of Intake," *J. Nutr.,* **75**:451–54, 1961.
György, P.: "The History of Vitamin B_6," *Am. J. Clin. Nutr.,* **4**:313–17, 1956.
Hines, J. D., and Harris, J. W.: "Pyridoxine-Responsive Anemia. Description of Three Patients with Megaloblastic Erythropoiesis," *Am. J. Clin. Nutr.,* **14**:137–46, 1964.
Linkswiler, H.: "Biochemical and Physiological Changes in Vitamin B_6 Deficiency," *Am. J. Clin. Nutr.,* **20**:547–57, 1967.
Prasad, A. S., *et al.:* "Effect of Oral Contraceptive Agents on Nutrients. II. Vitamins," *Am. J. Clin. Nutr.,* **28**:385–91, 1975.
Review: "Vitamin B_6 Deficiency Following Isoniazid Therapy," *Nutr. Rev.,* **26**:306–308, 1968.
Standal, B. R., *et al.:* "Early Changes in Pyridoxine Status of Patients Receiving Isoniazid Therapy," *Am. J. Clin. Nutr.,* **27**:479–84, 1974.

Vitamin B₁₂ and Folacin

Bianchi, A., *et al.:* "Nutritional Folic Acid Deficiency with Megaloblastic Changes in the Small-Bowel Epithelium," *N. Engl. J. Med.,* **282**:859–61, 1970.
Butterfield, S., and Calloway, D. H.: "Folacin in Wheat and Selected Foods," *J. Am. Diet. Assoc.,* **60**:310–14, 1972.
Halsted, C. H.: "The Small Intestine in Vitamin B_{12} and Folate Deficiency," *Nutr. Rev.,* **33**:33–37, 1975.
Herbert, V.: "Biochemical and Hematologic Lesions in Folic Acid Deficiency," *Am. J. Clin. Nutr.,* **20**:562–69, 1967.

————: "Nutritional Requirements for Vitamin B_{12} and Folic Acid," *Am. J. Clin. Nutr.*, **21:**743–52, 1968.

Herbert, V., and Jacob, E.: "Destruction of Vitamin B_{12} by Ascorbic Acid," *J.A.M.A.*, **230:**241–42, 1974.

Hoppner, K., *et al.:* "Folacin Activity of Frozen Convenience Foods," *J. Am. Diet. Assoc.*, **63:**536–39, 1973.

McCurdy, P. R.: "When Friends or Patients Ask About Vitamin B_{12} Shots," *J.A.M.A.*, **229:**703–704, 1974; **231:**289, 1975.

Mahmud, K., *et al.:* "The Importance of Red Cell B_{12} and Folate Levels After Partial Gastrectomy," *Am. J. Clin. Nutr.*, **27:**51–54, 1974.

Necheles, T. F., and Snyder, L. M.: "Malabsorption of Folate Polyglutamates Associated with Oral Contraceptive Therapy," *N. Engl. J. Med.*, **282:**858–59, 1970.

Paine, C. J., *et al.:* "Oral Contraceptives, Serum Folate, and Hematologic Studies," *J.A.M.A.*, **231:**731–33, 1975.

Review: "Cerebrospinal Folate Levels in Epileptics and Their Response to Folate Therapy," *Nutr. Rev.*, **32:**70–72, 1974.

————: "Folic Acid Absorption, Anticonvulsant and Contraceptive Therapy," *Nutr. Rev.*, **32:**39–41, 1974.

————: "Folic Acid and Pregnancy," *Nutr. Rev.*, **26:**5–8, 1968.

Stadtman, T. C.: "Vitamin B_{12}," *Science*, **171:**859–67, 1971.

Toskes, P. P., and Deren, J. J.: "Vitamin B_{12} Absorption and Malabsorption," *Gastroenterology*, **65:**662–83, 1973.

West, R.: "Activity of Vitamin B_{12} in Addisonian Pernicious Anemia," *Science*, **107:**398, 1948.

Phosphorus	1.52	gm
Iron	18.3	mg
Magnesium	339	mg
Vitamin A value	8200	I.U.
Thiamin	1.87	mg
Riboflavin	2.29	mg
Niacin	23.3	mg
Vitamin B_6	2.25	mg
Vitamin B_{12}	9.5	mg
Ascorbic acid	122	mg

13 Food Selection and Meal Planning For Healthy Persons

One instrument does not make up an orchestra; neither does one food, no matter how good it is, make up a well-balanced diet. The emphasis in the preceding chapters was on the metabolic roles of specific nutrients and on food sources that would supply these nutrients. Foods, however, are complex substances that make a variety of nutritive contributions and therefore should be evaluated in terms of their total composition and not only for single nutrients for which they may be outstanding. The discussion in this chapter aims to show how each food group contributes to the total nutritional intake, to describe a dietary pattern for the adult that is based upon the Four Food Groups, and to outline essential factors in meal planning.

The national food supply. Are national food supplies adequate for the population needs? What is the relative contribution that may be expected of each of the major food groups to the nutrient supplies? Answers to these questions are provided annually by the Economic Research Service of the U.S. Department of Agriculture. The per capita nutritive value of the available food supply in 1975 was as follows:[1]

Food energy	3160	kcal
Protein	99	gm
Fat	147	gm
Carbohydrate	369	gm
Calcium	0.91	gm

The percentage of total nutrients contributed by each of the major food groups is shown in Table 13–1. From this table it is easy to see the relative importance of each food group in supplying a given nutrient. This table also demonstrates how some food groups are important suppliers of several nutrients. The following statements represent a summary of the contribution made by each of the major food groups.

1. Milk and dairy products far exceed other food groups for calcium and riboflavin; they are second only to the meat group for the protein contribution.

2. The meat group, including eggs and dry beans, peas, and nuts as well as meat, poultry, and fish, ranks first as a source of protein, phosphorus, magnesium, iron, thiamin, niacin, vitamin B_6, and vitamin B_{12}. Because of the high level of consumption, this group ranks second for vitamin A and riboflavin.

3. Fruits and vegetables are the only important sources of ascorbic acid and contribute about half of the vitamin A; they supply roughly one fifth of the iron and about one fourth of the magnesium and vitamin B_6.

4. The flour-cereal group takes second place as a source of calories, iron, thiamin, and niacin. this group becomes increasingly important for these nutrients as the income is lowered and the consumption of them is increased.

5. Sugars and sweets and fats and oils each contribute about one sixth of the energy value of the diet but do not add appreciably to the protein, mineral, or vitamin levels.

MILK GROUP

Milk serves as the sole food for the young during the most critical period of life for some 8000 species. Although the milk of various mammals is used for

Table 13–1. Contribution of Major Food Groups to Nutrient Supplies Available for Civilian Consumption*

Food Group	Food Energy %	Pro-tein %	Fat %	Carbo-hydrate %	Cal-cium %	Phos-phorus %	Iron %	Magne-sium %	Vitamin A Value %	Thia-min %	Ribo-flavin %	Niacin %	Vitamin B₆ %	Vitamin B₁₂ %	Ascorbic Acid %
Dairy products, excluding butter	11.4	22.0	13.2	6.7	74.5	34.7	2.2	21.1	12.7	9.0	39.8	1.5	10.2	19.8	3.7
Meat (including pork fat cuts), poultry, and fish	19.9	41.6	34.1	0.1	3.8	27.6	29.5	13.5	21.9	26.4	25.1	46.9	44.8	70.5	1.1
Eggs	2.0	5.0	3.0	0.1	2.3	5.2	4.8	1.2	5.5	2.2	5.0	0.2	1.9	8.1	0
Dry beans and peas, nuts, soya flour and grits	3.1	5.6	3.7	2.3	3.0	6.3	6.7	12.1	†	6.1	2.0	7.0	4.5	0	†
Citrus fruits	1.1	0.5	0.1	2.2	1.0	0.8	0.8	2.5	1.6	3.2	0.6	1.0	1.3	0	27.6
Other fruits	2.4	0.6	0.3	5.1	1.3	1.2	3.4	4.1	5.5	1.9	1.6	1.8	5.8	0	11.2
Potatoes and sweet potatoes	2.9	2.4	0.1	5.6	1.0	3.9	4.4	7.2	5.3	6.2	1.8	7.2	11.3	0	17.5
Dark-green and deep-yellow vegetables	0.3	0.5	†	0.5	1.7	0.7	1.7	2.2	21.6	0.9	1.1	0.7	1.8	0	8.2
Other vegetables, including tomatoes	2.7	3.4	0.5	5.0	5.1	5.1	9.1	10.7	15.4	7.0	4.7	6.2	9.5	0	27.3
Flour and cereal products	19.9	17.8	1.4	35.9	3.4	12.5	27.7	18.1	0.4	36.9	17.7	23.7	8.9	1.6	0
Fats and oils, including butter	17.5	0.2	42.4	†	0.4	0.2	0	0.4	7.8	0	0	0	0.1	0	0
Sugars and other sweeteners	16.2	†	0	35.9	1.6	0.3	7.5	0.2	0	†	†	†	†	0	†
Miscellaneous‡	0.7	0.4	1.3	0.5	0.9	1.6	2.1	6.7	2.2	0.1	0.6	3.9	0.1	0	3.4
Total§	100.1	100.0	100.1	99.9	100.0	100.1	99.9	100.0	99.9	99.9	100.0	100.1	100.2	100.0	100.0

* Rearranged from Friend, B., and Marston, R.: "Nutritional Review," *National Food Situation*, NFS 154. Economic Research Service, U.S. Department of Agriculture, Table 10. November 1975. Preliminary data for 1975.

† Less than 0.05 per cent.

‡ Coffee and chocolate liquor equivalent of coca beans and fortification of products not assigned to a specific food group.

§ Components may not add to total due to rounding.

food, cow's milk is by far the most common. The milk group includes fresh and processed milks, cheese, and ice cream.

Importance of milk as a food. There is no adequate substitute for milk. No food has a wider acceptability or offers a greater variety of uses. Adults of all ages should include about 2 cups of fluid milk daily, or its equivalent as evaporated milk, dry milk, or hard cheese. This allowance should be raised to 3 cups or more for schoolchildren and pregnant women, and to 4 cups or more during the adolescent years and for the nursing mother.

Milk is a complex substance in which over 100 separate components have been identified.[2] It is fluid in spite of the fact that it contains more solids than many solid foods. Fresh cow's milk contains 87 per cent water and 13 per cent solids, whereas such foods, as cabbage, strawberries, and summer squash, to name but a few examples, are lower in solids content and higher in water content.

The exact composition of milk varies with the breed of cattle, the feed used, and the period of lactation. Pooled market milk has a uniform composition which may be varied slightly by local or state regulations for butterfat and solids content.

Energy. Too many people become concerned about the caloric value of milk and sometimes eliminate milk from their diets for this reason. From Figure 13–1 it may be seen that 2 cups of whole milk furnish about 16 per cent of the calories for the moderately active young woman, but the percentage contribution for most of the nutrients is considerably greater. By adjusting the fat level of milk, caloric modifications can be made for low-calorie and high-calorie diets.

> 1 cup skim milk = 90 kcal
> 1 cup 2 per cent milk = 145 kcal
> 1 cup whole milk = 160 kcal
> ½ cup whole milk + ½ cup light cream
>   = 330 kcal

Protein. One cup of whole, skim, or diluted evaporated milk contains 9 gm protein. Thus, 2 cups daily furnish about one third of the adult protein allowance.

Casein accounts for four fifths of the protein in milk, and various whey proteins, including lactalbumins and lactoglobulins, constitute the re-

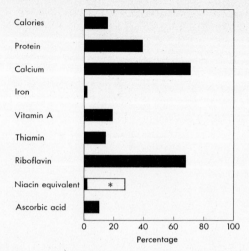

Figure 13–1. Percentage contributions of 2 cups of milk to the Recommended Dietary Allowances for the woman aged 23 to 50 years.

° Unshaded area represents niacin equivalent from tryptophan.

maining protein fractions. The essential amino acids present in milk proteins are supplied in almost ideal proportions for maximum tissue synthesis.

Milk supplements cereal proteins in an excellent fashion, for it supplies the amino acids lysine and tryptophan, which are low in the cereals. The biologic value of proteins in white wheat flour is only 50 per cent when used alone, but this is raised to 75 per cent when milk is used with the wheat flour.[3]

Fat. The fat of milk is highly emulsified and is easily digested. Milk fat contains a high proportion of short-chain fatty acids which are especially well tolerated. About 60 to 75 per cent of the fatty acids in milk are saturated, 24 to 40 per cent are monounsaturated, and 2 to 10 per cent are polyunsaturated. In modified-fat diets, when saturated fats must be kept to a minimum, skim milk may be substituted for whole milk.

Carbohydrate. Lactose is a carbohydrate occurring only in milk. This sugar is much less sweet, less soluble, and more stable than sucrose and other sugars. It gives to milk a bland flavor. Lactose favors the growth of lactic-acid-producing bacteria which are believed to retard or prevent the growth of putrefying bacteria. Lactose probably favors the absorption of calcium and phosphorus and the synthesis of some B-complex vitamins in the small intestine. Some persons, especially adults, have a lactase deficiency and therefore a poor tolerance for milk. (See Chapter 34.)

Minerals and vitamins. Only the milk group provides a practical basis for meeting the recommended allowance for calcium. Phosphorus occurs in correct proportions with calcium to support optimum skeletal growth. Milk contains appreciable amounts of sodium, potassium, and magnesium, but it furnishes very little iron, so that the infant's diet must be supplemented at an early age to prevent anemia.

Milk is an outstanding dietary source of riboflavin and also supplies fair amounts of vitamin A, thiamin, vitamin B_6, and vitamin B_{12}. It is low in niacin but is an excellent source of tryptophan, which functions as a precursor of niacin. About 85 per cent of market milk today is fortified with vitamin D to a level of 400 I.U. per quart. Milk furnishes only small amounts of ascorbic acid.

Cheese. The composition of cheese depends upon the kind of milk used—whole or skim—and the amount of water present. A pound of hard cheese contains the casein and fat of 1 gallon of milk. One ounce of Cheddar cheese is about equal to $3/4$ cup milk for its protein, calcium, and calories. The proteins (principally casein) in cheese contain all the essential amino acids and are therefore of high biologic value. Only a trace of the lactose present in milk remains in the cheese. Varying amounts of calcium, thiamin, and riboflavin are lost depending upon the method of preparation.

Soft cheeses vary widely in their composition. If made with skim milk, cottage cheese will contain as little as 1 per cent fat; the protein content is about 19 per cent. Creamed cottage cheese contains 4 per cent fat. The caloric values of creamed and uncreamed cottage cheeses do not differ greatly, being 120 and 98 kcal per $1/2$-cup serving, respectively. Cottage cheese is considerably lower than Cheddar cheese in its calcium content since some of the calcium is lost in the whey with acid coagulation. Almost 11 oz of cottage cheese are needed to provide the calcium of 1 cup of milk.

Cream cheese contains approximately 9 per cent protein and 37 per cent fat. It is therefore high in calories but is not a good substitute for cottage or hard cheese in terms of protein. Its calcium content is low.

Other milk products. Cultured milks have a nutritive value equal to that of the milk from which they are made. The fermentation of the milk results in the splitting of the lactose to lactic acid and in some coagulation of casein. Yogurt is prepared from whole, skim, or partially skimmed milk and is fermented with a mixed culture of microorganisms. It is available plain or in a variety of fruit flavorings.

Ice cream supplies the nutrients of cream, milk, and any fruits or nuts used in flavoring. Most ice creams contain about 10 per cent fat and furnish 130 kcal per half cup. About $1\frac{1}{2}$ cups ice cream furnish the calcium and protein equivalent to 1 cup milk. Ice milk contains 4 to 5 per cent fat and about 100 kcal per half cup.

Meat Group

The meat group includes beef, veal, mutton, lamb, pork, poultry, eggs, fish, legumes, and nuts. The daily recommendation from this group is two servings, the equivalents for one serving being:

2 or 3 oz edible portion lean cooked beef, veal, pork, lamb, poultry, or fish
2 eggs
1 cup cooked dry beans, peas, or lentils
4 tablespoons peanut butter

Place of meat in the diet. On the basis of available food supplies, the per capita consumption each year of meat is about 188 pounds; of poultry, 50 pounds; and of fish, 12 pounds.[1] About three fifths of the meat consumed is beef, and pork accounts for about one third. Veal, lamb, and mutton together account for less than 5 per cent of the meat consumed. (See Figure 13–2.)

The use of variety meats depends on family traditions and beliefs. The tongue, liver, brain, and heart of beef, lamb, veal, or pork, the sweetbreads or thymus gland of calves, and tripe of beef are highly nutritious meats.

Fish and poultry in the diet. Some reasons for the limited use of fish are the ideas held by some people that fish is inferior food because it is used on fast days; that it is food selected by the poor; that it has not always been available far away from the sea-coast, lake, or river regions; and that it is so often

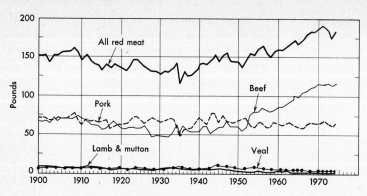

Figure 13–2. Per capita consumption of meat. (Courtesy, Economic Research Service, U.S. Department of Agriculture.)

poorly cooked and unpalatable. Fish is equal in nutritive value to meat except that the caloric value is usually lower by reason of the lower fat concentration.

Chicken and turkey, available year-round, have become more widely used in recent years because they have been lower in cost than most meats.

Acceptability of meat and fish. The often heard comment "It doesn't seem like a meal without meat" attests to the popular and psychologic importance of meat. The aromas and flavors provided by meat extractives stimulate the appetite. The protein and fat content increase the satiety value of the meal.

Eggs. As breakfast, luncheon, or dinner main dishes, eggs may be used in numerous ways. They are essential ingredients in many desserts and baked foods. In fact, the individual who is allergic to eggs soon discovers that an egg-free diet limits his choice of foods considerably.

Legumes and nuts. Dried peas, beans, and soybeans are not widely used in the United States, but they are of major importance in many of the developing countries. Soybeans are used in the manufacture of textured vegetable proteins. These products may be used in combination with meat, or may be flavored and shaped to simulate beef, ham, chicken, or fish. These fabricated foods are important in many vegetarian diets.

Peanuts, which are also leguminous seeds, are popular not only as a snack food but also in peanut butter. This class of foods is an excellent source of protein, iron, and niacin.

Nutritive values of the meat group. Variations in the composition of meat from one cut to another and from one kind to another are due largely to the proportion of lean and fat tissue. The nutritive value

of meat as consumed depends on whether (1) fat was trimmed off before cooking, (2) fat in drippings was used, and (3) surrounding fat on meat was eaten.

Based upon extensive analyses of cooked meat, Leverton and Odell[4] have suggested the following values as a guide in dietary planning:

	Energy	Protein	Fat
	(per 100 gm cooked meat)		
	kcal	gm	gm
Extremely lean portion	200	32	8
Lean-plus-marble portions	255	28	16

The extremely lean portion contains no visible traces of fat. The lean-plus-marble portion represents meat as it is more usually consumed (choice grade).

Leverton and Odell also found that no one kind of cooked meat or of lean-plus-marble meat was significantly different from other kinds. Cooked pork was no higher in fat than similar portions of beef, veal, or lamb. For most dietary purposes, the four kinds of meat may be used interchangeably on a protein, fat, and caloric basis.

Protein. On a cooked basis, 30 gm (1 oz) lean meat, one egg, ½ cup cooked dried beans or peas, and 2 tablespoons peanut butter furnish about 7 gm protein.

The proteins of eggs are so well proportioned in their amino acid composition that whole egg is used as a reference standard for computing the quality of proteins in other foods. The white and yolk of the egg are about equal in protein content.

Regardless of the species, the amino acid composition of the proteins in flesh foods is relatively constant and of such balance and quality that meats, fish, and poultry rank only slightly below eggs and milk in their ability to effect tissue synthesis. The protein differences between so-called red and white meats are insignificant.

The proteins in legumes and nuts are of somewhat lesser quality because the amounts of methionine and lysine are below optimum levels. When legumes are eaten with other foods such as milk, cheese, or eggs, or in combination with cereal grains, these deficiencies are corrected.

Fats. The fatty acids in beef, veal, and lamb are more saturated than those in pork, poultry, and fish. When the diet of pigs and poultry is high in linoleic acid, the fat contains appreciable amounts of linoleic acid. Fatty acids in fish are more highly unsaturated, with a more generous proportion of the polyunsaturated fatty acids.

Most peas and beans are very low in fat. Peanuts and soybeans contain significant amounts of fat; indeed these legumes are extensively used for their oils.

Animal foods contribute substantially to the cholesterol intake. Egg yolk, liver, brains, and some shellfish are high in cholesterol content. The lean and fat portions of meat supply approximately equal concentrations of cholesterol. Legumes, nuts, and egg white contain no cholesterol.

Minerals. The mineral elements of special importance in the meat group are iron and zinc, all foods of this group being valuable. Light meats, including fish and light meat of poultry, are somewhat lower in iron content than the red muscle meats of beef. Meats are also rich in phosphorus, magnesium, sulfur, and potassium, moderately high in sodium, and poor in their calcium content. Some shellfish and canned salmon with the bones contain appreciable amounts of calcium. Saltwater fish is a good source of iodine.

Vitamins. All foods of the meat group are good sources of the B-complex vitamins. Pork, liver, and other organ meats and legumes are excellent for their thiamin content; poultry, veal, peas, and peanuts are rich in niacin. Vitamin B_{12} is supplied by organ meats, muscle meats, and eggs, but it is not found in the legumes.

Liver is an outstanding source of vitamin A; other organ meats and egg yolk are good sources of vitamin A. Otherwise, meats do not provide vitamin A, and they are not a source of ascorbic acid.

Extractives and purines. Various nonprotein nitrogenous substances, especially the purines, give meat its characteristic flavor. They are readily extracted from meat with water, as in the preparation of broth. They have very little nutritive value.

VEGETABLE-FRUIT GROUP

No group of foods lends greater variety to the diet in terms of color, flavor, and texture than does the vegetable-fruit group. This group includes practically every part of the plant—leaves, stems, roots, tubers, bulbs, flowers, and seeds. Mature seeds of the grasses are included in the cereal group, and those of leguminous plants such as peas and beans are included in the meat group.

In order to ensure optimum vitamin and mineral contributions, the daily recommendation of four servings from the vegetable-fruit group should be governed as follows:

1 serving citrus fruit or other source of vitamin C
1 serving at least every other day of dark-green or deep-yellow vegetables for vitamin A
2 servings other vegetables and fruits, including potatoes

A serving is equivalent to $\frac{1}{2}$ cup cooked vegetable or a whole piece of vegetable or fruit such as a banana, an apple, or medium-sized potato. Teenagers should have larger servings of each, and young children may have smaller-size servings.

Nutritive characteristics. This group is unique for its contribution to the ascorbic acid value of the diet; it is the major source of vitamin A value; it makes an excellent contribution to the iron level of the diet; and it is a fair source of other minerals and B-complex vitamins. The composition of vegetables and fruits covers a wide range depending upon the part of the plant represented. Moreover, the handling of the food from farm to table may be so variable that the amounts of vitamins and minerals retained may be high or low. The vitamin concentration is affected by the season, the degree of maturity, and the temperature and length of storage.

Water. As the chief constituent of fruits and vegetables water constitutes 75 to 95 per cent of the weight. Foods relatively high in carbohydrate such as bananas and potatoes are lower in water content than those which are low in carbohydrate such as tomatoes, lettuce, and melons.

Energy. As a group, these foods are not important contributors to the caloric value of the diet, although potatoes and sweet potatoes when eaten in quantity make an appreciable contribution. Many vegetables such as tomatoes, celery, asparagus, salad greens, and others furnish no more than 20 kcal per serving. Potatoes, Lima beans, fresh corn, and bananas, for example, are slightly below 100 kcal per serving unit. Other vegetables and fruits range from 40 to 80 kcal per average serving.

Protein and fat. The protein concentration of most fresh vegetables ranges from 1 to 2 per cent and is even lower in fruits. Fresh peas and Lima beans are slightly above these levels. All foods of this group are extremely low in fat with the exception of avocados and olives.

Carbohydrate. The carbohydrate composition of this group ranges widely, being as low as 3 to 5 per cent for rhubarb, greens, summer squash, tomatoes, and others, to more than 30 per cent for a few foods such as sweet potatoes. Dried fruits contain about 65 per cent carbohydrate.

The exchange lists (Table A–4) provide a convenient classification for fruits and vegetables according to carbohydrate content. Fruits (list 3) are listed in the amounts required to furnish 10 gm carbohydrate. Vegetables are placed in three groups. Most vegetables (list 2) contain about 5 gm carbohydrate per half cup serving. Some vegetables such as raw celery, endive, lettuce, and green peppers in the amounts ordinarily eaten do not contribute significant amounts of energy or carbohydrate. The so-called starchy vegetables including Lima beans, corn, peas, potatoes, pumpkin, winter squash, and sweet potatoes are comparable to a slice of bread in carbohydrate, protein, and energy value. (See list 4.)

Starches, dextrins, sucrose, fructose, glucose, and cellulose occur in vegetables and fruits. The starch content of immature fruits is converted to sugars during ripening. The skins, seeds, and fibers of fruits and vegetables contribute variety to the textures of the diet and are also of value in the maintenance of normal gastrointestinal motility. Some fruits are also rich in pectin.

Minerals. Turnip greens, mustard greens, collards, kale, and broccoli are excellent sources of calcium. The calcium of spinach, poke, dock, beet greens, chard, and lamb's quarters is not nutritionally available because the oxalic acid of those plants combines with calcium to form insoluble salts that are not absorbed. Some fruits contribute small amounts of calcium, but the daily contribution cannot be considered important.

The dark-green leafy vegetables are fair-to-good sources of iron. Likewise, fresh and dried apricots, raisins, prunes, dates, figs, peaches, and berries are good sources of iron.

Fruits and vegetables are rich sources of potassium, but the sodium content is negligible except for a few vegetables such as beets, carrots, spinach, celery, and chard.

Fruits and vegetables contribute to an alkaline ash. The acid or sour taste of some fruits, including citrus fruits, peaches, and others, is accounted for by several organic acids (citric, malic, tartaric) which are fully oxidized in the body. The mineral content of these fruits is such that they also yield an alkaline ash. Plums, prunes, rhubarb, and cranberries, on the other hand, contain benzoic acid, which cannot be utilized by the body; hence, they contribute to an acid reaction.

Vitamins. Among the best contributors to ascorbic acid are the citrus fruits, fresh strawberries, cantaloupe and honeydew melon, broccoli, kale, spinach, turnip greens, sweet green peppers, and cabbage. Potatoes and sweet potatoes contain lesser concentrations of this vitamin, but the amounts eaten daily by some people may appreciably add to the total intake. Dried fruits supply little vitamin C.

Dark-green leafy vegetables and deep-yellow vegetables and fruits are outstanding for their carotene content. The concentration of the vitamin is directly proportional to the depth of the color. Lightly colored foods such as lettuce, cabbage, and white peaches are poor sources of the vitamin, although the outer green leaves of lettuce may contain 30 times as much vitamin A as the inner pale leaves.

Vegetables and fruits are fair sources of the B-complex vitamins.

BREAD-CEREAL GROUP

Today in nearly every country of the world some cereal grain is regarded as "the staff of life." Man's discovery thousands of years ago that he could cultivate the land and grow grains meant that he no longer had to lead the nomadic life of the hunter. The word *cereal* is derived from Ceres, the ancient Roman goddess of agriculture and harvest. Numerous references in the Bible attest to the importance of cereals. For example, in Psalm 65:13 we read, "The pastures are clothed with flocks; the valleys also are covered with corn: they shout for joy; they also sing." In the Bible and other early literature *corn* referred to grains such as wheat, millet, and barley.

By reason of its availability, high yield per acre, low production cost, and excellent keeping qualities, grain is used more abundantly than any other food material. The bread-cereal group includes breads, breakfast cereals, flours and meals, rice, and pastas (macaroni, noodles, and spaghetti). Four servings or more of enriched or whole-grain cereal foods are recommended daily.

Rice is the chief dietary staple for half the world's population and constitutes as much as 80 per cent of the calories for most of Asia's peoples. Wheat ranks second to rice in worldwide use but is the principal cereal grain used in the United States and in some European countries. Corn is widely used in Central and South America. Millet, sorghum, rye, and barley are important in some parts of the world.

Nutritional value of cereal foods. The seed or kernel of the cereal grain (see Figure 13-3) is divided into three parts, the bran, germ, and endosperm. The aleurone layer just below the bran layer is sometimes identified as a fourth part. Although cereal grains vary somewhat in their composition, the average percentage composition of the whole grain is protein, 12; fat, 2; carbohydrate, 75; water, 10; minerals, especially phosphorus and iron, and the B-complex vitamins, especially thiamin, 1. The mineral and vitamin compositions of market forms of cereal foods vary widely depending upon whether they are whole grain, enriched, or unenriched. Cereal grains contribute importantly to every nutrient need except calcium, ascorbic acid, and vitamin A.

Energy. Cereal foods, it is well known, are the primary source of energy for most of the world's people. Many people infer from this fact that cereals per se are fattening, and so they omit this group of foods from their diets. By such omission they lose the many nutrient benefits provided by whole-grain and enriched products. The average serving of a cereal food—1 slice bread, or ½ cup cooked cereal,

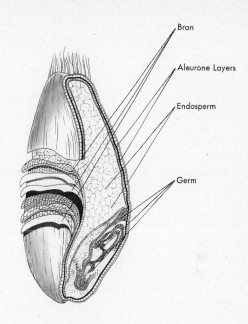

Figure 13-3. Whole wheat—cross section of grain. (Courtesy, the Ralston Purina Company.)

The Bran. The brown outer layers. This part contains:
1. Bulk-forming carbohydrates.
2. B vitamins.
3. Minerals, especially iron.

The Aleurone Layers. The layers located right under the bran. They are rich in:
1. Proteins.
2. Phosphorus, a mineral.

The Endosperm. The white center. This consists mainly of:
1. Carbohydrates (starches and sugars).
2. Protein.

This is the part used in highly refined white flours. Less refined flours and refined cereals are made from this part and varying amounts of the aleurone layer.

The Germ. The heart of wheat (embryo). It is this part that sprouts and makes a new plant when put into the ground. It contains:
1. Thiamin (vitamin B_1). Wheat germ is one of the best food sources of thiamin.
2. Protein. This protein is of value comparable to the proteins of meat, milk, and cheese.
3. Other B vitamins.
4. Fat and the fat-soluble vitamin E.
5. Minerals, especially iron.
6. Carbohydrates.

or 1 cup ready-to-eat cereal—furnishes from 75 to 100 kcal.

Protein. The protein of cereal grains is somewhat inferior to that of animal sources because some of the essential amino acids are present in less than needed amounts. Lysine is a limiting amino acid in wheat, rice, and corn, whereas tryptophan and threonine are present in too small amounts in corn and rice, respectively. The aleurone layer of the grain contains protein which is superior to that found in the endosperm, whereas that found in the germ compares favorably in biologic value with animal protein. Unfortunately, these better-quality proteins are removed when cereals are refined. However, when even small amounts of milk, cheese, eggs, or meat are fed simultaneously with cereal foods, either whole grain or refined, an economical protein intake of excellent biologic value results. Recent knowledge of the amino acid composition of foods is making it practicable to develop mixtures of cereals and other plant foods so that the protein approaches the quality of animal proteins.

Minerals and vitamins. The greater part of the minerals, iron and phosphorus, and of the B-complex vitamins occurs in the bran and germ of the grain. Consequently, most of these nutrients are lost when cereals are highly milled. Not only the American public, but people throughout the world, when given a choice, select white bread in preference to whole-grain breads. Whole-grain flours become rancid easily and are more subject to insect infestation if kept for any length of time so that a rapid turnover of this flour is essential. In view of these facts, it is of vast public health significance that refined cereals and breads be enriched (see page 277).

Cereal grains are poor sources of calcium. Breakfast cereals are ordinarily consumed with milk, and commercial breads commonly include certain calcium salts, which are yeast foods or dough conditioners, and calcium propionate, which is a mold inhibitor. The dough conditioners used in commercial breads furnish appreciable amounts of iodine.[5] Many commercial breads also contain 2 to 4 per cent nonfat dry milk resulting in further improvement of the calcium level as well as of the quality of the protein.

Nutritive efficiency of bread. The nutritive contribution of bread is illustrated in Figure 13–4. That bread is an important dietary constituent was convincingly demonstrated in a study reported by

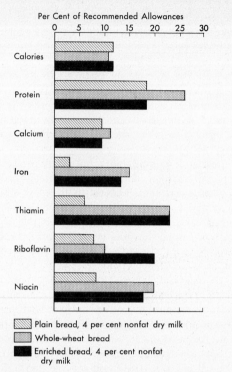

Figure 13–4. Percentage contribution of 4 slices (1/5 pound) of bread to Recommended Dietary Allowances for the woman of 23 to 50 years.

Widdowson and McCance.[6] These eminent British investigators observed the progress of 169 undernourished children, 4 to 15 years of age, for a year in a German orphanage at a time when food supplies were limited. The calories in the diets consumed by the children were distributed in these percentages: bread, 75; potatoes, 6; soups, vegetables, fruits, butter, margarine, 15; and milk, cheese, meat, fish, 4. Whole-wheat, enriched, and unenriched white breads were tested. The diets were not low in protein, but only 8 to 9 gm were derived from animal sources. Supplements of vitamins A, D, and C were included.

At the end of one year the children had made more rapid gains in height and weight than would be expected of normal children at the same age level; bone development was somewhat more rapid than normal; skin conditions had improved; and muscle tone had increased. The children were stated to be in excellent physical condition. No differences were observed in growth, development, or health with any of the breads tested, but the

B-vitamin reserves were somewhat better in those children who had eaten bread enriched to the whole-wheat levels. These results clearly demonstrated the nutritive efficiency of unusually large amounts of bread.

OTHER FOOD GROUPS

Fats and oils. Butter, margarine, hydrogenated fats, lard, and vegetable oils constitute the visible fats used in the diet. All the fats are concentrated sources of energy, but margarine and butter are the only fats that contain vitamin A. Margarine is fortified with 15,000 I.U. vitamin A per pound, thus equaling the year-round average for butter. Vegetable oils are good sources of vitamin E.

Butter, regular margarine, and hydrogenated fats contain higher proportions of saturated fatty acids than do the vegetable oils. Cottonseed, corn, soybean, sesame, and safflower oils are rich in linoleic acid, but olive and coconut oils are poor in this polyunsaturated acid.

Sugars and sweets. Cane and beet sugars comprise the primary source of sweets in America; corn sugar (glucose), corn syrup, molasses, honey, and maple syrup are other sweetenings of varying importance. Except for honey and maple syrup, they are relatively inexpensive sources of energy, but since they are almost 100 per cent carbohydrate they make no appreciable contribution to any other nutrient. Molasses is an exception in that it contains a fair concentration of iron; however, the quantities used in the average diet are too small to make this a contribution of significance.

Sugars and sweets are valued for the way in which they enhance the acceptability of some cooked fruits and their role in making possible the many desserts and baked goods we enjoy so much.

Beverages. Tea, coffee, and cocoa contain caffeine, theobromine, and theophylline, which are stimulants. Of these, caffeine is the most active stimulant and is also a mild diuretic. Coffee furnishes about 0.5 mg niacin per 200 ml beverage; tea, coffee, and cocoa contain about 15 to 20 mg magnesium and 45 to 65 mg potassium per cup of beverage. A cup of tea furnishes about 0.3 to 0.5 mg fluoride.

Alcoholic beverages furnish about 7 kcal per gram of alcohol metabolized. There are no nutrients supplied by distilled liquors. Although beer supplies some nutrients, one slice of bread furnishes more nutrients than a 12-ounce bottle of beer.[7]

A BASIC DIETARY PATTERN

Evaluation of the daily food guide. The Four Food Groups were described as a practical guide in Chapter 3, and were used in succeeding chapters to identify important sources of the nutrients. The calculations in Tables 13–2 and 13–3 summarize the nutritive values that may be expected when one selects the recommended amounts of food from each of the four groups. The calculations are average values for each food group, taking into consideration the per capita consumption of food in the United States. For example, the annual consumption of beef and pork is much higher than that for chicken and fish; hence, the values for the meat group are based upon a greater weighting for beef and pork.

The Four Food Groups were never intended to be a complete diet, but to serve as a foundation for dietary planning. It is evident from the calculations in Table 13–2 that the Basic Diet plan does not provide sufficient calories for men or women. The only serious nutrient shortcoming in this plan for the woman is iron, with the Basic Diet furnishing just over half of the recommended allowance. If a woman were to meet her full caloric needs with emphasis upon iron-rich foods, including liver, dried fruits, molasses, additional meat, and iron-fortified cereals, she might achieve the recommended allowance of 18 mg iron. If, however, fats and sugars make up most of the difference in calories, her diet will continue to be low in iron. (See Figure 13–5.)

For the man, the basic pattern is below recommended levels for thiamin and riboflavin. When a modest part of the additional calories is selected from the bread-cereal group and/or the meat group, these deficiencies are easily overcome. Although the niacin level appears to be low, it must be taken into account that the tryptophan available from the protein will yield an additional 12 mg niacin.

Other minerals and vitamins. Table 13–3 is a calculation of the Basic Diet for certain minerals and vitamins for which information at the present time is less complete and reliable. For some of these nutrients the Recommended Dietary Allowances

Table 13–2. Nutritive Value of a Basic Diet Pattern for the Adult in Health*

Food	Measure	Weight gm	Energy kcal	Protein gm	Fat gm	Carbohydrate gm	Minerals		Vitamins				
							Ca mg	Fe mg	A I.U.	Thiamin mg	Riboflavin mg	Niacin mg	Ascorbic Acid mg
Milk	2 cups	488	320	18	18	24	576	0.2	700	0.14	0.82	0.4	4
Meat Group													
Egg	1	50	80	6	6	tr	27	1.1	590	0.05	0.15	tr	0
Meat, fish, poultry (lean cooked)†	4 ounces	120	240	33	10	0	17	3.6	35	0.32	0.26	7.4	0
Vegetable-Fruit Group													
Leafy green or deep yellow	¼–⅓ cup‡	50	15	1	tr	3	14	0.5	3700	0.03	0.04	0.3	14
Other vegetable	¼–⅓ cups§	50	15	1	tr	3	10	0.4	240	0.03	0.03	0.3	7
Potato	1 medium	122	80	2	tr	18	7	0.6	tr	0.11	0.04	1.4	20
Citrus fruit‖	1 serving	100	40	1	tr	10	10	0.2	160	0.07	0.02	0.3	40
Other fruit#	1 serving	100	60	1	tr	16	12	0.5	600	0.04	0.04	0.4	9
Bread-Cereal Group													
Cereal, enriched or whole grain**	¾ cup	30 (dry)	105	3	tr	22	10	0.8	0	0.12	0.04	0.8	0
Bread, enriched or whole grain	3 slices	75	210	6	3	39	63	1.8	tr	0.18	0.15	1.8	tr
			1165	72	37	135	746	9.7	6025	1.09	1.59	13.1††	94
Recommended Dietary Allowances													
Woman (23–50 years)			2000	46				800	18	4000	1.0	1.2	13	45
Man (23–50 years)			2700	56				800	10	5000	1.4	1.6	18	45

*Values for foods in the meat, vegetable-fruit, and bread-cereal groups are weighted on the basis of the approximate consumption in the United States.

†Calculations based upon an average weekly intake for meat of 11 ounces beef, 7½ ounces pork, 6½ ounces poultry, 1½ ounces lamb and veal, and 1½ ounces fish.

‡Dark-green leafy and deep-yellow vegetables include carrots, green peppers, broccoli, spinach, endive, escarole, and kale. It is assumed that an average serving of ½ cup is eaten at least every other day.

§Other vegetables include tomatoes, lettuce, cabbage, snap beans, Lima beans, celery, peas, onions, corn, cucumbers, beets, and cauliflower. It is assumed that an average serving of ½ cup is eaten at least every other day.

‖Citrus fruit includes fresh, canned, and frozen oranges, orange juice, grapefruit, and grapefruit juice.

#Other fruit includes apples, peaches, pears, apricots, grapes, plums, prunes, berries, and bananas.

**Cereals include corn flakes, wheat flakes, macaroni, oatmeal, shredded wheat, and enriched rice.

††The protein in this diet contains about 720 mg trytophan, equivalent to 12 mg niacin; thus, the niacin equivalent of this diet is 25 mg.

Table 13-3. Additional Mineral and Vitamin Values for the Basic Diet Pattern*

Food	Measure	Weight gm	Minerals					Vitamins				
			Sodium† mg	Potassium mg	Phosphorus mg	Magnesium mg	Zinc gm	Vitamin E mg	Folacin mcg	Vitamin B$_6$ mcg	Vitamin B$_{12}$ mcg	Pantothenic Acid mcg
Milk	2 cups	488	240	691	446	62	1.9	0.19	5	192	1.9	1632
Meat Group												
Egg	1	50	61	65	103	6	0.5	0.23	3	55	1.0	800
Meat, fish, poultry (lean cooked)	4 ounces	120	79	471	319	33	5.4	0.26	9	589	1.6	839
Vegetable-Fruit Group												
Leafy green or deep yellow	1/4–1/3 cup	50	14	124	29	13	0.3	0.47	22	75	0	133
Other vegetable	1/4–1/3 cup	50	9	108	24	13	0.2	0.16	14	50	0	152
Potato	1 medium	122	2	348	51	14	0.3	0.05	9	212	0	320
Citrus fruit	1 serving	100	1	171	17	11	0.1	0.04	3	33	0	206
Other fruit	1 serving	100	2	204	18	13	0.2	0.22	5	100	0	174
Bread-Cereal Group												
Cereal, enriched or whole grain‡	3/4 cup	30 (dry)	1	60	51	21	0.5	0.22	15	39	0	166
Bread, enriched or whole grain‡	3 slices	75	15	135	121	38	0.8	0.21	17	78	0	446
			424	2377	1179	224	10.2	2.05	102	1423	4.5	4868
Recommended Dietary Allowances												
Woman (23–50 years)					800	300	15	12	400	2000	3.0	
Man (23–50 years)					800	350	15	15	400	2000	3.0	

*Values calculated on basis of same foods used for Table 13-2; see footnote descriptions. Table A-2 was used for the calculations. Values given are to be regarded as approximations because of limited availability of quantitative data.
† Sodium values are based upon foods processed and prepared without the addition of salt. As consumed in the ordinary diet, the sodium intake would range widely—about 2500 to 5000 mg.
‡ Average of whole-grain and enriched cereals.

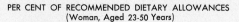

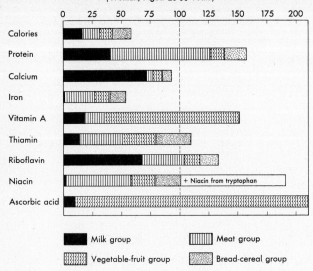

PER CENT OF RECOMMENDED DIETARY ALLOWANCES
(Woman, Aged 23-50 Years)

Figure 13-5. The Four Food Groups of the Basic Diet meet, or nearly meet, the recommended allowances for nutrients except calories and iron for the woman of 23 to 50 years. See Table 13-2 for calculations.

have only recently been set. The Food and Nutrition Board has pointed out that more research needs to be done upon which to base the allowances and that changes will be made as more information becomes available. It may be that some of the allowances have been set too high.

The tables of food composition for these nutrients are not as reliable as might be désired: (1) only a few analyses have been made for many of the foods; (2) methods used for analyses are not always in close agreement; for example, values for folacin will vary widely depending upon the forms of the vitamin that have been determined; (3) samples are not always fully described in the publications, and variations could occur because of raw or cooked forms; (4) wide variations exist from one sample to another, depending upon conditions of processing, storage, and cookery. Nevertheless, the calculations in Table 13-3 do give some information on the sources of these nutrients and the relative magnitude.

From Table 13-3 it becomes evident that the recommended servings of the Four Food Groups do not supply the daily allowances of magnesium, zinc, folacin, vitamin B_6, and vitamin E. If one observes the following guidelines, most of these deficiencies will be corrected.

1. To complete the caloric requirement select additional foods from the Four Food Groups. Include minimum amounts of sugars, sweets, and fats.

2. From day to day vary the choice of foods from each group, rather than depending upon a few favorite items. A variety of dark-green leafy vegetables are excellent sources of magnesium and folacin. Whole-grain breads and cereals are far superior to enriched white breads and cereals for magnesium, zinc, folacin, vitamin B_6, and vitamin E.

3. The Four Food Groups furnish very little vitamin E. Vegetable oils—corn, soybean, cottonseed, safflower—are excellent sources of vitamin E. One to two tablespoons of oil daily, used in cooking or in salad dressings, will furnish sufficient amounts of vitamin E.

ESSENTIALS OF MEAL PLANNING

In addition to meeting nutritive needs, successful meal planning depends upon many other factors which are summarized in Table 13-4. Food habits are discussed in further detail in Chapters 14 and 15, and food costs are considered more fully in Chapter 16.

Begin with a good breakfast. A large proportion of children as well as adults eat an inadequate breakfast or skip it altogether. Studies conducted by the Departments of Physiology and Nutrition at the

Table 13–4. Factors to Consider in Meal Planning

Essential Factors	Interpretation
Family composition	Adjust amounts for children, teen-agers, pregnant and lactating women. For persons with low energy requirements (women and elderly persons) select foods high in nutritive value
Food habits	Consider psychologic and cultural meanings of food. See Chapters 14 and 15 for full discussion
Food costs	Budgeting and food selection for economy are discussed in Chapter 16
Time for food preparation	Budget time for best use, by planning menus for several days; shopping once a week; planning for leftovers; using some convenience foods if homemaker is also employed outside the home
Variety in meals	*Four Food Groups:* establish menu pattern that includes recommended amounts of each group for each member of the family
	Variety of choice: vary the choice of foods within each group from day to day; do not use the same meats, vegetables, fruits every day
	Color: be sensitive to color combinations. Avoid meals that are all white, or all one color tone. Use garnishes for a touch of color; for example, paprika, pepper rings, radishes, parsley
	Texture: include some crisp and chewy foods with soft foods
	Flavor: combine bland foods with those that are more strongly flavored; do not use all spicy or all bland foods at one meal
	Preparation: use a variety of preparation methods; for example, boiling, roasting, baking, frying; with or without sauces; various combinations of foods
Season	Hearty foods such as stews and soups are favored in cold weather; lighter foods in hot weather, but including the same nutrients
Satiety	Provide some protein and fat in each meal to allay sense of hunger
Meal spacing	Arrange meal times so that family can be together whenever possible. Plan snacks to include nutrients for the day. Be discriminate in use of high-carbohydrate, high-calorie foods for snacks

State University of Iowa determined the effectiveness of various breakfast plans on physical and mental efficiency.[8] These studies showed that (1) efficiency in physiologic performance, as measured by bicycle ergometer, treadmill, and maximum grip strength, decreased in late morning hours when breakfast was omitted; (2) attitude toward school work and scholastic achievement was poorer when breakfast was omitted; (3) the content of the breakfast did not determine its efficiency so long as it was nutritionally adequate; (4) a breakfast providing one fourth of the daily caloric and protein allowances was superior to smaller or larger breakfasts for maintaining efficiency in the late morning hours; (5) a protein intake of 20 to 25 gm maintained the blood glucose level during the late morning hours; and (6) the omission of breakfast was of no value in weight reduction. In fact, those who omit breakfast while on a weight reduction regimen experience greater hunger in addition to being physiologically inefficient.

A change to better breakfast habits means (1)

planning simple, easy-to-prepare, but varied meals; (2) arising sufficiently early so that there is time for eating breakfast; (3) eating breakfast with the family group so that it, like other meals, has pleasant social associations.

Breakfast may include some protein food such as egg or milk, cereal or breadstuff, or both, and a beverage. Children and teen-agers should include milk for breakfast. If citrus fruit or another good source of ascorbic acid is included at breakfast, the day's allowance is assured. Cereal may be hot or cold; breads may vary from plain white enriched or whole grain to muffins, griddle cakes, waffles, or sweet rolls, as the occasion warrants. A breakfast may be light or heavy depending upon the individual's activity and preferences. (See Figure 13–6.)

Light Breakfast
Stewed prunes
Poached egg (1) on buttered toast
Coffee with cream and sugar
Milk for children

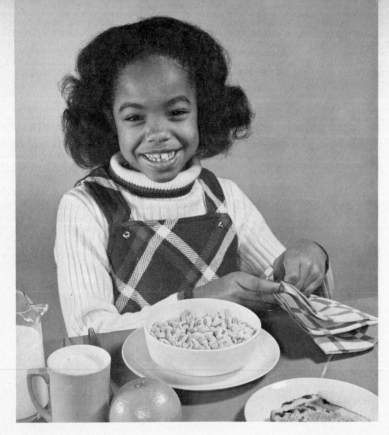

Figure 13-6. A good breakfast provides one fourth to one third of the recommended allowances. This easily prepared breakfast is appropriate for the schoolchild or adult. (Courtesy, Cereal Institute, Inc.)

HEAVY BREAKFAST
Cantaloupe
Griddle cakes with syrup
Sausages
Coffee with cream and sugar
Milk for children

Lunch is often neglected. Thousands of workers eat lunches in facilities that have a selection limited to sandwiches, pastries, and beverages. All too common a pattern is a sandwich, perhaps a piece of pie, and a glass of carbonated beverage or a cup of coffee. This pattern can be improved by including a salad and a glass of milk, or by carrying a piece of fruit from home. When the choice of food is restricted at lunch, the basic foods must be included in the morning and evening meals.

Through school food services lunches are made available to children and teen-agers in a large proportion of the nation's schools. These lunches are appetizing, nutritious, low in cost, and designed to improve the food habits. Many older Americans now receive a noon meal at centers for group feeding that provide one third of the recommended allowances.

Often the lunch eaten by homemakers and preschool children consists of a day-to-day monotony of sandwiches or leftovers because the homemaker does not take time for planning or adequate preparation. Such a practice sometimes leads to indiscriminate snacking throughout the day. Luncheons at home can be inexpensive, easy to prepare, tasty, and nutritionally adequate with a little foresight and planning. The following menus illustrate good luncheons or suppers that require a minimum of preparation time.

LUNCHEON OR SUPPER
Spanish omelet
Buttered green cabbage
Fresh fruit cup
Cookie
Milk

Salad bowl with mixed greens, diced ham, cheese, tomato
    wedges
French dressing
Whole-wheat muffin with butter and jelly
Pumpkin pie (leftover from dinner)
Milk

Dinner patterns. The evening meal is the only meal over which many homemakers have control. For many families it is the only time when all members are together. In many American homes this meal is much larger than the other two. To be sure, dinner must provide important nutrients that have not been included in breakfast or luncheon. However, an excessive intake of carbohydrate and calories at one time necessitates an additional load upon the normal metabolic mechanisms. Sometimes alternate pathways of metabolism are used which may favor the synthesis of adipose tissue and of cholesterol. (See Figure 5–5.)

Meat, fish, fowl, cheese, eggs, or legumes comprise the main dish at dinner. Potatoes or a starchy food and a green or yellow vegetable are generally included. If no salad has been provided in the luncheon, it should be served here. Dessert may consist of fruit, simple puddings, cake, ice cream, or pastries. Milk should be given to children. (See Figure 13–7.)

The meal pattern for dinner is the same for all members of the family, but adjustments in the size

of servings are made according to age, activity, and weight status.

Snacks. Most people eat two or three meals a day but also consume snacks and beverages between meals and in the evening. Active children often benefit by having a midmorning or midafternoon snack, provided that it is of such a nature that the appetite at mealtime is not lessened. Workers in industry, homemakers, students, young children— all experience a "lift" with a snack. Between-meal snacks, properly chosen, may actually aid some persons to maintain normal weight by reducing the tendency to overeat at mealtime.

Snacks should be planned as part of the total food intake for the day. Concentrated sweets or carbonated beverages contribute to the caloric intake but do not supply a corresponding proportion of needed nutrients. Fruits, fruit juices, milk, crackers and cheese, or a sandwich is a good snack of low to high caloric content. (See Figure 13–8.)

Meal patterns using the Four Food Groups. The basic diet pattern using the Four Food Groups is illustrated below:

Four Food Groups	Sample Menu Using Four Food Groups	Completed Menu with Typical Additions
BREAKFAST		
Citrus fruit	Orange juice	Orange juice
Cereal	Oatmeal	Oatmeal with milk and sugar
Bread—1 slice	Muffin	Muffin with margarine and jelly
Milk	Milk	Milk
		Coffee or tea for adults; cream and sugar
LUNCHEON		
Meat group—1 to 2 oz	Sandwich:	Sandwich:
Bread—2 slices	2 slices whole-wheat bread	Whole-wheat bread
	1 chopped egg	Chopped egg
		Celery
		Mayonnaise
Other vegetable	Lettuce and tomato	Lettuce and tomato
Other fruit	Fresh plums	Fresh plums
		Spice cupcake
Milk	Milk	Milk
DINNER		
Meat group—3 to 4 oz	Meat loaf	Meat loaf with gravy
Potato	Mashed potatoes	Mashed potatoes
Leafy green or deep-yellow vegetable	Carrots	Parsley carrots
Bread—1 slice	Dinner roll	Dinner roll
		Butter
		Lemon chiffon pie
		Coffee or tea
		Milk for children

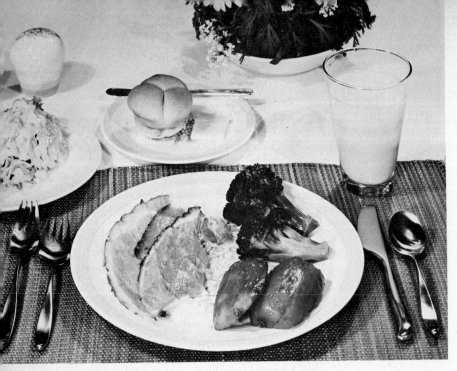

Figure 13-7. This colorful meal is rich in all nutrients and balances the day's meals. Dessert might be cake or pastry, but for those who need to watch their weight, fruits would be a better choice. (Courtesy, U.S. Department of Agriculture.)

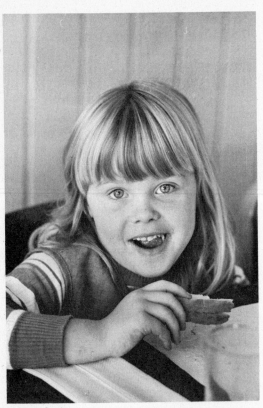

Figure 13-8. A snack such as a sandwich or milk and fruit are good choices for the active schoolchild. (Courtesy, U.S. Department of Agriculture.)

PROBLEMS AND REVIEW

1. *Problem.* Calculate the nutritive values for three foods that you eat regularly. Which of these foods provides the greatest nutritive value per 100 kcal?
2. *Problem.* Compare the nutritive values of 1 cup whole milk, 1 ounce Swiss cheese, 2 ounces cottage cheese, ⅛ quart ice cream, 1 ounce cream cheese. Use Table A–1.
3. *Problem.* Compare the nutritive values of 2 ounces lean roast beef, 2 ounces lean roast pork, 2 eggs, 4 tablespoons peanut butter, and 1 cup baked beans. Use Table A–1.
4. How does the protein quality of peanut butter and baked beans compare with that of meat?
5. *Problem.* Select a series of menus from a popular magazine. Check the menus against the Four Food Groups for dietary adequacy. Point out good examples of menu planning.
6. *Problem.* Plan breakfast and supper menus for three days for a woman who lives alone and who works in a department store. She is of normal weight and 47 years old. She eats a lunch consisting of soup, crackers, ice cream or pie, and coffee. She has a refrigerator at home, but only a two-burner hot plate on which to cook.
7. Plan a breakfast that includes foods from each of the Four Food Groups.
8. Why are each of the following combinations poor examples of meal planning? How could you change each combination to effect improvement?
   a. Meat loaf, mashed potatoes, mashed winter squash, baked custard
   b. Macaroni and cheese, roast beef, buttered spinach, cheese pie
   c. Broiled flounder, creamed onions, spicy cole slaw, pickles
9. Compare the nutritive value of a small bag (20 gm) potato chips with one apple. What conclusions can you draw regarding their value as snacks?

CITED REFERENCES

1. Friend, B., and Marston, R.: "Nutrition Review," *National Food Situation.* Economic Research Service, U.S. Department of Agriculture, Washington, D.C., November 1975.
2. Macy, I. G., *et al.: The Composition of Milks.* Pub. 254. National Academy of Sciences—National Research Council, Washington, D.C., 1953.
3. Brody, S., and Sadhu, D. P.: "The Nutritional Significance of Milk with Special Reference to Milk Sugar," *Sci. Month.,* **64:**5–13, 1947.
4. Leverton, R. M., and Odell, G. V.: *The Nutritive Value of Cooked Meat.* Misc. Pub. MP-49, Oklahoma Agricultural Experiment Station, Oklahoma State University, 1959.
5. Kidd, P. S., *et al.:* "Sources of Dietary Iodine," *J. Am. Diet. Assoc.,* **65:**420–22, 1974.
6. Widdowson, E. M., and McCance, R. A.: "Studies on the Nutritive Value of Bread and on the Effect of Variations in the Extraction Rate of Flour on the Growth of Undernourished Children," Her Majesty's Stationery Office, Privy Council, Medical Research Council Special Report Series No. 287, London, 1954.
7. Iber, F. L.: "In Alcoholism, the Liver Sets the Pace," *Nutr. Today,* **6:**2–9, Jan. 1971.
8. *Breakfast Source Book.* Cereal Institute, Chicago, 1959.

ADDITIONAL REFERENCES

Asprey, G. M., *et al.:* "Effect of Eating at Various Times on Free-Style Swimming Performance," *J. Am. Diet. Assoc.,* **47:**198–200, 1965.
Bauman, H. E.: "What Does the Consumer Know About Nutrition?" *J.A.M.A.,* **225:**61–62, 1973.
Hansen, R. G.: "An Index of Food Quality," *Nutr. Rev.,* **31:**1–7, 1973.
Henthorn, F. Y.: "Better Breakfasts," *Am. J. Nurs.,* **63:**98–100, Aug. 1966.
Ohlson, M. A., and Hart, B. P.: "Influence of Breakfasts on Total Day's Food Intake," *J. Am. Diet. Assoc.,* **47:**282–86, 1965.

Popkin, B. M., and Latham, M. C.: "The Limitations and Dangers of Commerciogenic Nutritious Foods," *Am. J. Clin. Nutr.*, **26**:1015–23, 1973.

Thornton, R., and Horvath, S. M.: "Blood Sugar Levels After Eating and After Omitting Breakfast," *J. Am. Diet. Assoc.*, **47**:474–77, 1965.

PUBLICATIONS FOR THE LAYMAN

Publications by the United States Department of Agriculture:
Beef and Veal in Family Meals, G 118.
Breads, Cakes, and Pies in Family Meals, G 186.
Cereals and Pastas in Family Meals, G 150.
Cheese in Family Meals, G 112.
Eat a Good Breakfast, Leaflet 268.
Eggs in Family Meals, G 103.
Family Fare: A Guide to Good Nutrition, G 1.
Food Guide for Older Folks, G 17.
Food for Families with School Children, G 13.
Food for Families with Young Children, G 5.
Food for the Young Couple, G 85.
Food for Us All. Yearbook of Agriculture 1969.
Fruits in Family Meals, G 125.
Lamb in Family Meals, G 124.
Milk in Family Meals, G 127.
Money Saving Main Dishes, G 43.
Nutrition: Food at Work for You, GS-1.
Nuts in Family Meals, G 176.
Pork in Family Meals, G 160.
Poultry in Family Meals, G 110.
Vegetables in Family Meals, G 105.

14 Factors Influencing Food Habits and Their Modification

Just as "you can lead a horse to water, but you can't make him drink," so the presentation of well-prepared, highly nutritious food to people does not mean that they will eat it. Food is a common denominator to all people throughout the world. Not only is it essential for their physiologic needs but it also fulfills social, psychologic, and emotional needs. Although food meets common needs for all people, food habits are infinitely complex, being derived from man's earliest experiences and being influenced by his family, as well as by the social, economic, geographic, ethnic, and religious environment. Thus, if one studies food habits one also learns much about the culture of a people. One cannot study the culture of any group of people without some understanding of the food habits.

To understand fully the factors that determine food acceptance requires the multidisciplinary approach of the anthropologist, physiologist, psychologist and psychiatrist, educator, social worker, and nutritionist. It is beyond the scope of a single chapter, such as this, to provide the depth of understanding of all factors influencing food acceptance. The objectives of the discussion that follows are (1) to create for the reader an awareness of the complexity of factors that determine food acceptance; (2) to provide some basis for understanding that the same food may have quite different meanings to different individuals; and (3) to develop attitudes of

respect and tolerance for individuals who may have food habits differing widely from those of others.

PHYSIOLOGIC BASES FOR FOOD ACCEPTANCE

Regulation of food intake. The theories for the regulation of food intake are based principally upon animal experiments, and involve these factors: regulation of the contractions and distention of the stomach, control of glucose levels in the blood, and regulation of body temperature, circulating amino acids, and the mass of adipose tissue. How these factors interact with each other is not fully understood.

Contractions of the stomach and a drop in blood sugar have long been associated with the sensation of hunger. Physiologic studies have established that the hypothalamus is the primary control center for the regulation of food intake. Two areas in the hypothalamus are often referred to as the "feeding" and the "satiety" centers. In experimental animals the bilateral destruction of the ventromedial nucleus leads to overeating and obesity. On the other hand, if an area lateral to the ventromedial nucleus is destroyed, eating stops and the animal will starve.

A model for a closed-loop system with a negative feedback has been described by Hamilton.[1] The nervous system carries information to the hypothalamus where comparisons are made with a "set point." For each of the factors that regulate food intake there is a set point. When there is a deviation from this point, forces come into play to correct the error.

Role of gastrointestinal tract. Walter B. Cannon and Anton Carlson, two famous physiologists early in this century, observed the relationship of the sensations of hunger to increases in contractions of the stomach, and the satiety effect of a filled stomach. There exists a neural link between the gastrointestinal tract and the hypothalamus. This link serves to inform the hypothalamus when the stomach is distended. Although this mechanism is useful to normal individuals, it should be remembered that persons who have had a gastrectomy still experience hunger and satiety, and that other controls must be in effect.

Glucostatic theory. One example of control is the regulation of the blood sugar. Insulin is secreted at a controlled rate when the glucose of the blood coursing through the pancreas is high. Conversely, other hormones such as glucagon, epinephrine, the glucocorticoids of the adrenal cortex, and the adrenocorticotropic and growth hormones of the pituitary can bring the glucose level back to its normal range when the blood concentration is too low. The maintenance of the blood sugar within physiologic limits obviously is a complex interaction involving the liver, pancreas, adrenal, and pituitary.

Mayer and his associates have shown that chemoreceptors in the ventromedial center of the hypothalamus have an affinity for glucose and are activated by it.[2] According to their GLUCOSTATIC THEORY, when glucose utilization is high, these receptors respond by acting as a brake upon the lateral nucleus (the feeding center) and also exercising some control over the hunger contractions of the stomach. When glucose utilization is low, these receptors are not stimulated and the sensation of hunger causes the individual to eat.

Theory of thermostatic control. According to Brobeck, food intake in certain conditions is part of the system of regulation of body temperature.[3] In the cold, food intake is increased and in hot environments intake is reduced. At an environmental temperature of 7° C rats consumed 126 kcal per day, but at 35° C they consumed only 18 kcal per day. If the rats were force-fed at the high temperature, they died of heat stroke. The area in the brain for this control is the preoptic anterior hypothalamus. When this area is destroyed in the rat, there is undereating in a cold environment and overeating in a hot environment.

Adipose tissue and food intake. All factors considered, it is quite remarkable that the body weight for most adults remains fairly constant. Another hypothesis regarding control of food intake asserts that the balance between energy intake and energy loss involves a regulation by body fat.[1] The theory is that some unknown metabolite related to the mass of adipose tissue is sensed by the central nervous system. In turn, the ventromedial hypothalamus in some way acts like a brake to prevent excessive weight gain. In one study rats that were fed excess calories by tube until they became obese consumed little food after tube feeding stopped. Their food intake returned to normal only after they had lost the extra body weight. In other words, the communication from the adipose tissue to the hypothalamus indicated a deviation from the body weight "set point," and correction of the increased body weight was brought about by reducing the food intake.

Sensations produced by food. The palatability of food is a composite of taste, smell, texture, and temperature. It is further conditioned by the surroundings in which food is consumed.

Sweet, sour, salty, and bitter are terms used to describe the sensations that result when foods placed in the mouth produce specific stimuli to the taste buds on the tongue. (See Figure 14–1.) The sense of taste is more highly developed in some individuals than in others; foods may be too salty for one individual and just right for another; or they may be too sweet for one, but not quite sweet enough for another. Some persons can detect slight differences in taste, others cannot. The number of taste buds varies not only from individual to individual, but also from age to age. Korslund and Eppright found that preschool children who had low taste sensitivities tended to accept more variety of foods than did those with high taste sensitivities.[4] As the taste buds diminish in number later in life, foods that are more highly flavored tend to be preferred, whereas children voluntarily select bland or sweet foods. Taste sensitivity is decreased in those who smoke tobacco.

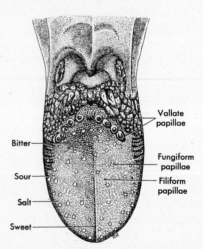

Figure 14–1. The upper surface of the tongue, showing kinds of papillae and areas of taste. (Courtesy, Miller, M. A., and Leavell, L. C.: *Kimber-Gray-Stackpole's Anatomy and Physiology,* 16th ed. Macmillan Publishing Co., Inc. New York, 1972.)

controlled rate when the glucose of the blood coursing through the pancreas is high. Conversely, other hormones such as glucagon, epinephrine, the glucocorticoids of the adrenal cortex, and the adrenocorticotropic and growth hormones of the pituitary can bring the glucose level back to its normal range when the blood concentration is too low. The maintenance of the blood sugar within physiologic limits obviously is a complex interaction involving the liver, pancreas, adrenal, and pituitary.

Mayer and his associates have shown that chemoreceptors in the ventromedial center of the hypothalamus have an affinity for glucose and are activated by it.[2] According to their GLUCOSTATIC THEORY, when glucose utilization is high, these receptors respond by acting as a brake upon the lateral nucleus (the feeding center) and also exercising some control over the hunger contractions of the stomach. When glucose utilization is low, these receptors are not stimulated and the sensation of hunger causes the individual to eat.

Theory of thermostatic control. According to Brobeck, food intake in certain conditions is part of the system of regulation of body temperature.[3] In the cold, food intake is increased and in hot environments intake is reduced. At an environmental temperature of 7° C rats consumed 126 kcal per day, but at 35° C they consumed only 18 kcal per day. If the rats were force-fed at the high temperature, they died of heat stroke. The area in the brain for this control is the preoptic anterior hypothalamus. When this area is destroyed in the rat, there is undereating in a cold environment and overeating in a hot environment.

Adipose tissue and food intake. All factors considered, it is quite remarkable that the body weight for most adults remains fairly constant. Another hypothesis regarding control of food intake asserts that the balance between energy intake and energy loss involves a regulation by body fat.[1] The theory is that some unknown metabolite related to the mass of adipose tissue is sensed by the central nervous system. In turn, the ventromedial hypothalamus in some way acts like a brake to prevent excessive weight gain. In one study rats that were fed excess calories by tube until they became obese consumed little food after tube feeding stopped. Their food intake returned to normal only after they had lost the extra body weight. In other words, the communication from the adipose tissue to the hypothalamus indicated a deviation from the body weight "set point," and correction of the increased body weight was brought about by reducing the food intake.

Sensations produced by food. The palatability of food is a composite of taste, smell, texture, and temperature. It is further conditioned by the surroundings in which food is consumed.

Sweet, sour, salty, and bitter are terms used to describe the sensations that result when foods placed in the mouth produce specific stimuli to the taste buds on the tongue. (See Figure 14–1.) The sense of taste is more highly developed in some individuals than in others; foods may be too salty for one individual and just right for another; or they may be too sweet for one, but not quite sweet enough for another. Some persons can detect slight differences in taste, others cannot. The number of taste buds varies not only from individual to individual, but also from age to age. Korslund and Eppright found that preschool children who had low taste sensitivities tended to accept more variety of foods than did those with high taste sensitivities.[4] As the taste buds diminish in number later in life, foods that are more highly flavored tend to be preferred, whereas children voluntarily select bland or sweet foods. Taste sensitivity is decreased in those who smoke tobacco.

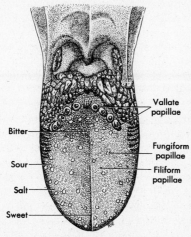

Bitter

Sour

Salt

Sweet

Vallate papillae

Fungiform papillae

Filiform papillae

Figure 14–1. The upper surface of the tongue, showing kinds of papillae and areas of taste. (Courtesy, Miller, M. A., and Leavell, L. C.: *Kimber-Gray-Stackpole's Anatomy and Physiology,* 16th ed. Macmillan Publishing Co., Inc. New York, 1972.)

PROBLEMS AND REVIEW

1. *Problem.* Calculate the nutritive values for three foods that you eat regularly. Which of these foods provides the greatest nutritive value per 100 kcal?
2. *Problem.* Compare the nutritive values of 1 cup whole milk, 1 ounce Swiss cheese, 2 ounces cottage cheese, ⅛ quart ice cream, 1 ounce cream cheese. Use Table A–1.
3. *Problem.* Compare the nutritive values of 2 ounces lean roast beef, 2 ounces lean roast pork, 2 eggs, 4 tablespoons peanut butter, and 1 cup baked beans. Use Table A–1.
4. How does the protein quality of peanut butter and baked beans compare with that of meat?
5. *Problem.* Select a series of menus from a popular magazine. Check the menus against the Four Food Groups for dietary adequacy. Point out good examples of menu planning.
6. *Problem.* Plan breakfast and supper menus for three days for a woman who lives alone and who works in a department store. She is of normal weight and 47 years old. She eats a lunch consisting of soup, crackers, ice cream or pie, and coffee. She has a refrigerator at home, but only a two-burner hot plate on which to cook.
7. Plan a breakfast that includes foods from each of the Four Food Groups.
8. Why are each of the following combinations poor examples of meal planning? How could you change each combination to effect improvement?
   a. Meat loaf, mashed potatoes, mashed winter squash, baked custard
   b. Macaroni and cheese, roast beef, buttered spinach, cheese pie
   c. Broiled flounder, creamed onions, spicy cole slaw, pickles
9. Compare the nutritive value of a small bag (20 gm) potato chips with one apple. What conclusions can you draw regarding their value as snacks?

CITED REFERENCES

1. Friend, B., and Marston, R.: "Nutrition Review," *National Food Situation.* Economic Research Service, U.S. Department of Agriculture, Washington, D.C., November 1975.
2. Macy, I. G., *et al.: The Composition of Milks.* Pub. 254. National Academy of Sciences—National Research Council, Washington, D.C., 1953.
3. Brody, S., and Sadhu, D. P.: "The Nutritional Significance of Milk with Special Reference to Milk Sugar," *Sci. Month.,* **64:**5–13, 1947.
4. Leverton, R. M., and Odell, G. V.: *The Nutritive Value of Cooked Meat.* Misc. Pub. MP-49, Oklahoma Agricultural Experiment Station, Oklahoma State University, 1959.
5. Kidd, P. S., *et al.:* "Sources of Dietary Iodine," *J. Am. Diet. Assoc.,* **65:**420–22, 1974.
6. Widdowson, E. M., and McCance, R. A.: "Studies on the Nutritive Value of Bread and on the Effect of Variations in the Extraction Rate of Flour on the Growth of Undernourished Children," Her Majesty's Stationery Office, Privy Council, Medical Research Council Special Report Series No. 287, London, 1954.
7. Iber, F. L.: "In Alcoholism, the Liver Sets the Pace," *Nutr. Today,* **6:**2–9, Jan. 1971.
8. *Breakfast Source Book.* Cereal Institute, Chicago, 1959.

ADDITIONAL REFERENCES

Asprey, G. M., *et al.:* "Effect of Eating at Various Times on Free-Style Swimming Performance," *J. Am. Diet. Assoc.,* **47:**198–200, 1965.
Bauman, H. E.: "What Does the Consumer Know About Nutrition?" *J.A.M.A.,* **225:**61–62, 1973.
Hansen, R. G.: "An Index of Food Quality," *Nutr. Rev.,* **31:**1–7, 1973.
Henthorn, F. Y.: "Better Breakfasts," *Am. J. Nurs.,* **63:**98–100, Aug. 1966.
Ohlson, M. A., and Hart, B. P.: "Influence of Breakfasts on Total Day's Food Intake," *J. Am. Diet. Assoc.,* **47:**282–86, 1965.

Popkin, B. M., and Latham, M. C.: "The Limitations and Dangers of Commerciogenic Nutritious Foods,"
    Am. J. Clin. Nutr., **26**:1015–23, 1973.
Thornton, R., and Horvath, S. M.: "Blood Sugar Levels After Eating and After Omitting Breakfast," *J. Am.
    Diet. Assoc.*, **47**:474–77, 1965.

PUBLICATIONS FOR THE LAYMAN

Publications by the United States Department of Agriculture:
Beef and Veal in Family Meals, G 118.
Breads, Cakes, and Pies in Family Meals, G 186.
Cereals and Pastas in Family Meals, G 150.
Cheese in Family Meals, G 112.
Eat a Good Breakfast, Leaflet 268.
Eggs in Family Meals, G 103.
Family Fare: A Guide to Good Nutrition, G 1.
Food Guide for Older Folks, G 17.
Food for Families with School Children, G 13.
Food for Families with Young Children, G 5.
Food for the Young Couple, G 85.
Food for Us All. Yearbook of Agriculture 1969.
Fruits in Family Meals, G 125.
Lamb in Family Meals, G 124.
Milk in Family Meals, G 127.
Money Saving Main Dishes, G 43.
Nutrition: Food at Work for You, GS-1.
Nuts in Family Meals, G 176.
Pork in Family Meals, G 160.
Poultry in Family Meals, G 110.
Vegetables in Family Meals, G 105.

14 Factors Influencing Food Habits and Their Modification

Just as "you can lead a horse to water, but you can't make him drink," so the presentation of well-prepared, highly nutritious food to people does not mean that they will eat it. Food is a common denominator to all people throughout the world. Not only is it essential for their physiologic needs but it also fulfills social, psychologic, and emotional needs. Although food meets common needs for all people, food habits are infinitely complex, being derived from man's earliest experiences and being influenced by his family, as well as by the social, economic, geographic, ethnic, and religious environment. Thus, if one studies food habits one also learns much about the culture of a people. One cannot study the culture of any group of people without some understanding of the food habits.

To understand fully the factors that determine food acceptance requires the multidisciplinary approach of the anthropologist, physiologist, psychologist and psychiatrist, educator, social worker, and nutritionist. It is beyond the scope of a single chapter, such as this, to provide the depth of understanding of all factors influencing food acceptance. The objectives of the discussion that follows are (1) to create for the reader an awareness of the complexity of factors that determine food acceptance; (2) to provide some basis for understanding that the same food may have quite different meanings to different individuals; and (3) to develop attitudes of respect and tolerance for individuals who may h[ave] food habits differing widely from those of oth[ers].

PHYSIOLOGIC BASES FOR FOOD ACCEPTANCE

Regulation of food intake. The theories for [the] regulation of food intake are based principally u[pon] animal experiments, and involve these factors: [reg]ulation of the contractions and distention of [the] stomach, control of glucose levels in the blood, [the] regulation of body temperature, circulating am[ino] acids, and the mass of adipose tissue. How t[hese] factors interact with each other is not fully un[der]stood.

Contractions of the stomach and a drop in b[lood] sugar have long been associated with the sensa[tion] of hunger. Physiologic studies have established [that] the hypothalamus is the primary control cente[r in] the regulation of food intake. Two areas in [the] hypothalamus are often referred to as the "feed[ing"] and the "satiety" centers. In experimental ani[mals] the bilateral destruction of the ventromedial [nu]cleus leads to overeating and obesity. On the o[ther] hand, if an area lateral to the ventromedial nu[cleus] is destroyed, eating stops and the animal will st[arve].

A model for a closed-loop system with a neg[ative] feedback has been described by Hamilton.[1] [The] nervous system carries information to the hypo[thal]amus where comparisons are made with a [set] point." For each of the factors that regulate [food] intake there is a set point. When there is a devi[ation] from this point, forces come into play to corre[ct the] error.

Role of gastrointestinal tract. Walter B. Ca[nnon] and Anton Carlson, two famous physiologists [early] in this century, observed the relationship o[f the] sensations of hunger to increases in contracti[on of] the stomach, and the satiety effect of a filled [stom]ach. There exists a neural link between the g[astro]intestinal tract and the hypothalamus. This [link] serves to inform the hypothalamus when [the] stomach is distended. Although this mechani[sm is] useful to normal individuals, it should be re[mem]bered that persons who have had a gastrec[tomy] still experience hunger and satiety, and that [other] controls must be in effect.

Glucostatic theory. One example of control [is the] regulation of the blood sugar. Insulin is secrete[d]

The taste and smell of foods are directly linked. If one were to hold the nose while eating a piece of fruit, much of the enjoyment would be lost. As a matter of fact, odor is the most important component of flavor, and an individual would derive limited pleasure from food if the tongue were the sole source of the sensations. The stimulation of the olfactory organs is brought about by certain volatile oils. Foods may be accepted because of their aromas, or they may be rejected because of their repulsive odors. No doubt, the odors of certain cheeses, for example, are the determinants in their acceptance by some and their rejection by others.

The sense of touch is highly developed in the tongue. Temperature, pain, and variations in texture or "feel" are experienced. Steaming hot foods are necessary to enjoyment by some, but children usually prefer foods that are lukewarm. A choice of ice cream may be influenced as much by its texture—smooth, creamy, and velvety, or crystalline and grainy—as by its other flavor qualities. Children may reject foods that are slippery such as baked custard or a gelatin dessert only later to learn to enjoy this texture sensation. The stringiness of certain vegetables, the stickiness of some mashed potatoes, the greasiness of fried foods may be important factors in rejection.

CULTURAL AND EMOTIONAL FACTORS INFLUENCING FOOD ACCEPTANCE

The studies on the physiologic and biochemical regulation described on pages 215–16 have been restricted principally to experimental animals. The principal control center is the hypothalamus. In humans the regulation of food intake is much more complex. For example, animals stop eating when satiated, but humans often continue to eat because they derive pleasure from the food. Social pressures, habits, prejudices, and the communications media are among the many factors that can obscure the hypothalamic mechanisms.[5]

Appetite and hunger. The words "appetite" and "hunger" are often used loosely. APPETITE is "a desire for food and drink."[*] There is often an appetite for specific foods. Appetite is related to pleasurable sensations associated with food intake.

HUNGER is a "compelling need or desire for food; the painful sensation or state of weakness caused by need of food."[*] With continued deprivation one passes from appetite to hunger.

Starving people will usually, but not always, accept anything edible that will fill the stomach. This might even be that which would normally be quite repellent. It is also true that people refuse food for the relief of acute hunger when religious or cultural taboos are strongly entrenched.

Man does not choose by instinct that which is best for him. In different environments, he eats what is available and sometimes learns through experience that some foods may be better for him than others. This method of trial and error, at best, is time consuming and may, in the meantime, jeopardize one's state of health. It could also lead to gross misconceptions concerning foods. Quite obviously the scientific planning of diets, rather than guidance by hunger and instinct, is the only sound basis for being sure that physiologic needs are being met.

Role of culture. Montagu,[6] Lee,[7] and many other writers have pointed out that the circumstances under which one eats are largely determined by one's culture. Used in this sense, CULTURE is "the sum total of ways of living built up by a group of human beings and transmitted from one generation to another."[*] Food habits may have existed among a given ethnic group for centuries, and such a heritage accounts for great conservatism in accepting change. These patterns reflect the social organization of the people, including their economy, religion, beliefs about the health properties of food, and attitudes toward the various members of the family. The emotional reactions to the consumption of certain foods may be so deeply rooted that effecting acceptance of them is almost impossible.

Food taboos and folklore. In every group of people customs have arisen concerning foods that should and should not be eaten. Although there is little or no scientific basis for these taboos, they are rigidly held so that change is likely to be resisted. Among people in the developing nations these taboos often accentuate malnutrition. For example, in one ethnic group in Nigeria children are rarely given meat or eggs. These are expensive foods, and it is thought that giving them to children will en-

[*] *The Random House Dictionary of the English Language,* unabridged edition, Random House, New York, 1966.

[*] *Ibid.*

courage them to steal. Coconut milk is taboo for children since it is believed to make them unintelligent. Similar taboos prevail for the pregnant woman. She should not eat snails so that her baby will not salivate too much. She should not eat pounded yams because the pounding is likely to have an effect on the child's brain. On the other hand, the pregnant woman is encouraged to eat food leftover by rats since this will help ensure an easy delivery such as rats are supposed to have![8]

An example of folklore is that held by many Chinese, especially those who are older.[9] These beliefs have their origin in Eastern philosophy, which holds that the universe is regulated by two opposing components, *yin* and *yang*. To maintain health these forces must be in balance. When illness is caused by an excess of yang, "cold" or yin foods should be used, and vice versa. Among the yin or "cold" foods are winter melon, white turnips, and bean sprouts; yang or "hot" foods include scrambled eggs and ginger root. The Zen macrobiotic diet is derived from this earlier folklore. (See page 56.)

The family. No influence upon food habits is greater than that existing within the home. The mother especially sets the pattern for the food habits that will be developed by the children, for she is the one who plans the meals, purchases the food, prepares it, and serves it. Her values have been developed in the environment in which she grew up and they are based upon income, geographic region from which she came, level of education, superstitions, and taboos.

The mother who creates within the home an atmosphere of security and contentment reinforces the positive values of food. On the other hand, in an environment of hostility, anger, and tension unpleasant images are created for food, often leading to their rejection. In this atmosphere, also, there may be excessive concern about "pure" foods, "pure" morals, and so on.[10]

Lewin in 1943 referred to the mother as one of the "gatekeepers" who controls the food that reaches the table.[11] In many families this role is diminishing because so many meals are eaten away from home, for example, school lunches, business lunches, and frequently dinner for business or pleasure. Schoolchildren also have money to purchase snacks or full meals away from home.

Meal patterns. Nutritional planning is usually based on a three-meal pattern. Although many people in the United States eat three meals a day, others eat only two, and still others four or five. The coffee break is prevalent in business and industry. This includes coffee, or coffee and doughnuts, pastry, or cookies, and is, for many, a replacement of breakfast. Midafternoon and evening snacks are commonplace.

Breakfasts tend to be light and informal. Family members often eat this meal at different times depending upon the time they must leave for work or school. Such a casual arrangement does not always provide the share of essential nutrients, nor is there the enjoyment that should be experienced at mealtime. In rural areas breakfast is still a substantial meal. Elderly people often enjoy breakfast more than other meals.

A good deal of ritual is part of the mealtime in some homes. Bread becomes the "staff of life" to some people; rice is the basic food for others, and corn to still others. (See Figure 14–2.) The meal would not be complete if these foods were not included. The art of food preparation is exercised, and food is highly valued for its many properties. Meals are to be enjoyed and relaxation is encouraged. A siesta following meals is customary in some countries. In other homes, mealtime is hurried. It may become the time when members of the family air their problems and when tensions are created.

Communications. The influence of the mass media on food habits can scarcely be overestimated. Those who enjoy an abundant variety of food can no longer be ignorant of the malnutrition and hunger that exist even in the United States as well as in the underdeveloped nations of the world. By these media the poor are also exposed to food products which they are unable to purchase. The affluent and the poor alike know that the distribution of food is decidedly uneven, and that the capability exists to feed all people better.[12]

Manufacturers usually create desires for their products by appealing to the emotions. Foods are pictured in forms highly appealing to the eye and in situations that suggest fun, social status, and group acceptance. Foods will consequently be purchased to fulfill these emotional needs rather than for their nutritional content.

Political-economic significance. Large food programs exist in the United States and throughout the world to help the poor meet their nutritional needs.

Such programs are important in determining agricultural policies and food prices, on the one hand, and impose regulations for participation by the poor, on the other hand. Each of these important groups influences legislation and has an effect on international diplomacy.

During a war food supplies may be rationed and people are forced to substitute one food for another. The scarcity of a given food sometimes creates a tremendous pressure to possess that food. The collapse of a government may indeed be brought about by its failure to provide food for its people.

Throughout history people have gone on "hunger strikes" to achieve some political goal. Gandhi, the great Indian leader, comes to mind for his many fasts. Not many years ago, some people who protested the involvement of the United States in the Vietnam war fasted for brief or long periods of time.

Food movements. Millions of Americans today have adopted eating patterns that differ widely from those of their childhood and that are at variance with so-called typical American diets. Among these groups are (1) those who are vegetarians for ecologic, philosophic, or religious reasons (see also pages 225–27); (2) those who oppose the use of any additives in foods or the use of chemical fertilizers, and who consume only "natural" or "organic" foods (see also pages 266–67); and (3) those who subscribe to the healthful properties of some foods and who proscribe other foods. These groups are often referred to as "faddists" but their adherence to the particular belief is no passing fancy. It is not always possible to change these beliefs, but the counselor for nutrition should recognize what is good in the individual's diet and should attempt to improve the diet within the framework of the beliefs.

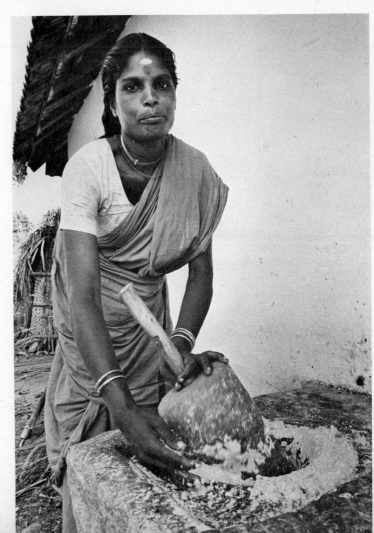

Figure 14–2. Indian homemaker preparing chappatties. In those parts of India where wheat is the staple grain, this unleavened bread forms an important part of the meal. The dough is baked in thin cakes. (Courtesy, The Rockefeller Foundation.)

Social values of food. "To break bread" together has been from time immemorial an act of friendship. One provides food for friends during a visit in the home; one likewise extends friendship to the stranger by inviting him to share food. The food served to guests is the best that one can afford and the table appointments are as beautiful as one can make them. Important family events are joyously celebrated with meals: the wedding breakfast or reception; birthday parties; Christmas dinner; a Fourth of July picnic. To eat together, whatever the occasion, is to provide friendly relaxation and conversation. The loneliness of eating by oneself, day after day, is not appreciated by those who have never tried it. (See Figure 14–3.)

Eating together also has connotations of status. Throughout history one's place at the table has been governed by his social standing. To be placed "above the salt" at a medieval banquet, to sit at the "head" table at a banquet today, and to be invited to eat at the captain's table while on board ship are marks of social distinction. In some societies women are considered to be inferior to men and must wait to eat until the men and boys have finished the meal. In other authoritarian situations, children may not be permitted to eat until the father has had his meal; in such a society, the father is always served the choicest foods. Many bonds of business or of politics are cemented at businessmen's luncheons or political dinners.

Prestige, it would appear, is ensured when one serves foods that are costly, difficult to obtain, distinctive in flavor, or time consuming in preparation. Caviar, lobster, filet mignon, champagne, flaming crepes suzette are examples of such prestige foods. In the nineteenth century, the purchase of white sugar and white flour conveyed the idea that one could afford to buy that which was refined and

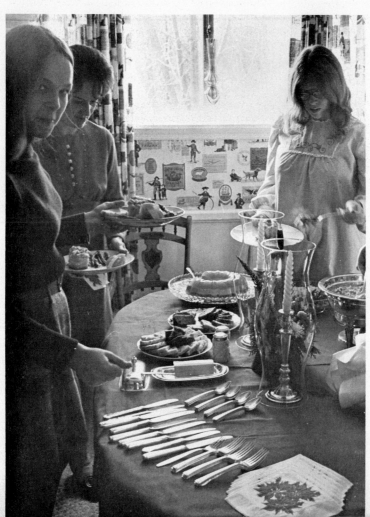

Figure 14–3. Holidays and anniversaries are occasions when specially prepared foods are enjoyed by relatives, friends, and coworkers. (Courtesy, University of Delaware, Newark.)

therefore "better." Is the purchase today of the more costly breads prepared from hand-ground flours an expression of status with respect to one's supposed knowledge of nutrition, or to one's ability to buy or bake that bread which is distinctive from the more commonly available loaf?

Children too are highly influenced by the foods that are popular with their peer groups. Sometimes they come to scorn certain foods that they have liked because they are different from the prevailing pattern of other children. On the other hand, they are also susceptible to the suggestions of their teachers and classmates and learn to like foods with which they have not been familiar in their homes.

Some foods are looked down upon by many people as lacking status; thus a delicious stew, or ground meat, or fish—no matter how good they may be—are considered by some to be food for the poor. However, these attitudes also are subject to change. Tourists to seacoast cities now seek out restaurants that specialize in seafoods and may be willing to spend considerable amounts of money for a specialty.

Some people delight in being epicures or gourmets. They derive a certain satisfaction from adventurous eating of food which is unusual, or which might be, in fact, unacceptable to most people—rattlesnake meat, for example. Others make a specialty of dining at unusual or expensive restaurants, or in becoming known for their ability to prepare complex, unusual dishes.

Religious and moral values attributed to foods. Almost all religions place some regulations on the use of foods. The association of a food with religion gives some clue to its importance in daily living. In the Middle East, bread becomes a symbol in the religious ceremonies of the people; to the Indians of Mexico, corn, the staple food, is invested with religious significance. Christians use bread and wine as symbols of Christ's body and blood in the Eucharist (Lord's Supper or Holy Communion). Religious significance is attached to a number of foods by the Jewish people. (See page 227.)

Certain foods are forbidden by religious regulation. Pork is forbidden to the Orthodox Jews and to the Islamites. Strict Hindus and Buddhists are vegetarians; they will eat no flesh of any animal, and many of them also abstain from eggs and milk. Seventh Day Adventists are lactovegetarians; that is, they will eat milk, cheese, eggs, nuts, and legumes but they eat no flesh foods. (See also Chapter 15.)

Fasting is common to most, if not all, religions. On fast days one food may be substituted for another or foods may be abstained from altogether. A substitute food, such as fish for meat, is likely to be associated with denying oneself, and so when one wishes enjoyment, he doesn't choose to eat fish!

Moral attributes—"good" and "bad"—are often ascribed to foods. A child may be told to eat liver even if he does not like it because it is "good" for him; he may also be told not to eat candy, which he does like, because it is "bad" for him. Or he might be told that he may have candy if he eats some liver!

Food is often used as a reward, punishment, or means of bribery. Thus, if a child has behaved well he is often rewarded with a prized food—candy, ice cream, cake; but if he has behaved badly he may be punished by being deprived of a food such as dessert. Adults, too, may reward themselves after a strenuous day or a trying experience by eating a special food or an expensive meal, often saying as they do so, "I certainly earned this today!" The family may feel a sense of reward, as well as the expression of a mother's love, when they sit down to a meal of their favorite foods; they may feel punished and unloved when the meal includes foods they dislike.

Age and sex influence food choices. Too often foods are categorized as being suitable for a given age group, or as more suitable for one sex than the other. Peanut butter, jelly, and milk are looked upon as foods for children, but olives and coffee are appropriate for adults! Teen-agers adopt current fashions in foods—hot dogs, hamburger, pizza, ice cream with many sauces and toppings. (See Figure 14-4.) Women are said to prefer light foods such as soufflés, salads, fruits, and vegetables, whereas filling meals such as meat, potatoes, and pie represent the more usual choice of men.

Emotional outlets provided by food. Eating provides gratification for life stresses—the difficult examination in school; the homely adolescent who has no date to take her to the movies; the quarrel with a friend; the frustration and loneliness of having no friends; the profound grief at the death of a dear one; and countless others.

Food is a symbol of security to many. Milk, the

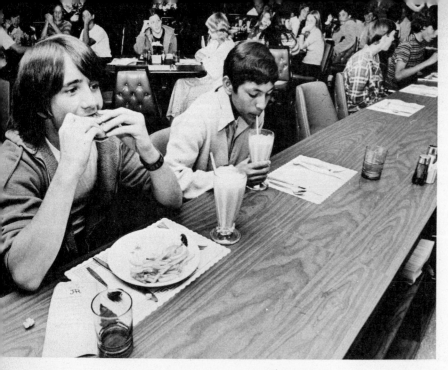

Figure 14–4. Hamburger on bun, French fries, and a milk shake are popular foods for teen-agers. They provide substantial amounts of energy and many nutrients. A salad such as coleslaw or a piece of fruit would furnish missing nutrients such as ascorbic acid. (Courtesy, U.S. Department of Agriculture.)

first food of the infant, is associated with the security of the infant held lovingly in his mother's arms. A person away from home, or ill, looks upon milk as expressing the comfort and security of the home; or, milk might be refused because the individual drinking it experiences a feeling of dependence which he does not want to admit, and so he says he does not "want to be treated like a baby."

Food may be used as a weapon. An insecure child refuses to eat food so that his mother will be concerned about him. The ill and the lonely impose dietary demands upon those caring for them in an effort to gain as much attention as possible.

Illness modifies food acceptance. Disease processes and drug therapy often modify the appetite. The anxiety of illness, the loneliness experienced if one eats from a tray alone, the lack of activity, and perhaps a modified diet are likely to interfere with food intake. (See also Chapter 25.)

REVIEW

1. How do you feel about food? List insofar as you are able the meanings which you clearly associate with foods. List the foods you especially like; those you especially dislike. Can you give any specific reason for placing the food in one category or another?
2. Note for one day the comments made by people around you about food. Do any of these fall within the physiologic or psychologic categories discussed in this chapter? Do they give you any clue concerning readiness to change food habits?
3. Suppose you were trying to introduce nonfat dry milk to a group of people who were entirely unfamiliar with it. How would you go about gaining their acceptance?
4. What is the difference between hunger and appetite?
5. Describe the physical factors in food acceptance.

CITED REFERENCES

1. Hamilton, C. L.: "Physiologic Control of Food Intake," *J. Am. Diet. Assoc.*, **62:**35–40, 1973.
2. Mayer, J.: "Why People Get Hungry," *Nutr. Today*, **1:**2–8, June 1966.

sufficient nitrogen. Diets that omit either legumes or grains can seriously deplete the protein reserves. Pure vegetarian diets for infants, children, and pregnant women can be dangerously deficient unless fortified soy milk is used. Young children do not always utilize legumes as well as adults.

Minerals. The omission of milk means that the calcium intake is often inadequate. Although large amounts of dark-green vegetables can furnish appreciable amounts of calcium, the daily ingestion in sufficient amounts is not likely. Soy milk fortified with calcium should be used to improve the calcium intake.

Vitamins. Vitamin B_{12} deficiency is characteristic of all pure vegetarian diets since vitamin B_{12} is found only in animal foods. The signs of deficiency are not likely to show up until several years of use of the diet, and then correction is often too late. Fortified cereals could correct this problem, but some Vegans refuse to use any fortified foods.

Vitamin D deficiency is likely unless there is ample exposure to sunshine since the diets do not include fortified milk. The Vegans usually refuse to use vitamin-D-rich fish oils.

Ordinarily, most of the riboflavin in diets is obtained from milk and meat. An abundance of green leafy vegetables, legumes, and whole-grain or enriched cereals will probably meet the need.

Typical Food Choices

By selecting a wide variety of foods from the following groups, nutritional adequacy can be achieved.

Milk Group

All milk and milk products for lactovegetarian diets; 2 cups or more for adults; 3 to 4 cups for children. Milk should be encouraged for infants, children, and pregnant women in pure vegetarian groups, but soy milk can be substituted.

Protein Group

Choose from dried beans: black, broad, kidney, Lima, mung, navy, pea, soy, white; dried peas: blackeye, chick, split; lentils; nuts: black walnut, Brazil, cashew, peanut, peanut butter, pistachio; seeds: sesame, sunflower; meat analogs, especially those processed to be nutritional replacement for meat. Combine legumes with nuts or cereal foods in the same meal.

Vegetable-Fruit Group

Generous use of vitamin A- and calcium-rich greens: collards, dandelion, kale, mustard, turnip; also broccoli, okra, rutabaga.

Citrus fruit daily or other good source of ascorbic acid.

Bread-Cereal Group

Preferably whole-grain breads and cereals: barley, buckwheat, bulgur, cornmeal, millet, oatmeal, rice, rye, wheat.

Supplements

Vitamin B_{12} for pure vegetarian diets; possibly vitamin D, calcium, and iodine.

Orthodox Jewish Food Habits

Outstanding characteristics. The description of the dietary pattern of the Jewish people presented here is based, in large part, on an article by Kaufman.[8] Orthodox Jews observe dietary laws based on Biblical and rabbinical regulations (the rules of Kashruth). These laws pertain to the selection, preparation, and service of food. Conservative Jews nominally observe the laws but make distinctions within and without the home, while Reform Jews minimize the significance of dietary laws. Food habits of the Jewish people are also influenced by the country of origin—for example, Russia, Poland, or Germany.

Milk and its products are never eaten in the same meal as meat. Usually two meals contain dairy products and one meal contains meat and its products.

Religious festivals include certain food restrictions. No food is cooked or heated on the Sabbath. Yom Kippur (Day of Atonement) is a 24-hour period of fasting from food and drink. The Passover, sometimes also referred to as "The Feast of Unleavened Bread," lasts for eight days and commemorates the release of the Israelites from the slavery of Egypt. During this period only unleavened bread is used (Exod. 12:15–20; 13:3–10; 23:15). Only utensils and dishes that have made no contact with leavened foods are used during this time. Thus, the Orthodox Jewish home would have four sets of dishes: one for meat and one for dairy meals during the Passover, and one for meat and one for dairy meals during the rest of the year when leavened breads and cakes may be used.

The Passover begins with the Seder when everyone sits down to a beautifully set table. On a platter are foods that commemorate the Exodus from Egypt: matzoth, the unleavened bread the Jews ate when they left Egypt; a bone as a reminder of the sacrifice of the lamb by the Jews; bitter herbs for the

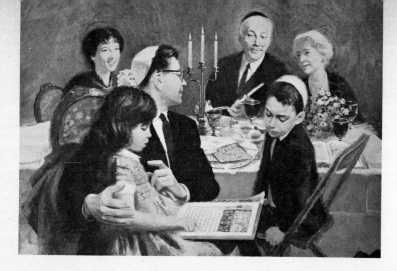

Figure 15–1. Jewish family at a Seder table. (Courtesy, the B. Manischewitz Company.)

bitterness of slavery; and *harosseth*, a mixture of apples, nuts, cinnamon, and wine to look like the clay of which the Jews made bricks in Egypt. (See Figure 15–1.)

The diet is generally rich in pastries, cake, many preserves, and relishes. Breads, cereals, legumes, fish, and dairy products are used abundantly. Encouragement should be given to the inclusion of more fruits and vegetables.

TYPICAL FOODS AND THEIR USES

Milk Group

Milk, cottage and cream cheese, sour cream used abundantly. Milk and its products may not be used at same meal as meat (Exod. 23:19; 34:26; Deut. 14:21). Milk may not be taken until six hours after eating meat. Separate dishes and utensils must be used for milk and meat dishes.

Meat Group

ALLOWED FOODS

All quadruped animals that chew the cud and divide the hoof (Lev. 11:1–3; Deut. 14:3–8): cattle, deer, goats, sheep. Organs of these animals may be used.

Animals must be killed in prescribed manner for minimum pain to animal, and for maximum blood drainage. Blood is associated with life and may not be eaten (Gen. 9:4; Lev. 3:17; 17:10–14; Deut. 12:23–27). Meat is made *kosher* (clean) by soaking it in cold water, thoroughly salting it, allowing it to drain for an hour, and then washing it in three waters.

Hindquarters of meat may be used only if the part of the thigh with the sinew of Jacob is removed (Gen. 32:33).

Poultry: chicken, duck, goose, pheasant, turkey. Chicken is common for Sabbath eve meal.

Fish with fins and scales (Lev. 11:9; Deut. 14:9–10): cod, haddock, halibut, salmon, trout, tuna, whitefish, etc.

Eggs. Fish and eggs may be eaten at both meat and milk meals.

Dried beans, peas, lentils, in many soups.

Corned beef, smoked meats, herring, *lox* (smoked, salted salmon) are well liked.

Cholent: casserole of beef, potatoes, and dried beans. Served on the Sabbath.

Gefillte fish: chopped, highly seasoned fish; a first course for the Sabbath meal.

Kishke: beef casings stuffed with rich filling and roasted.

Knishes: pastry filled with ground meat.

Kreplach: noodle dough filled with ground meat or cheese filling.

PROHIBITED FOODS

Animals which do not chew the cud or divide the hoof (Lev. 11:4–8): pork.

Diseased animals or animals dying a natural death (Deut. 14:21).

Birds of prey (Lev. 11:13–19; Deut. 14:11–18).

Fish without fins or scales (Lev. 11:10–12): eels, shellfish such as oysters, crab, lobster.

Egg with blood spot.

Vegetable-Fruit Group

All kinds used without restriction.

Cucumber, lettuce, tomato very frequently used.

Cabbage, potatoes, and root vegetables are often cooked with the meat.

Borsch: soup with meat stock and egg, or without meat stock and with sour cream; includes beets, spinach, cabbage.

Dried fruits are used in many pastries.

Bread-Cereals Group

All kinds used without restriction. Rye bread (pumpernickel), white seed rolls; noodles and other egg and flour mixtures.

Bagel: doughnut-shaped hard yeast roll.

Blintzes: thin rolled pancakes filled with cottage cheese, ground beef, or fruit mixture; served with sour cream.

Bulke: light yeast roll.

Challah: braided loaf or light white bread.

Farfel: noodle dough grated for soup.

Kasha: buckwheat groats served as cooked cereal or as potato substitute.

Kloese: dumplings, usually in chicken soup.

Latkes: pancakes.

Matzoth: flat, unleavened bread.

Other Foods

Unsalted butter preferred.

Chicken fat or vegetable oils for cooking.

Rich pastries are common.

Cheese cake.

Kuchen: coffee cake of many varieties.

Leckach: honey cake for Rosh Hashana (New Year).

Strudel: thin pastry with fruit, nut filling.

Teiglach: small pieces of dough cooked in honey, with nuts.

Sponge cake and macaroons at Passover.

Many preserves, pickled cucumbers, pickled green tomatoes, relishes.

Many foods are highly salted.

BLACK AMERICAN FOOD PATTERNS

Outstanding characteristics. The meals eaten by poor black and white people in southeastern United States were generally similar. For most black Americans in the South poverty was more extreme, and the diet was more restricted. They had small gardens if any at all, and canned less food.

"Soul food" is a term recently used to denote foods of the black culture, especially those foods that prevailed in the South. Many of these foods originated in pre-Civil War days. When black Americans migrate from the South to northern cities, they at first retain most of their favored southern dishes. In time they use more and more foods typical of the area in which they live, but usually retain some of their favorite dishes.

As the income improves, black Americans spend increasing amounts of money for meat. Too little money is spent for vegetables, fruits, and milk.[9] Although lactose tolerance is poor in many adults, most children can drink sufficient milk to meet their calcium needs without untoward symptoms.[10] Diets of many black Americans furnish too much pork fat, sweets, and starches, and too little green salads, milk, and eggs.

The traditional breakfast in the South consisted of fried meat, rice, grits, biscuits, gravy, fried sweet or Irish potatoes, coffee, or milk. In the North a more typical breakfast consists of eggs, bacon or sausage with eggs, biscuits (sometimes hot), and coffee.[9]

The traditional boiled dinner in the South was eaten in the early afternoon and consisted of a main dish such as boiled vegetables or legumes seasoned with meat, sweet or Irish potato, cornbread, sweet beverage or milk, and occasionally fruit. Enough food was prepared to be used also at the evening meal.

In northern cities the main meal of the day is usually eaten at night and includes two or three "boiling days" characteristic of the southern noon meal, and two or three "frying days" that were more typical of the fried breakfasts.[9]

TYPICAL FOODS AND THEIR USES

Milk Group

Little milk is consumed. Most children can tolerate milk well and should be given moderate amounts spaced throughout the meals for the day.

Meat Group

Fried chicken and fish are well liked; also catfish stew.

Meat from every part of the pig: bacon, ham hocks, pork chops, salt pork, spareribs (often barbecued); chitterlings (lining of pig stomach boiled and then fried); and pig's feet, tail, and ears.

Wild game when available: beaver, coon, possum, rabbit, squirrel.

Blackeyed peas with molasses and bacon or salt pork; kidney beans; marrow fat beans.

Vegetable-Fruit Group

Greens: collards, dandelion, kale, mustard, turnip—boiled in salt water with bacon or ham hocks or bits of salt pork; "pot likker" is consumed as well as the greens.

Stewed corn, okra, tomatoes; sweet potatoes.

Fruit sometimes used as snack; needs more emphasis.

Bread-Cereal Group

Baking powder biscuits, served hot.

Cornbread in many ways: crackling bread, hoecakes, hush puppies, spoon bread.

Hominy, hominy grits, rice.

PUERTO RICAN FOOD HABITS

Outstanding characteristics. Most of the Puerto Ricans now living in the mainland of the United States were born here, but many of them retain the food habits of their parents who came from the island. Because of unfamiliarity with the English language, expensive imported foods are often bought in stores managed by other Puerto Ricans.

Some familiarity with the American supermarket would help these people to obtain similar, if not identical, foods more in keeping with their limited income. The typical dietary pattern of the Puerto Rican has been described by Torres.[11]

Rice, legumes, and *viandas* (starchy vegetables) are basic to all diets. Dried codfish (*bacalao*) and milk are used as the income permits. Meat is well liked, but it is too expensive except for the well-to-do. Fruits on the island are abundant and provide ample ascorbic acid; green vegetables are also abundant. Neither fruits nor vegetables are eaten as much as they should be. The diet is high in carbohydrate and fat. Increased amounts of protein, vitamin A, and ascorbic acid should be provided.

A typical breakfast for the very poor consists of *café con leche* with or without bread; oatmeal and egg are included when income permits. Lunch in the rural areas is a plateful of viandas with codfish and oil; rice and stewed beans might be used in the city. Dinner in urban and rural areas consists of rice and beans, and viandas or bread. Between-meal eating is frequent.

Families with a more liberal income add meat to the daily meals. Chicken, pork, and beef are well liked. Desserts are not always used, but fruits cooked in syrup are especially well liked.

TYPICAL FOODS AND THEIR USES
Milk Group
Milk is well liked but very little is used. Nonfat milk solids well accepted; people must be shown how to use it.

Most of the milk is used in strong coffee (*café con leche*); 2–5 ounces milk per cup. Many drink this several times a day.

Cocoa and chocolate used widely.
Meat Group
Chicken, pork especially well liked. Seldom used by low-income groups, but liberally by the prosperous.

Chicken often cooked with rice (*arroz con pollo*).

Codfish used frequently; served with viandas.

Legumes (*granos*): chick peas, kidney beans, navy beans, dried peas, pigeon peas, and other varieties. Stewed and dressed with sauce (*sofrito*). About 3–4 ounces legumes eaten daily.
Vegetable-Fruit Group
Viandas (starchy vegetables): green bananas and green plantain most common; *batata amarillo* (yellow sweet potato); *batata blanca* (white sweet potato); ripe plantain; white *ñame*; white *tanier; panapen* (breadfruit) in some parts of the island; yautia; *yuca* (cassava), occasionally.

Viandas are boiled and served hot with oil, vinegar, and some codfish—often as a one-dish meal in rural areas.

Beets and eggplant most commonly used vegetables.

Carrots, green beans, okra, and tomatoes in small amounts.

Some spinach and chard but insufficient succulent vegetables eaten.

Yellow squash (*calabaza*) used in soups or fritters.

Fruits usually eaten between meals rather than at meals. Include: acerola (richest known source of vitamin C), cashew nut fruit, grapefruit, guava, mango, orange, papaya, pineapple.

Preference often shown for imported canned peaches, pears, apples, fruit cocktail.

In the United States, potatoes and sweet potatoes may be used instead of tropical viandas. Citrus fruits should be stressed.
Bread-Cereals Group
Rice (*arroz*) used once or twice daily by all (7 ounces per capita daily). Enriched by Puerto Rican law. May be boiled and dressed with lard or combined with legumes, chopped pork sausages, dry codfish, or chicken.

Cornmeal mush made with water or milk is popular.

Oatmeal may be cooked in thin gruel for breakfast.

Cornmeal may substitute for rice, and may be eaten with beans and codfish.

Wheat bread, noodles, spaghetti are widely used. Cream of Wheat and other cereals imported by the well-to-do.

In the United States suggest whole-grain and enriched cereals and potatoes for some of the rice.
Other Foods and Seasonings
Sofrito: sauce made of tomatoes, onion, garlic, thyme, and other herbs, salt pork, green pepper, and fat. This is basis for much of cooking.

Annato: yellow coloring used with rice.

Lard, oil, salt pork, or ham butts used in cooking. Lard is used on bread.

Sugar in large amounts in coffee, cocoa, chocolate; molasses.

Coffee (Mocha, never a blend) is very strong; consider American coffee to be very weak and dislike it. Coffee usually served with hot milk.

Carbonated beverages are being used more frequently.

MEXICAN-AMERICAN FOOD HABITS

Outstanding characteristics. The chief foods of the Mexican-Americans are dried beans, chili peppers, and corn, but wheat is gradually replacing corn. Many families eat one good meal daily at noon, such as lentil-noodle vegetable soup, and breakfast and supper consist of a sweet coffee or

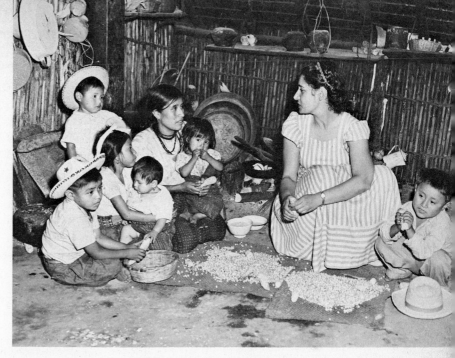

Figure 15-2. Corn is a staple food in southwestern United States and in Central America. An anthropologist studies the living habits in an Indian community as part of a nutrition survey. (Courtesy, Pan American Sanitary Bureau, World Health Organization.)

sometimes milk and tortillas. Those of low income use very little meat, usually for flavoring beans, soups, and vegetable stews.

The National Nutrition Survey in the Southwest showed that a high proportion of Mexican-Americans had low blood levels of vitamin A, riboflavin, and hemoglobin.[12] Deficiencies of thiamin, ascorbic acid, and protein were less frequent but of sufficient magnitude to constitute a problem. (See Figure 15-2.)

The diets of these people would be improved with greater emphasis on inexpensive variety meats, tomatoes, chili peppers, cheese, and evaporated milk.[12] Beans are an important source of protein but the people need to learn to supplement the beans with milk. Enriched flours and breads, citrus fruits, and cooking in iron pots are also recommended.

Typical Foods and Their Uses[12-13]

Milk Group

Very little milk is used; some evaporated milk for infant feeding.

Meat Group

Beef and chicken well liked; meat used only two or three times weekly.

Eggs: two or three times a week.

Fish: infrequently.

Pinto or calico beans: refried (*frijoles refritos*); used daily by some; two or three times weekly by others.

Chile con carne: beef with garlic seasoning, beans, chili peppers.

Enchiladas: tortilla filled with cheese, onion, shredded lettuce, and rolled.

Taco: tortilla filled with seasoned ground meat, lettuce, and served with chili sauce.

Tamales: seasoned ground meat placed on masa, wrapped in corn husks, steamed, and served with chili sauce.

Topopo: corn tortilla filled with refried beans, shredded lettuce, green or ripe olives.

Vegetable-Fruit Group

Corn: fresh or canned; *chicos*, corn steamed while green and dried on the cob; *posole*, similar to hominy.

Chili peppers: fresh, canned, or frozen are good source of ascorbic acid.

Beets, cabbage, many tropical greens, peas, potatoes, pumpkin, squash, string beans, sweet potatoes, turnips.

Bananas used frequently. *Chayotes* (cactuslike fruit), oranges.

Nopalitos: leaf or stem of prickly pear cactus; diced as vegetable.

Bread-Cereals Group

Corn is staple cereal with wheat gradually replacing it. Rice, macaroni, spaghetti. Some yeast bread; sweet rolls very popular. Increasing use of ready-to-eat cereals.

Atole: cornmeal gruel.

Masa: dried corn which has been heated and soaked in lime water, washed, and ground while wet into putty-like dough; contains appreciable amounts of calcium.

Sopaipillas: puffs of deep-fried dough. Use as bread or dessert, usually with honey.

Tortilla: thin, unleavened cakes baked on hot griddle, using masa; wheat now replacing lime-treated corn.

Other Foods and Seasoning

Ground red chili powder is essential to most dishes; garlic and onion very common; salt in abundance.

Cinnamon, coriander, lemon juice, mint, nutmeg, oregano, parsley, saffron.

Butter rarely used.

Coffee with much sugar used in large amounts.

Sugar and sweets in large amounts.

ITALIAN FOOD HABITS

Outstanding characteristics. The favorite foods for the Italian diet are readily available, and the nurse or dietitian should experience no difficulty in adapting the diet of a given locality to the Italian pattern. Cantoni[14] has summarized the prevailing pattern for Italian people in the United States.

Pastas, available in a great variety of shapes, are an important staple of the Italian diet. They are prepared from durum wheat of high-gluten content. Crusty white bread is widely used. The Italians use fruits, vegetables, and cheese liberally and should be encouraged in continuing to do so. Milk is not as widely used as it should be, although cheese will substitute in part. Dietary instruction should include emphasis on the use of enriched flour for bread and pastas.

The typical breakfast consists of fruit, Italian bread with butter, and coffee with hot milk and sugar. The main meal of the day comes at noon if all members of the family are at home but will come in the evening when some members are away from home all day. The main meal may consist of broth with noodles, meat or chicken or pasta with sauce, vegetables, green salad, bread without butter, fruit, and coffee with milk. The evening meal (or lunch) includes a substantial soup as a main dish, Italian bread, coffee with milk and sugar, sometimes cold cuts or cheese or salad, and sometimes wine.

TYPICAL FOODS AND THEIR USES

Milk Group

Goat milk is preferred. Most adults drink little milk; usually with coffee or chocolate; dislike plain milk.

American cheese disliked. Prefer expensive Italian cheeses: *Mozzarella* and *Ricotta* for cooking and with bread; *Parmesan* and *Romano* for grating; *Gorgonzola.*

Meat Group

Chicken: roast; baked with oil, garlic, salt, pepper; *cacciatora,* browned in oil, simmered in wine, tomato sauce.

Lamb.

Pork: roasted or fried sausages; baked or fried chops.

Veal: cutlets, *scallopine* or with tomato sauce.

Cold cuts: *coppa* (highly peppered), *mortadella* (bologna), *prosciutto* (cured ham), salami.

Meats often browned in salt pork or oil and simmered in a sauce with combinations of celery, garlic, onion, parsley, green pepper, tomato purée, wine; meat balls; meat loaf. Smaller quantities of meat eaten than by some other groups.

Fish: fresh preferred; canned: anchovies, sardines, tuna. Fish sauces (anchovy, clam, tuna) for spaghetti on fast days.

Chick peas, kidney beans, lentils, split peas in soups. *Pastafasiole:* bean soup. *Minestrone:* substantial soup of vegetables, chick peas, pasta.

Frittata: omelet with eggs, cheese, bread crumbs, seasonings.

Vegetable-Fruit Group

Favorite vegetables: artichoke, asparagus, broccoli, eggplant, escarole, peppers, squash (zucchini and others), string beans, tomatoes in sauce. Vegetables are cooked in water, drained, dressed with olive oil or oil and vinegar or lemon juice.

Insalata: salad of greens; may be mixed with celery, onions, green peppers, tomatoes. Dressed with olive oil, vinegar (often wine vinegar), garlic, pepper, salt.

Fruits are well liked and eaten abundantly when available: apricots, cherries, dates, figs, grapes, melons, peaches, plums, quinces.

Bread-Cereals Group

White crusty bread forms substantial part of meal. Made of high-protein flour, water, yeast, salt, and little if any fat. Flour not likely to be enriched except where state law requires it.

Pasta: includes macaroni, spaghetti, noodles in many forms and shapes. Used two to three times a week. Spaghetti is usual pasta of southern Italy, but rice, cornmeal, and noodles are more common in northern Italy.

Pastasciutta: pasta with gravy or sauce.

Noodle doughs filled with meat, vegetable, or cheese mixtures: *cannelloni, lasagne, manicotti, ravioli, tortellini.*

Polenta: thick cornmeal mush served plain, or in casserole with sausages, tomato sauce, grated cheese.

Risotto alla Milanese: rice cooked in broth, flavored with Parmesan cheese, onion, mushroom, saffron, wine.

Other Foods and Seasonings

Butter, olive oil, salt pork. Oil in cooking; preference for olive oil.

Pies and pastry used more in America than in Italy. *Cannoli:* filled pastries.

Farfalleti dolci: dough mixture fried in fat.

Torta: cake.

Zabaglione: soft custard with egg yolks, white wine, sugar.

Tutti-frutti ice creams.

Seasonings: basil, celery, garlic, nutmeg, onion, oregano, parsley, pepper, green pepper, hot peppers, rosemary, saffron, tomato purée, wine.

DIETARY PATTERNS OF THE NEAR EAST—ARMENIA, GREECE, SYRIA, TURKEY

TYPICAL FOODS AND THEIR USES[15]

Milk Group

Cow's, goat's, or sheep's milk; fermented preferred to sweet (yogurt); little used by adults. Often served hot and sweetened to children.

Soft and hard cheeses.

Meat Group

Lamb is preferred; also pork, poultry, mutton, goat, beef.

Fish: fresh, salted, or smoked; octopus, squid, shellfish, roe.

Eggs often used as main dish but not at breakfast.

Beans, peas, and lentils.

Nuts may be used with wheat and rice in place of meat; pignolias, pistachios.

Ground or cut meat often cooked with wheat or rice, or in stews with cereal grains and vegetables. For example:

Breast of lamb stuffed with rice, currants.

Squash stuffed with chopped meat, onions, rice, parsley.

Cabbage rolls with ground meat, rice, and baked in meat stock; served with lemon juice.

Barbecued meats on special occasions: skewered meats are broiled.

Shashlik: mutton or lamb marinated in garlic, oil, vinegar; roasted on skewers with tomato and onion slices.

Vegetable-Fruit Group

Eggplant, greens, onions, peppers, tomatoes; also cabbage, cauliflower, cucumbers, okra, potatoes, zucchini.

Vegetables cooked with olive oil and served hot or cold; cooked in meat or fish stews; stuffed with wheat, meat, nuts, beans; salads with olive oil, vinegar.

Grapes, lemons, oranges; also apricots, cherries, dates, figs, melons, peaches, pears, plums, quinces, raisins. Fresh fruits widely used in season; fruit compotes.

Bread-Cereals Group

Bread is staff of life; used at every meal. Baked on griddles in round, flat loaves.

Cracked whole wheat (*bourglour*) and rice used as starchy food, or with vegetables, or with meat (*pilavi*). (See Figure 15–3.)

Corn in *polenta.*

Other Foods and Seasonings

Olive oil and seed oils used in cooking. Butter is not much used.

Nuts (hazel, pignolia, pistachio) used for snacks, in desserts, pastries.

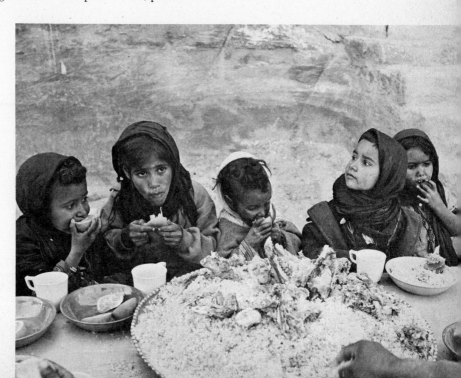

Figure 15–3. Traditional meal of Jordanian children is supplemented with milk. (Courtesy, UNICEF; photo by George Holton.)

Paklava: pastry with nuts and honey.

Black olives.

Herbs, honey, sugar, lemon juice, seeds of caraway, pumpkin, and sesame.

Apricot candy, Turkish paste.

Wine, coffee.

DIETARY PATTERNS OF THE CHINESE

TYPICAL FOODS AND THEIR USES

Milk Group

Milk and cheese are well liked but need to be emphasized. Soybean milk for children.

Meat Group

Pork, lamb, goat, chicken, duck, fish, and shellfish, eggs, and soybeans. Organ meats including brain and spinal cord, blood, and bone are used.

Egg rolls: shrimp or meat and vegetable filling rolled in thin dough, and fried in deep fat.

Egg foo yung: combination of eggs, chopped chicken, mushrooms, scallions, celery, bean sprouts cooked similar to an omelet.

Sweet and pungent pork: pork cubes coated with batter and fried in oil; then simmered in a sauce of green pepper, cubed pineapple, molasses, brown sugar, vinegar, and seasonings.

Chow mein: veal, chicken, shrimp, with celery, mushrooms, water chestnuts, bamboo shoots, in sauce; served with soy sauce. A popular dish made for American tastes.

Tofu: soybean curd; used in many dishes. An excellent source of protein, iron, and calcium if made with calcium salts.

Vegetable-Fruit Groups

Cabbage, carrots, onions, peas, cucumbers, many greens, mushrooms, bamboo shoots, soybean sprouts, sweet potatoes.

Vegetables are thinly sliced or chopped; cooked in a little oil for a short time before water is added to seal in flavor, preserve crispness, and fresh green color. Any juice remaining is served with the vegetable.

Bread-Cereals Group

Rice is staple food served with every meal.

Wheat and millet are widely used; noodles.

Other Foods and Seasonings

Lard, soy, sesame, and peanut oils used in cooking.

Soy sauce present in almost every meal contributes to high salt intake.

Almonds, ginger, sesame seeds, garlic, fresh herbs, for flavoring.

Tea is beverage of choice.

PROBLEM AND REVIEW

1. What factors must be kept in mind in teaching normal nutrition to people whose food habits differ widely from our own?
2. What technologic advances of the twentieth century have tended to eliminate regional differences in food patterns of the United States?
3. *Problem.* Select any one ethnic group and plan menus for one day including recipes for special dishes.
4. Make a survey of the ethnic groups represented in the class. List favorite dishes for each of these ethnic groups. Discuss the nutritive values of these dishes. What foods require emphasis in the patterns of these ethnic groups?
5. What problems in dietary adjustment would you expect to encounter for a Puerto Rican child; a student from India who is a strict vegetarian?
6. Compare the principal cereal foods and meats used by the Chinese, the Mexicans, and the Greeks.
7. What problems might arise owing to the bulk of the vegetarian diet?
8. Plan a menu for one day that would be nutritionally adequate for an adult who is a strict vegetarian. What supplements would be indicated?
9. What considerations must be kept in mind in dietary planning for the child whose parents are strict vegetarians?

CITED REFERENCES

1. Wenkam, N. S., and Wolff, R. J.: "A Half Century of Changing Food Habits Among Japanese in Hawaii," *J. Am. Diet. Assoc.*, **57:**29–32, 1970.
2. Register, U. D., and Sonnenberg, L. M.: "The Vegetarian Diet," *J. Am. Diet. Assoc.*, **62:**253–61, 1973.

3. Dwyer, J. T., *et al.*: "The New Vegetarians. Who Are They?" *J. Am. Diet. Assoc.*, **62:**503–509, 1973.

4. Dwyer, J. T., *et al.*: "The 'New' Vegetarians," *J. Am. Diet. Assoc.*, **64:**376–82, 1974.

5. Dwyer, J. T., *et al.*: "The New Vegetarians: The Natural High?" *J. Am. Diet. Assoc.*, **65:**529–36, 1974.

6. Erhard, D.: "The New Vegetarians. 1. Vegetarianism and Its Medical Consequences," *Nutr. Today*, **8:**4–12, Nov. 1973.

7. Erhard, D.: "The New Vegetarians. 2. The Zen Macrobiotic Movement and Other Cults Based on Vegetarianism," *Nutr. Today*, **9:**20–27, Jan. 1974.

8. Kaufman, M.: "Adapting Therapeutic Diets to Jewish Food Customs," *Am. J. Clin. Nutr.*, **5:**676–81, 1957.

9. Jerome, N. W.: "Changing Meal Patterns Among Southern-Born Negroes in a Midwestern City," *Nutr. News*, National Dairy Council, Chicago, Oct. 1968.

10. Committee on Nutrition, American Academy of Pediatrics: "Should Milk Drinking by Children Be Discouraged?" *Nutr. Rev.*, **32:**363–69, 1974.

11. Torres, R. M.: "Dietary Patterns of Puerto Rican People," *Am. J. Clin. Nutr.*, **7:**349–55, 1959.

12. Bailey, M. A.: "Nutrition Education and the Spanish-Speaking American," *J. Nutr. Educ.*, **2:**50–54, Fall 1970.

13. Hacker, D. B., and Miller, E. D.: "Food Patterns of the Southwest," *Am. J. Clin. Nutr.*, **7:**224–29, 1959.

14. Cantoni, M.: "Adapting Therapeutic Diets to the Eating Patterns of Italian-Americans," *Am. J. Clin. Nutr.*, **6:**548–55, 1958.

15. Valassi, K. V.: "Food Habits of Greek Americans," *Am. J. Clin. Nutr.*, **11:**240–48, 1962.

ADDITIONAL REFERENCES

Bass, M. A., and Wakefield, L. M.: "Nutrient Intakes and Food Patterns of Indians on Standing Rock Reservation," *J. Am. Diet. Assoc.*, **64:**36–41, 1974.

Berkowitz, P., and Berkowitz, N. S.: "The Jewish Patient in the Hospital," *Am. J. Nurs.*, **67:**2335–37, 1967.

Brown, P. T., and Bergan, J. G.: "The Dietary Status of "New" Vegetarians," *J. Am. Diet. Assoc.*, **67:**455–59, 1975.

Bruhn, C. M., and Pangborn, R. M.: "Food Habits of Migrant Farm Workers in California," *J. Am. Diet. Assoc.*, **59:**347–55, 1971.

Carey, R. L., *et al.*: *Common Sense Nutrition. A Guide to Good Health for Your Family.* Pacific Press Publishing Association, Mountain View, California, 1971. (Vegetarianism—Seventh Day Adventists.)

Chang, B.: "Some Dietary Beliefs in Chinese Folk Culture," *J. Am. Diet. Assoc.*, **65:**436–38, 1974.

Erhard, D.: "Nutrition Education for the 'Now' Generation," *J. Nutr. Educ.*, **2:**135–39, 1971.

Food Customs of New Canadians. Toronto Nutrition Committee, Toronto, Ontario, 1967.

Grivetti, L. E., and Pangborn, R. M.: "Origin of Selective Old Testament Dietary Prohibitions," *J. Am. Diet. Assoc.*, **65:**634–38, 1974.

Harwood, A.: "The Hot-Cold Theory of Disease," *J.A.M.A.*, **216:**1153–58, 1971.

Ho, G. P., *et al.*: "Adaptation of American Dietary Patterns by Students from Oriental Countries," *J. Home Econ.*, **58:**277–80, 1966.

Jerome, N. W.: "Northern Urbanization and Food Consumption Patterns of Southern-Born Negroes," *Am. J. Clin. Nutr.*, **22:**1667–69, 1969.

Jerome, N. W.: "Flavor Preferences and Food Patterns of Selected U.S. and Caribbean Blacks," *Food Technol.*, **29:**46–51, June 1975.

Kight, M. A., *et al.*: "Nutritional Influences of Mexican-American Foods in Arizona," *J. Am. Diet. Assoc.*, **55:**557–61, 1969.

Longman, D. P.: "Working with Pueblo Indians in New Mexico," *J. Am. Diet. Assoc.*, **47:**470–73, 1965.

Majumder, S. K.: "Vegetarianism: Fad, Faith, or Fact," *Am. Sci.*, **60:**175–79, 1972.

Marsh, A. G., *et al.*: *About Nutrition.* Southern Publishing Association, Nashville, Tenn. 1971. (Vegetarianism—Seventh-Day Adventists)

Natow, A. B., *et al.*: "Integrating the Jewish Dietary Laws into a Dietetics Program. Kashruth in a Dietetics Curriculum," *J. Am. Diet. Assoc.*, **67:**13–16, 1975.

Raper, N. R., and Hill, M. M.: "Vegetarian Diets," *Nutr. Rev.*, **32** (Suppl. 1):29–33, July 1974.

Sakr, A. H.: "Dietary Regulations and Food Habits of Muslims," *J. Am. Diet. Assoc.*, **58**:123–26, 1971.

Sakr, A. H.: "Fasting in Islam," *J. Am. Diet. Assoc.*, **67**:17–21, 1975.

Smith, E. B.: "A Guide to Good Eating the Vegetarian Way," *J. Nutr. Educ.*, **7**:109–11, 1975.

Soulsby, T.: "Russian-American Food Patterns," *J. Nutr. Educ.*, **4**:170–72, 1972.

Understanding Food Patterns in the United States of America. The American Dietetic Association, Chicago, 1969.

Vogel, M.: "Soul Food Is as American as Apple Pie," *What's New in Home Econ.*, **38**:12, March 1974.

16 Food Selection for Quality and Economy

food costs tremendously. Likewise family income has increased greatly so that one hour of labor today purchases a little more food than it did 10 years ago. It is not practical to describe food budgets based on a fixed expenditure. However, within groups of foods it is possible to provide general information on which foods are more costly and which are less so. This chapter will provide guidelines for the selection of foods based upon economy and quality.

Factors in food budgeting. Today's homemaker, in most instances in the United States, has more money to spend, spends less time in food preparation, and serves better meals than at any time in history. She has a better education and enjoys more leisure than did her mother. She lives longer and returns to the work force when her children are in school, if not sooner. During a given year she will purchase about one ton of food for each teen-ager and adult in her family. As individuals and families budget their money for food they must take a number of factors into account, including the following:

1. Number of family members, their age distribution, increased food needs during pregnancy, lactation, adolescence, or special food needs for modified diets.

2. Family income. On a national average about 16 per cent of income is spent for food. (See Figure 16–1.) When income is low the proportion of money spent for food is likely to be 25, 30, or 40 per cent or even more. The choices of food will be far more restricted when income is low. For example, there will be greater emphasis upon breads, cereals, and legumes, and less emphasis upon meats.

3. The availability of supplementary programs when income is limited. Free or reduced-cost school lunches, school breakfasts, congregate meal programs for the elderly, and food stamps are important ways to increase the effectiveness of the available income.

4. The location of markets. Supermarkets generally provide food at less cost than small, neighborhood markets, but transportation to large markets is sometimes a problem.

5. Whether foods are prepared in the home or are purchased as convenience foods; many but not all convenience foods are more expensive.

6. The choice of foods within each major group. Some kinds of foods are more expensive than others as described in the sections that follow.

THE FOOD BUDGET

Market systems and cost of food. In some societies, even today, agriculture is the chief occupation of most of the workers. Indeed, the agricultural methods may be so primitive that the time of almost all workers is occupied in meeting even minimal food needs of the population. In such societies the market system is a very simple one and is confined principally to foods that are locally produced.

In the United States and other highly developed countries the market system is complex. The foods eaten at any given meal have been grown in many parts of the country or may have been imported. In the United States a farmer produces enough food for about 45 people. The farmer's costs include the seed and fertilizer, feed for animals, housing for animals, storage for grains, farm equipment, and labor. Each increase in recent years for each of these items has greatly increased the farmer's cost of production. The farmer, on the average, receives about 39 per cent of each food dollar.

Before food reaches the consumer the added costs include processing, packaging, storage, distribution from farm to processor to wholesaler to retailer, and, in turn, the costs of the retailer. Many food products in today's market have entailed much preparation that was at one time performed in the home. The built-in services further increase food costs. The inflation of recent years has increased

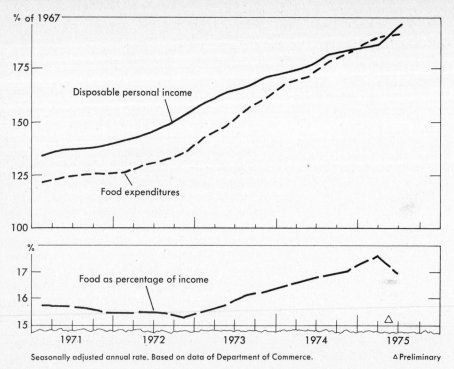

% of 1967

Figure 16–1. The amount of money spent for food has risen steadily, but the percentage of total income spent for food is about 17 per cent. At low-income levels, however, 30 per cent, or even more, of the total income must be spent for food to achieve an adequate diet. (Courtesy, U.S. Department of Agriculture.)

7. The amount of food that may be spent for snack items and beverages. This category can substantially increase the food expenditure if care is not taken to select items that make important nutritional contributions. (See Figure 16–2.)

Ten recommendations for effecting economy. Appreciable savings are possible if the following suggestions are observed.

1. Plan meals several days in advance. Use the Four Food Groups as the basis for menu planning to assure good nutrition.

2. Use eggs, cheese, fish, peanut butter, and legumes in place of meat for one or two main meals each week.

3. Eat meals at home or carry lunch whenever practical. Meals in restaurants generally cost more than twice as much as similar food prepared at home.

4. Read newspapers for reports of the U.S. Department of Agriculture on foods in plentiful sup-

ply. Watch advertisements for the items featured as specials for that week. (See Figure 16–3.)

5. Use a market list. Be prepared to make substitutions when other foods of equal nutritive value are cheaper. Avoid impulse buying.

6. Purchase foods that the family will eat. Uneaten foods are no bargain, but the wise homemaker introduces new foods attractively prepared from time to time so that her family learns to enjoy a wide variety.

7. Read labels. Look for information on dates and nutritive values. Check unit prices and compare costs of one product or brand with another. Purchase the grade appropriate to an intended use. The private label of a market is often less expensive than nationally advertised brands.

8. Buy large-size packages only if the price per unit is less, if there is space to properly store the food, and if the food can be used before it spoils.

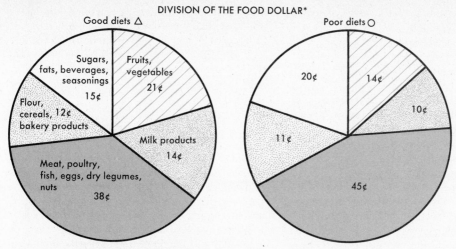

DIVISION OF THE FOOD DOLLAR*

Good diets △

Sugars,
fats, beverages,
seasonings
15¢

Fruits,
vegetables
21¢

Flour,
cereals, 12¢
bakery products

Milk products
14¢

Meat, poultry,
fish, eggs, dry legumes,
nuts
38¢

Poor diets ◯

20¢   14¢

10¢

11¢

45¢

*Based on 1965-66 U.S. household survey.
△Had recommended dietary allowances for 7 nutrients.
◯Had less than 2/3 RDA for 1 to 7 nutrients; is not synonymous with hunger and malnutrition

Figure 16-2. The quality of the diet is influenced by the allotment of the food dollar to various food groups. In good diets a larger share of the food dollar is spent for milk and fruits and vegetables; a smaller share of the dollar is spent for the meat group and for sugars, fats, and beverages. (Courtesy, U.S. Department of Agriculture.)

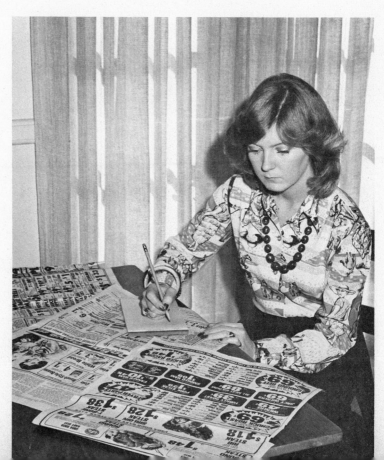

Figure 16-3. Before going to the market this homemaker checks against advertised food prices. Menu plans can be adjusted as the market list is prepared. (Courtesy, Department of Nutrition and Food Sciences, Texas Woman's University, Denton.)

9. Know the best storage conditions for each food and store foods accordingly.

10. Avoid home waste:
   a. Use food when it is at its peak of quality.
   b. Avoid loss of vegetables through excessive peeling.
   c. Cook vegetables in minimum quantities of water until just tender to preserve maximum nutritive value.
   d. Season foods and serve attractively so that they are well accepted.
   e. Use leftovers within 24 hours.

Convenience foods. Homemakers today take for granted the built-in services in many foods that have been cleaned, trimmed, and made ready for cooking, such as poultry, washed greens, and frozen foods. Canned soups, fruits, vegetables, and citrus juices, frozen orange juice and vegetables, and muffin, cake, and pudding mixes compare favorably in cost with home-prepared fresh products. Items that are appreciably more expensive are usually those that involve much preparation or that have a short shelf life, for example, ready-to-eat salads, packaged salad greens, ready-to-bake rolls, pastries, frozen entrées, and frozen vegetables in sauces. For some homemakers the somewhat higher costs may be less important than the appreciable savings in time that convenience foods afford. (See Figure 16–4.)

MILK GROUP

Market forms of milk. Among the kinds of milk available in the market, those described in the following paragraphs are the most common.

Homogenized milk is fresh milk that has been pasteurized and subjected to a process that breaks up the fat into very fine droplets and mixes them so completely as to make it impossible for the fat to rise as cream.

Skim milk is fresh pasteurized milk from which the fat has been removed. It contains all the nutrients of whole milk except fat and vitamin A. It is often fortified with vitamins A and D.

Figure 16–4. Nutritionist is beginning a lesson on budgeting for young homemakers. (Courtesy, Division of Nutrition, Pennsylvania Department of Health.)

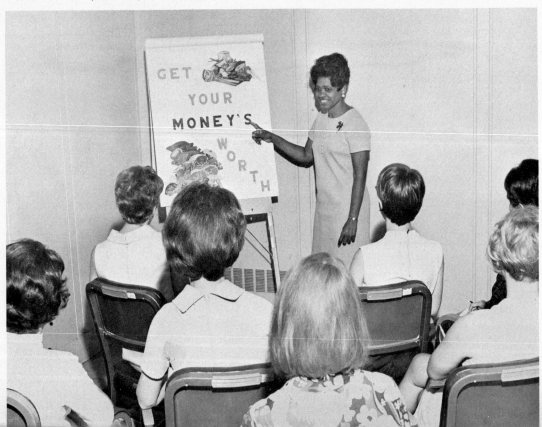

Two per cent milk is fresh pasteurized milk which contains only 2 per cent fat and up to 10 per cent milk solids to give a richer body and flavor than skim milk.

Fortified milks are those to which one or more nutrients have been added. Vitamin D is added to most evaporated and fresh whole milks to a level of 400 I.U. per quart. Vitamin A is sometimes added to skim milk. Multiple fortified milk incorporates multivitamin preparations including vitamins A, D, and the B complex; it must conform to local or state regulations.

Chocolate milk is whole milk to which chocolate syrup has been added, and *chocolate-flavored milk drink* is skim or partially skimmed milk to which the chocolate syrup has been added. The nutrients of milk are diluted in proportion to the amount of chocolate syrup used. The syrup adds caloric value without a corresponding addition of protective nutrients. These flavored milks are nutritious and wholesome, but they should not become the sole way in which milk is taken.

Cultured milks are prepared from pasteurized milk to which certain desirable microorganisms have been added. They have a nutritive value equal to that of the milk from which they are made. Buttermilk is produced by culturing skim milk, partly skimmed milk, or reconstituted nonfat dry milk with *Streptococcus lactis* and incubating it. Salt is usually added to bring out the flavor. *Acidophilus milk,* of very limited distribution, is cultured with *Lactobacillus acidophilus* under standard conditions. *Yogurt* is a pasteurized milk product of custardlike consistency which is fermented by using a mixed culture of organisms. It may be prepared from whole milk, skim milk, or partially skimmed milk.

Evaporated whole or skim milk is the product obtained from fresh milk after a little more than half the water has been removed. The protein is so changed that a softer, finer curd results. The milk is homogenized, fortified with vitamin D, and sterilized. When diluted with water to its original volume, it has a composition like that of fresh milk. Evaporated milk is easily digested, free from bacteria until the can is opened, and lends itself particularly well to the preparation of infant formulas.

Condensed milk is prepared by adding sugar to milk and reducing its water content by evaporation. It owes its keeping qualities to its high sugar content (42 per cent) rather than to the application of heat. It has found wide use in the preparation of desserts. It should not be used as a replacement for milk in the diets of infants and children.

Dried milk is made from fresh milk by spraying partially evaporated milk into warm dry air (spray process), thus removing 95 to 98 per cent of the water. *Nonfat dry milk* is made from skim milk and accounts for most of the dry milk in the market. The *instantizing* process produces a fine powder that dissolves instantly. One pound of nonfat dry milk is equivalent to 5 quarts fresh skim milk. Nonfat dry milk has excellent keeping qualities, requiring no refrigeration until it is diluted. Whole dried milk is subject to oxidation and consequent rancidity.

Filled milk is any milk or cream in which the butterfat has been removed and replaced with a vegetable fat (often coconut oil). The nutritive value is similar to that of whole milk.

Cream is the fat of milk which has been separated by centrifugation or by gravity. It is sold as light or "coffee" cream, which has a fat content of 18 to 20 per cent, and as heavy or "whipping" cream, which has a fat content of 35 to 40 per cent. *Half-and-half,* often used in high-calorie diets, consists of half milk and half light cream with a final fat content of about 11.5 per cent. *Sour cream* is light cream which has been cultured under controlled conditions.

Cheese. Cheese is produced by the action of rennet or of lactic acid on milk. As the casein coagulates and becomes semisolid, the whey separates out. The difference in varieties of cheese is due to the kind of milk used—cow (most common), goat, or sheep; the method used for curding the milk—rennet or lactic acid; the temperature and humidity for ripening; the amount of salt and seasonings used; the amount of moisture retained; and the type of bacteria or mold used for ripening.

More than 400 varieties of hard, semihard, and soft cheeses are marketed, but American, Cheddar, cottage, cream, and process cheeses account for the bulk of the consumption in this country. Cheeses with little curing are mild in flavor and less expensive; those cured for six months or longer are mellow to sharp in flavor. Good-quality cheese has a smooth, waxy texture, uniform color, and a nutty, slightly acid flavor. Cheeses that have been aged for six months or longer have better cooking qualities.

Process cheese consists of a blending of mild cheeses, followed by pasteurization. An emulsifying agent, such as disodium phosphate or sodium citrate, gives a smooth texture and keeps the fat from separating out. The process cheeses have a consistently uniform flavor and texture, and they keep well; they do not have the fine flavor of an aged Cheddar.

Purchase of milk and cheese. Whole milk purchased in half-gallon or gallon containers in supermarkets or dairy outlets is less expensive than milk delivered to the door. Nonfat dry milk costs about one half as much as fresh milk, and its use for cooking and as a beverage can result in worthwhile savings. Many people find that mixing one part reconstituted nonfat milk with one part whole milk gives a highly acceptable beverage. Evaporated milk is also less expensive than fresh milk and lends itself well to preparation of cooked dishes. American, Cheddar, process, and cottage cheese are economical buys. Among the expensive items in the dairy group are cream, ice cream, aged cheese, and imported cheeses.

Meat Group

Quality of meat. The standards for various grades of beef, veal, and lamb established by the U.S. Department of Agriculture are based upon the amount of surface fat and marbling (fat interspersed among the muscle fibers), color, firmness of flesh, texture, and maturity. (See Table 16–1.) No comparable grading standards have been set up for pork.

Prime beef, which is very tender and has a considerable amount of surface fat and generous marbling, is sold chiefly to hotels and restaurants. Many retail markets sell only one grade of meat—either choice or good, depending upon location. These

Table 16–1. Government Grades for Meat

Beef	Veal	Lamb
Prime	Prime	Prime
Choice	Choice	Choice
Good	Good	Good
Standard	Standard	—
Commercial	—	—
Utility	Utility	Utility
Cutter	Cull	Cull
Canner	—	—

grades are less generously marbled with fat than prime meat, but they are juicy and flavorful. Standard-grade beef has very little fat, is less tender and juicy, but is quite rich in flavor.

Americans have become accustomed to beef that is well marbled. To bring about marbling of beef, animals must be fed grains for a period of time before marketing. For each pound of beef protein produced, the animal must be fed about 20 pounds of grain protein. To many concerned people this is an extravagant use of grain in a world where severe shortages of food exist for some people.

Selection of meat for economy. By intelligent selection the homemaker can keep the expenditures for the meat group to reasonable proportions. When there is a choice of grades available, the good or standard grades for many purposes will yield delicious dishes. Rib roasts, steaks, and chops that are tender will be more costly than chuck roasts, round steak, and so on. When comparing costs per pound, one must consider the number of lean, edible portions. For example, 1 pound of spare ribs will serve only two persons, whereas 1 pound of lean round steak will serve three to four. (See Figure 16–5.)

Ground beef or hamburger is the least expensive of the ground meats, but is also higher in fat content. Even so, it is likely to provide more protein per dollar spent than other ground meats such as chuck, sirloin, or round. In some markets the percentage of fat in ground meat is indicated on the label, and this is a good guide when comparing costs per pound. (See Figure 16–6.)

Expenditure for meat can be reduced if the selection is made according to the market supply. Pork may be less costly at one time and beef at another. Poultry and fish have been good buys in recent years, although shellfish is a luxury item. Larger chickens and turkeys contain a smaller proportion of waste and are a better buy if the family can use the larger sizes. Buying whole birds is more economical than cut-up birds or pieces such as breast or leg.

Quality of eggs. A strictly fresh egg has a thick, gelatinous white, a round, firm, upstanding yolk, and gives a delicate flavor. As the egg ages, the yolk and white become more watery so that the egg flattens out over a large surface when broken. Eggs are graded as AA, the finest quality, new laid, especially good for poached or fried eggs where delicacy of flavor is desirable; A, of excellent quality for all

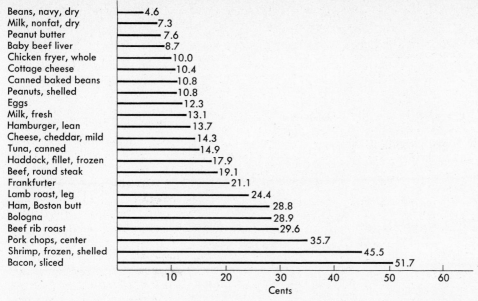

Figure 16–5. The cost of 10 grams of protein, based on supermarket prices in January 1976. This amount of protein furnishes about one sixth of the man's daily allowance and about one fifth of the woman's daily allowance. Although prices vary from week to week, the relative cost positions of these foods are not likely to shift greatly.

table use and cooking; B, useful for all cooking and some table purposes; C, with thin whites and weakened yolks which break easily, but quite suitable for baking and cooking. Cracked eggs are likely to be contaminated by *Salmonella* and should be used only in foods that are to be thoroughly heated. They are not suitable for table use or for foods such as custards cooked at low heat.

Selection of eggs for economy. The price of eggs is related to the grade, size, and color. For each size the following minimum weights have been set up:

Size	Minimum Weight Per Dozen
	ounces
Jumbo	30
Extra large	27
Large	24
Medium	21
Small	18
Peewee or pullet	15

Small eggs are often a better buy in the fall, whereas large eggs may cost only a few cents more during winter and spring months. A practical guide is this:

if the difference in cost is less than seven cents between one size and the next smaller size, the larger egg is a better buy.

People in some communities prefer brown eggs (Boston, for example), whereas others prefer white eggs (New York and Philadelphia). The color of the shell has nothing to do with the nutritive values; so there is no merit in paying an additional amount for eggs of one color or another.

Legumes. Dried peas and beans, lentils, cowpeas, chickpeas, and peanuts or peanut butter are inexpensive alternates for meat. They require long cooking to make them palatable. A cup of cooked legumes or 4 tablespoons peanut butter furnish about 15 gm protein, the amount of protein in 60 gm meat. Small amounts of milk, cheese, or eggs should be served at the same meal to furnish the amino acids that are lacking in the legumes.

VEGETABLE-FRUIT GROUP

Quality of vegetables and fruits. Fresh, canned, frozen, and dehydrated vegetables and fruits provide a broad selection on a year-round basis.

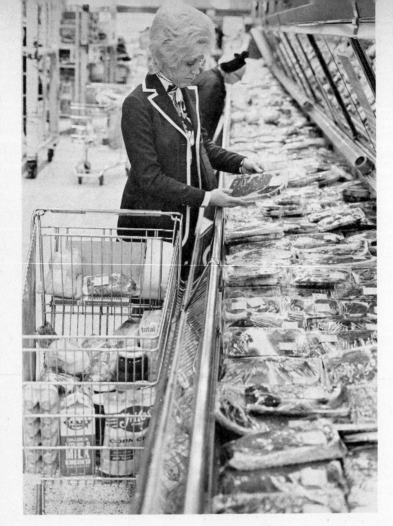

Figure 16–6. In today's supermarket the consumer must make selection from 6 to 10 thousand items. The cost of meat is an important part of the total money spent for food. (Courtesy, U.S. Department of Agriculture.)

Crisp, ripe, but not overmature vegetables that are firm in texture and free from blemishes should be selected. As vegetables become too mature, the lignocellulose that is formed gives the characteristic stringy or woody texture which cannot be overcome by cookery. Wilted vegetables are lower in carotene and ascorbic acid content than crisp vegetables. Vegetables deteriorate rapidly in palatability and nutritive value unless proper storage facilities are provided.

Fruits improve in flavor and aroma with ripening. As the fruit ripens, there is an increase in the sugar content and the volatile flavoring compounds and a decrease in the starch and organic acid. Unripe fruits lack flavor, and the sugar content will not have been fully developed. Some fruits such as peaches and pears bruise so easily that they are customarily picked before fully ripe. They should be allowed to ripen fully at room temperature before refrigeration.

Bananas are high in starch content when green. During the ripening at room temperature, this starch is changed to more digestible sugars. Bananas have the best flavor when the skin shows speckles of brown (not bruised or decayed spots). A tinge of green at the stem end of a banana is an indication that the fruit is not sufficiently ripe for use in its raw form.

Canned fruits and vegetables are usually sold by grade. Grade A products are of excellent quality, uniform in color and size of pieces, practically free of blemishes, and of the proper degree of maturity. When serving fruits or vegetables in a way where size and color are important, this grade is the preferable choice. Grade B fruits and vegetables are of less uniform color and size of pieces, slightly less tender, and less free of defects. They are just as nutritious as grade A vegetables.

Commercially canned fruits and vegetables closely approximate cooked fresh products in their nutritive values since vacuum closure of the cans reduces the rate of oxidation. There is some unavoidable loss of ascorbic acid and thiamin.

The water-soluble nutrients distribute themselves in canned foods so that the concentration is about equal in the liquid and solid phases. Thus, if the contents are in the proportion of two-thirds solid and one-third liquid, two thirds of the vitamin C, for example, would be in the solids and one third in the liquid. If the liquid is not used, one third of the original vitamin C value would be lost. When vegetables are used, the liquid should be drained off first into a saucepan and reduced in volume by heating before the solids are added.

The nutritive values of the frozen products are equal to those of the fresh foods; in fact, frozen fruits and vegetables that have been packed immediately after harvesting may be superior to fresh foods that have been improperly handled from farm to market to consumer. Frozen foods require storage at 0° F, and thus a freezer or a separate freezing compartment in the refrigerator is essential if the foods are to be kept for more than a few days. When frozen foods are to be used within a week, it is satisfactory to keep them in the ice-cube section of the refrigerator. The consumer should select frozen foods only in markets which appear to use care in the display of these foods. If foods are stored above the freezing line indicated in the cabinet, or if frozen foods have thawed, they will lose some of the qualities of texture and may even spoil because of the growth of organisms.

Purchase of vegetables and fruits. Fresh fruits and vegetables locally grown and in season are usually less expensive. Apples, cabbage, and root vegetables in fall, citrus fruits in winter, and peaches, tomatoes, and melons in midsummer to fall represent examples of good buys. The cost of canned and frozen products should be compared with the cost of fresh food in terms of edible portions per purchase unit. Fresh peas, for example, will yield about two servings per pound, and even in season are likely to be more expensive than frozen or canned peas.

Canned foods should be selected according to use.

For service as dessert, peach halves may be preferred, but pieces will serve as well at less cost in a fruit cup or salad.

Fruits and vegetables are highly perishable, so that they should be used before deterioration takes place. The liberal use of these foods in their raw state ensures maximum nutritive values.

BREAD-CEREAL GROUP

Flour. Because of its high gluten content, wheat is superior to other flours in giving a light, porous quality to leavened products and is consequently the grain of first importance in the United States. The wheat flour used in the United States is usually a 70 per cent extraction; this means that 70 per cent of the grain, namely the endosperm, is used, and the bran and germ layers are discarded for animal feeds. Practically all of the flour sold in retail markets is now enriched.

The ancient civilizations of the Incas in Peru, the Mayas in Mexico, and the Indians of North America used corn or maize—a food unknown to the Spanish adventurers and the English colonists. Even today cornmeal is widely used in the southern and southwestern states, Puerto Rico, and Central and South America. It is used in porridge, corn bread, spoon bread, and, in the Southwest especially, in tortillas.

Rye and barley flours are used much more extensively in Europe than in America. These flours produce a heavier loaf of bread than that of wheat.

The flours of potato, soybean, oats, and rice find usefulness in specialty breads, but wheat flour is the principal ingredient in order to give the porous, elastic quality to the finished product.

Kinds of bread. The Food and Drug Administration has established standards of identity for five kinds of bread: white, enriched, milk, raisin, and whole wheat. Under these regulations specified levels of certain ingredients must be included for bread offered for interstate sale. For numerous other breads on the market no standards of identity have been developed. However, interstate trade requires that the ingredients of such breads be listed on the label in the order of the amounts used in the formula.

About 85 per cent of all white bread and rolls sold to the American public are enriched. The B vitamins and iron are included at levels to equal whole-wheat bread.

Whole-wheat flour is the only flour that may be used in bread labeled as "whole-wheat," "graham," or "entire-wheat" bread. This bread accounts for only a small proportion of bread sold in America today. Many people buy breads labeled as "cracked wheat," "wheaten," "wheat," and "rye" in the mistaken belief that they are made with the whole grain. These breads, in fact, are made with white flour and varying proportions of cracked-wheat, whole-wheat, or rye flours, as the case may be.

Specialty breads are often advertised as possessing special nutritional qualities. Soy flour, wheat germ, molasses, and nonfat milk increase the nutritive value in relation to the amounts used in the bread formula. The soy flours, wheat germ, and nonfat milk also improve the quality of the protein. When claims are made for nutritional properties, these must be indicated on the label according to the labeling requirements of the Food and Drug Administration.

Breakfast cereals. Hot or cold, enriched or whole grain, from wheat, corn, rice, or oats, cereals are a mainstay of the breakfast. Cereals also find usefulness as ingredients in many desserts, as extenders for main dishes such as meat loaf, as crumb toppings for casserole dishes, and in place of part of the flour in quick breads and yeast breads.

Cereals vary widely in their protein, mineral, and vitamin content. Most ready-to-eat cereals are now fortified to supply substantial proportions of the daily allowance for vitamins and iron; others are improved in the quantity and quality of protein that they contain. A wide variety of sugar-coated cereals—some fortified, some not—is intended to appeal particularly to children's tastes.

Breakfast cereals vary widely in cost per serving, and the cost is not, of itself, always related to the nutritive value. Labels need to be read and interpreted with care in order to determine which products are the best buy in nutritional value. Generally, cereals that require cooking are more economical than ready-to-serve cereals. Almost all cereals are now of the quick-cooking variety and require only a few minutes of cooking. Among the more costly cereals are: ready-to-eat, sugar-coated, "natural," and precooked instant cereals, as well as those packaged in individual portions.

Bulgur. This has been a popular staple among people of the Near East for centuries. Large quantities of bulgur have been donated by the government in the Food for Peace Program. Bulgur is a wheat product of whole or cracked grains with a nutlike flavor and a slightly chewy texture. The wheat is parboiled and dried, and some of the bran is removed. Present methods of processing retain 75 per cent or more of the minerals and vitamins in the wheat.

Pastas. A special kind of hard wheat flour—durum—is used in the manufacture of some 150 different shapes of pastas, including macaroni, spaghetti, vermicelli, and noodles. The pastas are used in many side dishes for the main meal or as a main dish in combination with cheese, meat, fish, or poultry.

Rice. About 95 per cent of the world's rice is grown in the Orient. Rice was first introduced into South Carolina in 1685 and is an important crop in Louisiana, Texas, Arkansas, and California.

Brown rice is the whole-grain rice with the hull and a little of the bran removed. White rice is milled to remove the hull, bran, and germ. In the milling some of the minerals and vitamins are removed. Since white (polished) rice is a staple for so many of the world's people, enrichment is of major importance. Rice may be enriched by coating the kernels with a premix of vitamins. It should not be washed prior to cooking. The amount of cooking water should be no more than can be absorbed by the rice kernels.

Parboiled rice is steamed by a special process so that the thiamin and other vitamins and minerals are distributed throughout the kernel with only a slight loss taking place in washing and cooking. *Converted rice* is parboiled by a patented process. *Precooked rice* requires the addition of hot water and a short period of standing before it is ready to be served; it is more costly than uncooked rice.

OTHER FOODS

About 15 to 20 per cent of the food expenditure is for fats, sweets, beverages, and foods other than those included in the Four Food Groups.

Fats. Regular margarines cost somewhat less than butter, but those margarines high in polyunsaturated fats are almost as expensive as butter. Hydrogenated fats, lard, and oils are suitable for cooking and frying. Corn, cottonseed, soybean, and safflower oils have the advantage of being high in linoleic acid. Olive oil, prized by some for its flavor, is not a good source of linoleic acid and its cost is greater than that of other oils.

Sweets. Cane and beet sugars, corn syrup, and corn sugar are relatively inexpensive sources of calories. Confectioners' and brown sugars are slightly more expensive than granulated sugar. Colored sugars for cookie decoration and cinnamon sugar sold in shakers as a convenience item can be easily prepared in the home at a fraction of the cost. Honey, maple sugar, maple syrup, candies, cake icings, and preserves are among the more costly items in the sweets category.

Beverages and condiments. Coffee, tea, cocoa, and carbonated beverages are included in the budget allotment for beverages. It goes without saying that a high consumption of carbonated beverages adds greatly to the grocery bill while yielding no nutritional values other than carbohydrate and calories. The sugar-free beverages furnish only flavored water and a few calories per container.

Spices, herbs, pickles, and relishes add interest and variety to meals. Spices and herbs lose much of their flavor if kept too long; therefore, the smallest size container should be purchased and should be kept tightly sealed.

FABRICATED FOODS

Numerous products variously referred to as *fabricated, engineered,* or *simulated* foods are available in today's market. These foods usually simulate a conventional food in color, texture, and flavor. Many of them have been widely accepted by consumers, and their numbers will undoubtedly increase in the next decade.

Imitation milk is a product resembling milk but it contains no milk products such as skim milk or nonfat dry milk. Typical constituents of imitation milk are a protein source such as sodium caseinate or soy protein, corn syrup solids, sugar, and a vegetable fat (usually coconut oil). Additives for color, flavor, and stability are normally present. The nutritive values vary from brand to brand, but they are generally lower in protein, calcium, and vitamins than milk and are not a replacement for whole milk.

Coffee whiteners contain a protein source such as casein, vegetable fat (usually coconut oil), corn syrup solids, emulsifiers, stabilizers, and coloring.

Textured vegetable proteins are the basis for a number of meat analogs. To produce textured vegetable protein, the protein is extracted from grains or legumes, soy protein being widely used. The protein is solubilized and forced through spinnerets to form fibers, which are then coagulated. The fibers are further processed to simulate beef, pork, ham, chicken, or fish by appropriate flavorings, coloring, and texture modification. Minerals and vitamins may be added to correspond to the composition of the product it replaces.

Nutritive values of fabricated foods. If fabricated foods comprise only a small part of the diet, there need be no great concern pertaining to nutritive values except in diets that are marginal in quality. However, as the number and variety of these products increase and they become a greater proportion of the total diet, some regulation of nutritive content becomes essential.

One way to measure the nutritive value of simulated foods is to make comparisons with the foods that they would replace in the diet. This information would be available from the labeling of the product. (See regulations for labeling, Chapter 18.) For example, does the breakfast beverage that replaces orange juice contain the same amounts of ascorbic acid and carbohydrate that are present in orange juice? Does the meat analog supply the same amounts and quality of protein as the conventional meat product? Does it also supply the important minerals and vitamins found in meat in the same proportions? Many of the products are being brought to the nutritional equivalence of the food they replace. Nevertheless, a present area of concern are the numerous compounds found in conventional foods but lacking in fabricated foods because there is insufficient information on daily requirements—for example, some of the trace minerals.

MASTER FOOD PLANS

Although the Four Food Groups are a convenient tool for planning diets that will be nutritionally satisfactory, they do not provide a quantitative basis necessary for estimating the full cost of a diet. Nutritionists, nurses, and other health workers must be able to help families set up food plans that will provide nutritionally adequate diets within their incomes. To establish the cost of adequate diets in terms of the available food supply at varying levels of income, it is necessary to have information on the amounts of specific food groups that must be provided. Such quantitative information for various age-sex categories also provides the basis for setting the amount of money to be included in the welfare allowances for the poor.

The Consumer and Food Economics Institute of the U.S. Department of Agriculture has set up master food plans at these cost levels: low cost; moderate cost; and liberal cost.[1] The plans include the recommendations for 15 food groups for each of 14 age-sex categories. The low-cost and moderate-cost plans are shown in Tables 16–2 and 16–3.

The plans take into account the typical patterns of food consumption by most groups of people in the United States. For each category the amounts of food to be brought into the kitchen are listed. Based upon surveys showing practices in typical households at varying levels of income, allowances have been made for waste in preparation, losses of nutrients in cooking, and plate waste. On the low-cost plan 10 per cent waste is allowed and on the moderate-cost plan 20 per cent waste.

Compared with the moderate-cost plan, the low-cost plan calls for more bread, flour, and cereals, but smaller amounts of milk, cheese, ice cream; meat, poultry, and fish; fruits and vegetables other than potatoes; and bakery products. On the low-cost plan it is also necessary to select the less expensive foods within each group. The moderate-cost plan permits more frequent use of expensive cuts of meat and out-of-season foods. The latter also provides greater variety and can make use of more bakery products and other convenience foods.

Periodically the Consumer and Food Economics Institute determines the cost of food for each age-sex category for each plan, and releases this information to the communications media. In September 1974 the low-cost plan for a family of four, including two school-age children, cost $45.60 for a week; the moderate-cost plan for the same family, $57.10; and the liberal-cost plan, $68.50. Although the costs will obviously change from time to time, the percentage differences will not fluctuate a great deal. Thus, it may be expected that the moderate-cost plan will cost about 25 per cent more than the low-cost plan, and the liberal-cost plan about 50 per cent more.

Each of the plans was designed to furnish the Recommended Dietary Allowances as the foods are actually consumed. However, if the higher standards proposed by the Food and Drug Administration for iron enrichment of breads, flours, and cereals are not adopted, the food allowances will not furnish the level of iron recommended for girls and women and possibly for teen-age boys. It is also emphasized that iron-fortified cereals and iron-fortified formulas should be used during the first year of life.

The food allowances do not furnish the full RDA for magnesium and vitamin B_6. To meet these allowances it would be necessary to eat two to three times as much of vegetables, fruits, and cereals. To expect that most people would do this is unreasonable. Peterkin[1] has pointed out that data for magnesium and vitamin B_6 contents in foods are very limited.

The food plans take some account of the desirability to restrict fats and cholesterol. The total fat content is 40 per cent or less, representing a slight reduction from typical American diets. Eggs, the primary source of cholesterol, are restricted to not more than four per week.

PROBLEMS AND REVIEW

1. Prepare a chart that shows the kinds of milk available in a supermarket near your home. Include the following information: size of container; price; principal characteristics of each kind. Write a summary of your study.
2. *Problem.* Assuming that a given family requires 3 quarts of milk per day, calculate the cost of milk for one month, using current prices and purchasing the milk in these ways: (1) as fresh, grade A homoge-

Table 16–2. Low-Cost Food Plan: Amounts of Food for One Week*†

Family Member	Milk, Cheese, Ice Cream‡ qt	Meat, Poultry, Fish§ lb	Eggs No	Dry Beans and Peas, Nuts‖ lb	Dark-Green, Deep-Yellow Vegetables lb	Citrus Fruit, Tomatoes lb	Potatoes lb	Other Vegetables, Fruit lb	Cereal lb	Flour lb	Bread lb	Other Bakery Products lb	Fats, Oils lb	Sugar, Sweets lb	Accessories** lb
Child															
7 months to 1 year	5.70	0.56	2.1	0.15	0.35	0.42	0.06	3.43	0.71#	0.02	0.06	0.05	0.05	0.18	0.06
1–2 years	3.57	1.26	3.6	0.16	0.23	1.01	0.60	2.88	0.99#	0.27	0.76	0.33	0.12	0.36	0.68
3–5 years	3.91	1.52	2.7	0.25	0.25	1.20	0.85	2.95	0.90	0.30	0.91	0.57	0.38	0.71	1.02
6–8 years	4.74	2.03	2.9	0.39	0.31	1.58	1.10	3.67	1.11	0.45	1.27	0.84	0.52	0.90	1.43
9–11 years	5.46	2.57	3.9	0.44	0.38	2.13	1.41	4.81	1.24	0.62	1.65	1.20	0.61	1.15	1.89
Male															
12–14 years	5.74	2.98	4.0	0.56	0.40	1.99	1.50	3.90	1.15	0.67	1.88	1.25	0.77	1.15	2.61
15–19 years	5.49	3.74	4.0	0.34	0.39	2.20	1.87	4.50	0.90	0.75	2.10	1.55	1.05	1.04	3.09
20–54 years	2.74	4.56	4.0	0.33	0.48	2.32	1.87	4.81	0.93	0.71	2.10	1.47	0.91	0.81	2.11
55 years and over	2.61	3.63	4.0	0.21	0.61	2.38	1.72	4.92	1.02	0.62	1.73	1.23	0.77	0.90	1.16
Female															
12–19 years	5.63	2.55	4.0	0.24	0.46	2.17	1.17	4.57	0.75	0.63	1.44	1.05	0.53	0.88	2.44
20–54 years	3.02	3.21	4.0	0.19	0.55	2.34	1.40	4.17	0.71	0.55	1.31	0.94	0.59	0.72	2.13
55 years and over	3.01	2.45	4.0	0.15	0.62	2.54	1.22	4.57	0.97	0.58	1.24	0.86	0.38	0.64	1.11
Pregnant	5.25	3.68	4.0	0.29	0.67	2.80	1.65	4.99	0.95	0.66	1.52	1.06	0.55	0.78	2.56
Nursing	5.25	4.16	4.0	0.26	0.66	2.99	1.67	5.33	0.78	0.61	1.55	1.16	0.76	0.91	2.70

*Peterkin, B.: "USDA Family Food Plans, 1974." National Agricultural Outlook Conference, Washington, D.C., Dec. 12, 1974.

†Amounts are for food as purchased or brought into the kitchen from garden or farm. Amounts allow for discard of about one tenth of the *edible* food as plate waste, spoilage, etc. Amounts of foods are shown to two decimal places to allow for greater accuracy, especially in estimating rations for large groups of people and for long periods of time. For general use, amounts of food groups for a family may be rounded to the nearest tenth or quarter of a pound.

‡Fluid milk and beverages made from dry or evaporated milk. Cheese and ice cream may replace some milk. Count as equivalent to a quart of fluid milk: Natural or processed Cheddar-type cheese, 6 ounces; cottage cheese, 2½ pounds; ice cream, 1½ quarts.

§Bacon and salt pork should not exceed ⅓ pound for each 5 pounds of this group.

‖Weight in terms of dry beans and peas, shelled nuts, and peanut butter. Count 1 pound of canned dry beans—pork and beans, kidney beans, etc.—as 0.33 pound.

#Cereal fortified with iron is recommended.

**Includes coffee, tea, cocoa, punches, ades, soft drinks, leavenings, and seasonings. The use of iodized salt is recommended.

Table 16-3. Moderate-Cost Food Plan: Amounts of Food for One Week*†

Family Member	Milk, Cheese, Ice Cream‡ qt	Meat, Poultry, Fish§ lb	Eggs No	Dry Beans, and Peas, Nuts‖ lb	Dark-Green, Deep-Yellow Vegetables lb	Citrus Fruit, Tomatoes lb	Potatoes lb	Other Vegetables, Fruit lb	Cereal lb	Flour lb	Bread lb	Other Bakery Products lb	Fats, Oils lb	Sugar, Sweets lb	Accessories** lb
Child:															
7 months to 1 year	6.46	0.80	2.2	0.13	0.41	0.49	0.06	3.98	0.64#	0.02	0.06	0.05	0.05	0.19	0.08
1–2 years	4.04	1.69	4.0	0.15	0.29	1.24	0.59	3.44	1.03#	0.26	0.81	0.33	0.12	0.28	0.79
3–5 years	4.74	1.88	3.0	0.22	0.30	1.46	0.85	3.51	0.74	0.27	0.82	0.73	0.41	0.81	1.42
6–8 years	5.79	2.60	3.3	0.34	0.37	1.94	1.17	4.39	0.84	0.39	1.14	1.11	0.56	1.03	1.97
9–11 years	6.68	3.31	4.0	0.38	0.45	2.61	1.40	5.76	1.03	0.51	1.47	1.51	0.66	1.31	2.63
Male:															
12–14 years	7.02	3.77	4.0	0.48	0.48	2.44	1.52	4.66	0.94	0.56	1.69	1.54	0.85	1.34	3.65
15–19 years	6.65	4.65	4.0	0.29	0.47	2.73	2.00	5.45	0.80	0.67	1.98	1.82	1.05	1.15	4.41
20–54 years	3.38	5.73	4.0	0.29	0.59	2.92	1.94	5.93	0.76	0.65	1.97	1.65	0.95	0.96	2.95
55 years and over	2.97	4.64	4.0	0.19	0.70	2.91	1.69	5.88	0.89	0.53	1.58	1.45	0.87	1.05	1.50
Female:															
12–19 years	6.22	3.32	4.0	0.24	0.53	2.62	1.21	5.38	0.68	0.56	1.34	1.22	0.56	0.97	3.36
20–54 years	3.35	4.12	4.0	0.19	0.62	2.84	1.35	4.94	0.54	0.49	1.28	1.08	0.65	0.81	2.89
55 years and over	3.35	3.21	4.0	0.14	0.72	3.09	1.17	5.50	0.81	0.52	1.20	0.98	0.45	0.73	1.39
Pregnant	5.44	4.57	4.0	0.25	0.91	3.52	1.60	6.13	0.73	0.83	1.77	1.28	0.46	0.85	3.50
Nursing	5.31	5.01	4.0	0.26	0.91	3.76	1.73	6.52	0.74	0.81	1.84	1.42	0.69	1.00	3.79

*Peterkin, B.: "USDA Family Food Plans, 1974." National Agricultural Outlook Conference, Washington, D.C., Dec. 12, 1974.

†Amounts are for food as purchased or brought into the kitchen from garden or farm. Amounts allow for a discard of about one sixth of the *edible* food as plate waste, spoilage, etc. Amounts of foods are shown to two decimal places to allow for greater accuracy, especially in estimating rations for large groups of people and for long periods of time. For general use, amounts of food groups for a family may be rounded to the nearest tenth or quarter of a pound.

‡Fluid milk and beverage made from dry or evaporated milk. Cheese and ice cream may replace some milk. Count as equivalent to a quart of fluid milk: Natural or processed Cheddar-type cheese, 6 ounces; cottage cheese, 2½ pounds; ice cream, 1½ quarts.

§Bacon and salt pork should not exceed ⅓ pound for each 5 pounds of this group.

‖Weight in terms of dry beans and peas, shelled nuts, and peanut butter. Count 1 pound of canned dry beans—pork and beans, kidney beans, etc—as 0.33 pound.

#Cereal fortified with iron is recommended.

**Includes, coffee, tea, cocoa, punches, ades, soft drinks, leavenings, and seasonings. The use of iodized salt is recommended.

250

nized milk; (2) as fresh milk for half of the supply and nonfat dry milk equivalent to half of the supply.

3. Determine the kinds of cheeses available in your market. Have you tasted all of these at one time or another? What are their characteristics?

4. What factors determine the grading of eggs? What changes occur in eggs with age?

5. Obtain the prices of various grades and sizes of eggs in local markets and discuss the relative economy of each.

6. List the factors that determine the quality of meat.

7. Why are not all so-called cheap cuts of meat economical?

8. *Problem.* Complete the following table:

	Cost per pound	Protein per Pound as Purchased, Grams	Cost per 100 Grams Protein
Lamb chop		83	
Lamb neck		66	
Pork shoulder		59	
Pork loin chop		70	
Beef rib roast		69	
Beef round		88	
Frankfurter		65	
Frying chicken		69	

9. *Problem.* Calculate the cost of 25 mg ascorbic acid from each of five fresh fruits available in your market.

10. *Problem.* Compare the cost of three brands of canned peaches, canned peas, canned tomatoes. Note labeling information concerning grade. How do you account for the differences?

11. *Problem.* Obtain the prices and weights of family-size packages of ready-to-eat cereals, including the following: cornflakes; puffed wheat; rice flakes; two brands of sugar-coated cereals; two brands of cereals that are fortified with vitamins and minerals. Calculate the cost per ounce. Tabulate the nutritive values stated for one ounce on the label. What conclusions can you draw from this study?

12. *Problem.* Compare the label information and cost per pound for five kinds of bread available in your local market.

CITED REFERENCE

1. Peterkin, B.: "USDA Family Food Plans," Consumer and Food Economics Institute, National Agricultural Outlook Conference, Washington, D.C., Dec. 12, 1974.

ADDITIONAL REFERENCES

Captain, O. B., and McIntire, M. S.: "Cost and Quality of Food in Poverty and Nonpoverty Urban Areas," *J. Am. Diet. Assoc.*, **55**:569–71, 1969.

Economic Research Service: *What Makes Food Prices.* ERS 308, U.S. Department of Agriculture, Washington, D.C., 1969.

Moore, M. L.: "When Families Must Eat More for Less," *Nurs. Outlook*, **14**:66–69, April 1966.

Meyers, T.: "Food Goes to Market," *J. Home Econ.*, **58**:337–41, 1966.

Review: "Nutritional Quality and Food Product Development," *Nutr. Rev.*, **31**:226–27, 1973.

Watson, K. R., and Kilgore, L. T.: "Fat, Moisture, and Protein in 'Ground Beef' and Ground Chuck," *J. Am. Diet. Assoc.*, **65**:545–47, 1974.

PUBLICATIONS FOR THE LAYMAN

Publications of the U.S. Department of Agriculture, available from Government Printing Office, Washington, D.C.

Family Food Budgeting for Good Meals, G 94.
How to Buy Beef Roasts, G 146.
How to Buy Beef Steaks, G 145.
How to Buy Cheddar Cheese, G 128.
How to Buy Dry Beans, Peas, and Lentils, G 177.
How to Buy Eggs, G 144.
How to Buy Fresh Fruits, G 141.
How to Buy Poultry, G 157.
How to Buy Fresh Vegetables, G 143.
How to Use U.S.D.A. Grades in Buying Foods, PA 708.
More Food, Better Diets for Low-Income Families, PA 930.
Your Money's Worth in Foods, G 183.

17 Safeguarding the Food Supply

ILLNESS CAUSED BY FOOD

Following the exodus of the Jews from Egypt, the people had a great craving for meat. When quails were brought in large numbers by winds from the sea, the people gathered them and ate them. This is what happened:°

While the meat was yet between their teeth, before it was consumed, the anger of the Lord was kindled against the people, and the Lord smote the people with a very great plague. Therefore the name of that place was called Kibrothhattaavah,† because there they buried the people who had the craving.

Recently among some people living on the island of Lesbos (Greece) a syndrome has been observed following the eating of quail.[1] The symptoms include muscular pain, paralysis of used muscles, excretion of myoglobin in the urine, and oliguria. Apparently this illness occurs only in persons who have some enzymatic abnormality and who have become physically fatigued before eating the quail. It is theorized that the eating of quail elicits the abnormality in these persons, thus producing the symptoms. The author of this report believes that this twentieth-century syndrome is the same as that which afflicted the Jews during the exodus.

°*The Holy Bible*, Numbers 11:33–34.
†Graves of craving.

The ancient Egyptians realized that the meat of animals that had died a natural death was unfit for human food. Greek records of many centuries ago note that the wife, daughter, and two sons of the Greek poet Euripides died after having eaten poisonous fungi. For centuries kings were protected against poisoning by employing official food tasters. Thus, history records on numerous occasions the role of food in producing illness.

Illness resulting from the eating of food may be caused (1) by contamination of the food by bacteria, molds, and fungi, (2) by the presence of some natural toxicant in the food, (3) by the contamination of food by a toxic chemical, or (4) by sensitivity of a given individual to one or more foods. Bacterial, parasitic, and chemical contaminations are considered in this chapter.

Food-borne diseases as a public health problem. When one considers the total population of the United States and the amount and variety of foods consumed each day, it becomes evident that the reported incidence of outbreaks of illness from the food supply is indeed very low. In 1966 the National Communicable Disease Center instituted a program for the control of food-borne diseases. During the first two years the "big three" reported as causes of illness were *Salmonella, Clostridium perfringens,* and *Staphylococci*.[2] The number of cases reported is believed to represent not more than 1 to 2 per cent of the total number of persons who became ill as a result of food poisoning.[3] Thus, millions of persons experience some food-borne illness each year.

For most people in good health an outbreak of food poisoning from the organisms listed above results in an illness of short duration leading to discomfort and absence from work or school. But for the very young, the elderly, and those who are debilitated from other illness, these seemingly mild infections can lead to serious complications or even death. The outbreak of an infection in a child-care institution or in a nursing home is especially life threatening. Therefore, to protect the vulnerable, every precaution must be taken to minimize the occurrence of infection among the more vigorous who in turn become the agents for transmission of organisms.

Other diseases transmitted by foods are typhoid fever, bacillary dysentery, tuberculosis, scarlet fever, streptococcic sore throat, botulism, undulant fever, amebic dysentery, trichinosis, infectious hepatitis, and cholera.

Food-borne diseases result from eating food (1) from an animal or plant that has been infected, (2) that has been contaminated by organisms transmitted by insects, flies, roaches, or rodents, (3) that has had contact with sewage-polluted water (shellfish, for example), or (4) that has been contaminated by a food handler who has not observed good personal hygiene or acceptable food-handling practices.

Some illnesses are enteric in that the symptoms are confined to the gastrointestinal tract with mild to severe nausea, vomiting, abdominal pain, and diarrhea. Other food-borne diseases are systemic; that is, the organisms invade the circulation and produce symptoms in organs and tissues.

Bacterial food infections. A bacterial *infection* results from the ingestion of food that has been contaminated with large numbers of bacteria. The bacteria continue to grow in the favorable intestinal environment and produce irritation of the mucosa with symptoms occurring in 12 to 36 hours after ingestion of the food.

Salmonellosis. About 1300 serotypes of the *Salmonella* genus have been identified, each of which is capable of causing infection in man.[4] The organisms are easily killed by boiling for 5 minutes, but survive in foods that are inadequately heated. Paratyphoid fever (enteric fever) occurs frequently. The symptoms usually last for two or three days, but the organisms may be eliminated for two or three weeks thereby providing a continuing source of contamination for others.

Typhoid fever, fortunately rare in the United States, is the most serious of the *Salmonella* infections. The symptoms of the gastrointestinal tract may be severe with ulcerations of the mucosa occurring. Unlike most infections by *Salmonella,* typhoid fever is systemic. The organisms particularly affect the liver and gallbladder, but they may also localize in the bone marrow, kidney, spleen, and the lungs where bronchitis and pneumonia may result.

Meat, poultry, fish, eggs, and dairy products that are eaten raw or that have been inadequately heated are most frequently implicated in salmonellosis. Contaminated cake mixes, bakery foods, coloring agents, powdered yeast, and chocolate candy have also caused outbreaks of the infection.

Animals including cattle, swine, poultry, fish, dogs, and birds harbor the organisms. They are usually infected by contact of one animal with another or by animal feeds. A single egg that is infected can contaminate a whole batch of eggs being frozen or dried. A butcher block or kitchen counter with which infected meat has been in contact is a source of contamination for any food placed upon it. Flies and rodents coming in contact with feces of animals or man are responsible for contamination of food. Food handlers who do not observe good personal hygiene or who do not follow essential directions in the preparation of food are a major source of contamination of the food supplies.

Shigellosis (bacillary dysentery). The *Shigella* genus includes pathogenic organisms widely distributed and capable of producing severe illness. Bacillary dysentery is characterized by fever, abdominal pain, vomiting, and diarrhea. The intestinal mucosa may become ulcerated, and stools often contain blood and mucus. Fatalities from the infections are ordinarily low, but in tropical countries where sanitation is poor and malnutrition is prevalent the disease is fatal to as many as 20 per cent of persons affected.

Infected human feces are the source of the infection, which is transmitted by the direct fecal-oral route or through contamination of food or water.

Clostridium perfringens, the gas gangrene organism, ordinarily inhabits the intestinal tract and in usual numbers does not produce illness. However, when a food is consumed which has been contaminated with large numbers of bacteria, illness results. In 1968 this food-borne illness accounted for 28 per cent of all outbreaks reported to the National Communicable Disease Center.[5]

Clostridium perfringens appears normally in the soil, in the intestinal tract of man and animals, and in sewage. The bacteria are destroyed by heat, but the spores they produce will survive boiling for as long as five hours. If foods are allowed to remain at temperatures between 10° and 60° C (50° and 140° F) for several hours, the spores germinate and prodigious numbers of bacteria are then present in the food. Refrigeration of food immediately after heating will prevent rapid germination of the spores. However, a large mass of food cools so slowly even at refrigerator temperatures that considerable bacterial growth occurs.

Bacterial food intoxication. Food poisoning frequently results from the ingestion of a food in which a bacterial toxin has been produced. The preformed toxin is responsible for the symptoms, which may be mild to severe. Usually the symptoms are apparent from one to six hours following a meal.

Staphylococcal poisoning occurs abruptly after the ingestion of food containing the enterotoxin. The gastrointestinal symptoms are often severe but usually the illness lasts for only one to three days.

Staphylococci are found in the air and occur especially in infected cuts and abrasions of the skin, boils, and pimples. They may be present in the nose and throat of food handlers. Food becomes contaminated through failure to observe rules of hygiene. Rapid growth of the bacteria occurs in contaminated food if it is held at temperatures ranging between 10° and 60° C (50° and 140° F) for three to four hours. Semisolid foods such as custards, cream fillings in pastries, cream puffs, cream sauces, mayonnaise, chicken and turkey salads, croquettes, potato salad, ice cream, poultry dressing, ham, ground meat, stews, and fish provide the ideal culture media for bacterial growth.

Staphylococci are killed at high temperatures, but the toxin is not inactivated with temperatures ordinarily used in food preparation. The contaminated food usually does not smell, taste, or appear to be spoiled. The best safeguard against staphylococcal poisoning is prompt refrigeration of food so that bacterial growth is retarded and toxin formation does not take place.

Botulism is an extremely rare type of food poisoning but of such serious consequences that it captures the attention of the news media. Each year there are 10 to 20 outbreaks of botulism in the United States with two to five deaths.[6] The illness has been attributed to inadequately processed nonacid vegetables, fish and fish products, soup, meats, and other undetermined sources.

The symptoms of botulism occur 8 to 72 hours after ingestion of the contaminated food and usually begin in the gastrointestinal tract. The principal hazard is the effect on the nervous system. When the toxin enters the circulation, the nerve endings become blocked. Headache, dizziness, double vision, difficulty in swallowing, and paralysis occur. Death is usually the result of respiratory paralysis and cardiac failure. When botulism is suspected

early and treatment with antitoxin is initiated, the death rate is about 25 per cent.[6] Failure to initiate early treatment increases the death rate to about 65 per cent.

Clostridium botulinum is present in soils all over the world and in the sediment at the bottom of rivers and lakes. Consequently, vegetables grown on these soils and fish become contaminated. The bacteria do not grow in the presence of oxygen; that is, they are anaerobic. They will grow within a few millimeters below the surface of the foods, however. The bacteria are sporeformers which are resistant to ordinary boiling temperature. As the spores germinate the deadly neurotoxin is produced.

Most instances of botulism are traced to the ingestion of home-canned nonacid vegetables and meats. A few outbreaks in recent years have been reported from commercially processed tuna fish, whitefish, and soup. When measured against the 29 billion cans of food prepared each year, the incidence is remarkably small.[6]

Canned foods that contain little or no acid (pH above 4.6) such as meat, beans, asparagus, corn, and peas are very good media for the growth of the bacillus botulinus, whereas acid-containing foods such as tomatoes and certain fruits are not favorable to growth. The use of sterilization with steam under pressure is absolutely necessary in the home for any nonacid food products, as well as for those processed commercially.

Botulinus-infected foods do not necessarily taste or smell spoiled, so home-canned vegetables should be brought to a vigorous boil and kept boiling for 10 minutes. Any toxin that may be present will thereby be inactivated. Any can of food that shows gas production, change in color or consistency, bulging ends, or leaks should be discarded without even tasting. "When in doubt, throw it out" is a good axiom. The foods must be disposed of so that animals do not have access to them since they too might be poisoned.

Parasitic infestations of food. Many protozoa and helminths (worms) gain admission to the body by means of food and parasitize the bowel, thereby causing injury to the intestinal lining. Some of them also invade other tissues of the body.

Among the parasitic protozoa are *Endamoeba histolytica*, which causes amebic dysentery. The source of infection is human feces, and infection is transmitted by a food handler who is a carrier or by contaminated water supplies. The symptoms may be acute, chronic, or intermittent. Erosion of the intestinal mucosa sometimes occurs with profuse bloody diarrhea. The individual with a chronic infection may experience only mild discomfort of diarrhea or constipation. The liver, lung, brain, and other tissues may be infected and abscesses may form. Preventive measures include maintenance of sanitary controls of the water supply and sewage disposal, as well as supervision of public eating places by health agencies.

The helminths that frequently invade the intestinal tract include *nematodes* (roundworms), *cestodes* (tapeworms), and *trematodes* (liver, intestinal, and lung flukes). Trichinosis, one of the more serious infestations, results from the ingestion of raw or partially cooked pork infected with *Trichinella spiralis*, a very minute roundworm barely visible to the naked eye. In the intestinal tract the larvae are set free from their cysts during digestion of the meat and develop into adults within a few days. The females deposit larvae in the mucosa and invade the lymph and blood circulation. The muscles of the diaphragm, the thorax, the abdominal wall, the biceps, and the tongue are frequently involved, there being muscular pain, chills, and weakness.

Trichinella is destroyed by cooking pork until no trace of pink remains. The recommended internal temperature for cooked pork is 77° C (170° F), which allows a margin of about 17° C (30° F) above the lethal point of the organisms. *Trichinella* is also destroyed by freezing at −18° C (0° F) or below for at least 72 hours. Government inspection does not include examination for *Trichinella* at the present time. The cooking of all garbage fed to hogs will go a long way toward reducing *Trichinella* infestation.

Hookworm infestation is a serious problem in children in tropical countries of the world, and in some parts of the United States. The larvae penetrate the exposed skin and reach the lymphatics and blood circulation. They are carried to the lungs and migrate into the alveoli, trachea, epiglottis, and pharynx and are swallowed. They may also be carried from soil to hands to mouth.

It has been estimated that a single hookworm removes almost 1 ml blood per day as it carries on its blood-sucking activity in the intestine. The loss of blood produces an anemia with symptoms of

weakness, fatigue, and growth retardation. Usually the infestation is present in children who also are malnourished. A good nutritious diet is always important for these children, but the eradication of hookworm infestation depends upon sanitary measures for disposal of feces so that the cycle of parasite growth in the soil is broken.

Naturally occurring toxicants in foods. Foods are exceedingly complex mixtures of chemicals that probably number in the hundreds of thousands.[7] For example, potatoes, often considered to be a simple food, contain at least 150 chemical substances including not only the nutritionally important protein, carbohydrate, minerals, and vitamins, but also oxalic acid, tannins, solanine, arsenic, and nitrate.[8]

Two terms must be defined when considering the possible danger from food components. TOXICITY is the capacity of a substance when tested by itself to harm living organisms. HAZARD is the capacity of a chemical to produce injury under conditions of use.[7] For example, vitamin A is potentially toxic, but it is a hazard only when ingested over a period of time in amounts that are 10 to 20 times the recommended allowances. Salt is potentially toxic; it is a hazard when ingested in three to five times normal amounts. For hypertensive patients salt may be hazardous at much lower levels of intake.

Foods contain thousands of compounds that are potentially toxic. The hazards are minimal because of several factors: (1) the body has metabolic mechanisms for degrading, detoxifying, and eliminating some substances; (2) some toxic substances are modified by processing—for example, the heating of soybeans to destroy trypsin inhibitor; and (3) some toxic compounds are antagonistic to other toxic compounds, and the net effect is one of neutralization. Molybdenum, an essential nutrient, is toxic in excess; copper, another essential nutrient, also toxic, is antagonistic to molybdenum, thus reducing the toxicity of the pair.

Poisoning from natural food toxicants often occurs in times of stress such as famine or war when abnormally large amounts of single foods containing toxic materials are ingested daily for prolonged periods of time.

Alkaloids. The alkaloids such as strychnine, atropine, scopolamine, solanine, and others have long been known as poisonous compounds. Varieties of hemlock have been mistaken for parsley, horseradish, or wild parsnip and eaten in salads and soup only to produce immediate, often fatal, illness. Monkshood, foxglove, and deadly nightshade have from time to time been mistaken for edible plants and have caused violent illness.

Solanine, representing a series of glycosides, occurs in the stems and leaves of the potato plant and in the green part of sprouting potatoes. When potatoes are stored in bright light, significant amounts of solanine are produced in the skin, evidenced by greening. When ingested in sufficient amounts, solanine produces pain, vomiting, jaundice, diarrhea, and prostration. Ordinarily the green parts of the potato are removed with the peel.

Legumes and seeds. Because legumes are important sources of protein and energy in some parts of the world, the presence of toxic factors in them is of nutritional and economic importance. Soybeans are a most valuable source of protein when they are heated. Raw soybeans contain a trypsin inhibitor and probably some other factors that interfere with the metabolism and with growth in animals. In addition, the phytic acid content of soybeans binds zinc so that animals fed a diet in which soybeans are the source of protein develop a severe zinc deficiency. This can be corrected by supplementing the diet with zinc. Soybeans also contain a goitrogen but this is not believed to be a factor in endemic goiter.

Cassava and Lima beans contain *linmarin,* a glycoside that can be split to hydrocyanic acid. People in West Africa, Jamaica, and Malaysia consume up to 750 gm cassava daily. It is thought that the incidence of blindness and tropical ataxic neuropathy, a degenerative disease, may be caused by chronic cyanide poisoning from the cassava.

Lathyrism has been known since the time of Hippocrates. It is observed in India and in Mediterranean countries following the ingestion of large amounts of the seeds of *Lathyrus sativus,* a legume, for six months or more. These legumes grow under adverse conditions of drought and hence they may be ingested extensively during a famine. Lathyrism is a neurologic disease characterized by weakness of the leg muscles, dragging of the feet, loss of sensation of heat and pain, and spinal cord lesions.

Favism is an inherited sensitivity to fava or broad beans and is fairly common in the Mediterranean area, and in Asia and Formosa. Sensitive individuals have a deficiency of glucose-6-phosphate dehydrogenase and reduced glutathione content of the red blood cells. An unidentified substance in the fava beans leads to hemolysis of the red blood cells and thus hemolytic anemia in the sensitive individuals.

Gossypol is a toxicant in cottonseed that must be removed before the meal can be used in protein mixtures. Some strains of cottonseed are now being developed that are free of this toxic substance.

Mushroom poisoning. A few species of mushrooms are so toxic that eating them may be fatal, others are mildly toxic, and many species are harmless and greatly enjoyed. The *Amanita* is the most poisonous of the mushrooms and produces severe abdominal pain, prostration, jaundice, and death in more than half the people who ingest it. This source of poisoning can be eliminated if people will use only the commercially grown mushrooms.

Mycotoxins. In medieval times a poisoning known as "St. Anthony's Fire" was a terrible scourge.[7] It was caused by ergot, a toxic fungus, growing on cereal grains. Ergotism is almost unknown today. Deaths of thousands of people in Russia in times of war and famine have been attributed to the consumption of moldy millet.[7]

Many molds growing on grains and nuts can produce illness in animals and probably in man. A class of substances of extreme toxicity to swine, cattle, poultry, and laboratory animals is the aflatoxins produced by the mold *Aspergillus flavus.*[9] The aflatoxins are potent hepatocarcinogens. Much attention has been focused on peanuts, Brazil nuts, and grains that are subject to mold growth when they are allowed to remain on damp ground or when they are stored without sufficient drying. The only practical way to prevent the development of the mold growth is through prompt drying of grains and nuts to a moisture content not over 15 per cent. Allowing crops to remain in fields over winter invites mold growth.

Interference with nutritive properties. The adverse effect of some chemical substances is an interference with the utilization of a nutrient and thus the imposition of a deficiency. One of the best-known examples of this is the oxalic acid content of certain green leafy vegetables such as spinach, beet tops, and chard that interferes with the absorption of calcium. The occasional use of these vegetables with an adequate calcium intake is of no concern whatsoever. However, if the calcium intake is low and the vegetables are eaten frequently, a problem of calcium deficiency could arise. Rhubarb leaves are so high in oxalic acid content that their ingestion leads to gastrointestinal upsets, and in severe intoxications to hematemesis, hematuria, noncoagulability of the blood, and convulsions.

Goiter is a major public health problem affecting 200 million people throughout the world. Goitrogens, which are antithyroid compounds, are held responsible for about 4 per cent of the goiter incidence, representing a total of 8 million persons.[7] Goitrogens are found in broccoli, Brussels sprouts, cabbage, cauliflower, kale, kohlrabi, rutabagas, and turnips. There is no adverse effect when eating normal amounts of these vegetables, but when they become a major part of the diet for extended periods of time, the antithyroid effect becomes evident. Additional iodine does not counteract this effect.

Thiaminase, an enzyme antagonistic to thiamin, is present in bracken fern, raw fish, and a variety of fruits and vegetables. In an ordinary mixed diet this is of no concern. The enzyme is destroyed by heat.

Excess of nutrients. The toxic effects of vitamins A and D are well known. The ingestion of seal or polar bear liver leads to symptoms of acute vitamin A toxicity, inasmuch as 1 pound of the liver contains about 10 million I.U. of vitamin A. On a practical basis in the United States the hazards of vitamin A toxicity relate to the indiscriminate use of vitamin supplements and not to excesses in the diet itself. If several foods that are fortified with vitamin D are consumed each day, the intake could be in excess of requirements, and hypercalcemia is a possible outcome. (See Chapter 10.)

Selenium, a nutritional essential in trace amounts, is toxic to animals that graze in pastures with selenium-rich soils. People living in seleniferous areas also appear to have a higher incidence of dental caries.[10]

Tyramine toxicity. Cheddar cheese and Chianti wine contain appreciable amounts of tyramine, which is produced by the decarboxylation of tyrosine. Tyramine is a potent vasopressor substance but it is normally metabolized in the body by the action of monoamine oxidase. Patients with depressive states are frequently treated with monoamine oxidase inhibitor because of its ability to produce euphoria. Since the inhibitor interferes with the metabolism of tyramine, the ingestion of tyramine-containing foods leads to nausea, vomiting, headache, and severe hypertension, and sometimes death. A glass of Chianti wine or as little as 1 ounce of Cheddar cheese contains enough tyramine to produce some toxic effects, and large amounts may be dangerous for some.

Chemical poisoning. Lead, mercury, and cadmium are serious environmental pollutants. Excesses of copper, beryllium, zinc, and silver also interfere with metabolic processes. These metals modify metabolism in several ways: (1) by inactivating enzymes such as ribonuclease, alkaline phosphatase, catalase, and others; (2) by chelating with a nutrient so that the latter is unavailable; (3) by altering cell permeability; and (4) by replacing a structural element—for example, lithium in place of sodium.

Lead is a particularly serious contaminant since it accumulates in the body and results in chronic illness characterized by severe anemia and changes in the arteries and kidneys, with death occurring in some instances. A minute quantity of lead occurs naturally in food and is ingested daily, but when the daily intake is 1 mg or more, the eventual accumulations may become toxic. Food becomes contaminated with lead when it is exposed to dust containing lead or when it is kept in containers in which solders, alloys, or enamel containing lead have been used. The canning industry has long since devised containers that are entirely safe for food.

At least 100,000 children are affected by lead poisoning. Most of them are black and live in ghetto areas.[11] The primary source of the lead is the layers of old paint in the interior of houses. Children from 18 to 30 months chew paint from the woodwork, and a daily ingestion of 3 mg can lead to elevated blood levels in three to four months. A number of cities are now making a concerted effort to correct the problem by educating parents, by emphasizing the removal of old paint, and by screening children through blood lead determinations in areas where there is hazard.

A few years ago there was great concern about the mercury content of fish. Strong,[7] an authority on food toxicants, believes the danger was overemphasized and that serious contamination takes place only in areas of pollution by industrial wastes. The mercury in tuna fish appears to be nontoxic because of its interaction with selenium which is also present.

Accidental poisonings occur when chemicals have been mistaken for powdered milk, flour, or baking powder. Some years ago in a state institution 47 deaths resulted when roach powder containing sodium fluoride was mistaken for dry milk powder and used as such.[12] In another instance boric acid was mistaken for lactic acid for the preparation of infant formulas, again resulting in infant deaths. It goes without saying that insecticides, lye, mothballs, and numerous other poisons should be well labeled, kept away from foodstuffs, and out of the reach of small children.

The metals used in cooking utensils and in food containers have been a source of much controversy. Many studies have shown that glass, stainless steel, aluminum, agate, and tin are suitable containers for food since these materials are practically insoluble or, when dissolved to a slight degree, are not harmful to health. Acid foods may dissolve some of the tin from cans so that a change of flavor results from the iron underneath the tin coating, but the ingestion of these foods is not harmful. It is recommended that acid foods be transferred from the can to a covered glass container if the food is to be refrigerated after opening. The intentional use of chemicals in foods is discussed on pages 264–66.

Radioactive fallout. Man has always been exposed to the radiation of naturally occurring radioisotopes in the environment. With the advent of the nuclear bomb the amount of such exposure has increased, although to date the annual exposure of the population from this source is very small when compared to that which occurs naturally. No change in food habits is currently indicated by the amounts of radioactive contamination.

Following a nuclear detonation there are several pathways by which the radionuclides eventually are ingested by man. (See Figure 17–1.) For example, contaminated plants may be eaten by cows; much of the element is excreted in the urine of the cow, but some will be secreted in the milk which, in turn, is consumed by man. Some of the consumed element will be excreted in the feces of man, but some will enter the metabolism in a manner similar to that of the element with which it is related. Strontium-90 is related to calcium and is deposited chiefly in the bones; cesium-137, like potassium, is distributed throughout the body in the soft tissues; and within 48 hours of ingestion iodine-131 is accounted for in the thyroid gland and in the urine. Excessive depos-

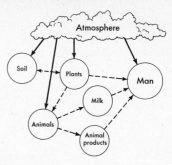

Figure 17–1. Pathways of radioactive fallout. (Courtesy, National Dairy Council.)

its of radioactive elements carry the threat of cancer—of the thyroid with iodine-131, and of the bone with strontium-90.

Each radioisotope has a specific *physical half-life.* This is the amount of time that elapses before half of the element is decayed. The element thus emits radiations to the external environment with consequent exposure of man, animals, and plants over this period of time. The *biologic half-life* refers to the length of time before half of the element is excreted from the body. Thus, some elements may be rapidly excreted causing little harm, whereas others are retained. Strontium-90 and cesium-137 have a physical half-life of 28 years. Strontium-90 is of much more serious biologic consequence since its rate of turnover is slow in the body, whereas cesium-137 has a biologic half-life of about 140 days.

The Federal Radiation Council has established guidelines which define the potential hazards of radiation.[13] The U.S. Public Health Service, Atomic Energy Commission, and U.S. Department of Agriculture are among the groups that periodically analyze foods from all over the country to determine levels of radioactivity. About one third to one half of the dietary strontium-90 is present in milk; however, the high calcium intake helps to ensure a preferential use of calcium rather than strontium by the body. The current levels in foods present no risks whatsoever. (See Figure 17–2.)

PRESERVATION OF FOODS

Factors contributing to food spoilage. Foods are made unsafe to eat or become aesthetically undesirable or both by the actions of bacteria, yeasts, and

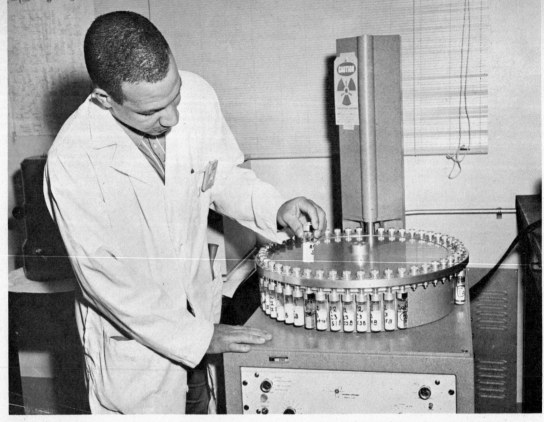

Figure 17-2. Samples of milk are tested for radiostrontium contamination. Fifty samples of milk are loaded into this automatic scintillation counter which counts and automatically records data. (Courtesy, U.S. Department of Agriculture.)

molds; by enzymatic action; by chemical or physical changes; and by contact with insects and rodents. In food spoilage these factors often coexist. Unsafe foods do not necessarily show any changes in appearance and palatability, and hence the danger from them is great. Foods that are rancid, moldy, or rotting are less likely to be consumed and therefore may not be a direct threat to health, but the economic waste is considerable.

Temperature and growth of organisms. Bacteria, yeasts, and molds grow rapidly at temperatures of 10° to 60° C (50° to 140° F); within this range the rate of growth increases tenfold for each 10° C (18° F) increase in temperature. Thus, the bacteria produced in a food left at room temperature for three or four hours can reach astronomical numbers.

Growth of microorganisms is retarded at refrigerator temperatures and is stopped at freezing temperatures. Many molds and some bacteria known as *psychrophils* grow even at refrigerator temperatures, leading to spoilage of food. Pathogenic bacteria

do not grow at these temperatures. Many bacteria are not killed by freezing—an important fact to remember when frozen foods are thawed and allowed to stand at room temperatures. (See Figure 17-3.)

Some bacteria known as *thermophils* thrive at relatively high temperatures. They are responsible for the "flat sour" which occurs in some home-canned foods.

Many bacteria produce spores that are very resistant to heat. In fact, several hours of boiling do not destroy them. Under favorable conditions such spores will germinate rapidly.

Physical and chemical changes. Appearance, texture, flavor, and the chemical constituents of foods are modified by the influence of air, heat, light, moisture, and time. These changes are accelerated by enzyme action and by the presence of minute traces of mineral catalysts such as copper and iron. All plant and animal tissues contain enzymes that are highly active at room temperatures and above.

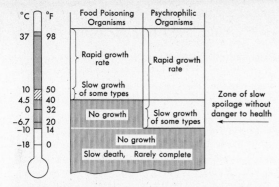

Figure 17–3. Low-temperature limits on growth of food poisoning and psychrophilic organisms. (Courtesy, Dr. Horace K. Burr and the *Journal of the American Medical Association,* **174**:1178–80, 1960.)

The rate of chemical change doubles for each 10° C (18° F) rise in temperature. Rancidity of fats is one example of undesirable oxidation and contributes to the deterioration of flavor even in foods that contain only small amounts of fat. Oxidation also leads to loss of ascorbic acid.

Plant and animal tissue fibers are softened, and the surface of cut nonacid fruits is oxidized and becomes darkened as a result of enzyme action, thereby changing the texture, color, and nutritive value. Some nutrients may be lost by discarding fluids in which they have been dissolved. The exposure of milk to sunlight leads to a tallowy flavor and loss of riboflavin and vitamin B_6. With storage, changes in texture also occur: sugar may crystallize out of jellies; ice cream becomes gummy and granular; and frozen meats and poultry become dry.

Food preservation. The criteria for successful food preservation, whether it be for a day or two or for months, are these: (1) safety from contamination by pathogenic organisms or toxicity through chemicals; and (2) maintenance of optimum qualities of color, flavor, texture, and nutritive value.

Methods of food preservation that destroy bacteria are *bactericidal;* these include the application of heat by cooking, canning, preserving, and irradiation sterilization. Other methods such as dehydration, freezing, treatment with antibiotics, salting, and pickling retard the growth of bacteria, molds, and yeasts; they are *bacteriostatic.*

Pasteurization. Of all foods, milk is most susceptible to contamination. The inspection of cows,

barns, milk handlers, and dairy-processing plants is essential to the production of milk of high quality. Cattle diseases such as brucellosis, tuberculosis, and mastitis are now rare because of testing and vaccination programs and prompt isolation and treatment of infected animals. Pasteurization, nevertheless, is essential not only for milk but also for the preparation of cheese, butter, and ice cream.

Milk is pasteurized by (1) the *holding* process in which milk is heated to at least 62° C (143° F) and kept at that temperature for at least 30 minutes, or by (2) the *high-temperature short-time* method in which milk is heated to 71° C (160° F) and kept at that temperature for at least 15 seconds.

Milk may be sterilized by boiling it for a specified time as in the preparation of infant formulas or by heat as in the processing of evaporated milk. Pasteurization does not appreciably change the color or flavor of milk, but sterilization deepens the color and gives to milk a slightly carmelized flavor.

Cooking and baking. Boiling temperature (100° C), if maintained sufficiently long for heat to completely penetrate the food, will kill bacteria. When low-heat cookery is used as in the preparation of custards or when heat penetrates food masses very slowly as in casseroles or stuffed poultry, bacteria are not killed. Such foods may cause food poisoning if they have been carelessly handled prior to cookery.

The spores of *Clostriduim perfringens* and *Clostridium botulinum* are highly resistant to heat, and temperatures above boiling, as with a pressure cooker, are necessary to destroy them. The enterotoxin produced by staphylococci is not inactivated by boiling; on the other hand, botulin is inactivated by boiling for at least 10 minutes. Cooked foods that are improperly handled are rapidly subject to spoilage.

Canning. Commercial firms now employ standard methods for canning each food. Sterilization is brought about by means of steam under pressure. By means of agitation of the cans during processing, heat penetration of the can contents is accelerated and the heating time is shortened with a great improvement in flavor and in color.

Some nutritive losses, especially of heat-labile vitamins, occur during canning, but the newer techniques have reduced these losses considerably. The manner of storage is probably the major factor in nutrient retention or loss. As much as 25 per cent of ascorbic acid and thiamin may be lost from fruits and vegetables stored for a year at 27° C (80° F), but with storage at 18° C (65° F) these losses are reduced to 10 per cent. Meats, likewise, lose 20 to 30 per cent of their thiamin content after six months' storage at 21° C (70° F), but the riboflavin content is not adversely affected. Carotene losses in fruits and vegetables are small even after months of storage. Water-soluble nutrients distribute themselves evenly throughout the solids and liquids; thus, if the solids constitute two thirds of the total, one third of these water-soluble nutrients will be lost if the liquid is not used.

Home canning. When foods are canned in the home, a pressure canner should always be used for low-acid foods, including most vegetables, poultry, and meat, in order to destroy bacteria and their heat-resistant spores. Fruits and tomatoes, being acid foods, may be safely canned at boiling temperatures.

Cool storage and refrigeration. Modern refrigeration has been largely responsible for the tremendous variety of foods available all over the country, in season and out. By means of it foods can be kept for long periods of time in commercial cold-storage rooms at the proper humidity, or may be transported from coast to coast without danger of loss from spoilage or freezing, or may be kept in the home refrigerator to reduce the number of trips the homemaker makes to the market.

Fruits except bananas and vegetables are kept just above the point at which they will freeze. Butter and meats may be kept at much lower temperatures.

Cool storage is being gradually extended to canned and dehydrated foods to retain optimum color, flavor, and nutritive values.

Freezing. In the quick freezing of foods, first developed as a practical method of processing some 40 years ago, bacteria are unable to grow and enzymes are inactivated. Today an almost endless variety of frozen foods is available—fruits, vegetables, juices, meats, poultry, fish, pies, cakes, cookies, rolls, stews, casseroles, and complete meals.

Foods to be frozen must be carefully selected for quality and maturity. No frozen product is ever any better than the raw materials from which it was frozen. Because ready-to-eat foods involve mixtures

and are subject to more handling prior to freezing, special care must be taken to enforce the most rigid sanitary practices. Some foods such as raw salad vegetables and tomatoes cannot be frozen satisfactorily because of texture changes. Fruits are softened by the freezing process.

Before freezing, vegetables are blanched to inactivate the oxidative enzymes. The darkening of fruits is prevented by immersion in a sugar syrup or by using ascorbic acid. Foods are packed in consumer-size moisture-vapor-proof containers and placed between metal plates at −40° C where freezing begins almost immediately and is complete within an hour. Pieces of foods such as shrimp, green beans, peas, and carrots may also be spread on a wire mesh belt that is moved slowly through a freezing tunnel and subsequently packaged. In a modification of this method, known as "fluidized freezing," a current of air is passed through the belt thus lifting the food up into the air and quickly freezing it on all sides.

Cryogenic freezing utilizes liquid nitrogen (−186° C), liquid or solid carbon dioxide (−78° C), or some other refrigerant. With this method some foods can be frozen that were not satisfactory with sharp freezing, for example, tomatoes, watermelon, onion rings, and green pepper. Liquid nitrogen systems are in extensive use for the transportation of frozen foods.

Because frozen foods still contain bacteria and enzymes, it is essential that foods be maintained at −18° C (0° F), or lower, until they are to be used. Bacteria begin to multiply and enzymes begin to bring about oxidative changes as soon as foods begin to thaw.

With freezing the ascorbic acid losses are greater than those for other nutrients. Orange juice held at 0° C (32° F) for a year loses no more than 5 per cent of its ascorbic acid content, but nonacid foods lose an appreciable amount at −18° C (0° F) and much lesser amounts at −23° to −28° C (−10° to −20° F). Frozen foods should be kept for only a few days in the freezing compartment of a refrigerator.

If frozen foods are allowed to stand for some time at room temperature subsequent to their thawing, microorganisms multiply rapidly. Fully thawed foods should not be frozen again because further deterioration will take place. Fruits retain the best color if they are thawed in the container before it is opened. Most vegetables are cooked by dropping the frozen vegetable directly into a small quantity of boiling water and rapidly returning it to the boiling point. Meats may be cooked while still frozen or may be thawed prior to cooking; the former procedure requires a considerable increase in the cooking time.

Dehydrofreezing, a relatively new process, consists in evaporating about half the water from fruits and vegetables and then freezing the product. The costs of packaging, shipping, and storage are thus reduced. Water is added to reconstitute the food when it is cooked.

Freeze-drying consists in placing the frozen food under a vacuum to remove the water and packaging in the presence of an inert gas such as nitrogen. The product retains its original volume and shape and rehydrates readily. Freeze-dried coffee is probably the most widely used product prepared by this technique. Seafoods, beef, pork, chicken, soups, and several food mixtures have been found acceptable in taste tests conducted by the U.S. Department of Agriculture. They rated somewhat lower than frozen or canned foods but possessed the advantages of long shelf life and light weight.

Dehydration. Drying of foods is an effective means of avoiding spoilage since microorganisms cannot grow in the absence of water. Dried foods possess the special advantages of light weight and small volume and are easily transported and stored. The dehydration of certain fruits such as prunes, peaches, apricots, apples, figs, dates, and raisins, as well as meat, fish, and legumes, has been practiced for centuries. Every market today features numerous dried foods: nonfat dry milk; quick bread, yeast bread, cake, cookie, and pudding mixes; dehydrated soups; instant coffee; instant mashed potatoes; citrus juice powders; precooked rice and beans; cereals; and many others. Dried whole eggs and egg whites are used extensively in the baking industry.

Chemical preservation. Sugar is employed in high concentrations for the preparation of jams, jellies, and preserves. The water is made unavailable to the microorganisms, and hence spoilage will not occur. However, molds will grow on the surface of these foods if sterility is not maintained. Sodium chloride and vinegar are also good preservative agents as employed in brining and pickling.

The number of chemicals that may be used for preservation is now strictly limited by government regulations. Sodium benzoate is used in some foods up to a concentration of 0.1 per cent if labels specifically indicate its use. Sulfur dioxide is used in the drying of apples to lessen darkening. Meats may be cured with smoke that contains phenols. Older methods of curing meat employed considerable amounts of salt so that preservation was possible at ordinary room temperature. Recent processes employ less salt and more uniform though shorter curing periods, but it is important to emphasize that hams so cured are perishable and require refrigeration. Failure to refrigerate hams has caused a number of outbreaks of food poisoning in recent years. Spices such as cloves and cinnamon have been much overrated for their preservative properties, since concentrations sufficient to inhibit bacterial growth would render food inedible. (See also food additives on page 264.)

Antibiotics in food preservation. The uncontrolled use of antibiotics in foods or as drugs is a potential hazard to approximately 10 per cent of the population who react unfavorably to contact with them with symptoms ranging from a mild skin rash to fatal anaphylactic shock.[14] The repeated ingestion of antibiotics may produce an immunity in other individuals so that they do not respond to therapeutic doses required in the treatment of disease conditions. It is, therefore, a prime requirement that the food supply that may have had any contact with antibiotics contain no residues when eaten.

Antibiotics are used in food production. The farmer adds antibiotics to feeds to stimulate the growth of swine and poultry, or he may employ antibiotics to prevent and treat illness in animals. Crops are sometimes sprayed with antibiotics. Since no residues of the antibiotics are present in the foods as eaten, these practices constitute no health hazard. One possible source of antibiotic residues has been milk from cows which have been treated for mastitis. Regulations of the Food and Drug Administration now specify that milk obtained for three days following treatment for mastitis with antibiotic drugs must not be used for human consumption.

For some years chlortetracycline (Aureomycin) and oxytetracycline (Terramycin) were used in the cooling water for dressed poultry and in the ice slush for packing raw fish and shellfish, thereby increasing the shelf life for several days. The cooking of poultry and fish destroys any antibiotic residues remaining in the flesh. With improved methods of food handling the Food and Drug Administration has recommended that the use of antibiotics to prolong shelf life be prohibited.

Preservation of foods by irradiation. One of the potential peacetime uses of atomic energy is in the radiation preservation of foods. Microorganisms can be destroyed by using gamma rays or high-speed electrons, both types of radiation being referred to as ionizing radiations. The unit of absorbed dose is the *rad*, which is the energy absorption of 100 ergs per gram. One million rad will increase the temperature of a food by only about 2° C; therefore, the term *cold sterilization* is applied to radiation processing.

Low-level irradiation. Ionizing radiation at dosages between 5000 and 20,000 rad is sufficient to depress the sprouting of potatoes, onions, and similar foods. With 25,000 to 50,000 rad insects that infest grains are destroyed. Presently, other methods are used to control these problems because of their lower cost and their known reliability. A dosage of 750,000 rad will eliminate *Trichinella* in pork, but 20,000 rad suffice to prevent maturation of the worm larvae.

At somewhat higher levels of irradiation, that is, 100,000 to 1,000,000 rad, most microorganisms are destroyed but the product is not sterile. Fruits and vegetables may be kept for a longer time; and meats, poultry, and fish may be kept under refrigeration for appreciable lengths of time without deterioration. Radiopasteurization with doses of less than 500,000 rad holds promise of market application in the not-too-distant future.

To effect sterilization, that is, complete destruction of bacteria, 4.8 to 6.0 million rad are required, the spores of *Clostridium botulinum* being especially resistant. The inactivation of enzymes requires such high levels that it appears some heat treatment, such as blanching prior to radiation, is the only practical solution. At high dosages of radiation such as are required for sterilization, adverse changes occur in color, flavor, and texture so that many products are no longer acceptable. Moreover, modifications of nutritive value also occur. Vitamins A and E, ascorbic acid, and thiamin are especially sensitive.

Irradiation does not make the food radioactive. Irradiated foods are not presently available in the market, nor are they approved for sale by the Food and Drug Administration. Many technologic problems must be overcome before irradiation becomes practical for commercial use. Long-term studies are being conducted by the Armed Forces Food and Container Institute at Natick, Massachusetts.

FOOD ADDITIVES

More than 2000 additives are used for foods. Yet they make up only a small fraction of 1 per cent of the weight of food.[8] Many of the additives are normal constituents of foods, for example, the nutrients, some natural coloring compounds, flavors, spices, and inorganic and organic salts of sodium, potassium, calcium, and magnesium.[8] Additives are broadly classed as *intentional* and *incidental*.

Intentional additives. An INTENTIONAL ADDITIVE is a substance of known composition that has been added to a food to improve the quality in some way. Among the many functions additives perform are these: enhance the flavor; improve the color; stabilize and improve texture by emulsifying, retaining moisture, thickening, binding, leavening, preventing caking or hardening or sticking; enrich or fortify with minerals and vitamins; prevent oxidation and spoilage; act as a propellant for food in pressurized cans. Some additives perform a single function and others perform several. For example, salt is both a preservative and flavoring agent. Ascorbic acid prevents the discoloration of cut fruit and also adds to the nutritive value. Table 17–1 lists some examples of additives and the functions they perform.

If additives are used, the benefit must outweigh any possible risk. If the risks are high in proportion to the benefit derived, the use of the additive would be contraindicated. For example, the improvement of color, flavor, or consistency would not be justified if a substance had a known risk, even though slight. The regulations for the use of additives are described in Chapter 18.

The nitrite dilemma. Of the additives currently being studied, nitrates and nitrites have been the subject of heated controversy. Nitrates and nitrites are used in the curing of bacon, frankfurters, sausage, ham, and smoked fish as preservatives, coloring

Table 17-1. Typical Uses of Some Intentional Additives

Function	Chemical Compounds	Examples of Food
Acids, alkalies, buffers		
Enhance flavor	Acetic acid	Cheese, catsup, corn syrup
	Sodium hydroxide	Pretzel glaze
Leavening	Baking powder, baking soda	Cakes, cookies, quick breads, muffins
Antioxidants		
Prevent darkening	Ascorbic acid	Fruit to be frozen
	Sulfur dioxide	Apples, apricots, peaches to be dried
Prevent rancidity	Butylated hydroxyanisole (BHA); butylated hydroxytoluene (BHT)	Lard, potato chips, meat pies, cereals, crackers
	Lecithin	Margarine, candy
	Tocopherol	Candy, oils
Coloring	Annatto; carotene	Butter, margarine
	Certified food colors	Baked goods, soft drinks
Flavoring (over 300 compounds in use)	Aromatic chemicals, essential oils, spices	
Nutritional fortification	Mineral salts, vitamins	Iodized salt; enriched breads and cereals; fortified milk and margarine; see p. 278
Preservatives	Sodium chloride	Dried pickles, salted meats
	Sodium benzoate	Dried codfish; maraschino cherries
	Chlortetracycline	Antibiotic dip for fish and dressed poultry
Inhibit mold	Calcium propionate	Bread, rolls
	Sorbic acid	Cheese wrappers
Sweeteners, nonnutritive	Saccharin	Dietetic foods and beverages
Texture	Alum	Firm pickles
Anticaking agents, retain moisture, emulsifiers, give body, jelling, thickening, binding	Disodium orthophosphate	Evaporated milk, cheese
	Mono- and diglycerides	Margarine, chocolate
	Sodium alginate	Cream cheese, ice cream
	Pectin	Jelly, French dressing
Whipping agents	Carbon dioxide	Whipped cream in pressurized can
Yeast foods and dough conditioners	Calcium phosphate; calcium lactate	Bread

agents, and flavorings. Consumer advocates have indicted nitrosamines as potent carcinogens. Government regulators of the food industry claim that the elimination of nitrates and nitrites in cured meats would pose a real danger of botulism, and they are unwilling to risk this hazard. An expert panel of the National Research Council further states that there is no existing evidence in the world literature that nitrosamines have been the cause of carcinoma in humans.[15]

What are nitrosamines? Under certain conditions amines in meats and in the human stomach can combine with nitrites to form NITROSAMINES. When fed to laboratory animals these compounds have carcinogenic, mutagenic, and teratogenic proper-

ties. Under controlled conditions it has been found that nitrosamines were formed in sausages only when the concentration of nitrite was ten times that normally used. It has also been demonstrated that the inclusion of sodium ascorbate in bacon blocked the formation of nitrosamines.[15]

Infants under three months of age are sensitive to nitrites present in processed meats and fish.[16] Broccoli, beets, celery, collards, radishes, and spinach have a high concentration of naturally occurring nitrate. The low acidity of the gastrointestinal tract of the young infant favors the growth of bacteria that change nitrates to nitrites. The nitrites, upon absorption, change some of the hemoglobin to methemoglobin. Young infants lack two enzymes necessary for the conversion of methemoglobin to hemoglobin. Consequently, some reduction in oxygen transport takes place. This is not a widespread problem at the present time.

Toxicity to nitrites is rarely reported in adults. The "hot-dog headache" syndrome occurs sometimes after eating cured meats. It has been reproduced experimentally by ingesting sodium nitrite, a vasodilator.[17]

The expert panel of the National Research Council has recommended that the nitrite level in cured meats and fish be restricted to 156 ppm, a level that protects against botulism yet is sufficiently low to prevent the formation of nitrosamines. Further studies on this dilemma are in progress.

Incidental additives. Foods sometimes contain minute traces of a chemical as a result of contact with a substance used in its production, processing, or packaging. Since its presence serves no useful purpose in the final food product, such a chemical is considered to be an INCIDENTAL ADDITIVE. For example, food may have picked up a substance from a wrapper or container, either through dissolving it out or by abrasion from the container into the food. Or food may contain a residue of detergents remaining on dishes, or a residue of pesticides used in crop control. Dirt, hairs, and insect fragments are also classed in this group.

The farmer uses chemicals that destroy insects, control plant diseases, and kill weeds. Without the use of these pesticides it is doubtful that enough food could be produced to feed the population. Nevertheless, these chemicals if improperly used pose some hazards.

By their very nature the chemicals used are toxic to some forms of life or they would not be effective in controlling the pests that peril crops. It is essential that the pesticide residues remaining on foods be at levels that do not constitute any danger to health of the consumer either immediately or through gradual buildup in the body over a long period of time. It is equally important that there be no appreciable increase from year to year in the concentration of pesticides in the environment to endanger animal, fish, or bird life or to increase the levels in soils and water so that future food supplies contain levels that are toxic. Some pesticides meet these criteria but others do not. The kinds and amounts of pesticides that may be used and the residues that may remain in foods are established by

regulations formulated by the Food and Drug Administration, the U.S. Department of Agriculture, and the U.S. Department of Interior. (See page 273.)

Polychlorinated biphenyls. A group of compounds known as POLYCHLORINATED BIPHENYLS (PCBs) has recently gained the attention of toxicologists. PCBs are synthetic organic compounds widely used in industry because they are fire resistant and water insoluble. They are used in paints, rubber, plastics, asphalt, adhesives, lubricants, and electrical insulators. They enter the food chain through industrial accidents or improper disposal. A random sample of people in the United States showed that 30 per cent had significant amounts (over 1 ppm) of PCBs in adipose tissue.[18] The cumulative effect is not known.

Several hundred individuals in Japan developed a serious disease called "Yusho disease" after consuming rice bran oil that was accidentally contaminated with PCBs.[19] An acne-type skin lesion difficult to cure resulted. It was not established that the condition was caused by the PCBs or by other contaminants. Monkeys fed diets containing 300 ppm PCBs for three months developed hyperplasia of the gastric mucosa together with skin and liver changes.[18] The dosage used was ten times the concentration reported by the Food and Drug Administration present in milk and fish. Environmental control of these compounds is essential, and much study is required to determine the possibility of hazard to man.

Misinformation concerning additives. A widespread and often exaggerated consumer concern is related to the use of additives in foods, whether intentional or incidental. This has led many people to use only "organically grown" foods or "natural foods." The terms are often used interchangeably although they are not synonymous.

"Organically grown" foods are those grown on soils enriched with compost and manure and in the absence of any chemical fertilizers. That foods are organically grown is a misconception. Manures and composts used to enrich the soil must be degraded by bacteria to inorganic phosphates and nitrates since the plant utilizes only the inorganic substances just as it would from the commercial fertilizer. The nutritive values of foods grown on soils enriched in either way are of equal value, and the foods are equally safe and wholesome.

"Natural foods" are those that have been grown

without benefit of chemical fertilizers or pesticides, and in which no additives have been used whatsoever. The very words "chemical" and "additive" strike unreasoning fear in some people who are not informed about the safety and indeed the necessity for them in the food supply. These people forget that their own bodies and the world in which they live constitute a fantastic environment of chemical substances. They become alarmed whenever they note from labeling of a food that some chemical substance has been used in the processing. Many of these substances are normal constituents of some foods.

Four points should be made concerning additives: (1) no harm to human health has been clearly demonstrated through the legitimate use of additives in foods;[8] (2) synthetic chemicals and naturally occurring chemicals in foods react identically in the body—e.g., synthetic or naturally occurring ascorbic acid; (3) the food supply would be drastically reduced in the United States if commercial fertilizers and pesticides were not available; and (4) the safety of each new additive—intentional for foods, or incidental through pesticide residues—must be established beyond any doubt by the manufacturer before the Food and Drug Administration or the U.S. Department of Agriculture will permit use. The regulations pertaining to the use of additives are discussed further in Chapter 18.

Emergency Feeding

Following a natural or man-made disaster, the goals of emergency feeding are "to keep people alive, to restore and maintain morale, and to provide adequate and familiar food that will keep people at work or enable them to return to work."[*] The American Red Cross assumes responsibility for emergency feeding in a natural disaster such as a flood, and the civil defense and welfare services carry out feeding during disaster from war.

Problems associated with emergency feeding. Disruption of one or more utilities may make it impossible to cook foods or to use water. Stockpiles must be so planned that some foods not requiring heating are available. The lack of water limits the

*Bovee, D. L.: "Emergency Feeding in Disaster," *Am. J. Clin. Nutr.*, 6:77, 1958.

kinds of foods which can be cooked and seriously interferes with cleaning and waste disposal.

The dietary needs of special groups require preplanning. Infants and young children are especially vulnerable to the lack of food, and parents are likely to become panic stricken if their children are not cared for. Supplies of dry or evaporated milk or commercial formulas are vital for infants and children. When no water is available for formula preparation, canned fruit juices and even carbonated beverages might be used. The ill and the aged should also be considered. Most patients on modified diets can survive a short period when some foods needed by them are not available. Every diabetic patient should be fully instructed on what to do when he is unable to get his food or his insulin.

The worker in a disaster—fire fighter, rescue worker, or the person restoring facilities—must receive sufficient food allowances so that he can keep his work at a maximum output; this may require 3000 to 3500 kcal daily.

A disaster is no time to give unfamiliar foods, since the stress of the emergency will usually lead to refusal. Therefore, local foods which are familiar and well liked should be used.

During the first few days following a disaster, food to allay hunger and to sustain morale takes precedence over meeting nutritional needs. A cup of hot coffee to the adult and milk to the child given as soon as possible are tangible evidence that someone is caring for them and that some community facilities are functioning. When an emergency is of more than a few days' duration, nutrient needs must be considered. The recommended allowances, however, are likely to provide unrealistic goals when there are food shortages; rationing priorities must be defined.

Safety of food supplies. Following a nuclear attack, the hazards of radioactive contamination of food and water must be appreciated. Foods which are in sealed, unbroken packages or in cans are safe for use, as are those in a refrigerator or freezer which has remained closed. However, the outside of the food container or utensil for cooking and eating must first be washed in detergent solution to remove the radioactive substances. Wash water and cloths used for cleaning must be buried.

If no refrigeration facilities are available, food spoilage occurs rapidly and food poisoning may affect large numbers of people. Infant formulas may be prepared from dry milk just before use if they cannot be refrigerated.

GUIDE FOR AN EMERGENCY SHELF FOR THE FAMILY*

General Considerations

1. Allow about 2 quarts liquid per person per day—fruit and vegetable juices, bottled water, soft drinks. Allow 2 additional quarts water for personal care.

2. Plan menus in advance using foods the family likes, and keeping these situations in mind: (1) no fuel available and water is limited; (2) no fuel available but there is sufficient water; (3) cooking facilities but little water; (4) cooking facilities and ample water.

3. Stock foods on the basis of menus planned. Avoid those foods which increase thirst. A two-week supply of foods is recommended.

4. Rotate food supplies at least every six months so that stock is always fresh.

5. Use only airtight containers—metal, plastic, or heav-ily waxed cardboard. Glass is not satisfactory since it may shatter.

6. Consider emergency cooking facilities.

Suitable Foods from Which to Select (all in airtight containers)

LIQUIDS: fruit juices including citrus juices; vegetable juices; carbonated beverages; water

MILK: nonfat dry and evaporated

CANNED FOODS: fruits; vegetables; soups; stews; baked beans; spaghetti and other pastes with sauces; chicken, meatballs, seafood, pressed pork; peanut butter; cheese; oils; shortening; jelly, jam, preserves

DRIED FOODS: dried fruits; legumes

CEREALS AND BREADS: dry cereals; ready-to-eat cereals; spaghetti, macaroni, rice, noodles; flour; canned or frozen breads; cookies

INFANT FOODS: dry milk, cereals, fruits, vegetables, strained meats

MISCELLANEOUS FOODS: instant coffee, tea, salt, pepper, sugar, candy, pickles

SUPPLIES: cooking and eating utensils, paper dishes, matches, candles, bottle and can openers, covered cans for waste disposal, water containers, paper towels and napkins, detergent powder

*Adapted from "Confidentially Speaking—A Report on Emergency Feeding," Nutrition Section, Louisiana Department of Health, August 1957.

REVIEW

1. Understanding of the following terms will help you in your review of factors affecting food safety:

aflatoxin	lathyrism
alkaloid	mycotoxin
amebic dysentery	nematode
bactericidal	nitrosamine
bacteriostatic	PCBs
cestode	protozoa
favism	psychrophil
gossypol	solanine
half-life, biologic	thermophil
hazard	toxicity
helminth	trematode
	tyramine

2. List several ways by which bacterial diseases are transmitted by foods.
3. Give two examples of bacterial infections transmitted by food; two examples of bacterial intoxication.
4. What organisms are responsible for most cases of summer food poisoning?
5. Explain what is meant by botulism. Which types of foods are most likely to contain botulinus toxin? What measures are necessary to eliminate this hazard?
6. Describe the effects of *Trichinella* infestation. How can it be avoided?
7. Name several plants that are poisonous to man. What types of chemical compounds produce this poisoning?
8. Lead and mercury are especially toxic to man. What are some ways by which they contaminate food?
9. What are the causes of food spoilage?
10. Why are commercially canned foods likely to be superior to home-canned foods in their vitamin content?
11. Which method of canning is recommended for home use? Why?

12. Name three chemical agents frequently used for food preservation.
13. What are the time and temperature requirements for the pasteurization of milk?
14. Read the labels of a variety of packaged foods and list the additives. Try to determine the reason for each additive. What objections can you see to the use of additives? Would it be advisable to eliminate all additives from foods? Defend your answer fully.
15. What is strontium-90? Why is a liberal intake of milk protective against its effects?
16. What purposes are served by nitrates and nitrites in cured meats? What is the dilemma faced by food processors in their use?
17. Based upon your reading of this chapter, set up practical rules that you would expect a food handler to observe.
18. Prepare a menu for three days that could be used following a disaster when cooking facilities are available but the water supply is lacking. List the foods that would be necessary in the family stockpile for these menus.

Cited References

1. Ouzounellis, T.: "Some Notes on Quail Poisoning," *J.A.M.A.*, **211**:1186–87, 1970.
2. Woodward, W. E., *et al.*: "Foodborne Disease Surveillance in the United States, 1966 and 1967," *Am. J. Public Health*, **60**:130–37, 1970.
3. Foster, E. M.: "Microbial Problems in Today's Foods," *J. Am. Diet. Assoc.*, **52**:485–89, 1968.
4. Foltz, V. D.: "Salmonella Ecology," *J. Am. Oil Chem. Soc.*, **46**:222–24, 1969.
5. "Clostridium Perfringens," *FDA Papers*, **4**:19–22, Feb. 1970.
6. Kauter, D. A., and Lynt, R. K., Jr.: "Botulism," *Nutr. Rev.*, **31**:265–71, 1973.
7. Strong, F. M.: "Toxicants Occurring Naturally in Foods," *Nutr. Rev.*, **32**:225–31, 1974.
8. Coon, J. M.: "Natural Food Toxicants—A Perspective," *Nutr. Rev.*, **32**:321–32, 1974.
9. Campbell, A. D.: "Natural Food Poisons," *FDA Papers*, **1**:23–27, Sept. 1967.
10. Hadjimarkos, D. M.: "Geographic Variations of Dental Caries in Oregon," *J. Pediatr.*, **48**:195–201, 1956.
11. Guinee, V. F.: "Pica and Lead Poisoning," *Nutr. Rev.*, **29**:267–69, 1971.
12. Lidbeck, W. L., *et al.*: "Acute Sodium Fluoride Poisoning," *J.A.M.A.*, **121**:826–27, 1943.
13. Dunning, G. M.: "Radioactivity in the Diet," *J. Am. Diet. Assoc.*, **42**:17–28, 1963.
14. Welch, H.: "Problems of Antibiotics in Foods," *J.A.M.A.*, **170**:2093–96, 1959.
15. IFT Expert Panel on Food Safety and Nutrition: "Nitrites, Nitrates, and Nitrosamines in Foods—A Dilemma," *J. Food Sci.*, **37**:989–92, 1972.
16. Raab, C. A.: "The Nitrite Dilemma: Pink and Preserved?" *J. Nutr. Ed.*, **5**:8–9, 1973.
17. Editorial: "One Man's Cured Meat," *J.A.M.A.*, **224**:1756, 1973.
18. Allen, J. R., and Morback, D. H.: "Polychlorinated Biphenyl- and Triphenyl-induced Gastric Mucosal Hyperplasia in Primates," *Science*, **179**:498–99, 1973.
19. Olcott, H. S.: "Mercury, DDT, and PCBs in Aquatic Food Resources," *J. Nutr. Ed.*, **4**:156–57, 1972.

Additional References

Anderson, E. C., and Nelson, D. H., Jr.: "Surveillance for Radiological Contamination," *Am. J. Public Health*, **52**:1391–1400, 1962.
Armstrong, R. W.: "Type E Botulism from Home-canned Gefillte Fish," *J.A.M.A.*, **210**:303–305, 1969.
Bird, K.: "The Food Processing Front of the Seventies," *J. Am. Diet. Assoc.*, **58**:103–108, 1971.
Brooke, M. M.: "Epidemiology of Amebiasis in the U.S.," *J.A.M.A.*, **188**:519–21, 1964.
Bryan, F. L.: "Microbiological Food Hazards Today Based on Epidemiological Information," *Food Technol.*, **28**:52, Sept. 1974.
Expert Panel on Food Safety and Nutrition, Institute of Food Technologists: *"Phthalates in Food,"* *Nutr. Rev.*, **32**:126–28, 1974.
Food Protection Committee, National Academy of Sciences: "The Use of Chemicals in Food Production, Processing, Storage and Distribution," *Nutr. Rev.*, **31**:191–98, 1973.

Hodges, R. E.: "The Toxicity of Pesticides and Their Residues in Food," *Nutr. Rev.*, **23**:225–30, 1965.

Jukes, T. H.: "Estrogens in Beefsteaks," *J.A.M.A.*, **229**:1920–21, 1974.

Jukes, T. H.: "Fact and Fancy in Nutrition and Food Science: Chemical Residues in Foods," *J. Am. Diet. Assoc.*, **59**:203–11, 1971.

Longrée, K.: "Sanitation in Food Vending," *J. Am. Diet. Assoc.*, **54**:215–20, 1969.

Marshall, W. E.: "Health Foods, Organic Foods, Natural Foods," *Food Technol.*, **28**:50, Feb. 1974.

Merson, M. H., *et al.*: "Current Trends in Botulism in the United States," *J.A.M.A.*, **229**:1305–1308, 1974.

Moses, W. R., and Pippin, H. N.: "Chemical Preservatives," *FDA Papers*, **4**:25–28, Feb. 1970.

Review: "Nitrosamines and Cancer," *Nutr. Rev.*, **33**:19–20, 1975.

Review: "Patulin, a Carcinogenic Mycotoxin Found in Cider," *Nutr. Rev.*, **32**:55–56, 1974.

Schroeder, S. A., *et al.*: "Epidemic Salmonellosis in Hospitals and Institutions," *N. Engl. J. Med.*, **279**:674–78, 1968.

Somers, E.: "The Toxic Potential of Trace Metals in Foods," *J. Food Sci.*, **39**:215, 1974.

Taylor, A., Jr.: "Botulism and Its Control," *Am. J. Nurs.*, **73**:1380–82, 1973.

Tschirley, F. H.: "Pesticides: Relation to Environmental Quality," *J.A.M.A.*, **224**:1157–59, 1973.

Werrin, M., and Kronick, D.: "Salmonella Control in Hospitals," *Am. J. Nurs.*, **65**:528–31, 1965.

PUBLICATIONS FOR THE LAYMAN

Available from Consumer Information, Manufacturing Chemists Association, 1825 Connecticut Ave., N.W. Washington, D.C.:
Everyday Facts About Food Additives
Food Additives: What They Are. How They Are Used, 1972.
Why Chemicals? 1973.
Keeping Food Safe to Eat, HG 162, Government Printing Office, Washington, D.C.
We Want You to Know about Protecting Your Family from Foodborne Illness, FDA Pub. 74–2003, Government Printing Office, Washington, D.C.

18 Controls for the Safety and Nutritive Value of the Food Supply

You shall not eat anything that dies of itself.
DEUT. 14:21

You shall not have in your bag two kinds of weights, a large and a small. You shall not have in your house two kinds of measures, a large and a small. A full and just weight you shall have, a full and just measure you shall have.
DEUT. 25:13–15

These Biblical quotations are but two of the many laws concerning the use of food set down by Moses and others. Although examples may be found throughout history of efforts to exercise some controls over the food supply, the major advances have come in the present century.

NEED FOR FOOD LAWS

Changing national environment. The growth of an urban society and the revolutionary developments in science and technology have necessitated numerous controls to protect consumers. In the early days of this nation consumers, for the most part, were also the producers. They grew the crops, raised the cattle, preserved the food by methods then available, and cooked the food in their own homes. By and large, those not engaged in agriculture purchased food from sellers who were known on a personal basis. Even in colonial history, however, one can find examples of laws designed to protect consumers against fraud.

With the industrial development and movement to cities people became dependent upon growers, manufacturers, and distributors for the food supply. Not all practices were honest. In fact, the conditions for sanitation in food processing and marketing by the end of the nineteenth century were often described as appalling. Far too common were fraudulent practices whereby the products were diluted with some cheap and unsafe ingredient so that a greater profit could be realized. Over these unsavory practices the consumer had little control.

Advances in science and technology. The twentieth-century developments in microbiology have provided the rationale for good practices in handling food and have served as the basis for setting up controls which might be exercised for a safe food supply. The chemists' laboratory has opened hitherto undreamed-of possibilities for variety in the food supply, preservation, and improvement of nutritional quality, but it has also created vast problems in controls from farm, to factory, to warehouse, and to market. Today's farmer fertilizes his soil with products purchased from a chemical plant; he dusts and sprays his crops; he uses hormones to accelerate the growth of animals. The manufacturer chooses from hundreds of chemical products to improve the color, flavor, texture, nutritional quality, and keeping properties of his product. Chemicals of some sort enter into the numerous steps in food production—from the sanitation of the plant machinery to the package in which the food is sold. Without these aids from the chemical industry, this country could not produce its abundant supply of high-quality food.

Role of the food industry. Much credit for the remarkable improvements in the food supply must be given to responsible growers, manufacturers, and distributors. A visit to a modern food plant can be an exciting experience. One is impressed with the systems developed for the quality grading of food as it is received, the complex machinery for handling food from raw product to package, the continuous emphasis upon sanitation, and the attractiveness of the finished product. The laboratories in such a plant are at the very center of the successful operation. On the one hand, they are concerned with quality control; on the other, they are developing products for tomorrow's market basket. Many specialists are employed in the maintenance of controls and development of new products—agricultural specialists, food scientists, chefs, microbiologists, chemists, biochemists, nutritionists, and home economists, to name but a few.

Good laws aid industry, for they provide guidelines for good manufacturing practice and protect against unfair competition through dishonest labeling and adulteration. Federal agencies of the Department of Agriculture and of Health, Education, and Welfare work closely with manufacturers on problems which arise in food production.

Consumer interest. During the 1960s many groups of people became concerned about the environment and the appropriate uses to which finite resources were being put. Major influences in the thinking were the book *Silent Spring* by Rachel Carson and environmental organizations such as the Sierra Club, National Audubon Society, and Environmental Defense Fund. Although Dr. Carson in her book and these groups took an exaggerated position, they also alerted responsible scientists to the need for additional research to establish effective controls.

In the late 1960s a television documentary and especially the Ten-State Nutrition Survey indicated that malnutrition was more prevalent in the people of the United States than had been generally believed. The White House Conference on Food, Nutrition, and Health in 1969 engaged not only professional persons in nutrition and health fields but representatives from industry and many consumer groups. The public has become sensitized to the issues of nutrition as never before and has requested an accounting, as it were, from industry and also from governmental agencies. One of the major recommendations made at this conference pertained to the establishment of regulations concerning nutrition information, based upon the consumer's "right to know."

FOOD, DRUG, AND COSMETIC ACT

One of the principal crusaders in the movement to secure legislation for a wholesome food supply was Dr. Harvey W. Wiley, who was a chief chemist for the U.S. Department of Agriculture. Through his writings and his public appearances he sought the cooperation of women's groups and was instrumental in the enactment in 1906 of the first "pure food" law, the Food and Drug Act. The law, signed by President Theodore Roosevelt, has been represented by some as the most significant peacetime legislation in the history of the country.

Food, Drug, and Cosmetic Act. With rapid advances in food technology and industry, the manufacture and distribution of food became increasingly complex and broader in scale so that the original law became inadequate. Many consumer pressures in the 1930s led to the enactment of the Food, Drug, and Cosmetic Act of 1938. The objectives of the law have been summarized as "safe, effective drugs, and cosmetics; pure, wholesome foods; honest labeling and packaging."[1] The Food and Drug Administration (FDA) is an agency of the Department of Health, Education, and Welfare charged with the responsibility for the enforcement of this act and its amendments.

Additive amendments. The Food, Drug, and Cosmetic Act has been amended a number of times to meet new problems of control as they have arisen. Although additives are essential for high-quality food in sufficient supply for a rapidly expanding population, the introduction of thousands of such products on the market necessitates legal controls for safety and usefulness. For such protection, these amendments to the 1938 law have been enacted:

1954: Pesticides Amendment.
1958: Food Additives Amendment, including intentional and incidental additives.
1960: Color Additive Amendments.

An important regulation in the additives amendment is the Delaney clause. This states that an additive is prohibited if at any level of feeding whatsoever it induces cancer in an experimental animal.

The GRAS list. At the time the Food Additives Amendment was enacted about 600 substances were excluded from testing since they had been used over long periods of time and they were "generally recognized as safe" (GRAS). Among the items on the GRAS list are salt, baking powder, baking soda, spices, and minerals and vitamins for nutritional purposes. The GRAS list is continually being reevaluated. As new research is completed items may remain on the list or may be removed. The removal of cyclamates a few years ago is an example.

Before an additive may be marketed approval must be secured from the Food and Drug Administration, which has spelled out in some detail the requirements that must be met. Essentially, these amendments place the burden of proof for usefulness and safety of a food additive upon the manufacturer, who is required to submit full data which includes name, chemical properties, methods for manufacture, quantities to be used, the conditions for use, the effect of additions on the food, methods for detecting residues in foods, safety, and recommended tolerances. Data pertaining to safety must include toxicity tests on two or more species of animals, usually for a two-year period; estimates of the maximum amounts which might be consumed in a day; and the cumulative effects upon the body.

The Food and Drug Administration may conduct further tests after examination of the manufacturer's data. Approval will include specific limits for amounts and conditions of use. If a request is denied, the manufacturer may appeal the decision, submit additional data, and request a hearing.

Regulation of pesticides. The public concern about pesticides in the early 1960s led to the appointment by President Kennedy in 1963 of a Science Advisory Committee which later issued a report recognizing the advantages that pesticides had played in food production and disease control, but also calling for "orderly reduction in the use of persistent pesticides."[*] Intensive study of the effects of pesticides has been conducted by toxicologists and public health officials. In March 1969 the Food and Drug Administration found that shipments of coho salmon from Lake Michigan contained DDT far in excess of safe tolerances. This was a threat to public health and also to the fishing industry, and a commission was appointed to study the problem. In November 1969 the Commission on Pesticides set forth these principles:

1. Chemicals, including pesticides used to increase food production, are of such importance in modern life that we must learn to live with them;
2. In looking at their relative merits and hazards we must make individual judgments upon the value of each

chemical, including the alternatives presented by the nonuse of these chemicals. We must continue to accumulate scientific data about the effects of these chemicals on the total ecology; and
3. The final decision regarding the usage of these chemicals must be made by those governmental agencies with the statutory responsibilities for the public health, and for pesticides regulations.[*]

The Commission made 14 recommendations to the Secretary of Health, Education, and Welfare.[2] Some of these have been implemented and others require legislative action. Among the recommendations are these:

Close cooperation between the Departments of Agriculture, Health, Education, and Welfare, and Interior.

Elimination of the use of DDT and DDD within two years except where essential for human health and welfare.

Restriction on the use of other persistent pesticides.

Development of standards for pesticide content of foods, water, and air so that the public is protected from hazards, but also recognizing the need for an optimum food supply.

Reviewing adequacy of legislation pertaining to the labeling and instructions for use of pesticides, the packaging and transportation to avoid spillage and contamination of other materials, and control of effluents from plants manufacturing pesticides; and others.

Fair Packaging and Labeling Act. In 1966 the Congress authorized the FDA to set up requirements for complete information in labeling and for packaging that is not deceptive in terms of the contents. This act supplements the 1938 law. Included are these label regulations:[3]

1. A statement of identity of a food, under its usual or common name such as *peaches* or *beets*, must appear in bold type on the principal display panel. If a standard of identity (see page 276) has been established for the product, the name shall appear as it is stated in the standard. When a food is packed in various forms such as whole, sliced, or chopped, the form shall be prominently shown with the name of the product except when a see-through container is used.
2. The name and full business address of the manufacturer, packer, or distributor shall be conspicuously shown, indicating "packed for" or "distributed by" if the name is not that of the manufacturer.
3. A statement of the net contents separated from other

[*] Ramsey, L. L.: "A Twilight for Persistent Pesticides," *FDA Papers*, 4:14–18, Feb. 1970.

[*] *Ibid.*, pp. 16–17.

label information shall appear in legible boldface type within the bottom 30 per cent of the principal display panel.

4. When a label includes a statement of the number of servings, the usual size of that serving shall be stated, for example, in cups or tablespoons.

5. When ingredient listing is required, the information shall appear in a single panel listing by common name in decreasing order of predominance.

Meat and Poultry Inspection Acts

The "pure food" law of 1906 did not include meat and meat products. The Meat Inspection Act, passed in 1906, is enforced by the Meat Inspection Division of the Agricultural Research Service in the U.S. Department of Agriculture. The Poultry Inspection Act passed in 1957, with regulations similar to the Meat Inspection Act, requires the inspection of poultry and poultry products that enter interstate commerce. These laws provide for (1) the inspection of animals intended for slaughter; (2) the inspection of carcasses and all meat products; (3) enforcement of sanitary regulations; (4) guarding against the use of harmful preservatives. Federal inspection stamps (see Figure 18–1.) are placed upon the surface of the carcass if the meat is wholesome. The flesh of an animal that is diseased is stamped "inspected and condemned" and the carcass must be destroyed or may be used for nonfood purposes if warranted. (See Figure 18–2.)

Two laws recently enacted are the 1967 Federal Wholesome Meat Act and the 1968 Federal Wholesome Poultry Products Act.[4] These laws give authority to the U.S. Department of Agriculture to seize meat and poultry products that are moved illegally or that have become adulterated or misbranded after leaving official premises. An important part of these laws sets up a cooperative arrangement between state and federal inspection programs. This provides better protection for the consumer of meat and poultry products within a given state. Preventive sanitation is an important part of the inspection program.

Law Enforcement and Specific Regulations

Food and Drug Administration. The enforcement of the Food, Drug, and Cosmetic Act is the responsibility of the Food and Drug Administration of the U.S. Public Health Service. One aspect of the program is research by specialists to determine the physical and chemical characteristics of products and to develop improved methods to detect deviations from the standards that have been set up. For this work pharmacologists, microbiologists, entomologists, chemists, biochemists, veterinarians, and physicians are involved.

The Food and Drug Administration also conducts educational programs pertaining to voluntary compliance activities directed to the manufacturer. More recently nutritionists and dietitians have been appointed to serve as consumer consultants. The educational activities are especially important for the recently adopted regulations on nutrition labeling. (See page 278.)

The federal laws cover thousands of establishments that process foods which enter interstate commerce and foods which are imported. Inspectors visit factories, warehouses, and stores to see that the laws are being complied with. They are concerned with the raw materials used, the processes of manufacturing, the packaging and storage practices, and plant sanitation. (See Figure 18–3.)

If inspectors find violations of the law they may remove the food from the market or require that the labeling be revised. Depending on the circumstances, the food may be destroyed, or it may be reclaimed and relabeled under the supervision of the inspectors.

Court proceedings become necessary for those who flagrantly violate the laws. Fines or imprisonment, or both, may be imposed for each violation.

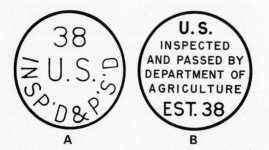

Figure 18–1. (A) Seal appearing as purple stamp on cuts of meat passed by the U.S. Department of Agriculture inspector. (B) Seal appearing on labels of prepared meat products. (Courtesy, U.S. Department of Agriculture.)

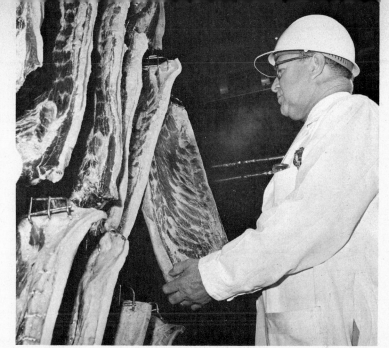

Figure 18–2. U.S. Department of Agriculture meat inspectors check for the wholesomeness of all meat products and meat produced in plants dealing in interstate or foreign commerce. An inspector examines bacon during processing at a smokehouse to make sure the processing is done according to approved formulas and procedures. (Courtesy, U.S. Department of Agriculture.)

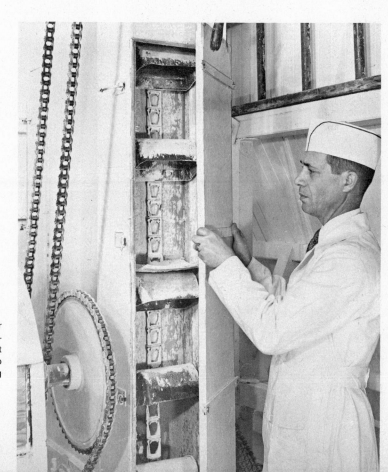

Figure 18–3. The FDA inspector knows that the interior of the elevator is a common place for insect development if flour is allowed to remain. (Courtesy, Food and Drug Administration.)

Injunctions may be issued by the court to prevent repetition of a violation.

Adulteration and misbranding. Under the law, definitions of adulteration and misbranding have been developed.

Adulteration of food has occurred if it contains any substance injurious to health; it contains any filthy, putrid, or decomposed substance; it is prepared, handled, or stored under unsanitary conditions; diseased animals have been used in preparation; the container is made of a poisonous substance which will render the contents harmful; valuable constituents have been omitted; substitutes have been used to conceal inferiority; it contains coal-tar colors other than those permitted by law; it contains pesticide residues or additives not recognized as safe.

Misbranding has occurred if the label is false or misleading; the food is sold under another name; imitations are not clearly indicated; the size of the container is misleading; statement of weight, measure, or count is not given or is wrong; manufacturer,

packer, or distributor is not listed on the package forms; it is below standard without indication of substandard quality on the label; it fails to list nutrient information when nutrients have been added or when claims are made for nutritional properties; it fails to list artificial colorings, flavorings, and preservatives.

Standards. A *standard of identity* establishes what a product really is. A product which has been so defined must include specified ingredients, often with amounts restricted to designated minimum-maximum ranges. For example, the standard of identity for Cheddar cheese specifies a minimum of 50 per cent milk fat (on a moisture-free basis) and not more than 25 per cent moisture. Fruit jelly and preserves must contain not less than 45 parts by weight of fruit or fruit juice to 55 parts total sweetener. Optional ingredients listed in the standard may be used, but any ingredients that are not mentioned in the standard are forbidden. (See Figure 18–4.)

The standards are set up after consultation with

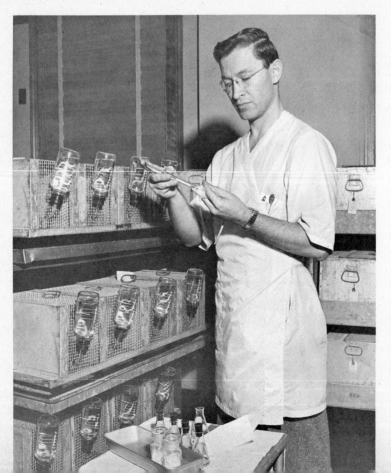

Figure 18–4. An FDA chemist checks the vitamin D content of milk by feeding a test dose to a laboratory animal. After a given period of time the bone calcification will be measured by the line test shown in Figure 10–5. (Courtesy, Food and Drug Administration.)

numerous sources for the customary practices in manufacture and preparation. Proposals for new standards are published in the Federal Register. Opportunity is then given for interested parties, including manufacturers and consumers, to study the proposed regulations and to recommend changes. If there is any controversy, public hearings may be held.

The label for a food for which a standard of identity has been set does not need to include a listing of required ingredients since these are defined within the standard. However, a recently proposed regulation would require the listing of ingredients as for other nonstandardized products. Such listing would be of great assistance to many consumers who have allergies to some food substance or who require some kind of modified diet.

Among the products for which standards of identity have been established are: chocolate and cocoa products; cereal flours and related products; macaroni and noodle products; bakery products; milk and cream; cheese and cheese products; frozen desserts; dressings for foods—mayonnaise, French dressing, salad dressing; canned fruit and canned fruit juices; fruit butters—jellies, preserves; shellfish; canned tuna; eggs and egg products; oleomargarine—margarine; vegetables and vegetable products.

Standards of quality indicate the minimum quality below which foods must not fall. Foods that do not meet the quality specifications must be labeled "Below Standard in Quality" followed by a statement such as "Good Food—Not High Grade" or "Excessively Broken," etc. Canned foods that do not meet standards of quality are seldom seen on the market.

Standards for fill aim to protect the customer against deception through the use of containers that appear to contain more food than they actually do. Specifications are set up for foods that tend to shake down in the package, or for number of pieces of food within a container.

Other regulations. The Food and Drug Administration has proposed many regulations including (1) principles governing nutrient additions to food; (2) nutritional quality guidelines for fortified foods (hot breakfast cereals, ready-to-eat cereals, formulated meal replacements, breakfast beverages); (3) uniform listing of ingredients on food labels and prohibition of misleading vignettes; (4) ingredients and

nutrition information for heat-and-serve dinners; (5) labeling of fats and oils with respect to their sources (e.g., peanut); (6) standard serving sizes for breakfast beverages, cereals, milk beverages, formulated meal replacements; (7) uniform method of declaring percentages of ingredients in foods.[5]

ENRICHMENT POLICIES AND REGULATIONS

General policies. In 1961 the Food and Nutrition Board of the National Research Council and the Council on Foods and Nutrition of the American Medical Association adopted jointly a statement of general policy regarding addition of specific nutrients to foods. This statement was revised and reaffirmed in 1968 and again in 1973. The following continue to be endorsed:

The enrichment of flour, bread, degerminated cornmeal, corn grits, wholegrain cornmeal, white rice, and certain other cereal grain products with thiamin, riboflavin, niacin, and iron; the addition of vitamin D to milk, fluid skim milk, and nonfat dry milk; the addition of vitamin A to margarine, fluid skim milk, and nonfat dry milk; and the addition of iodine to table salt. The protective action of fluoride against dental caries is recognized and the standardized addition of fluoride to water in areas in which the water supply has a low fluoride content is endorsed.[°]

The addition of nutrients to foods is endorsed when all of the following criteria are met:

1. The intake of the nutrient(s) is below the desirable level in the diets of a significant number of people;
2. The food(s) used to supply the nutrient(s) is likely to be consumed in quantities that will make a significant contribution to the diet of the population in need;
3. The addition of nutrient(s) is not likely to create a dietary imbalance;
4. The nutrient(s) added is stable under customary conditions of storage and use;
5. The nutrient(s) is physiologically available from the food;
6. The enhanced levels attained in the total diet will not be harmfully excessive for those who may employ the foods in varying patterns of use; and
7. The additional cost is reasonable for the intended consumer.[†]

° "General Policies in Regard to Improvement of Nutritive Quality of Foods," *Nutr. Rev.*, **31**:324–26, 1973.

† *Ibid.*, p. 325.

With the introduction of numerous formulated foods and also fabricated foods additional guidelines are necessary. A FORMULATED FOOD is a mixture of two or more ingredients such as many convenience foods. A FABRICATED FOOD is a complex mixture of ingredients that may or may not resemble an existing conventional food, for example, a soy protein analog of meat. If one serving of such foods furnishes 5 per cent or more of the RDA for calories, it becomes an important part of the diet. It is recommended that additions of nutrients to such foods should be "according to a concept of a calculated nutrient density."° For example, if a serving of food furnishes 240 kcal or 10 per cent of the recommended allowance, then the nutrient content should also furnish approximately 10 per cent of the recommended allowances.

If a product replaces a meal—for example, a frozen dinner—it should furnish 25 to 50 per cent of the nutrients except calories. Fabricated foods that are analogs to conventional foods should supply the same variety and quantities of essential nutrients that are present in the foods they replace.

Enrichment standards. The enrichment of foods is not required by federal law, but approximately 85 to 90 per cent of cereals, flours, and breads are now enriched. When enrichment nutrients are added to foods, they must comply to standards established by the Food and Drug Administration. A revision of the standards was recently proposed so that increased amounts of iron would be included. Table 18–1 presents the proposed standards.

° Council on Foods and Nutrition: "Improvement of the Nutritive Quality of Foods. General Policies," *J.A.M.A.*, **225:**1116, 1973.

The standards for other voluntary additions of nutrients to food include:

1. Vitamin A fortification of margarine: 15,000 U.S.P. units per pound to compare with the year-round average for butter.

2. Vitamin fortification of milk: 400 U.S.P. units per quart or tall can of evaporated milk. Most fluid and evaporated milk is now fortified.

NUTRITION LABELING

One of the major recommendations of the White House Conference on Food, Nutrition, and Health in 1969 was that the label on food products should contain nutrition information. Experts from the Food and Nutrition Board of the National Research Council, the American Dietetic Association, the American Institute of Nutrition, the American Home Economics Association, the Institute of Food Technology, the food industry, and consumers have been consulted by the Food and Drug Administration to determine the uses to which labeling might be put and to formulate the standards for such labeling.

Purposes served. The principal reason for nutrition labeling is that the consumer has a right to know what is in the foods he purchases so that he can make better decisions for his own well-being and that of his children. A consumer can compare one product with another to determine which product offers the best nutritive values for the money. One important result of such comparisons is that the consumer gradually becomes aware of the good and poor sources of nutrients. Labeling also leads food

Table 18–1. Standards of Identity for Enriched Flour, Bread, Rolls, and Buns*

	Thiamin mg/lb	Riboflavin mg/lb	Niacin† mg/lb	Iron mg/lb
Enriched flour‡	2.9	1.8	24	40
Enriched self-rising flour‡	2.9	1.8	24	40
Enriched bread, rolls, or buns‡	1.8	1.1	15	25

*"Standards of Identity," *Nutr. Rev.*, **32:**29, 1974.

† Niacin equivalents as derived from tryptophan equivalents shall not be used in determining total niacin content.

‡ Calcium is an optional addition. A claim on the label as an included nutrient can only be stated if the calcium content is 960 mg per pound for flour or 600 mg per pound for bread, rolls, or buns.

Table 18-2. United States Recommended Daily Allowances (U.S. RDA)

Mandatory Nutrients		Optional Nutrients	
Protein		Vitamin D	400 I.U.
Protein quality equal to or		Vitamin E	30 I.U.
greater than casein	45 gm	Vitamin B_6	2.0 mg
Protein quality less than casein	65 gm	Folic acid (folacin)	0.4 mg
Vitamin A	5000 I.U.	Vitamin B_{12}	6 mcg
Vitamin C (ascorbic acid)	60 mg	Phosphorus	1.0 gm
Thiamin (vitamin B_1)	1.5 mg	Iodine	150 mcg
Riboflavin (vitamin B_2)	1.7 mg	Magnesium	400 mg
Niacin	20 mg	Zinc	15 mg
Calcium	1.0 gm	Copper	2 mg
Iron	18 mg	Biotin	0.3 mg
		Pantothenic acid	10 mg

processors to be constantly aware of the nutritive values of the foods that they produce. Nutrition labeling is a useful teaching tool in the classroom and in education of the public. Labeling will help persons who require modified diets to select those foods appropriate for their needs. One urgent reason for labeling is the identification of the nutritive values of the numerous fabricated foods that food technology has made possible. With such information the consumer can decide whether the fabricated food is an appropriate replacement for an ordinary food.

Regulations for labeling. For many processed foods labeling is *voluntary*. The manufacturer may choose to include nutrition information because it places his product in fair competition with others. There are two circumstances when labeling is *mandatory*:

1. If any nutrient is added to a food, even if that nutrient is only replacing one taken out in processing; thus, enriched or fortified foods must be labeled.

2. If any claim is made for nutritional properties on the label or in advertising; all foods for special dietary use would require labeling. (See page 281.)

The labeling standard. The Food and Drug Administration has developed the United States Recommended Dietary Allowances (U.S. RDA). (See Table 18-2.) This standard replaces the Minimum Daily Requirements (MDR) used for many years in the labeling for vitamin and mineral supplements, breakfast cereals, and so on. The U.S. RDA for

adults and children over four years of age is based upon the Recommended Daily Allowances of the Food and Nutrition Board. It represents the amounts of nutrients needed daily by healthy adults, plus approximately 30 to 50 per cent margin to allow for individual variations. Many adults need only two thirds to three fourths of the U.S. RDA and many children about half.[6] The standards include some nutrients not listed in the Recommended Dietary Allowances but for which requirements have been estimated. The nutrient information listed by the manufacturer on a label must be based upon laboratory analyses of the product; calculations of nutritive values are not adequate.

Labeling standards have also been set up for infants under 12 months and for children under four years for the labeling of baby foods and vitamin-mineral supplements. Another standard has been set up for pregnant and lactating women pertaining especially to the mineral and vitamin supplements often recommended for use.

Labeling format. Nutrition labeling must follow a standard format. (See Figure 18-5.) The information shall be placed on a panel to the right of the principal panel. The kinds of information required and the sequence are as follows:

1. Serving size and number of servings in container
2. Calories in one serving
3. Protein, carbohydrate, and fat in grams per serving

NUTRITION INFORMATION
(PER SERVING)
SERVING SIZE = 1 OZ.
SERVINGS PER CONTAINER = 12

CALORIES	110
PROTEIN	2 GRAMS
CARBOHYDRATE	24 GRAMS
FAT	0 GRAM

PERCENTAGE OF U.S. RECOMMENDED DAILY
ALLOWANCES (U.S. RDA)*

PROTEIN	2
THIAMIN	8
NIACIN	2

*Contains less than 2 percent of U.S. RDA for vitamin A, vitamin C, riboflavin, calcium and iron.

NUTRITION INFORMATION
(PER SERVING)
SERVING SIZE = 8 OZ.
SERVINGS PER CONTAINER = 1

CALORIES	560
PROTEIN	23 GM
CARBOHYDRATE	43 GM

FAT (PERCENT OF CALORIES 53%) ..... 33 GM
POLYUNSATURATED* ..... 2 GM
SATURATED ..... 9 GM
CHOLESTEROL* (20 MG/100 GM) .... 40 MG
SODIUM (365 MG/ 100 GM) ..... 830 MG

PERCENTAGE OF U.S. RECOMMENDED DAILY
ALLOWANCES (U.S. RDA)

PROTEIN	35	RIBOFLAVIN	15
VITAMIN A	35	NIACIN	25
VITAMIN C (ASCORBIC ACID)	10	CALCIUM	2
		IRON	25
THIAMIN (VITAMIN B_1)	15		

*Information on fat and cholesterol content is provided for individuals who, on the advice of a physician, are modifying their total dietary intake of fat and cholesterol.

This is the minimum information that must appear on a nutrition label.

A label may include optional listings for cholesterol, fats, and sodium.

Figure 18–5. Regulations for labeling for nutrition information have been established by the Food and Drug Administration. (Courtesy, Food and Drug Administration.)

4. Percentages of the U.S. RDA provided by one serving for protein, vitamins A and C, thiamin, riboflavin, niacin, calcium, and iron.

Optional information may be included in the panel. If it is used it must follow the recommended format and must comply with the U.S. RDA standards:

1. Fat and cholesterol content, including
   a. Per cent of calories from fat
   b. Polyunsaturated fatty acids and saturated fatty acids in grams per serving
   c. Cholesterol in milligrams per serving and per 100 gm of food
   d. Footnote which reads as follows: "Information on fat and cholesterol is provided for individuals who, on the advice of a physician, are modifying their total dietary intake of fat and cholesterol."
2. Vitamins D, E, B_6, folacin, vitamin B_{12}, phosphorus, iodine, magnesium, zinc, copper, biotin, and pantothenic acid.

What labeling does not do. People could add up the percentages for each nutrient from various foods and thus conclude that their diets were fully adequate if the total were 100 per cent or more for each listed nutrient. Such a conclusion might, in fact, be justified if the totals resulted from a wide variety of ordinary foods. However, if the choice is restricted to a few food items or if an important part of the intake consists of fabricated foods, it is quite likely that the combinations will not furnish all of the 45 to 50 nutrients required by man even though the percentages for the listed nutrients all add up to 100 or more. As fabricated foods become more prominent in the diet, the danger of nutritive inadequacy increases. Although the manufacturer of such products may indeed be producing a food that is high in the listed nutrients, some trace elements about which relatively little is known could be omitted, for example, chromium, selenium, molybdenum, and manganese. Labeling does not require listing of sodium and potassium, both of which are essential. Ordinarily the diet contains more than enough sodium, but the margin of potassium may not be great. In other words, the best advice for dietary planning still is the selection of a wide variety of foods from all of the important food groups.

Special dietary foods. All foods used for modified diets must be labeled with full nutrition information according to the format described above. In addition, five prohibitions have been set up for the labeling of these foods:°

1. With certain exceptions, it prohibits any claim or promotional suggestion that products intended to supplement diets are sufficient in themselves to prevent, treat, or cure disease.
2. It prohibits any implication that a diet of ordinary foods cannot supply adequate nutrients.
3. It prohibits all claims that inadequate or insufficient diet is due to the soil in which a food is grown.
4. It prohibits all claims that transportation, storage, or cooking of foods may result in inadequate or deficient diet.
5. It prohibits nutritional claims for nonnutritive ingredients such as rutin, other bioflavonoids, para-aminobenzoic acid, inositol, and similar ingredients, and prohibits their combination with essential nutrients.

OTHER AGENCY ACTIVITIES

Federal Trade Commission. Many consumer groups have been very critical of food advertising, especially that which appears on children's programs on television. The Federal Trade Commission in November 1974 proposed regulations for food advertising that closely follow the principles of nutrition labeling.[7] These regulations define the conditions under which claims can be made for nutrients present in a food and the conditions under which terms such as "loaded with ———," "nutritious," "wholesome," and "nourishing" may be used. When one product is compared with another, the basis must be equal-size servings of food. Adver-

° "The New Look in Food Labels," DHEW Pub. (FDA) 73–2036, Washington, D.C., 1973.

tising regulations are also set up for "organic" foods; "natural" foods; fats, fatty acids, and cholesterol; special diet foods; and health and health-related claims.

U.S. Public Health Service. One of the concerns of the Public Health Service is the effect of diet on nutritional status and health, and it has sponsored research to make these determinations. The safety of the food supply is another concern that leads to the promulgation of sanitary codes and ordinances. During outbreaks of food poisoning the Public Health Service conducts tests to determine the source and nature of the poisoning.

The Public Health Service has defined standards for milk production and quality that provide the basis for the codes used in most states and communities. It also certifies interstate milk shippers.

Food Protection Committee. To study the legitimate uses of chemical additives, the Food Protection Committee was established in 1950 as a permanent committee of the Food and Nutrition Board. The membership of the committee includes specialists who are qualified to establish criteria for the evaluation of additives on the basis of their chemical and physical properties, their toxicologic aspects when tested in several species, and their metabolic and nutritional aspects.

The Food Protection Committee acts as a clearing house for information on pesticides and intentional additives; it reviews the information and makes it available; it assists in the integration and promotion of research on foods; it aids regulatory agencies such as the Food and Drug Administration in the formulation of principles and standardized procedures; it aids in the dissemination of accurate information to the public.

State and local regulations. Food that is produced and sold within state boundaries does not come under control of federal agencies. Therefore, states and communities must establish their own regulations for the safety and quality of foods. The identity of foods, the labeling, and the inspection of plants, markets, and public eating places are subject to controls set up by the state departments of agriculture and health. Some cities and states require periodic medical examination of food handlers. Most of the regulations are patterned after those of federal laws, but considerable variations exist, nevertheless, from state to state.

PROBLEMS AND REVIEW

1. What reasons can you give for the need for federal legislation concerning the food supply?
2. What is the aim of the Food, Drug, and Cosmetic Act? Under its provisions what is meant by misbranding? Adulteration?
3. What provisions are included in the Meat Inspection Act?
4. Where does the primary responsibility for proving the safety of an additive rest? What information is essential for establishing this safety?
5. What purposes are served by nutrition labeling?
6. Compare the nutrition labeling for three brands of ready-to-eat cereals. Which is the best buy? Why?
7. Compare two margarines that carry nutritional labeling for fat and cholesterol. Which supplies the greater amount of polyunsaturated fatty acids? On the basis of cost is such a difference justified?
8. *Problem.* Watch television advertising for three food products. Note especially the words used to describe products and the claims for the products. Look for labels on the packages of these products in a market. What conclusions can you make regarding this advertising?
9. Determine the governmental agency in your community that is responsible for controlling the sale of milk; the sale of meat within your state; the inspection of public eating places.
10. *Problem.* Prepare a short paper (about 300 words) that describes the activities of any one of the following organizations in promoting a safe food supply: Food Protection Committee; your state department of health; your state department of agriculture; the U.S. Public Health Service; the Federal Trade Commission.

CITED REFERENCES

1. Larrick, G. P.: "The Role of the Food and Drug Administration in Nutrition," *Am. J. Clin. Nutr.,* **8:**377–82, 1960.
2. Ramsey, L. L.: "A Twilight for Persistent Pesticides," *FDA Papers,* **4:**14–18, Feb. 1970.
3. Friedelson, L.: "Fair Packaging," *FDA Papers,* **1:**21–24, Oct. 1967.
4. "New Meat Inspection Laws for Consumer Protection," *Public Health Rep.,* **84:**214, 1960.
5. "Food Labeling: Phase IV," *J. Nutr. Educ.,* **6:**86–87, 1974.
6. "Nutrition Labels and U.S. RDA," U.S. Department of Health, Education, and Welfare, FDA Pub. 73–2042, Washington, D.C., 1973.
7. "FTC Issues Initial Proposals on Food Advertising," *J. Am. Diet. Assoc.,* **66:**70, 1975.

ADDITIONAL REFERENCES

Anderson, O. E.: *The Health of a Nation: Harvey W. Wiley and the Fight for Pure Food.* University of Chicago Press, Chicago, 1958.

Bauman, H. E.: "What Is the Food Industry Doing on Nutritive Problems?" *Bull. N.Y. Acad. Med.,* **47:**601–605, 1971.

Chadwick, D. R.: "The Public Health Role in Controlling Radiation," *Am. J. Public Health,* **55:**731–37, 1965.

Cooke, J. A.: "Nutritional Guidelines and the Labeling of Foods," *J. Am. Diet. Assoc.,* **59:**99–101, 1971.

Darby, W. J.: "Man—His Environment and Health. Part II. Pesticides: A Contribution to Agriculture and Nutrition," *Am. J. Public Health,* **54** (Supplement):18–23, Jan. 1964.

Food and Nutrition Board: "General Policies in Regard to Improvement of Nutritive Quality of Foods," *Nutr. Rev.,* **31:**324–26, 1973.

Food Technologists' Expert Panel on Food Safety and Nutrition: "Nutrition Labeling," *Nutr. Rev.,* **32:**251–55, 1974.

Food Protection Committee, Food and Nutrition Board, Selected Publications:
   Chemicals Used in Food Processing, Pub. 1274, 1965.

An Evaluation of Public Health Hazards from the Microbiological Contamination of Foods, Pub. 1195, 1964.

Evaluating the Safety of Food Chemicals, Pub. 1859, 1970.

Johnson, O. C.: "The Food and Drug Administration and Labeling," *J. Am. Diet. Assoc.,* **64**:471–75, 1974.

Meyer, W.: "Role of Industry in Implementing Good Nutritional Practice," *Bull. N.Y. Acad. Med.,* **47**:644–46, 1971.

Moore, J. L., and Wendt, P. F.: "Nutrition Labeling—A Summary and Evaluation," *J. Nutr. Educ.,* **5**:121–25, 1973.

Patterson, M. I., and Marble, B.: "Dietetic Foods," *Am. J. Clin. Nutr.,* **16**:440–44, 1965.

Review: "Nutrition Labeling—II," *Nutr. Rev.,* **31**:133–34, 1973.

————: "Nutrition Labeling—III," *Nutr. Rev.,* **31**:260–64, 1973.

————: "Standards of Identity," *Nutr. Rev.,* **32**:29–30, 1974.

Ross, M. L.: "What's Happening to Food Labeling?" *J. Am. Diet. Assoc.,* **64**:262–67, 1974.

Stewart, G. F.: "Food Quality—A Focus for Togetherness for Food Scientists and Nutritionists. Commentary," *J. Nutr. Educ.,* **5**:9–10, 1973.

Vinz, G. L.: "The Compleat Inspector," *FDA Papers,* **2**:4, Sept. 1968.

Wodicka, V. O.: "The Role of Government in Implementing Good Nutritional Practice," *Bull. N.Y. Acad. Med.,* **47**:641–43, 1971.

Publications for the Layman

Bauer, W. W.: "Why Today's Bread Is Better," *Today's Health,* **44**:60–64, Dec. 1966.

Deutsch, R.: "Where You Should Be Shopping for Your Family," *Today's Health,* **50**:16, April 1972.

Earl, H. G.: "Food Poisoning: The Sneaky Attacker," *Today's Health,* **43**:64, Oct. 1965.

Food and Drug Administration, U.S. Department of Health, Education, and Welfare:

Additives in Our Foods, Pub. 43.

Metric Measures in Nutrition Labels, Pub. 74–2022.

FDA—What It Is and Does, Pub. 1.

How Safe Is Our Food? Pub. 41.

The New Look in Food Labels, Pub. 73–2036.

Nutrition Labeling—Terms You Should Know, Pub. 74–2010.

Nutrition Labels and U.S. RDA, Pub. 73–2042.

We Want You to Know About the Laws Enforced by FDA, Pub. 73–1031.

We Want You to Know About Nutrition Labels on Food, Pub. 74–2039.

19 Nutrition During Pregnancy and Lactation

The concept of maternal care is described as follows by the World Health Organization:[*]

The object of maternity care is to ensure that every expectant and nursing mother maintains good health, learns the art of child care, has a normal delivery, and bears healthy children. Maternity care in the narrower sense consists in the care of the pregnant woman, her safe delivery, her postnatal care and examination, the care of her newly born infant, and the maintenance of lactation. In the wider sense, it begins much earlier in measures aimed to promote the health and well-being of the young people who are potential parents, and to help them to develop the right approach to family life and to the place of the family in the community. It should also include guidance in parentcraft and in problems associated with infertility and family planning.

The Committee on Maternal Nutrition of the Food and Nutrition Board has recently issued a comprehensive report on the role of nutrition in human reproduction.[1] Two summaries of this report may be read with profit by the student who does not have time to study the detailed report.[2,3]

Some vital statistics. Maternal deaths in the United States decreased from 367 per 100,000 live births in 1940 to 20.8 in 1974.[1,4] These remarkable

[*]World Health Organization: *The Organization and Administration of Maternal and Child Health Services.* Fifth Report of the World Health Organization Expert Committee on Maternal and Child Care, WHO Tech. Rep. Ser. No. 428, Geneva, 1969.

improvements in the maternal mortality rate are not evenly distributed throughout the population. The mortality rate is higher in nonwhite women and appears to be associated with low income; when white and nonwhite women of similar income were compared there was little difference. Maternal deaths are highest in the teen-age groups.

In the United States for 1974 there were 16.5 infant deaths for each 1000 live births. This reflects steady improvement from decade to decade. For white infants there were 14.7 deaths per 1000 live births, and for nonwhite infants the rate was 24.6 deaths per 1000 live births. About two thirds of the infant deaths occur within the first month of life. Again, the mortality rate is higher for infants born to mothers of low income and to teen-age mothers. These differences reflect the adverse effects of low income, limited education, faulty nutrition, and other environmental factors.

The infant with a birth weight of less than 2500 gm has less chance of survival than does the infant who is larger. About 1 in 12 infants has a birth weight below this level. Even when low-birth-weight infants survive, there remains a long period of costly care and a continuing concern about establishing normal growth and development patterns.

NUTRITIONAL STUDIES

Folklore and diet in pregnancy. Since earliest times the diets of pregnant women have been considered to be of importance. The foods eaten by the pregnant woman were believed to convey to the unborn child not only certain physical characteristics but also desirable or undesirable attributes of behavior. Consequently, various societies set up rigid rules for the pregnant woman, including the foods she could eat, the foods she must not eat, and even the foods she must not touch lest she contaminate them for the rest of the community. Even today superstitions about foods and their desirability for the pregnant woman prevail among some people.

Some of the theories relating to nutrition that have been practiced by physicians are now known to be incorrect: the semistarvation of the mother with the view of a smaller baby and easier delivery;

the restriction of salt and fluids to reduce the incidence of toxemia; and the theory the maternal organism will produce a healthy baby reagardless of the mother's own state of nutrition.[3]

Factors influencing the outcome of pregnancy. On a probability basis, a mother who is well nourished prior to and during pregnancy is likely to have an uncomplicated pregnancy and to deliver a healthy infant. A poorly nourished woman is more likely to have complications during pregnancy and to bear a small infant in poor physical condition. There are, of course, exceptions. Some well-nourished mothers have problems during pregnancy and may not bear a healthy infant. Also, some poorly nourished mothers may have a successful pregnancy. Such exceptions are understandable when one considers the numerous factors influencing the outcome of pregnancy. (See Figure 19–1.)

The Committee on Maternal Nutrition has listed the following factors of importance in the incidence of low-birth-weight infants and the related neonatal mortality: "socioeconomic status of the mother, . . . biological immaturity (under 17 years of age), high parity, short stature, low prepregnancy weight for height, low gain in weight during pregnancy, poor nutritional status, smoking, certain infectious agents, chronic disease, complications of pregnancy, and a history of unsuccessful pregnancies."° Many of these factors will be considered in more detail in the discussion that follows.

Prematernal nutrition. The PERINATAL CONCEPT[5] assumes that the mother is in a good nutritional state prior to conception, and that this status will be maintained throughout pregnancy, labor, and the period after birth. Fewer complications in pregnancy, fewer premature births, and healthier babies result when the mother is well nourished prior to conception.

The influence of the quality of prematernal nutrition was strikingly demonstrated in World War II.[6] In Holland food rations were severely restricted from October 1944 to May 1945 so that pregnant women early in 1945 had less than 1000 kcal and 30 to 40 gm protein available. Prior to this period women had ingested diets that were reasonably adequate. The babies conceived before the hunger

° Committee on Maternal Nutrition: *Maternal Nutrition and the Course of Pregnancy: Summary Report.* Food and Nutrition Board, National Academy of Sciences—National Research Council, Washington, D.C., 1970, p. 4.

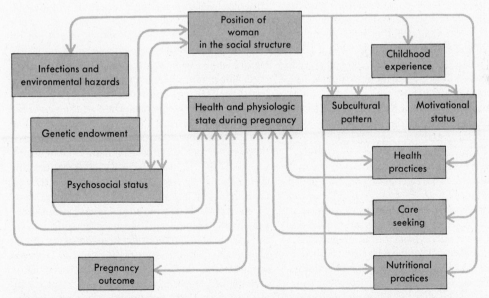

Figure 19–1. Factors influencing pregnancy outcome: a theoretical model. Reprinted with permission of *Nutrition Today,* Copyright Summer 1970 by Nutrition Today, Inc.; chart adapted by permission of the Food and Nutrition Board.)

period and born during the hunger period were shorter and had lower birth weights than those born before this time, this being a direct result of the mother's diet during the latter half of pregnancy. However, there was no increase in the rate of still births, prematurity, and malformations but the rate of conception fell off markedly during the hunger period.

During the siege of Leningrad acute food shortages occurred between August 1941 and February 1942. Prior to this time the food supplies had been inadequate so that women were chronically undernourished. During 1942 the birth rate fell off markedly, the stillbirth rate was twice as high, and prematurity had increased 41 per cent. The infants had low vitality, had poor resistance to infection, and did not suckle well. The better outcome in Holland was directly related to the better diets of women prior to conception.

Tompkins' studies in Philadelphia showed that women who are underweight at the time of conception have the greatest probability of premature labor and toxemia. He found a strikingly high incidence of prematurity in infants born of mothers who were both underweight and anemic.[7]

Difficult deliveries are more frequent in short than in tall women, according to studies reported from Scotland.[8] The more frequent occurrence of "flat pelvis" in short women was believed to be related to inadequate diet in childhood. Thus, a short stature may mean that a woman has not achieved the full genetic possibilities of body structure because of dietary inadequacies.

Prenatal nutrition. One of the classic studies of the importance of nutrition during pregnancy was conducted by Burke and her coworkers in Boston.[9] They studied 216 pregnant women over an extended period during which the women were examined and their diets were rated as excellent, good, fair, poor, and very poor.

These studies indicated that a woman who has a poor or a very poor diet during pregnancy will in all probability have a poor infant; that is, prematurity, congenital defects, and stillborn infants occurred almost entirely in this group. On the other hand, the women who had good-to-excellent diets almost invariably bore infants in good physical condition. The mother's protein intake correlated well with the infant's physical condition, weight, and length.

Inadequate nutrition resulted in relatively greater harm to the fetus than to the mother. No cases of eclampsia were noted in those women having excellent or good diets, whereas 50 per cent of those receiving poor or very poor diets developed toxemia of varying degrees of severity.

The Vanderbilt cooperative study of 2338 pregnant white women of low income showed the effects of weight status and hemoglobin levels of the mother on the infant.[10] Underweight women (less than 85 per cent of standard) produced smaller babies, prematurity occurred more frequently, and artificial feeding was more common. The overweight group (120 per cent of standard) had more stillborn children and a threefold increase in preeclampsia. Women who gained too much, especially during the second trimester, had more toxemia.

Low intakes of iron and ascorbic acid were correlated with lower hemoglobin levels and blood levels of vitamin C. However, during the first year of life the infants of these mothers maintained hemoglobin levels equal to those whose mothers had higher hemoglobin levels, showing that appropriate infant feeding practices can make up for the deficient infant stores of iron.

The Vanderbilt study did not fully establish nutritional deficiency as a primary causative factor in metabolic diseases of pregnancy. The investigators point out that the patient cannot be assured of freedom from complications simply through a satisfactory intake of nutrients. They did observe that diets which contained less than 50 gm protein and less than 1500 kcal resulted in a greater frequency of complications of pregnancy and of the newborn, but they felt that the low levels of intake were a result of the complications rather than the cause.

Nutrition and brain development. The development of the brain and resulting behavior are dependent upon the interaction of genetic and environmental factors including nutrition, illness, psychologic factors, and cultural variables. Interference with learning and behavior could occur in three ways: (1) abnormalities of the biochemical and physiologic characteristics of the brain; (2) reduced exposure and stimulation because of the unfortunate social-familial environment; and (3) interruptions in learning because of emotional, personality, and behavioral changes in the child.[11] Intrauterine malnutrition can result from a poor maternal diet before and/or during pregnancy or from insufficiency of the placenta.

In the development of the fetus and of the infant for the first few months after birth, severe malnutrition can lead to reduced brain weight, cell numbers, cell size, and myelin formation. In early postnatal life myelin formation is affected with reduced levels of cholesterol, phospholipids, and gangliosides. The activity of enzymes required for myelin formation is also reduced. The effects of moderate malnutrition on brain development have not been established. In most instances malnutrition coexists with reduced social and cultural stimulation.[11]

The mental performance of men born during the severe famine in Holland (see page 285) was studied when they enrolled for military service.[12] There was no difference in the mental performance of men from western Holland where the famine was severe and men from other parts of Holland not subjected to the severe food privations. This study does not support the view that severe undernutrition during pregnancy will affect the intellectual development. It must be remembered that the mothers were generally well nourished prior to the famine and thus their bodies were a reasonable reserve for the fetus. On the other hand, in the developing countries where prematernal as well as prenatal nutrition is extremely poor, the effect on intellectual ability could indeed be adverse.

Teen-age pregnancies. Each year in the United States there are about 200,000 live births to girls under 17 years of age. In every category the risks are greater for these young mothers and their babies. Toxemia occurs three to four times more frequently in teen-age pregnancies and is higher in younger girls than in older girls.[13] Fetal losses, low birth weights, neonatal deaths, and deaths of mothers are substantially higher in girls under 16 years than in older girls and women. The risk is greater for nonwhite girls than for white girls. Those from low-income families have less successful pregnancies than those from higher-income families.

Many factors enter into the high risk in teen-age pregnancies. The nutritional needs of the girl during the period of maturation are considerable, but often are not met because many adolescents regardless of socioeconomic status are known to have unsatisfactory, often bizarre diets. When the nutritional demands of pregnancy are superimposed upon the immature girl who is inadequately nourished, the outcome for mother and infant may well be poor. Young girls who become pregnant may also be under severe emotional stress, especially if the pregnancy is out of wedlock. Under stress nutrient balances such as nitrogen and calcium are often negative even when an adequate diet is consumed. Many teen-age pregnancies occur in low-income families where there is the least understanding of the nutritional needs during pregnancy, the least money to purchase foods for an adequate diet, and the least prenatal care.

In recent years an increasing number of multidisciplinary programs have provided food supplements when needed together with opportunities to continue education. There is special emphasis upon nutrition for the well-being of the girl herself and upon the essentials of child care.[14]

PHYSIOLOGIC AND BIOCHEMICAL CHANGES IN PREGNANCY

Three stages of pregnancy. Pregnancy may be considered in three stages:[5]

1. The preimplantation period, about two weeks following conception. The fertilized ovum becomes implanted in the wall of the uterus and the placenta begins to develop.

2. The period of organ formation, about two to eight weeks. All the major organs—heart, kidneys, lungs, liver, and skeleton—are formed during this period. Studies on experimental animals have shown that congenital malformations occur when the pregnant animal has had a diet grossly deficient in vitamins, for example vitamin A or riboflavin.[15] However, it is difficult to correlate poor nutrition with malformations sometimes seen in humans.

3. The period of rapid growth of the fetus and the establishment of the maternal reserves in preparation for labor, the puerperium, and the production of milk from the eighth week to term.

The placenta. This is the organ to which the fetus is attached by means of the umbilical cord and by which the nutrition of the fetus is maintained. The placenta achieves its maximum size early in gestation. Its large surface area is estimated to be between 10 and 13 sq m. By active transport as well as by diffusion, nutrients and hormones are taken up from the maternal circulation and transferred to the fetal circulation. Likewise, carbon dioxide and catabolites are transferred from the fetal circulation to the maternal circulation. The placenta also has synthetic functions and regulates selectively the transfer of nutrients and hormones according to the changing needs of the fetus. Many drugs such as tranquilizers, sedatives, and some antibiotics can be transmitted to the fetal circulation. Thus, the mother must have the advice of her physician concerning this possible danger.

Hormones. Progesterones, the estrogens, and the gonadotropins are the hormones primarily involved in reproduction. Progesterone is secreted by the corpus luteum and brings about increased secretion by the endometrium, as well as developing glycogen and lipid stores. It also inhibits contraction of the uterine smooth muscle layers thereby preventing expulsion of the embryo. In these ways progesterone has prepared for the implantation of the fertilized ovum and its early growth. Between the second and third months of gestation the formation of progesterone is taken over by the placenta.

Gonadotropins are especially concerned with organ formation up to about the fourth month of pregnancy and with fetal growth. Chorionic gonadotropin is produced by the *trophoblastic* cells (outer layer of cells of the dividing ovum) and has the same effects on the corpus luteum as the luteinizing hormone and the luteotropic hormone from the pituitary gland. It keeps the corpus luteum from degenerating and keeps it secreting large quantities of estrogen and progesterone. The endometrium remains in the uterus and is gradually phagocytized by the growing fetal tissues, thereby furnishing a major portion of the nutrition to the fetus during the first weeks of pregnancy.

Estrogen production increases appreciably after about the one-hundredth day of gestation. Estrogen and progesterone stimulate the growth of the mammary glands and also inhibit the lactogenic function of the pituitary gland until birth of the infant.

Steroid hormones are produced in greater amounts with the result that water and sodium are more readily retained in the body. The thyroid gland is less active during the first four months of pregnancy, and thereafter is somewhat more active than normal.

Blood circulation. A gradual increase in blood volume up to about 25 per cent by the end of pregnancy occurs. This increase is required in order to carry the essential nutrients to the placenta and also to remove the increased level of metabolic wastes. There is a corresponding increase in cardiac output, heart rate, and pulse pressure. The blood flow through the kidney is increased and this increases the elimination of the waste products.

With the increase in blood volume there is a corresponding dilution of the blood constituents. For example, the hemoglobin concentration of healthy young women averages 13.7 gm per 100 ml blood with a range from 12.0 to 15.3 gm.[3] During pregnancy, women who have received supplemental iron have an average hemoglobin of 12.0 gm per 100 ml. This change is sometimes referred to as the "physiologic anemia of pregnancy." A level of 11.0 gm hemoglobin per 100 ml blood is considered to be the border below which a true anemia exists. The plasma albumin is also lowered during pregnancy. On the other hand, the serum alkaline phosphatase is increased considerably.

Gastrointestinal changes. Most women have an increase in appetite and thirst during the first trimester, although morning nausea may temporarily interfere with eating. Some women have cravings for certain foods and aversions to others. Pica, an appetite for such things as starch, clay, and chalk, is present in a surprising number of women and these abnormal items are sometimes consumed in large amounts.

Less acid and pepsin are produced by the stomach, and regurgitation of stomach contents into the esophagus (heartburn) sometimes occurs. The reduced motility of the intestinal muscles may contribute to constipation. However, there is no apparent impairment of absorption.

Weight gain. The gain in weight for the healthy woman who enters pregnancy at her desirable weight level should average 11 kg (24 lb). Gains in weight vary widely, being somewhat greater in young women than in those who are older, and greater in those who are having their first babies. (See Figure 19–2.)

The Committee on Maternal Nutrition has indicated that appropriate weight gain during the first trimester is 0.7 to 1.4 kg (1.5 to 3.0 lb). Thereafter, a steady gain of 0.25 to 0.45 kg per week is satisfactory.

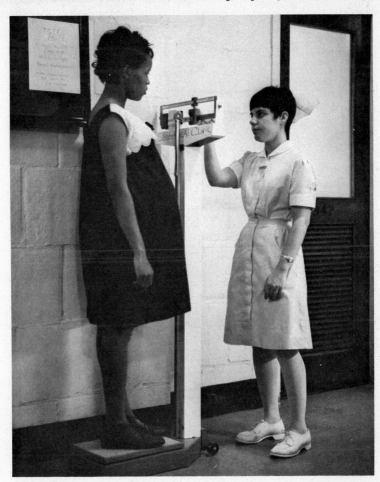

Figure 19–2. Weight is checked at each clinic visit. After the first trimester the weekly gain should be about 0.25 to 0.45 kg (average 0.8 pound). (Courtesy, School of Nursing, Thomas Jefferson University, Philadelphia.)

The weight gain is accounted for by the weight of the full-term infant, the increase in size of the uterus, the placenta, amniotic fluid, breast tissue, expanding blood circulation, and the reserves of nitrogen and lipids that help to meet the needs during parturition and lactation. (See Table 19–1.)

NUTRITIONAL CONSIDERATIONS

Energy. Blackburn and Calloway observed a 17 per cent increase in the basal metabolism of adolescent girls by the last trimester.[16] This increase was accounted for entirely by the increase in weight. Others have reported an increase in basal metabolism as great as 25 per cent by the last trimester.

The total caloric cost of producing the fetus, the placenta, and other maternal tissues and of establishing reserves is about 80,000 kcal. Part of this is made up by the reduction in activity especially during the last trimester. For most women an extra allowance of 300 kcal daily will permit satisfactory weight gain.[17] An allowance of at least 36 kcal per kilogram pregnant weight is needed for satisfactory utilization of protein.[18]

Adolescent girls who were extremely sedentary required an increased intake of about 150 kcal to cover the growth needs and the development during pregnancy. When the work pace must be kept up, the calorie needs could substantially exceed the recommended allowance, for example, the woman who has several children and many household duties

Table 19–1. Average Components of Weight Gain in Pregnancy*

	Cumulative Gain (kg) at End of Each Trimester		
	First	Second	Third
Fetus	Negligible	1.0	3.4
Placenta	Negligible	0.3	0.6
Amniotic fluid	Negligible	0.4	1.0
(Fetal subtotal)		(1.7)	(5.0)
Increased uterine size	0.3	0.8	1.0
Increased breast size	0.1	0.3	0.5
Increased blood volume	0.3	1.3	1.5
Increased extracellular fluid	0	0	1.5
(Maternal subtotal)	(0.7)	(2.4)	(4.5)
Total gain accounted for	0.7	4.1	9.5

*Pitkin, R. M., et al.: "Maternal Nutrition. A Selective Review of Clinical Topics," Obstet. Gynecol., **40**:777, 1972.

or the woman whose employment involves entire body movement. (See Table 19–2.)

Protein. About 925 gm protein is deposited in the fetus and maternal tissues during pregnancy. The rate of deposit in these tissues averages 0.6, 1.8, 4.8, and 6.1 gm daily during the four quarters of the pregnancy. Protein may be stored in the body at a uniform rate during the entire pregnancy and is made available to the specialized tissues as needed. The recommended allowance during pregnancy is increased by 30 gm.[17]

Minerals. The efficiency of absorption of minerals such as calcium and iron improves during pregnancy, but the demands of the fetus and other developing tissues necessitate increases in the diet during the second and third trimesters. The full-term fetus contains about 28 gm calcium. Some calcium and phosphorus deposition takes place early in pregnancy, but most of the calcification of bones occurs during the last two months of pregnancy. The first set of teeth begins to form about the eighth week of prenatal life, and they are well formed by the end of the prenatal period. The six-year molars, which are the first permanent teeth to erupt, begin to calcify just before birth.

If the mobile reserve of calcium is lacking in the mother, the demands of the fetus can be met, perhaps inadequately, only at severe expense to the mother. For many women it is advisable to increase the calcium intake early in pregnancy even though fetal calcification does not occur until later. The phosphorus allowance should be about equal to that for calcium and will be readily supplied through the calcium-rich and protein-rich foods.

Iron. The amount of iron in the full-term fetus is about 300 mg. For the maternal tissues and for the increase in blood volume an additional 500 mg is required. Thus, the iron need during pregnancy is just under 1 gm, most of which is added during the last half of gestation.[19]

Although some iron is saved by the cessation of menstruation, the typical diet takes care of only the daily losses from the skin, and in the urine and stools. The prematernal stores are about 300 mg iron, and often less than this. The recommended allowance is over 18 mg, and the Committee on Maternal Nutrition has recommended a daily supplement of 30 to 60 mg iron.

Iodine. The daily allowance of 125 mcg iodine is easily met by using iodized salt. If sodium restriction is required for any reason, the physician may prescribe a supplement.

Sodium. Studies by Pike on experimental animals have shown that sodium restriction has adverse effects.[20,21] During pregnancy the total sodium content of the body will increase to take care of the fetal needs, the enlarging maternal tissues, and the expanding blood volume. There is no convincing evidence that sodium restriction has any effect on the incidence of preeclampsia. On the other hand,

Table 19–2. Recommended Dietary Allowances Before and During Pregnancy and Lactation

Nutrient	11–14 Years	15–18 Years	19–22 Years	23+ Years	Pregnancy	Lactation
Energy, kcal	2400	2100	2100	2000	+300	+500
Protein, gm	44	48	46	46	+30	+20
Vitamin A, R.E.	800	800	800	800	1000	1200
I.U.	4000	4000	4000	4000	5000	6000
Vitamin D, I.U.	400	400	400	400	400	400
Vitamin E, I.U.	12	12	12	12	15	15
Ascorbic acid, mg	45	45	45	45	60	80
Folacin, mcg	400	400	400	400	800	600
Niacin, mg	16	14	14	13	+2	+4
Riboflavin, mg	1.3	1.4	1.4	1.2	+0.3	+0.5
Thiamin, mg	1.2	1.1	1.1	1.0	+0.3	+0.3
Vitamin B_6, mg	1.6	2.0	2.0	2.0	2.5	2.5
Vitamin B_{12}, mcg	3.0	3.0	3.0	3.0	4.0	4.0
Calcium, mg	1200	1200	800	800	1200–1600*	1200–1600*
Phosphorus, mg	1200	1200	800	800	1200–1600*	1200–1600*
Iodine, mcg	115	115	100	100	125	150
Iron, mg	18	18	18	18	18+	18
Magnesium, mg	300	300	300	300	450	450
Zinc, mg	15	15	15	15	20	25

*The higher levels are indicated for the teen-age girl.

some women tolerate restriction poorly. The woman should be allowed to salt food to her taste.[22]

Vitamins. The thiamin, riboflavin, and niacin allowances are slightly increased to correspond to the increase in calories. There is also an increased allowance for vitamin A, and 400 I.U. vitamin D is recommended.

Pregnancy apparently imposes an additional demand for folacin. Megaloblastic anemia occurs in a small number of women especially during the last trimester. This may be caused by dietary deficiency or by some metabolic alteration. Vitamin B_6 levels in the blood are often low in the pregnant woman. Although supplementation with vitamin B_6 will restore blood levels to the normal range, there is no evidence that such supplementation confers any physiologic advantage.

DIETARY COUNSELING

The basic diet. The Basic Diet plan (Table 13–2) provides ample allowances for protein, vitamin A, and ascorbic acid. The caloric level of this plan is just over half that needed by the pregnant woman. (See Figure 19–3.) When 1½ to 2 cups milk are added, the calcium, thiamin, and riboflavin needs are fully met. Vitamin D will be provided by using fortified milk. Except for iron and iodine other minerals and vitamins will be provided in sufficient amounts by the recommended amounts of foods. (See Table 19–3.)

For the pregnant teen-ager the food allowances are the same as for the pregnant woman except that the intake of milk should be 5 to 6 cups daily.

Dietary management. Nutrition education may be especially effective during pregnancy, for the mother-to-be is usually anxious that her baby have the best opportunity for a healthy life. The father is also concerned about the well-being of his wife, and in encouraging her proper diet he may also improve his own food habits.

The pregnant teen-ager who is a happy homemaker is quite receptive to nutrition counseling, but when a pregnancy is unwanted, especially out of wedlock, the teen-ager may resist many efforts to help. She may use food as an outlet for

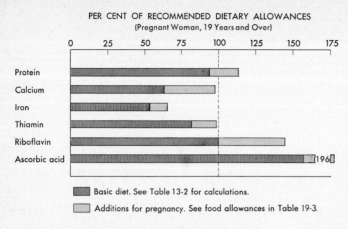

PER CENT OF RECOMMENDED DIETARY ALLOWANCES
(Pregnant Woman, 19 Years and Over)

Protein
Calcium
Iron
Thiamin
Riboflavin
Ascorbic acid   196

■ Basic diet. See Table 13-2 for calculations.

□ Additions for pregnancy. See food allowances in Table 19-3.

Figure 19–3. The Basic Diet provides ample vitamin A and niacin (not shown in chart) as well as protein, riboflavin, and ascorbic acid to meet the needs of the pregnant woman. The addition of 1 to 2 cups of milk supplies the needed calcium. The iron intake can be increased by including liver weekly and by eating more meat, dark-green leafy vegetables, and enriched bread. An iron supplement prescribed by the physician will be less costly than these additional amounts of food, and will not increase the calorie intake.

her emotions, but in so doing she often selects those foods rich in calories but having little else to recommend them nutritionally. The motivation for better nutrition for this girl may be in terms of her own well-being.

As in all dietary counseling the dietary pattern must be based upon the woman's present food habits and her cultural and socioeconomic circumstances. (See Figure 19–4.) Women who are pregnant for the first time will require more counseling than those who have had successful

pregnancies. Those whose incomes are low may need help in budgeting their food expenditures. This means help for the entire family, for a mother is not likely to improve her own diet at the expense of that of other children in the family.

Some women dislike milk and find it difficult to consume the 3 cups or more that are required. The inclusion of milk in soups, puddings, and sauces may be suggested. Part of the milk may be used as nonfat dry milk in cooked foods or as a

Table 19–3. Food Allowances for Pregnancy and Lactation

	Pregnant Woman	Pregnant Teen-Age Girl	Lactating Woman
Milk	3–4 cups, whole	5–6 cups, whole	6 cups, whole
Meat, fish, poultry (liver once a week), cooked weight	4 ounces	4 ounces	4 ounces
Eggs	3 to 4 per week	3 to 4 per week	3 to 4 per week
Vegetables, including:			
Dark green leafy or deep yellow	½ cup	½ cup	½ cup
Potato	1 medium	1 medium	1 medium
Other vegetables	½–1 cup	½–1 cup	½–1 cup
One vegetable to be raw each day			
Fruits, including:			
Citrus	1 serving	1 serving	1 serving
Other fruit	1 serving	1 serving	1 serving
Cereal, whole grain or enriched	1 serving	1 serving	1 serving
Bread, whole grain or enriched	5 slices	5 slices	5 slices
Butter or fortified margarine	To meet caloric needs	To meet caloric needs	To meet caloric needs
Desserts, cooking fats, sugars, sweets			
Vitamin D supplement (or use fortified milk)	400 I.U.	400 I.U.	400 I.U.
Iodized salt	Daily	Daily	Daily

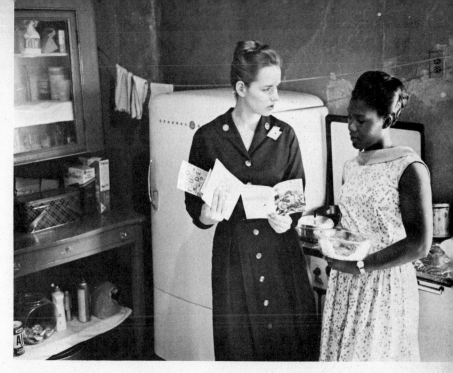

Figure 19–4. Within the home a public health nurse can provide practical suggestions for a satisfactory diet for the mother-to-be. Should any problems of planning arise, the nurse may consult a nutritionist. (Courtesy, United Fund and Community Nursing Services, Philadelphia.)

reinforcement of the fresh whole milk that is taken. Milk may be flavored with fruit or chocolate, vanilla, or molasses. Cheddar cheese may be substituted for part of the milk, using 1 ounce as an equivalent for 1 cup of milk.

As sources of protein, poultry, fish, legumes, and peanut butter are less expensive than meat. When legumes or peanut butter is used, the meal should include part of the day's allowance of milk so that all the essential amino acids will be available.

Canned or frozen citrus juices are less expensive ways to include ascorbic acid for the day. Fresh fruits in season—for example, cantaloupe—may be inexpensive sources of ascorbic acid.

Many women are especially concerned about maintaining their slender figures and may be reluctant to include such foods as milk, bread, and potatoes because of the belief that these foods are fattening. Some instruction concerning the caloric value of foods may be useful.

Supplements. Multiple vitamin supplements combined with calcium and iron are prescribed as a routine measure by some physicians. Are they really necessary? Except in situations where there is an intolerance, the calcium allowance is easily met by an adequate intake of milk. For iron, on the other hand, it is difficult to meet the recommended allowance even when a conscientious effort is made to select iron-rich foods. A supplement of 30 to 60 mg iron daily is recommended.

All vitamins except possibly folacin are readily supplied by a good diet, and the use of multiple supplements is unnecessary except when there are clinical and biochemical evidences of an existing deficiency. The increased need for folacin suggests the desirability of a supplement of 200 to 400 mcg.[23]

Multiple vitamin-mineral supplements can give a false sense of confidence so that little effort is made to improve the diet. The diet during pregnancy should, in fact, establish a pattern for nutritive adequacy that can be sustained in the years ahead.

COMPLICATIONS OF PREGNANCY

Mild nausea and vomiting. During the first trimester, the physiologic and biochemical balances are often disturbed, possibly because of excessive hormone production. Gastrointestinal upsets, including loss of appetite, nausea, and vomiting, are relatively frequent; loss of weight occasionally takes place because of inability to eat sufficient food.

Mild early morning nausea may usually be overcome by the use of high-carbohydrate foods such as crackers, jelly, hard candies, and dry toast before arising. Frequent small meals rather than three large ones are preferable. Fluids should be taken between meals rather than at mealtime. Fatty, rich foods such as pastries, desserts, fried foods, excessive seasoning, coffee in large amounts, and strongly flavored vegetables may be restricted or eliminated if the nausea persists or if the patient complains of heartburn or gastric distress.

Pernicious vomiting. Severe and persistent vomiting requires close supervision by the physician, and hospitalization may become necessary. Intravenous or tube feedings to provide some fluid, electrolytes, and calories are occasionally indicated. When oral feedings are resumed, it is of the utmost importance to proceed gradually with the kinds and amounts of foods which are offered.

High-carbohydrate, low-fat foods are best tolerated and include dry toast with jelly, crackers with jelly, baked potato, plain gelatin, cereal with milk and sugar, tomato juice, hard candy, and broth. Fasting aggravates the condition, and therefore feedings of 3 to 6 ounces should be offered every two hours. Dry foods are more likely to be retained than liquid foods. However, dehydration must be guarded against.

The psychologic factor is of some importance and little is gained by urging the woman to eat foods that do not appeal to her. She should be consulted about her likes and dislikes; a food that appeals to her is more likely to be retained.

When the high-carbohydrate foods are satisfactorily taken, the diet is gradually liberalized to include the foods customarily allowed on first a soft and then a normal diet. Generally speaking, foods high in fat, pastries, rich desserts, fried foods, and cream are poorly tolerated. Highly seasoned foods and strongly flavored vegetables may also cause some distress. It is usually desirable to give only dry foods at meals and to allow liquids one to two hours after meals.

Constipation. The occurrence of constipation especially during the latter half of pregnancy is common. The amount of pressure exerted by the developing fetus on the digestive tract, the limitation of exercise, and insufficient bulk may be contributing factors in its causation. The normal diet outlined on page 292 provides a liberal allowance of fruits, whole-grain cereals, and vegetables, and consequently of fiber. It is also necessary to stress the importance of adequate fluid intake and of regular habits of exercise, elimination, sleep, and recreation.

Overweight. Although obesity represents an added risk during pregnancy, the stress of weight loss should not be superimposed upon the stress of pregnancy.[1] It is recommended that the emphasis be placed upon a consistent rate of weight gain during pregnancy and that weight loss be postponed until after the pregnancy has come to term.

Anemia. Iron-deficiency anemia is relatively common and it is corrected by prescribing oral iron supplements. The diet should be liberal in its protein content to furnish the essential amino acids for globin formation.

Megaloblastic anemia is not common in pregnant women in the United States. It is corrected by prescribing a supplement of folacin.

Toxemia. By toxemia is meant that combination of symptoms including hypertension, edema, and albuminuria. Preeclampsia is the appearance of hypertension, edema of the face and hands, and/or albuminuria about the twentieth week of pregnancy. It should be suspected when there is a sudden gain in weight, indicating fluid retention rather than tissue building. Eclampsia is the end result of preeclampsia; it includes the earlier symptoms but may culminate in convulsions.

The treatment of toxemias is highly controversial. In fact, toxemia has been called the "disease of theories."[1] Protein and calorie restriction are no longer recommended, and sodium restriction should be used with caution.

LACTATION

Nutritive requirements. McGanity and his associates[10] found that women who had high intakes of calcium, phosphorus, and riboflavin from their diets nursed their babies more frequently than did women who drank less than 3 glasses of milk daily and who had calcium supplements. When one considers the nutritive value of human milk, and that the nursing mother will produce 20 to 30 ounces each day, it becomes apparent that the requirements for protein, minerals, vitamins, and calories are even greater than they were during pregnancy. The recommended allowances for the various nutrients have been listed in Table 19–2.

The need for protein is greatest when lactation has reached its maximum, but it is a need which should be anticipated and planned for during pregnancy. An increase of 20 gm protein is recommended during the period of lactation.

Each 100 ml breast milk supplies 67 to 77 kcal. The average milk production is about 850 ml, representing about 600 kcal. The conversion of energy to milk energy is about 80 per cent efficient, thus necessitating about 750 kcal.[24] If weight gain averaged 11 kg during pregnancy, the fat deposits will furnish 200 to 300 kcal for the first 100 days, or roughly one third of the increased caloric need. An added allowance of 500 kcal is therefore recommended.

Even liberal intakes of calcium may not be successful in completely counteracting a negative calcium balance. Consequently, a high level of calcium intake and the building of considerable reserves

throughout pregnancy cannot be overemphasized. The baby is born with a relatively larger reserve of iron since milk is not a good source of iron. A good allowance of iron in the mother's diet during lactation does not convey additional iron to the infant. Nevertheless iron-rich foods are essential for the mother's own health, and supplements are included early in the infant's diet.

Selecting the daily diet. The pattern of diet used during pregnancy (page 292) may be used during lactation, provided the following additions are made: (1) 1 pint of milk; (2) foods as desired to provide the additional calories. Weight gain, beyond that desirable for body build, should be avoided. When the baby is weaned, the mother must reduce her food intake in order that obesity may be avoided.

The choice of foods during lactation may be wide. There are no foods that require restriction, except where distress may occur in individual cases following the taking of a particular food such as strongly flavored vegetables or highly seasoned or spicy foods. Successful lactation is dependent not only upon an adequate diet, but also upon sufficient rest for the mother, freedom from anxiety, and a desire to nurse the baby.

PROBLEMS AND REVIEW

1. What evidence exists that diet is of importance in the development of the fetus and the health of the mother?
2. What physiologic changes occur during the course of pregnancy?
3. Name the hormones which are especially important in controlling the changes occurring during pregnancy? What is the effect of an excess production?
4. In what way do the nutritional practices of teen-age girls affect the outcome of pregnancy?
5. What weight increases are recommended for each trimester? What are the dangers of underweight or insufficient weight gain?
6. What foods are especially important for their protein content in the diet during pregnancy and lactation?
7. What mineral elements require especial attention during pregnancy? What changes occur in the rate of absorption of calcium and iron?
8. Discuss the need for an increased vitamin intake. What foods would you recommend for this?
9. Mrs. A. does not like milk and is taking calcium gluconate to correct calcium deficiency. Why is this less desirable than taking milk? List ways by which she could incorporate milk into her diet.
10. What recommendations can you make to a woman with complaints of nausea, vomiting, and gastric distress?
11. What instructions are in order for the woman who complains of constipation?
12. What is meant by the "physiologic anemia of pregnancy"? What are the hazards of iron-deficiency anemia? What measures are essential for its prevention and treatment?

13. A woman secretes 800 ml milk daily. What amount of protein is here represented? What allowances must be made in the diet for protein?

14. *Problem.* Plan a low-cost diet for a woman of moderate activity during the second half of pregnancy. Calculate the nutrients in this diet and compare them with the recommended allowances.

15. *Problem.* Modify the diet in problem 14 for a woman who is lactating.

CITED REFERENCES

1. Committee on Maternal Nutrition, Food and Nutrition Board: *Maternal Nutrition and the Course of Pregnancy.* National Research Council—National Academy of Sciences, Washington, D.C., 1970.

2. Committee on Maternal Nutrition, Food and Nutrition Board: *Maternal Nutrition and the Course of Pregnancy, Summary Report.* National Research Council—National Academy of Sciences, Washington, D.C. 1970.

3. Shank, R. E.: "A Chink in Our Armor," *Nutr. Today,* **5:**3–11, Summer 1970.

4. *Vital Statistics Report,* Annual Summary for the United States 1974. National Center for Health Statistics, U.S. Department of Health, Education and Welfare, Washington, D.C., May 30, 1975.

5. Macy, I. G.: "Metabolic and Biochemical Changes in Normal Pregnancy?" *J.A.M.A.,* **168:**2265–71, 1958.

6. Stearns, G.: "Nutritional State of the Mother Prior to Conception," *J.A.M.A.,* **168:**1655–59, 1958.

7. Tompkins, W. T., and Wiehl, D. G.: "Nutritional Deficiencies as a Causal Factor in Toxemia and Premature Labor," *Am. J. Obstet. Gynecol.,* **62:**898–919, 1951.

8. Thomson, A. M., and Hytten, F. E.: "Nutrition in Pregnancy and Lactation," in *Nutrition, a Comprehensive Treatise, Vol III.* G. H. Beaton and E. W. McHenry, eds. Academic Press, New York, 1966, pp. 103–45.

9. Burke, B. S., *et al.:* "Nutrition Studies During Pregnancy," *Am. J. Obstet. Gynecol.,* **46:**38–52, 1943.

10. McGanity, W. J., *et al.:* "Vanderbilt Cooperative Study of Maternal and Infant Nutrition. XII. Effect of Reproductive Cycle on Nutritional Status and Requirements," *J.A.M.A.,* **168:**2138–45, 1958.

11. Subcommittee on Nutrition, Brain Development and Behavior, Food and Nutrition Board: "The Relationship of Nutrition to Brain Development and Behavior," *Nutr. Today,* **9:**12–17, July 1974.

12. Review: "Effect of Famine on Later Mental Performance," *Nutr. Rev.,* **31:**140–42, 1973.

13. Gold, E. M.: "Interconceptional Nutrition," *J. Am. Diet. Assoc.,* **55:**27–30, 1969.

14. Weigley, E. S.: "The Pregnant Adolescent," *J. Am. Diet. Assoc.,* **66:**588–92, 1975.

15. Warkany, J.: "Production of Congenital Malformations by Dietary Measures (Experiments in Mammals)," *J.A.M.A.,* **168:**2020–23, 1958.

16. Blackburn, M. L., and Calloway, D. H.: "Energy Expenditure of Pregnant Adolescents," *J. Am. Diet. Assoc.,* **65:**24–30, 1974.

17. Food and Nutrition Board: *Recommended Dietary Allowances,* 8th ed. National Research Council—National Academy of Sciences, Washington, D.C., 1974.

18. Oldham, H., and Sheft, B. B.: "Effect of Caloric Intake on Nitrogen Utilization during Pregnancy," *J. Am. Diet. Assoc.,* **27:**847–54, 1951.

19. Pitkin, R. M., *et al.:* "Maternal Nutrition. A Selective Review of Clinical Topics," *Obstet. Gynecol.,* **40:**773–85, 1972.

20. Pike, R. L.: "Sodium Intake during Pregnancy," *J. Am. Diet. Assoc.,* **44:**176–81, 1964.

21. Pike, R. L., and Gursky, D. S.: "Further Evidence of Deleterious Effects Produced by Sodium Restriction during Pregnancy," *Am. J. Clin. Nutr.,* **23:**883–88, 1970.

22. Lindheimer, M. D., and Katz, A. I.: "Sodium and Diuretics in Pregnancy," *N. Engl. J. Med.,* **288:**891–94, 1973.

23. Cooper, B. A., *et al.:* "The Case for Folic Acid Supplements During Pregnancy," *Am. J. Clin. Nutr.,* **23:**848–54, 1970.

24. Thomson, A. M., *et al.:* "The Energy Cost of Human Lactation," *Br. J. Nutr.,* **24:**565–72, 1970.

ADDITIONAL REFERENCES

Anderson, E. H., and Lesser, A. J.: "Maternity Care in the United States. Gains and Gaps," *Am. J. Nurs.*, **66:**1539–44, 1966.

Bartholomew, M. J., and Poston, F. E.: "Effect of Food Taboos on Prenatal Nutrition," *J. Nutr. Educ.*, **2:**15–17, Summer 1970.

Beal, V. A.: "Nutritional Studies during Pregnancy. 1. Changes in Intake of Calories, Carbohydrate, Fat, Protein, and Calcium," *J. Am. Diet. Assoc.*, **58:**312–20, 1971.

———: 2. Dietary Intake, Maternal Weight Gain, and Size of Infant," *J. Am. Diet. Assoc.*, **58:**321–26, 1971.

Coursin, D. B.: "Maternal Nutrition and the Offspring's Development," *Nutr. Today*, **8:**12–18, 1973.

Harrill, I., *et al.:* "Nutritive Value of Foods Selected During Pregnancy," *J. Am. Diet. Assoc.*, **63:**164–67, 1973.

Hytten, F. E., and Leitch, I.: *The Physiology of Human Pregnancy*, 2nd ed. F. A. Davis Company, Philadelphia, 1971.

Jacobson, H. N.: "Maternal Nutrition," *Mod. Med.*, **39:**102–105, Oct. 18, 1971.

Miller, G. L., and Gerald, L.: "Diabetes Increases Risk in Pregnancy," *Postgrad. Med.*, **43:**91–95, 1968.

Review: "The Caloric Cost of Pregnancy," *Nutr. Rev.*, **31:**177–79, 1973.

Review: "Fetal Malnutrition," *Nutr. Rev.*, **31:**179–81, 1973.

Review: "Maternal Dietary Supplementation and Infant Birth Weight," *Nutr. Rev.*, **31:**45–47, 1973.

Review: "Starvation in Pregnancy: Metabolic Changes," *Nutr. Rev.*, **31:**82–83, 1973.

Seifrit, E.: "Changes in Beliefs and Food Practices in Pregnancy," *J. Am. Diet. Assoc.*, **39:**455–66, 1961.

Thompson, M. F., *et al.:* "Nutrient Intake of Pregnant Women Receiving Vitamin-Mineral Supplements," *J. Am. Diet Assoc.*, **64:**382–85, 1974.

Woody, N. C., and Woody, H. B.: "Management of Breast Feeding. How to Be a Grandmother," *J. Pediatr.*, **68:**344–50, 1966.

Zackler, J., *et al.:* "The Young Adolescent as an Obstetric Risk," *Am. J. Obstet. Gynecol.*, **103:**305–12, 1969.

20 Nutrition During Infancy

Growth and development of the infant. Each infant's physical growth and development are determined by the characteristics acquired from his ancestors, the quality of the nutrition of his mother during pregnancy, and the adequacy of the breast feeding or formula and supplements offered throughout infancy. The development of personality patterns begins at birth and is closely related to feeding habits. The importance of satisfying feeding relationships between the mother and infant from the earliest days after birth can scarcely be overemphasized.

Each infant is individual and he best serves as his own control in the measurement of his progress. Although it is often useful to make comparisons with stated norms, such as height and weight, it is also dangerous to expect every infant to conform exactly to such norms. No single criterion of physical status is indicative of the quality of nutrition, but a series of measurements over a period of time are likely to be reliable indicators.

Several criteria may be applied to determine whether an infant is well nourished, namely: steady gain in height and weight, but some weekly fluctuations are to be expected; sleeps well, is vigorous and happy; firm muscles and a moderate amount of subcutaneous fat are developed; teeth begin to erupt within five to six months, and from 6 to 12 teeth have come through by the end of the year; and elimination is normal for the type of feeding.

The breast-fed baby usually has two to three soft, yellow stools each day and the formula-fed infant has one to two yellow, somewhat firmer stools.

During the first year the infant will grow and develop more rapidly than at any other time of life. At a weekly gain ranging from 140 to 225 gm (5 to 8 ounces) he will double his birth weight in the first five months. The weekly gain slows down to 110 to 140 gm (4 to 5 ounces) for the remainder of the year, and he will have tripled his birth weight by the time he is 10 to 12 months old.

The baby will increase his birth length of 50 to 55 cm (20 to 22 inches) by another 23 to 25 cm (9 to 10 inches) during the first year. At birth he has a large head in proportion to the rest of his body, but his short arms and legs will grow especially rapidly in the next 12 months.

The infant's body contains a much higher proportion of water than that of older children and adults; the muscles are poorly developed and the amount of subcutaneous fat is limited. Since the skin surface area is high in proportion to the total body weight, the loss of body water and of body heat is also relatively high. The skeleton contains a high percentage of water and cartilage and will be only gradually mineralized throughout childhood and adolescence. At birth the calcium content of the body is about 25 to 28 gm, and by the end of the first year this has tripled.

The gastrointestinal system of the full-term infant is able to digest protein, emulsified fats, and simple carbohydrates. The enzymes that digest starches and fats develop gradually during the first few months.

The kidneys reach their full functional capacity by the end of the first year. During the first few months the glomerular filtration rate is somewhat lower, and therefore the excretion of a high concentration of solutes is more difficult. Young infants also excrete greater amounts of some amino acids, apparently because of lower ability to reabsorb them from the tubules.[1] The reabsorption of other amino acids, such as phenylalanine, is high; thus, 97 to 98 per cent of phenylalanine may be reabsorbed even though blood levels may be high, as in phenylketonuria, one of many genetic diseases.

The hemoglobin level of the full-term infant at birth is about 17 to 20 gm per 100 ml. This level is gradually lowered as the infant grows and his blood circulation expands, but the levels remain satisfactory until about the third month when iron-rich foods should be introduced.

The brain develops rapidly in fetal life and during infancy and early childhood. By the age of four years the brain has reached 80 to 90 per cent of its adult size. The increase in the number of brain cells is most rapid during fetal life and in the first five to six months after birth, and thereafter the rate slows down markedly. If malnutrition is unusually severe during pregnancy and during the first few months of life, as in the marasmic infant, the number of the brain cells may be greatly reduced. It has not been established, however, that brain development is in any way impaired when the level of undernutrition is less severe. (See also Chapter 19.)

NUTRITIONAL REQUIREMENTS

The Food and Nutrition Board has recognized that human milk is the best food for infants and will meet the nutritive requirements early in life when it is supplied in sufficient quantity. In order to plan formulas using cow's milk or other substitutes, the nutrient allowances are stated in Table 20-1.

Energy. The caloric requirement of the infant is high in terms of his body weight. The allowance of 120 kcal per kilogram for the infant at birth is accounted for approximately as follows: basal metabolism, 60; specific dynamic action, 5; growth, 15; activity, 35; and fecal loss, 5. Since the activity of infants varies widely, an allowance that is correct for one infant may be too high or too low for others who are more or less active. During rapid growth the caloric storage is greater than during slow growth.

The wide spread of caloric requirements for large and small babies at a given age is shown in Figure 20-1. If the total formula is restricted, large babies will require supplementary foods at an earlier age than will small babies in order to meet their caloric needs.

Protein. The infant adds about 3.5 gm protein to his body daily during the first four months and thereafter about 3.1 gm per day for the rest of the year. The allowances are based on the protein furnished by the amounts of milk needed to provide a satisfactory growth rate.[2] When proteins are used

Table 20-1. Recommended Allowances for Normal Infants*

Nutrient	0–6 Months	6–12 Months
Weight, kg	6	9
lb	14	20
Height, cm	60	71
in	24	28
Energy, kcal	kg × 117	kg × 108
Protein, gm	kg × 2.2	kg × 2.0
Vitamin A, R.E.†	420	400
I.U.	1400	2000
Vitamin D, I.U.	400	400
Vitamin E, I.U.	4	5
Ascorbic acid, mg	35	35
Folacin, mcg	50	50
Niacin, mg	5	8
Riboflavin, mg	0.4	0.6
Thiamin, mg	0.3	0.5
Vitamin B_6, mg	0.3	0.4
Vitamin B_{12}, mcg	0.3	0.3
Calcium, mg	360	540
Phosphorus, mg	240	400
Iodine, mcg	35	45
Iron, mg	10	15
Magnesium, mg	60	70
Zinc, mg	3	5

*Food and Nutrition Board: *Recommended Dietary Allowances,* 8th ed. National Academy of Sciences—National Research Council, Washington, D.C., 1974.

† Assumed to be all as retinol in milk during the first six months of life. All subsequent intakes are assumed to be one-half retinol and one half as β-carotene when calculated from international units. As retinol equivalents, three fourths are as retinol and one fourth as β-carotene.

that are of lesser quality than milk protein, the allowances should be increased somewhat.

A comparison has been made of breast milk, cow's milk formula, and soy isolate formula supplemented with methionine. Growth rates were comparable on the three formulas, and it was suggested that the protein requirement be stated in terms of grams per 100 kcal; a level of 1.62 gm per 100 kcal was satisfactory for infants 8 to 112 days old.[3]

Fat. The intake of fat is important to maintain caloric adequacy. About 1 to 2 per cent of the caloric intake should be supplied as linoleic acid to maintain the integrity of the skin and normal growth.[2] Human milk supplies about 6 to 9 per cent of its calories as linoleate. Whole cow's milk formu-

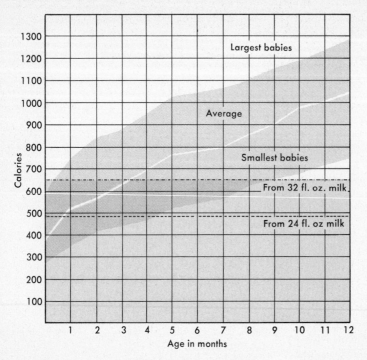

Figure 20-1. Spread of daily calorie requirements during the first year. Note that the largest babies would require a supplement to the formula by the end of the first month to meet their caloric requirements. For smaller babies a formula of 24 to 32 ounces (720 to 960 ml) per day would suffice for the caloric need for several months. Excessive weekly weight gains should be avoided. (Courtesy, Gerber Products Company.)

las will furnish satisfactory levels. In some premodified formulas part of the butter fat has been replaced by vegetable fats high in linoleic acid.

Skim milk formulas that are sometimes used need to be concentrated to supply sufficient calories, but such concentration presents an undesirable renal solute load. When babies are gaining too rapidly, a milk with 2 per cent fat level is preferable to skim milk.

Water. The normal daily turnover of water by the infant is about 15 per cent of his body weight. The water loss from the skin is large because of the greater surface area in relation to body weight. The ability of the kidneys of the young infant to concentrate urine is much less than that of older children or adults. Hence, to excrete a given amount of solute, chiefly urea and sodium chloride, a larger volume of fluid is required. The osmolar load of breast milk is well within the excretion capacity of the kidney, but more concentrated formulas could present an excessive osmolar load.

Infants require about 150 ml water per 100 calories. This requirement is met by breast milk, and by formulas containing 5 to 10 per cent sugar and enough water to give a concentration of 65 to 70 kcal per 100 ml (20 kcal per ounce).

Minerals. A recent study has shown that infants receiving human milk absorbed 50 to 60 per cent of the total calcium, whereas those receiving a commercial formula absorbed about 25 to 30 per cent of the total calcium.[4] Inasmuch as the formula contained about twice as much calcium as human milk, the total amount of calcium absorbed was about equal. A calcium-to-phosphorus ratio of 1.5 to 1 is recommended in early infancy to offset the tendency to hypocalcemia.

The circulating hemoglobin of the well-nourished infant is ample during the first three months, after which foods providing iron must be added in order to meet the needs of the expanding blood volume. The incidence of anemia is high in infants, usually appearing by the age of six months unless there has been iron supplementation. It is especially prevalent in premature infants and in twins; for such infants supplementation is recommended from the first few weeks of life. The use of either iron-fortified cereals or milk is recommended up to 18 months of age.[5]

The infant requires about 1.0 to 1.5 mEq sodium daily for growth and losses from the skin and excretions are about 1 to 2 mEq daily. The total sodium needs are estimated to be 2 to 5 mEq (46 to 115 mg) daily.[6]

Although many trace elements are needed by the infant, the exact requirements have not been determined. It is safe to assume that human milk or cow's milk formulas will supply adequate amounts. The use of fluoridated water for the dilution of infant formulas is recommended.

Vitamins. A supplement containing 400 I.U. vitamin D should be provided to the breast-fed infant. If the formula is prepared from vitamin D milk, no further supplementation is required. Human milk or whole cow's milk will furnish sufficient vitamin A without further supplementation. Vitamin K is routinely administered to the infant at birth by intramuscular injection of 0.5 to 1.0 mg to prevent hemorrhage.

The vitamin E requirement is ordinarily met by the milk feeding. Increased amounts of polyunsaturated fatty acids in the formula plus the addition of 12 to 13 mg iron per liter have led to vitamin E deficiency in premature infants. The presence of iron leads to lipid peroxidation, anemia, reticulocytosis, and thrombocytosis.[7,8]

Human milk from the well-nourished mother supplies sufficient ascorbic acid for the infant's needs, although supplements are generally introduced early. Infants who are fed high-protein formulas early in life require as much as 50 mg ascorbic acid in order to avoid tyrosinemia and tyrosinuria.

The allowances for thiamin, riboflavin, and niacin have been set up proportionate to the caloric intake. These allowances are easily met by human milk or the formula with the gradual addition of supplementary foods.

The infant is born with a store of vitamin B_6 that protects him during the neonatal period inasmuch as human milk is very low in this vitamin. When the protein intake increases, the vitamin B_6 intake must also increase. An intake of 0.015 mg vitamin B_6 per gram of protein, or 0.04 mg per 100 kcal, is adequate. Symptoms of vitamin B_6 deficiency have been observed in infants who were fed by undernourished mothers or who received formulas in which vita-min B_6 had been destroyed by overheating. (See page 182.)

BREAST FEEDING

Approximately 87 per cent of all mothers can supply their infants with enough milk to justify the continuation of nursing if there is proper management.[9] In the United States, however, less than 20 per cent of all mothers breast-feed their babies. No doubt there are many reasons for this, including in some instances the mother's early return to work. If breast feeding is to be successful, the advantages must be sold to the mother early in pregnancy. An adequate diet, exercise, rest, and freedom from anxiety are important during the prenatal period as well as during lactation.

Advantages of breast feeding. Human milk is the natural food for the infant. Breast feeding gives a safe and protected feeling to the infant and a sense of satisfaction to the mother. In lower economic groups breast-fed infants have a consistently lower mortality rate, probably because there is no problem of sanitation. As a rule, there are fewer and less serious illnesses and feeding problems among breast-fed infants; constipation also occurs less frequently. On a practical basis breast feeding eliminates preparation of a feeding; the milk is available at proper temperature; and errors in calculation and in formula preparation are avoided.

The encouragement of breast feeding is of great importance in many developing countries when income is insufficient to purchase the formula supplies, where water supplies are contaminated, and where a high rate of illiteracy makes it difficult for mothers to prepare satisfactory formulas.[10] (See Figure 20–2.)

Contraindications to breast feeding. If the mother can supply less than half of the infant's needs, breast feeding is usually not practical. It must be discontinued when (1) chronic illnesses are present in the mother, such as cardiac disease, tuberculosis, severe anemia, nephritis, and chronic fevers; (2) another pregnancy ensues; (3) it is necessary for the mother to return to employment outside the home; or (4) the infant is weak or unable to nurse because of cleft palate or harelip. Temporary

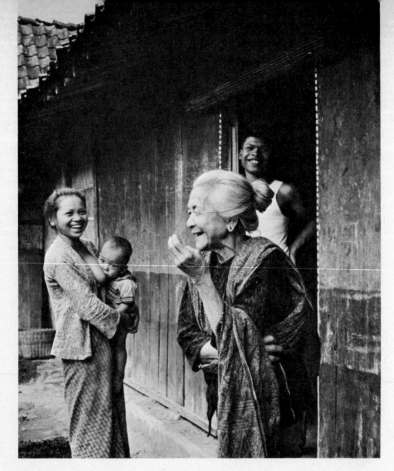

Figure 20–2. Health programs in developing countries need to emphasize the advantages of breast feeding of the infant. (Courtesy, UNICEF; photo by Jack Ling.)

cessation is also indicated when the mother acquires an acute infection which the infant has not yet acquired; in such a situation the mother's breasts should be completely pumped at regular intervals so that the milk supply will not dwindle.

Colostrum. The clear, yellowish secretion from the breast during the first few days after delivery is not mature milk, but a substance richer in protein and in vitamin A than the milk secreted later. The levels of carbohydrate, fat, niacin, pantothenic acid, biotin, and riboflavin are low initially and reach mature milk levels by the tenth day. Both colostrum and mature milk contain the same levels of ascorbic acid.

The infant receives only 10 to 40 ml of colostrum during the first two to three days, but by the end of the first week the supply of milk will usually satisfy the full nutrient needs. Although the nutritive contribution of colostrum seems to be small, the secretion apparently confers an immunity to certain infections during the first few months and aids in the development of the digestive enzymes.

Technique of feeding. Whether the baby is breast fed or bottle fed, the feeding satisfies at the same time the baby's needs for food, a feeling of safety and warmth, and love. The mother, likewise, gains a sense of satisfaction and a feeling of closeness to the baby. If these important needs are to be met, the mother must be comfortable and relaxed; she not only feeds the baby but talks and smiles. Anxiety or tension, on the other hand, are also communicated to the baby.

Breast feeding should be initiated within 24 to 48 hours after birth since the sucking of the hungry infant stimulates the flow of milk. At first the mother will probably hold the baby against the breast while reclining and supported by pillows. Later she should sit in a comfortable chair with armrests—perhaps a rocker. A footstool to support the feet is also helpful.

A publication by the Children's Bureau, *Infant Care*, gives practical advice to the new parents in an interesting, easy-to-understand manner. For example, to initiate breast feeding:

To get the baby started, press a little milk onto the baby's lips. If he's frantically nuzzling about, stroke the cheek nearest the nipple and he will turn toward it. If you touch the opposite cheek he will turn away automatically.*

The baby may get enough food by emptying one breast but if he is still hungry he should be offered the other breast. At the next feeding the breast not emptied should be offered first.

When the baby stops sucking he should be held over the shoulder and patted on the back to release any air which may have been swallowed. Some babies "burp" best if they are laid across the knee, abdomen down, and patted. Some babies require two or three "burpings" for each feeding.

Intervals of feeding. Healthy infants will establish, after a few weeks, schedules of their own which are reasonably regular from day to day if they are fed when they indicate that they are hungry. This is sometimes referred to as *self-demand feeding.*

The success of self-demand feeding depends upon the mother's ability to determine when the child is hungry. The infant who cries at intervals much shorter than three hours may be underfed, may have swallowed too much air at the previous feeding, or may be crying because of other discomforts.

The very young infant may require as many as 10 or 12 feedings at first, but he soon establishes a rhythm of feeding which falls into approximately three- to four-hour intervals. After the second month, the night feeding usually may be discontinued. By the end of the fourth or fifth month, the infant sleeps through the night and will no longer require a feeding around 10 P.M.

Adequacy of feeding. About 150 to 165 ml human milk per kilogram body weight (2.5 ounces per pound) result in satisfactory weight gain. The baby is getting enough milk if he is satisfied at the end of a 15-to-20-minute feeding, if he falls asleep promptly and sleeps quietly for several hours thereafter, and if he makes satisfactory gains from week to week. The infant should be weighed once a week in the same amount of clothing each time.

Insufficient milk intake is indicated when the infant is not satisfied at the completion of the feeding, when he is restless and fails to fall asleep

* *Infant Care,* Children's Bureau Pub. No. 8, U.S. Department of Health, Education, and Welfare, Washington D.C., 1963, p. 14.

quickly after nursing, when he awakens frequently if he does go to sleep, and when his gains are not satisfactory. In such cases, the physician may advise adding a supplementary food, or replacing one or more of the breast feedings with bottle feedings.

Even human milk is low in some nutrients required by the growing baby so that it is necessary to supplement the diet of the breast-fed infant according to the routine suggested in Table 20–3 (page 309).

Weaning the baby. As a rule, weaning is started during the fifth to the ninth month by substituting a cup feeding for the breast at any convenient interval. When the baby has become accustomed to this—after about four to five days—the second cup feeding is offered and so continued in this way until the baby is entirely weaned. Weaning usually requires a period of two to three weeks. The transfer from breast to cup should be gradual.

If breast feeding must be terminated at an earlier age, it is usually necessary to substitute bottle feeding and subsequently to proceed with weaning to the cup. Breast feeding after nine months has no special advantages for the infant and may lead to serious depletion of the mother.

BOTTLE FEEDING

Although breast feeding is highly desirable and should be encouraged, the fact remains that most babies are now bottle fed. Who is to say that one method is greatly superior to another? The circumstances for each family must be considered in making the choice, and no mother should ever be made to feel guilty if she chooses bottle feeding instead of breast feeding.

Comparison of human and cow's milk. The most widely used substitute for human milk is cow's milk. Goat's milk is used in some countries, and occasionally in the United States when the infant is allergic to cow's milk. Milk of other mammals such as the water buffalo, llama, camel, and sheep is used in countries where such milk is available. Table 20–2 gives a comparison of the nutritive values of human, cow's, and goat's milk.

Cow's milk contains about three times as much protein as human milk. About 60 per cent of the protein in human milk is lactalbumin and the re-

Table 20–2. Composition of Human, Cow's, and Goat's Milk* (per 100 gm milk)

	Human†	Cow's	Goat's		Human	Cow's	Goat's
Water, gm	85.2	87.4	87.5	Sodium, mg	16	50	34
Energy, kcal	77	65	67	Potassium, mg	51	144	180
Protein, gm	1.1	3.5	3.2	Vitamin A, I.U.	240	140	160
Fat, gm	4.0	3.5	4.0	Thiamin, mg	0.01	0.03	0.04
Carbohydrate, gm	9.5	4.9	4.6	Riboflavin, mg	0.04	0.17	0.11
Total ash, gm	0.2	0.7	0.7	Niacin, mg	0.2	0.1	0.3
Calcium, mg	33	118	129	Ascorbic acid, mg	5	1	1
Phosphorus, mg	14	93	106				
Iron, mg	0.1	tr	0.1				

*Watt, B. K., and Merrill, A. L.: *Composition of Foods—Raw, Processed, Prepared*. Handbook No. 8, U.S. Department of Agriculture, 1964, p. 39.

†U.S. samples.

mainder is casein. In cow's milk only 15 per cent of the protein is lactalbumin, with the remainder being casein. The efficiency of the proteins in the two milks is about equal. Human milk forms fine flocculent curds and the emptying time of the stomach is more rapid than for cow's milk. The curd from cow's milk is larger, tougher, and more slowly digested; it is modified by heating the milk, by homogenization, or by acidification.

The full-term infant utilizes well the fat of both human and cow's milk. Cow's milk, however, contains a larger proportion of volatile, short-chain fatty acids (such as butyric acid), which are somewhat more irritating than the long-chain fatty acids (such as oleic acid) found in human milk. Human milk contains almost twice as much lactose as cow's milk. Both kinds of milk provide about 70 kcal per 100 ml (20 kcal per ounce).

The total ash content is more than three times as high in cow's milk, almost all of this being accounted for by the higher contents of calcium, phosphorus, sodium, and potassium. Some healthy full-term infants fed cow's milk have a syndrome of convulsions known as *neonatal tetany* about the sixth day of life.[11] This is believed to be due to the high blood phosphorus and low blood calcium levels observed in these infants and attributed to the high phosphorus level of cow's milk. Some dilution of the milk is desirable to reduce the phosphorus content.

Because of the lesser capacity of the infant's kidneys to excrete wastes, the high ash content of cow's milk may present too high a solute load. By dilution of the milk, this problem is corrected.

The vitamin contents of human and cow's milk

vary considerably. Human milk from a well-nourished mother can meet the infant's ascorbic acid requirements, but cow's milk will need to be supplemented. Neither milk contains sufficient vitamin D or iron to meet the infant's needs for the first year.

Proprietary premodified formulas. About 90 per cent of formula-fed infants are now being given commercially prepared formulas. Some of these are concentrated, requiring dilution with an equal volume of water; some are ready-to-use to be measured into the bottle, or available in disposable nursing bottles; and some are available in dry form to be mixed with water.

For healthy babies these formulas are modified to simulate human milk. They have a low curd tension, are homogenized, and appropriate adjustments have been made for nutrient content. Their cost is moderate, although the packaging in disposable bottles for each feeding increases the cost considerably.

The typical modifications in the formulas are as follows:

Protein content is usually lowered; the protein is treated to produce a fine, flocculent, easily digested curd.

Butterfat is removed, and vegetable oils, such as corn oil, are substituted to increase the linoleic acid content.

Lactose or other carbohydrate is added.

Calcium level is reduced by dilution.

Vitamins A, D, and ascorbic acid are usually added.

Iron may be added; iron-fortified formulas should be encouraged as cup feedings after the infant is weaned.

Home-prepared formulas. Studies have shown that a formula prepared in the home from evaporated vitamin D milk, cane sugar, and ascorbic acid tablets is least expensive.[12,13] The formula cost was increased when fresh whole milk, special sugars such as Dextri-maltose, and fresh orange juice were used. In the studies cited, premodified formulas cost slightly more than the fresh-milk fomulas, and about half again as much as the evaporated-milk formulas.

Although some savings can be effected by preparing the formula in the home, the families that can most benefit from these savings are sometimes least able to understand the importance of sanitary preparation or of proper measurements.

The following guidelines may be used for a satisfactory formula using evaporated milk.

Amount of milk. About 50 to 65 ml per kilogram of body weight of evaporated milk ($\frac{3}{4}$ to 1 oz per pound).

Sugar. Sucrose and corn syrup are inexpensive, easily digested, and lend themselves readily to formula preparation. Lactose, the sugar of milk, is expensive and seldom used. Dextri-maltose is less sweet than sugar and sometimes used.

During the first two weeks about 15 gm ($\frac{1}{2}$ oz) sugar added to the day's formula is sufficient. Thereafter, 30 gm (1 oz) is sufficient. Sugar is discontinued at the time the baby is taking appreciable amounts of other foods.

Liquid. At two months the infant will take about 120 ml (4 oz) of formula. This is increased about 30 ml each month until the infant is taking a maximum of 240 ml at approximately six months of age.

Intervals of feeding. As with breast feeding, the number of feedings and the amount taken at each feeding should be flexible. Formula-fed babies should not, as a rule, be fed at less than three-hour intervals since the cow's milk remains for a longer time in the stomach.

Calculation of the formula. The calculation of a formula using evaporated milk is as follows:

Infant, 5 months old, weighs 7 kg
Number of feedings . . . . 5 (assuming approximately 4-hour intervals)
Volume of feeding: 210 ml (7 oz)
Total volume of formula: 5 × 210 ml = 1050 ml (35 oz)
Evaporated milk: 7 × 55 ml = 385 ml (13 oz)
Water: 1050 − 385 = 665 ml (22 oz)
Sugar: 30 gm (2 tablespoons)

This formula provides 527 kcal from milk and 120 kcal from sugar, or a daily intake of 92 kcal per kilogram of body weight. Food supplements given at this age will increase the caloric intake to the desired level. (See Table 20–1, and page 309.) The formula contains 27 gm protein, or about 3.8 gm per kilogram of body weight.

Sterilization of formula. Terminal sterilization of the formula is preferred. The steps are as follows: (1) Pour measured amount of formula into thoroughly washed bottles. (2) Put nipples on bottles and test the flow of milk. (3) Cover loosely with nipple covers. (4) Place bottles on rack in sterilizer and add water to halfway level of bottles. (5) Cover sterilizer, bring water to boiling, and maintain boiling for 25 minutes. (6) Remove bottles as soon as they can be handled, and cool slightly. (7) Store in refrigerator.

Technique of feeding. The feeding is usually warmed to body temperature, but no adverse effects have been noted when it is given cold. As with breast feeding the baby should be held in a semi-reclining position. He should never be propped up and allowed to feed himself. (See Figure 20–3.)

An overly large hole in the nipple leads to rapid

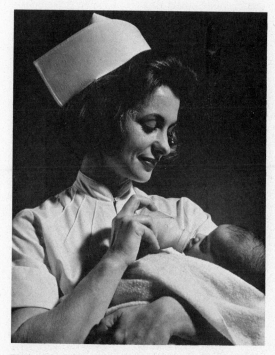

Figure 20–3. The young infant experiences security and comfort as he is held while being fed. (Courtesy, Ross Laboratories.)

taking of the formula and excessive swallowing of air, discomfort, and perhaps regurgitation. On the other hand, a very small hole in the nipple will necessitate too long a period of feeding. During the feeding the nipple should be filled with fluid, and not air, so that less air is swallowed. Even so, the infant will need to be "burped" one or more times as experience shows to be necessary.

The baby should not be expected to finish the entire amount of formula in the bottle at each feeding. The mother soon learns how much the baby will usually take at each feeding and can adjust the amounts of formula in the bottle. Any formula remaining at the end of each feeding must be discarded.

NUTRITION FOR THE PREMATURE INFANT

Developmental problems. The premature infant is one whose gestational age is less than 38 weeks and who weighs less than 2500 gm (5½ lb). He is born with poorly developed muscle tissues, very little body fat, low stores of iron, and an inadequately mineralized skeleton. Because there is very little fat and practically no glycogen, the energy stores are minimal and hypoglycemia, hyperbilirubinemia, and starvation result unless calories are supplied early.[14] The energy needs are high because the surface area is proportionately great, and because the extremely small deposits of subcutaneous fat result in a higher rate of heat loss.

The capacity of the stomach is about 5 ml at birth and increases to about 20 ml per kilogram by the end of the first week. The activity of sucrase, maltase, and lactase is reduced or may be nonexistent. Lactose intolerance is not uncommon during the first weeks of life. The digestion of fats is reduced, but some fat excretion is not harmful. The digestion of protein is adequate.

Because the kidneys are immature there is a reduced capacity to excrete wastes and consideration must be given to the concentration of nitrogenous constituents and electrolytes. When there is evidence of growth, the renal solute load is reduced because of the storage of nitrogen and minerals in the body.

The infant of less than 34 weeks has poor sucking and swallowing reflexes, and regurgitation of feedings is common. Aspiration and pneumonia are ever-present dangers.

Nutritional requirements. Premature infants are especially vulnerable to the effects of inadequate nutrition. Weight loss during the first few days should not exceed 5 to 10 per cent of body weight, and the birth weight should be regained in one to two weeks.[15] Infants that weigh 1 to 2 kg should then gain about 20 gm a day. The estimated requirements are as follows:

Energy: 110 to 125 kcal per kilogram
Protein: 3 to 4 gm per kilogram

Supplements. In addition to the formula, supplements of iron and of the fat-soluble and water-soluble vitamins are indicated.[15] Anemia is common in premature infants and a daily supplement of 2 mg iron is advisable. Larger iron supplements can lead to vitamin E deficiency and increased hemolytic effects. Not only are the vitamin E stores in the infant low, but the absorption of the vitamin is also likely to be reduced.[7,8] The multivitamin supplement includes 5 I.U. vitamin E and 50 mcg folacin. The infant has reduced ability to metabolize the aromatic amino acids, phenylalanine and tyrosine, and to correct this defect 60 mg ascorbic acid is recommended. Because of the increased tendency to rickets, 400 I.U. vitamin D is also included; some pediatricians recommend vitamin D dosages from 1000 to 2000 I.U.[16]

Selection of formula. The formula must be appropriate for the nutritional requirements, the gastrointestinal osmotic load, and the renal osmotic load. For premature infants the protein content of the formula can be 16 per cent of the calories. Protein levels at 5 to 6 gm per kilogram may present an excessive renal solute load. Concentrated formulas increase the gastrointestinal osmotic load and can lead to loose stools and diuresis. Rickard and Gresham[15] suggest that human milk and several commercial formulas° avoid excessive osmotic load when fed at a concentration of 85 kcal per 100 ml (24 kcal per ounce) or less. When the concentration of the formula is increased, the specific gravity of the urine should be watched closely.

Techniques of feeding. Babies who are unable to suck may be given gavage feedings every two or three hours. Such feedings must be reduced or discontinued if there is distention, regurgitation, or

---

° Enfamil, Mead Johnson Laboratories, Evansville, Indiana. Similac, Isomil (soy-based formula), Ross Laboratories, Columbus, Ohio.

diarrhea. Continuous intragastric drip has been used with some success, as has also transpyloric feeding.[15,17]

Intravenous alimentation by peripheral vein may be used for short periods of time, using glucose, synthetic amino acids, multivitamins, and minerals. Such feedings cannot meet the caloric requirements for growth. When oral feeding is not possible for prolonged periods of time, alimentation through an indwelling catheter in the superior vena cava permits greater caloric intake and satisfactory levels of nutrients.

Schedule of feeding. The schedule suggested by Rickard and Gresham is as follows:[15]

First day. Give 65 to 150 ml per kilogram of 10 per cent glucose intravenously with multivitamin supplement and iron.

Second day. By gavage or nipple give 3 ml per kilogram of a formula providing 70 kcal per 100 ml (20 kcal per ounce). Give feedings every two hours for the smallest babies. At every other feeding increase the amount of formula by 1 to 2 ml, provided there are no adverse effects. Include oral multivitamins and iron. Continue the intravenous glucose, allowing a total volume, including the formula, of 80 to 150 ml per kilogram.

Third day. Increase the strength of the formula to 85 kcal per 100 ml (24 kcal per ounce). Gradually increase the size of the feedings as on day 2. Continue the multivitamins and iron. Continue the intravenous glucose allowing a total volume of intake, including the formula, that ranges between 100 to 200 ml per kilogram.

By the fourth day the caloric intake should reach 90 kcal per kilogram, and by the seventh day 100 kcal per kilogram. If the caloric intake is less, it becomes necessary to consider intragastric infusions or transpyloric feeding.

SUPPLEMENTARY FOODS DURING THE FIRST YEAR

Practices vary widely concerning the time when solid foods are introduced. Many infants are now given some solid food as early as six weeks, whereas others are fed the first solid foods at about three months or so. No clear advantage can be ascribed to one or the other, since babies thrive on either.

Introduction of new foods. A number of practical suggestions are offered for the introduction of new foods.

1. Introduce only one new food at a time. Allow the infant to become familiar with that food before trying to give another.

2. Give very small amounts of any new food—teaspoonfuls or even less—at the beginning.

3. Use a very thin consistency when starting solid foods. Gradually the consistency is made more solid as the infant learns how to use his tongue in propelling the food back. A small spoon is put into the baby's mouth so that the food is placed on the middle of the tongue and swallowing is more readily accomplished. The fact that a baby spits out his first feedings of solid food may indicate that he has not yet learned the tongue movements rather than that he does not like the food.

4. Never force an infant to eat more of a food than he takes willingly.

5. If, after several trials, it is apparent that a baby has an acute dislike for a food, omit that item for a week or two and then try it again. If the dislike persists it is better to forget about that food for a while and substitute another.

6. Food should be only slightly seasoned with salt. Other seasonings are avoided.

7. Use foods of smooth consistency at first—strained fruits, vegetables, and meats.

8. When the baby is able to chew, gradually substitute finely chopped fruits and vegetables for puréed foods—usually at eight to nine months.

9. Infants may object to taking some foods by themselves but will take them willingly if they are mixed with another food. For example, egg may be mixed with formula, cereal, or vegetable; again, vegetables may sometimes be made into a soup with a little milk until the baby becomes accustomed to the new flavor.

10. Variety in choice of foods is important. The baby, like older persons, tires of the repetition of certain foods, especially cereals and vegetables.

11. The mother or anyone feeding the infant must be careful to avoid showing in any way a dislike for a food which is being given. (See Figure 20–4.)

Proprietary and home-prepared baby foods. Commercially prepared baby foods are convenient to use, bacteriologically safe, moderate in cost, and offer a considerable variety for the baby. Unless an iron-fortified formula is being used, the iron-fortified

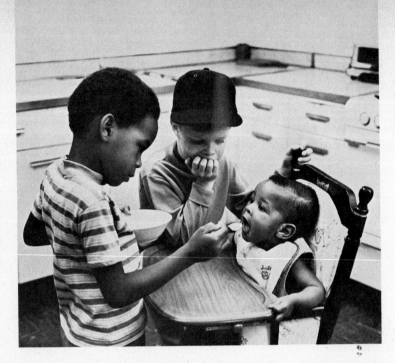

Figure 20-4. Feeding is also a means whereby happy relationships are established with others. (Courtesy, The Equitable Life Assurance Society of the United States.)

infant cereals are preferable to home-cooked cereals. Strained meats furnish considerably more protein than do the meat dinners.

Modified food starches have been added to dinners, high-meat dinners, fruits, and desserts in order to retain proper texture, consistency, and uniformity of ingredient distribution. These starches, contrary to popular opinion, are utilized satisfactorily by the infant and do not constitute an excessive proportion of the total caloric intake. In a study of 430 infants ranging in age from 1 to 14 months, the average daily intake of starch was 5.7 gm, equivalent to 23 kcal, or 2.3 per cent of the total caloric intake. In only four infants of this study was the starch intake equivalent to as much as 10 per cent of the total caloric intake.[18]

With a little expenditure of time the mother can prepare satisfactory foods for the infant, usually at lower cost. A blender is useful to give the fine texture needed for the vegetables, fruits, and meats. When a freezer is available, individual-size servings of food may be kept frozen for several weeks.

Sequence of additions. No uniformity of opinion exists concerning the time and sequence at which supplements are added. Some pediatricians introduce cereals, egg yolk, strained meats, fruits, and vegetables very early. In many infants the swallowing reflex is not fully established until the third or fourth month, and too early feeding, especially if forced, could lead to resistance and rebellion later on. The outline in Table 20-3 for feeding during the first year is typical of many.

Vitamins. Premodified formulas usually supply vitamins A and D and ascorbic acid without requiring further supplementation. When fortified evaporated or fresh milk is used for the preparation of the formula in the home, no further vitamin A or D is ordinarily required.

If, for any reason, vitamins A and D are prescribed as a supplement, the water-miscible preparation is preferable because of the lessened danger of aspiration. Since both vitamins are toxic when taken in excessive amounts, great care must be taken to see that the exact prescribed dosages are used.

Synthetic ascorbic acid is usually preferred initially because some babies may show an intolerance to orange juice. The ascorbic acid is added to the formula just before it is given to the baby, or it may be given separately in a bottle of water. After several weeks orange juice is gradually introduced. One teaspoonful of strained orange juice (frozen, canned, or fresh) is diluted with an equal amount of boiled water. Gradually the amount is increased until the baby is taking 3 ounces of undiluted juice daily, at about three months of age. Grapefruit juice or to-

Table 20–3. Typical Feeding Schedules for Normal Babies During the First Year*

Hour	Food	1 Month	3 Months	6 Months	10–12 Months
6 A.M.	Formula†	3–4 oz	5–6 oz	7–8 oz	6 A.M.
					Orange juice, 3 oz
8 A.M.	Orange juice	1 oz	3 oz	3 oz	Zwieback, ½ piece
	Vitamin D‡	400 I.U.	400 I.U.	400 I.U.	
					Breakfast, 7:30 A.M.
10 A.M.	Formula	3–4 oz	5–6 oz	7–8 oz	Cereal, 2–5 tbsp
	Cereal		¼–2 tbsp	2–4 tbsp	Milk, 8 oz‖
2 P.M.	Formula	3–4 oz	5–6 oz	7–8 oz	Chopped fruit, 1–2 tbsp
	Egg yolk			1 yolk	Vitamin D, 400 I.U.
	Vegetable			2–3 tbsp	
					Dinner, 11:30–12
6 P.M.	Formula	3–4 oz	5–6 oz	7–8 oz	Meat, ½–1 oz, or
	Cereal			2–4 tbsp	Egg, 1 whole
	Fruit			¼–2 tbsp	Potato, 2–4 tbsp
					Chopped vegetable, 2–4 tbsp
10 P.M.	Formula	3–4 oz	5–6 oz	Discontinued	Milk, 8 oz
2 A.M.	Formula	3–4 oz	Discontinued		Supper, 5:30 P.M.
					Cereal or potato, 2–5 tbsp
					Milk, 8 oz
					Chopped fruit, 1–2 tbsp
					Toast or zwieback

*Feeding intervals, amounts of food, and age at which supplements are given are subject to individual variation.
†Formula or breast milk.
‡Vitamin D should be given as a supplement if breast-fed; vitamin D is usually included in formulas.
‖Iron-fortified formula should be continued to the end of the first year; if plain milk is given, use iron-enriched cereal.

mato juice may be used, but the latter must be given in twice as great amounts to provide the equivalent amount of vitamin C. The mother must be cautioned not to boil the juices.

Cereal foods. Cereals are often the first semisolid foods given to the baby, at approximately two to four months. Specially formulated dry infant cereal foods possess the distinct advantage of enrichment with iron, thus bolstering the iron intake when body reserves have reached a low point. These cereal foods are mixed with a portion of the warm formula to the desired consistency.

Crisp toast, zwieback, and graham crackers may be given when the teeth begin to appear, about five to eight months.

Egg yolk. By the third to fifth month egg yolk is introduced. Hard-cooked egg yolk may be mashed and mixed with part of the formula, cereal, or vegetable. Only ¼-teaspoon amounts should be given initially since some infants are allergic to egg protein. Soft custard is also a suitable way by which to introduce the egg yolk. Egg white leads to allergic manifestations more frequently and is not given until the infant is at least 8 to 10 months old. At that time it is introduced cautiously.

Fruits. Ripe banana and strained orange or grapefruit juice are the only raw fruits permitted during the first year. Cooked or canned prunes, pears, applesauce, peaches, and apricots are the fruits with which an infant first becomes acquainted, usually by the third to fourth month. These fruits are strained for the first few months they are offered, but they are chopped by the end of the first year. Most babies accept fruits very well.

Vegetables. Strained carrots, green beans, spinach, squash, peas, asparagus, and tomatoes are all suitable for the infant from the fourth month or earlier. The first feeding of less than 1 teaspoon is gradually increased to 3 or 4 tablespoons daily by the end of the year. Chopped vegetables are substituted for strained vegetables at 10 to 12 months. Baked or mashed potato may be included occasionally by the seventh month.

Meats. Canned strained baby meats may be used as early as the second month, although they are more usually introduced at the fifth to seventh month. When the baby is accustomed to strained meats and meat soups, he may be given ground meat including beef, lamb, lean pork, thoroughly boned fish, chicken, and liver. The baby who is teething often enjoys a piece of crisp bacon.

Other foods. In some areas such as the Southwest, a variety of beans are widely used. They are a good source of protein, iron, and B-complex vitamins and may be cooked and sieved for the infant. The infant may be given simple puddings toward the end of the first year. It is desirable that the amounts of sugar used in the preparation of fruits and puddings be kept small so that the infant does not develop a special craving for sweets.

Overnutrition During Infancy

Rapid growth of a baby and the early introduction of supplementary foods are taken as signs of good development by many people. Parents often boast of the early feeding of solid foods. Such feedings are believed to accelerate the rate of growth, to reduce the likelihood of anemia, and to satisfy the appetite so that the baby sleeps well at night. There are, however, some hazards to be considered in overnutrition, whether from the formula or from added foods.

Some babies are susceptible to allergies. The early introduction of food could initiate an allergy before adequate defenses have been established. Moreover, very young infants have functionally immature kidneys so that the additional electrolytes in solid foods could present an undesirable renal solute load.

Obesity. Infants who gain excessive weight could be setting a pattern for obesity in later years. A recent study showed that there was a close correlation between excessive weight gains at 6 weeks, three months, and 6 months and overweight or obesity at 6 to 8 years of age.[19] In the first year of life there is a rapid increase in cell numbers, including adipose cell numbers. Thereafter the increase in the number of adipocytes is much more gradual. There is also an increase in adipose cell size from birth to age 6, and little change from 6 to 13 years. Extremely obese persons were found to have 3.5 times as many adipose cells as nonobese persons.[20] Weight loss later in life was found to be accompanied by a reduction in cell size but not in cell numbers. The final number of adipose cells can be influenced only early in life.

Salt. Babies will accept unsalted and salted foods equally well, and much of the salt added to infant foods seems to be a response to the mother's—and not the infant's—taste. The healthy baby excretes salt readily and apparently adapts to wide variations in intake. Several investigators have expressed concern about the large amount of salt ingested by many infants, believing that it could lead to hypertension in later life.[21-23] Although the salt content of infant foods has been reduced since 1970, the amount of sodium ingested by infants from formulas and foods substantially exceeds the requirement.

Problems and Review

1. Select an article from the list of references pertaining to breast feeding and on the basis of your reading prepare a 200-word summary of viewpoints on breast feeding.
2. What vitamins are customarily prescribed for breast-fed infants?
3. Describe the procedures to follow to ensure satisfactory weaning.
4. What advantages can be claimed for the use of commercially prepared formulas?
5. Compare the composition of human and cow's milk. What adjustments can be made so that cow's milk simulates human milk?
6. *Problem.* Calculate a formula using evaporated milk for an infant who weighs 5.5 kg and is four months old.
7. *Problem.* Examine the labeling of four popular brands of premodified formulas. How much of each would

be required daily for the four-month infant weighing 5.5 kg? Are any supplements required? Calculate the cost for the formula for one day, and compare with the cost of the formula calculated in problem 6.

8. What explanations might there be for the failure of an infant to gain weight at a satisfactory rate?
9. List the supplementary foods that are customarily introduced during the first year. What are the important nutritive contributions of each food added? At what approximate age is each usually introduced?
10. What functions, other than nutrition, are provided by the inclusion of supplementary foods during the first year? What are some guidelines you could give to the young mother for the satisfactory introduction of new foods?
11. Why is egg white customarily omitted from the infant's diet?
12. *Problem.* Outline a day's diet for an infant of seven months.
13. How do the nutritive requirements of premature infants differ from those of full-term infants? What feeding progression is recommended for these infants?
14. What are some of the possible consequences of overfeeding in infancy?

CITED REFERENCES

1. Brodehl, J., and Gellissen, K.: "Endogenous Renal Transport of Free Amino Acids in Infancy and Children," *Pediatrics*, **42**:395–404, 1968.
2. Food and Nutrition Board: *Recommended Dietary Allowances*, 8th ed. National Research Council—National Academy of Sciences, Washington, D.C., 1974.
3. Fomon, S. J., *et al.:* "Requirements for Protein and Essential Amino Acids in Early Infancy," *Acta Paediatr. Scand.*, **62**:33–45, 1973.
4. Hanna, F. M., *et al.:* "Calcium-Fatty Acid Absorption in Term Infants Fed Human Milk and Prepared Formulas Simulating Human Milk," *Pediatrics*, **45**:216–24, 1970.
5. Committee on Nutrition: "Iron Balance and Requirements in Infancy," *Pediatrics*, **43**:134–42, 1969.
6. Filer, L. J.: "Salt in Infant Foods," *Nutr. Rev.*, **29**:27–30, 1971.
7. Hassan, H., *et al.:* "Syndrome in Premature Infants Associated with Low Plasma Vitamin E Levels and High Polyunsaturated Fatty Acid Diet," *Am. J. Clin. Nutr.*, **19**:147–57, 1966.
8. Williams, M. L., *et al.:* "Role of Dietary Iron and Fat on Vitamin E Deficiency Anemia of Infancy," *N. Engl. J. Med.*, **292**:887–90, 1975.
9. Review: "The Vitamin Composition of Human Milk," *Nutr. Rev.*, **4**:134, 1946.
10. Jelliffe, D. B., and Jelliffe, E. F. P.: "The Urban Avalanche and Child Nutrition," *J. Am. Diet. Assoc.*, **57**:111–18, 1970.
11. Oppé, T. E., and Redstone, D.: "Calcium and Phosphorus Levels in Healthy Newborn Infants Given Various Types of Milk," *Lancet*, **1**:1045–48, 1968.
12. Heseltine, M. M., and Pitts, J. L.: "Economy in Nutrition and Feeding of Infants," *Am. J. Public Health*, **56**:1756–84, 1966.
13. Division of Nutrition: "Infant Formula Feeding," *Nutrition News*, Pennsylvania Department of Health, Fourth Issue, 1969.
14. Smallpiece, V., and Davies, P. A.: "Immediate Feeding of Premature Infants with Undiluted Breast Milk," *Lancet*, **2**:1349–52, 1964.
15. Rickard, K., and Gresham, E.: "Nutritional Considerations for the Newborn Requiring Intensive Care," *J. Am. Diet. Assoc.*, **66**:592–600, 1975.
16. Snyderman, S. E., and Holt, L. E., Jr.: "Nutrition in Infancy and Adolescence," in Goodhart, R. S., and Shils, M. E.: *Modern Nutrition in Health and Disease*, 5th ed. Lea & Febiger, Philadelphia, 1973, pp. 659–80.
17. Valman, H. B., *et al.:* "Continuous Intragastric Milk Feeds in Infants of Low Birth Weight," *Br. Med. J.*, **3**:547–50, 1972.
18. Filer, L. J., Jr.: "Modified Food Starches for Use in Infant Foods," *Nutr. Rev.*, **29**:55–59, 1971.
19. Eid, E. E.: "Follow-up Study of Physical Growth of Children Who Had Excessive Weight Gain in First Six Months of Life," *Br. Med. J.*, **2**:74–97, 1970.

20. Hirsch, J., and Knittle, J. L.: "Cellularity of Obese and Non-obese Human Adipose Tissue," *Fed. Proc.*, **29:**1516–21, 1970.
21. Dahl, L. K., *et al.:* "High Salt Content of Western Infants' Diet: Possible Relationship to Hypertension in the Adult," *Nature*, **198:**1204–1205, 1963.
22. Guthrie, H. A.: "Infant Feeding Practices—A Predisposing Factor in Hypertension?" *Am. J. Clin. Nutr.*, **21:**863–67, 1968.
23. Committee on Nutrition: "Salt Intake and Eating Patterns of Infants and Children in Relation to Blood Pressure," *Pediatrics*, **53:**115–21, 1974.

ADDITIONAL REFERENCES

Abrams, C. A. L., *et al.:* "Hazards of Overconcentrated Milk Formulas," *J.A.M.A.*, **232:**1136–40, 1975.
Beal, V. A., *et al.:* "Iron Intake, Hemoglobin and Physical Growth during the First Two Years of Life," *Pediatrics*, **30:**518–39, 1962.
Brown, R. E.: "Breast Feeding in Modern Times," *Am. J. Clin. Nutr.*, **26:**556–62, 1973.
Fomon, S. J.: *Infant Nutrition*, 2nd ed. W. B. Saunders Company, Philadelphia, 1974.
Gerrard, J. W.: "Breast Feeding: Second Thoughts," *Pediatrics*, **54:**757–64, 1974.
Lloyd-Still, J. D., *et al.:* "Intellectual Development After Severe Malnutrition in Infancy," *Pediatrics*, **54:**306–11, 1974.
Maslansky, E., *et al.:* "Survey of Infant Feeding Practices," *Am. J. Public Health*, **64:**780–85, 1974.
Murdaugh, Sr. Angela, and Miller, L. E.: "Helping the Breast-feeding Mother," *Am. J. Nurs.*, **72:**1420–22, 1972.
Newton, M.: "Psychologic Differences Between Breast and Bottle Feeding," *Am. J. Clin. Nutr.*, **24:**993–1004, 1971.
O'Grady, R. S.: "Feeding Behavior in Infants," *Am. J. Nurs.*, **71:**736–39, 1971.
Review: "Feeding the Baby of Low Birth Weight," *Nutr. Rev.*, **31:**14–15, 1973.
Review: "Growth of the Human Brain," *Nutr. Rev.*, **33:**6–7, 1975.
Review: "Infant Protein Needs Provided by a Soy-based Formula," *Nutr. Rev.*, **32:**42–44, 1974.
Review: "Overfeeding in the First Year of Life," *Nutr. Rev.*, **31:**116–18, 1973.
Robson, J. R. K., *et al.:* "Zen Macrobiotic Dietary Problems in Infancy," *Pediatrics*, **53:**326–29, 1974.
Schmitt, M. H.: "Superiority of Breast Feeding—Fact or Fancy?" *Am. J. Nurs.*, **70:**1488–93, 1970.

21 Nutrition for Children and Teen-agers

Growth and development. The term *growth* refers to an increase in size because of cell multiplication; the term *development* denotes an increase in the complexity of function. The latter, for example, not only refers to the increasing ability to metabolize nutrients and to coordinate motor skills, but it also refers to the complex mental and behavioral changes that occur. The outstanding fact to remember is that each person is unique in every way. Although many factors influence his life, he is physically, biochemically, mentally, and emotionally like no other person.

Neither growth nor development occurs at a uniform rate. The rapid growth in overall size that occurred in fetal life and during infancy is followed by a long period of very gradual growth that accelerates again in the adolescent years. In organ development cellular growth occurs in three phases: (1) rapid cell division occurs (hyperplasia); (2) cell division slows down but protein synthesis continues so that the cells increase in size (hypertrophy); and (3) cell division ceases but protein synthesis continues for a time with further increase in size.[1] Eventually growth ceases. These phases follow a chronologic schedule for each organ, but the timing of development differs for the organs and tissues of the body. Although the number of adipocytes has been largely determined by the end of the first year, the size of adipose cells increases about threefold from birth to six years. The nervous system shows rapid growth early in life with the brain having achieved 80 to 90 per cent of its maximum size by the age of four years. However, the complexity of function continues to develop. On the other hand, the growth and development of the reproductive organs are negligible until the beginning of the adolescent years. Since each organ has a critical time for its development, it should be evident that interference with the supply of nutrients at any given period can be serious for the development of specific organs and systems as well as the organism as a whole.

Food habits and development. Food influences each stage of physical, mental, and emotional growth and development. The infant's earliest relationships are associated with food, and throughout the growing years food continues to be a major factor in the development of the whole person. Food becomes a language of communication; it has cultural and social meanings; it is intimately associated with the emotions; and its acceptance or rejection becomes highly personal.

The environment in which the child lives determines the quality of nutrition. Sims and Morris[2] have studied environmental factors by considering the family as one ecosystem and the child as a second ecosystem. The family has responsibility for the child's food, controls the child's access to the foods, and establishes the emotional climate. Interacting factors within the family include the family composition, income, general education, the stability of the family, the quality of housing, the attitudes toward food, parental knowledge of nutrition, attitudes toward child rearing—authoritarian or nonauthoritarian—and others.

The child is the second ecosystem. From the family ecosystem he uses information, materials, and energy and his nutrient intake is the output of the family ecosystem. The nutrient supply is processed by the child to the output of his own ecosystem, namely his own development and nutritional status.

Good food habits have several characteristics. First, the pattern of diet permits the individual to achieve the maximum genetic potential for his physical and mental development. Second, the food habits are conducive to delaying or preventing the onset of degenerative diseases that are so prevalent in American society today. Third, the food habits are part of satisfying human relationships and contribute to social and personal enjoyment. The development of food habits is a continuous process in which each year builds upon what has gone before. The responsibility of parents and all who work with children goes far beyond assuring the ingestion of specified levels of nutrients. It requires the application of knowledge from the fields of human behavior and development, psychology, sociology, and anthropology. (See Figure 21–1.)

Nutritional Status of Children

Assessment of nutritional status. The determination of nutritional status can be made only by specialists qualified to give comprehensive physical and dental examinations, to make biochemical studies of the blood and urine, and to evaluate patterns of growth and measurements of body size. (See Chapter 23.) However, every mother, teacher, or nurse should be aware of these characteristics of the well-nourished child:

SENSE OF WELL-BEING: alert; interested in activities usual for the age; vigorous; happy.

VITALITY: endurance during activity, quick recovery from fatigue; looks rested; does not fall asleep in school, sleeps well at night.

WEIGHT: normal for height, age, and body build.

POSTURE: erect; arms and legs straight; abdomen pulled in; chest out.

TEETH: straight, without crowding in well-shaped jaw.

GUMS: firm, pink; no signs of bleeding.

SKIN: smooth, slightly moist; healthy glow; reddish-pink mucous membranes.

EYES: clear, bright; no circles of fatigue around them.

HAIR: lustrous; healthy scalp.

MUSCLES: well developed; firm.

NERVOUS CONTROL: good attention span for his age; gets along well with others; does not cry easily; not irritable and restless.

GASTROINTESTINAL FACTORS: good appetite; normal, regular elimination.

Nutritional status of children. Numerous studies have shown that the nutritional status of most children in the United States is good. Because some of these studies have been limited to children from middle-income groups, the problems of undernutrition or malnutrition often seemed less serious than they, in fact, are. Longitudinal studies in Denver and Boston have shown that children of a given age set up their individual patterns of growth, which may vary widely, just as their intakes of nutrients vary.[3,4]

Growth retardation and iron-deficiency anemia are considered to be the primary nutritional problems of American children.[5] The incidence of anemia reported in some areas is as low as 5 to 10

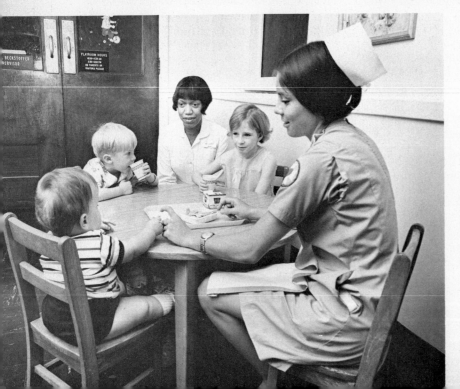

Figure 21–1. The playroom in a hospital provides opportunity at snack time for young children to develop good food habits by observing other children and through the guidance of adults who care for them. (Courtesy, Medical College of Virginia, Health Sciences Division, Virginia Commonwealth University, Richmond.)

per cent and in other areas as high as 25 per cent, and is influenced not only by the low iron intake but also by the presence of intestinal parasites. Many children who have normal hemoglobin and hematocrit values have a low saturation of transferrin. Such children thus have poor stores of iron that could be drawn upon for any stress. The incidence of anemia and growth retardation is seen more often in children from low-income families and from homes where parents have had only a limited education. Preschool children are the most vulnerable to these effects. The presence of anemia increases the likelihood of infections, and also increases the severity of such infections.

In addition to the high incidence of anemia and growth retardation, the Ten-State Nutrition Survey showed that dental decay was almost universal.[6] Although the number of severe deficiency diseases was low, one might ask why kwashiorkor, rickets, goiter, and other preventable deficiencies should occur.

Common dietary errors. Studies of food habits of children have shown repeatedly that the foods requiring particular emphasis for the improvement of diets are milk, dark-green leafy and deep-yellow vegetables, and whole-grain or enriched breads and cereals. Among the food habits that contribute to these deficiencies are these:

POOR BREAKFAST OR NONE AT ALL: lack of appetite; getting up too late; no one to prepare breakfast; monotony of breakfast foods; no protein at breakfast, meaning that the distribution of good quality protein is poor even though the day's total may be satisfactory; too little fruit, meaning that ascorbic acid often is not obtained.

POOR LUNCHES: failure to participate in school lunch program; poor box lunches; spending lunch money for snacks or other items; unsatisfactory management of school lunch program with resultant poor menus, poor food preparation, excessive plate waste.

SNACKS: account for as much as $\frac{1}{4}$ of calories without providing significant amounts of protein, minerals, and vitamins; often eaten too near to mealtime thus spoiling the appetite. (See also page 318.)

OVERUSE OF MILK, ESPECIALLY BY YOUNGER CHILDREN: other foods are not eaten so that the intake of iron and certain vitamins may be low.

SELF-IMPOSED DIETING, ESPECIALLY BY TEEN-AGE GIRLS: caloric restriction but no consideration given to protein, minerals, and vitamins.

IRREGULAR EATING HABITS: few meals with the family group; no adult supervision in eating; children often prepare own meals without guidance.

NUTRITIONAL REQUIREMENTS

Changes in growth and development. Height and weight changes follow a general pattern throughout childhood, but the chronologic age at which these changes occur varies considerably; hence, a child cannot be compared with others of the same age. Growth often occurs in spurts, and a temporary drop in the appetite and the growth is of no concern. Weight gains are generally more rapid in the fall and winter.

By the end of the first year the growth rate has slowed considerably. The toddler gains 3 to 4 kg during the second year, approximately quadrupling the birth rate. Thereafter, the yearly gains approximate 2 to 3 kg up to the preadolescent period. Boys are taller and heavier at each age than girls, except about 11 to 12 years when girls are usually heavier. The percentage of body fat increases more in girls than boys, being about $1\frac{1}{2}$ times as high at age 20.

For a year or two before adolescence and during adolescence the growth rate accelerates. The most rapid changes occur in girls between 11 and 14 years and in boys between 13 and 16 years. The rapid spurt in growth usually covers a period of two to three years. There are tremendous variations in the age at which maturation occurs so that the nutritional requirements for an 11-year-old girl who is maturing early, for example, will be quite different from those of the 11-year-old girl who has not yet begun to show these rapid changes.

The number, size, and composition of the bones change from birth to maturity. The skeleton has reached its full size in girls by the age of 17 years, and in boys at 20 years. The water content of the bones gradually diminishes as the mineralization increases. Provided that the diet remains good, bone mineralization continues for several years after the attainment of full size.

Dietary allowances. Because the anabolic activities are considerable during the entire period of childhood, the nutritional requirements in proportion to body size are much higher than they will be in the adult years. Moreover, childhood and adolescence are times of considerable physical activity and hence the energy requirement is greater. The Recommended Dietary Allowances are those levels of nutrients that are believed to support optimum growth and development (see Table 3–1). When using these allowances it is important to interpret them in terms of the child's size as well as with reference to age category.

Energy. The very young child has a high basal metabolic rate incident to intensive cellular activity and to a proportionately high surface area. Year by year the rate of metabolism decreases, then accelerates somewhat during adolescence, after which it again declines to the adult level. The basal metabolism of boys is higher than that of girls owing to the greater muscle mass.

The 1- to 3-year-old needs about 1300 kcal daily; the 7- to 10-year-old should have 2400 kcal, which is more than his mother is likely to need; and the 15- to 18-year-old boy requires 3000 kcal. Based upon body weight, the caloric requirement decelerates from about 100 kcal per kilogram at 1 to 3 years to about 50 kcal per kilogram at age 15. Boys engaged in competitive athletics or heavy labor must have considerably more calories if they are to grow satisfactorily. Macy and Hunscher[7] have shown that a deficit of as little as 10 kcal per kilogram body weight resulted in failure to grow and depression of nitrogen retention even though the protein intake had been satisfactory.

Protein. The protein allowance for children at one to three years is 23 gm and increases to 36 gm for the 7- to 10-year-old. The allowance for teenagers is approximately that of adult males and females. Based on body weight, the allowance decelerates from 1.8 gm per kilogram for the one- to three-year-old to 0.9 gm per kilogram for the teenager. About 12 to 15 per cent of the total calories should normally be obtained from protein.

Minerals. The recommended calcium and phosphorus allowances are 800 mg for children from 1 to 10 years. During the teen years the allowance for boys and girls is 1200 mg. The greatest retention of calcium and phosphorus precedes the period of rapid growth by two years or more, and liberal intakes of these minerals before the age of 10 are a distinct advantage. Children whose diets have been poor require a good diet for as long as six months before they can equal the calcium and phosphorus retention of children on a good diet.[8] Such a lag in retention can be a special hazard for the poorly nourished teen-age girl who becomes pregnant.

Adequacy of calcium intake is directly correlated with the intake of milk or milk foods. All nonmilk foods can be expected to yield only 0.2 gm calcium in the diet of young children, and 0.3 gm calcium in the diet of older children.

The data on magnesium requirements are limited, and hence the daily allowances are estimates based upon amounts of magnesium contained in milk.[9] For children the allowances range from 150 mg at one to three years to 250 mg at 7 to 10 years. Boys from 11 to 18 years should receive daily allowances of 350 to 400 mg and girls should receive 300 mg. One quart of milk furnishes about 120 mg magnesium, and dark-green leafy vegetables are also good sources. Many diets that are reasonably adequate in other nutrients may be somewhat lower than these allowances in magnesium; however, symptoms of magnesium deficiency have not been demonstrated on such intakes.

The recommended allowances of iron—from 10 to 18 mg, depending upon age—can be satisfied only when consistent emphasis is placed upon the inclusion of enriched or whole-grain cereals and breads, meats of all kinds, legumes, fruits, and green leafy vegetables. Far too often children of all ages consume minimum amounts of fruits and vegetables, thus leading to suboptimal iron intakes. Milk, which is low in iron, may be consumed in excessive amounts by some children, thus crowding out other essential foods.

Throughout childhood, but especially during adolescence, the use of iodized salt should be encouraged because the high-energy metabolism increases the activity of the thyroid gland and the corresponding likelihood of simple goiter.

Vitamins. The vitamin requirements of children have not been extensively studied. Throughout childhood and adolescence 400 I.U. vitamin D should be provided—an allowance easily met by using fortified milk. The vitamin A needs are related to body weight, and the allowance increases from 2000 I.U. at one to three years to 5000 I.U. for boys and 4000 I.U. for girls. Milk, butter and margarine, egg yolk, dark-green leafy and deep-yellow vegetables, and fruits are good sources.

The allowances for ascorbic acid range from 40 mg for the one- to three-year-old to 45 mg for the

11- to 18-year-old boy and girl. Thiamin and niacin allowances are 0.5 mg and 6.6 mg, respectively, per 1000 kcal. Allowances for riboflavin range from 0.8 to 1.2 mg for children from 1 to 10 years; teen-age boys need up to 1.8 mg and girls 1.4 mg. The allowance for vitamin B_6 ranges from 0.6 mg for the toddler to 1.2 mg by 10 years of age. Teen-age boys and girls need 1.6 to 2.0 mg vitamin B_6.

Although allowances have been established for vitamin E, the data pertaining to requirements for children are limited. An increased intake of polyunsaturated fats increases the need for vitamin E. When diets are adequate in protein, minerals, ascorbic acid, and thiamin, the dietary allowances for folacin, vitamin B_{12}, and vitamin B_6 are likely to be met.

Diet for the Preschool Child

Food selection correlated with behavioral changes. The nutritional requirements of the child cannot be satisfied apart from an understanding of behavioral changes which occur. During the second year the appetite tapers off corresponding to the slower rate of growth. Beal[10] found that healthy, well-nourished girls reduced their milk intake as early as six months and returned to higher intakes at two to three years of age. Boys also reduced their milk intake at about nine months, but started to increase their consumption between one and two years. An intake of 2 cups or less is not uncommon for a period of time. Some children's appetites improve by five years or earlier, but other children have poor appetites well into the school years.

Many mothers must be reassured that the child will remain well nourished provided that foods abundant in protein, minerals, and vitamins are offered, and that feeding does not become an issue between mother and child. Some compensation for the reduced consumption of milk may be made by incorporating milk into foods such as simple puddings. The occasional use of flavorings such as molasses or cocoa may increase milk acceptance. Children are sometimes encouraged to drink milk if they are permitted to pour it for themselves from a small pitcher. Cottage cheese and mild American cheese are often well liked and help to increase the calcium intake as well as the protein.

Because young children have a high taste sensitivity they prefer mildly flavored foods. Generally they like meat, chicken, and milk. Fruits are well liked but vegetables are frequently disliked. Plain foods are preferred to mixtures such as casserole dishes, creamed dishes, and stews. Preschool children do not like extremes of food temperatures, and may seem to dawdle until the mashed potatoes are lukewarm or the ice cream is beginning to melt.

The feel of food is important to young children, and they enjoy foods that can be picked up with the fingers such as pieces of raw vegetables, small sandwiches, strips of cheese or meat, and narrow wedges of fruit. The ability to chew food should determine the textures that are given. Toddlers may be given chopped vegetables and ground meat, whereas the three- to five-year-old can manage diced vegetables and minced or bite-size pieces of tender meat. Foods that are stringy such as celery, sticky such as some mashed potatoes, or slippery such as custard are often disliked because the child is not familiar with the texture. (See Figure 21–2.)

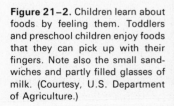

Figure 21–2. Children learn about foods by feeling them. Toddlers and preschool children enjoy foods that they can pick up with their fingers. Note also the small sandwiches and partly filled glasses of milk. (Courtesy, U.S. Department of Agriculture.)

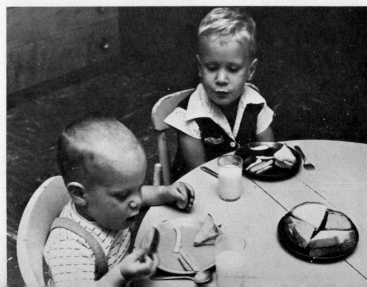

The gastrointestinal tract of the preschool child is easily irritated by very sweet or rich foods, and fried foods. Foods of this nature also displace dietary essentials and it is advisable to omit them in the diet of one- to three-year-olds, and to use them seldom for older preschool children.

Food jags are not uncommon, especially between the ages of two and four years. The child may shun all but a few foods, such as milk or peanut-butter-and-jelly sandwiches. Such occurrences do not last too long, if the parent does not show concern, and if the foods which constitute the child's preference at the moment are nutritious in general.

The preschool child is almost constantly active. His interest is readily diverted from food. If he becomes overtired or excessively hungry, his appetite may lag a great deal.

Meal patterns. The Four Food Groups constitute a sound basis for planning the daily meals. Children of this age should consume each day:

2 cups milk
3–4 eggs per week
1–3 ounces chopped meat, fish, or poultry
   4 ounces orange juice or other source of ascorbic acid
2–4 tablespoons other fruit such as banana, peaches, pears, apple, apricot, prunes
2–4 tablespoons vegetables, including deep yellow and dark green leafy
   1 potato
   1 raw vegetable such as carrot sticks, cabbage slices, lettuce, tomato
$\frac{1}{3}$ to $\frac{2}{3}$ cup enriched dry or cooked cereal
1–3 slices enriched or whole-grain bread
400 I.U. vitamin D, either as fortified milk or as a concentrate

The following meal patterns for a child from one to six° show that little adjustment needs to be made from the adult menu.

BREAKFAST
Fruit or juice
Cereal with milk
Toast
Butter or margarine
Milk

° *Your Child from 1 to 6.* Children's Bureau Pub. 30, Welfare Administration, U.S. Department of Health, Education, and Welfare, Washington, D.C., 1963.

LUNCH OR SUPPER
Main dish—mainly meat, eggs, fish, poultry, dried beans or peas, cheese, peanut butter
Vegetable or salad
Bread
Butter or margarine
Dessert or fruit
Milk

DINNER
Meat, poultry, or fish
Vegetable
Relish or salad
Bread
Butter or margarine
Fruit or pudding
Milk

Snacks. Most young children with a limited capacity for food are more likely to obtain all the dietary essentials if they are fed something in the middle of the morning and the afternoon. Moreover, very active children become excessively fatigued and hungry if they are not fed between meals. Snacks should make a liberal contribution to one or more of the nutrient needs. (See Figure 21–3.) Some which are suitable for preschool children are:

Fruit juices without sugar
Milk and milk beverages
Fruit of any kind; raw vegetables
Small sandwiches; crackers with peanut butter
Molasses, oatmeal, or peanut butter cookies
Dry cereal from the box or with milk
Cheese wedge
Fruit sherbert or ice cream

Establishing good food habits. Suggestions have been made in the preceding chapter for the establishment of good food habits in the infant. In addition, the following considerations are conducive to the development of good food habits in the preschool child.

Meals should be served at regular hours in a pleasant environment. The child should be comfortably seated at a table. Deep dishes permit the child to get his food onto the fork or spoon with greater ease. A fork, such as a salad fork with blunt tines, and a small spoon can be handled comfortably. A small cup or glass should be only partially filled with liquid to minimize spilling; however, the coordina-

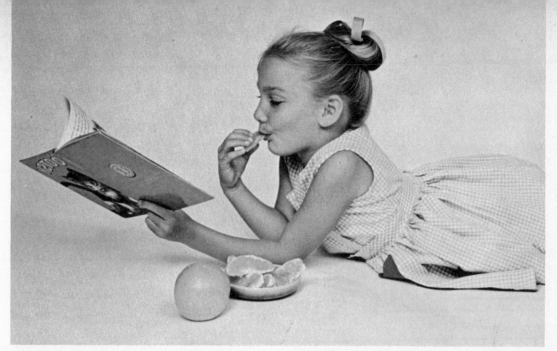

Figure 21-3. Snacks can provide valuable nutrients such as ascorbic acid. (Courtesy, Sunkist Growers.)

tion of eye, hand, and mouth is difficult and some spilling is to be expected. (See Figure 21-4.)

Children enjoy colorful meals just as adults do. Their appetites also vary from day to day, and like adults they react strongly to portions that are too large. It is much better to serve less than the child is likely to eat and to let him ask for more.

Even favorite foods should not be served too often. Breakfasts do not need to be stereotyped. A hamburger or sandwich and an orange cut in sections to be picked up with the fingers is just as satisfactory as a juice, cereal, and egg breakfast.

Fewer difficulties are likely to be encountered if new foods are given at the beginning of the meal when the child is hungry. A food is more likely to be accepted if it is given in a form which can be easily handled, which can be chewed, and if some favorite food is also included in the same meal. The parent should assume that the child will also take some responsibility in accepting the offered food.

Whether or not the preschool child should eat with other members of the family or alone is a matter that each mother must determine for the child's greatest good and the family's convenience. In most situations the young child should eat with the rest of the family because the interactions between family members are a part of normal development. If, however, the father returns from work at

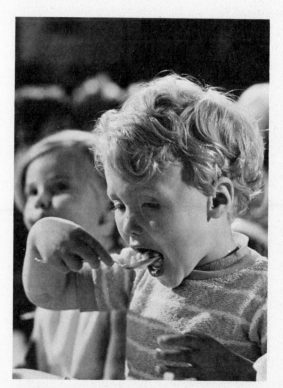

Figure 21-4. The young child learns finger dexterity by feeding himself. A word of encouragement now and then is helpful. (Courtesy, U.S. Department of Agriculture.)

such an hour that the evening meal must be late, if the child becomes overexcited about the family doings, or if the child is expected to live up to a code of behavior beyond his young years, it is better that he be allowed to eat before the rest of the family in a pleasant, quiet atmosphere with his mother nearby. Even so, an occasional meal with the family is a treat for the child and parent if tension can be avoided. Since children are great imitators, they enjoy doing just as Daddy or Mother or the other children are doing.

The child may well learn early in life that he is expected to eat foods prepared for him, but this does not mean that nagging or bribery will accomplish anything. Children, like adults, enjoy attention, and they are quick to realize that food can be a powerful weapon for gaining such attention. A display of concern or the use of force in getting a child to drink milk or to take any other food can have nothing but unfavorable effects. When a child refuses to take a food, the unwanted item should be calmly removed without comment after a reasonable period of time. If the child is refusing to eat because he thereby attracts attention, the mother should make certain that the child receives his full share of affection and companionship at other than mealtimes. By so doing the child will lose interest in using food as a weapon.

DIET FOR THE SCHOOLCHILD

Characteristics of food acceptance. Elementary-school children are usually better fed than preschool children or adolescents. Group acceptance is extremely important at this time, and the child needs to be able to keep up with his classmates and to have a sense of accomplishment. When the child goes to school for the first time he makes acquaintance with food patterns that may be different from those he knows at home. He learns that certain foods are acceptable to the peer group, whereas other foods from a different cultural pattern may be looked upon with disdain; as a result he may be unwilling to accept these foods at home—good though they may be. On the other hand, within a group he is willing to try foods with which he is unacquainted and which he would not try alone.

Schoolchildren have relatively few dislikes for food except possibly for vegetables, which are usually not eaten in satisfactory amounts. By the time children reach 8 to 10 years of age the appetite is usually very good. Feeding problems are more likely to result because parents are unduly concerned with behavior at mealtime which does not come up to adult standards. Most children of this age are in a hurry, and do not like to take time for meals. Breakfast, especially, is likely to be skipped.

Schoolchildren are subject to many stresses which affect the appetite. Communicable diseases occur often in this age group. They reduce the appetite on the one hand, but they increase body needs on the other. Schoolwork, class competition, and emotional stresses in getting along with many children may have adverse effects on appetite, as may also an unbalanced program of activity and rest.

Choice of foods. Table 21–1 lists the kinds and amounts of foods which may be taken in a day by healthy schoolchildren. A number of other equally satisfactory patterns could be devised for different cultural groups. A diet for adults which places emphasis first on the inclusion of protein, minerals, and vitamins is also a good one for schoolchildren. The amount of milk given to children should be greater than that for the adult. Although no foods need to be forbidden to this age group, it is extremely important that high-carbohydrate and high-fat foods not be allowed to replace essential items of the diet.

Food habits. The suggestions concerning good food habits for preschool children also apply to schoolchildren. A good school lunch program (see page 322) may introduce new foods in a setting where the child is anxious to conform to the group. The elementary teacher should integrate nutrition education with the total classroom experience so that good food habits are strengthened.

Since children are likely to be in a hurry, it is often wise to require that a certain time be spent at the table—say 15 or 20 minutes—so that the child will take time to eat. Children learn good manners by imitation of adults, and not by continuous correction at the table. During the elementary-school years, little can be gained by overemphasis on manners. In fact, the food intake may be adversely affected.

Table 21–1. Foods to Meet Nutritional Needs of Elementary-School Children and Teen-agers

Food	6 to 10 Years	10 to 12 Years	12 to 16 Years
Milk	2–3 cups	3–4 cups	4 cups or more
Eggs	3–4 per week	3–4 per week	3–4 per week
Meat, poultry, fish	2–3 ounces (small serving)	3–4 ounces (average serving)	4 ounces
Dried beans, peas, or peanut butter	2 servings each week. If used as an alternate for meat, allow $\frac{1}{2}$ cup cooked beans or peas or 2 tablespoons peanut butter for 1 ounce meat		
Potatoes, white or sweet (occasionally spaghetti, macaroni, rice, noodles, etc.)	1 small or $\frac{1}{3}$ cup	1 medium or $\frac{1}{2}$ cup	1 large or $\frac{3}{4}$ cup
Other cooked vegetable (green leafy or deep yellow 3 to 4 times a week)	$\frac{1}{4}$ cup	$\frac{1}{3}$ cup	$\frac{1}{2}$ cup or more
Raw vegetable (salad greens, cabbage, celery, carrots, etc.)	$\frac{1}{4}$ cup	$\frac{1}{3}$ cup	$\frac{1}{2}$ cup
Vitamin C food (citrus fruit, tomato, cantaloupe, etc.)	1 medium orange or equivalent	1 medium orange or equivalent	1 large orange or equivalent
Other fruit	1 portion or more, as: 1 apple, 1 banana, 1 peach, 1 pear, $\frac{1}{2}$ cup cooked fruit		
Bread, enriched or whole grain	3 slices or more	3 slices or more	4–6 slices or more
Cereal, enriched or whole grain	$\frac{1}{2}$ cup	$\frac{3}{4}$ cup	1 cup or more
Vitamin D	400 I.U. at all ages, using fortified milk or vitamin D concentrate		
Additional foods	Butter or margarine, sweets, desserts, etc., to satisfy energy needs		

Diet for the Teen-ager

Adolescent dietary problems. Even boys and girls who have had an excellent dietary pattern are likely to succumb to bizarre, unbalanced diets during the adolescent years. Teen-agers have many concerns about their development such as the size and shape of the body, their attractiveness, skin conditions, their vitality, sexual development, and social approval by their peers. They feel independent and seek freedom to make their own decisions. It is a period in which family conflict is likely to increase.

Failure to maintain normal weight is a frequently recurring problem. Studies on approximately 4000 teen-agers showed that girls were more often overweight and boys were more frequently underweight, the degree of overweight or thinness increasing with age.[11] The caloric intake by overweight girls is, surprisingly, not as great as that of girls of normal weight; however, the activity of the overweight girls has been less.[12,13]

The teen-ager himself is concerned about his weight.[14,15] Most girls want to weigh less; they want smaller hips, smaller thighs, and smaller waists but larger busts. Most boys want to weigh more and they equate overweight with muscle development which is desirable. They want a larger upper torso and arms, an indication of strength.

Stresses of various kinds have an adverse effect on nutrition. The incidence of tuberculosis is higher than it should be in adolescent years and in early adulthood and is believed to occur more frequently in those who have inadequate diets, especially with respect to protein and calcium. Many teen-age girls become pregnant before they have completed their own body growth and maturation. The stress of pregnancy can have serious effects on the girl who has had a poor intake of protein, calcium, and iron during the preceding years. (See page 287.)

Emotional difficulties often stem from the feeling of social inadequacy or the pressures of schoolwork. When there is conflict within the home because of the teen-ager's food choices, failure to accept responsibilities, the use of money, dating hours, and so on, the emotions not only determine the food intake but also modify nutrient utilization. Students who were taking examinations and young women who were upset about a pregnancy were found to have negative nitrogen and mineral balances.[8,16]

Selection of foods. Because of their high energy requirements boys are more likely to meet their nutrient needs than are girls. Emphasis upon green leafy and deep-yellow vegetables is necessary for both boys and girls. In addition girls need to increase their intake of milk and whole-grain or enriched breads and cereals. The list in Table 21–1 serves as a starting point for the planning of meals.

Snacks furnish about one fourth of the energy requirement. They should also furnish an equivalent amount of the day's allowances for protein, minerals, and vitamins. Thus, sandwiches, hamburgers, pizza, fruit, and milk are types of snacks to be encouraged. A study by Thomas and Call based upon the Ten-State Nutrition Survey has shown that typical teen-age snacks are better nutritionally than many people have believed them to be.[17] For each 100 kcal supplied by the snacks they found substantial contributions of protein, calcium, iron, vitamin A, thiamin, riboflavin, and ascorbic acid. Rather than making broad generalizations about excessive intake of "empty calorie" foods, the parent or educator should review the actual intake of between-meal foods to determine whether some change in direction is required.

Diets for athletes. The protein, mineral, and vitamin needs of athletes are similar to those of the more sedentary individuals of the same body size. The energy requirements, however, are considerably increased, depending upon the amount of exertion, and may be 4000 kcal or more. With such an increase in energy requirement, it is preferable that the fat intake be moderate with proportionate increases in the carbohydrate intake. The foods ingested to meet the caloric requirement will normally provide the additional amounts of thiamin, riboflavin, and niacin that are needed for the increased energy metabolism.

The athlete needs additional amounts of water and sodium to replace losses that occur during vigorous activity. During excessive heat the losses from perspiration are great and dehydration not only leads to increased fatigue but can result in heat stroke.[18]

Athletes should eat three meals a day, but five meals are sometimes preferable for the individual who is training for a long-endurance event. During the event itself, sugar is often taken to provide a quick source of energy. The last meal before an athletic event should contain only a moderate amount of protein, a low amount of fat—especially fried foods—and a high amount of carbohydrate thus ensuring rapid digestion. It should be eaten at least three to four hours prior to game opening to allow time for maximum digestive activity.

Coaches often impose rigorous dietary rules upon athletes. Many of these rules are based upon personal experience rather than on sound nutrition information. Physical education majors in colleges hold many misconceptions, seldom have a nutrition course, and yet will be influencing students in the schools.[19] One unfounded belief is that athletes require a high-protein intake with emphasis upon beef. Typical food selections to meet the energy requirement also increase the protein intake. The additional protein intake furnishes the psychologic satisfaction of the meal but is not necessary for muscle development; there is no particular merit in a high meat intake. Some coaches forbid milk on the day of an event in the belief that milk causes a dry mouth and mucus formation in the respiratory tract, thus reducing endurance; this belief is unfounded. Other coaches recommend high-protein supplements, vitamin-mineral supplements, or wheat germ—none of which is needed when the diet itself is planned to meet recommended allowances.

CHILD NUTRITION PROGRAMS

National School Lunch Program. The school lunch program has experienced rapid growth since the 1930s when surplus commodities were first distributed following the passage of a federal law in 1935. In 1946 the National School Lunch Act was passed to provide participating schools with (1) cash assistance; (2) donation of surplus food commodities; and (3) technical assistance in the purchase and use of foods and in the management and equipment of the school lunchroom. Nutrition education has always been regarded as an important component of the lunch program. (See Figure 21–5.)

To participate in the program, a school must agree to: operate the program on a nonprofit basis; provide free or reduced-price lunches for needy children; serve all children regardless of race, color, or national origin; serve nutritious lunches that meet the requirement for type A lunches as established by the Secretary of Agriculture; provide kitchen and dining facilities. No discrimination must be shown in any way to children who are eligible for free or reduced-price meals; that is, they must not be identified by placing them in separate lines, requiring them to sit in places set apart, or requiring them to provide service as a reimbursement for the meal. On a typical day in 1974 lunches were served to 24.9 million children, with about 39 per cent of these being free or reduced-price meals.[20]

Type A lunch. The Type A lunch includes:

1. Fluid milk, ½ pint, served as a beverage.
2. Protein-rich food such as: 2 ounces cooked or canned lean meat, fish, poultry; 2 ounces cheese; 1 egg, ½ cup cooked dry beans or peas; 4 tablespoons peanut butter; or an equivalent of any combination of these in a main dish.

3. Vegetables and fruits, at least ¾ cup, consisting of two or more servings. One serving of full-strength juice may be counted as not more than ¼ cup of the requirement.

4. Whole-grain or enriched bread, 1 slice; or muffins, cornbread, biscuits, rolls made of enriched or whole-grain flour.

5. Butter or fortified margarine, 1 teaspoon, as a spread, as a seasoning, or in food preparation.

Nutritive value of lunches. In planning menus to meet dietary allowances, a vitamin-C-rich food should be served daily and a vitamin-A-rich food at least twice a week. When foods are served in the amounts specified for the type A lunch, and additions are made to satisfy the appetite, the nutrient contributions are equivalent to one third of the recommended allowances for children of 10 to 12 years. Larger portions must be provided for older

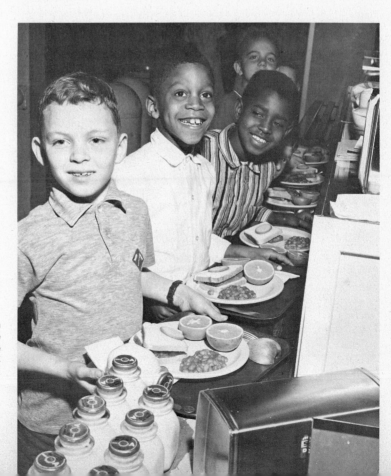

Figure 21–5. These boys in a Louisville, Kentucky, school are obviously ready to enjoy their type A lunch. (Courtesy, U.S. Department of Agriculture.)

children. Since the child eats only five meals in the school each week, the contribution represents about one fourth of the total weekly nutritive needs.

Alternate plans for building menus without necessarily adhering to the type A lunch format are under investigation. One of the concerns about some meals served in schools is the high percentage of calories derived from fat.[21] In view of the excessive intakes of saturated fat in the United States and the correlation with atherosclerosis, menus that supply not more than 35 per cent of calories from fat would be preferable.

There is an increasing trend in schools to permit the installation of vending machines that dispense soft drinks, candy, pretzels, crackers, and cakes. This is unfortunate inasmuch as these foods contribute little except calories to the child's nutritional needs, and because the child's money intended for lunch may be used instead for these attractive snacks. The American Dietetic Association, the American Medical Association, and the National Congress of Parents and Teachers have opposed the sale of candies and soft drinks within the schools.[22,23]

School breakfast program. In 1974 breakfasts were served in about 12,000 schools to an average of 1.34 million children each day. About 1 million of these meals were served free or at reduced price.[20] A breakfast includes:

1. One-half pint milk.
2. One-half cup fruit, or fruit or vegetable juice.
3. One serving bread or cereal; may be 1 slice of whole-grain or enriched bread, or an equivalent amount of cornbread, biscuits, or muffins; or ¾ cup of whole-grain or enriched or fortified cereal.
4. As often as practicable, a serving of protein-rich food such as 1 egg, or 1 oz meat, fish, or poultry, or 1 oz cheese, or 2 tablespoons peanut butter.

Additional foods to round out the breakfast and to satisfy the appetite may include foods of popular appeal such as doughnuts, potatoes, or bacon; sweeteners; butter or margarine.

Figure 21–6. Child-care centers throughout the world are an effective means whereby the nutrition of preschool children can be improved. In such centers children also learn about new foods. This group of children in Brazil is provided with a thick soup and milk. (Courtesy, UNICEF; photo by Jean Speiser.)

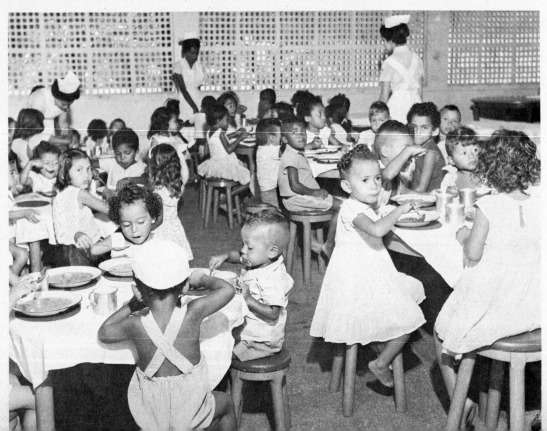

The standards for participation in the breakfast program are similar to those of the National School Lunch Program.

Special food service program. Federal legislation provides assistance to day-care centers, recreation centers, settlement houses, and summer day camps. The program administered by the U.S. Department of Agriculture provides meals for preschool children on a year-round basis, and to children over three years during the summer months. The guidelines for meals are similar to those for the school lunch. (See Figure 21–6.)

Special milk program. Reimbursement to schools, child-care centers, and camps is provided from federal funds to defray part of the cost of milk served. Because the milk can be sold at low cost to the child, milk drinking is encouraged. In schools where there are many needy children the full cost of the milk is reimbursed.

PROBLEMS AND REVIEW

1. What criteria, other than height and weight, may be used to determine nutritional status?
2. What average yearly gains may be expected from the end of the first year until maturity is reached? How do these vary for boys and girls?
3. Compare the protein and caloric needs of the one- to three-year-old; 7- to 10-year-old; 11- to 14-year-old; and 15- to 18-year-old boy with those of the adult.
4. Why would you expect the calcium, phosphorus, and iron needs to be especially high during childhood?
5. How long should vitamin D supplementation be provided? Why?
6. In terms of food habits, what can be expected at each of these ages: 18 months to 2 years; 5 years; 7 years; 10 years; 15 years?
7. Discuss the role of cultural pressures on food habits and attitudes to food.
8. In what way may disturbances in the mother-child relationship be reflected in feeding difficulties?
9. What is meant by the type A lunch?
10. Why is skipping breakfast a serious problem? What factors may interfere with the child's appetite for breakfast?
11. What objections may there be to the use of fried foods in the diet of preschool children? To the sale of soft drinks and candy on school premises?
12. *Problem.* Record the food intake of a child for one day, and calculate the nutritive values. Are all the nutrients provided at recommended levels? What suggestions can you make for the improvement of the diet?
13. Plan three menus for packed lunches for an eight-year-old boy. Do these lunches provide ⅓ of the day's recommended allowances?
14. A mother asks you about the advisability of allowing her children to eat between meals. What suggestions can you make to her?
15. *Problem.* Plan a menu for one day for a family consisting of father, mother, 16-year-old boy, 13-year-old girl who tends to be overweight, eight-year-old girl, and three-year-old boy. Indicate in table form the approximate amounts of food for each, and include any modifications in preparation which may be required.
16. *Problem.* List several ways in which a school nurse could assist in bringing about the improvement of food habits of schoolchildren.

CITED REFERENCES

1. Winick, M.: "Nutrition and the Ultimate Makeup of Various Tissues," *Food and Nutrition News,* National Livestock and Meat Board, Chicago, April 1969.
2. Sims, L. S., and Morris, P. M.: "Nutritional Status of Preschoolers. An Ecologic Perspective," *J. Am. Diet. Assoc.,* **64**:492–99, 1974.
3. Beal, V. A.: "Dietary Intake of Individuals Followed Through Infancy and Childhood," *Am. J. Public Health,* **51**:1107–17, 1961.

4. Burke, B. S., *et al.*: "Longitudinal Studies on Child Health and Development, Harvard School of Public Health, Series II, No. 4. Calorie and Protein Intakes of Children Between One and Eighteen Years of Age," *Pediatrics*, 24:922–74, 1959.
5. Nichaman, N. Z.: "Developing a Nutritional Surveillance System," *J. Am. Diet. Assoc.*, 65:15–17, 1974.
6. Schaefer, A. E., and Johnson, O. S.: "Are We Well Fed? The Search for the Answer," *Nutr. Today*, 4(1):2–11, 1969.
7. Macy, I. G., and Hunscher, H. A.: "Calories—A Limiting Factor in the Growth of Children," *J. Nutr.*, 45:189–99, 1951.
8. Ohlson, M. A., and Stearns, G.: "Calcium Intake of Children and Adults," *Fed. Proc.*, 18:1076–85, 1959.
9. Food and Nutrition Board: *Recommended Dietary Allowances*, 8th ed. National Academy of Sciences—National Research Council, Washington, D.C., 1974.
10. Beal, V. A.: "Nutritional Intake of Children. II. Calcium, Phosphorus and Iron," *J. Nutr.*, 53:499–510, 1954.
11. Morgan, A. F., *et al.*: *Nutritional Status, U.S.A.* Bull. 769, California Agricultural Experiment Station, Berkeley, 1959.
12. Eppright, E. S., *et al.*: "Very Heavy and Obese School Children in Iowa," *J. Home Econ.*, 48:168–72, 1956.
13. Johnson, M. L., *et al.*: "Relative Importance of Inactivity and Overeating in the Energy Balance of Obese High School Girls," *Am. J. Clin. Nutr.*, 4:37–44, 1956.
14. Huenemann, R. L., *et al.*: "A Longitudinal Study of Gross Body Composition and Body Conformation and Their Association with Food and Activity in a Teen-age Population. View of Teen-Age Subjects on Body Conformation, Food and Activity," *Am. J. Clin. Nutr.*, 18:325–38, 1966.
15. Dwyer, J. T., *et al.*: "Adolescent Attitudes Toward Weight and Appearance," *J. Nutr. Educ.*, 1 (No. 2):14–19, Fall 1969.
16. Stearns, G.: "Nutritional State of the Mother Prior to Conception," *J.A.M.A.*, 168:1655–59, 1958.
17. Thomas, J. A., and Call, D. L.: "Eating Between Meals—A Nutrition Problem Among Teen-agers?" *Nutr. Rev.*, 31:137–39, 1973.
18. Committee on Nutritional Misinformation, Food and Nutrition Board: "Water Deprivation and Performance of Athletes," *Nutr. Rev.*, 32:374–75, 1974.
19. Cho, M., and Fryer, B. A.: "What Foods Do Physical Education Majors and Basic Nutrition Students Recommend for Athletes?" *J. Am. Diet. Assoc.*, 65:541–44, 1974.
20. Bunting F., and Reese, R.: "USDA Food and Nutrition Programs—A Progress Report," *National Food Situation*, Economic Research Service, U.S. Department of Agriculture, Washington, D.C., Feb. 1975, pp. 34–42.
21. Head, M. K., *et al.*: "Major Nutrients in the Type A Lunch. 1 Analyzed and Calculated Values of Meals Served," *J. Am. Diet. Assoc.*, 63:620–25, 1973.
22. Council on Foods and Nutrition: "Confections and Carbonated Beverages," *J.A.M.A.*, 180:1118, 1962.
23. Martin, E. A.: *Roberts Nutrition Work with Children.* University of Chicago Press, Chicago, 1954.

ADDITIONAL REFERENCES

American Dietetic Association: "Position Paper on Child Nutrition Programs," *J. Am. Diet. Assoc.*, 64:520–21, 1974.
Arena, J. M.: "Nutritional Status of China's Children. An Overview," *Nutr. Rev.*, 32:289–95, 1974.
Bergstrom, J., and Hultman, E.: "Nutrition for Maximal Sports Performance," *J.A.M.A.*, 221:999–1006, 1972.
Beyer, N. R., and Morris, P. M.: "Food Attitudes and Snacking Patterns of Young Children," *J. Nutr. Educ.*, 6:131–33, 1974.
Chenoweth, A. D.: "Standards and Progress in Day Care Center Programs," *J. Am. Diet. Assoc.*, 60:197–200, 1972.
Christakis, G., *et al.*: "A Nutritional Epidemiologic Investigation of 642 New York City Children," *Am. J. Clin. Nutr.*, 21:107–26, 1968.
Committee on Nutrition, American Academy of Pediatrics: "Should Milk Drinking by Children Be Discouraged?" *Nutr. Rev.*, 32:363–69, 1974.

Futrell, M. F., *et al.:* "Nutritional Status of Black Preschool Children in Mississippi," *J. Am. Diet. Assoc.*, **66:**22–27, 1975.

Gaines, E. G., and Daniel, W. A., Jr.: "Dietary Iron Intakes of Adolescents," *J. Am. Diet. Assoc.*, **65:**275–80, 1974.

How Children Grow. Clinical Research Advances in Human Growth and Development. Pub. 73-166, National Institutes of Health, Bethesda, Md., 1972.

Huenemann, R. L., *et al.: Teenage Nutrition and Physique.* Charles C Thomas, Springfield, Ill. 1974.

Johnson, C. C., and Futrell, M. F.: "Anemia in Black Preschool Children in Mississippi," *J. Am. Diet. Assoc.*, **65:**536–41, 1974.

Knittle, J. L.: "Obesity in Childhood. A Problem in Adipose Tissue Cellular Development," *J. Pediatr.*, **81:**1048–59, 1972.

Leverton, R. M.: "The Paradox of Teen-age Nutrition," *J. Am. Diet. Assoc.*, **53:**13–16, 1968.

Martin, H. P.: "Nutrition: Its Relationship to Children's Physical, Mental, and Emotional Development," *Am. J. Clin. Nutr.*, **26:**766–75, 1973.

"School Athletics Food Facts and Myths," *Today's Health*, **44:**85, Sept. 1966.

Schuchat, M. G.: "The School Lunch and Its Cultural Environment," *J. Nutr. Educ.*, **5:**116–18, 1973.

Stunkard, A., *et al.:* "Influence of Social Class on Obesity and Thinness in Children," *J.A.M.A.*, **221:**579–84, 1972.

Thompson, R. J., and Palmer, S.: "Treatment of Feeding Problems. A Behavioral Approach," *J. Nutr. Educ.*, **6:**63–66, 1974.

PUBLICATIONS FOR THE LAYMAN

American Heart Association: *Healthy Eating for Teenagers*, 1969.

Children's Bureau, U.S. Department of Health, Education and Welfare, Washington, D.C.:
The Adolescent in Your Family.
Your Child from 1 to 3.
Your Child from 3 to 4.
Your Child from 1 to 6.

Nutrition Foundation: *Food Choices: The Teen-age Girl.*

U.S. Department of Agriculture, Washington, D.C.:
Food for the Family with Young Children, HG 5.
Food for the Families with School Children, HG 13.

22 Nutrition in Later Maturity

Some characteristics of aging. One person in ten today in the United States is 65 years or older, thus accounting for some 22 million individuals. The average life-span for a girl born today is 75 years, and for a boy it is 68 years. Most of the increase in life-span since the first years of this century has resulted from the greatly reduced infant mortality and not from the lengthening of the life-span during the later years. Having reached the age of 65 years, an individual has a life expectancy of another 14 years; at age 70, the expectancy is another 10 years.

Aging is a continuous process that begins with conception and ends with death. The Greek word for *old man* is *geron* and that for *treatise* is *logos*: therefore, the term GERONTOLOGY means the study of the aging process. The suffix *-iatrics* means *the treatment of;* thus, GERIATRICS is the specialty in medicine concerned with the prevention and treatment of disease in older persons.

Persons in later maturity fall into three subgroupings: those in middle age are likely to be at the peak of their careers and the fulfillment of their hopes, but are beginning to think about retirement; those for whom retirement has become a fact rightfully should be able to live up to high expectations; those in old age experience a decline with increasing dependency based upon state of health, economics, and social change. Vast differences may become apparent from one decade to another, but it is dangerous to generalize. It is just as wrong to place all persons over 65 years into one category as

it is to consider all individuals under 21 years in the single category of children. One individual in his 80s may well fit into a group characteristic of the 60s, whereas another in his 60s can be "older than his years."

An individual may enter upon the later years of his life with sufficient income for the necessities and some of the amenities of life; good physical and mental health; the love and support of a wife or husband and children; a role in the community; satisfying hobbies and interests to keep him busy; outlets for recreation; a sense of security and a feeling of being needed; and strong personal goals and spiritual values. He who has these blessings is indeed fortunate. But, for the majority of persons in the later years one or more of these characteristics is missing. The older person often comes to resent the designation "golden age" or "senior citizen," for reality is far removed from these connotations.

Socioeconomic factors. One third of all persons over 65 years have an income below the poverty level. Most of those who are rated above the poverty level are concerned about loss of income that may result from catastrophic illness. Retirement from one's occupation brings reduced income, with the majority of persons dependent upon small pensions (or none at all) and upon Social Security. Relatively small numbers of older persons have savings to provide income or to meet emergencies. In the recent inflationary years, the older person with a fixed income has had an increasingly difficult time providing for his needs. Technologic changes have also led to earlier retirement for many people; the man who is retired at 60 years, or even 55 years, has had less time to accumulate savings and finds it difficult to find other employment in our youth-oriented culture.

Loneliness is the complaint of millions of older persons. The active, productive individual upon retirement often finds that he has been "put on the shelf"; he is no longer consulted for advice; he seldom sees his former coworkers, and when he does he experiences a feeling of condescension—real or imagined. Loneliness also results from a change in the family situation. Children are often located in distant cities, and there is less communication with them. Most devastating of all is the loss of one's husband or wife. One of the major aspects of aging is that a larger and larger proportion of the older population consists of women who are widowed and living alone. There are 143 women over 65 years for every 100 men. (See Figure 22–1.)

Housing is a major problem for many older persons. Most older people remain in their own homes but they find it increasingly difficult to maintain repairs and to pay for expensive utilities and ever-increasing taxes. Those who live in apartments find that they cannot afford the increasing rents so they are forced to move to less desirable places. Many live in neighborhoods where they are afraid to walk on the streets because they might be robbed or physically assaulted. Living in a single room with no facilities for food preparation is the lot of a very large number of the elderly.

Transportation to shopping facilities, physician, dentist, and churches is a serious problem for many older people. Some cannot afford to drive an automobile and others have lost the ability to drive safely. Even those who live near public transportation find it difficult to manage bags of groceries while boarding or getting off vehicles.

PHYSIOLOGIC AND BIOCHEMICAL CHANGES

Cellular changes. For each species there appears to be a built-in limitation of the life-span. The forces that bring this about are by no means clear, but investigations of the aging process at the molecular level are beginning to shed some light on the process.

At least in part the changes in function that occur with aging are believed to be caused by a loss in the number of functioning cells.[1] The cells of the liver, gastrointestinal mucosa, skin, and hair continue to divide and reproduce throughout life. On the other hand, muscle and nerve cells do not have this capacity, thereby leading to gradual decrease in function. The changes that occur in the glomerular filtration rate and renal blood flow are caused, at least in part, by a reduction in the number of functioning nephrons.

The changes in connective tissue, which is so abundant in the human body, are of especial note. Collagen is one of the fibrous materials found in tendons, ligaments, skin, and blood vessels. With aging the amount of collagen increases and becomes more rigid; the skin loses its flexibility, the joints creak, and the back becomes bent.

The causes of aging are not known, but among the theories that have been set forth are these:[2,3] (1) there is a deterioration of the DNA molecule or a failure of the DNA repair mechanism so that protein synthesis is reduced; (2) a defect may occur in the RNA assembly of amino acids for protein synthesis; (3) a breakdown of immunologic processes could result in a failure to counteract damage by

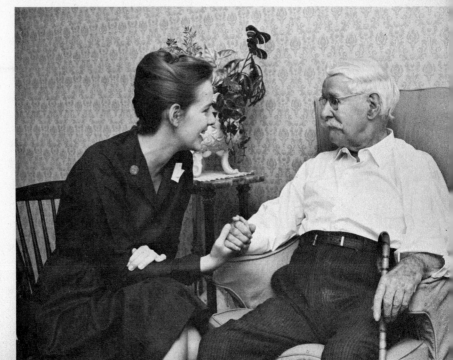

Figure 22–1. This public health nurse's warmth and genuine interest are important qualities for making diet instruction more likely to be followed. (Courtesy, The United Fund and Community Nursing Service, Philadelphia.)

harmful substances; and (4) highly reactive molecular fragments known as free radicals could lead to deterioration of collagen, elastin, and lipids. Free radicals can react with polyunsaturated fatty acids to form peroxidation products that could be the "mainspring of the aging process."[4] Lipid peroxidation is believed to bring about disintegration of the cell mitochondria, which are the energy powerhouse; thus, the ability to bring about electron transport and phosphorylation is lost. In addition, the lysosome membranes are broken, and the enzymes contained in these "suicide bags" bring about the hydrolysis of the cell.

Function of the gastrointestinal tract. The senses of taste and smell are less acute in later life, thus interfering with the appetite for many foods. Less saliva is secreted and the swallowing of food is sometimes difficult. The loss of natural teeth and a seeming inability on the part of the individual to become accustomed to dentures make it difficult to chew food properly or to eat with comfort. Consequently, more and more carbohydrate-rich foods which require a minimum of chewing may be selected, leading to seriously deficient intakes of protein, minerals, and vitamins.

Digestion in later years is affected in a number of ways. A reduction of the tonus of the musculature of the stomach, small intestine, and colon leads to less motility so that the likelihood of abdominal distention from certain foods is greater, as is also the prevalence of constipation. The volume, acidity, and pepsin content of the gastric juice are often reduced, achlorhydria being observed in 35 per cent of those 65 years and older. A reduction in acidity is known to have an adverse effect on the absorption of calcium and iron, and may also explain the lower vitamin B_{12} levels of blood observed in many older persons.

Fats are often poorly tolerated because they further retard gastric evacuation, because the pancreatic production of lipase is inadequate for satisfactory hydrolysis, and because chronic biliary impairment may reduce the production of bile or interfere with the flow of bile to the small intestine.

Energy metabolism. After maturity is reached, the energy metabolism decreases about 2 per cent for each decade. There is an increasing proportion of body fat to protoplasmic tissue, lesser muscle tension, and sometimes a diminution of thyroid activity. The rate of basal metabolism was found to

be higher in a group of vigorous, healthy women of middle age than it was for less active women of the same age.[5]

In the population as a whole the weight increases steadily throughout the years of maturity until it plateaus at the decade of 65 to 74 years. Thereafter, a gradual decline takes place. In general the incidence of overweight and underweight after 65 years follows the pattern of the population as a whole. Undoubtedly, obesity increases the susceptibility to the degenerative diseases of middle age, becomes an extra burden on weight-bearing joints, and increases the likelihood of accidents.

Carbohydrate metabolism. Usually the fasting blood sugar is normal. Likewise, the absorption of carbohydrate is not impaired. However, when a carbohydrate load is presented, as in the glucose tolerance test, the blood sugar remains elevated for a longer period of time than it does in younger persons. Following exercise, the levels of blood lactic acid and pyruvic acid are often above normal limits.

Fat metabolism. With increasing age the blood cholesterol and blood triglyceride levels gradually increase. The kind and amount of fat and carbohydrate in the diet, the degree of overweight, the stresses of life, and many other factors are believed to be responsible for these changes.

Health problems. In their later years many people experience one or more health problems that are related to their present or past nutritional status. (See Figure 22–2.) Anemias reflect several kinds of nutritional deficiency. Hypochromic, microcytic anemia characteristic of iron deficiency is surprisingly common in older persons. It could reflect a life-long inadequacy of iron intake, or, not infrequently, it is caused by a small, undetected chronic loss of blood from the gastrointestinal tract. Folacin lack is also fairly common and leads to a macrocytic anemia. Pernicious anemia results from a lack of intrinsic factor in the gastric juice and failure to absorb vitamin B_{12}.

Hormonal imbalances occur frequently. These lead to disturbances in nitrogen and calcium metabolism, and in turn to osteoporosis or bone loss. Osteoporosis is highly prevalent in women after age 50 and in men after age 60, with fractures occurring often. It occurs more frequently in people who have been poor milk drinkers throughout their lives.[6]

Disorders of the gastrointestinal tract are ex-

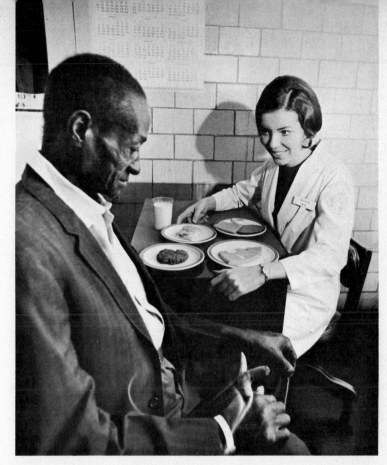

Figure 22-2. Inadequate income and declining health are major concerns of many older Americans. The dietitian or nurse must take these problems into consideration when giving guidance for a better diet. (Courtesy, Medical College of Virginia, Health Sciences Division, Virginia Commonwealth University, Richmond.)

tremely common, ranging from functional disorders such as irritable colon, to hiatus hernia, to pathologic changes such as diverticulitis and colon cancer. One of the etiologic factors is believed to be the low fiber content of the diet.[7]

The highest incidence of cardiovascular diseases occurs in those who are over 45 years, and these diseases account for the majority of deaths in the nation. There are many risk factors, of which a diet high in calories, saturated fat, and cholesterol over a lifetime is one. Adult-onset diabetes is seen especially in obese women after age 50, and its presence increases the susceptibility to atherosclerosis.

Crippling arthritis or a stroke interferes with the ability to shop, to prepare meals, and sometimes even to feed oneself.

Nutritional Requirements

Dietary deficiencies. Man's nutrition at age 60, 70, or 80 is the product of the influences of heredity, environment, and nutrition in the entire preceding years. Consequently, the variations in nutritional status are likely to be even more diverse than they are in the younger age groups which have been subject to the influences for a shorter period of time.

The individual who has had a lifetime of poor nutritional habits is not likely to be in as good health as the one who has enjoyed the benefits of a good diet. Good diet in later years cannot completely make up for the years of inadequacy or correct irreversible tissue changes. Furthermore, an older individual cannot completely change his whole pattern of eating. Nevertheless, even the individual with poor food habits who is in a poor state of nutrition can benefit greatly through the application of the principles of good nutrition.

The Ten-State Nutrition Survey showed that the nutrient density of food eaten by older persons was fairly good, and that the adequacy of protein, iron, thiamin, and vitamin A intakes depended upon the amount of food eaten.[8] On the other hand, ascorbic acid and riboflavin inadequacies were frequent and reflected the failure to choose foods rich in these nutrients. The diets of Spanish-Americans and blacks were less satisfactory than those of whites.

Recommended allowances. Although some clinicians prescribe increased levels of some nutrients for the older person, there is no convincing evidence that the requirements for protein, minerals, and vitamins are increased.[1]

Energy. For each decade after 25 years the caloric allowance is reduced. After 50 years, the allowance for a man is 2400 kcal and for a woman it is 1800 kcal. Inasmuch as the allowances for other nutrients are not reduced, women especially must choose their diets with care lest they exceed their caloric requirements. The Basic Diet (see Table 13–2) furnishes about three fourths of the woman's caloric need, so that in a given day approximately 500 kcal can be obtained from foods that are often favorite dishes of older people.

Protein. A daily intake of 0.8 gm protein per kilogram body weight is satisfactory.

Minerals. The allowance for calcium is the same as that for younger adults, whereas the iron allowance for men and women is 10 mg. Because anemia is a common occurrence in many men and women, iron supplements are sometimes prescribed. A diet liberal in calcium is believed to reduce bone loss but it will not reverse osteoporosis that has already occurred. Moderate restriction of salt intake is encouraged.

Vitamins. The allowances for vitamins are the same as those for younger adults. Because the energy requirement is lower, a slight reduction in niacin and riboflavin allowances is listed; this is proportionate to the caloric requirement.

Water and fiber. About 6 to 8 glasses fluid is as essential for the older person as it is for the younger individual. The kidneys can function more adequately when there is sufficient fluid with which to eliminate the waste solids. Water stimulates peristalsis and thus aids in combating constipation. When nocturia is a problem, the individual should be encouraged to take as much water as possible early in the day.

Many older persons select diets that are smooth in character. This choice, together with an inadequate fluid intake, can lead to persistent constipation and often to the use of harmful laxatives and mineral oil. Older persons, like younger individuals, should eat foods that provide fiber. Because fiber has the ability

to absorb water, normal laxation is encouraged and the transit time of wastes through the intestinal tract is reduced.

DIETARY MANAGEMENT

Food habits. The older person tends to follow dietary patterns of his earlier years. He has been influenced by the many factors which determine food acceptance from infancy throughout life (see Chapter 14). By the time he reaches middle age and later maturity, his pattern has become fixed and it is indeed difficult to introduce new foods or markedly to change the patterns of eating.

With increasing years the individual sees and hears less well, moves more slowly, and may be troubled by chronic illness. The frustrations and isolation from the people and work one loves and the feelings of being rejected and unwanted may be expressed by complaints against food and refusal to eat, or, on the other hand, by self-indulgence in favorite foods such as sweets.

Good food served in pleasant circumstances by people who care indicates to the older person that someone cares for him and that he is important. Attention to holiday customs, for example, bolsters the morale and the food intake. On the contrary, food poorly prepared or carelessly served may be associated with lack of love and thus will be refused.

Older persons who live alone often have no incentive to cook. They may eat carbohydrate foods to excess because they are easy to chew, require no preparation, and are inexpensive. Milk is taken poorly by many because of erroneous ideas concerning its value for adults, its supposed constipating or gas-producing effects, and its cost. Vegetables may be considered as too difficult to chew and too expensive. Fruits are often thought to be too "acid." Many older persons labor under the mistaken notion that their food needs are small because they no longer have growth needs, and because they are inactive.

Older persons are particularly susceptible to the claims of the food faddists. Having lost some sense of well-being they are likely to be misled by claims of unscrupulous persons concerning "miracle" diets and drugs. Although the foods recommended by these faddists may not in themselves be harmful, the undue emphasis placed upon them may mean that the necessary foods for nutritional adequacy are neglected and that the individual delays too long in seeking medical advice for his ills.

Daily meal plans. The Basic Diet outlined for the younger adult (Table 13–2) serves also as the foundation for the diet after 50 years. For the woman with her lower caloric requirements the remaining foods must be chosen with care lest the caloric intake be excessive. The following are two examples of a day's menus:*

BREAKFAST
Prune juice
French toast with powdered sugar
Coffee
  MIDDAY MEAL
Meat loaf
Au gratin potatoes
Broccoli
Cornbread with butter or margarine
Butterscotch pudding
Tea
  EVENING MEAL
Salmon salad
Tomato-green pepper salad
Bread with butter or margarine
Apricots
Milk
  SNACK
Toast
Tea

Second Menu
  BREAKFAST
Tangerine
Scrambled eggs
Toast with butter or margarine
Coffee
  MIDDAY MEAL
Macaroni and cheese
Brussels sprouts
Orange-grapefruit salad
French dressing
Bread with butter or margarine
Tapioca pudding
Milk
  EVENING MEAL
Fish chowder
Carrot and raisin salad

* Walker, M. A., and Hill, M. A.: *Food Guide for Older Folks.* HG 17, U.S. Department of Agriculture, Washington, D.C., 1972.

Bread with butter or margarine
Apple crisp
Milk
  SNACK
Toast
Tea

DIETARY COUNSELING

Most persons beyond 65 years live in their own homes and are able to take care of themselves. Any plans for the diet must give consideration to the individual's income, the facilities for food preparation, the physical ability to shop for food and prepare it, the social and cultural background, and the individual attitudes toward food together with the motivations for obtaining an adequate diet. With increasing age, the problems of meal management are greater. (See Figure 22–3.)

Many people will improve their diets if they are given assistance in planning simple meals that meet their nutritional requirements; advice concerning best food buys for the money; recipes suitable for one or two people; and suggestions for simple food preparation. Because many older people fall prey to "health food" hucksters, nutrition education is essential pertaining to the nutritional values of foods available in food markets in relation to their specific needs. Many older people do not need mineral or vitamin supplements. Those who do are identified only by medical examination, following which a prescription for the specific supplements should be given. The following suggestions may enhance the enjoyment of meals:

1. Serve colorful foods attractively on a tray if eating alone.

2. Eat leisurely in pleasant surroundings.

3. Eat four or five light meals instead of three heavier meals.

4. Include essential foods first. Sweets may be taken in moderate amounts but excess may cause discomfort and lead to overweight.

5. Eat a good breakfast to start the day right.

6. Fats may retard digestion. If there is discomfort, avoid fatty meats and fish; fried foods;

gravies, sauces, and salad dressings; rich cakes, doughnuts, pastries, and puddings.

7. Certain foods cause distress for some people. A given food should not be arbitrarily omitted just because a few cannot tolerate it.

8. Eat the heaviest meal at noon rather than at night if sleeping is difficult.

9. Avoid coffee and tea late in the day if insomnia is a problem.

Many older people are unable to chew their food well. Nevertheless, ground meats and puréed foods are quite unpopular. Older people in nursing homes were found to prefer roasts and chops even though they could not chew well, but they disliked steaks because they were difficult to cut and to chew; they also disliked ground meats.[9] With a sharp scissors or knife it is possible to finely mince meats and other foods for ease in swallowing and rapid digestive action. The following suggestions may help the person who has chewing difficulty to obtain a more adequate diet.

Milk as a beverage
Cottage or cream cheese; American cheese in sauces or casserole dishes
Eggs, soft cooked, scrambled, poached

Tender meat, or poultry, finely minced or ground; flaked fish; finely diced meat in sauces often taken more readily
Soft raw fruits as banana, berries; canned or cooked fruits; fruit juices
Soft-cooked vegetables, diced, chopped, or mashed. Raw vegetables such as tomatoes can often be eaten if finely chopped—skin and seeds removed
Cooked and dry cereals with milk
Bread, crackers, and toast with hot or cold milk
Desserts: diced cake with fruit sauce; fruit whips; gelatin; ice cream and ices; puddings; pie, if crust is tender and cut up

Community services. The Older Americans Act of 1965 established state and local agencies to develop comprehensive and coordinated service systems for the elderly. Within the past few years, under the act, nutrition programs variously known as *congregate meals* and *group feeding* have been initiated in many communities throughout the nation.[10,11] (See Figure 22–4.) These programs provide at least five hot meals a week, with each meal planned to furnish one third of the recommended allowances. Any person over 60 years is eligible to participate in the program, but priority is given to those who are over 75 years, who have a low income, who have a health problem and find meal

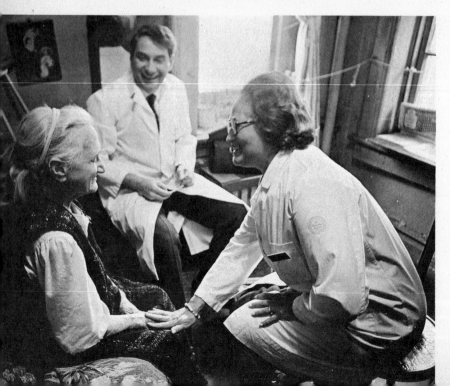

Figure 22–3. A visit by the physician and nutritionist gives reassurance to this homebound person, and establishes the need for meals delivered through the Meals-on-Wheels program. (Reprinted from *Hospitals, J.A.H.A.,* Dec. 16, 1973, and Courtesy, Mt. Sinai School of Medicine of the City University of New York.)

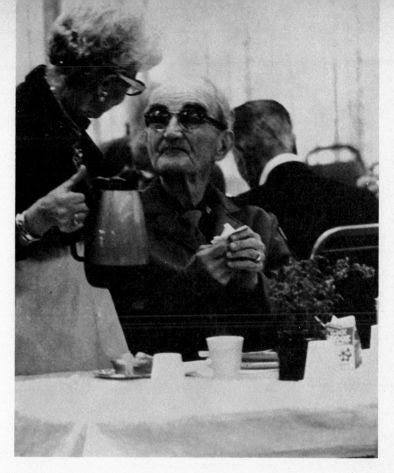

Figure 22–4. Group dining provides a meal meeting one third of the recommended allowances for older Americans in many communities, as well as offering opportunities for socialization. Many older Americans serve as volunteers in this program. (Courtesy, *The Evening and Sunday Bulletin,* Philadelphia; and Delaware County Nutritional Program for the Elderly, Community Nursing Service, Chester, Pennsylvania.)

preparation to be difficult, or who belong to a minority group. The program does more than provide a meal. Nutrition education is required, and there is opportunity for socialization, development of hobby interests, entertainment, and assistance in referral to specific agencies when there are problems of one kind or another. Senior citizens are encouraged to contribute to the cost of the meal, but a meal is not denied to a person who is unable to do so.

Under the Older Americans Act meals may be provided to home-bound persons. The meals are packaged at the group feeding site and delivered by volunteers. Another program, Meals on Wheels, has been in existence for many years under the auspices of volunteer organizations. This program furnishes a hot noon meal and a packaged supper five days a week.

PROBLEMS AND REVIEW

1. What changes occur with aging which may modify the digestion of foods?
2. Compare the nutritional needs of the adult of 25 years with one of 65 years.
3. What reasons can you give for the difficulty many older women experience in the healing of a bone?
4. What are the dangers of overweight in the middle aged?
5. A widow has no cooking facilities in her room and eats dinner in a restaurant. Her income is limited. What are some foods she could eat at home which require no cooking, but which would be nutritionally valuable?
6. *Problem.* Plan menus for two days which could be prepared with only a single gas burner available for cooking.

7. *Problem.* Using the low-cost plan on page 249 plan a week's menus for a man and woman 65 years old.
8. Consult the suggestions for effecting economy in food purchasing in Chapter 16. Which of these might not be practical for a single person or an older couple? Why?
9. Determine what nutrition programs are available for older persons in your community. How many persons are served? What are the requirements for participation in the program?

CITED REFERENCES

1. Shock, N. W.: "Physiologic Aspects of Aging," *J. Am. Diet. Assoc.*, **56**:491–96, 1970.
2. Krehl, W. A.: "The Influence of Nutritional Environment on Aging," *Geriatrics*, **29**:65–76, May 1974.
3. Marx, J. L.: "Aging Research. I. Cellular Theories of Senescence," *Science*, **186**:1105–1107, 1974.
4. Tappel, A. L.: "When Old Age Begins," *Nutr. Today*, **2**:2–7, Dec. 1967.
5. Roberts, P. H., *et al.*: "Nutritional Status of Older Women—Nitrogen, Calcium, Phosphorus Retentions of Nine Women," *J. Am. Diet. Assoc.*, **24**:292–99, 1948.
6. Lutwak, L.: "Continuing Need for Dietary Calcium Throughout Life," *Geriatrics*, **29**:171–78, May 1974.
7. Burkitt, D. P., and Painter, N. S.: "Dietary Fiber and Disease," *J.A.M.A.*, **229**:1068–74, 1974.
8. Young, C. M.: "Nutritional Counseling for Better Health," *Geriatrics*, **29**:83–91, May 1974.
9. Lane, M. M.: "Stereotyped Ideas About Food," *Nurs. Homes*, **16**:27, Dec. 1967.
10. Wells, C. E.: "Nutrition Programs Under the Older Americans Act," *Am. J. Clin. Nutr.*, **26**:1127–32, 1973.
11. Pelcovits, J.: "Nutrition Education in Group Meals Programs for the Aged," *J. Nutr. Educ.*, **5**:118–20, 1973.

ADDITIONAL REFERENCES

American Dietetic Association: "Position Paper on Nutrition and Aging," *J. Am. Diet. Assoc.*, **61**:623, 1972.
Ball, I. M.: "The World's Oldest Commune," *Nutr. Today*, **8**:13–16, Sept. 1973.
Dreizen, S., ed.: "Symposium on Nutrition," *Geriatrics*, **29**:55–178, May 1974.
Elwood, T. W.: "Nutritional Concerns of the Elderly," *J. Nutr. Educ.*, **7**:50–52, 1975.
Foster, H. A.: "Understanding the Senior Citizen," *Nurs. Care*, **6**:27–31, June 1973.
Frenay, Sr. A. C.: "Helping Students Work with the Aging," *Nurs. Outlook*, **16**:44–46, July 1968.
Goldstein, S.: "Biological Aging. An Essentially Normal Process," *J.A.M.A.*, **230**:1651–52, 1974.
Johnston, H., and Holmen, C.: "Nutrition for the Aged and Handicapped," *Nurs. Care*, **6**:12–15, Sept. 1973.
Luhrs, C. E.: "Feeding the Elderly," *Am. J. Clin. Nutr.*, **26**:1150–52, 1973.
Mann, G. V.: "Relationship of Age to Nutrient Requirements," *Am. J. Clin. Nutr.*, **26**:1096–97, 1973.
Mayer, J.: "Aging and Nutrition," *Geriatrics*, **29**:57–59, May 1974.
Rao, D. B.: "Problems of Nutrition in the Aged," *J. Am. Geriatr. Soc.*, **21**:362–67, 1973.
Schlenker, E. D., *et al.*: "Nutrition and Health of Older People," *Am. J. Clin. Nutr.*, **26**:1111–19, 1973.
Sherwood, S.: "Sociology of Food and Eating. Implications for Action for the Elderly," *Am. J. Clin. Nutr.*, **26**:1108–10, 1973.
Stone, V.: "Give the Older Person Time," *Am. J. Nurs.*, **69**:2124–27, 1969.
Weinberg, J.: "Psychologic Implications of the Nutritional Needs of the Elderly," *J. Am. Diet. Assoc.*, **60**:293–96, 1972.

PUBLICATIONS FOR THE LAYMAN

Food Guide for Older Folks, HG 17, U.S. Department of Agriculture, Washington, D. C., 1972.
Irwin, T.: *Better Health in Later Years.* Pamphlet 446, Public Affairs Committee, Inc., New York, 1970.
May, E. E., *et al.*: *Homemaking for the Handicapped.* Dodd, Mead, and Company, New York, 1966.

23 National and International Problems in Nutrition

that exist in official and voluntary organizations for working with these problems; to provide a few examples of nutrition programs in action; and to develop a sense of individual responsibility toward the improvement of nutrition and health.

SCOPE OF MALNUTRITION

The nature of malnutrition. Malnutrition is an inclusive term that involves the lack, imbalance, or excess of one or more of some 40 or so nutrients that are required by the body. Although some nutritional deficiencies are encountered in the United States and the countries of western Europe, the principal nutritional problems are obesity, dental caries, and some diseases such as cardiovascular diseases, and gastrointestinal disorders in which dietary excesses and imbalances appear to be among the risk factors implicated. In the Asian, African, and Latin American countries calorie and protein deficits are the chief problems of nutrition. Usually these deficits are associated with vitamin and mineral deficiencies as well.

An overview of the principal nutritional problems in the United States and throughout the world was presented in Chapter 1. The nutritional deficiencies arising from lack of specific nutrients, the nutritional problems encountered at various stages of the life cycle, and the effects of disease upon nutrition are discussed in detail in appropriate chapters of this text. Table 23–1 summarizes the principal nutritional deficiencies on the world scene today and includes a cross-reference to the chapters within this text where a fuller description is available.

Nutritional deficiencies. In the initial stages of development a deficiency is so mild that physical signs are absent and biochemical methods generally cannot detect the slight changes. As tissue depletion continues the biochemical changes can be measured in body fluids and tissues. With further depletion the physical signs become apparent until finally the full-blown signs of the predominating classic deficiency can be recognized.

Nutritional deficiencies rarely occur singly inasmuch as an inadequacy of food almost always reduces the intake of more than one nutrient. Moreover, the metabolic interdependence of nutri-

Focus on community nutrition. The term PUBLIC HEALTH NUTRITION is generally understood to be concerned with those problems of nutrition that affect large numbers and that can be solved most effectively through group action. The term COMMUNITY may be used to refer to any group of people—small or large; it might be, for example, a closely knit group such as the student community, or it might be certain areas of a city, state, or nation.

Physicians, nurses, dietitians, nutritionists, social workers, and teachers in their respective roles must be informed citizens regarding the nutritional concerns of the local community, the state, the nation, and even the world. Some of them will pursue careers in governmental or private agencies whose primary function is better health through better nutrition. All professional workers in health and education have a responsibility to assume leadership in finding solutions to nutritional problems of the community whether it be support of agencies that are providing services, expansion of educational programs in nutrition, committee activities to develop new programs, or taking a position on proposed legislation that affects the nutritional well-being of the population.

The purposes of this chapter and Chapter 24 are to give the reader an appreciation of the scope of nutrition problems in the nation and throughout the world; to create an awareness of the many resources

Table 23–1. Summary of Diseases of Malnutrition

Principal Disease Conditions	Nutrient Imbalances
Deficiencies	
Underweight	Calorie deficit (Chapter 29)
Protein-calorie malnutrition	
Kwashiorkor	Principally protein lack (page 347)
Marasmus	Calorie-protein lack (page 347)
Dental caries	Calcium, phosphorus, fluorine, vitamins A and D (Chapters 8, 10)
Anemia, microcytic, hypochromic	Iron (Chapters 8 and 43)
Macrocytic in infancy, pregnancy, malabsorption	Folacin (Chapters 12 and 43)
Pernicious (absorptive defect)	Vitamin B_{12} (Chapters 12 and 43)
Goiter, endemic	Iodine (Chapter 8)
Osteoporosis	Possibly calcium, vitamin D; endocrine factors (Chapter 38)
Osteomalacia	Vitamin D, calcium, phosphorus (Chapter 10)
Scurvy; hemorrhagic tendency; inflamed gums; loose teeth	Ascorbic acid (Chapter 11)
Beriberi; polyneuritis; circulatory failure; emaciation; edema	Thiamin (Chapter 12)
Pellagra; glossitis; dermatitis; diarrhea; nervous degeneration; dementia	Niacin (Chapter 12)
Cheilosis; scaling of skin; cracking of lips; light sensitivity; increased vascularization of eyes	Riboflavin (Chapter 12)
Growth failure, anemia, convulsions in infants	Vitamin B_6 (Chapter 12)
Night blindness; keratomalacia; xerophthalmia; blindness	Vitamin A (Chapter 10)
Rickets; bone deformities	Vitamin D (Chapter 10)
Hemorrhagic tendency in infants	Vitamin K (Chapter 10)
Excesses	
Obesity	Calorie excess (Chapter 29)
Toxicity: changes in skin, hair, bones, liver	Vitamin A excess (Chapter 10)
Hypercalcemia, calcification of soft tissues	Vitamin D excess (Chapter 10)
Dental caries	Sticky sugars (Chapter 5)
Atherosclerosis: cardiovascular and cerebrovascular disease*	Too much saturated fat, cholesterol; ?simple sugars (Chapter 40)
Hypertension*	Calorie excess; ?too much salt (Chapter 41)
Diverticulosis; irritable colon*	Excessively refined diets (Chapter 33)
Cancer of the colon*	?Excessively refined diets; ?excess of fat leading to excess metabolites of sterols and bile acids (Chapter 33)

*In these diseases diet is only one of a number of risk factors that must be considered; more research is needed to fully establish the role of diet.

ents means that a lack of one will interfere with the proper utilization of another, many examples of which have been cited in Chapters 4 through 12.

Primary nutritional deficiencies are those that are caused by inadequate or imbalanced intake of food.

These conditions are the result of many environmental factors, some of which are discussed more fully on page 340.

Secondary deficiencies are those that result from some fault in digestion, absorption, and metabolism so that tissue needs are not met even though the ingested diet would be adequate in normal circumstances. Thus, the restoration and maintenance of good nutrition are important concerns in clinical nutrition.

Some signs of nutritional deficiencies. Classic deficiency diseases are diagnosed relatively easily because the physical and biochemical findings are prominent and specific. Nevertheless, the diagnosis of even these may be missed when the disease is seldom seen by clinicians, as is the case in the United States.

Many of the physical signs that suggest nutritional lack are also the result of other factors. For example, a student who obtains only five or six hours of sleep may complain that he is unable to concentrate well, is irritable, and always feels tired. These symptoms are also characteristic of a continuing dietary lack of B-complex vitamins. A differential diagnosis and correct treatment can be arrived at only when there is a correlation of a complete medical and dietary history, a thorough physical examination, and laboratory studies. The latter include the blood concentration of many substances such as hemoglobin, plasma proteins, minerals, and vitamins, the urinary excretion of metabolic end products, and bone x-rays.

By being observant a teacher, nurse, or nutritionist can detect many signs in schoolchildren and in adults that suggest the possibility of nutritional deficiency and can hasten referral to a physician for diagnosis. These signs, of themselves, do not warrant a diagnosis of general or specific deficiency, and much harm can result when treatment is recommended by those not fully qualified to do so. Among the signs and complaints to which teachers and nurses may be alert are these:

Attendance: frequent absences from school or work.

Growth: deviation from standards by more than 10 per cent; appearance of excessive obesity or thinness; failure to grow in stature or gain in weight.

Behavior: easily fatigued; listless; apathetic; depressed; nervous; irritable; inability to concentrate; complaints of insomnia; lowered work capacity.

Skin: pallor; dermatitis; scaling around the nose and ear; wounds that fail to heal; bed sores.

Hair: dull, lifeless, thin; easily pulled out.

Eyes: swollen, congested eyelids; itching, burning; increased vascularization; poor vision in dim light.

Mouth: swollen, red lips; fissuring at the corners of the lips; sore, inflamed tongue; pale mucous membranes.

Teeth: dental caries; poor chewing; sore, bleeding gums.

Skeletal deformities: poor posture; deformities of the long bones, bones of the chest, spine, and pelvis.

Neuromuscular: poor coordination; flabby muscles; sore, painful muscles; muscle weakness.

Thyroid: enlarged.

Infections: frequent colds and other infections.

Gastrointestinal: poor appetite; diarrhea; fear of eating many foods.

Economic cost of malnutrition. The maintenance of health and the treatment of disease are important not only for humanitarian reasons but also in economic terms. What is good nutrition really worth? Can a preventive program in nutrition be economically justified? The answers are not easy to obtain.

Programs to prevent nutritional deficiencies, excesses, or imbalances must emphasize lifelong attention to diet. The costs of such preventive action include a vast educational program for the public, assistance to the poor, and the services of health and welfare agencies. Effective preventive programs can be expected to reduce the costs of medical services including hospital care, extended-care services, physician's fees, laboratory studies, drugs, and other expenses. Illness also means loss of income through absence from work and loss of time in school. In the marginally ill and the physically and mentally handicapped it means reduced efficiency at work, reduced ability to learn, and the ability to perform only a limited range of tasks.

Child wastage because of malnutrition has been singled out as being especially restrictive in an economic sense.[1] Children comprise up to half of the population in many developing countries, but most of them will never reach maturity. The costs involved in their short lives include extra food consumed by the mother during pregnancy, the costs of childbirth, the food, clothing, and shelter consumed by the child while living, and even the costs of burial. These malnourished children are consumers without ever reaching the status of producers and their own brief existence has usually been miserable.

When malnourished children survive to adulthood their stunted growth, retarded mental development, lessened ability to learn, reduced work efficiency, and physical defects including blindness are among the handicaps that beset them.

Factors Contributing to Undernutrition

The causes of undernutrition are complex. They include conditions that preexist within the individual—the *host*, the quality of the *environment*, and the specific *agents* that provoke the problem. Each element of this triad interacts with others. For example, many people in the United States suffer from some degree of malnutrition but the food supply, water, and waste disposal meet high standards of sanitation and safety so that health remains relatively good. On the other hand, people in some developing countries suffer the same degree of undernutrition but are exposed to grossly contaminated food and water so that life-threatening illness results.

Susceptibility of the individual. Within a given environment some individuals are more susceptible than others to malnutrition. Normal adults can usually survive moderate nutritional deficits rather well. Among the vulnerable groups are these:

1. Infants and preschool children: their nutritional requirements are high during rapid growth. When nutrients are not available for a given stage of development, the physical or mental retardation may be irreversible.

2. Pregnant women: inadequate diets compromise the development of the fetus and also the mother's own nutritional status and her freedom from the complications of pregnancy.

3. The elderly: malnutrition results from chronic ill health and long-standing nutritional deficiency; endocrine imbalances; inability to chew; physical handicaps that prevent adequate shopping or food preparation; loneliness and lack of interest in eating; and misconceptions concerning diet.

4. The sick: poor appetites; psychiatric disorders that prevent eating; infections; fevers and metabolic disorders that increase nutritional requirements; allergy; blood losses; injuries; gastrointestinal disorders that lead to fear of eating; diarrhea; malabsorption; and so on. (See Chapter 30.)

The vulnerability of these groups to malnutrition is considered when priorities are assigned to food assistance and to educational programs.

Environmental factors that favor malnutrition. In the United States and throughout the world poverty and ignorance are leading causes of malnutrition. Lack of available food is a principal cause of malnutrition in the underdeveloped and the developing countries of the world, but not in North America, Europe, and Oceania.

Poverty. Two billion people live in about 100 poor underdeveloped nations of the world. Two thirds of these people live in Asia. In most African and Latin American countries the per capita income ranges from moderate to extreme poverty.

Even in the United States approximately 30 million people are living at or below the poverty level. They are to be found in the slums of the cities and in rural areas as well. Minority groups including blacks, Puerto Ricans, Spanish-Americans, American Indians, and many people living in Appalachian regions constitute important segments of the poor population. The plight of no group in the United States is less favorable than that of the migrant farm workers who have few if any roots in a community and who often do not have the services of agencies that can provide assistance.

Inflationary food costs in recent years have worsened the plight of the poor. Poverty means too few dollars to spend for food; competition between food and other necessities of life as well as things that give personal satisfaction for the available income; lack of food storage and preparation facilities; inability to purchase foods under the most favorable price conditions; and crowded, often unsanitary housing. Poverty results in a vicious cycle: poverty—inadequate diet—undernutrition—illness—inability to work—poverty. (See Figure 23–1.)

Population growth. At present the food supply in the developing countries is just about keeping pace with the growth in population. (See Figure 23–2.) Half of the world's population live in the Far East but only one fourth of the world's food supply is produced there. If the entire world food supply could be evenly distributed, it would just about meet the energy needs of the people.

By the year 2000 a population of 6.5 to 7 billion persons is predicted. Thus, it becomes necessary within a quarter century to almost double the food supply even at the present inadequate standards.

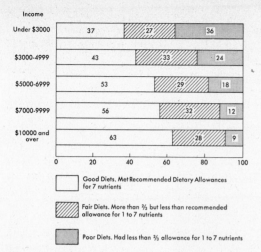

Income

Income			
Under $3000	37	27	36
$3000-4999	43	33	24
$5000-6999	53	29	18
$7000-9999	56	32	12
$10000 and over	63	28	9

0   20   40   60   80   100

☐ Good Diets. Met Recommended Dietary Allowances for 7 nutrients

▨ Fair Diets. More than ⅔ but less than recommended allowance for 1 to 7 nutrients

▦ Poor Diets. Had less than ⅔ allowance for 1 to 7 nutrients

Figure 23–1. With each decrease in income, the percentage of poor diets increases. Even at liberal income levels, however, 1 diet in 10 is poor, and 3 in 10 are fair. (Courtesy, U.S. Department of Agriculture.)

There is, however, a finite limit to the acreage available for agriculture, for water resources, and for fertilizers to increase crop yields. Control of population growth is especially difficult to achieve in countries where infant and child mortality is high and each couple wants survivors who can care for them in their old age.

Lack of education. People of all income classes and at all educational levels lack knowledge regarding the essentials of an adequate diet. (See Figure

23–1.) Those who are ignorant concerning nutrition are particularly susceptible to food faddism, superstition, and nutritional quackery.

A limited education exacts a particularly severe toll from those who are also poor. It is, for many of them, the cause of their poverty inasmuch as people with minimal education and technical skills are unable to secure employment to earn a satisfactory living wage. Somehow, the poor must use each dollar more carefully but they have too little consumer information to help them. Moreover, inasmuch as the amount and quality of food available to them are limited, they need to employ the best techniques in food preparation to preserve nutritive values—but they lack the facilities and skills to do so. (See Figure 23–3.)

Cultural factors. Malnutrition sometimes results because people refuse to eat foods prohibited by religious beliefs or taboos and superstitions, those that lack prestige value, and those that are unfamiliar.

The taking of life is prohibited by some religions and no flesh foods may be eaten. This restriction excludes even eggs and milk for some. The prohibition against the taking of life may also mean that pesticides will not be used against rodents, thus resulting in high food losses in some countries. In India the sacred cows still compete seriously for the food supply of humans.[2]

Social customs, taboos, and superstitions interfere with adequate food intake, especially by vulnerable

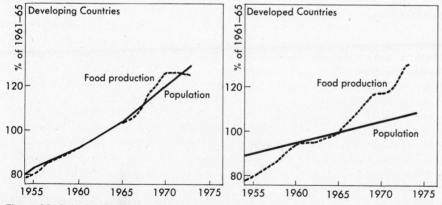

Figure 23–2. In the developing countries food production barely keeps pace with the population growth. The developed countries produce food in excess of population growth and can, therefore, meet emergency needs. As population increases there will be less ability to meet food needs. (Courtesy, Economic Research Service, U.S. Department of Agriculture.)

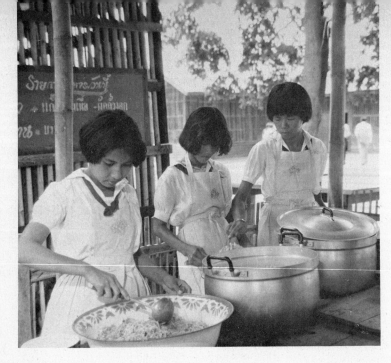

Figure 23–3. Young students in a village in Thailand learn about nutrition by preparing meals. (Courtesy, UNICEF; photo by Jack Ling.)

groups. In some of the developing countries the father and other men in the family eat first and are given the choicest share of food. When food is scarce, women and children may get less than they need. Many primitive people believe that foods are endowed with specific qualities that can influence the personality of the unborn child or that can mark him physically. Thus, animal foods in particular may be taboo for pregnant and lactating women.

To be accepted food must be familiar. People to whom rice is the staple do not quickly change to a diet consisting principally of wheat. Even a change in a familiar food will reduce its acceptability. The new high-yielding varieties of rice and corn are less well liked by the people who use them because they are slightly different in color and texture and have somewhat different cooking qualities.[3]

Plentiful foods may be ignored because they lack status value even though they are of excellent nutritive quality, whereas other foods of more marginal value may be selected because of their prestige value. Poor people often resent gifts of food that are classed as surplus. In the developing countries spices, fats, oils, sweets, tea, coffee, and cola beverages are often purchased because they are equated with a higher standard of living.[2]

Urbanization. Jelliffe[4] has described the flood of rural dwellers to the cities that is now occurring throughout the entire world as "disurbanization"

because the influx is too rapid to accommodate people in terms of employment, housing, food, and services. The shanty towns and ghettos provide surroundings that are often worse than the rural areas left behind. Because they need cash to purchase food, people find themselves with diets that are more meager than their rural fare.

Infants and children suffer most from this trend. Infants are often weaned early, partly because the mother seeks employment and partly because she is trying to emulate the women of the Western world who do not breast-feed their babies. Unfortunately, the substitute feedings for the baby are insufficient in quantity, often poor in quality, and likely to be grossly contaminated with bacteria. Jelliffe deplores the use of highly advertised expensive proprietary infant formulas because few people in the developing countries can afford them and mothers use too little of the formula to meet the baby's needs.

Inadequate supply of food. Since 1972–1973 there has been a deepening food crisis throughout the world. Natural disasters such as the floods in Bangladesh and India and the severe droughts for several years in the Sahel, Africa, have severely curtailed food production thus leading to starvation for millions of people. World food resources at the end of the crop year in 1974 were down to 27 days, a dangerously low level if crop failures were to occur in food surplus countries such as the United States and Canada. People in affluent countries are demanding more and more animal foods, especially meat, and thereby excessive amounts of grain are fed to animals rather than directly as human food.

Tremendous increases in oil prices have made it impossible for farmers in developing countries to adopt modern methods of agriculture that depend upon energy resources, or to purchase fertilizers that are dependent upon oil for their production. (See Figure 23–4.) Food spoilage is excessively high because of lack of processing, storage, and distribution facilities. Where agriculture is most primitive the diets are almost always at the subsistence level. Thus, there is no food left over for an emergency. In the developing countries governments are usually unable to finance the irrigation programs needed for crops, the industrial plants for food processing and storage, and the roads for food distribution.

Food Faddism and Nutritional Quackery

About 1 billion dollars is spent annually in the United States for food fads. There are at least 3000 "health food" stores, and a great number of super-markets stock "natural," "organic," and "health" foods.[5]

A FAD is a fashion of the moment—here today and gone tomorrow. Thus it is with many food fads. A teen-age girl often follows a fad diet to lose weight whereas the boy relies upon fad diets to give him athletic prowess. The elderly individual looks to a food or fad diet as a panacea for poor health. Food fads stem from ignorance about food properties and the essentials of nutritionally adequate diets. They are subscribed to by the rich and poor, and the young and old.

NUTRITIONAL QUACKERY refers to the misrepresentation and fraud practiced for financial gain by those who pose as authorities in nutrition but who have little or no preparation for their practice.

Types of food fads. Among the numerous fallacies foisted upon the unwary public are these.

1. *Fallacy.* So-called "health" foods are believed to have specific properties in promoting health or in curing disease beyond the values expected from their nutritive composition. For example, honey and vinegar is held to be useful in treating arthritis, and garlic is believed to reduce hypertension.

Facts. No single food has unique health-giving

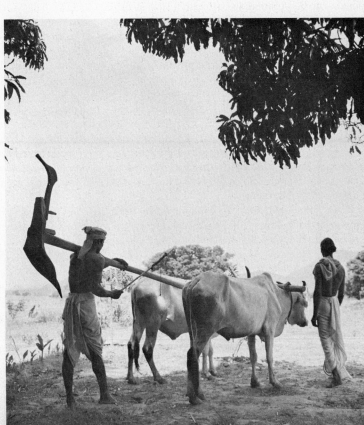

Figure 23–4. Primitive methods of agriculture restrict the amount of land that can be tilled and the yield per acre. (Courtesy, UNICEF; photo by Jack Ling.)

properties. To designate some foods as "health" foods implies that conventional foods one might purchase in a market are not healthful. This is not so. Good nutritional status requires that the proper balance and quantities of essential nutrients be obtained from a mixed diet of many possible food combinations.

Diseases have numerous causes, among which poor diet may be contributory, as in the nutritional deficiencies. No food is known to cause arthritis, nor is any specific food helpful in its treatment. Arthritic patients, like others, require a nutritionally adequate diet and should avoid becoming overweight. Chronic degenerative diseases such as cancer, diabetes, and others are not cured by specific foods. In some endocrine diseases such as diabetes mellitus a controlled diet planned to meet individual needs is essential therapy, but these pathologic conditions require medical advice and meticulous counseling by professionally qualified personnel.

2. *Fallacy.* Organically grown foods are nutritionally superior. The designation "organic foods" generally refers to those grown on soils fertilized only with manures and composts.

Facts. All foods are organic in that they are composed of carbon-containing compounds such as proteins, fats, and carbohydrates. Before the manures and composts can be used by plants they must be degraded by bacteria to inorganic compounds. Whether grown on soils fertilized by chemical fertilizers or by manures, the foods are equally high in nutritive value. The amount of manures and composts available is totally inadequate to meet the farmer's needs to obtain maximum yields from his lands.

3. *Fallacy.* Pesticides should never be used on crops, nor should additives be used in processing. These chemical compounds are toxic and can lead to diseases such as cancer.

Facts. Some pesticides, to be sure, have been shown to constitute a health hazard, and their use is prohibited. The Food Protection Committee of the Food and Nutrition Board, the Food and Drug Administration, and the U.S. Department of Agriculture are concerned with setting standards for pesticides, testing new products, and developing safe controls for their use. Without some control of insects and plant diseases, the food supply in many

parts of the world would be so seriously threatened that the effects of food shortages and famine would far outweigh the possible hazards of pesticides.

Many additives are useful for food preservation, for improvement of nutritional value, and for enhancement of quality. (See page 264.)

4. *Fallacy.* Foods used in their "natural" state, that is, without refinement, processing, or the use of additives, are more healthful. Processed foods are devoid of nutritive value. White bread, white sugar, canned foods, and pasteurized milk are held to be nutritionally impoverished.

Facts. Most white bread is now enriched with iron, thiamin, niacin, and riboflavin to whole-grain levels (See Figure 13–4.) Although white sugar provides no protein, minerals, or vitamins, its moderate use in the diet can be justified. (See page 73.) Brown sugar, raw sugar, and honey are also good sources of carbohydrate and calories, but they are more expensive than white sugar. They contain insignificant traces of some minerals and vitamins.

All food processing has some effect on nutritive values, but modern techniques in the food industry maintain high nutritive values. In fact, vegetables and fruits frozen or canned at the peak of their quality may be superior to the fresh product that has been poorly handled from farm to market.

5. Reducing fads are so numerous that one may wonder whether some popular publications could survive without them! Their proponents often reap generous incomes from them before the unsuspecting public realizes that weight loss is simply a matter of adjusting calories below the energy requirement on an otherwise adequate diet. See Chapter 29.

6. Extreme forms of vegetarianism such as the Zen macrobiotic diet will lead to nutritional deficiencies and to serious illness. See pages 56 and 227.

7. Many people believe that megadoses of vitamins will convey some superior health benefit. Excessive intakes of vitamins A and D are toxic (see pages 155 and 158). Vitamin E does not possess the many curative properties ascribed to it (see page 160), and the influence of ascorbic acid in the prevention or mitigation of the effects of common colds is controversial (see page 169).

Identifying the quack. The food faddist or charlatan is not always identified with ease, but he may have some of these characteristics and may employ some of these techniques.

He sells something—special foods, a dietary plan, cooking utensils, cookbooks, magazines, and books describing dietary regimens, or a series of lectures.

He appeals to the emotions rather than to the intellect. He plays upon the fears and hopes of people. Either he scares people about the dire consequences of failing to consume certain foods or to use certain products, or he makes fantastic claims for cure of disease, or for beauty, vitality, and long life.

He claims that he is persecuted by medical and nutritional groups. He generally attacks the medical profession, regulatory federal agencies, agricultural practices, and the food industry.

He glibly uses scientific terminology to confuse his audience and to impress upon them that he is learned in the science of nutrition. He often quotes reputable nutrition authorities, lifting their writings out of context.

He usually has no academic preparation in college or in a professional school that qualifies him to be an expert in nutrition, but he makes claim to diplomas, degrees, titles, and experience.

The products sold by the nutrition quack are dispensed through "health food" stores, by door-to-door sales, and through the mails. The advertising for their products is characterized by exaggerated claims, by money-back guarantees, and by testimonials.

How to combat food faddism and quackery. A program of nutrition education in the schools and for the adult population could immeasurably reduce the dangers of faddism but it is naïve to believe that faddism could be altogether avoided. There are always people who like to think that some special food or product can effect some miracle in their lives.

Several federal agencies are empowered to combat food faddism, but these powers are restricted to materials that cross state lines. Many states have also set up regulations comparable to those of federal groups. Among the legal channels to reduce food faddism are the regulations against adulteration and misbranding set up by the Food and Drug Administration. (See page 276.)

The U.S. Post Office can prosecute individuals who solicit money through the mails by fraudulent advertising. The Federal Trade Commission is empowered to issue orders of cease and desist, and to prosecute those who engage in deceptive advertising through public communications media.

Protein-Calorie Malnutrition—A World Concern

Protein-calorie malnutrition (P-CM), the world's most serious nutritional problem, to some degree affects up to 70 per cent of infants and preschool children in the developing countries of Africa, the Middle East, southeastern Asia, and Central and South America. Millions die annually and millions more will go through life stunted in their physical growth and unable to achieve their potential mental development. P-CM is an inclusive term that embraces mild deficiency, kwashiorkor, and marasmus. (See Figure 23–5.)

Etiology. Dr. Cicely Williams, a pediatrician, in the 1930s observed a syndrome in infants and children in Ghana which was called kwashiorkor. This is "the disease the deposed baby gets when the next one is born."[6] In the developing countries babies are usually breast fed for 18 to 24 months, and sometimes longer. Upon the birth of another child, the older child is deposed from the breast and subsists largely on a high-carbohydrate low-protein diet provided by the staple foods of the country. The symptoms become apparent about three to four months after the child has been weaned and have their highest incidence between two and five years of age.

In Africa the staples to which the child is weaned are manioc, cassava, plantain, and millet; in Central America and South America they are corn and beans; and in Asia, rice and some legumes. These foods do not provide sufficient amino acids for the rapid growth needs of the infant. The ignorance of the mother concerning food needs of the baby may further reduce the intake of protein. In Iran, for example, many babies are given tea sweetened with as much as 40 gm sugar daily.[7] Condensed milk has been substituted for evaporated milk in some instances, thereby providing a high-carbohydrate

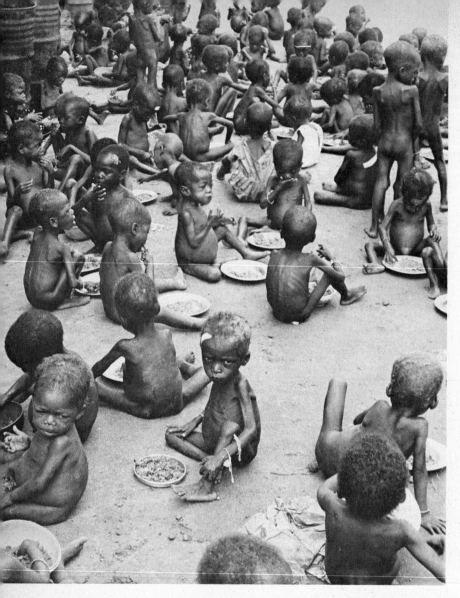

low-protein formula. When diarrhea is present, the concerned mother often resorts to feeding of dilute gruels for extended periods of time.

Marasmus results from a deficiency of calories as well as protein. It occurs at an earlier age than does kwashiorkor and is usually evident by the second half of the first year. The incidence of marasmus is increasing with urbanization in the developing countries because infants are being weaned at a very early age. The low-protein formulas and other staple foods, poverty, poor sanitation, and cultural patterns all contribute to the high incidence. The occurrence of P-CM in mild to severe stages accelerates rapidly in countries afflicted by drought, floods, and war.

Synergism between malnutrition and infection. When a diet is nutritionally inadequate but the sanitation is good and infections are minimal, the onset of deficiency symptoms is gradual. Likewise, when a well-nourished child succumbs to an infection, the period of illness is usually short, the residual effects are few, and the mortality rate is low. Conversely, the coexistence of malnutrition and infection vastly increases the severity of both; that

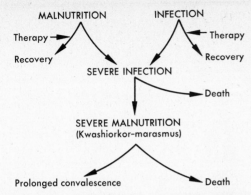

Figure 23–6. The prognosis in malnutrition or infection occurring independently is good if appropriate therapy is instituted. When malnutrition and infection interact, the severity of both is greatly increased and the prognosis is guarded.

is, a synergism exists between the two. (See Figure 23–6.) The child with prekwashiorkor rapidly advances to kwashiorkor if he also has gastroenteritis, measles, or some other infection. Infections that are ordinarily mild become so severe in the malnourished that the resulting death rate is high. In some countries the mortality from measles is 400 times greater than in the United States—not because of increase in virulence but because of coexisting malnutrition.[8]

Mild deficiency. Most infants and preschool children in the developing countries suffer from mild deficiency of calories or protein or both. The outstanding characteristic is growth retardation or growth failure. The deficiency is not always detected unless one determines the age of the child, since the height and the weight may be proportionate. There is delayed maturation of the bones and other biologic systems. Anorexia, mental apathy, infections, and diarrhea are common findings.

Kwashiorkor. Moderate to severe growth failure is present in kwashiorkor. For the first few months of life the breast-fed infant in the developing countries grows at a rate that is comparable to that of well-fed infants in the Western world. Thereafter, the increase in stature and in tissue development is increasingly retarded. The muscles are poorly developed and lack tone. Edema is usually severe resulting in a large pot belly and swollen legs and face and masking the muscle wasting that has occurred. (See Figure 23–5.) Anorexia and diarrhea are common. In fact, poor sanitation is likely to be the cause of the diarrhea, which, in turn, rapidly advances the child from moderate malnutrition to severe kwashiorkor.

One of the more striking features of the deficiency is the profound apathy and general misery of the child. He whimpers but does not cry or scream. He is not interested in or curious about his surroundings, but remains seated wherever he is put down. When he again begins to smile he is said to be on the road to recovery.

Pathologic and biochemical changes. Fatty infiltration of the liver is usually extensive. The serum levels of triglycerides, phospholipids, and cholesterol are reduced indicating an inability of the liver to manufacture and release these substances to the circulation. Atrophy of the pancreas results in a lessened production of amylase, lipase, and trypsin.

The total serum protein and albumin fractions are markedly reduced thus accounting for the severe edema that is present. Hemoglobin levels are low, especially if parasitism is also present. The serum vitamin A levels are usually reduced; profound vitamin A deficiency is a serious complication leading to blindness and death in some children.

Marasmus. Severe growth failure and emaciation are the most striking characteristics of the marasmic infant. The wasting of the muscles and the lack of subcutaneous fat are extreme. As in kwashiorkor, the incidence of diarrhea is high. (See Figure 23–7.)

Marasmus differs from kwashiorkor in several important respects: the onset is earlier, usually within the first year of life; growth failure is more pronounced; there is no edema and the blood protein concentration is reduced less markedly; skin changes are seen less frequently; the liver is not infiltrated with fat; and the period of recovery is much longer.

Mental development. Possibly the most serious problem of P-CM is in the mental retardation that may occur. It must be emphasized that the effects of malnutrition on mental development and learning are exceedingly difficult to measure. As a rule, the malnourished child is also exposed to environmental influences that interfere with rapid learning. Moreover, the methods for testing children in one cultural environment are not applicable in an entirely

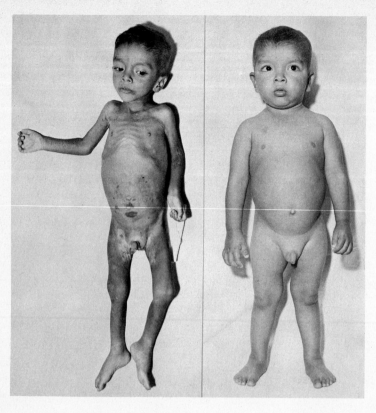

Figure 23–7. Severe protein-calorie malnutrition. Two-year-old child two weeks after admission and 10 weeks after treatment with IN-CAPARINA. (Courtesy, Institute of Central America and Panama, and the *Journal of the American Dietetic Association.*)

different cultural setting. If brain development is irreversibly retarded, this could mean that nations with large numbers of malnourished children might be unable to achieve their economic and social equality with the rest of the world.

Malnutrition can have two effects on the child's potential mental development. First, if the nutrients required for multiplication and growth of the brain cells are lacking during the period of most rapid development, it appears highly unlikely that the deficiency can be corrected by improved nutrition once the time cycle for brain development has gone by. It would be expected that the effects would be most profound in severe malnutrition during the first year of life. If nutrition is satisfactory during infancy and subsequently deteriorates, the effects are less devastating.

The second effect of malnutrition in the preschool years may be on the interference of learning that normally occurs in healthy preschool children at a truly fantastic rate. The apathy, lack of curiosity,

and reduced activity of the malnourished child over a protracted period of time will greatly reduce the amount of learning. Thus, the development of behavioral characteristics expected of the normal child at any given age may be delayed for months or years and may sometimes never be fully corrected.

Prevention and treatment of P-CM. The most practical approach to the prevention of P-CM is to improve the food supply of the entire family because this is the best way to ensure that the preschool child will receive his needed share. Such a goal involves a major improvement in locally available food supplies, income, and education. The realization of such an objective obviously is not of much help to the child in immediate need. Food mixtures that contain sufficient quantities of essential amino acids to meet the growth needs of the child have been developed in a number of countries. See Chapter 24 for further discussion. An indirect approach of considerable importance is the improvement of sanitation and programs of immunization so that the incidence of infections is greatly reduced.

A milk formula, when properly planned and administered, is curative of mild malnutrition. At later stages, a milk formula or food mixtures bring about weight gain, a return of the appetite, and increased interest in surroundings. The liver and pancreas rapidly return to normal and the blood proteins are replaced. The adverse effects of brain development are less likely to be reversed, unless therapy is instituted early enough.

The prognosis for children with alterations in fluid and electrolyte balance is not good. A deficit of potassium is usually present in severe malnutrition

and this may lead to cardiac failure if food therapy is too vigorous in the beginning. Also, an excess of sodium in the feedings can precipitate cardiac failure.

When electrolyte imbalance is present, the initial therapy should be directed to restoration of electrolyte and fluid balance. Thereafter, a half-strength formula of skim milk is fed, with gradual increases to normal concentration. Anemia and vitamin A deficiency become more apparent as growth resumes and blood volume increases. These complications can be prevented by using formulas that are fortified with vitamins A and D, and with iron and folacin.

REVIEW

1. What problems of malnutrition are you aware of in your community? What factors may be contributing to these problems?
2. If the nutritional needs of the community are not known, how could you go about finding out?
3. On the basis of their records of food intake for three days, a teacher tells her pupils that many of them have nutritional deficiencies, especially of vitamin C. In what ways is this conclusion misleading?
4. What are some characteristics that a teacher might observe in the children in her class that would indicate the need for referral to a physician?
5. List some superstitions regarding food with which you are familiar. What facts can you cite to refute these ideas?
6. Examine some popular publications to see if you can find examples of food misinformation. Or visit a "health food" store or the "health food" department of a supermarket to determine what claims are being made for the products being sold.
7. Describe the differences between marasmus and kwashiorkor.
8. For what reasons is a dilute formula used in the early treatment of protein-calorie malnutrition?
9. The rapid urbanization of the world's population can be especially devastating to infants and preschool children. Explain why this is so.
10. What is meant by the synergism between malnutrition and infection?

CITED REFERENCES

1. Cook, R.: "The Financial Cost of Malnutrition in the Commonwealth Caribbean," *J. Trop. Pediatr.*, **14**:60–65, June 1968.
2. Devadas, R. P.: "Social and Cultural Factors Influencing Malnutrition," *J. Home Econ.*, **62**:164–71, 1970.
3. Altschul, A. M.: "Food: Proteins for Humans," *Chem. Eng. News*, **47**:69–81, Nov. 24, 1969.
4. Jelliffe, D. B., and Jelliffe, E. F. P.: "The Urban Avalanche and Child Nutrition," *J. Am. Diet. Assoc.*, **57**:111–18, 1970.
5. McBean, L. D., and Speckmann, E. W.: "Food Faddism: A Challenge to Nutritionists and Dietitians," *Am. J. Clin. Nutr.*, **27**:1071–78, 1974.
6. Williams, C. D.: "Kwashiorkor. A Nutritional Disease Associated with a Maize Diet," *Lancet*, Nov. 16, 1935, p. 1151; reprinted in *Nutr. Rev.*, **31**:350–51, 1973.
7. Review: "Childhood Malnutrition in Iran," *Nutr. Rev.*, **27**:69–71, 1969.
8. Gordon, J. E.: "Nutritional Science and Society," *Nutr. Rev.*, **27**:331–38, 1969.

ADDITIONAL REFERENCES

Food Faddism

American Dietetic Association: "Position Paper on Food and Nutrition Misinformation on Selected Topics," *J. Am. Diet. Assoc.*, **66:**277–80, 1975.

Bruch, H.: "The Allure of Food Cults and Nutrition Quackery," *J. Am. Diet. Assoc.*, **57:**316, 1970; reprint, *Nutr. Rev.*, **32** (Suppl. 1): 62–66, 1974.

Calvert, G. P., and Calvert, S. W.: "Intellectual Convictions of 'Health' Food Consumers," *J. Nutr. Educ.*, **7:**95–98, 1975.

Council on Foods and Nutrition: "Zen Macrobiotic Diets," *J.A.M.A.*, **218:**397, 1971.

Darby, W. J.: "The Unicorn and Other Lessons from History," *Nutr. Rev.*, **32** (Suppl. 1):57–61, July 1974.

Deutsch, R.: "Where You Should Be Shopping for Your Family," *Nutr. Rev.*, **32** (Suppl. 1):48–52, July 1974.

Food Facts Talk Back, Revised. The American Dietetic Association, Chicago, 1975.

Frankle, R. T., and Heussenstam, F. K.: "Food Zealotry and Youth: New Dimensions for Professionals," *Am. J. Public Health*, **64:**11–18, 1974.

Henderson, L. M.: "Programs to Combat Nutritional Quackery," *J. Am. Diet. Assoc.*, **64:**372–75, 1974.

Jukes, T. H.: "The Organic Food Myth," *J.A.M.A.*, **230:**276–77, 1974.

Rynearson, E. H.: "Americans Love Hogwash," *Nutr. Rev.*, **32** (Suppl. 1):1–14, July 1974.

Schafer, R., and Yetley, E. A.: "Social Psychology of Food Faddism," *J. Am. Diet. Assoc.*, **66:**129–33, 1975.

Wolff, R. J.: "Who Eats for Health?" *Am. J. Clin. Nutr.*, **26:**438–45, 1973.

NUTRITIONAL ASSESSMENT

Christakis, G., ed.: "Nutritional Assessment in Health Programs," *Am. J. Public Health*, **63** (Suppl.), Nov. 1973.

Huenemann, R. L.: "Interpretation of Nutritional Status," *J. Am. Diet. Assoc.*, **63:**123–24, 1973.

Langham, R. A.: "A State Health Department Assesses Undernutrition," *J. Am. Diet. Assoc.*, **65:**18–23, 1974.

Nichaman, M. Z.: "Developing a Nutritional Surveillance System," *J. Am. Diet Assoc.*, **65:**15–17, 1974.

Sabry, Z. I., *et al.*: "Nutrition Canada," *Nutr. Today*, **9:**5–13, Jan. 1974.

Sabry, Z. I., *et al.*: "Nutrition Canada—A National Nutrition Survey," *Nutr. Rev.*, **32:**105–11, 1974.

WORLD NUTRITION

Brown, L. R.: "Death at an Early Age," *UNICEF News*, Issue 85, 1975/3, pp. 3–9.

Cobos, L. F., *et al.*: "Will Improved Nutrition Help to Prevent Mental Retardation?" *Prev. Med.*, **1:**185–94, 1973.

Goldsmith, G. E.: "Nutrition and World Health," *J. Am. Diet. Assoc.*, **63:**513–18, 1973.

Harrar, J. G.: "Nutrition and Numbers in the Third World," *Nutr. Rev.*, **32:**97–104, 1974.

Holdren, J. P., and Ehrlich, P. R.: "Human Population and the Global Environment," *Am. Scientist*, **62:**282–92, 1974.

Review: "Brain Growth in Kwashiorkor," *Nutr. Rev.*, **33:**107–10, 1975.

Review: "Calorie Supplementation and Growth of Pre-School Children," *Nutr. Rev.*, **32:**141–43, 1974.

"A Special Number Marking the Eightieth Year of Cicely D. Williams," *Nutr. Rev.*, **31:**330–84, 1973.

24 Nutrition Education and Services Through Community Action

National nutrition policy. Unemployment, poverty, worldwide inflation, dwindling food stockpiles, rapid developments in food technology, regulation of food quality and safety, concerns about diet and health—all of these and others point to the need for a nutrition policy at the highest levels of government. The United States has never had, and still does not have, a national nutrition policy. The need for such a policy has been expressed by nutritionists, health workers, food producers, and consumers, but there is a lack of agreement on what should be included in such a policy. For example, economists and food producers do not always agree with nutritionists on the food needs for the nation.

Recently a consortium of professional organizations was formed including the American Dietetic Association, American Institute of Nutrition, American Society of Clinical Nutrition, and Institute of Food Technologists. They have developed "guidelines for a national nutrition policy" that was used for the hearings in June 1974 of the Senate Select Committee on Nutrition and Human Needs.[1] These guidelines state that a national nutrition policy should aim "to provide an adequate diet at a reasonable cost to every person within the United States." This need has heretofore never been met in any nation, including the United States.

To achieve the goals of an adequate diet, a nutrition policy must include provision of a wholesome food supply; systems of controls for the safety and quality of food; sufficient food to meet emergency needs; education of the public in nutrition and food; and support for research and education. The published guidelines list in some detail the measures and programs that will be needed to achieve these goals.[1]

Role of health professionals. Public health nutritionists, dietitians, nurses, home economists, and social workers have direct roles to fulfill in implementing many of the community programs required for the improvement of nutrition. In addition they must be informed about programs involving research, legislation, food technology, and so on and lend their support to them. A few of the numerous activities designed to help people toward better nutrition will be described in this chapter.

MANY DOORS OPEN TO BETTER NUTRITION

Nature of services. In the hospital or clinic the nurse and dietitian give direct service to the individual. Nutrition services of the community are also provided on an individual basis, especially at the city-county level. For example, such direct services are given by a public health nurse, or a homemaker from a welfare agency, or a volunteer who delivers a hot meal to an aged person.

Community programs in nutrition seek to improve nutrition through research, education, improvement of the food supply, and feeding. (See Figure 24-1.) The individual reaps the rewards of activities such as these: legislation which makes funds available for feeding vulnerable groups and which protects the food supply; research concerning the preventive and therapeutic aspects of diet with respect to disease; methods for preserving the food supply; the development of new and better foods through food technology; a more abundant food supply because of research on plant varieties, soil conservation, pest control; education for an adequate diet—and so on.

Facilities of the community. The problems of food production and of nutrition are being met by a large number of groups that work either cooperatively or independently. The partial listings in Tables 24-1 and 24-2 give the student some idea of the scope of efforts being made by many groups at

351

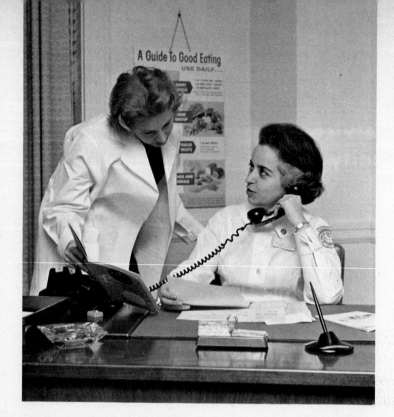

Figure 24-1. The Dial-a-Dietitian program in many cities provides reliable answers to questions about food and nutrition asked by the public. (Courtesy, the Nutrition Foundation, New York.)

Table 24-1. A Partial List of Organizations at Local and State Levels Concerned Directly or Indirectly with Nutrition Problems

Official
Department of agriculture (state)
Department of health
  Food sanitation
  Nutrition
  Regional medical programs
  Area agencies for aging
Department of welfare
Board of education
  Day care centers
  Health education and services
  Home economics
  Nutrition education
  School food services
Extension services
Public libraries
State universities

Voluntary
Educational groups
  Private elementary and secondary schools
  Private colleges and universities; home economics, medicine, nursing
  Parent-teachers associations
  Libraries

Voluntary (cont.)
Social agencies: church and community support
  Children's aid
  Community nursing
  Family service
  Salvation Army
  Settlement houses
  Welfare
Institutions:
  Children's camps, day nurseries
  Hospitals, nursing and convalescent homes
  Homes for the aged
  Correctional institutions
Professional organizations: see Table 24-2
Civic groups:
  Chambers of commerce
  Service organizations
  Women's clubs
Industry-sponsored groups
  Health centers and hospitals
  Plant cafeterias and restaurants
  Demonstration programs of stores and utility companies

Table 24-2. A Partial List of Organizations at the National Level Concerned Directly or Indirectly with Nutrition Problems

Official	*Voluntary*
Department of Agriculture	American Red Cross
Agricultural Research Service	National Academy of Sciences—National Research
Consumer and Marketing Service	Council
Cooperative State Research Service	Food and Nutrition Board: committees on dietary
Economic Research Service	allowances; clinical nutrition; food protection; food
Federal Extension Service	science and technology; nutrition, brain develop-
Foreign Agricultural Service	ment, and behavior; nutritional misinformation;
International Agricultural Development Service	nutrition and dental health; international nutrition;
Department of Health, Education, and Welfare	and others
Administration on Aging	Professional societies and voluntary health associations
Children's Bureau	American Academy of Pediatrics
Food and Drug Administration	American Dental Association
Maternal and Child Health Services	American Diabetes Association
Office of Education	American Dietetic Association
Public Health Service	American Heart Association
National Institutes of Health: allergy and infection,	American Home Economics Association
arthritis and metabolic, cancer, heart, mental	American Institute of Nutrition
National Nutrition Program	American Medical Association Council on Foods and
Department of the Interior	Nutrition
Bureau of Commercial Fisheries	American Nurses' Association
Bureau of Indian Affairs	American Public Health Association
Department of State	American School Food Service Association
Agency for International Development	American Society of Clinical Nutrition
	Institute of Food Technologists
	Nutrition Today Society
	Society for Nutrition Education
	Foundations
	Ford Foundation
	Kellogg Foundation
	National Vitamin Foundation
	Nutrition Foundation
	Rockefeller Foundation
	Williams-Waterman Fund of the Research Corporation
	Industry-sponsored groups
	American Institute of Baking
	Cereal Institute
	National Dairy Council
	National Livestock and Meat Board

local, state, and national levels. A number of categories are included: official agencies constitute those which have been authorized by the government and which are tax supported; voluntary agencies are supported by private funds, such as the United Fund, foundations, and other means; professional organizations; and industrial groups, especially from the food industry.

NUTRITION EDUCATION

Scope of educational programs. Education means change of behavior. It moves the individual from lack of interest and ignorance to increasing appreciation and knowledge and finally to action. Nutrition education offers a great opportunity to individuals to learn about the essentials of nutrition for health and to take steps to improve the quality of their diets and thus their well-being.

Nutrition education must become an essential component of the curriculum in elementary and secondary schools. The classroom instruction finds application in the meals provided through school food services. The implementation of nutrition education necessitates the development of coordinated, sequential curricula from kindergarten through high school. Also essential is the initiation of college and in-service courses in nutrition for the nation's teachers.

Nutrition education must continue throughout the individual's life in order to accommodate for developments in nutrition science and for changing economic circumstances, health requirements, and the new food products being developed for the nation's markets. To reach the millions of citizens requires a greatly expanded use of the mass media, and the involvement of governmental and private agencies, universities, and food industries. Educational activities at the community level in health centers, maternal and child-care centers, day-care centers, programs for the elderly, Head Start and Get Set programs, youth organizations, and women's clubs are also needed to reach the citizenry.

What knowledge is essential? The Interagency Committee on Nutrition Education developed basic concepts on the nutrition information needed to make wise choices of food for individuals and families. The concepts are not facts to be memorized as such, but they serve as guidelines for the selection of content, learning experiences, and teaching materials in a program of education.

BASIC CONCEPTS IN NUTRITION[*]

1. Nutrition is the food you eat and how the body uses it.

We eat food to live, to grow, to keep healthy and well, and to get energy for work and play.

2. Food is made up of different nutrients needed for health and growth.

All nutrients needed by the body are available through food. Many kinds and combinations of food can lead to a well-balanced diet. No food, by itself, has all the nutrients needed for full growth and health. Each nutrient has spe-

[*]Hill, M. M.: "I.C.N.E. Formulates Some Basic Concepts in Nutrition," *Nutrition Program News,* Sept.—Oct. 1964, U.S. Department of Agriculture, Washington, D.C.

cific uses in the body. Most of the nutrients do their best work in the body when teamed with other nutrients.

3. All persons, throughout life, have need for the same nutrients, but in varying amounts.

The amounts of nutrients needed are influenced by age, sex, size, activity, and state of health. Suggestions for the kinds and amounts of food needed are made by trained scientists.

4. The way food is handled influences the amount of nutrients in food, its safety, appearance, and taste.

Handling means everything that happens to food while it is being grown, processed, stored, and prepared for eating.

Dietary excesses. In addition to stressing a sufficiency of all nutrients to meet the metabolic needs of the individual throughout the life cycle, nutrition educators must emphasize the importance of avoiding excesses of calories, saturated fats, simple sugars, refined foods, and salt. These excesses over the course of a lifetime lead to obesity and dental caries and are considered to be risk factors in heart disease, hypertension, diabetes mellitus, and various gastrointestinal disorders. (See pages 447, 492, and 527.)

Some guidelines for family counseling. Dietitians, nutritionists, and nurses devote a great deal of time to counseling individuals and families. Certain important principles must guide the counselor throughout the process.[2,3] They apply to education for normal nutrition under varying cultural and economic situations, and also to the guidance essential for a modified diet. (See also Chapter 26.)

Become acquainted. The nurse or nutritionist must establish an environment of warmth, kindness, and genuine interest. The person needs to know that you are there to help him, that you think he can learn, and that he is worth something. What does the individual say first? How intense are his feelings? Ample time must be allowed to let him voice his problems without the frustration of interruptions.

Before you can help people with their food problems you must know something about their present food practices—what foods they use, how these foods are prepared, the facilities for food preparation, the meanings of food in terms of social, ethnic, and religious factors, the adequacy of income for the purchase of food, their concept of the importance of food to their total life style. The list of items for the dietary history on page 382 can be adapted to the interview for family counseling. (See Figure 24–2.)

Build upon that which is good. Every diet has some good features about it, and the counselor should capitalize upon these. A negative, critical attitude toward current practices is rarely helpful.

Focus on a specific problem. People often feel overwhelmed by many problems and are unable to progress toward solving any of them. A small problem that seems urgent to the individual and toward which some success can be anticipated should be singled out for attention. Then, with time, other problems are attacked.

Establish realistic goals. Although the counselor suggests possible goals, the decision for action must be made by the individual. Sometimes the goals may seem to be quite limited and of no great importance; for example, learning how to cook a one-dish meal may be a genuine accomplishment to an unskilled homemaker. Each person being helped needs to feel that something is expected of him and that

he can achieve the goals he has chosen. He needs to have a clear understanding of what he is to do before the next interview.

Learn to communicate effectively. Professional people must modify the scientific terminology they use so easily to the level of education of the individual. Homemakers want to know what foods their families should eat. They are less likely to talk in terms of diets that are "nutritious" or "balanced."[4] Counseling means talking together with the individual being helped—not lecturing; it means listening and answering questions as well as asking them; it means showing and doing as well. Learning has been described this way:

Each remembers *best* what he does,
Next best, what he *sees*,
Least well what he hears.°

°Project Head Start: *Nutrition Instructors Guide*, 3 B. Office of Child Development, U.S. Department of Health, Education, and Welfare, Washington, D.C., 1967, p. 8.

Figure 24–2. Students observe the application of nutritional principles to dietary planning, giving consideration to palatability, psychologic influences, cultural factors, and economy. (Courtesy, Medical College of Virginia, Health Sciences Division, Virginia Commonwealth University, Richmond.)

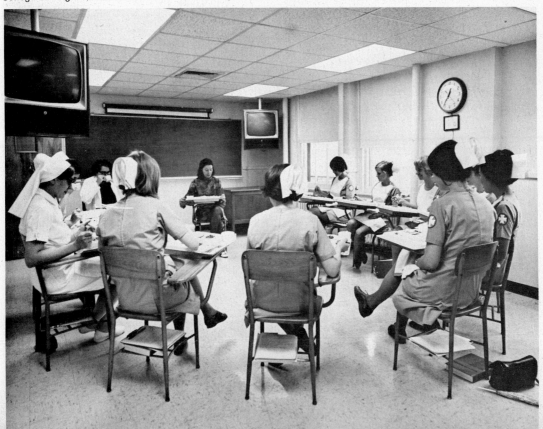

There is almost a surfeit of leaflets, bulletins, posters, slides and film strips, and movies available for family and group counseling. Most of these materials have been developed for middleclass families and are not useful to poor people who have little education. Films that portray affluence and lavish displays of food may create resentment rather than conveying information.

Printed materials are a supplement to counseling, never a substitute for it. Usually it is better to introduce only one leaflet or bulletin at a time, and to supplement this at later interviews if needed.

Maintain continuity. Whenever possible the same person should follow through with an individual or family. This helps the person to know that someone is really concerned and looking after his welfare, and it helps to avoid misunderstandings.

Evaluate the results. An evaluation indicates to the counselor whether her techniques are satisfactory, or whether some changes will increase her effectiveness. Sometimes the evaluation may show that an individual cannot be helped or does not want to be helped; this, too, should be recognized. From time to time the person being helped should evaluate his own progress, for by so doing he can reassess his goals and, if need be, change his direction.

HELPING PEOPLE WITH LOW INCOMES

Characteristics of the poor. The poor are often thought of as a single group that can be described in terms of a "culture of poverty." Although certain characteristics of behavior are enforced upon them by reason of poverty, it is a serious error to regard the poor as a homogeneous group.[2]

Variations in environment and culture. Poor people living in Appalachia, the Mexican-Americans of the Southwest, the Puerto Ricans, the American Indians, the black people in city ghettos, and many people in cities and in rural areas have one thing in common—lack of sufficient income to meet their basic needs. Their cultures, however, have little in common. Moreover, within each of these groups, individuals and families differ from one another in their values, aspirations, and style of living just as people of the more affluent society differ from one another. Some poor people come from families that have been poor for generations and have never known any other way of life; other people are poor because of changed circumstances brought about by unemployment, inflation, and health costs. Some of the poor have a fair level of education, whereas others are illiterate. Some homemakers are good managers and do a remarkable job in keeping the family together, whereas others lack even the simplest skills in homemaking and in child care. Some constantly strive for a better way of life, whereas others regard their present status as permanent and about which they can do little.

The limitations of poverty. A limited income restricts people to living in declining neighborhoods with deteriorating houses, inadequate sanitation, crowding, and lack of privacy. There is a constant fear of eviction because of loss of income and failure to pay the rent.

The poor are isolated from society. They move about from place to place—usually not by choice but by necessity—and therefore establish no roots in the community. Their participation in community activities is minimal and their contact with the outside world through newspapers and magazines is small. This isolation encourages suspicion of the motives of those who may try to help them; it also means that they are poorly equipped to cope with emergencies because they do not know what resources are available to them.

The poor must live from day to day and are unable to plan ahead. The future is uncertain, they are fatalistic about what is to come, and setting goals for the future seems pointless.

Lacking education, the poor may not be able to make the best use of the little money they have. They are often at the mercy of credit schemes that, over a period of time, exact large interest payments.

Poor people have known little success. They feel that people look down upon them and have little concern for them. They will often place more confidence in the advice of a neighbor, a faith healer, or a practitioner of folk medicine—all of whom are attuned to their way of living.

Social problems are not unique to the poor but they are likely to be more frequent. Many of the families have only one parent, usually the mother. Men in many households are unable to fulfill their roles as providers, and they leave their homes so that their families can qualify for public assistance.

Poverty and diet. The income is often inadequate to cover the period for which it is intended. At the beginning of the pay period the family may eat fairly well, even enjoying an occasional luxury. But as days go on the diet becomes more monotonous and inadequate, including inexpensive foods that may be good sources of calories but that are poor sources of protein, minerals, and vitamins.

The homemaker may lack transportation to a supermarket if one is not nearby and therefore food is purchased from a neighborhood grocer at prices that are almost certainly higher. Often the local grocer belongs to the same ethnic group, is someone to whom they can turn for advice, and is willing to extend credit.

Homemakers are unable to take advantage of bulk purchases or to stock their cupboards when food specials are advertised. It is sometimes said that the poor cannot afford to be thrifty.

Food preparation facilities are often limited. To tell people how to prepare foods that require an oven is not useful if there is only a hot plate. Sometimes the homemaker is unable to read a recipe and lacks even the simplest skills in food preparation.

Many homemakers are employed outside the home and children are left to fend for themselves. Sometimes the food supply is limited, but even with an adequate amount of food available children are not likely to select the foods that they need.

Better nutrition for the poor. Adequate income is basic to an adequate diet. Before you can tell people what foods they require and how to prepare them, there must be food in the home to prepare or money with which to purchase it. A recent study has shown that the welfare allowances in many states do not provide a sufficient allowance for food to provide the amounts of foods recommended for the low-cost plan (see page 249).[5]

Food Stamp Program. The concept on which this program is based is that low-income families should be able to buy a nutritionally adequate diet without spending more than 30 per cent of their net income for food. If they have little or no income, they should be able to get the adequate diet at no cost.[6] In late 1974 households receiving public assistance accounted for 48 per cent of all participants. Households that met other criteria of low income, limited assets, and so on accounted for 52 per cent of the participants at this time. More than 17 mil-

lion persons were receiving food stamps in 1974 compared with 2.9 million persons in 1969.

Purchases can be made with food stamps in any retail market that has been approved to accept stamps. Welfare workers, public health nurses, and nutritionists must be prepared to help families interpret the regulations for the use of the stamps and learn how to make the most effective use of them. Many people who are not receiving public assistance but who are living at subsistence levels do not realize that they can also purchase the stamps.

Nutrition education for the poor. An adequate income alone does not guarantee improvement in nutrition. When incomes are supplemented, only a small fraction of the increase in money is usually spent for food; even that small amount may be spent for a luxury item rather than one that improves the diet.

In an effort to reach low-income families the Cooperative Extension Service of the U.S. Department of Agriculture developed an *Expanded Nutrition Education Program.* This program uses program aides who are mature nonprofessional women selected from the community in which the people who are to be helped live. The program aide is given a period of intensive training by home economists and nutritionists from county extension services and is supervised on the job by staff aides and professionals. (See Figure 24–3.)

Program aides work with homemakers on an individual basis in their homes and give assistance on the problems associated with foods, child care, housekeeping and management, clothing repair, and so on. The assistance for better nutrition is on such practical points as how to prepare simple dishes, how to make the best use of food money, what to look for on a label, how to use the Daily Food Guide, and easily prepared breakfasts. The teaching includes the use of very simple booklets and demonstrations.

Because she comes from the community the program aide is aware of the problems of the family. She is able to make better contacts with people because she knows from experience what it means to have little money to spend for food. Her assistance is less likely to be viewed with suspicion than is that of a helper who comes from a middle-class environment with different standards and values, and with little understanding of the poor.

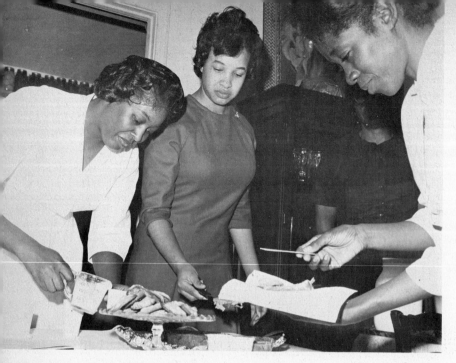

Figure 24–3. Nutrition aides prepare foods to be used in a demonstration in a home. (Courtesy, Kevin Shields and U.S. Department of Agriculture.)

SOME COMMUNITY PROGRAMS FOR NUTRITION EDUCATION AND SERVICES

State nutrition programs. A nutrition program in a state department of health is constantly adapted to the needs of the population of that state. Nutritionists in state programs work closely with physicians, nurses, dentists, dental hygienists, social workers, administrators of institutions, food service managers, dietitians, and others. The activities below are representative of those included in state nutrition programs.

1. Define the place of nutrition in program areas.
   a. Conduct surveys of community needs.
2. Provide materials on nutrition information.
   a. Analyze and interpret findings of science.
   b. Prepare leaflets on topics such as: weight control; meal planning; infant feeding; food misinformation; diet patterns for various cultural groups; teen-agers; senior citizens.
   c. Prepare diet manuals, food value charts, exhibits, newspaper, magazine, radio, and television releases.
3. Consultant service to agencies and institutions: child care, nursing homes, small hospitals, mental hospitals, homes for the elderly.
   a. Planning food service facilities.
   b. Personnel training; budgeting; menu planning; purchasing; sanitation; preparation and service of food; therapeutic diets.

4. Work with schools: elementary, secondary, college, medical, nursing, allied health.
   a. Plan and conduct dietary surveys as part of research program.
   b. Assist in developing programs in nutrition education.
   c. Conduct workshops for school faculty.
   d. Assist in training programs for school food service personnel; help to interpret educational value of school meals.
5. Cooperate with other health groups in rehabilitation and in chronic disease programs: cardiovascular disease, diabetes, tuberculosis, arthritis, cerebral palsy, orthopedic disabilities, mental retardation, etc.
   a. Preparation of materials for professional and lay instruction.
   b. Conduct of institutes for staff education of nurses, nutritionists, physicians.
6. Work with patients (usually on a demonstration basis with allied health personnel).
   a. Clinics: child health, crippled children, cardiovascular, diabetes, prenatal, tuberculosis.
   b. Food budgets.
   c. Home visits.
7. Work with other groups:
   a. Social and welfare agencies on dietary standards and budgets.
   b. Public instruction.
8. Assist in programs of research with schools of home economics, medical schools, departments of health, federal and private agencies.

Day care centers. Through public and private schools, community agencies, and industrial groups, day care centers are provided for children of mothers who work.[7] These programs are funded by parent fees, by subsidies from companies, and by local, state, and federal taxation. They care for preschool children during the day and for schoolchildren before and after school hours and during the summer months. (See Figure 24–4.)

Children are given breakfast, lunch, and mid-morning and midafternoon snacks so that 75 to 80 per cent of the nutritional needs are supplied. Food service and nutrition education have a symbiotic relationship.[7] For example, serving oneself with food helps the child to make decisions about what he can eat. The scraping of dishes, which might

seem like only a household chore, helps the child to achieve manual dexterity.

Through conversation at the table with the children, the teacher is able to build on their interests. For example, the question "How does corn get into bread?" can lead to a series of learnings about corn—how it grows, how it is cooked, and some recipes that might use it.[7] (See Figure 24–5.)

WIC program. A supplemental food program for women, infants, and children (WIC) is administered in projects throughout the country by the Food and Nutrition Service of the U.S. Department of Agriculture.[6] Pregnant and lactating women, infants, and children under four years of age who are nutritionally at risk and who have limited incomes are given vouchers for the purchase of foods to supple-

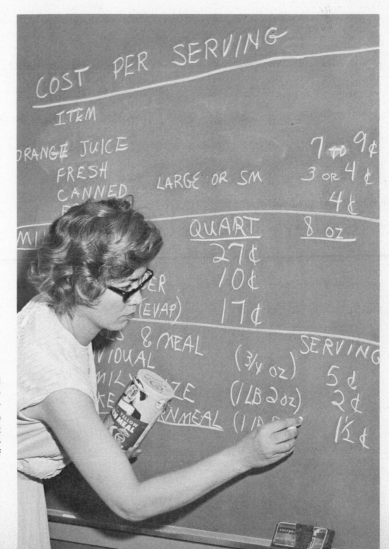

Figure 24–4. A leader in a Head Start Program shows mothers how to compare costs of foods per serving by using label and price information. (Courtesy, Project Head Start, Office of Child Development, U.S. Department of Health, Education, and Welfare.)

ment their inadequate diets. This program aims through dietary supplementation to increase birth weight of infants, thereby reducing the incidence of infant mortality, birth defects, mental retardation, and slow learning.

Women are considered to be at nutritional risk if they are obese, underweight, or stunted, if they are known to have inadequate diets, if they have anemia, or if they have frequent miscarriages or premature births.[8] Infants and children at nutritional risk are those with diets known to be inadequate, who are anemic, or who have deficient growth patterns. The nutritional needs are determined by medical examination or by nutritional interview by a physician, dietitian, nutritionist, registered nurse, or other medically trained health officials competent to evaluate risks.

The food supplements are high in calories, protein, calcium, iron, ascorbic acid, and vitamins A and D. The foods must meet nutritional standards of the U.S. Department of Agriculture. For example, each 100 ml of formula must supply 67 kcal and 10 mg iron. The supplements for a month are as follows:

Pregnant and Lactating Women and Children
2½ dozen eggs
31 qt milk
4 8-oz packages cereal
6 46-fluidounce cans juice

Infants
31 13-fluidounce cans concentrated formula
3 8-oz packages cereal
2 46-oz cans juice

Heart disease control programs. The Food and Nutrition Board and the Council on Food and Nutrition of the American Medical Association recommend that individuals who are at high risk for coronary or cerebrovascular disease be identified early, and that recommendations for dietary modification be made as well as control of hypertension and elimination of smoking.[9] They state that most American men and women have blood lipid levels that are higher than desirable.

The American Heart Association, the American Health Foundation, and the Intersociety Commission for Heart Disease Resources recommend that all persons in the United States should bring about moderate changes in the diet including: calories to maintain normal weight (weight loss, if obese); fat at not more than 35 per cent of calories; saturated fat at not more than 10 per cent of calories; cholesterol restriction to 300 mg daily; complex, rather than simple carbohydrates; and moderate salt restriction.[10-12] (See also Chapter 40.) Such diets are held to be preventive and should be initiated early in life before biochemical changes take place. On a practical basis the recommendations involve moderate reduction in the intake of animal foods, especially

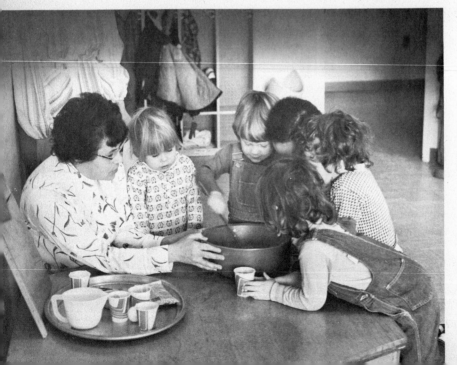

Figure 24–5. Nursery school children enjoy food preparation. They learn about food and develop muscle coordination. (Courtesy, University of Delaware, Newark.)

those meats high in saturated fat, not more than 3 to 4 eggs per week, and more emphasis upon vegetables, fruits, legumes, and cereal foods.

INTERNATIONAL AGENCIES FOR NUTRITION

Food and Agriculture Organization. The Food and Agriculture Organization of the United Nations (FAO) was founded in Quebec, Canada, in October 1945 the aims being:

To help the nations raise the standard of living;
To improve the nutrition of the people of all countries;
To increase the efficiency of farming, forestry, and fisheries;
To better the condition of rural people;
And, through these means, to widen the opportunity of all people for productive work.°

The headquarters office of FAO is in Rome where the work of the organization is supervised by a director-general. FAO provides assistance to about 120 member states by maintaining an intelligence service which gathers, analyzes, and distributes information on which action can be based, and by acting in an advisory capacity to help governments decide what action to take.

Technical assistance is provided by participating countries in agriculture, economics, fisheries, forestry, and nutrition to member countries. The diversified projects have included development of food storage, processing, and marketing facilities; land reclamation through irrigation and drainage; control of animal diseases; development of grains of higher nutritive value; increased yields of crops and greater resistance to disease; inland fish culture in ponds and rice fields; establishment of home economics programs in colleges; school feeding; and many others.

World Health Organization. The World Health Organization (WHO) was created in 1948 and is administered by a director-general with headquarters in Geneva, Switzerland, and with six regional offices, one of which is in Washington, D.C.

WHO is "the directing and coordinating author-ity for international health work." It is governed by two principles defined in its constitution:

UNIVERSALITY: The health of all peoples is fundamental to the achievement of peace and security. The enjoyment of the highest attainable standard of health is one of the fundamental rights of every human being without distinction of race, religion, political belief, economic or social condition.
CONCEPT OF HEALTH: Health is a state of complete physical, mental and social well-being and not merely the absence of disease or infirmity.°

The assistance which WHO renders to government includes:

. . . strengthening national health services; establishing and maintaining epidemiological and statistical services; controlling epidemic and endemic diseases; maternal and child health; promotion of mental health to foster harmonious human relations; improvement of sanitation and of preventive and curative medical services.°

Major efforts of WHO have been directed to the eradication of malaria, tuberculosis, venereal diseases, and yaws. These crippling diseases yearly reduce by thousands the number of workers available to produce food; the return of these people to productivity has incalculable effects on improving the food supply. The improvement of the sanitary standards—pure water supplies, pure milk and other food, insect control, housing, waste disposal—is likewise concerned with the improvement of nutrition.

United Nations Children's Fund. To children in different countries UNICEF means different things. It may mean an injection to cure them of yaws, a crippling disease, or vaccination to protect against tuberculosis; or protection against blindness caused by lack of vitamin A; or food to stave off starvation.

Organized in 1947, UNICEF continued the emergency feeding in war-devastated countries of Europe, with emphasis upon protein-rich foods, especially milk. Now, in developing countries all over the world, programs are directed to infants, children, and pregnant and lactating women. Although UNICEF continues to provide emergency

---

° *Food and Agriculture Organization—What It Is—What It Does—How It Works.* Leaflet, Food and Agriculture Organization, Rome, 1956.

° *World Health Organization—What It Is—What It Does—How It Works.* Leaflet, World Health Organization, Geneva, 1956.

relief, most of its funds are now diverted to long-range programs, for it is realized that countries must be able to solve their own nutritional problems.

United States responsibility in world nutrition. Each nation justifies its participation in programs to solve world nutrition problems on the basis of economic and political considerations as well as humanitarian concerns. The needs were identified at the World Food Conference held in Rome in 1974 as capital, technology, fertilizers, insecticides, and energy.[13] "The penalty of failure is a spectre of want, of need and starvation of inconceivably disastrous proportions."°

The first role of the United States must be to assume leadership and to set an example for helping to solve world nutrition problems. It must gain the cooperation of other nations including western Europe, the Soviet Union, and the oil-rich countries to set up adequate food reserves against crop failures and disasters, to provide technical assistance, and to help developing countries with capital funds to make the needed change in its food production and distribution.

The people of the United States can set an example by modest changes in their own food habits so that there is less demand for meat from grain-fed animals. (See pages 9 and 360.) Much food is wasted each day in the United States, and in the homes as well as institutions this can be greatly reduced.[14]

Food must be a vehicle for promoting peace and not a political tool used only at high levels of government. Public Law 480, first called the Food for Peace Program and more recently known as the Food for Freedom Program, was adopted by the Congress in 1954 as a means of using agricultural surpluses for feeding the world's needy people. The program has been administered by the Agency for International Development (AID) in the Department of State.

Throughout the years the program has provided food through UNICEF, CARE, and other relief agencies working in maternal and child health centers. (See Figure 24–6.) Food has been available for refugees and to feed people in disasters such as floods, hurricanes, and crop failures. Food has also been used as part payment for laborers working on

° Darby, W. J.: "Nutrition, Food Needs and Technologic Priorities: The World Food Conference," *Nutr. Rev.*, 33:233, 1975.

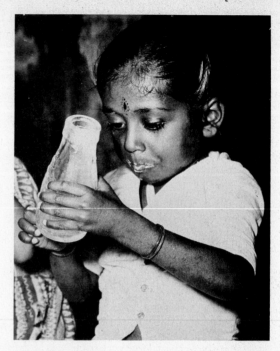

Figure 24–6. Undernourished children receive a daily ration of milk supplied by UNICEF. (Courtesy, UNICEF; photo by Jack Ling.)

development programs: irrigation projects, dams, roads, drainage, and so on. Assistance has been given to business investors by providing guarantees against losses of investments in developing countries through war, revolution, and expropriation. Loans have been made to the development of food industry in various countries including dairy plants, bakeries, fertilizer plants, and tractor manufacture.

INCREASING THE WORLD FOOD SUPPLY

Priorities. The rapid increase in the world's population without a comparable increase in wealth and in the production of food has been described by Altschul[15] as a "derangement of our ecosystem." At least 20 per cent of the people in less developed countries receive far too few calories and 60 per cent receive diets of poor quality.

Altschul lists three priorities for people who are poor and for whom the food supply is scarce. In descending order of need they are: (1) sufficient calories to sustain life; (2) protein of adequate quality and amount; and (3) aesthetic qualities to satisfy social as well as nutritional needs of even the poorest people.

Important enterprises of AID and foundations such as the Ford and Rockefeller Foundations have included the development of better agricultural practices, improved strains of plants, and protein mixtures of high nutritive value. In turn the skills of the agriculturist, food technologist, nutrition scientist, marketing expert, anthropologist, and many others have been involved in the governmental research programs, in universities, and in the food industries.

Potential sources of food. Cereal grains today comprise the principal source of food for the world's people and will, undoubtedly, continue to rank first throughout the world. In recent years agricultural scientists have brought about the so-called "green revolution."[16] In many less developed countries high yields of cereals are being achieved by using improved strains of rice, wheat, and corn, and by emphasizing modern agricultural practices including fertilizers and equipment. If it were not for dramatic improvements in crop yields and quality, there would have been a decline in per capita food supplies. The green revolution buys time, but eventually food production will not be able to keep up with the present rapid growth in population.[16]

Improved cereal quality. Cereal grains are deficient in one or more of the essential amino acids and thus do not meet the needs for rapid synthesis of proteins required for growth. (See page 56.) An outstanding example of an improved cereal grain is opaque-2 corn, a hybrid variety that has been developed in which the lysine and tryptophan content of the endosperm is 50 per cent higher than in regular varieties.[15,17] Also, the leucine content is lower so that the balance with isoleucine is improved. This development is of considerable significance to Central American, Latin American, and some African nations where corn is a staple food. In 1973 two varieties of high-lysine sorghum were developed. Eventually, this will be of benefit in arid regions of Asia and Africa where sorghum is a staple food.

Triticale is a man-made grain, combining the properties of wheat and rye. It contains a higher quality of protein than other grains, and it is more resistant to drought and cold than is wheat.

Amino acid supplementation. To improve the protein quality of wheat requires additional lysine; rice needs lysine and threonine; and legumes require methionine. The addition of lysine and methionine to low-cost foods is now economically feasible and it is expected that the cost of tryptophan will become sufficiently low in the not too distant future to make its use practical.

Nutrition scientists have been cautious about amino acid supplementation because an excess of certain amino acids can create an increased need for the next most limiting amino acid. Amino acid imbalances in low-protein diets can result in growth failure and other metabolic problems. *Modern Bread* was developed in India to include fortification with lysine, minerals, and vitamins. Now that the donated supply of lysine has been exhausted, this bread includes soya and peanut flours to maintain the protein quality.[16]

Other plant sources. Legumes, including chick peas, peanuts, and many varieties of beans, are important sources of protein and calories in Central America, Africa, and India. Soybeans contain protein of superior quality and probably have not been utilized for human food as much as they might be. Cottonseed is a useful source of protein when the toxic pigment, gossypol, is removed.

Soybean, wheat, cottonseed, and peanuts can be processed to provide protein-rich foods that simulate chunks of beef, chicken, ham, or bacon bits. (See page 247.) These products find wide use in restaurants and institutions. Meat dishes used in school food services may contain up to 30 per cent of such products.

Fish. Japan leads the world with an annual per capita consumption of 32 kg fish. In the Soviet Union the per capita intake is 10 kg and in the United States 6 kg. In recent years fishing has exceeded the capacity to regenerate the seas, and since 1970 there has been a steady decline in the catch of fish. Much competition exists today between nations concerning fishing rights. Another serious problem is the pollution of the seas by oil, and agricultural, industrial, and municipal wastes. Polluted waters may kill fish, interfere with their reproduction, or render fish unfit to eat, for example, the mercury poisoning that has been traced to fish in isolated instances in Japan.

Fish protein concentrate is a low-fat, bland powder produced from whole fish. It contains in excess of 80 per cent protein, but problems of production and palatability have prevented wide use of this product.

Food mixtures. Many food mixtures that apply the principle of the supplementary value of the proteins of various foods have been developed, particularly for the relief of protein-calorie malnutrition in children. These mixtures do not yet account for a sizable proportion of the world's protein needs. Among the mixtures that have been shown to be nutritionally satisfactory, economically feasible, and acceptable to the consumers are these:[15,18]

C.S.M.: corn, soy, milk blend; developed for use in U.S. AID programs

INCAPARINA: the first mixture to be developed; cottonseed and corn flours, vitamins, minerals, and torula yeast; protein efficiency equal to milk; 26 per cent protein; Central America.

BAL AHAR: a farina-like blend of bulgur wheat, peanut flour, nonfat dry milk, vitamins, minerals; 22 per cent protein; India.

GOLDEN ELBOW MACARONI (*General Foods*): corn, soy, and wheat flours; calcium carbonate, calcium phosphate, iron, B vitamins; 20 per cent protein; Brazil.

LECHE ALIM: a cereal food of toasted wheat flour, fish protein concentrate, sunflower meal, skim milk powder; 27 per cent protein; Chile.

PUMA (MONSANTO); SACI (COCA-COLA); AND VITASOY (LO): beverages containing vegetable protein, sugar, vitamins; compete with soft drinks in price and are well accepted; 2.5 to 3 per cent protein; Brazil, Guiana, Hong Kong.

Food for the future. Leaves of plants such as alfalfa and single-celled plants, including yeasts, fungi, and algae, may become important sources of food in the more distant future. The techniques for producing them at low cost are not yet known, and major problems remain in developing products that are aesthetically acceptable. The high nucleic acid content leads to increased uric acid production and subsequent problems of excretion.

PROBLEMS AND REVIEW

1. List the public and private agencies in your own community that work for better nutrition in one way or another. If possible, arrange for an interview to learn more about the activities of one of these.
2. *Problem.* Plan a 20-minute discussion-demonstration for a group of parents of underprivileged preschool children on one of these topics: menus for preschool children; taking care of the food in the home; developing good food habits in children.
3. List a number of learning experiences that could be used for children in a program.
4. *Problem.* Plan a lesson on one of these topics to help a homemaker who has a low income:
   a. How to obtain and use food stamps.
   b. How to use nonfat dry milk in some cooked foods.
   c. What to look for on labels of packages.
   d. Buying some economical cuts of meat.
5. *Problem.* Determine the current regulations for assistance through food stamps in your community.
6. *Problem.* Determine the current public assistance allowance for food in your community for:
   a. A man and his wife who are over 65 years.
   b. A mother with four children: girls, 6 and 10 years; and boys, 4 and 14 years. According to the current cost of food under the low-cost plan for this family, are these allowances adequate?
7. Write a 1000-word paper on any one of these topics, using at least four references in addition to the text:
   Nutritional status in the United States.
   Protein-calorie malnutrition.
   Economic factors in malnutrition.
   Cultural factors in malnutrition.
   Food mixtures for better protein.
   Program aides in nutrition education.

CITED REFERENCES

1. National Nutrition Consortium: "Guidelines for a National Nutrition Policy," *Nutr. Rev.*, **32**:153–59, 1974.

2. Shoemaker, L.: *Parent and Family Life Education for Low-Income Families.* Children's Bureau Pub. 434–1965. U.S. Department of Health, Education, and Welfare, Washington, D.C.

3. Matthews, L. I.: "Principles of Interviewing and Patient Counseling," *J. Am. Diet. Assoc.,* **50:**469–74, 1967.

4. Ikeda, J. P.: "Expressed Nutrition Information Needs of Low-Income Homemakers," *J. Nutr. Educ.* **7:**104–106, 1975.

5. Calloway, D. H.: "Malnutrition: Poverty or Education," *J. Nutr. Educ.,* **1:**9–12, Spring 1970.

6. Bunting, F., and Reese, R.: "USDA Food and Nutrition Programs—a Progress Report," *National Food Situation,* U.S. Department of Agriculture, Feb. 1975, pp. 34–42.

7. Juhas, L.: "Nutrition Education in Day Care Programs," *J. Am. Diet. Assoc.,* **63:**134–37, 1973.

8. "The WIC Program," *Nutrition News,* Nutrition Services, Pennsylvania Department of Health, Harrisburg, Fourth Issue, 1975.

9. Food and Nutrition Board, National Research Council and Council on Food and Nutrition, American Medical Association: "Diet and Coronary Heart Disease," *J. Am. Diet. Assoc.,* **61:**379–80, 1972.

10. Committee on Nutrition, American Heart Association: "Diet and Coronary Heart Disease," *Nutr. Today,* **9:**26–27, May 1974.

11. American Health Foundation: "Position Statement on Diet and Coronary Heart Disease," *Prev. Med.,* **1:**255–86, 1972.

12. Intersociety Commission for Heart Disease Resources: "Primary Prevention of the Atherosclerotic Diseases," *Circulation,* **42**(6):A55–95, 1970.

13. Darby, W. J.: "Nutrition, Food Needs and Technologic Priorities: The World Food Conference," *Nutr. Rev.,* **33:**225–34, 1975.

14. Harrison, G. G., *et al.:* "Food Waste Behavior in an Urban Population," *J. Nutr. Educ.,* **7:**13–16, 1975.

15. Altschul, A. M.: "Food: Proteins for Humans," *Chem. Eng. News,* **47:**68–81, Nov. 24, 1969.

16. Brown, L. R., with Eckholm, E. P.: *By Bread Alone.* Praeger Publishers, New York, 1974.

17. Clark, H. E.: "Meeting Protein Requirements of Man," *J. Am. Diet. Assoc.,* **52:**475–79, 1968.

18. "Fortified Foods: the Next Revolution," *Chem. Eng. News,* **48:**36–43, Aug. 10, 1970.

ADDITIONAL REFERENCES

Community Nutrition

Batchelor, T. M., *et al.:* "A Comprehensive Health Care Program in the Community," *J. Am. Diet. Assoc.,* **60:**112–13, 1972.

Frankle, R. T., and Christakis, G.: "Community Nutrition Teams," *Hospitals,* **47:**56–60, Dec. 16, 1973.

Goldberg, J. F.: "Some Community Nutrition Services in a Boston Program," *J. Am. Diet. Assoc.,* **62:**537–39, 1973.

Hallstrom, B. J., and Lauber, D. E.: "Multidisciplinary Manpower in the Nutrition Component of Comprehensive Health Care Delivery," *J. Am. Diet. Assoc.,* **63:**23–29, 1973.

Hinkle, M. M., and Fessler, E. G.: "A Decade of Dial-a-Dietitian in Columbus, Ohio," *J. Am. Diet. Assoc.,* **66:**48–50, 1975.

Kallen, D. J.: "Nutrition and Society," *J.A.M.A.,* **215:**94–100, 1971.

Nichaman, M. Z., and Collins, G. E.: "Nutrition Programs in State Health Agencies," *Nutr. Rev.,* **32:**65–67, 1974.

Spodnik, J. P.: "Nutrition in the Health Maintenance Organization," *J. Am. Diet. Assoc.,* **61:**163–65, 1972.

Low-Income Families

Inano, M., and Pringle, D. J.: "Dietary Survey of Low-Income, Rural Families in Iowa and North Carolina," *J. Am. Diet. Assoc.,* **66:**366–70, 1975.

Kaufman, M., *et al.:* "Florida Seasonal Farm Workers. Follow-Up and Intervention Following a Nutrition Survey," *J. Am. Diet. Assoc.,* **66:**605–609, 1975.

Krumdiek, C. L.: "The Rural-to-Urban Malnutrition Gradient. A Key Factor in the Pathogenesis of Urban Slums," *J.A.M.A.,* **215:**1652–54, 1971.

Walter, J. P.: "Two Poverties Equal One Hunger," *J. Nutr. Educ.,* **5:**129–33, 1973.

National Nutrition Policy

Dwyer, J. T., and Mayer, J.: "Beyond Economics and Nutrition: The Complex Basis of Food Policy," *Science*, **188:**566–70, 1975.

Hegsted, D. M.: "Food and Nutrition Policy—Now and in the Future," *J. Am. Diet. Assoc.*, **64:**367–71, 1974.

Manchester, A. C.: "Some Current Food Policy Issues," *National Food Situation*, U.S. Department of Agriculture, May 1975, pp. 33–35.

Nutrition Education and Diet Counseling

Andrew, B. J.: "Interviewing and Counseling Skills. Techniques for Their Evaluation," *J. Am. Diet. Assoc.*, **66:**576–80, 1975.

Bosley, B.: "Nutrition, Human Welfare, and Economics," *J. Am. Diet. Assoc.*, **67:**104–106, 1975.

Dillon, H. L.: "Improvement of the Quality of Life Through a Food and Nutrition Project," *J. Am. Diet. Assoc.*, **67:**129–31, 1975.

Editorial: "Nutrition Education Is Survival Education," *J. Nutr. Educ.*, **6:**84, 1974.

Emmons, L., and Hayes, M.: "Nutrition Knowledge of Mothers and Children," *J. Nutr. Educ.*, **5:**134–39, 1973.

Johnson, M. J., and Butler, J. L.: "Where Is Nutrition Education in the Public Schools?" *J. Nutr. Educ.*, **7:**20–21, 1975.

Leverton, R. M.: "What Is Nutrition Education?" *J. Am. Diet. Assoc.*, **64:**17–18, 1974.

Spitze, H. T.: "Innovative Techniques for Teaching Nutrition," *J. Nutr. Ed.*, **2:**156–59, 1971.

World Nutrition

Berg, A., and Muscat, R.: "An Approach to Nutrition Planning," *Am. J. Clin. Nutr.*, **25:**939–54, 1972.

Berg, A., *et al.*: *Nutrition, National Development and Planning.* The MIT Press, Cambridge, 1975.

Cottam, H. R.: "The World Food Conference," *J. Am. Diet. Assoc.*, **66:**333–37, 1975.

Mayer, J.: "Stopping Famines Before They Start," *UNICEF News*, Issue 85 (3):18–20, 1975.

Schertz, L. P.: "Nutrition Realities in the Lower Income Countries," *Nutr. Rev.*, **31:**201–206, 1973.

Wade, N.: "World Food Situation: Pessimism Comes Back into Vogue," *Science*, 181:634–38, 1973.

Wade, N.: "Green Revolution. I. A Just Technology Often Unjust in Use," Science, **186:**1093–96, 1974.

Part Two
Therapeutic Nutrition

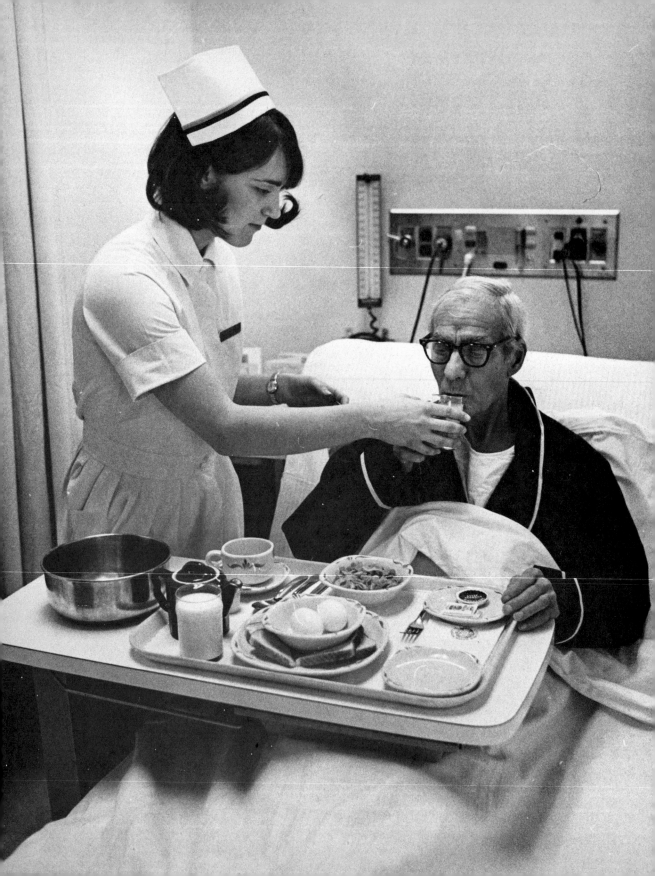

25 Therapeutic Nutrition: Factors in Patient Care

The best doctors in the world are Doctor Diet, Doctor Quiet, and Doctor Merryman.

JONATHAN SWIFT

Nutritional care of the patient. Man has probably always associated food, in one way or another, with health or illness. In fact, many of the ideas held by people for preventing or curing disease are based on food folklore. Some of these ideas are so firmly fixed that they may interfere with satisfactory food intake. Regardless of the diagnosis, the satisfactory intake of food by the patient is essential for the maintenance of tissue structures and body functions so that recovery from illness is not impeded.

The failure to ingest an adequate supply of the proper nutrients, or inability to digest, absorb, or metabolize foodstuffs, sooner or later leads to nutritional deficiency. This, in turn, may initiate or aggravate diseases of nonnutritional origin because of the body's lowered resistance. Many illnesses such as infections, injuries, and metabolic disturbances lead to deficiencies even in persons normally possessing good nutritional status because the individual is unable to ingest sufficient food or because the disease process imposes greatly increased demands for most, if not all, of the nutrients. Thus, a vicious cycle of disease, malnutrition, and prolonged convalescence is created.

The attributes of good nutrition and the principles and practices for achieving them have been discussed for all age categories in Part One of this text. The adaptation of the normal diet to the needs of individuals with some pathologic conditions is the objective of Part Two. For many patients no dietary modification is required. Good nutritional care for them consists in supplying a normal diet that furnishes the patient's nutritional, psychologic, and aesthetic needs, and in taking appropriate measures to enable him to consume it. Modified diets are the principal therapeutic agents in some metabolic diseases such as diabetes mellitus and phenylketonuria. In other instances diet therapy serves in supporting the overall therapeutic program; for example, a sodium-restricted diet may be prescribed together with diuretics to maintain water balance. Modified diets are also used as preventive measures. One example of this is the fat-controlled diet believed to be beneficial to those individuals who have genetic, physical, and biochemical characteristics that predispose to coronary disease.

The purposes of diet therapy are (1) to maintain good nutritional status, (2) to correct deficiencies that may have occurred, (3) to afford rest to the whole body or to certain organs that may be affected, (4) to adjust the food intake to the body's ability to metabolize the nutrients, and (5) to bring about changes in body weight whenever necessary.

Team approach to nutritional care. Meeting the patient's nutritional needs involves the coordination of the medical, nursing, and dietary staff. (See Figure 25–1.) The physician prescribes the diet and should also give the patient some information concerning the reasons why a modified diet has been

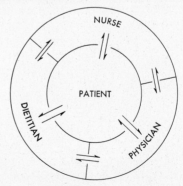

Figure 25–1. Lines of communication must be kept open between patient, dietitian, nurse, and physician.

ordered. The dietitian is the specialist who is uniquely qualified to plan and direct the activities related to the patient's nutritional care. She interprets the physician's order in terms of daily meal patterns that have been individualized according to the patient's food habits as well as modified according to the therapeutic needs. The dietitian is responsible for the preparation and service of food to the patient, the evaluation of the patient's response to his diet, and the subsequent counseling of the patient and his family if a home diet is required. (See Figure 25–2.)

What, then, is the role of the nurse in meeting the patient's nutritional needs? Fundamentally, nutritional care is an integral part of—not apart from—nursing care of the patient. The nurse is the member of the health team who has the most constant and intimate association with the patient, and the direct services she gives to the patient differ from those of the physician and the dietitian. In a large hospital the nurse maintains liaison between the patient, physician, and dietitian, gives assistance to the patient at mealtimes, observes the patient's response to his meals, and interprets the diet to the patient. The counseling of patients as well as the overall management of dietary services is provided by the dietary staff. In some small hospitals, nursing homes, and community nursing services the professional nurse may be responsible for planning modified diets, for supervising their use, and for patient

counseling. Usually a dietitian is available for consultation in these situations.

The specific activities related to nutritional care that may be expected of the nurse include the following:

1. To maintain lines of communication with the physician and dietitian regarding the patient's dietary needs:
   a. Obtaining a diet prescription if there is none, and arranging for food service to the patient.
   b. Providing the dietitian and physician with information regarding the patient's response to his diet.
   c. Serving as liaison between the patient and the physician and dietitian.
2. To assist the patient at mealtimes:
   a. Providing a pleasant environment conducive to eating.
   b. Preparing the patient for the meal.
   c. Giving assistance to the patient as needed, including feeding.
   d. Helping the handicapped to adjust to self-feeding.
   e. Giving encouragement and support to the patient.
3. To interpret the diet to the patient:
   a. Explaining the reasons for a modified diet and what may be expected of the diet.

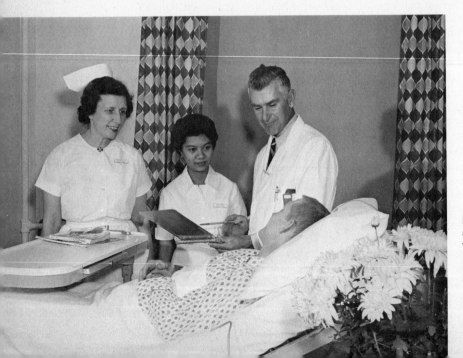

Figure 25–2. Physician, dietitian, and nurse discuss dietary changes with patient. (Courtesy, Miss Ruth Dickie and University Hospitals, University of Wisconsin Medical Center, Madison.)

b. Answering questions about the diet.
4. To observe, record, and report the patient's response to diet:
   a. Eliciting information regarding food habits, likes and dislikes, and attitudes toward diet.
   b. Noting adequacy of food intake.
   c. Reporting patient's response to dietitian and physician.
5. To plan for home care:
   a. Identifying needs for outside assistance.
   b. Arranging for counseling regarding home diet with member of family as well as patient.
   c. Providing detailed counseling regarding the home diet. (This is given by the clinical or ambulatory services dietitian in many hospitals.)

Factors to consider in the study of diet therapy. In order to assume the roles described above in patient care, certain understandings and abilities must be developed. An appreciation and knowledge are required of (1) the underlying disease conditions which require a change in diet, (2) the possible duration of the disease, (3) the factors in the dietary which must be altered to overcome these conditions, and (4) the patient's tolerance for food by mouth.

The planning of a modified diet implies the ability to adapt the principles of normal nutrition to the various regimens for adequacy, accuracy, economy, and palatability. This may necessitate the calculation of one or more nutrients. Also essential is a recognition of the need for dietary supplements such as vitamin and mineral concentrates when the nature of the diet imposes severe restrictions, the patient's appetite is poor, or absorption and utilization are impaired.

A correctly planned diet is successful only if it is eaten. The dietitian and nurse must be able to apply the principles pertaining to the preparation and service of appealing, palatable, and nutritious food. They must have the necessary understanding of the psychologic and emotional factors influencing food acceptance.

Patient care includes planning for his full rehabilitation. For some patients a modified diet may be required for weeks, months, or even a lifetime; for others, guidance may be desirable in the improvement of a normal diet. Such planning necessitates consideration of social, religious, and cultural patterns, availability of foods, cost of food, suitable methods of food preparation, and so on. (See Chapter 26.)

EFFECT OF ILLNESS ON FOOD ACCEPTANCE AND UTILIZATION

The physiologic, psychologic, and emotional factors governing food acceptance have been discussed in Chapter 14. Likewise, a number of cultural food patterns have been presented in Chapter 15. Illness may modify or accentuate the influence of any of these factors.

The stress of illness. The sick person has many fears: those relating to the outcome of the illness itself; economic concerns for himself and his family; emotional adjustments to having to depend on others during the illness; anxiety about loss of love and self-esteem.

These problems are compounded when hospitalization becomes necessary. Some patients adjust easily to a hospital routine, but for others it is difficult. The patient is subjected to seemingly endless questions, physical examinations, laboratory tests, and ministrations of therapy by a parade of specialists and auxiliary workers who, too often, do not explain what is happening, thus causing much needless anxiety. On the other hand, the patient often experiences long delays when he requires attention to his personal needs. It is not surprising that patients feel that there is no specific person who has the primary concern and responsibility for his care. The loss of privacy is an especial embarrassment and even shock to an elderly individual who has never before been in a hospital. Likewise the loss of independence to eat when and what he wishes, to get out of bed or not, to come and go as he wishes, and so on, can be frustrating. Each member of the health care team should be concerned that the patient is treated with dignity and that his rights are observed. The American Hospital Association has prepared a bill of rights for patients in the interest of better patient care.[1]

Nutritional stress. Immobilization is a stressful situation in which nitrogen and calcium excretions are elevated. In long-term illness, immobilization may be responsible for serious demineralization of bones.

Any trauma to the body such as bone fracture,

wound injury, or infection increases the losses of nitrogen and various electrolytes. The secretion of several hormones is often increased, thereby elevating the needs for vitamins required to carry on metabolic processes.

Balance studies on healthy young people have shown that emotional stress, such as the taking of examinations or a pregnancy for an unmarried girl, leads to increased losses of nitrogen and calcium. In fact, persons under such stress may achieve balances only with considerable difficulty. One may reasonably assume that the anxiety concerning illness may also accentuate such losses.

Effect of drugs. Drug therapy may have profound effects on nutritional status by interfering with food intake, decreasing nutrient absorption, or altering metabolic responses. Frequent gastrointestinal manifestations of drug intolerance are anorexia, nausea, and diarrhea. A listing of some commonly used drugs and some of the often reported nutritional effects is shown in Table 25–1. In the chapters that follow specific situations in which drug therapy may interfere with nutrient utilization are described. For further detail on the interrelationships involved, references at the end of the chapter may be consulted.[2-11]

Illness modifies food acceptance. The disease process itself may have a profound effect on food acceptance. Some foods may produce marked anorexia, others may be distending, and still others may be irritants to the gastrointestinal tract. Food preferences may revert back to those of earlier years.[12] These may be bland foods of childhood, but they might be the special dishes associated with one's ethnic origin.

When illness takes the individual from the home to the hospital, food acceptance becomes much more difficult. When the patient most needs the comfort and companionship of family and friends, he is relegated to eating alone. Perhaps the meal hours are different from those to which he is accustomed; the foods appearing on his tray may be unlike those he usually eats with respect to choice, or flavoring, or size of portion; a single food to which he has a strong aversion may so upset him that he is unable to eat anything served with it; managing a tray and the utensils for eating may be awkward when one is in bed; his expressed needs are often minimized or brushed aside.

Modified diets impose additional problems. When a patient is confronted with the need for a therapeutic diet, he may respond with comments such as these: "I just can't get it down." "This food is tasteless." "I can't afford such food when I go home." "Who is going to prepare my food at home?" "I can't buy these foods at work." These reactions and many others must be met by the nurse or dietitian during instruction by providing help in budgeting, arrangements for preparation, suggestions for palatability, and other useful advice.

Remarks such as the above also imply many responses to the diet: unwillingness to accept change; anger at those associated with the diet—nurse, dietitian, physician, or even mother or wife who has nagged about the food habits at home; fear of having to eat disliked foods or those foods to which he has a strong aversion; sense of deprivation with respect to choice of foods; fear of loss of social status and self-esteem; and the feeling that diet is, in some way, a punishment of him.

The patient may express fear by being angry, self-conscious, talkative or reticent, uneasy, depressed, indifferent, impatient, hostile, apologetic for his failure, or resentful.[13] Some patients may use diet as a means of gaining the attention from hospital personnel and later from the family who must provide this food. They may insist upon meticulous attention to the minutest of details, in order to gain this attention. They may actually enjoy the trouble this may be to others, and the release of responsibility for their welfare to others. Occasionally, one may actually prefer not to get well!

INTERPERSONAL RELATIONSHIP WITH THE PATIENT

The needs of the patient. Each patient has physical, psychologic, social, and spiritual needs. The pathophysiologic aspects of illness are the immediate reason for care by the health team, but other needs must not be overlooked. Each member of the health team has a unique contribution to make in providing for these needs. Some examples relating to nutritional care follow.

1. Each person wants to be treated as an individual. He has specific needs and values that are unique for him, and his care should be personalized rather than making him fit into a general mold.

Table 25–1. Some Effects of Drug Therapy of Nutritional Significance

Drug Group	Effects of Nutritional Significance	Proposed Mechanism
Adrenocortical Steroids		
ACTH	Gastric inflammation, ulcer	Breaks gastric mucosal barrier
Glucocorticoids	Gastric inflammation, erosion, ulcer with bleeding; pancreatitis; ↓ calcium, iron	↓ Active transport; stimulates pancreatic secretion in partially obstructed gland; breaks gastric mucosal barrier
Prednisone	Gastrointestinal hemorrhage; ↑ liver fat; ↓ muscle protein; peptic ulcer; ↓ glucose tolerance; iron-deficiency anemia	
Alcohol	Inflammation of gastric mucosa; interferes with activities of liver and pancreas; ↑ magnesium excretion; ↓ absorption: folic acid, B_{12}, thiamin hydrochloride	Mucosal blockade; direct toxic effect on pancreas
Antacids		
Nonsystemic		
Aluminum hydroxide	Constipation; nausea, vomiting; ↓ absorption vitamin A; phosphate depletion (with anorexia, weakness, progressive debility) in persons on low-phosphate diets; hypomagnesemia; if severe: urinary calculi, osteomalacia, osteoporosis, muscle weakness	
Calcium carbonate	Constipation; nausea; hypercalcemia with alkalosis, calcinosis, and azotemia in chronic use, especially with milk-alkali syndrome; acid rebound; electrolyte imbalance	
Magnesium hydroxide	Cathartic effect; flatulence	
Systemic		
Sodium bicarbonate	Belching; sodium retention; alkalosis; milk-alkali syndrome if taken with milk	
Antibiotics and Other Antiinfective Agents		
Ampicillin	Oral lesions; diarrhea	
Chloramphenicol	↓ Lactose absorption; ↓ protein synthesis; aplastic anemia	Inhibits disaccharidases
Lincomycin	Glossitis; stomatitis; nausea, vomiting, diarrhea	Irritant; stimulates myenteric nerve reflexes
Neomycin	Steatorrhea; binds bile acids; ↓ absorption: glucose, sucrose, d-xylose, nitrogen, iron, electrolytes, carotene, fat-soluble vitamins; ↓ synthesis of folic acid and vitamin K; ↓ serum cholesterol	Binds bile acids; precipitates fatty acids; produces histologic changes in mucosa (clubbing of villi, etc.), toxic effect on mucosa
Penicillins	↑ Malabsorption syndrome; nausea; diarrhea	
Tetracyclines	Stomatitis; esophagitis; nausea, vomiting; colitis; diarrhea; gastric ulcer; ↓ absorption fat, protein, glucose, d-xylose, lactose, carotene, ferrous sulfate, sodium; binds calcium → hypoplasia; ↓ absorption B_6, B_{12}	Reduces protein synthesis in body cells; may block normal carrier function of proteins; direct toxic effect on liver

Table 25–1. Some Effects of Drug Therapy of Nutritional Significance (Cont.)

Drug Group	Effects of Nutritional Significance	Proposed Mechanism
Sulfonamides	Hepatitis; pancreatitis; ↓ bacterial synthesis of folate and B vitamins	
Anticoagulants		
Coumarin	↑ Prothrombin activity with green leafy vegetables	
Heparin	Intestinal bleeding	
Anticonvulsants		
Phenytoin	Anorexia, nausea, vomiting; gingival hyperplasia; osteomalacia; ↓ absorption: B_{12}, folic acid, *d*-xylose	Inhibits folic acid conjugase
Phenobarbital	Osteomalacia; ↓ activity of folic acid and B_{12}	
Antidepressants		
MAO inhibitors	React with tyramines in foods → headache, hypertensive crises; diarrhea	
Tricyclic	Substantial weight gain	
Antihypertensives		
Diuretics	Gastrointestinal irritation; many types → hypokalemia	
Chlorothiazide	Sodium and water losses; large doses → pancreatitis	Unknown
Ethacrynic acid	Fluid and electrolyte imbalance; ↓ carbohydrate tolerance; interference with amino acid transport; ↓ serum sodium	Unknown
Furosemide	Fluid and electrolyte imbalance; hyperglycemia; hyperuricemia; ↓ serum potassium	
Guanethidine	Diarrhea	Augments parasympathetic activity
Hydralazine	Nausea and vomiting	
Methyldopa	Gastrointestinal upset	
Reserpine	Gastric inflammation, ulcer with bleeding	Breaks gastric mucosal protective barrier
Antimetabolites		
Aminopterin	↓ Absorption: B_{12}, folic acid, *d*-xylose	Mucosal damage
Fluorouracil	Sore mouth; oral ulcers; esophagitis; gastrointestinal bleeding; diarrhea	
Methotrexate	↑ Prothrombin; ↓ absorption: B_{12}, folic acid, *d*-xylose	Inhibits dihydrofolate reductase; mucosal damage
Antipyretics		
Acetylsalicylic acid	Nausea, vomiting; gastric ulcer; pancreatitis; ↓ absorption: glucose, amino acids	Unknown
Indomethacin	Anorexia, nausea; mucosal ulceration	
Phenylbutazone	Nausea, vomiting; epigastric distress; peptic ulcer; stomatitis; anticoagulant effect; edema; diarrhea	
Antituberculars		
Aminosalicylic acid	Anorexia, nausea, vomiting; abdominal distress; peptic ulcer; steatorrhea; ↓ absorption: *d*-xylose, cholesterol, iron, B_{12}	Unknown
Isoniazid	Dry mouth; epigastric distress; hepatitis; antipyridoxine effect	
Ganglionic Blockers		
Atropine	Bitter taste; dry mouth; nausea; vomiting; heartburn; constipation; occasional diarrhea; ↓ gastric secretion, motor activity of gastrointestinal tract	

Table 25-1 (Cont.)

Drug Group	Effects of Nutritional Significance	Proposed Mechanism
Ganglionic Stimulators		
Nicotine	↑ Tone and motor activity of bowel; occasional diarrhea	
Hypocholesterol- emic Agents		
Cholestyramine	Nausea; constipation; steatorrhea; osteomalacia; ↓ absorption of fat-soluble vitamins	Binds bile acids
Clofibrate	Unpleasant or altered taste sensation; occasional nausea, diarrhea; ↓ absorption: sugar, iron, electrolytes, B_{12}	↑ Fecal neutral sterol excretion; ↓ carbohydrate enzyme activity
Nicotinic acid	Dyspepsia; vomiting; diarrhea; peptic ulcer	
Laxatives		
Bisacodyl Cascara Phenolphthalein	Chronic use: mild steatorrhea, protein-losing enteropathy, osteomalacia; ↓ absorption; glucose, *d*-xylose, calcium, electrolytes	"Intestinal hurry"
Mineral oil	↓ Absorption: fat-soluble vitamins	Unknown
Oral Contraceptives		
Estrogen and progesterone compounds	↓ Serum folate levels	Inhibits folic acid conjugase enzyme secondary to underlying malabsorption
Oral Hypoglycemic Agents		
Biguanides Metformin Phenformin	↓ Serum cholesterol; ↓ absorption: glucose, ? fats, amino acids, B_{12}	Enhanced insulin action on tissues; interferes with oxidative phosphorylation in mitochondria; intestinal glucose malabsorption
Sulfonylureas Tolbutamide	Nausea; vomiting; cholestasis; peptic ulceration or perforation	
Others		
Colchicine	Nausea; vomiting; abdominal pain; diarrhea; ↓ serum cholesterol; high doses ↓ absorption: amino acids, fats, sterols, bile acids, lactose, glucose, *d*-xylose, iron, electrolytes, carotene, B_{12}	Damages mucosal enzymes; inhibits mitosis
Digitalis	Nausea; vomiting	Stimulates central or peripheral nerve receptors
Ferrous sulfate	Nausea; vomiting	Gastric irritation
Griseofulvin	Unpleasant or altered taste sensation; absorbed better with fatty meal	
Potassium chloride	Nausea; vomiting; ↓ absorption: B_{12}	Gastric irritation; ileal acidification
Levodopa	Anorexia; nausea; vomiting	Stimulates central or peripheral nerve receptors
Probenecid	Gastrointestinal irritation	Unknown
Triparenol	↓ Absorption: fat, glucose	Mucosal damage

Listening. She who cares for the patient must learn to listen carefully—not only to the words themselves but also to their tone and inflection. By taking time to listen, she may be made aware of a legitimate complaint about something wrong with the meals a patient receives—for example, cold coffee, an egg not cooked to his liking, or a vegetable he thoroughly dislikes. Such details are relatively easy to correct, and the patient is thereby made quite comfortable and satisfied. The seemingly casual conversation with the patient may bring to light that the past diet has been inadequate for a long period of time because of lack of teeth, poor health, inadequate income, or the inability to prepare food. Permitting the patient to talk about other things as well as the diet will often reveal that the problems encountered in food acceptance are actually a by-product of the deep anxieties caused by other problems; through understanding, the patient can often be helped.

2. Each person has a right to know what he should expect from the health team and what is expected of him. If a modified diet is prescribed, the patient should be given some understanding of the reasons for it and what he may expect by way of needed change in food habits. Reassurance with respect to the diet is essential, but it must be realistic in terms of the difficulties of adjustment to it and its legitimate role in the total therapeutic program. To illustrate, appropriate diets for obesity and diabetes are basic to treatment, but some patients may find the adjustment to the restrictions extremely difficult; to minimize the problems involved is to invite failure. A fat-restricted diet may be helpful to the patient with gallstones, but it should never be held as a guarantee that surgery would not be required at a later time. Likewise, benefit may accrue to a patient with cardiovascular disease who is placed on a diet with modification of the amount and nature of the fat, but success is so variable that promises of marked improvement would be ill-advised and rash.

3. Each patient should be helped to participate in his own care. A selective menu can be a useful tool to help him make good choices for a normal as well as a modified diet. If instruction concerning a diet is begun early, each meal helps the patient to learn what changes he will need to make in his diet when he goes home. A patient who has a physical handicap should be helped to feed himself insofar as he is able, thereby increasing his independence.

4. Each person expects that his behavior during his illness will be accepted as part of his illness. The modification of food acceptance during illness as described on page 372 is an important expression of the change in behavior.

5. Each person expects to be treated with kindness, thoughtfulness, and firmness. The work of the dietitian, nurse, or homemaker is often more successful if she can place herself in the patient's role, although she must guard against overidentification; if she becomes too close to the patient, she may accept his reactions as being always so reasonable that she is unable to do anything about changing them.

Recognition of attitudes. How does the nurse or dietitian feel about the patient who does not eat his food, who eats too much, or who complains about his food a great deal? When the patient expresses resentment or hostility toward her, does she realize that this may be against the restrictions the diet puts upon him and not against her as an individual? It is important that she recognize her own attitudes toward the patient, lest she give the impression that she is pitying, superior, intolerant, resentful, or critical of him. Moreover, she must avoid an expression of any negative attitudes she may have toward food.

FEEDING THE PATIENT

Environment for meals. Time and effort directed toward creating an atmosphere conducive to the enjoyment of food are well spent. Such an environment implies that the surrounding areas are orderly and clean; that ventilation is good; and that distracting activities such as treatment of patients and doctors' rounds are not occurring at mealtime except as emergencies may arise.

Patients who are ambulatory enjoy eating with others. In some hospitals a dining room is provided for patients, and in others food service may be easily arranged at small tables set up in the patients' lounge.

Readiness of the patient. The patient should be ready for his meal whether he is in bed or ambulatory. This may entail mouth care, the washing of the hands, and the positioning of the patient so that he can eat with comfort. If tests or treatment unavoidably delay a meal, arrangements must be made to hold trays so that the food can be fresh and appetizing when the patient is ready to eat.

The patient's tray. The appearance of the tray is of the utmost importance since the patient's consumption of the food presented to him is the goal to be achieved. Some of the items listed below which describe standards for tray service are the primary responsibility of the dietary department, but others require the maximum cooperation of nursing and medical staffs with the dietary department.

1. Variations in color, flavor, and texture for appeal to the senses would be expected as essentials in menu planning and food preparation. (See Chapter 13.)

2. The tray should be of a size suitable for the food to be served—small trays for liquid nourishment and large trays for full meals.

3. The tray cover and napkins should be of suitable size for the tray, immaculately clean, and unwrinkled.

4. Everything on the tray must reflect cleanliness—sparkling glassware, shining silver, clean china.

5. The tray should be set with the most attractive china available.

6. The tray should be symmetrically arranged for the greatest convenience. All necessary silver and accessories should be included.

7. Foods should be attractively served, with the size of portions not being overlarge. Spilled liquid or sloppy serving of food is inexcusable. Garnishes help to make foods more appealing.

8. Meals should be served on time. This requires careful planning so that foods will be prepared in the proper sequence.

9. Foods should be served at the proper temperature. Hot foods should be served on hot plates, protected with a cover, and cold foods should be served on chilled dishes.

10. A final check of the tray should establish that it fully meets the requirements of the diet order, and that the patient's preferences have been implemented. (See Figure 25–3.)

Assistance in feeding. Some patients may require assistance in the cutting of meat or other foods, the pouring of a beverage, or the buttering of a piece of toast. Very ill or infirm patients must be fed. The nurse should sit down while she feeds the patient so that she can be at ease and avoid undue haste. Food will be enjoyed more if it can be eaten with reasonable leisure and if there is some conversation. Obviously, if the nurse is responsible for feeding several patients, she will make arrangements to delay tray service or to keep foods hot for those who must await their turn.

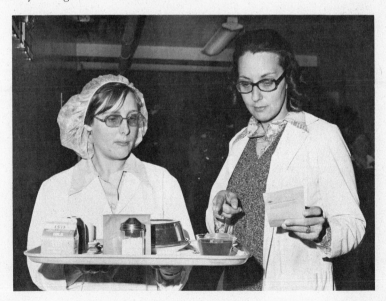

Figure 25–3. Nursing and dietary personnel work closely together to assure satisfactory meal service to the patient. Here the nurse makes a last-minute check of the tray before it is delivered to the patient. (Courtesy, University of Minnesota Health Sciences Center, Minneapolis.)

Problems and Review

1. What purposes are served by diet therapy?
2. Discuss the role of diet in total patient care.
3. How can you be sure that the diet prescribed for your patient is meeting his needs?
4. *Problem.* Keep a record of comments that your patients make about their meals.
   On the basis of these comments what can you do to ensure that your patients enjoy maximum comfort and optimum therapy insofar as their diets are concerned?
5. Discuss reasons why a patient's nutritional status may be unsatisfactory when he comes to the hospital.
6. A patient complains to you that his food is always cold. What steps can you take to correct this?
7. If a patient is having laboratory studies which will extend beyond the lunch hour, what arrangements will you make for the service of his meal?

Cited References

1. American Hospital Association: "Statement on a Patient's Bill of Rights," *Hospitals,* **47**:41, Feb. 16, 1973.
2. Bartelink, A.: "Drug-Induced Disease of the Gastrointestinal Tract," in *Drug-Induced Diseases.* Vol. 4, edited by Meyler, L., and Peck, H. M., Excerpta Medica, Amsterdam, 1972.
3. Berman, P. M., and Kirsner, J. B.: "Recognizing and Avoiding Adverse Gastrointestinal Effects of Drugs," *Geriatrics,* **29**:59–62, June, 1974.
4. Beutler, E.: "Drug-Induced Anemia," *Fed. Proc.,* **31**:141–46, 1972.
5. Christakis, G., and Miridjanian, A.: "Diets, Drugs, and Their Interrelationships," *J. Am. Diet. Assoc.,* **52**:21–24, 1968.
6. Faloon, W. W.: "Drug Production of Intestinal Malabsorption," *N.Y. State J. Med.,* **70**:2189–92, 1970.
7. Goodman, L. S., and Gilman, A., eds.: *The Pharmacological Basis of Therapeutics,* 5th ed. Macmillan Publishing Co., Inc. New York, 1975.
8. Lambert, M. L., Jr.: "Drug and Diet Interactions," *Am. J. Nurs.,* **75**:402–406, 1975.
9. Longstreth, G. F., and Newcomer, A. D.: "Drug-Induced Malabsorption," *Mayo Clin. Proc.,* **50**:284–93, 1975.
10. Morrissey, J. F., and Barreras, R. F.: "Antacid Therapy," *N. Engl. J. Med.,* **290**:550–54, 1974.
11. Stewart, R. B., and Cluff, L. E.: "Gastrointestinal Manifestations of Adverse Drug Reactions," *Am. J. Dig. Dis.,* **19**:1–7, 1974.
12. Chappelle, M. L.: "The Language of Food," *Am. J. Nurs.,* **72**:1294–95, 1972.
13. Young, C. M.: "Teaching the Patient Means *Reaching* the Patient," *J. Am. Diet. Assoc.,* **33**:52–54, 1957.

Additional References

Abdellah, F., and Levine, E.: "What Patients Say About Their Nursing Care," *Hospitals,* **31**:44–48, Nov. 1, 1957.
Beland, I. L.: *Clinical Nursing. Pathophysiological and Psychosocial Approaches,* 3rd ed. Macmillan Publishing Co., Inc., New York, 1975, pp. 1–19.
Bonnell, M.: "The Growth of Clinical Nutrition," *J. Am. Diet. Assoc.,* **64**:624–29, 1974.
Brown, E. L.: *Newer Dimensions of Patient Care.* Part 1. The Use of Physical and Social Environment of the General Hospital for Therapeutic Purposes. Part 2. Improving Staff Motivation and Competence in the General Hospital. Part 3. Patients as People. Russell Sage Foundation, New York, 1961, 1962, 1964.
Davies, G. J., *et al.:* "Special Diets in Hospitals: Discrepancy Between What Is Prescribed and What Is Eaten," *Br. Med. J.,* **1**:200–202, 1975.
Dodge, J. S.: "Factors Related to Patients' Perceptions of Their Cognitive Needs," *Nurs. Res.,* **18**:502–13, 1969.

Dolan, P. O., *et al.:* "Patients' Coffee Hour," *Am. J. Nurs.,* **74:**479–80, 1974.

Dumouchel, N.: "Are We Really Meeting Our Patients' Needs?" *Can. Nurse,* **66:**39–43, Nov. 1970.

Etzwiler, D. D.: "The Patient Is a Member of the Medical Team," *J. Am. Diet. Assoc.,* **61:**421–23, 1972.

Glew, G.: "Food Preferences of Hospital Patients," *Proc. Nutr. Soc.,* **29:**339–43, 1970.

Houston, C. S., and Pasanen, W. E.: "Patients' Perceptions of Hospital Care," *Hospitals,* **46:**70-74, Apr. 16, 1972.

Johnson, D.: "The Dietitian—A Translator of Nutritional Information," *J. Am. Diet. Assoc.,* **64:**608–11, 1974.

Kravitz, L.: "Patient Care Conferences," *Hospitals,* **48:**55–57, July 16, 1974.

Lebow, J. L.: "Consumer Assessment of the Quality of Medical Care," *Med. Care,* **12:**328–37, 1974.

Luckmann, J., and Sorensen, K. C.: "What Patients' Actions Tell You About Their Feelings, Fears and Needs," *Nursing '75,* **5:**54–61, Feb. 1975.

McKenzie, J.: "The Impact of Economic and Social Status on Food Choice," *Proc. Nutr. Soc.,* **33:**67–73, 1974.

Pender, N. J.: "Patient Identification of Health Information Received During Hospitalization," *Nurs. Res.,* **23:**262–67, 1974.

Phillips, H. T., and Larkin, M. C.: "Staff Education for Continuity of Care," *Hospitals,* **46:**54–57, Feb. 16, 1972.

Robinson, L.: "The Newly Admitted Patient," in *Liaison Nursing. Psychological Approach to Patient Care.* F. A. Davis Company, Philadelphia, 1974, Chap. 8.

Schiller, S. M. R., and Vivian, V. M.: "Role of the Clinical Dietitian," *J. Am. Diet. Assoc.,* **64:**284–87; 287–90, 1974.

Simonds, S. K.: "Psychosocial Determinants of Dietitians' Listening Patterns," *J. Am. Diet. Assoc.,* **63:**615–19, 1973.

26 Counseling and Coordinated Nutritional Services for Patients

Comprehensive care—a challenge. Chronic illnesses including cardiovascular diseases, neoplasms, diabetes, and arthritis are leading causes of illness in the United States. These diseases account for a large share of hospital admissions and place severe burdens of care, loss of income, and heavy medical costs on families who are often ill prepared to cope with these problems. The security and well-being of all members of the family may well be threatened.

Chronic diseases afflict the elderly more frequently, but younger people are not altogether immune to them. Many patients remain in hospitals longer than their therapy requires because there is no one in the home to adequately care for them, or because the other adult in the family is also the wage earner. Nursing homes sometimes provide for the transition from hospital to home. If single or multiple services are available within the home, the patient's rehabilitation is likely to be hastened in the happier environment of the home and the costs of care may be considerably reduced.

On a given day it has been estimated that 500 persons of each 100,000 are homebound because of illness or disability. Of these 500 persons, 20 could use some aspect of home care, and 40 would benefit most through coordinated home-care services. On the basis of a population of over 200 million persons, the total number of homebound persons who could benefit by some home-care services is staggering.

Federal legislation has greatly expanded the opportunities for better health care of the population. Especially significant are Medicare, children and youth programs, and regional medical programs. Undoubtedly further legislation will be enacted for programs designed to promote the maintenance of health of the entire population as well as care during illness. As the expectations of people for better health care increase, so it will become necessary to develop new approaches in the health disciplines to meet these needs.

Nutritional care is an essential and dynamic component of comprehensive health care. In fact, the ability to deliver the needed nutritional services and the quality of nutrition that the patient can maintain are often the decisive factors in restoring health or in maintaining it. In a survey of 200 agencies[1] respondents were asked to list those subjects for which increased teaching-aid material would be required as a result of the Medicare legislation. Of more than 30 subjects listed, nutrition ranked second only to rehabilitation.

This chapter is concerned with (1) dietary counseling as a sound approach to patient rehabilitation, and (2) dietary aspects of home-care services.

DIETARY COUNSELING

The plan for rehabilitation of many patients includes counseling to effect improvement of a normal diet or adjustment to a modified diet. Brandt[2] has suggested that the term *home diet* is more appropriate than the term *discharge diet*, in that the former immediately establishes the setting of the diet.

Responsibility for counseling. Dietitians, nutritionists, nurses, and physicians share responsibility for dietary counseling. Within the hospital the dietitian may provide the formalized instruction for the patient's home diet or she may have supervisory responsibility for nurses who give instruction to selected patients. The physician has an obligation to the patient to discuss the reasons why he has ordered a given diet, and what the patient may expect in terms of health as a result of adherence to the diet.

Numerous opportunities arise within the hospital for informal instruction by the nurse. It goes without saying that all who provide guidance should be in common agreement about the essentials of the patient's diet. The nurse who does not know the answer to a question should seek the correct information from the dietitian or ask the dietitian to see the patient, if the problem is complex. Nothing is more confusing to the patient than to receive information from several sources which varies widely or is contradictory.

Counseling begins early. For the in-patient, dietary counseling should be planned well in advance, for little can be accomplished when the home diet is given just as the patient is ready to leave the hospital and is concerned about his trip home, the medicines he is to take, and his readjustment to normal activities. The process of instruction, in fact, is part of the daily care of the patient. For example, the diabetic tray becomes, at each meal, a lesson in the use of the meal exchange lists; a complaint about unsalted food provides opportunity to tell about the use of other flavoring aids. Such informal instruction provided day by day gives the patient an opportunity to get used to the idea of the diet, to reflect on it, and to ask questions when they occur to him.

Establishing rapport. The nurse and dietitian have ample opportunity for establishing good rapport with the patient in the hospital, but in the clinic the patient may be seen for only a short time. The interviewer, then, must make every effort to make the patient feel comfortable and at ease before proceeding with the instruction. She must be cheerful, genuinely interested, and inspire confidence.

A quiet, pleasant room where privacy can be assured is essential. The patient and interviewer should be comfortably seated, preferably at a table or desk.

In establishing rapport, the interviewer gradually encourages the patient to talk about himself. Initial questions may well be of a general nature, such as the patient's address, occupation, height, weight, or age. The conversation is then directed to the food habits and should bring out the home situation and possibly give some clues to the patient's emotional state.

Timing is important. Choosing the right time of day for the interview and counseling is important. Just before or during meals, the patient is directed to familiar foods which have satisfied his hunger in the past, and he will resist efforts to divert him from them. Immediately following the satisfaction of hunger, he will have little interest in, and may even be nauseated by, the further mention of food. Therefore, some time should elapse after the meal when food can be discussed objectively. Instruction should come at a time when the patient need not be interrupted for routine care, treatments, etc. The counselor must have sufficient time for calm, unhurried teaching.

The diet history. In order to individualize the nutritional services to the patient and to make the necessary adjustments for the home diet a good deal of information regarding the patient's food habits is essential. The nurse and dietitian will obtain as much information as possible from the patient's chart. They will also be alert to the comments the patient makes about his food from time to time and will record these. Nevertheless, an interview with the patient will usually be required to elicit further information. Effective dietary counseling requires a good deal of experience in communicating purposefully with people and much insight into the behavior of people. Guidelines for effectiveness in diet counseling have been outlined by the Diet Therapy Section of the American Dietetic Association.[3]

The interview will be more successful if the following points are observed.

1. For the patient in the hospital assess the patient's willingness to talk about his diet. A patient who is fatigued and uncomfortable may not be as cooperative as required. Sometimes a family member may supply some or all of the information.

2. Use a conversational and casual approach rather than one that is bound to a structured form. Note, however, that a form may be helpful to you in planning your interview.

3. Use open-ended questions that permit the patient to respond fully. Avoid questions answered "Yes" or "No," or that suggest a correct answer. For example, "Tell me what you usually eat for breakfast"—*not* "Do you eat eggs for breakfast?"

4. Ask only those questions that are relevant to success in dietary counseling. Patients generally resent questions that appear to have nothing

to do with the diet and consider them to be an invasion of privacy. For example, although adequate income is essential, the nurse and dietitian can almost always obtain this information without direct questioning.

5. Give the patient time to think and to respond. Older people, especially, may be somewhat slow in responding.

The following items suggest the kinds of information that may be sought, but not every item will be required for every patient nor will direct questioning be necessary for all of them.

Socioeconomic History

Occupation: hours for work, travel time to and from work

Family relationships

Residence: house, apartment, room

Recreational activities: type, how often

Ethnic background

Religious beliefs regarding food

Medical History

Present illness: chief complaints, especially those relating to nutrition; diagnosis

Weight: any recent changes, comparison with desirable weight

Appetite: any recent changes

Digestion: ability to swallow, anorexia, vomiting, distention, cramps

Elimination: regular, constipation, diarrhea

Handicaps related to feeding: inability to chew, need for self-help devices in eating, inability to prepare food

Dietary History

Meals: where eaten, when, with whom

Meals skipped: which, how often

Food preparation: by whom, facilities

Meals away from home: which, how often, type of facility (lunch counter, cafeteria, school lunch, restaurant, vending machines)

Typical day's meals: 24-hour recall

Cross-check of day's meals: frequency of use of important food groups in a week, for example, milk, eggs, breakfast cereals

Snacks: how often, types, amounts

Mineral-vitamin supplements: type, how often, reasons for use

Food likes and dislikes: food intolerance, food allergies

Food budgeting: kinds of fruits, vegetables, meats purchased; sources of budget information; menu planning

Previous dietary restrictions: reasons for, type, how long, response to modified diet

Sources of nutrition information: use of advertising, popular publications, books

Dietary counseling based on patient needs. A fundamental tenet is to begin where the patient finds himself. Something good can be found in every diet, and every effort should be made to impose as few changes as necessary—not a complete discarding of the old pattern. The instruction should be in simple terms readily understood by the layman. Some judgment concerning the amount of detail which may be included is essential, for a weary patient may remember little when he gets home.

The patient will require guidance with respect to choice of foods, methods of preparation, kinds of seasonings which may be used, amounts of food allowed, the number of meals, and time for meals. A written meal pattern which has been developed with the patient is helpful. Printed menus that have little or no regard for individual preferences are of doubtful value.

Although the emphasis should always be directed to the foods the patient may have, in some instances, such as the sodium-restricted diets, it may be desirable also to provide a list of foods that are contraindicated. Printed aids such as the food exchange lists are useful and time saving, but they should always be accompanied with appropriate explanation. Illustrations, posters, and food models are helpful in clarifying instruction; even films may be used where group instruction is used as for pregnant women, the obese, diabetics, and others.

Other members of the family must often be included in the instruction. The wife or mother of the patient may not understand the reasons for the diet, may feel that the diet is an imposition upon her, and may not understand the methods for preparing the necessary foods unless she is present at the time of instruction. For some patients it is necessary to plan a food budget, to make arrangements for meals carried to work, to make suggestions for a conference with the employer, or to provide guidelines for eating meals away from home.

Continuity of guidance. Dietary counseling is time consuming. The effort is often wasted when no opportunity is given for follow-up of the instruction given. The outpatient clinic and home visits serve to extend and clarify the instruction itself, to provide reassurance, to check progress, and to recognize any tensions which are building up in the patient.

Initial counseling may have been provided by a clinical dietitian or sometimes a nurse in the hospital, but it is quite likely that follow-up of the patient is the responsibility of an outpatient clinic dietitian, a nutritionist, or a public health nurse. Insofar as possible, each follow-up visit should be scheduled with the same person. Obviously, an important element of such continuing guidance is an adequate record of what has been presented to the patient initially.

Teaching machines have been used with some success for instruction of patients with diabetes mellitus. Their use in hospitals, clinics, and health centers serves to reinforce the personalized instruction which has been given and to save instructional time. Programmed instruction through booklets pertaining to modified diets also merits attention. These aids allow the patient to progress at his own speed; they are not intended to replace individualized instruction, however.

Group instruction. In a food clinic or health center, classes may be held for groups with similar diet problems: pregnant women, mothers with preschool children, diabetic patients, those requiring sodium restriction, weight-control groups, and so on. Economy of time for the professional worker is an apparent advantage of using group instruction. Many patients are helped by this approach inasmuch as they learn to appreciate that others have similar problems and that they can share experiences with one another. The person who is given to much self-

pity may receive encouragement toward a more positive outlook on his problems if proper guidance is provided in the group setting. Group instruction may be supplemented by individual teaching, particularly with respect to problems of finance and emotional reactions to the diet.

Group instruction must be a democratic process in which everyone feels free to participate. The nurse or dietitian cannot be authoritarian, the talkative patient should not monopolize all of the time, and the self-conscious, shy patient should not be made uncomfortable by having to respond when he is not ready. Verbal instruction should be coordinated with visual aids, including dietary lists, leaflets, posters, food models, and films as the occasion may warrant. The leader of the group cannot change the individual or the group; she can only help them to recognize their own goals and to make their own decisions for change.

COMPREHENSIVE CARE SERVICES

Concepts of comprehensive care. The provision of all necessary health services so that the patient can maintain or be restored to independent living is implied in the term *comprehensive care.* Although such a goal has long been held by professional health workers, its achievement through continuing services from hospital to home has been limited.

Hallstrom has described the components of comprehensive health care as screening, assessment, intervention, and follow-up.[4] Careful evaluation and reevaluation of the client's physical, psychologic, economic, and social needs are required so that referral is made to the appropriate personnel in essential services. The services may be provided on an in-patient basis, including hospital care for the acutely ill, a minimum-care facility within a hospital, or convalescent care in a nursing home. Care may be furnished through an out-patient clinic, utilizing a single service in a physician's office or multiple services provided by a clinic or health center. Home care, of course, implies services provided in the home, and can range from a single service such as nursing to coordinated services by many disciplines that could include medical, nursing, dental, dietetic, social, occupational therapy, physical therapy, and others.

Many home-care programs are now being developed in communities, some of which are sponsored by the hospital whereas others are directed by a public or voluntary health agency. Such services will require the assistance of a variety of technicians so that the services of the professional nurse, dietitian, and others may be most effectively used. A brief discussion of some elements of home care is given below.

Home-delivered meals. Many individuals or couples with physical limitations can remain in their own homes rather than be institutionalized if some provision can be made for their meals. Others who are temporarily disabled by illness but who are ambulatory and can feed themselves may find it possible to return to their homes at an earlier time if they can procure their meals.

A service described as "Meals-on-Wheels" was first offered by The Lighthouse in Philadelphia in 1954 and is now available in many communities though still on a limited basis. Most programs have been operated by women's clubs, church groups, family service organizations, and so on. Dietitians, nutritionists, or home economists usually serve as consultants, giving particular attention to menu planning, food purchasing, and food preparation. Paid employees and volunteers share the responsibility for the actual purchase, preparation, packing, and delivery of meals.

Usually a hot noon meal and a packaged evening meal are delivered by a volunteer on a five-day basis. The recipient pays a fee for these meals, with gradations according to ability to pay. One important benefit of the service is the daily contact which the homebound person has with the volunteer who delivers the meals.

Homemaker services. The purpose of this service is to maintain the family in a healthful setting when no one in the family can fulfill the homemaking function. For example, the mother may be ill or convalescing from physical or mental illness; an aging person or couple is unable to perform the necessary tasks in the home, but could remain at home at less expense with homemaker assistance; death of the mother in a home with young children presents a major problem to the working father unless relatives help out or homemaker service is available.

The sponsoring organization may be a public or voluntary agency such as the welfare division, the family service organization, or the community nursing service. The organizations recruit, define duties, provide formalized training and in-service programs of education, and provide supervision on the job. Social workers, public health nurses, home economists, and others have participated in these duties.

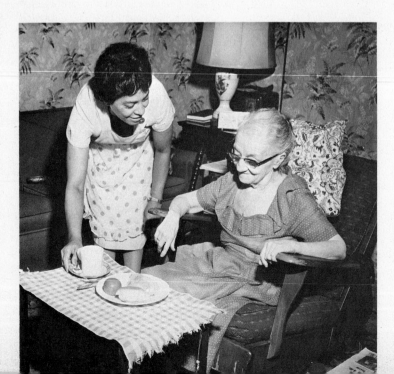

Figure 26–1. A home health aide adapts to the facilities within the home providing meals that will be satisfying to the older American. (Courtesy, Community Nursing Service, Philadelphia.)

The terms *homemaker, home health aide, house-keepers,* and *visiting homemakers* are used with some variations of duties depending upon the sponsoring agency. Generally speaking, homemakers are mature women who have had responsibility for raising their own families, who like to help other people, and who can follow instructions. Among the responsibilities pertaining to nutrition are meal planning, marketing, food preparation, and food service. (See Figure 26–1.) One of the problems may be that of getting children to eat regular meals; another may relate to a modified diet; a common problem is that of stretching the food dollar. The homemaker must be an adaptable individual who adjusts to the facilities within the home, whatever they may be. She must respect the wishes of the family and adhere to their socioeconomic and cultural values. She will accomplish little if in doing her job she creates antagonism and jealousy in any member of the family.

PHYSICAL HANDICAPS, REHABILITATION, AND NUTRITION

Physical handicaps. Millions of Americans have physical handicaps that restrict their ability to care for themselves and to work. Physical disabilities cover a wide range: the individual who has lost a hand or an arm, or who is hemiplegic and has the use of only one arm; arthritics with stiff, swollen, painful joints and who have a limited range of motion; those with cerebral palsy, Parkinson's disease, or multiple sclerosis and for whom incoordinated movements are a constant trial; those bound to a wheelchair; the blind; those who have limited cardiac and respiratory reserves such as patients with cardiac disease or emphysema; and many others.

Nutrition of the physically handicapped. Adequate nutrition is essential in restoring a patient to his potential capacity for independence, yet the handicap itself may be the principal factor that favors malnutrition even though the supply of food is plentiful.[5] The use of only one arm, or stiff, painful joints, or incoordinated movements present tremendous difficulties in feeding oneself and may limit the performance of simple kitchen tasks such as opening packages, cutting foods, peeling vegetables, and using appliances.

The energy balance is an important consideration. Some handicapped individuals have an increased energy requirement because they must exert a tremendous effort to complete tasks. The increased requirement, on the one hand, and the difficulties experienced in eating, on the other hand, lead to excessive weight loss and to tissue depletion. Other individuals confined to wheelchairs and who exert little effort may become obese and require a diet restricted in calories. (See Chapter 29.)

Good protein nutrition is essential for restoration of body tissues, to reduce the incidence of infection, and to maintain the integrity of the skin. For immobilized individuals decubitus ulcers are a frequent problem. During the early stages of immobilization the nitrogen losses from the body greatly exceed the intake. The accelerated catabolism of protein tissues appears to run a time sequence that is not wholly reversed in the early stages even though a high-protein diet may be used. Nevertheless, the replacement of these losses requires a high-protein diet over an extended period of time. (See Chapter 30.)

Excessive losses of calcium from the bones may lead to urinary calculi. A liberal fluid intake is essential to facilitate the excretion of calcium, and some restriction of the calcium intake is often prescribed. (See Chapter 42.)

Constipation is a frequent complication of those who are immobilized. Its prevention or correction requires a liberal intake of fluids, a diet containing sufficient bulk, and regular habits of elimination. (See Chapter 33 for further details.)

The nature of rehabilitation. Rehabilitation is the return of a handicapped individual to his maximum potential—to what he will be able to do in the future. It is an individualized process in which therapy is designed specifically in terms of the patient's handicap, his psychologic problems, his family situation, and his economic circumstances. It is individualized in that each patient's progress is measured against his own possibilities, not against some normal standard.

Rehabilitation may occur in a rehabilitation center, in a school for handicapped children, or in the home. The economic consideration is important inasmuch as rehabilitation is costly in terms of weeks or months in a rehabilitation center, and the involvement of many specialists in the process. In addition, when the homemaker is handicapped, additional costs for her substitute in the home are likely to be appreciable.

The handicapped individual experiences help-lessness, defeat, frustration, and even neglect. To surmount his difficulties becomes a constant uphill battle. Rehabilitation itself is usually slow, some-times painful, and fatiguing both physically and emotionally. The patient needs the support of every member of the rehabilitation team.

The rehabilitation team. The skills and techniques in physical medicine, physical therapy, occupa-tional therapy, nursing, home economics, nutrition, social work, and psychology are utilized in rehabili-tation. The patient is not only the focus of these specialized skills but he is part of the team and participates in the plans for his restoration—as do members of his family. Each member of the team

Figure 26–2. This patient is learning to use a universal cuff to become independent in self-feeding activities. A bowl with suction cups adheres to the table and prevents slipping. This will be used to make learning less difficult and will be replaced with regular utensils when the skill is perfected. (Courtesy, Allied Services for the Handi-capped, Inc., Scranton, Pennsylvania.)

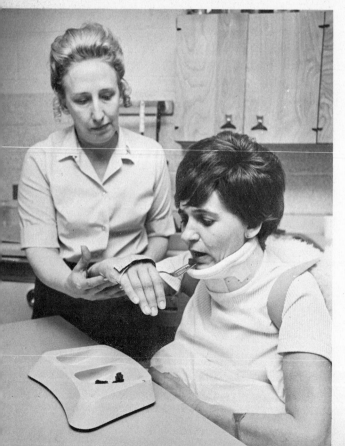

contributes his skills in a way that complements but does not overlap or duplicate the efforts of another. The nurse is usually the coordinator of these ser-vices in the rehabilitation center. For a full descrip-tion of the specialized roles of the team members the student is referred to texts and articles listed in the references.

Self-help devices for eating. Numerous devices for daily activities have been designed at the Institute of Rehabilitation Medicine of the New York Univer-sity Medical Center. In addition, publications such as the *Mealtime Manual for the Aged and Handi-capped* are valuable.[6] Many of the devices can be made in the home, and others are available at mod-erate costs. A few of the devices that are helpful to those who have only one arm or who have difficulty in holding articles or bringing food to the mouth are described below. (See Figure 26–2.)

Jointed handles for spoons and forks. When the motions of the arm and wrist are restricted, the joints of the utensil permit an angle that can ap-proach the mouth.

Knife for cutting. A knife needs a firm support, and cutting is difficult for persons with the use of only one arm. A cuff fitted over the hand permits the knife to be held firmly. A serrated edge is better than one with a smooth edge.

Plate guards. These are placed at the edge of the plate; they keep food from spilling and pro-vide a surface against which food can be pushed. A deep dish with straight sides is also helpful. The plate can be kept from sliding by placing it in a support constructed to hold it, or by setting it on a sponge.

Buttering bread. A right-angle ledge affixed to the corner of the breadboard will hold a piece of bread in place while it is being buttered.

Drinking glass and tube. A drinking glass can be fitted with a holder that has a wide handle easily grasped by the hand. If it is difficult to bring the glass to the mouth, a wooden block into which a hole has been cut to hold a standard-size glass will hold the glass firmly on the table. A piece of plastic tubing bent at an angle for approach to the mouth can be used. To keep the plastic tube from slipping, a bulldog clip can be fastened to the edge of the glass and the tubing can be placed through the hole of the handle of the clip.

Aids in food preparation. Homemaking is the

single most frequent occupation of the physically handicapped.[5] The rehabilitation of the homemaker in terms of food preparation skills and in overall homemaking activities benefits the entire family. Home economists, occupational therapists, and dietitians have specialized skills by which they are able to help the homemaker in simplification of procedures in food preparation and in more convenient kitchen arrangements.

The handicapped homemaker will find that each task requires a longer time to complete. As much food preparation should be completed in advance as possible so that there are few last-minute tasks. Arthritics fatigue easily and they should not attempt tasks that cannot be interrupted for a rest period. For many homemakers a list of things to be done is helpful.

Electric mixers, blenders, wedge-shape jar openers, electric can openers, long-handled tongs to reach packages and equipment out of reach, turntables in cupboards to hold supplies, sliding racks, magnetized equipment holders, and carts on wheels are among the pieces of equipment that facilitate work for the handicapped homemaker.

The person who has the use of only one arm needs firm support for devices. For example, a board with two stainless steel nails serves as a holder for vegetables to be peeled. (See Figure 26–3.) A sponge underneath a bowl helps to keep it from sliding. Boxes can be held firmly between the knees and a scissors can be used with one hand to cut off tops.

For those who will be confined to a wheelchair indefinitely or who must sit while working, a redesign of the kitchen is essential. Counter surfaces need to be lowered so that work can be done while

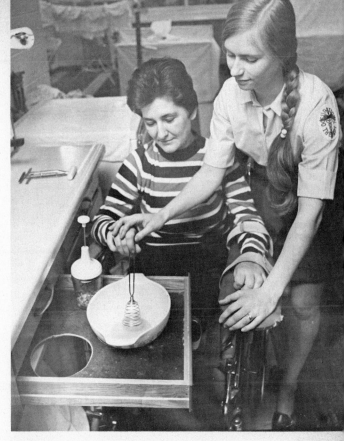

Figure 26–3. One-handed kitchen activities are learned in occupational therapy to enhance independence in the home. Illustrated are a one-handed egg beater, a one-handed nut chopper, and a simple method of holding the bowl steady. (Courtesy, Allied Services for the Handicapped, Inc., Scranton, Pennsylvania.)

sitting. Kneehole spaces are needed so that the chair or wheelchair can be partially underneath the work surface. Equipment and storage shelves must be within reach.

PROBLEMS AND REVIEW

1. Why is the term *discharge diet* undesirable?
2. Keep a record for a week of questions which relate to diet asked by patients under your care. How did you answer these questions?
3. *Problem.* Obtain a diet history from one of your patients who is receiving a normal diet. Use a form available in your hospital or develop one of your own. Evaluate the adequacy of the patient's diet according to the Four Food Groups. What recommendations can be made to the patient? How would you plan for this counseling?
4. Define these terms: coordinated home-care services; patient evaluation; homemaker service; programmed instruction; rehabilitation.

5. *Problem.* Determine the services available in your community for home care of patients. List the ways in which these services include nutritional care.

6. If you were asked to provide some guidelines for a group in your community which is setting up a meals-on-wheels service, what are the categories you would consider? What consultants would be desirable for this group?

CITED REFERENCES

1. "What 200 Agencies Are Saying About Medicare," *Nurs. Outlook*, **14:**30–32, June 1966.
2. Brandt, M. B.: "Perspective on Diet Manuals," *J. Am. Diet. Assoc.*, **47:**121–23, 1965.
3. Myers, M., *et al.:* "Guidelines for Diet Counseling," *J. Am. Diet. Assoc.*, **66:**571–75, 1975.
4. Hallstrom, B. J., and Lauber, D. E.: "Multidisciplinary Manpower in the Nutrition Component of Comprehensive Health Care Delivery," *J. Am. Diet. Assoc.*, **63:**23–29, 1973.
5. Rusk, H. A.: "Nutrition in the Fourth Phase of Medical Care," *Nutr. Today*, **5:**24–31, Autumn 1970.
6. Klinger, J. L., *et al.: Mealtime Manual for the Aged and Handicapped.* Simon and Schuster, Inc., New York, 1970.

ADDITIONAL REFERENCES

"The American Dietetic Association Position Paper on Child Nutrition Programs," *J. Am. Diet. Assoc.*, **64:**520–21, 1974.

"The American Dietetic Association Position Paper on Food and Nutrition Services in Day-Care Centers," *J. Am. Diet. Assoc.*, **59:**47, 1971.

"The American Dietetic Association Position Paper on the Nutrition Component of Health Services Delivery Systems," *J. Am. Diet. Assoc.*, **58:**538–40, 1971.

"The American Dietetic Association Position Paper on Nutrition Education for the Public," *J. Am. Diet. Assoc.*, **62:**429–30, 1973.

"The American Dietetic Association Position Paper on Nutrition Services in Health Maintenance Organizations," *J. Am. Diet. Assoc.*, **60:**317–20, 1972.

Christopherson, V. A., *et al.: Rehabilitation Nursing. Perspectives and Applications.* McGraw-Hill Book Company, New York, 1974.

Danish, S. J.: "Developing Helping Relationships in Dietetic Counseling," *J. Am. Diet. Assoc.*, **67:**107–10, 1975.

Egan, M. C., and Hallstrom, B. J.: "Building Nutrition Services in Comprehensive Health Care," *J. Am. Diet. Assoc.*, **61:**491–96, 1972.

Juhas, L.: "Nutrition Education in Day Care Programs," *J. Am. Diet. Assoc.*, **63:**134–37, 1973.

Kocher, R. E.: "Monitoring Nutritional Care of the Long Term Patient. I. Policies and Systems that Support the On-Going Evaluation of Care," *J. Am. Diet. Assoc.*, **67:**45–46, 1975.

Smith, C. E.: "New Federal Regulations for Skilled Nursing Homes," *J. Am. Diet. Assoc.*, **64:**467–69, 1974.

27 Adaptations of the Normal Diet for Texture

Normal, Soft, and Fluid Diets

Therapeutic nutrition begins with the normal diet. Normal and therapeutic diets are planned to maintain, or restore, good nutrition in the patient. In diet manuals the normal diet may be designated as *regular, house, normal,* or *full diet.* It consists of any and all foods eaten by the person in health. Fried foods, pastries, strongly flavored vegetables, spices, and relishes are not taboo, but good menu planning means that these foods are used judiciously. The normal diet satisfies the nutritional needs for most patients and also serves as the basis for planning modified diets.

The nutritive contributions of a basic diet composed of recommended levels from each of the Four Food Groups were discussed in Chapter 13 and are summarized in Table 13–2. One of the many ways by which such a foundation diet may be amplified to provide meal patterns that are typical in many hospitals is shown in Table 27–1. In the suggested additions to the basic list of foods an additional cup of milk is included because it provides important amounts of several nutrients that are likely to be needed in increased amounts by many patients.

Contrary to the opinion held by some, milk is one of the best-accepted foods in the hospital dietary.

To use the normal diet as the basis for therapeutic diets is sound in that it emphasizes the similarity of psychologic and social needs of those who are ill with those who are well, even though there may be differences in quantitative or qualitative requirements. Insofar as possible the patient is provided a food allowance that avoids the connotation of a "special" diet that sets him apart from his family and friends. Moreover, in the home, food preparation is simplified when the modified diet is based upon the family pattern, and the number of items requiring special preparation is reduced to a minimum.

Although it is desirable that the normal diet provide the basis for planning modified diets, it must be remembered that the nutritional requirements of patients are likely to vary widely. The Recommended Dietary Allowances are designed to meet the nutritional needs for almost all healthy persons in the United States, and they should not be interpreted as being appropriate allowances during illness. For any given patient the nutritional requirements depend upon his nutritional status, modifications in activity, increased or decreased metabolic demands made by the illness, and the efficiency of digestive, absorptive, and excretory mechanisms.

Many adaptations to the plan presented in Table 27–1 could be devised for varying cultural and socioeconomic circumstances. The calculated values for the basic plan are useful in determining the effects of the omission or addition of foods to such a plan. For example, if a patient is allergic to milk, the plan shows that adjustment would need to be made especially for calcium, riboflavin, and protein. Or, if the intake of vegetables and fruits were to be curtailed, it is obvious that there would be a deficiency of vitamin A and ascorbic acid and that a supplement of vitamins should be prescribed.

REGULAR OR NORMAL DIET

Include These Foods, or Their Nutritive Equivalents, Daily:
2–3 cups milk
   4 ounces (cooked weight) meat, fish, or poultry; cheese, additional egg or milk, or legumes may substitute
    in part

1 egg (3 to 4 per week)
3–4 servings vegetables including:
    1 medium potato
    1 serving dark-green leafy or yellow vegetable
    1–2 servings other vegetable
    One of the above vegetables to be served raw
 3 servings fruit including:
    1 serving citrus fruit, or other good source of ascorbic acid
    2 servings other fruit
 1 serving enriched or whole-grain cereal
 3 slices enriched or whole-grain bread
Additional foods such as butter or fortified margarine, soups, desserts, sweets, salad dressings, or increased
   amounts of foods listed above will provide adequate calories. See calculation in Table 27–1.

Meal Pattern	**Sample Menu**
BREAKFAST	
Fruit	Sliced banana in orange juice
Cereal, enriched or whole grain	Oatmeal
Milk and sugar for cereal	Milk and sugar
Egg	Soft-cooked egg
Whole-grain or enriched roll or toast	Whole-wheat toast with butter
Butter or margarine	
Hot beverage with cream and sugar	Coffee with cream and sugar
LUNCHEON OR SUPPER	
Soup, if desired	
Cheese, meat, fish, or legumes	Cheese soufflé
Potato, rice, noodles, macaroni, spaghetti, or vegetable	Buttered peas
Salad	Lettuce and tomato salad
Enriched or whole-grain bread	Russian dressing
Butter or margarine	Hard roll with butter
Fruit	Royal Anne cherries
Milk	Milk
DINNER	
Meat, fish or poultry	Meat loaf with gravy
Potato	Mashed potato
Vegetable	Buttered carrots
Enriched or whole-grain bread	Enriched white, rye, or whole-wheat bread with butter
Butter or margarine	
Dessert	Apple Betty
Milk	Milk
Coffee or tea, if desired	

Therapeutic modifications of the normal diet.
The normal diet may be modified (1) to provide change in consistency as in fluid and soft diets to be described below; (2) to increase or decrease the energy values; (3) to include greater or lesser amounts of one or more nutrients, for example, high-protein and sodium-restricted diets; (4) to increase or decrease bulk—high- and low-fiber diets; (5) to provide foods bland in flavor; (6) to include or exclude specific foods, as in allergic conditions; and (7) to modify the intervals of feeding.

Rationale for modified diets. The principles for diet therapy in many pathologic conditions are well established, and dietary regimens are based upon a sound rationale. In such regimens the food allowances may vary according to ethnic and socioeconomic factors. It is to be expected that differences in interpretation will be found in the detailed descriptions of diet that are presented in the diet manuals of hospitals. Some of these differences are caused by the fact that some modified diets have only an empiric basis. Research to establish the

Table 27-1. Nutritive Value of the Normal Diet Pattern as a Basis for Therapeutic Diets.*

Food	Measure	Weight gm	Energy kcal	Protein gm	Fat gm	Carbohydrate gm	Minerals		Vitamins				
							Ca mg	Fe mg	A I.U.	Thiamin mg	Riboflavin mg	Niacin mg	Ascorbic Acid mg
Milk	2 cups	488	320	18	18	24	576	0.2	700	0.14	0.82	0.4	4
Meat Group													
Egg	1	50	80	6	6	tr	27	1.1	590	0.05	0.15	tr	0
Meat, fish, poultry (lean, cooked)	4 ounces	120	240	33	10	0	17	3.6	35	0.32	0.26	7.4	0
Vegetable-Fruit Group													
Leafy green or deep yellow	½–⅔ cup	100	30	2	tr	6	28	1.0	7400	0.06	0.08	0.6	28
Other vegetable	½–⅔ cup	100	30	2	tr	6	20	0.8	480	0.06	0.06	0.6	14
Potato	1 serving	122	80	2	tr	18	7	0.6	tr	0.11	0.04	1.4	20
Citrus fruit†	1 serving	100	40	1	tr	10	10	0.2	160	0.07	0.02	0.3	40
Other fruit	2 servings	200	120	2	tr	32	24	1.0	1200	0.08	0.08	0.8	18
Bread-Cereal Group													
Cereal, enriched or whole grain	¾ cup	30 (dry)	105	3	tr	22	10	0.8	0	0.12	0.04	0.8	0
Bread, enriched or whole grain	3 slices	75	210	6	3	39	63	1.8	tr	0.18	0.15	1.8	tr
			1255	75	37	157	782	11.1	10,565	1.19	1.70	14.1	124
Additional Foods													
Milk	1 cup	244	160	9	9	12	288	0.1	350	0.07	0.41	0.2	2
Butter or margarine	4 pats	28	200	tr	24	tr	6	0	940	—	—	—	—
Sugars, sweets	3 tablespoons	33	120	0	0	33	0	0	0	0	0	0	0
Dessert§	1 serving	varies	190	4	6	30	70	0.3	190	0.03	0.10	0.1	tr
Bread	3 slices	75	210	6	3	39	63	1.8	tr	0.18	0.15	1.8	0
Total nutritive value			2135	94	79	271	1209	13.3	12,045	1.47	2.36	16.2‡	126

*The nutritive values of the foods listed for the normal diet, pages 389–90, have been calculated using Table A–1 in the Appendix. The additional foods listed at the bottom of the table suggest one of many ways to complete the diet.

†Other ascorbic-acid-rich foods such as cantaloupe and strawberries are also included.

‡The tryptophan content of this diet is about 940 mg, equivalent to 15.7 mg niacin, thus providing a niacin equivalent of 31.9 mg.

§Desserts include plain gelatin, cake with icing, custard, ice cream, cookies, and plain pudding.

merits of a particular regimen as opposed to another is difficult to control because of the numerous physiologic and psychologic variables in human beings. Fortunately, a number of widely varying dietary programs may be equally effective because of the remarkable response of the human body.

Probably no diets are more subject to criticism than those modified for fiber and flavor. In order to reduce the fiber content of a diet, meats may be ground and vegetables and fruits strained. Yet, experience has shown that few patients consume such foods in satisfactory amounts, and the harm to nutritional status is likely to be greater than the possible insult to the mucosa of the gastrointestinal tract.

Some patients experience heartburn, abdominal distention, and flatulence following the ingestion of strongly flavored vegetables, dry beans or peas, and melons. Other patients refuse to eat these foods simply because they have been told that they are poorly digested. There is no evidence that justifies the omission of these foods for all patients.[1,2] Although dietitians and nurses have a responsibility to correct food misinformation whenever it is encountered, little is gained by coercing someone who is ill into eating a food that he dislikes intensely or against which he has a prejudice.

Diet manuals and dietary patterns. Numerous manuals are available as guides in the standardization of dietary procedures for a given hospital. The best of these manuals have been prepared by committees including representatives of the various medical specialties, nursing, and dietary departments. The manual generally includes statements concerning principles of diet, food allowances with detailed lists of foods to use and to avoid, typical meal patterns, and nutritive evaluations. They serve as a guide for the physician in prescribing a diet, a reference for the nurse, a procedural manual for the dietary department, and a teaching tool for professional personnel.

Although a manual achieves standardization in procedures, it does *not* mean that every patient on a given diet must have exactly the same food allowances as every other patient. In fact, within the guide ample opportunity is provided for individualization of a given patient's regimen. The diet manual is *not* an instructional guide for the patient for whom individualized and more detailed aids are necessary. It may, however, serve as the basis for the development of such teaching aids.

Throughout this text dietary regimens which are representative of those used in many hospitals are presented. Each description includes a statement of characteristics, lists of foods to include, detailed lists of foods permitted and contraindicated, a typical meal pattern, and a sample menu. The student will learn much by comparing one regimen with another and will begin to understand the rationale for diet therapy and how the goals may be achieved in a number of ways.

Nomenclature of diets. Insofar as possible, the nomenclature used in this text will describe the modification in consistency, in nutrients, or in flavor; thus *bland* diet, *1200-kcal* diet, etc. When the quantity of one or more nutrients is important to the success of the diet, it is essential that these quantities be specified in the diet prescription. Thus, the term *diabetic diet* has little meaning, but a prescription for 200 gm carbohydrate, 90 gm protein, and 70 gm fat can be accurately interpreted. Likewise, a *sodium-restricted* diet gives no indication of the exact level of restriction required, but the designation *500-mg sodium diet* leaves no room for misinterpretation.

Several undesirable practices have been, and still are, common in the naming of diets. The literature is replete with illustrations of diets named for their originators. The Sippy diet is a classic example, but there have been others from time to time. Unfortunately, such nomenclature tells nothing about the diet, and the practice should be discouraged.

Others have used the name of a disease condition to specify a given diet, such as ulcer, ambulatory ulcer, ulcer discharge, cardiac, and gallbladder diets. Psychologically, this is not good practice, for the patient should not need to be reminded of his condition every time he looks at a diet on a tray card. Moreover, the diets used for many of these conditions have multiple uses, and the uninitiated may overlook the full usefulness of a given regimen with such disease-oriented terminology.

Frequency of feeding. Research on experimental animals and on humans has shown that more than three meals daily may be desirable for some patients. When the patient eats five, six, or more meals a day which are approximately balanced for protein, fat, and carbohydrate, the metabolic load at a given time is less, and the nutrients can be more effectively utilized. It is well known that protein is inefficiently used if the day's allowance is more or less concentrated in one meal. Large amounts of carbohydrate at a given meal require the use of alternate metabolic pathways which favor the deposition of fat.

Irwin has described guidelines for health care facilities using menu patterns with four or five meals daily. Each meal provides at least three menu items and 10 per cent or more of calories as protein. Between-meal snacks are not considered as meals. In compliance with federal guidelines the time lapse between the last meal of one day and the first meal of the next is not more than 14 hours. From 20 to 50 per cent of total calories are given in consecutive five-hour periods between 7 A.M. and 10 P.M.[3]

Sometimes it is desirable to adapt home diets of patients to a six- or seven- meal program. Some protein, fat, and carbohydrate should be given at each meal. Thus, milk or a protein sandwich may be useful for interval feedings, but juices or sweets alone do not satisfy the requirements. The interval between meals should be $1\frac{1}{2}$ to 3 hours, with meals spread throughout the waking hours. Any of the modified diets might be presented in more than three meals. A judicious choice of bedtime snacks apparently does not modify sleep. (See Figure 27–1.)

Mechanical soft diet. Many persons require a soft diet simply because they have no teeth. It is neither desirable nor essential to restrict the patient to the selection allowed on the customary soft diet (page 394) employed for a postoperative patient or for a patient with a gastrointestinal disturbance. For example, stewed onions, baked beans, and apple pie are foods considered to be quite unsuitable for the latter patients but which may be enjoyed by those who simply require foods that are soft in texture. The terms *mechanical soft* and *dental soft* are used in some diet manuals to describe such a dietary modification. The following changes in the normal diet will usually suffice for individuals without teeth:

Meats should be finely minced or ground.
Soft breads are substituted for crusty breads.
Cooked vegetables are used without restriction, but dicing

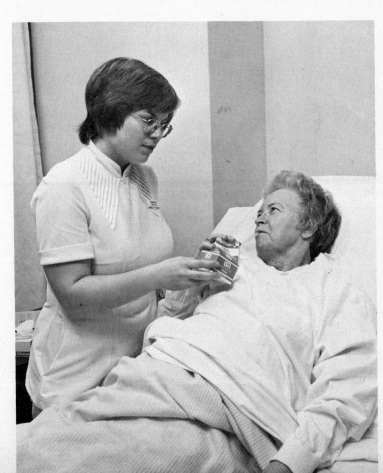

Figure 27–1. Milk is well accepted by most patients and provides important nutrients for liquid diets or between-meal feedings. (Courtesy, University of Minnesota Health Sciences Center, Minneapolis.)

or chopping may be desirable for some; for example, diced beets, chopped spinach, corn cut from cob.

Most raw vegetables are omitted; raw tomatoes, cut finely, may usually be used. Sometimes finely chopped lettuce in a sandwich may be accepted.

Many raw fruits may be used: banana, orange, grapefruit, soft berries, soft pear, apricots, peaches, grapes with tender skins.

Hard raw fruits such as pineapple and apple are usually avoided; but finely diced apple in fruit cup may be used.

Tough skins should be removed from fruits: raw, soft pear, or baked apple, etc.

Nuts and dried fruits, when used in desserts or other foods, are acceptable if finely chopped.

Soft diet. This diet represents the usual dietary step between the full fluid and normal diet. It may be used in acute infections, some gastrointestinal disturbances, and following surgery. The diet is soft in consistency, easy to chew, made up of simple, easily digestible food, and contains no harsh fiber, no rich or highly flavored food. It is nutritionally adequate when planned on the basis of the normal diet.

SOFT DIET

Include These Foods, or Their Nutritive Equivalents, Daily:

2–3 cups milk

    4 ounces (cooked weight) very tender or ground meat, fish, or poultry; soft cheese, legumes, or additional milk may substitute in part

    1 egg (3 to 4 per week)

3–4 servings vegetable including:

    1 medium potato

    1 serving dark-green or yellow vegetable—tender chopped or strained

    2 servings other vegetable—tender chopped or strained

3 servings fruit including:

    2 servings citrus fruit or juice

    1 serving banana, cooked fruit without skin or seeds, or strained cooked fruit

1 serving enriched or strained whole-grain cereal

3 slices enriched or fine whole-grain bread

Additional foods such as butter or fortified margarine, soups, desserts, sweets, or increased amounts of the above will provide adequate calories.

Nutritive value. See calculation for the normal diet in Table 27–1.

Foods Allowed

All beverages

Bread—white, fine whole wheat, rye without seeds; white crackers

Cereal foods—dry, such as cornflakes, Puffed Rice, rice flakes; fine cooked, such as cornmeal, farina, hominy grits, macaroni, noodles, rice, spaghetti; strained coarse, such as oatmeal, Pettijohn's, whole wheat

Cheese—mild, soft, such as cottage and cream; Cheddar; Swiss

Desserts—plain cake, cookies; custards; plain gelatin or with allowed fruit; Junket; plain ice cream, ices, sherbets; plain puddings, such as bread, cornstarch, rice, tapioca

Eggs—all except fried

Fats—butter, cream, margarine, vegetable oils and fats in cooking

Foods to Avoid

Bread—coarse dark; whole-grain crackers; hot breads; pancakes; waffles

Cereals—bran; coarse unless strained

Cheese—sharp, such as Roquefort, Camembert, Limburger

Desserts—any made with dried fruit or nuts; pastries; rich puddings or cake

Eggs—fried

Fats—fried foods

Fruits—raw: ripe avocado, banana, grapefruit or orange sections without membrane; canned or cooked: apples, apricots, fruit cocktail, peaches, pears, plums—all without skins; Royal Anne cherries; strained prunes and other fruits with skins; all juices

Meat—very tender, minced, or ground; baked, broiled, creamed, roast, or stewed: beef, lamb, veal, poultry, fish, bacon, liver, sweetbreads

Milk—in any form

Soups—broth, strained cream or vegetable

Sweets—all sugars, syrup, jelly, honey, plain sugar candy without fruit or nuts, molasses
Use in moderation.

Vegetables—white or sweet potato without skin, any way except fried; young and tender asparagus, beets, carrots, peas, pumpkin, squash without seeds; tender chopped greens; strained cooked vegetables if not tender; tomato juice

Miscellaneous—salt, seasonings and spices in moderation, gravy, cream sauces

Fruits—raw except as listed; stewed or canned berries; with tough skins

Meat—tough with gristle or fat; salted and smoked meat or fish, such as corned beef, smoked herring; cold cuts; frankfurter; pork

Soups—fatty or highly seasoned

Sweets—jam, marmalade, rich candies with chocolate

Vegetables—raw; strongly flavored, such as broccoli, Brussels sprouts, cabbage, cauliflower, cucumber, onion, radish, sauerkraut, turnip; corn; dried beans and peas; potato chips

Miscellaneous—pepper and other hot spices; fried foods; nuts; olives; pickles; relishes

Meal Pattern

BREAKFAST
Fruit or fruit juice
Cereal—strained, if coarse
Milk and sugar for cereal
Egg
Soft roll or toast
Butter or fortified margarine
Hot beverage with cream and sugar

LUNCHEON OR SUPPER
Strained soup, if desired
Mild cheese, tender or ground meat, fish, or poultry
Potato without skin, rice, noodles, macaroni, or spaghetti; or
Cooked vegetable
Enriched bread
Butter or fortified margarine
Fruit
Milk
Coffee or tea, if desired

DINNER
Orange, grapefruit, or tomato juice
Tender or ground meat, fish, or poultry
Potato, any way except fried
Cooked vegetable
Enriched bread
Butter or fortified margarine
Dessert
Milk
Hot beverage with cream and sugar, if desired

Sample Menu

Orange sections and banana slices
Oatmeal
Milk and sugar for cereal
Soft-cooked egg
Buttered toast

Coffee

Cream of tomato soup
Cheese soufflé

Tender peas
Soft roll
Butter
Royal Anne cherries
Milk
Coffee or tea, if desired

Grapefruit juice
Meat loaf (no onion or pepper) with gravy
Mashed potato
Buttered carrots
Rye bread without seeds
Butter
Baked apple without skin; cream
Milk
Tea with sugar and lemon

Liquid diets. Fluid diets are used in febrile states, postoperatively, or whenever the patient is unable to tolerate solid foods. The degree to which these diets are adequate will depend upon the type of liquids permitted.

Clear-fluid diets. Whenever an acute illness or surgery produces a marked intolerance for food as may be evident by nausea, vomiting, anorexia, distention, and diarrhea, it is advisable to restrict the intake of nutrients. A clear-fluid diet is usually used for one to two days, at the end of which time the patient is usually able to utilize a more liberal liquid diet.

Tea with lemon and sugar, coffee, fat-free broth, carbonated beverages, and cereal waters are the usual liquids permitted. In addition, strained fruit juices, fruit ices, and plain gelatin are often in-cluded. A more liberal clear-fluid diet permits the addition of egg white, whole egg, and gelatin to strained fruit juices and other beverages.

The amount of fluid in a given feeding on the clear-fluid diet is usually restricted to 30 to 60 ml per hour at first, with gradually increasing amounts being given as the patient's tolerance improves. Obviously, such a diet can accomplish little beyond the replacement of fluids.

Full-fluid diet. This diet is indicated whenever a patient is acutely ill or is unable to chew or swallow solid food. It includes all foods liquid at room temperature and at body temperature. It is free from cellulose and irritating condiments. When properly planned, this diet can be used for relatively long periods of time. However, iron is provided at inadequate levels.

FULL-FLUID DIET

General Rules

Give six or more feedings daily.

The protein content of the diet can be increased by incorporating nonfat dry milk in beverages and soups. Strained canned meats (used for infant feeding) may be added to broths.

The caloric value of the diet may be increased by: (1) substituting 10 per cent cream for part of the usual milk allowance; (2) adding butter to cereal gruels and soups; (3) including glucose in beverages; (4) using ice cream as dessert or in beverages.

If a decreased volume of fluid is desired, nonfat dry milk may be substituted for part of the fluid milk.

Include These Foods, or Their Nutritive Equivalents Daily:

  6 cups milk
  2 eggs (in custards or pasteurized eggnog)
1–2 ounces strained meat
  $\frac{1}{2}$ cup fine or strained whole-grain cooked cereal for gruel
  $\frac{1}{4}$ cup vegetable purée for cream soup
  1 cup citrus fruit juices; plus other strained juices
  $\frac{1}{2}$ cup tomato or vegetable juice
  1 tablespoon cocoa
  3 tablespoons sugar
  1 tablespoon butter
  2 servings plain gelatin dessert, Junket, soft or baked custard, ices, sherbets, plain ice cream, or plain cornstarch pudding
Broth, bouillon, or clear soups
Tea, coffee, carbonated beverages as desired
Flavoring extracts, salt

Nutritive values of foods listed in specified amounts: kcal, 1950; protein, 85 gm; calcium, 2.1 gm; iron, 7.7 mg; vitamin A, 7150 I.U.; thiamin, 1.1 mg; riboflavin, 3.2 mg; niacin equivalents, 19.1 mg; ascorbic acid, 160 mg.

Meal Pattern	Sample Menu
BREAKFAST	
Citrus juice	Orange juice
Cereal gruel with butter, sugar	Cream of wheat with milk, butter, and sugar
Milk	
Beverage with cream, sugar	Coffee with cream and sugar
MIDMORNING	
Fruit juice with egg	Lemonade with egg white
or	
Milk, plain, malted, chocolate, or eggnog (pasteurized)	
LUNCHEON OR SUPPER	
Strained soup	Beef broth with strained meat
Tomato juice	Tomato juice
Custard, Junket, ice cream, sherbet, ice, gelatin dessert or plain pudding	Maple Junket
Eggnog, milk, or cocoa	Milk
Tea with sugar, if desired	Tea with sugar and cream
MIDAFTERNOON	
Same as at midmorning	Pineapple eggnog (pasteurized)
DINNER	
Strained cream soup	Cream of carrot soup
Citrus juice	Grapefruit juice
Custard, Junket, ice cream, ice, sherbet, or gelatin dessert	Vanilla ice cream
Milk or cocoa	Cocoa
Tea, if desired	Tea with sugar and lemon
EVENING NOURISHMENT	
Same as at midmorning	Hot malted milk

Other methods of feeding. Food by mouth is the method of choice when the patient can eat, digest, and absorb sufficient food to meet his nutritive requirements. In illness, however, it is occasionally necessary to augment the oral intake by giving parenteral feedings of one type or another.

When the patient is unable to chew or swallow because of deformity or inflammation of the mouth or throat, corrosive poisoning, unconsciousness, paralysis of the throat muscles, etc., tube feeding is used (see page 482.)

Synthetic low-residue diets are used in situations in which it is desirable to have a minimum of residue in the intestine. These preparations are administered orally or by tube and may be used for extended periods.

Intravenous feeding is used when it is necessary to rest the patient's stomach completely. Fluids given by such means include solutions of glucose, amino acids, salts, and vitamins. Transfusions of whole blood or of plasma are commonly used. For selected patients who are seriously depleted nutritionally, total parenteral nutrition is used.

PROBLEMS AND REVIEW

1. What is meant by routine house diets?
2. Why is the normal diet used as a basis for planning therapeutic diets?
3. What are the advantages of using a diet manual for planning diets? What are the limitations?
4. What objections can you see to the following examples of dietary nomenclature: nephritic diet; Kempner diet; low-protein diet; ulcer discharge diet? Examine the nomenclature used for diets in your hospital, and suggest ways for improvement.

5. *Problem.* Write a menu for one day for a patient to receive a regular diet. Modify this pattern for a patient who is unable to chew foods well.

6. *Problem.* Prepare a table that shows the food intake for one day by a patient receiving a full-fluid diet. Calculate the protein, energy, and ascorbic acid intake.

7. *Problem.* Prepare a chart that shows the dietary orders for five patients. On this chart include a statement concerning the reasons for the diet order and the patient's acceptance of his diet.

CITED REFERENCES

1. Weinstein, L., *et al.*: "Diet as Related to Gastrointestinal Function," *J.A.M.A.*, **176**:935–41, 1961.
2. Koch, J. P., and Donaldson, R. M.: "A Survey of Food Intolerances in Hospitalized Patients," *N. Engl. J. Med.*, **271**:657–60, 1964.
3. Irwin, E. R.: "Alternate Menu Patterns—Survey and Nutritional Guidelines," *J. Am. Diet. Assoc.*, **65**:291–93, 1974.

ADDITIONAL REFERENCES

Barnes, R. H.: "Doctors' Dietary Antics," *Nutr. Today*, **3**:21–25, Sept. 1968.
Brandt, M. B.: "Perspective on Diet Manuals," *J. Am. Diet. Assoc.*, **47**:121–23, 1965.
Galbraith, A. L., and Hatch, L.: "Diet Manual in a Large Teaching Hospital: Philosophy and Purpose," *J. Am. Diet. Assoc.*, **62**:643–44, 1973.
Ohlson, M. A.: "Uses of the Dietary Manual to Promote Communication," *J. Am. Diet. Assoc.*, **62**:534–37, 1973.
Robinson, C. H.: "Updating Clinical Dietetics: Terminology," *J. Am. Diet. Assoc.*, **62**:645–48, 1973.

28 Dietary Calculation Using the Food Exchange Lists

Need for quick methods of dietary calculation. To provide for the nutritional needs of the patient the nurse and dietitian are frequently expected to make quick, yet reasonably accurate, estimations of nutritive values of diets. Some therapeutic diets must be planned within a stated maximum of one or more nutrients, for example, the fat-restricted diet. For other diets, such as that used for diabetic patients, carbohydrate, protein, and fat levels must be kept within relatively narrow allowances in the prescription. Sometimes a physician may request that the intake of protein or calories be charted from day to day for patients who are presenting nutritional problems.

The uses of Table A–1 have been described in Chapter 3, so that the student undoubtedly has had some experiences with dietary calculation on the basis of this table. It soon becomes evident that day-to-day calculations of all the listed nutrients—or even for selected nutrients—are much too time consuming for the nurse or dietitian with many responsibilities. Such detailed calculations are not justified unless great care is also taken in controlling the preparation procedures, and accurately measuring or weighing all food served to the patient and likewise all food which is returned on the tray. Moreover, the body itself varies from day to day in its net utilization of food, depending upon activity, endocrine balance, and the proportions of nutrients presented to it. Thus, it is evident that dietary calculation should be directed to reasonable assurances of control without time-wasting paper work. To this end, a short method of dietary calculation will be discussed here.

FOOD EXCHANGE LISTS

Evolution of the food exchange lists. Probably the classic example requiring rapid dietary calculations is afforded by the diet used for the diabetic patient. At one time these calculations were time consuming. Far too much faith was placed on decimal point calculations, with too little understanding of the variability of food composition and of body utilization. Many short tables of food composition were developed for the calculation of diets, but to the patient the variations existing in them were confusing to say the least. Incorporating the best features of several methods in use, food exchange lists were evolved and published in 1950 by a joint committee of the American Dietetic Association, the American Diabetes Association, and the United States Public Health Service.[1] The 1976 revision of these lists is shown in Table A–4.[2]

These lists are now used for most diets for diabetic patients. With some experience the nurse and dietitian find that calculations can be made rapidly. Patients soon learn how to use the lists for planning a wide variety of menus within their daily food allowances. The wide use of the exchange method of dietary planning means that patients can move from one community to another without experiencing the frustrations of using different and often contradictory lists. The food exchange lists not only are used for calculating diets for diabetic patients, but have many applications in the planning of other diets that require control of calories, protein, fat, and/or carbohydrate.

More recently other lists have been developed for specialized needs such as the sodium-restricted diet (pages 544–46) and the fat-controlled diet (pages 530–36). The overall groupings of foods in these lists are similar but differences in food selection within the lists soon become obvious. The general procedure for dietary calculation described below is also applicable to these diets.

Six exchange lists. An exchange list is a grouping of foods in which specified amounts of all the foods listed are of approximately equal carbohydrate, protein, and fat value. Specific foods within the lists may differ slightly in their nutritive value from the averages stated for the group. (See Table 28–1.) These differences in composition tend to cancel out because of the variety of foods selected from day to day. Thus, any food within a given list can be substituted or exchanged for any other food in that list. In the fruit list, for example, 1 small apple, or ½ banana, or 2 prunes, or ½ cup orange juice would contain 10 gm carbohydrate.

Milk list. One cup of skim milk is the basis for this list. If 2 per cent fortified skim milk is used in place of skim milk, an adjustment must be made. For each cup of 2 per cent milk one fat exchange should be omitted from the diet. If whole milk is used regularly, the milk allowance is calculated to provide 12 gm carbohydrate, 8 gm protein, and 9 gm fat per cup.

Note that cheeses are listed with meat exchanges; cream, cream cheese, and butter are listed as fat exchanges.

Vegetable lists. An exchange of most vegetables in this list is ½ cup and provides 5 gm carbohydrate and 2 gm protein. Vegetables high in carbohydrate are included in the bread list. A few salad greens and radishes may be used as desired.

Fruit list. Each fruit in the amount stated supplies 10 gm carbohydrate. Many of the fruits are in average-size servings, but some are not. For example, 2 prunes, 1 fig, and ¼ cup grape juice would be smaller-than-average servings. It is important, therefore, not to use the terms *exchange* and *serving* interchangeably.

Bread list. One slice of bread is the basis for the exchanges in this list. Included are biscuits, muffins, and rolls; dry and cooked breakfast cereals; grits, macaroni, noodles, spaghetti, and rice; crackers; and a number of vegetables—corn, Lima beans, baked beans, cooked dry beans, peas, white potato, and lentils, winter squash, sweet potato, and others.

Meat list. Meats are listed in three groups: low, medium, and high fat. Protein sources in the low-fat group are used for planning diets low in saturated fat and cholesterol (see Chapter 40). One ounce of cooked medium-fat meat, poultry, or fish is used as the basis for the next list. On a raw-weight basis this is equivalent to about 1⅓ ounces of edible portion; thus, one would need to purchase 4 ounces of raw meat, edible portion to equal a 3-ounce serving of cooked meat. It is assumed that the visible fat is trimmed off, but a wide selection of meat cuts including those marbled with fat is permissible.

Luncheon meats, canned fish, shellfish, Cheddar, American, Swiss, and cottage cheese, eggs, and peanut butter in the amounts listed are exchanges for meat.

Fat list. This list is based upon 1 teaspoon of margarine. It includes butter, solid fats and oils used in cooking, bacon, light and heavy cream, cream cheese, salad dressings, nuts, avocado, and olives.

Miscellaneous list. Coffee, tea, broth, spices, herbs, and some other items are insignificant for their nutritive values but they lend interest to the diet. They may be included in dietary plans without calculation.

Supplementary lists. Several groups have calculated the carbohydrate, protein, and fat content of

Table 28–1. Composition of Food Exchange Lists*

Food Exchange	Measure	Weight gm	Carbohydrate gm	Protein gm	Fat gm	Energy kcal
Milk, nonfat	1 cup	240	12	8	—	80
Milk, whole	1 cup	240	12	8	9	160
Vegetables	½ cup	100	5	2	—	25
Fruit	Varies		10	—	—	40
Bread	Varies		15	2	—	70
Meat, low fat	1 ounce	30	—	7	2.5	50
medium fat	1 ounce	30	—	7	5	75
high fat	1 ounce	30	—	7	7.5	95
Fat	1 teaspoon	5	—	—	5	45

*Consult Table A–4 for food selections for each of the exchange lists.

various commercial products and have determined the amount of the food that can be substituted for items in the traditional exchange lists. References are listed at the end of this chapter. In using these supplementary lists, it is well to remember that it is not possible to have an up-to-date, accurate list of products because of the rapidity with which new products are introduced and because formulations may change from time to time.

Assuring mineral and vitamin adequacy. Since the exchange lists do not provide information on mineral and vitamin values it becomes evident that some degree of discretion must be used in establishing the daily food allowances and in selecting specific menus. For example, 2 cups of milk daily will supply sufficient calcium and riboflavin for the adult; 3 to 4 cups of milk would be included in the diet plan of children and pregnant or lactating women. At least two fruit exchanges are included daily, one of these being selected from those fruits rich in ascorbic acid. Fruits that are good sources of this vitamin are marked with an asterisk in the listing. Vegetables are often neglected in dietary planning or are restricted to a few choices. Those that are dark green or deep yellow are excellent sources of vitamin A, and one of these should be included daily. Note that vitamin-A-rich vegetables have been indicated in the vegetable lists.

Procedure for calculation. The calculation of a diet requires only the nutritive values of Table 28–1. Let us suppose that the following diet prescription is to be calculated: carbohydrate, 225 gm; protein, 75 gm; and fat, 65 gm. A daily food allowance for this prescription is shown in Table 28–2, using the procedures described below.

1. Estimate the amounts of milk, vegetables, and fruits to be included. The allowances are dictated somewhat by the preferences of the patient, but the following amounts are minimum levels that should ordinarily be included:

Milk—2 cups for adults; 3 to 4 cups for children and for pregnant or lactating women
Vegetables—2 exchanges
Fruit—2 exchanges

2. Fill in the carbohydrate, protein, and fat values for the tentative amounts of milk, vegetables, and fruits.

3. To determine the number of bread exchanges: Total the carbohydrate value of the milk, vegetables, and fruit. Subtract this total from the total amount of carbohydrate prescribed. Divide the remainder by 15 (the carbohydrate value of one bread exchange). Use the nearest whole number of bread exchanges. Fill in the carbohydrate and protein values.

4. Total the carbohydrate column. If the total deviates more than 3 or 4 gm from the prescribed amount, adjust the amounts of vegetable, fruit, and bread. No diet should be planned with fractions of an exchange since awkward measures of food would sometimes be encountered.

5. To determine the number of meat exchanges: Total the protein value of the milk, vegetable, and bread. Subtract this total from the amount of protein prescribed. Divide the remainder by 7 (the protein value of one meat exchange). Use the nearest whole number of meat exchanges. Fill in the protein and fat values.

6. To determine the number of fat exchanges: Total the fat values for milk and meat. Subtract this total from the amount of fat prescribed. Divide the remainder by 5 (the fat content of one fat exchange). Fill in the fat value.

7. Check the entire diet for the accuracy of the computations. Divide the daily food allowance into a meal pattern suitable for the individual. For some diets the distribution of food may be specified in the prescription.

The following menu illustrates one way that the day's food allowance for the diet shown in Table 28–2 could be used. Another menu is shown on page 499 in the adaptation for a patient with diabetes.

BREAKFAST
Stewed prunes—2
Dry cereal—¾ cup
Skim milk—1 cup
Toast, whole wheat—2 slices
Butter or margarine—2 teaspoons
  LUNCHEON
Tomato juice—½ cup
Saltines—6
Sandwich
  Rye bread—2 slices
  Sliced ham—1 thin slice (1 ounce)
  Swiss cheese—1 slice

Table 28–2. Calculation of Diet Using Food Exchange Lists (*Carbohydrate, 225 gm; Protein, 75 gm; Fat, 65 gm*)

List	Food	Measure	Weight gm	Carbohydrate gm	Protein gm	Fat gm
1	Milk, skim	2 cups	480	24	16	—
2	Vegetables	3 exchanges	300	15	6	—
3	Fruit	5 exchanges	Varies	50	—	—
				89		
4	Bread	9 exchanges	Varies	135	18	—
					40	
5	Meat, low fat	2 exchanges	Varies	—	14	5
	medium fat	3 exchanges	Varies	—	21	15
						20
6	Fat	9 exchanges	Varies	—	—	45
				224	75	65

225 gm carbohydrate prescribed total

 89 gm carbohydrate from milk, vegetables, and fruit

136 gm carbohydrate to be supplied from bread exchanges

$$136 \div 15 = 9 \text{ bread exchanges}$$

75 gm protein prescribed total

40 gm protein from milk, vegetable, and bread exchanges

35 gm protein to be supplied from meat exchanges

$$35 \div 7 = 5 \text{ meat exchanges}$$

65 gm fat prescribed total

20 gm fat from meat exchanges

45 gm fat to be supplied from fat exchanges

$$45 \div 5 = 9 \text{ fat exchanges}$$

Lettuce
Mayonnaise—2 teaspoons
Celery and radishes
Olives—5 small
Honeydew melon—¼ medium
DINNER
Skewered lamb and vegetables
   Lamb—3 ounces (4 ounces raw)
   Onions—4 small
   Tomato wedges
   Mushroom caps
   Green-pepper strips
Oil—2 teaspoons for basting meat and vegetables while
   cooking
Rice—½ cup
Dinner roll—1
Butter or margarine—2 teaspoons
Fruit cup (2 exchanges fruit)
   Banana, small—½
   Blueberries—⅓ cup
   Grapes—6
EVENING SNACK
Skim milk—1 cup
Graham crackers—2

PROBLEMS AND REVIEW

1. How do you explain the fact that Cheddar and cottage cheese are listed as meat exchanges, but that they are included in the milk group of the Four Food Groups (page 35)?
2. Which vegetables are especially rich in vitamin A? In iron? In ascorbic acid?
3. Explain the placement of potatoes, corn, Lima beans, and baked beans in the bread exchange list.

4. *Problem.* Plan a menu for a lunch that permits the following exchanges: one milk; two vegetables; one fruit; three bread; two meat; three fat.
5. *Problem.* Write three breakfast menus based upon the following exchange requirements: one milk; one fruit; two bread; two meat; and three fat.
6. *Problem.* Keep a record of your food intake for one day and calculate the carbohydrate, protein, fat, and caloric value with the exchange lists.

CITED REFERENCES

1. Caso, E.: "Calculation of Diabetic Diets," *J. Am. Diet. Assoc.,* **26:**575–83, 1950.
2. American Dietetic Association and American Diabetes Association: *Exchange Lists for Meal Planning.* Chicago/New York, 1976.

ADDITIONAL REFERENCES

"Bingo Game Teaches Meal Planning to Diabetics," *Hospitals,* **49:**15, Mar. 1, 1975.
Cinnamon, P. A., and Swanson, M. A.: *Everything You Always Wanted to Know About Exchange Values for Foods.* Univ. Cities Diabetes Education Program, Moscow, Idaho, 1973.
Convenience Foods for Calculated Diets, 3rd ed. Department of Nutrition. Lutheran General Hospital, Park Ridge, Ill., 1970.
Dwyer, L. S., *et al.:* "Simplified Meal Planning for Hard-to-Teach Patients," *Am. J. Nurs.,* **74:**664–65, 1974.
Simpson, J., and Schoberg, M.: *Food Values of Special Products for the Diabetic Diet.* Department of Dietetics, Indiana University Medical Center, 1969.

29 Overweight and Underweight

Low-Calorie and High-Calorie Diets

IMPORTANCE OF WEIGHT CONTROL

Hazards of obesity. The prevention and treatment of obesity are among the most perplexing problems facing the physician, the nutritionist, and, most especially, the patient himself. The incidence and mortality from degenerative diseases are significantly greater for those who are obese than those who are lean. The popular saying "The longer the belt, the shorter the life" is far too true.

Excessive weight is closely associated with cardiovascular and renal diseases, diabetes, degenerative arthritis, gout, and gallbladder disease. The obese frequently have elevated blood triglycerides and cholesterol, and a reduced carbohydrate tolerance. Obesity entails a respiratory cost in normal persons by increased work of breathing, a decrease in lung volume, and pulmonary hypertension. In any person with chronic pulmonary disorders such as emphysema and asthma obesity greatly increases the respiratory stress.[1] The hazards of surgery and of pregnancy and childbirth are multiplied in the presence of excessive adipose tissue.

Overweight is a physical handicap as well as a primary health hazard. Obese people are more uncomfortable during warm weather because the thick layers of fat serve as an insulator. More effort must be expended to do a given amount of work because of the increase in body mass. Because of their lessened agility, obese people are more susceptible to accidents. Fatigue, backache, and foot troubles are common complaints of the obese.

Emotional and psychologic problems may be the cause or result of obesity. The obese individual may be the butt of jokes, considered greedy or as having no will power, or may experience social humiliation and inability to get a job. He may lose his self-esteem and may withdraw from others in order to avoid embarrassment. Such attitudes may reinforce the conditions that led to the obesity.

Obesity and faddism. The preoccupation with slimness on the part of many young women is in itself—surprising as it may seem—a major problem. Too many people resort to fad diets, pills, and gadgets which result in nutritive inadequacy, economic loss, and sometimes serious effects on health. Medical supervision is bypassed and weight reduction is undertaken even though it might be contraindicated. Many people resort to one merry-go-round after another of reducing diets, losing a little only to regain it, thus submitting themselves to repeated body stresses that accompany weight loss.

Reducing pills range from those that are nothing more than vitamin pills to those that are laxatives and diuretics, thus upsetting the water balance but being ineffective in loss of adipose tissue. So-called "reducing candies" are combinations of sugars, nonfat dry milk, some mineral salts, and vitamins.

Fad diets are numerous. The fact that a different one appears practically every month in some popular magazine as the answer to weight-losing problems is in itself an indication that the solution to obesity is poorly understood. Many of these diets include some bizarre food combinations, whereas others emphasize a single food or combination of foods. Some of the diets are nutritionally adequate but many are not. None possesses any magic qualities for weight loss, and seldom do they accomplish the essential lifetime change required to maintain a lower level of weight. Among the popular fad diets in recent years have been: "Drinking Man's Diet," "Ice Cream Diet," "Steak and Grapefruit Diet," "Low-Carbohydrate Diet," and many others.

Problems of underweight. Much less attention has been directed to the problems of underweight although many people in all age categories are not enjoying optimum health because of the undernutrition associated with extreme underweight. Both the National Nutrition Survey[2] and HANES[3] indicated that a significant number of children from low-income families had not achieved normal growth. Fatigue and lowered resistance to infections are corollaries of underweight. Tuberculosis, especially, is found more frequently among young people whose weight is considerably below normal. Underweight at the beginning of pregnancy and the failure to gain at a sufficient rate during pregnancy increases the likelihood of prematurity.[4]

EVALUATION OF WEIGHT STATUS AND BODY COMPOSITION

Desirable weight. The best weight for a given individual's height, age, bone structure, and muscular development is not exactly known. On the basis of life insurance statistics the most nearly ideal weight to maintain throughout life is that which is proper at age 25 for one's height and body build. Generally, the best weight is likely to be that at which one both looks and feels his best. Although a large number of people continue to gain weight until late middle life, this is not physiologically desirable nor need it be inevitable.

Height-weight tables (see Table A–10) currently classify people as having a large, average, or small frame. Unfortunately, there is no simple guide by which an individual's body frame can be classified. The person who is stocky may be 5 to 10 per cent

above the weight for average build without being considered overweight, whereas the individual who has a small frame should weigh 5 to 10 per cent less than the desirable weight for average build.

Recognizing the limitations of height-weight tables, a deviation of not more than 10 per cent above or below the desirable weight for a given individual is not considered to be significant. The term *overweight* is applied to persons who are 10 to 20 per cent above desirable weight. *Obesity* is applied to persons 20 per cent or more over desirable weight. *Underweight* denotes those individuals who are more than 10 per cent below the established standards; those more than 20 per cent below these standards are considered to be seriously underweight.

Body composition. Gross obesity is easily identified by visual observation alone, but errors in making a diagnosis of moderate obesity are frequent by reference to height-weight tables. The concern in obesity, from a clinical point of view, is the excessive amount of adipose tissue and not overweight per se. A football player may be overweight by the usual height-weight standards but he has a well-developed musculature and does not have excessive fat deposits, and therefore is not classified as obese.

Many clinicians now measure body fatness by determining the thickness of subcutaneous tissues at designated body locations by means of calipers (see Figure 29–1). A number of anthropometric meas-

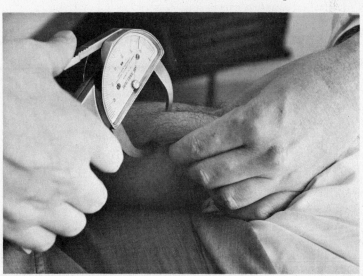

Figure 29–1. A skinfold measurement is made by means of a caliper. This determines the amount of subcutaneous fat of an individual and is an indicator of total body fat. (Courtesy, *Roche Medical Image,* Hoffmann La Roche, Inc.)

urements may also be used. These include the circumference of the chest, abdomen, buttocks, thigh, calf, ankle, biceps, forearm, and other body locations as measured with a flexible steel tape. Bony widths can be measured with a caliper, and the diameters of joints and the thickness of fat pads determined by x-ray.

Research centers employ precise measurements for the degree of adiposity but these tests are too complex for routine use in clinical practice. They include determination of the body density by underwater weighing, by measurement of total body water, by determination of lean body mass using a scintillation counter to assay body potassium, and by determination of the total body fat based upon the amounts of fat-soluble gases retained.

Hirsch has described two types of obesity: *hyperplastic*, characterized by an excess number of fat cells, and *hypertrophic*, in which adipose cells are greatly enlarged.[5] The degree of obesity correlates more closely with the hyperplastic type. This type is seen in childhood, and the hypertrophic type is more common in adult-onset obesity. The age at which cell number is determined is not yet known. Once formed, however, the number of adipose cells is not altered by weight loss. The size of these cells can be decreased with weight reduction. Hirsch's hypothesis is that hyperplasia of adipose cells at an early age sets the stage for later obesity which is refractory to treatment.

Estimation of weight gain or loss. Adipose tissue consists of about 72 per cent fat, 23 per cent water, and small amounts of protein and mineral salts.[6] Each kilogram of adipose tissue represents 7700 kcal (1 pound = 3500 kcal). An individual who consumes 100 kcal in excess daily ingests an excess of 3000 kcal by the end of one month. This would result in a weight gain of 0.4 kg monthly, or 4.8 kg (about 10 pounds) in a year. The weight gain from consistently overeating by this amount over a 5- to 10-year period would be considerable. It requires about 2 teaspoons of butter, or two 1-inch squares of fudge, or an oatmeal cookie to supply the additional 100 kcal each day.

Conversely, the loss of 1 kilogram of adipose tissue means that the diet would be deficient by 7700 kcal for the total time period of the weight loss. A young woman requiring 2000 kcal a day to meet her energy needs who consumes a diet that supplies only 1200 kcal has a weekly deficit of 5600 kcal, and the adipose tissue loss would be 5600 ÷ 7700, or 0.7 kg (1.6 pounds).

Weight gain and weight loss do not always follow the predicted straight line because of variations in water balance. Also, weight gain and weight loss are not explained solely on the basis of changes in adipose tissue; some changes in protein-rich tissues are likewise taking place.

OBESITY

Incidence. The exact incidence of obesity is not known, but it does not take much people-watching to become aware of the high numbers of most age groups who exceed their desirable weight. On the basis of percentage of body composition as fat, Buskirk has suggested that about 40 per cent of adults are obese.[7] The HANES data, based on triceps skinfold thickness, indicates that a substantial number of adults in the United States are obese; the incidence is higher in females than in males.[8] (See Table 29-1.) Estimates of the prevalence in children vary from 3 to 20 per cent.[9] The incidence is higher in girls than in boys. Contrary to popular opinion, most children do not outgrow their overweight; they remain obese throughout life and are particularly resistant to treatment later in life.

Causes. Obesity is invariably caused by an intake of calories beyond the body's need for energy. Such a statement, however, tends to oversimplify the problem of obesity, for one might infer that it could

Table 29-1. Prevalence of Obesity in Adults in the United States, 1971-1972.*

Years		White	Black
		Per Cent	
Males,	20-44	16.0	10.6
	45-74	13.4	7.7
Females,	20-44	18.9	29.2
	45-74	24.7	32.4

*Source of data: Abraham, S., *et al.*: *Preliminary Findings of the First Health and Nutrition Examination Survey, United States, 1971-1972: Anthropometric and Clinical Findings.* U.S. Department of Health, Education, and Welfare Publication 75-1299, 1975.

be easily corrected by bringing the energy intake and expenditure into balance. The reasons for an existing imbalance are many and complex, and some understanding of the problems of the individual must be gained before therapy can be effectively instituted. A thorough physical examination, a dietary history, and an investigation of habits relating to activity, rest, and family and social relationships are indicated.

Food habits. Eating too much becomes a habit for many people. Sometimes this is the result of ignorance of the calorie value of food. The amounts of food are not necessarily excessive, but it is the extra foods, beyond the calorie need, that account for the gradual increase in weight, for example, the extra pats of butter, the spoonful of jelly, the second roll, the preference for a rich dessert, or the TV snack. Eating too much may result from having to maintain social relationships including rich party foods in addition to usual mealtime eating. Excessive amounts of carbohydrate-rich foods are sometimes eaten because they are cheaper than lower-calorie fruits and vegetables. (See Figure 29–2.)

Activity patterns. Many persons continue to gain weight throughout life because they fail to adjust their appetites to reduced energy needs. The many laborsaving devices in homes and in industry reduce the energy requirement. Most people enjoy sports as spectators rather than as participants. Riding rather than walking to school or work is common practice

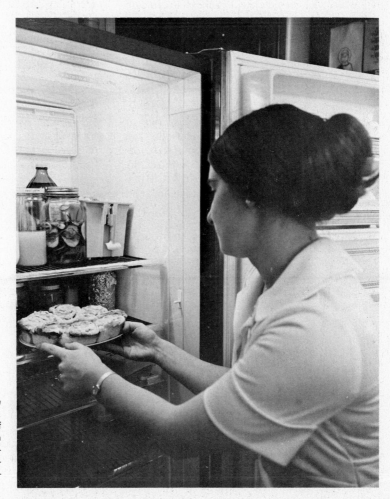

Figure 29–2. Almost everyone enjoys a snack from time to time. Do they provide a good balance of nutrients? Are they in line with caloric need? (Courtesy, Department of Human Ecology, Marywood College, Scranton, Pennsylvania.)

even for short distances. Other circumstances may further reduce the energy needs: (1) basal metabolism is gradually decreased from year to year (see Chapter 7); (2) changes in occupation may result in reduced activity; (3) the middle years of life sometimes bring about a repose and consequent reduction of muscle tension; (4) periods of quiet relaxation and sleep may be increased; and (5) disabling illness such as arthritis or cardiac disease may reduce markedly the need for calories.

Psychologic factors. Eating is a solace and a pleasure to the individual who is bored, feels lonely or unloved, has become discontented with his family, social, or financial standing, has experienced deep sorrow, or needs an excuse to avoid the realities of life. Such an individual often eats because he has nothing else to do or has no motivation to seek another outlet for his problems.

Genetic influences. Several investigators have shown that there is a high correlation between obesity in parents and their children. Mayer noted that if both parents are of normal weight, only 7 per cent of children will be obese; if one parent is obese, the incidence in children is 40 per cent, and it climbs to 80 per cent if both parents are obese.[10] His observations led him to conclude that food habits alone do not explain these differences; further, he found a correlation between obesity and body build.

The *endomorphic* or round, soft individual gains weight readily, whereas the *ectomorphic* or slender, wiry person rarely becomes overweight.[11] This does not mean that obesity is inevitable for the endomorph, but it does mean that constant vigilance is required to avoid it. (See Figure 29–3.)

Metabolic abnormalities. Many people would like to place the blame for their obesity on endocrine disorders, but only a small percentage of all obese individuals do have such disturbances. A deficiency of the thyroid gland can reduce the basal metabolism, but overweight from this cause can be prevented if the diet is sufficiently restricted in calories.

In experimental animals damage to the area of the hypothalamus that regulates feeding leads to excessive eating and obesity. Whether there is interference with the regulation of appetite by the hypothalamus in humans has not been proven. In fact, many obese persons actually have a lower intake of calories than those of normal weight, but they have become obese because of greatly decreased activity.[11]

Another explanation offered for obesity is overloading of the metabolic pathways for carbohydrate and fat so that lipogenesis is favored. When rats are restricted to forced feeding twice a day instead of being allowed to nibble, they become obese.[12] According to this hypothesis, the individual who skips breakfast, eats little lunch, and then consumes a

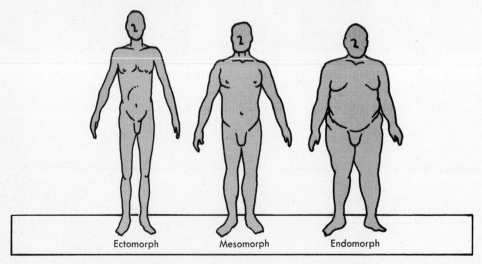

Figure 29–3. Types of body build.

large dinner might be overloading the metabolic pathways at one time. Some obese patients have shown alterations in blood lipids that suggest the possibility of increased formation of fatty tissue.[13]

Some impairment of carbohydrate tolerance is common in obese persons. The hypertrophic adipocytes are resistant to the action of insulin; however, they become more sensitive to insulin when the size of the fat cells lessens as the individual loses weight.

PREVENTION OF OBESITY

Identifying those who are likely to become obese. The most vigorous efforts to prevent obesity should be directed to those individuals who are most susceptible, namely children of obese parents and children who have stocky frames. Certain periods of life are also likely to bring about obesity. Men of normal weight often begin to gain weight in the late 20s and early 30s, and women are more likely to gain in the 40s and 50s. Following pregnancy weight gain is common. If these trends are recognized, the individual can elect to reduce his caloric intake, or increase his exercise, or both.

Education for prevention. The best hope for the prevention of obesity is through greatly expanded programs of nutrition education directed particularly to schoolchildren, teen-agers, and mothers. The pattern for obesity is often set in infancy when the mother overfeeds the baby in the erroneous belief that a "fat baby is a healthy baby." Sometimes overeating becomes a habit with a child following an illness because the mother keeps urging food upon the child through her concern for his state of nutrition. During adolescent years food is often used to submerge the many problems that face the boy and girl. By recognizing these trends, the mother can do much to redirect the food habits. The education of the mother in terms of weight control for her family and the education of the child in the elementary and secondary school can be effective.

Increased activity. In these times of affluence, mechanization, and automation many individuals become overweight because of lack of exercise. A pattern of activity is best taught during childhood and must also be emphasized during the school years. Too often competitive sports exclude the child who most needs the exercise. Physical educa-

tion should be directed to those activities that are likely to carry over into adult life.

Public health approach. The Bureau of Nutrition of New York City since 1952 has used public health methodology in the control and treatment of obesity.[14] This approach deserves trial on a larger scale.

TREATMENT OF OBESITY

Two criteria must be satisfied if the treatment is to be considered successful: (1) weight loss must be such that desirable weight according to body frame and state of health is achieved; and (2) the desired weight must be maintained. The essential components of treatment are diet, activity, adequate dietary counseling, and psychologic support.

Assessment of the patient. The treatment of obesity is a frustrating problem to the physician, nutritionist, and nurse because failures are so frequent. To a patient a failure can be demoralizing. Therefore, it is important that each patient be evaluated in terms of his medical and dietary history and his emotional stability. Weight reduction should be guided by a physician since the physiologic and psychologic stresses of weight loss are not equally tolerated by all.

Some persons lose weight satisfactorily when shown how to keep the calorie intake within prescribed limits; others benefit from group methods or behavior modification; still others have such deep emotional problems that psychiatric help is needed before weight loss is attempted.

In general, results of dietary treatment of obesity have been disappointing in the majority of patients. In a review of the literature, Stunkard noted that only 25 per cent of patients were able to lose as much as 20 pounds and only 5 per cent lost as much as 40 pounds.[15] For some persons, self-help groups for weight control provide the incentive needed to adhere to a diet.

Behavior modification is based on the premise that excessive food intake is a learned response that can be changed. By means of this technique the individual learns to focus attention on the environmental factors that influence his food intake and gradually to modify these so that a change in eating habits and subsequent weight loss occurs.[16]

Survey findings of patients seen in an obesity

clinic have shown that: (1) weight loss is more difficult to achieve as the duration of obesity and the degree of obesity increase; (2) married persons were more successful than single persons in effecting weight loss; (3) many women had onset of obesity associated with the first pregnancy; and (4) women over 40 years reduced more successfully than those who were younger. Men and women were equally able to reduce, level of education had no effect on success of reaching normal weight, and group methods supervised by the physician and nutritionist were more successful than individual instruction.[14]

Calorie-restricted diets. Many widely accepted nutritionally sound diets are available and are designed to bring about steady weight loss, to establish good food habits, and to promote a sense of wellbeing. Such diets must be palatable, must fit into the framework of family food habits, and must not require additional expense or long preparation time. Basic considerations in planning weight reduction diets include the following:

Energy. A diet that provides 800 to 1000 kcal below the daily energy requirement leads to a loss of 3 to 4 kg (6 to 8 pounds) monthly. This gradual loss does not result in severe hunger, nervous exhaustion, and weakness that often accompany drastic reduction regimens. For most men 1400 to 1600 kcal is a satisfactory level, and for women 1200 to 1400 kcal are indicated. Diets that supply 1000 kcal or less are rarely necessary except for individuals who are bedfast.

Protein. Although 0.8 gm protein per kilogram desirable body weight is sufficient, an allowance of $1\frac{1}{2}$ gm per kilogram improves the satiety value of the diet. Most dietary plans can include 70 to 100 gm protein daily.

Fat and carbohydrate. Many diets drastically restrict the fat intake and allow a moderate carbohydrate intake. (See the 1000-kcal diet in Table 29–2.) Some patients prefer a more liberal fat intake and a reduced carbohydrate level. In the high-protein moderate-fat 1500-kcal diet, Table 29–2, about half the calories are provided by fat.

Minerals and vitamins. A multivitamin preparation, iron salts, and possibly calcium are indicated for diets containing 1000 kcal or less. Calorie-restricted diets for obese children and for pregnant women must be planned with the increased mineral and vitamin requirements in mind. For these reasons the diets used for them are usually less restricted.

Daily meal patterns. The diets in Table 29–2 have been calculated with the food exchange lists (Table A–4). The mineral and vitamin values equal or exceed the recommended allowances. (See page 391.)

These diets include 3 cups of milk, thus enhanc-

Table 29–2. Food Allowances for Calorie-Restricted Diets

Food for the Day	Normal Protein, Moderate Carbohydrate, Low to Moderate Fat			High Protein, Low Carbohydrate, Moderate Fat
	1000 kcal	1200 kcal	1500 kcal	1500 kcal
Milk, whole, cups	3 (skim)	3	3	3
Vegetable, raw	1 cup	1 cup	1 cup	1 cup
cooked	$\frac{1}{2}$ cup	$\frac{1}{2}$ cup	$\frac{1}{2}$ cup	$\frac{1}{2}$ cup
Fruit, unsweetened, exchanges	4	3	4	2
Bread, exchanges	2	2	4	2
Meat, medium fat, exchanges	5	5	5	9
Fat, exchanges	1	1	3	2
Nutritive Value				
Protein, gm	67	67	71	95
Fat, gm	30	57	67	82
Carbohydrate, gm	116	106	146	96
Kcal	1000	1205	1470	1500

ing the calcium intake, and also providing a convenient bedtime snack, if desired. Some adults will prefer 2 cups of milk and more meat. This can be arranged by substituting one meat exchange for 1 cup of skim milk. The caloric exchange for 1 cup of whole milk would be two meat exchanges, thus giving a slightly higher protein intake.

A great deal of flexibility in food choices is possible with the exchange lists. One important consideration is the satiety value of the diet. Inasmuch as proteins and fats remain in the stomach longer, the protein and fat allowance should be divided approximately equally between the three meals.

Some plans permit six meals a day instead of three; in these, some protein should be provided at each feeding. Part of the success of a reducing diet depends upon learning to be content with smaller portions of food and less concentrated foods.

Foods to restrict or avoid. The patient who learns to select his foods in appropriate amounts from the exchange lists does not require specific lists of foods to avoid. For some persons, however, it may help to create calorie consciousness if listings of concentrated foods are provided. Some of the foods listed below are permitted in specified amounts in the exchange lists, but others are best avoided altogether.

High-fat foods: butter, margarine, cheese, chocolate, cream, ice cream, fat meat, fatty fish, or fish canned in oil, fried foods of any kind such as doughnuts and potato chips, gravies, nuts, oil, pastries, and salad dressing

High-carbohydrate foods: breads of any kind, candy, cake, cookies, corn, cereal products such as macaroni, noodles, spaghetti, pancakes, waffles, sweetened or dried fruits, legumes such as Lima beans, navy beans, dried peas, potatoes, sweet potatoes, honey, molasses, sugar, syrup, rich puddings, sweets

Beverages: all fountain drinks, including malted milks and chocolate, carbonated beverages of all kinds, rich sundaes, alcoholic drinks, sweetened drink mixes

Other dietary regimens. Commercial low-calorie meal substitutes, as *formulas* in liquid or powder form, cookies, and combination dishes are popular. Generally, they are nutritionally adequate and possess the advantages of convenience and strict calorie control. Some persons find them useful initially while they are learning the essentials of dietary

Sample Meal Patterns

Normal Protein, Moderate Carbohydrate, Moderate Fat
  1500 kcal
  BREAKFAST
Unsweetened citrus fruit—1 exchange
Egg—1
Bread—1 slice
Butter—1 teaspoon
Milk, whole—1 cup
Coffee or tea
  LUNCH
Meat, poultry, or fish—2 ounces
Vegetable, raw or cooked—1 serving
Milk, whole—1 cup
Bread—1 slice
Butter—1 teaspoon
Unsweetened fruit—1 exchange
  DINNER
Meat, poultry, or fish—2 ounces
Potato—1 small
Vegetable, cooked—½ cup
          raw—1 serving
Milk, whole—1 cup
Bread—1 slice
Butter—1 teaspoon
Unsweetened fruit—2 exchanges
Coffee or tea, if desired

High Protein, Low Carbohydrate, Moderate Fat
  1500 kcal

Unsweetened citrus fruit—1 exchange
Eggs—2
Bread—1 slice
Butter—1 teaspoon
Milk, whole—1 cup
Coffee or tea

Meat, poultry, or fish—4 ounces
Vegetable, raw or cooked—1 serving
Milk, whole—1 cup

Meat, poultry, or fish—3 ounces
Potato—1 small
Vegetable, cooked—½ cup
          raw—1 serving
Milk, whole—1 cup

Butter—1 teaspoon
Unsweetened fruit—1 exchange

planning. Others substitute these preparations for one meal a day.

The principal disadvantages of the formula diets are these: (1) they do not retrain the individual to a new pattern of food habits that must be followed once the weight is lost; (2) they are monotonous if used for a long period of time; and (3) they may be constipating for some patients, whereas others occasionally experience diarrhea.

Ketogenic diets. Low-carbohydrate ketogenic diets have been widely publicized in recent years as a revolutionary aid to rapid weight reduction. Advocates of these diets claim that one need not be concerned about calorie intake as long as carbohydrate is sharply restricted or even eliminated from the diet; and that the diet will produce more rapid weight loss than more conventional calorie-restricted diets. The American Medical Association has pointed out some of the facts and fallacies concerning ketogenic weight reduction diets.[17] There is no scientific evidence that this type of diet is any more effective than better balanced diets in promoting weight reduction. Weight loss is attributed to a decrease in calorie intake as a result of the high satiety value of the diet, and to increased urinary excretion of water and sodium. Potential adverse effects include elevations in serum lipids and increased blood uric acid levels.

Starvation. Partial or total starvation for weeks or months has been used in treatment of persons who fail to achieve weight loss by conventional methods. The overall results are disappointing in that most patients regain the weight lost.[18]

Exercise and weight loss. Moderate exercise on a consistent daily basis is an important aid in weight loss. It results in increased pulmonary and cardiovascular efficiency, better muscular tone, and a sense of well-being. It does not lead to increased appetite; conversely, a diminution of activity does not lead to a corresponding decrease in appetite. The exercise program should be determined by the physician on the basis of the patient's age, state of health and physical condition, and activity preferences.

Gwinup studied the effect of exercise alone, in the form of walking, on weight control. Walking for longer than 30 minutes daily for a year or more was associated with an average weight loss of 22 pounds in 11 obese women who were not on calorie-restricted diets.[19] The importance of exercise can be illustrated by calculating the energy equivalents of foods in terms of various kinds of activity. Six foods shown in Figure 29–4 illustrate the wide ranges of time required to utilize the energy provided by various foods at sedentary to moderate activities.

Role of hormones and drugs. Most overweight persons have no deficiency of endocrine secretions and should not be led to believe that they have glandular disturbances, nor should they be exposed to the increased nervousness and irritability that

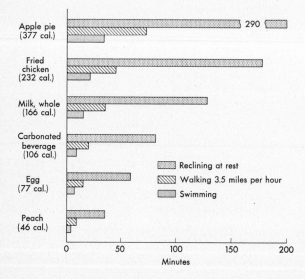

Figure 29–4. The energy value for foods expressed as number of minutes of activity for three levels of energy expenditure. (Data from Konishi, F.: *J. Am. Diet. Assoc.,* **46**:187, 1965.)

result from such medication. Thyroid deficiency should be treated only by a physician.

Anorexigenic drugs such as amphetamine sulfate are sometimes prescribed by a physician because of their ability to dull the appetite. They may produce insomnia, excitability, dryness of the mouth, gastrointestinal disturbances, and other toxic manifestations. For some patients they are a crutch and for others they have no effect on decreasing the appetite. The Food and Drug Administration has cautioned that these drugs are of limited value in the treatment of obesity and should be used with great care because of the possibility of dependence and abuse. The label must state that they are for short-term use, and only when a calorie-restricted diet is also used.[20]

Surgical treatment. Surgical treatment of obesity has been used for selected patients who are more than 100 pounds over their ideal weight and who meet certain other criteria. Both jejunoileal shunts and gastric bypass are used. By these procedures about 90 per cent of the small bowel is bypassed, thereby reducing both the absorptive surface and transit time for foods. For most patients steady weight loss occurs for one to two years following the surgery, after which weight stabilizes at substantially lower, but still obese, weights. The functioning small bowel tends to hypertrophy with time, thereby lessening the malabsorption and weight loss. Besides malabsorption, serious electrolyte disturbances and liver disease are frequent postoperative sequelae.[21]

Dietary considerations. Diarrhea is a major problem once oral food intake is resumed following the surgery. Excesses of dietary fat or of fibrous foods aggravate the diarrhea. A high-protein, low-fat, low-carbohydrate diet is given in six small feedings.[22] Fluids are permitted between meals rather than with the meal, and may be restricted to less than 1 liter daily initially. Calcium, magnesium, and potassium losses may be substantial and good food sources of these minerals should be emphasized. Multivitamins are generally recommended.

DIETARY COUNSELING

Success in weight reduction is dependent upon effective motivation and suitable knowledge.

Motivation and psychologic support. A diet prescription is worthless unless the patient has some motivation for losing weight, such as the maintenance or recovery of health, the ability to win friendship, admiration, and affection, or the importance of normal weight in being able to earn one's livelihood or in being considered for occupational advancement, as the case may be. The patient must have the capacity for self-discipline, patience, and perseverance.

Although the motivation must come from within the patient, the physician, nurse, and dietitian can be of immeasurable help toward initiating this motivation, and subsequently by providing encouragement and guidance at frequent follow-up visits. The patient needs to understand that a calorie intake in excess of his needs is the cause of his overweight, and that weight loss is accomplished only when the calorie intake is reduced below his energy needs. But this explanation is not enough. He also needs to gain insight into the reasons why he is overeating, and to work at correcting these.

Obesity is not a moral issue but a clinical problem and it is important that all who work with obese patients keep this in mind. Threatening the patient with the dire consequences of failing to lose weight or chiding him because he has not adhered to his diet rarely accomplishes anything. On the contrary, each patient must be helped to maintain his self-esteem and deserves treatment with dignity.

Counseling and group sessions. Individual counseling is essential to determine the goals that are realistic for the patient and to initiate a dietary regimen that is appropriate for the patient's food habits and patterns of living. (See also Chapter 26 and Figure 29–5.)

Group sessions are effective in that people compare their progress, share their problems in adhering to diets, and exchange ways to vary their diets. When groups are formed it is important that professional guidance be available from a physician, dietitian, or nurse. Each individual joining such a group should first be evaluated by his physician to determine his fitness for weight reduction.

Essential knowledge. Most people are quite ignorant of the calorie values of foods. Each of

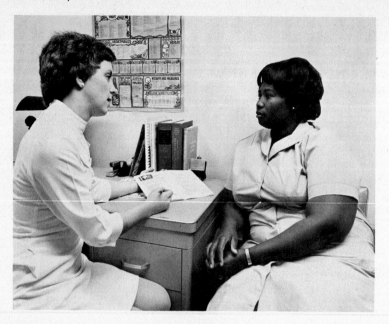

Figure 29–5. Tailoring a diet to the individual's life style is an important part of the counseling process for patients who need modified diets for weight control. (Courtesy, University of Minnesota Health Sciences Center, Minneapolis.)

the food exchange lists (Table A–4) provides a variety of foods that have approximately equal calorie values, and their consistent use helps to develop awareness of nutritive values. Many other tables of calorie values of foods are also available. Keeping a record of the daily calorie intake is useful, at least for a period of time. However, it is important that clear distinctions be made between the calorie values of foods that also supply protein, minerals, and vitamins and those foods that are principally carbohydrate and fat.

Portion control, taught by means of measuring cups, spoons, food models, or actual foods, is essential. Although a given diet is planned for a specific calorie level, it must be expected that the daily calorie intake may vary by as much as 200 to 300 kcal because of variations in food composition as well as in the precision of measurements.

Few dietetic foods are necessary. When fresh fruits are expensive or unavailable, water-packed canned fruits may be used. Artificial sweetening may be used if desired. Many low-calorie beverages currently available provide less than half the calories contained in regular beverages. The calorie information on the label should be checked if these beverages are used.

Some patients ask about including cocktails and wine in their diets. If the physician permits these beverages, the patient needs to know that each gram of alcohol supplies 7 kcal and that the calorie value of the beverage must be taken into consideration. A glass of dry table wine provides fewer calories than a cocktail. Usually an alcoholic beverage is restricted to one serving daily. (See Table A–7 for caloric values of alcoholic beverages.)

A single dinner in a restaurant can nullify careful adherence given to a diet for several days. Usually it is possible to select a clear soup, broiled or roasted meat without sauces, vegetables without sauces, and salad without dressing. Meat portions are likely to be larger than those allowed and the dieter will need to restrict his intake to that allowed. The diet will not be exceeded too much if one foregoes the rolls, butter, and dessert.

What does the dieter do when he has many dinner invitations? For every dieter there are occasions when the limitations of the diet are exceeded, and such breaks in the dieting pattern should be anticipated. Each day gives an opportunity to begin again toward the goal of desired weight. Nevertheless, the person who has many social engagements will find it difficult to make the progress he would like to make. Occasionally, when one knows that the social event will make it difficult to keep within dietary restrictions, the intake at the preceding meal can be kept especially light. Most hostesses are very understanding if the guest tells her that he is on a diet and is therefore restricting the size of portions or letting some of the foods pass by without partaking of them.

Maintenance of weight. To lose weight is not easy; to maintain the desirable level of weight is even more difficult. The calorie-restricted diet planned with regard for the patient's pattern of living also provides the basis for building a maintenance diet. The patient must learn that a change in food habits is essential not only for weight loss, but that such a change must also continue throughout life if desirable weight is to be maintained. Thus, additions of foods should be made judiciously until weight is being kept constant at the desired level. It is important for the patient to weigh himself at weekly intervals or so in order to be sure that the foods added are in appropriate amounts.

If foods added for maintenance are also selected from the Four Food Groups, the quality of the diet with respect to protein, minerals, and vitamins is thereby enhanced. On the other hand, the additions of concentrated high-calorie foods may be more difficult to control in amounts suitable for maintenance. For example, the sedentary person of middle age must continue to forego rich desserts and sweets except on rare occasions.

UNDERWEIGHT

Causes. Underweight results when the energy intake does not fully meet the energy requirements. Not infrequently this occurs in people who are very active, tense, and nervous, and who obtain too little

rest. Sometimes irregular habits of eating and poor selection of foods are responsible for an inadequate caloric intake.

Just as psychologic factors have been noted as contributing to overeating, so they may contribute to eating too little food. Some patients with mental illness reject food to such an extent that severe weight loss results; this condition is referred to as *anorexia nervosa*. (See Chapter 39.)

Underweight also occurs in many pathologic conditions such as fevers in which the appetite is poor but the energy requirements are increased; gastrointestinal disturbances characterized by nausea, vomiting, and diarrhea; and hyperthyroidism in which the metabolic rate is greatly accelerated.

Modifications of the diet. Before weight gain can be effected, the direct cause for the inadequate caloric intake must be sought. As in obesity, these causes in relation to the individual must be removed and a high-calorie diet provided. (See Figure 29-5.)

Energy. Approximately 500 kcal in excess of the daily needs will result in a weekly gain of about 0.5 kg (1 pound). For moderately active individuals diets containing 3000 to 3500 kcal will bring about effective weight gain. Somewhat higher levels are required when fever is high, or gastrointestinal disturbances are interfering with absorption, or metabolism is greatly increased.

Protein. A daily intake of 100 gm protein or more is usually desirable since body protein as well as body fat must be replaced.

Minerals and vitamins. If the quality of the diet resulting in weight loss was poor, considerable body deficits of minerals and vitamins may likewise have occurred. Usually the high-calorie diet will provide liberal levels of all these nutrients. When supplements are prescribed, it is important that the patient understand that they are in no way a substitute for the calories and protein provided by food.

Planning the daily diet. A patient cannot always adjust immediately to a higher caloric intake. It is better to begin with the patient's present intake and to improve the diet both qualitatively and quantitatively day by day until the desired caloric level is reached. Nothing is more conducive to loss of appetite than the appearance of an overloaded tray of food.

The caloric intake may be increased by using additional amounts of foods from the Four Food

Groups, thus increasing the intake of protein, minerals, and vitamins. For example, 500 kcal might be added to the patient's present intake as follows:

1 glass milk, ½ cup ice cream, 1 small potato, 1 small banana; *or*

2 slices bread, 2 ounces meat, 1 ounce cheese, ½ cup Lima beans.

The judicious use of cream, butter, jelly or jam, and sugars will quickly increase the caloric level, but excessive use may provoke nausea and loss of appetite.

Some patients make better progress if given small, frequent feedings; but for many patients midmorning and midafternoon feedings have been found to interfere with the appetite for the following meal. Bedtime snacks, however, may be planned to provide 300 to 800 kcal, thus making it possible to follow a normal pattern for the three meals.

The following list of foods illustrates one way in which the Four Food Groups may be adapted to a high-calorie level. The meal patterns outlined for the high-protein diet (page 423) suggest suitable arrangements of these foods.

3 to 4 cups milk
1 cup light cream
5 to 7 ounces meat, fish, poultry, or cheese
1 egg
4 servings vegetables including:
    1 serving green or yellow vegetable
    2 servings white or sweet potato, corn, or beans
    1 serving other vegetable
2 to 3 servings fruit, including one citrus fruit
1 serving whole-grain or enriched cereal
3 to 6 slices whole-grain or enriched bread
4 tablespoons or more butter or fortified margarine
High-calorie foods to complete the caloric requirement:
    cereals such as macaroni, rice, noodles, spaghetti; honey, molasses, syrups; hard candies; glucose; salad dressings; cakes, cookies, and pastry in moderation; ice cream, puddings, sauces

PROBLEMS AND REVIEW

1. What are the hazards of obesity to health?
2. List eight situations that may account for obesity.
3. Mr. Reese's calorie requirement is 2600, but he is restricting his diet to 1800 kcal. How much weight might he expect to lose in a month?
   a. As part of his weight reduction program, Mr. Reese has increased his activity by walking each day. If he uses 285 kcal per hour, how many hours will it take him to lose 1 pound of adipose tissue?
   b. The physician has indicated that Mr. Reese may include alcoholic beverages not to exceed 150 kcal each day. By consulting Table A–7 prepare a list of several choices that come within this allowance. What adjustments would be necessary in the 1500-kcal diet in Table 29–2 to include the beverage?
   c. What are some important factors to consider in order that maximum cooperation of this patient may be achieved?
4. Mrs. Aston has adhered to her 1500-kcal diet for the past three weeks but has lost no weight. What possible explanations may there be for her failure to lose weight?
   a. Write menus for two days for the 1500-kcal moderate-fat diet listed in Table 29–2.
   b. Mrs. Aston has brought her weight to the desired level. What measures are now important so that this weight level will be maintained?
5. A teen-age girl is 25 pounds underweight and needs some help in planning a diet to bring about weight gain. She is now averaging 55 gm protein and 1800 kcal daily.
   a. Plan some additions to her diet that would increase calories to about 2600 with a minimum of bulk.
   b. What are some factors that may contribute to underweight?
   c. Using the food exchange lists, calculate the protein, fat, and carbohydrate value of the list of foods suggested for weight gain in the right column above. How many calories are provided?
   d. Plan three bedtime snacks that will each provide 500 kcal.

CITED REFERENCES

1. Wilson, R. H. L., and Wilson, N. L.: "Obesity and Respiratory Stress," *J. Am. Diet. Assoc.,* **55:**465–69, 1969.
2. ———: "Highlights from the Ten State Nutrition Survey," *Nutr. Today,* 7:4–11, July–Aug. 1972.

3. Abraham, S., *et al.: Preliminary Findings of the First Health and Nutrition Examination Survey, United States, 1971–1972: Dietary Intake and Biochemical Findings.* U.S. Department of Health, Education, and Welfare. Publication (HRA) 74-1219-1, 1974.

4. Tompkins, W. T., and Wiehl, D. G.: "Nutritional Deficiencies as a Causal Factor in Toxemia and Premature Labor," *Am. J. Obstet. Gynecol.,* **62:**898–919, 1951.

5. Hirsch, J.: "Adipose Cellularity in Relation to Human Obesity," *Adv. Intern. Med.,* **17:**289–300, 1971.

6. West, E. S., *et al.: Textbook of Biochemistry,* 4th ed. Macmillan Publishing Co., Inc., New York, 1966, p. 416.

7. Buskirk, E. R.: "Obesity: A Brief Review with Emphasis on Exercise," *Fed. Proc.,* **33:**1948–51, 1974.

8. Abraham, S., *et al.: Preliminary Findings of the First Health and Nutrition Examination Survey, United States, 1971–1972: Anthropometric and Clinical Findings,* U.S. Department of Health, Education, and Welfare Publication (HRA) 75-1229, 1975.

9. Knittle, J. L.: "Obesity in Childhood. A Problem in Adipose Tissue Cellular Development," *J. Pediatr.,* **81:**1048–59, 1972.

10. Mayer, J.: "Obesity: Causes and Treatment," *Am. J. Nurs.,* **59:**1732–36, 1959.

11. Mayer, J.: *Overweight: Causes, Cost, and Control,* Prentice-Hall, Inc., Englewood Cliffs, N.J., 1968.

12. Leveille, G. A., and Romsos, D. R.: "Meal Eating and Obesity," *Nutr. Today,* **9:**4–9, Nov.–Dec. 1974.

13. Sjöstrom, L., and Björntorp, P.: "Body Composition and Adipose Tissue Cellularity in Human Obesity," *Acta Med. Scand.,* **195:**201–11, 1974.

14. James, G., and Christakis, G.: "New York City's Bureau of Nutrition. Current Programs and Research Activities," *J. Am. Diet. Assoc.,* **48:**301–306, 1966.

15. Stunkard, A., and McLaren-Hume, M.: "The Results of Treatment for Obesity," *Arch. Intern. Med.,* **103:**79–85, 1959.

16. ———: "New Therapies for the Eating Disorders," *Arch. Gen. Psychiatry,* **26:**391–98, 1972.

17. Council on Foods and Nutrition: "A Critique of Low-Carbohydrate Ketogenic Weight Reduction Regimens," *J.A.M.A.,* **224:**1415–19, 1973.

18. Innes, J. A., *et al.:* "Long Term Follow Up of Therapeutic Starvation," *Br. Med. J.,* **2:**356–59, 1974.

19. Gwinup, G.: "Effect of Exercise Alone on the Weight of Obese Women," *Arch. Intern. Med.,* **135:**676–80, 1975.

20. *FDA Drug Bulletin,* Rockville, Md., Food and Drug Administration, Dec. 1972.

21. Chandler, J. G.: "Surgical Treatment of Massive Obesity," *Postgrad. Med.,* **56:**124–33, Aug. 1974.

22. Swenson, S. A., and Oberst, B.: "Pre- and Postoperative Care of the Patient with Intestinal Bypass for Obesity," *Am. J. Surg.,* **129:**225–28, 1975.

ADDITIONAL REFERENCES

Flatt, J. P., and Blackburn, G. L.: "The Metabolic Fuel Regulatory System: Implications for Protein-Sparing Therapies During Caloric Deprivation and Disease," *Am. J. Clin. Nutr.,* **27:**175–87, 1974.

Gopalan, C., *et al.:* "Effect of Calorie Supplementation on Growth of Undernourished Children," *Am. J. Clin. Nutr.,* **26:**563–66, 1973.

Heydmann, A. H.: "Intestinal Bypass for Obesity," *Am. J. Nurs.,* **74:**1102–1104, 1974.

Mann, G. V.: "The Influence of Obesity on Health," *New Engl. J. Med.,* **291:**178–85; 226–32, 1974.

Orkow, B. M., and Ross, J. L.: "Weight Reduction Through Nutrition Education and Personal Counseling," *J. Nutr. Educ.,* **7:**65–67, 1975.

Sohar, E., and Sneh, E.: "Follow-Up of Obese Patients 14 Years After a Successful Reducing Diet," *Am. J. Clin. Nutr.,* **26:**845–48, 1973.

Tullis, I. F.: "Rational Diet Construction for Mild and Grand Obesity," *J.A.M.A.,* **226:**70–71, 1973.

Worthington, B. S., and Taylor, L. W.: "Balanced Low-Calorie vs. Low-Protein-Low-Carbohydrate Reducing Diets," *J. Am. Diet. Assoc.,* **64:**52–55, 1974.

INSTRUCTIONAL MATERIALS FOR THE PATIENT

Calories and Weight—the USDA Pocket Guide. Home and Garden Bull. 153, U.S. Department of Agriculture, Washington, D.C., 1968.

Leverton, R. M.: *A Girl and Her Figure.* National Dairy Council, Chicago, 1956.

Obesity and Health. Pub. Health Service Pub. 1485, U.S. Department of Health, Education, and Welfare, Washington, D.C., 1966.

Page, L., and Finch, L. J.: *Food and Your Weight.* Home and Garden Bull. 74, U.S. Department of Agriculture, Washington, D.C., 1960.

Washbon, M. B., and Harrison, G. G.: "Overweight, and What It Takes to Stay Trim," in *Food for Us All—Yearbook of Agriculture 1969,* U.S. Department of Agriculture, Washington, D.C., pp. 304–14.

30 Protein Deficiency

High-Protein Diets

Incidence and etiology. Protein deficiency resulting primarily from lack of dietary protein is extremely rare in the United States—at least in a degree of severity that it can be diagnosed. Moreover, dietary surveys provide little or no evidence that such deficiencies would be expected. (See Figure 1–5.) Under certain conditions the dietary intake of protein may be inadequate. An emphasis upon excessive thinness and ill-advised reduction regimens, especially by young women, can lead to gradual depletion of tissue proteins. Chronic alcoholism and drug addiction also interfere with a satisfactory food intake, in part because the cost of the habit often leaves insufficient money for the purchase of an adequate diet. Ignorance of the essentials of an adequate diet and child neglect are contributing factors to malnutrition in children. Protein-calorie malnutrition as a principal world health problem in children has been discussed in Chapter 23.

Protein undernutrition as a complication that requires attention during illness and injury is by no means unusual. In two recent studies, fully one third of medical patients and one half of surgical patients in two municipal hospitals were found to have protein malnutrition.[1,2] Many pathologic conditions are aggravated by nutritional deficiency, and, conversely, an existing deficiency is likely to become more severe during illness.

1. Disturbances of the gastrointestinal tract frequently initiate nutritional deficiency because of interference with intake, digestion, or absorption of foods. Anorexia, nausea, vomiting, the discomfort of ulcers, the abdominal distention present in many illnesses, and the cramping associated with diarrhea preclude a satisfactory food intake. Many patients are afraid to eat and restrict their choice to a few foods that do not meet nutritional requirements.

Even though the food intake may be adequate under normal circumstances, increased motility that accompanies some disturbances does not permit sufficient time for digestion and absorption so that excessive amounts of nutrients are lost. In the malabsorption syndrome—sprue, for example—a reduction in the digestive enzymes and in the absorptive surfaces leads to great losses of all nutrients from the bowel.

2. Excessive protein losses result from proteinuria in certain renal diseases, from hemorrhage, from increased nitrogen losses in the urine during the catabolic phase accompanying injury and immobilization, and from exudates of burned surfaces or draining wounds. The increased catabolism that follows immobilization is not fully understood, but is related, at least in part, to an increased production of adrenocortical hormones. Following an injury healthy individuals show greater nitrogen losses than do persons who have more limited reserves. During the acute stage of catabolism high-protein high-calorie diets seem to have little effect on reducing the losses. Eventually, of course, such losses must be replaced.

3. An increased metabolic rate in fevers and in thyrotoxicosis is accompanied by increased destruction of tissue proteins.

4. In diseases of the liver the synthesis of plasma proteins may be reduced even though the supply of amino acids is satisfactory.

Clinical and biochemical signs of protein undernutrition. Fatigue, loss of weight, and lack of resistance to infection are among the symptoms presented by patients with protein deficiency. Because these are common to many pathologic conditions they are of little diagnostic value. Nutritional edema, reduced levels of plasma proteins, a history of inadequate protein intake, and disorders of digestion, absorption, or metabolism help to establish the presence of protein malnutrition. None of these, however, is particularly useful in detecting deficiency in a mild stage when it can be easily corrected.

Underweight together with a history of weight loss is of particular concern in many disease conditions. The loss of weight has been at the expense of tissue proteins as well as adipose tissue. Recovery from illness is often slow, and wound healing is prolonged because the essential amino acids for tissue repair are lacking. Anemia is sometimes observed because of a reduced synthesis of the protein globin. Likewise antibodies are not manufactured in sufficient quantity and infections are more likely to occur.

The presence of nutritional edema supports a diagnosis of protein deficiency. When edema occurs it is necessary to rule out impaired circulation and excretion that occur in cardiac or renal failure. Nutritional edema does not become evident until the protein deficiency has advanced to a relatively severe level. Moreover, it is a rather inconstant finding that is not directly related to the plasma protein level. Thus, an individual may be severely depleted of proteins and show no signs of edema.

Following prolonged protein deficiency the concentration of the plasma proteins and the circulating blood volume are decreased. The principal deficit is in the plasma albumin fraction; the globulins are not appreciably reduced. Since plasma albumin is particularly important for the maintenance of osmotic pressure, the hypoalbuminemia has an adverse effect on the fluid balance between the extracellular and intracellular compartments. Sometimes the plasma protein concentration is essentially normal but a reduction in the total blood volume and hence the total circulating protein has taken place so that any stress could bring about circulatory failure.

Although the liver has an amazing ability to carry out its functions even under adverse conditions, a prolonged nutritional deficiency gradually reduces the regeneration of liver cells as well as the synthesis of many regulatory compounds. A deficit in the lipotropic factors and of the lipoproteins leads to a decreased mobilization of fats from the liver, and thus fatty infiltration reduces the efficiency of the organ. The liver is less able to neutralize the effects of toxic substances and its cells may be damaged—sometimes beyond repair.

Severity of tissue protein depletion. When the supply of amino acids from dietary sources is inadequate, tissues such as muscle, liver, and others are depleted in order to furnish amino acids for the synthesis of the vital regulatory proteins including the plasma proteins. The protein reserves of the tissues are seriously reduced before the concentration of plasma proteins is decreased. One estimate places the tissue protein loss at 30 gm for every gram by which the plasma proteins are reduced. For example, if the total plasma protein concentration has been reduced from 7 gm per 100 ml to 6 gm per 100 ml, and the total circulating plasma volume is 3000 ml, the reduction in circulating protein would be 30 gm. The tissue loss would be about 900 gm (30 × 30 gm). To replace these losses the diet would need to include 930 gm "ideal" protein over and above the maintenance requirement. If the efficiency of the protein in a typical diet is assumed to be 70 per cent,[3] the dietary requirement is increased to 1329 gm (930 ÷ 0.70). Suppose the patient consumes a diet that is adequate in calories and that supplies 25 gm of protein in excess of the daily maintenance level; about 57 days would be required at this level of intake for full repletion to occur (1329 ÷ 25).

Nitrogen balance studies have also shown that extensive depletion of tissue proteins takes place following immobilization, bone fractures, burns, or surgery. In one study the nitrogen loss following fracture of both legs was 137 gm in a 10-day period.[4] This is equivalent to 856 gm protein.

The above examples emphasize that protein repletion cannot be accomplished by giving a patient a high-protein diet for a few days, but that a diet adequate in calories and somewhat liberalized in protein is essential for several weeks to several months.

Just as the degree of protein deficiency is difficult to assess, so it is also hard to determine when full replacement of protein deficits has been made. The concentrations of the plasma protein fractions are poor indicators inasmuch as normal levels are reached long before tissue proteins are fully replaced. Weight gain is a useful, but not infallible, indicator that the protein and calorie deficits are being reversed. But the changes in body weight must be interpreted in relation to other findings. A sudden gain in weight could be caused by increased fluid retention. On the other hand, as improvement in the protein content of tissues is taking place, edema fluids are released and the patient shows weight loss rather than gain. If changes in fluid balance can be ruled out, any gain in weight suggests, at the very least, that protein tissue is not being further catabolized for energy. If the weight gain is correlated with a liberal protein intake, it is fairly safe to assume that it includes the replacement of protein as well as adipose tissue.

Modification of the diet. A high-protein diet furnishes 100 to 125 gm protein and includes at least 2500 kcal. The calorie ratio from protein is about 16 to 20 per cent, thus permitting a selection of foods that is typical of American diets. When higher protein and calorie levels are necessary, the diet order should specify the amounts required.

Protein and calories. The levels of protein and calories are equally important in achieving satisfactory tissue synthesis. A British team studied high-protein diets in 152 hospitals and concluded that too much emphasis is placed on protein intake and not enough on the calorie level.[5] Too often a high-protein diet is ordered but the protein is used largely for energy because the caloric intake is inadequate. These investigators believe that there is no advantage in giving more than 14 per cent of the calories as protein until the patient's daily caloric intake is at least twice his daily basal metabolism. Thus, at 2500 kcal an intake of 350 protein calories or about 90 gm protein would be as satisfactory as a higher level of protein. When the caloric intake is more than twice the basal requirement, protein levels as high as 18 to 20 per cent of the total calorie level may be beneficial.

Management of the diet. To consume a diet containing 100 to 125 gm protein and at least 2500 kcal is not difficult for an individual with a good appetite. Most patients who require these liberal diets have had an impaired appetite for some time, and only the continuous and determined effort on the part of the nurse and others working with the patient can help the patient toward the goal of adequate intake. Some patients prefer small meals with between-meal feedings whereas for others three meals and an evening snack are more suitable. High-protein beverages aid in achieving maximum protein intake with a minimum increase in volume. They may be prepared by combining milk, nonfat dry milk, and eggs and using a variety of flavorings.

A number of palatable, inexpensive, and convenient proprietary compounds using nonfat dry milk and casein as the principal sources of protein are also available.

For emaciated patients the amount of food and the concentration of protein are increased gradually until the gastrointestinal tract again becomes accustomed to handling more food, and until the heart and circulatory system can cope with the additional demands made on it. When the food intake by these patients is rapidly increased, circulatory failure and even death can occur.

DIETARY COUNSELING

Dietary counseling is initiated by an evaluation of the patient's present meal pattern and food intake. The patient needs to know why adequate calorie and protein intakes are essential. Practical suggestions are given for increasing the calorie intake (see page 416) and the protein intake. With a list of protein equivalents from which to choose, the patient is guided toward developing a meal pattern that more nearly meets his needs. (See Figure 30–1.)

Protein Equivalents (6–8 gm protein per unit)
1 cup milk or buttermilk
1/3 cup nonfat dry milk
1 ounce American type cheese
1/4 cup cottage cheese
1 egg
1 ounce meat, fish, or poultry
2 tablespoons peanut butter
8 ounces ice cream
2/3 cup milk pudding

From such a list patients select a combination that will be acceptable to them. Some will prefer additional amounts of milk, whereas others find larger portions of meat to be more acceptable. A high-protein diet need not strain the food budget since nonfat dry milk can be used in substantial amounts. Most patients, and those who cook for them, need practical suggestions, including recipes, for incorporating dry milk into eggnogs, milk shakes, custards, puddings, cream soups, and other prepared foods.

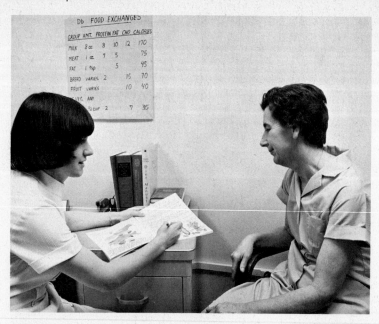

Figure 30–1. Dietetic intern uses food exchange lists and illustrated booklet to assist patient in planning meals for good sources of protein. (Courtesy, University of Minnesota Health Sciences Center, Minneapolis.)

The individual who requires a high-protein high-calorie diet is likely to be one who finds it difficult to consume a large volume of food. One who has a daily intake of 55 gm protein and 1600 kcal does not readily consume 120 gm protein and 2500 kcal. The physician, nurse, and dietitian can help the patient to recognize his needs, but only the patient can set goals that are realistic for him. Perhaps a regular meal pattern requires emphasis; skipping breakfast, for example, makes it difficult to consume enough food for the rest of the day. Possibly a high-protein high-calorie beverage can be substituted for a low-calorie beverage, or an additional portion of dessert can be eaten at bedtime.

Patients need to know whether their efforts are successful. Probably one of the better guides for the patient is gradual weight gain—1 to 2 pounds per week being a reasonable expectation. With improvement in the state of protein nutrition the patient will experience a greater sense of well-being.

High-Protein Diet

Characteristics and General Rules

Select ½ to ⅔ of the day's protein allowance from complete protein foods. Include some complete protein at each meal.

Divide the protein allowance as evenly as practical among the meals of the day.

To increase the protein content of liquid milk add 2 to 4 tablespoons nonfat dry milk to each cup of milk.

For a soft high-protein diet consult the list of foods for a soft diet, page 394.

Include These Foods, or Their Nutritive Equivalents, Daily:

    4 cups (1 quart) milk

7–8 ounces (cooked weight) meat, fish, poultry, or cheese

    2 eggs

    4 servings vegetables including:

        1 serving green or yellow vegetable

1 to 2 servings potato
1 to 2 servings other vegetable
One vegetable to be eaten raw daily
2 servings fruit including:
1 serving citrus fruit—or other good source of ascorbic acid
1 serving other fruit
1 serving whole-grain or enriched cereal
5 slices whole-grain or enriched bread
Additional foods including butter or fortified margarine, sugars, desserts, or more of the listed foods to meet caloric needs.

Nutritive value: On the basis of specified amounts of foods above: protein, 125 gm; kcal, 2500. All vitamins and minerals in excess of normal diet—see page 391.

Meal Pattern	Sample Menu
BREAKFAST	
Fruit	Half grapefruit
Cereal	Oatmeal
Egg—1	Fried egg
Bread, whole grain or enriched	Whole-wheat toast
Butter or margarine	Butter
Milk to drink and for cereal	Milk
Beverage	Coffee
LUNCHEON OR SUPPER	
Meat or substitute of egg, cheese, fish, or poultry—large serving	Chicken soufflé
	Mushroom sauce
Potato, macaroni, spaghetti, noodles, or vegetable	Buttered green beans
Salad with dressing	Shredded carrot and raisin salad
Bread with butter or margarine	Whole-wheat roll and butter
Fruit	Fresh peaches
Milk—1 glass	Milk
DINNER	
Meat, fish, or poultry—large serving	Broiled trout with parsley garnish
Potato	Creamed potato
Vegetable	Buttered spinach
Bread with butter or margarine	Rye bread with butter
Dessert	Lemon-flake ice cream
	Brownies
Milk	Milk
Beverage	Tea with lemon
EVENING NOURISHMENT	
Eggnog—1 glass	Chocolate eggnog
Sandwich with cheese or equivalent	American cheese and tomato sandwich

HIGH-PROTEIN FLUID DIET

Characteristics and General Rules

From 2 to 4 tablespoons nonfat dry milk may be added to each cup of milk or it may be used in custards or cream soups.

Eggs are sometimes contaminated with *Salmonella*. Pasteurized eggnogs may be purchased and are preferable to those made with raw eggs.

The calorie intake is increased by adding butter to gruels and cream soups; adding sugar to beverages; and substituting light cream for part of the milk allowance.

Include These Foods or Their Nutritive Equivalents Daily:
 6 cups milk
 ⅔ cup nonfat dry milk
 4 eggs
1–2 ounces strained meat
 ½ cup strained cereal for gruel
 1 cup citrus juice
 ½ cup tomato juice
 ¼ cup vegetable purée for cream soup
 2 servings plain dessert—gelatin, Junket, custard, cornstarch pudding, ice cream, sherbet
2–3 tablespoons sugar
1–2 tablespoons butter or margarine
Cream for coffee, for gruel, and in milk
Tea, coffee, decaffeinated coffee, cocoa powder, carbonated beverages
Flavoring extracts

Nutritive value: Protein, 110 gm; kcal, 2100.

Meal Pattern
 BREAKFAST
Citrus fruit juice
Cereal gruel with milk and sugar
Poached or soft-cooked egg
Hot beverage with cream, sugar
 MIDMORNING
Fruit juice with egg white
 LUNCHEON OR SUPPER
Cream soup with butter
Tomato juice
High-protein milk, plain or flavored
Fruit-juice gelatin, cornstarch pudding, ice cream, or custard
 MIDAFTERNOON
Malted milk or eggnog
 DINNER
Broth with strained meat
Strained fruit juice
Milk, high-protein milk, or eggnog
Ice cream, Junket, custard, gelatin or plain pudding
 EVENING
Eggnog, milk shake, or plain milk
Ice cream, gelatin, or custard

PROBLEMS AND REVIEW

1. When the availability of protein for tissue synthesis is reduced, what functions of protein will be affected? What clinical and biochemical changes result?
2. In what pathologic conditions is protein deficiency likely to be a problem? Why?
3. Why is a liberal calorie intake essential for effective use of a high-protein diet?
4. *Problem.* The normal diet (page 391) furnishes about 94 gm protein and 2100 kcal. Develop three plans whereby this pattern could be supplemented with 25 gm protein and 500 kcal.
5. *Problem.* Plan a meal pattern for a 17-year-old boy who is allergic to eggs and who needs 150 gm protein and 4000 kcal.

6. A patient's food intake averages 50 gm protein and 1700 kcal. What are some things you need to know about this patient before you can give him guidance for a high-protein high-calorie diet?

CITED REFERENCES

1. Bollet, A. J., and Owens, S.: "Evaluation of Nutritional Status of Selected Hospitalized Patients," *Am. J. Clin. Nutr.,* **26:**931–38, 1973.
2. Bistrian, B. R., *et al.:* "Protein Status of General Surgical Patients," *J.A.M.A.,* **230:**858–60, 1974.
3. Food and Nutrition Board: *Recommended Dietary Allowances,* 8th ed. National Academy of Sciences— National Research Council, Washington, D.C., 1974, p. 46.
4. Albanese, A. A., and Orto, L. A.: "The Proteins and Amino Acids," in Goodhart, R. S., and Shils, M. E., eds.: *Modern Nutrition in Health and Disease,* 5th ed. Lea & Febiger, Philadelphia, 1973, p. 75.
5. Eddy, T. P., and Pellett, P. L.: "Protein-Calorie Intakes of Hospital Patients," *Br. J. Nutr.,* **18:**555–66, 1964.

ADDITIONAL REFERENCES

Baertl, J. M., *et al.:* "Serum Proteins and Plasma Free Amino Acids in Severe Malnutrition," *Am. J. Clin. Nutr.,* **27:**733–42, 1974.

Butterworth, C. E.: "The Skeleton in the Hospital Closet," *Nutr. Today,* **9:**4–8, Mar.–Apr. 1974.

Cravioto, J., and DeLicardie, E. R.: "The Long-Term Consequences of Protein-Calorie Malnutrition," *Nutr. Rev.,* **29:**107–11, 1971.

Gopalan, C., *et al.:* "Effect of Calorie Supplementation on Growth of Undernourished Children," *Am. J. Clin. Nutr.,* **26:**563–66, 1973.

Isaksson, B.: "Clinical Nutrition. Requirements of Energy and Nutrients in Diseases," *Bibl. Nutr. Dieta,* **19:**1–10, 1973.

Kühnau, J.: "Hospital Food and Possibilities of Its Improvement," *Bibl. Nutr. Dieta,* **19:**80–85, 1973.

Latham, M. C.: "Nutrition and Infection in National Development," *Science,* **188:**561–65, 1975.

Payne, P. R.: "Safe Protein-Calorie Ratios in Diets," *Am. J. Clin. Nutr.,* **28:**281–86, 1975.

Review: "FAO/WHO Handbook on Human Nutritional Requirements, 1974," *Nutr. Rev.,* **33:**147–51, 1975.

31 Diet in Fevers and Infections

Nutrition and infection. Resistance to infection is maintained by a number of mechanisms that may be adversely affected by poor nutrition. The skin and mucous membranes provide an important barrier to the invasion of bacteria. Deficiencies of vitamin A, niacin, riboflavin, vitamin B_6, and ascorbic acid lead to characteristic skin lesions which serve as entry points for bacteria and subsequent infections. A deficiency of protein and some of the B-complex vitamins leads to reduced formation of antibodies. Nutritional deficiencies probably also interfere with phagocytosis and with the development of other mechanisms of resistance.

Persons who are chronically undernourished succumb to infections more readily and have a longer period of recovery than do the well nourished. In the United States the vulnerable groups are the elderly who are poor or who lack incentive to eat properly, the chronically ill who have poor appetite, the young child living in a low-income area, and the teen-ager who follows a poor pattern of food intake. In the developing countries infants and preschool children are the most vulnerable. The effects of infection and malnutrition are synergistic. Infections are more severe in the poorly nourished, and the presence of an infection seriously aggravates an existing malnutrition. (See also page 346.)

Classification of fevers. Fever is an elevation of temperature above the normal and results from an imbalance between the heat produced in the body and the heat eliminated from the body. Fevers may be (1) acute or of short duration such as in colds, tonsillitis, influenza, pneumonia, measles, chickenpox, scarlet fever, and typhoid fever, or (2) chronic such as in tuberculosis lasting for years, or intermittent such as in malaria. Infectious hepatitis varies widely in that it is scarcely recognized in some and is severe in others, leading to permanent liver damage if nutrition is not rigorously maintained over a long period of time (see page 468). The acute phase of rheumatic fever is of short duration, but the nutritional problems may be prolonged. The high temperatures that accompany some fevers such as typhoid and malaria are extremely debilitating.

Metabolism in fevers. The metabolic effects of fevers are proportional to the elevation of the body temperature and the length of time the temperature remains elevated. Among these effects are:

1. An increase in the metabolic rate amounting to 7 per cent for every degree Fahrenheit rise in body temperature; an increase also in the restlessness and hence a greatly increased calorie need.

2. Decreased glycogen stores and decreased stores of adipose tissue.

3. Increased catabolism of proteins, especially in typhoid fever, malaria, typhus fever, poliomyelitis, and others; the increased nitrogen wastes place an additional burden upon the kidneys.

4. Accelerated loss of body water owing to increased perspiration and the excretion of body wastes.

5. Increased excretion of sodium and potassium.

6. Modified motility of the gastrointestinal tract. In some infections motility is reduced and nausea and vomiting may seriously interfere with the intake of food. In other infections the motility is increased and diarrhea interferes with the absorption of nutrients.

General dietary considerations. The diet in fevers and infections depends upon the nature and severity of the pathologic conditions and upon the length of the convalescence. In general it should meet the following requirements:

Energy. The caloric requirement may be increased as much as 50 per cent if the temperature is high and the tissue destruction is great. Restlessness also increases the caloric requirement. Initially, the patient may be able to ingest only 600 to 1200 kcal daily, but this should be increased as rapidly as possible.

426

Protein. About 100 gm protein or more is prescribed for the adult when a fever is prolonged. This will be most efficiently utilized when the calorie intake is liberal (see Chapter 30). High-protein beverages may be used as supplements to the regular meals.

Carbohydrates. Glycogen stores are replenished by a liberal intake of carbohydrates. Any sugars such as glucose, corn syrup, and cane sugar may be used. However, glucose is less sweet than some other sugars and consequently more of it can be used. Furthermore, it is a simple sugar which is absorbed into the bloodstream without the necessity for enzyme action. Lactose, used by some, is relatively expensive, dissolves poorly in cold solutions, and may increase fermentation in the small intestine resulting in diarrhea.

Fats. The energy intake may be rapidly increased through the judicious use of fats, but fried foods and rich pastries may retard digestion unduly.

Minerals. A sufficient intake of sodium chloride is accomplished by the use of salty broth and soups and by liberal sprinklings of salt on food. Generally speaking, foods are a good source of potassium, but a limited food intake might result in potassium depletion whenever fever is high and prolonged. Fruit juices and milk are relatively good sources of this element. Iron supplementation is often required to correct the anemia that results from some parasite infections.

Vitamins. Fevers apparently increase the requirements for vitamin A and ascorbic acid, just as the B-complex vitamins are needed at increased levels proportionate to the increase in calories; that is, 0.5 mg thiamin, 0.6 mg riboflavin, and 6.6 mg niacin equivalents per 1000 additional kcal. Oral therapy with antibiotics and drugs interferes with synthesis of some B-complex vitamins by intestinal bacteria, thus necessitating a prescription for vitamin supplements for a short time.

Fluid. The fluid intake must be liberal to compensate for the losses from the skin and to permit adequate volume of urine for excreting the wastes. From 2500 to 5000 ml daily are necessary, including beverages, soups, fruit juices, and water.

Ease of digestion. Bland, readily digested foods should be used to facilitate digestion and rapid absorption. The food may be soft or of regular consistency. Although fluid diets may be used initially there are some disadvantages: (1) most fluid diets occupy bulk out of all proportion to their caloric and nutrient values, so that reinforcement of liquids is essential; (2) a liquid diet sometimes increases abdominal distention to the point of acute discomfort, whereas solid foods may be better tolerated; (3) many patients experience less anorexia, nausea, and vomiting when they are taking solid foods.

Intervals of feeding. Small quantities of food at intervals of two to three hours will permit adequate nutrition without overtaxing the digestive system at any one time. With improvement, many patients consume more food if given three meals and a bedtime feeding.

Diet in fevers of short duration. The duration of many fevers has been shortened by antibiotic and drug therapy, and nutritional needs are usually met without difficulty. During an acute fever the patient's appetite is often very poor, and small feedings of soft or liquid foods as desired should be offered at frequent intervals (see Chapter 27). Sufficient intake of fluids and salt is essential. If the illness persists for more than a few days, high-protein, high-calorie foods will need to be emphasized. See High-Protein Diet (Chapter 30).

Diet in typhoid fever. Improved sanitation has greatly reduced the incidence of typhoid fever, and antibiotic therapy has shortened the acute stage of the disease. Nevertheless, short and uneventful convalescence is determined to an important degree by adequate nutrition.

The febrile period may cause loss of tissue protein amounting to as much as $\frac{1}{2}$ to $\frac{3}{4}$ pound of muscle a day. The body store of glycogen is quickly depleted, and a probable upset in water balance occurs.

The intestinal tract becomes highly inflamed and irritable, and diarrhea, which is a frequent complication, interferes with the absorption of nutrients. The ulceration may be so severe that hemorrhage and even perforation of the intestines may occur.

The dietary considerations outlined on page 426 apply as in other fevers. Special emphasis must be placed upon a caloric intake of 3500 or more and a protein intake in excess of 100 gm. Because of the intestinal inflammation, great care must be exercised to eliminate all irritating fibers. The high-protein fluid diet may be used as a basis in dietary planning. In addition, low-fiber foods including white breads and crackers, refined cooked and dry cereals, eggs, cheese, tender meat, fish, and poultry, potato, and plain desserts may be used. A representative meal pattern is as follows:

BREAKFAST
Orange juice with glucose
Cream of Wheat with cream and sugar
Poached egg on
Buttered white toast
Cocoa
   MIDMORNING
Eggnog made with cream
   LUNCHEON OR SUPPER
Cream of tomato soup
Roast chicken
Baked potato (no skin) with butter
Buttered white toast
Vanilla ice cream
High-protein milk
   MIDAFTERNOON
Orange juice
Baked custard
   DINNER
Consommé with gelatin
Soft-cooked egg
Boiled rice with sugar and cream
Buttered white toast
Tapioca cream
Milk
   BEDTIME
Chocolate malted milk
Cream cheese sandwich on white bread

Diet in rheumatic fever. Rheumatic fever is one of the leading causes of chronic illness in children. It will permanently damage the heart if it is not recognized early and treated promptly. Rheumatic fever follows *Streptococcus* infections and is more common among poorer classes of people. However, all attempts to correlate the incidence of the disease with specific nutrient deficiencies have so far failed.

The soft and liquid diets described in Chapter 27 are suitable during the acute phase of rheumatic fever. When cortisone or ACTH therapy is used, the diet must be mildly restricted in sodium to avoid sodium retention and edema formation (see Chapter 41).

The acute stage may last only a few weeks, but absolute bed rest is essential for many weeks or months. The chief problem in nutrition is that of maintaining an adequate intake of nutrients during the prolonged period of bed rest. Because the appetite may be poor, cereal foods and sweets should probably be restricted as a means of ensuring adequate intake of milk, meat, fish, poultry, citrus fruits, and other essential foods. The diet is planned according to the principles of the normal diet described in Chapter 21.

Diet in tuberculosis. Tuberculosis is a major cause of illness and death worldwide. In spite of a sharp decline in incidence in the United States over the past 50 years, some 16 million persons in this country have the disease, with an estimated 70,000 new cases occurring each year.[1] The reduced incidence has been attributed to more effective chemotherapeutic agents, better housing, and improved nutrition; yet there is still concern in areas where poverty and poor sanitation prevail.

Pulmonary tuberculosis is an inflammatory disease of the lungs accompanied by a wasting of the tissues, exhaustion, cough, expectoration, and fever. In its acute form it resembles pneumonia, because the temperature is high and the circulation and respiration are increased. In the chronic phase of tuberculosis the fever is low grade and the metabolic rate is lower than in the acute fevers. Even in the chronic phase the wasting may be considerable because of the protracted illness. The following modifications of the normal diet are usually indicated:[2]

Energy. Satisfactory weight is maintained, as a rule, at 2500 to 3000 kcal. It is not desirable to gain weight beyond 10 per cent above the desirable weight for body frame.

Protein. From 75 to 100 gm protein help to regenerate the serum albumin levels, which are often low in cases of long standing.

Minerals. Calcium requires particular emphasis to promote the healing of the tuberculous lesions. At least a quart of milk should be taken daily. Iron supplementation may be necessary if there has been hemorrhage.

Vitamins. Carotene appears to be poorly converted to vitamin A so that the diet should provide as much preformed vitamin A as possible. In addition, a vitamin A supplement may be necessary. Ascorbic acid deficiency is frequently present, and additional amounts of citrus fruits or ascorbic acid supplementation are essential.

Chemotherapeutic agents used in treatment of tuberculosis may have an adverse effect on certain of the B-complex vitamins. Isoniazid is an antagonist of vitamin B_6 and may inhibit the folate-dependent interconversion of glycine and serine. Low serum folate and megaloblastic anemia have been noted in patients receiving this therapy. Supplements of vitamin B_6 are indicated to prevent the peripheral neuritis characteristic of B_6 deficiency. Other drugs, such as para-aminosalicylic acid, may cause malabsorption of vitamin B_{12}.[3]

Selection of foods. During the acute stage of the illness, a high-protein high-calorie fluid diet may be given as in other acute fevers, progressing to the soft and regular diets when improvement occurs. Most patients have very poor appetites. For some a six-meal routine is best, whereas others eat better if they receive three meals and a bedtime feeding. The individuals responsible for planning meals should respect the patient's food idiosyncrasies. To this end, a selective menu from which the patient chooses his foods each day is helpful. Other patients may eat better when they are not consulted in advance about their diets, thus introducing an element of surprise. Needless to say, every attention must be given to making meals as appetizing in appearance and taste as possible. The high-protein and high-calorie diets described in Chapters 29 and 30 may be adapted to the individual patient's needs.

DIETARY COUNSELING

Failure of the patient to follow the prescribed drug regimen leads to great increase in recurrence and repeated hospitalization. Good nutrition is likewise important in preventing recurrence.[2] The characteristics of a normal diet, with special emphasis on a liberal milk intake, protein-rich foods, fruits, and vegetables, must be pointed out. To increase the calcium and protein intake, 3 to 5 tablespoons of nonfat dry milk may be added to each 8 ounces of whole milk. If desired, fruit flavors or chocolate syrup may be added. This beverage supplementation is conveniently prepared, provides substantial nutritive value at minimum bulk, and is low in cost.

Because many of the patients with tuberculosis have low incomes, some assistance is necessary in providing practical measures to purchase the necessary foods. This entails not only additional welfare allowances in some instances but guidance in budgeting the food money. In families with low incomes it may not be practical to improve the diet of the patient alone, for additional allowances of money may be spent for the children's diet rather than for the patient. In such situations the best prophylaxis may well be the improvement of the diet of all members of the family.

Emphysema. This is a pathologic enlargement or overdistention of the alveoli of the lung brought about by a number of causes, including bronchitis, asthma, infection, and cigarette smoking. Patients with emphysema often complain of abdominal distress, and peptic ulcers occur frequently. In early stages some patients may be obese, and the distress in breathing is further accentuated. Some improvement is noted when weight is brought within desirable levels.

Shortness of breath places a severe limitation upon the ability to ingest an adequate diet, with the result that weight loss and tissue wasting are common. Not infrequently the purchase and preparation of food, or seeking a place to eat a·meal, require more effort than the patient can expend. Because the patient is unable to work, there may be insufficient income to purchase adequate food. Chewing and swallowing require further effort and the patient often stops short of satisfactory intake.

A soft high-calorie diet is usually indicated. Patients are especially short of breath after a night's sleep and experience difficulty in eating breakfast. Small, frequent feedings of concentrated foods should be used. High-protein commercial supplements are useful because they are concentrated, palatable, easy to prepare, and easy to ingest. Too many fibrous fruits and vegetables or meats requiring much chewing may necessitate an energy expenditure beyond that justified by the nutrient values obtained. The patient will eat very slowly, and should refrain from talking while eating since the swallowing of air is responsible for much of the discomfort.

For a discussion of infectious hepatitis see page 468; for a discussion of infections from food poisoning, see page 254.

PROBLEMS AND REVIEW

1. What is the effect of nutritional status on the incidence of infections?
2. How great is the increase in energy metabolism brought about by fever? What other changes in metabolism of nutrients take place during fever? In view of these changes how do you view the widely held belief "Starve a fever"?
3. Give examples of foods that can be used to reinforce the protein and calorie level of the diet.
4. *Problem.* Plan a fluid diet in six meals that eliminates milk. Calculate the calorie value.
5. *Problem.* Plan a full fluid diet in six meals to include 80 gm protein and 2500 kcal.
6. *Problem.* Plan a diet for a 12-year-old boy with rheumatic fever. What techniques can you use to help the boy accept the diet?
7. What are the principles of dietary management in typhoid fever?
8. Outline a plan of dietary counseling for a 34-year-old woman with healed tuberculosis. She has three children under the age of 10 years and is receiving welfare assistance. You will need to determine the amount of money available through welfare in your community to this family of four.
9. *Problem.* Keep a record of the food intake for two days by a patient with an infection. What factors enter into this patient's acceptance of food? Develop recommendations for any improvement that may be required.
10. What are the problems encountered in feeding a patient with emphysema? How would you try to solve them?

CITED REFERENCES

1. Bates, J. H.: "Treatment of TB," *Adv. Intern. Med.,* **20**:1–23, 1975.
2. Mayer, J.: "Nutrition and Tuberculosis," *Postgrad. Med.,* **50**:53–56, Dec. 1971.
3. Stebbins, R., *et al.:* "Drug-Induced Megaloblastic Anemias," *Semin. Hematol.,* **10**:235–51, 1973.

ADDITIONAL REFERENCES

Barstow, R. E.: "Coping With Emphysema," *Nurs. Clin. North Am.,* **9**:137–45, 1974.
"Current Status of Tuberculosis in the United States," *Stat. Bull. Metropol. Life Ins. Co.,* **55**:9–11, Jan. 1974.
Fagerhaugh, S. Y.: "Getting Around with Emphysema," *Am. J. Nurs.,* **73**:94–99, 1973.
Faulk, W. P., *et al.:* "Some Effects of Malnutrition on the Immune Response in Man," *Am. J. Clin. Nutr.,* **27**:638–46, 1974.
Gordis, L., and Markowitz, M.: "Prevention of Rheumatic Fever Revisited," *Pediatr. Clin. North Am.,* **18**:1243–53, 1971.
Gordon, J. E., and Scrimshaw, N. S.: "Infectious Disease in the Malnourished," *Med. Clin. North Am.,* **54**:1495–1508, 1970.
Heineman, H. A.: "The Clinical Syndrome of Malaria in the United States," *Arch. Intern. Med.,* **129**:607–16, 1972.
Latham, M. C.: "Nutrition and Infection in National Development," *Science,* **188**:561–65, 1975.
Rodnan, G. P., ed.: "Rheumatic Fever," *J.A.M.A.,* **224** (Suppl. 5):736–39, 1973.
Solomon, D. A., and Gracey, D. R.: "Modern Concepts in Treating Tuberculosis," *Geriatrics,* **29**:110–14, July 1974.
Standal, B. R., *et al.:* "Early Changes in Pyridoxine Status of Patients Receiving Isoniazid Therapy," *Am. J. Clin. Nutr.,* **27**:479–84, 1974.
WHO Expert Committee on Malaria, 16th report, *WHO Tech. Rep. Ser.,* **549**:1–89, 1974.

32 Diet in Diseases of the Esophagus, Stomach, and Duodenum

Bland Fiber-Restricted Diet in Three Stages

Modified diets are commonly prescribed for many disorders of the digestive tract, including hiatal hernia, peptic ulcer, gastritis, diarrhea, constipation, malabsorption syndrome, cirrhosis of the liver, cholecystitis, and pancreatitis, among others. Much controversy exists over the role of diet in the treatment of gastrointestinal disturbances. In certain conditions there is a physiologic basis for dietary modification; in others, a sound rationale is lacking and diets traditionally used are of unproven value. For the latter more objective evidence is needed before sound conclusions can be reached in regard to beneficial effects of dietary modification.

DIAGNOSTIC TESTS IN GASTROINTESTINAL DISEASE

Disorders of the gastrointestinal tract are classified as *functional* or *organic* in nature. Functional disturbances involve no alterations in structure. In organic diseases, on the other hand, pathologic lesions are seen in tissue, as in ulcers or carcinoma. Both types of disorders are characterized by changes in secretory activity and motility. A number of factors including diet are believed to influence these changes. (See Table 32–1.)

Studies of motility and secretion, together with radiologic evidence and, in some instances, biopsy specimens of the affected mucosa, are used in the diagnosis of gastrointestinal disease.

Measurement of motility. X-ray and fluoroscopic examinations are widely used to determine the emptying time and motility of the intestinal tract, and to locate the site of the disturbance. Following an overnight fast the patient is given a "barium swallow" consisting of a pint of buttermilk or malted milk in which barium sulfate has been mixed. The progress of this opaque "meal" along the intestinal tract can then be visualized by means of fluoroscopy. X-rays taken before and after the meal are studied for filling defects and other abnormalities. (See Figure 32–1.)

In GASTRIC ATONY, due to lack of normal muscle tone of the stomach, contractions are not of sufficient strength to move the food mass out of the stomach at a normal rate. Larger pieces or fragments of food are not adequately disintegrated and mixed with the stomach juices.

Increased action of the musculature of the stomach and intestine is known as HYPERPERISTALSIS. It may be brought on by excessive amounts of fibrous foods, psychologic factors such as worry or fear, or nervous stimulation.

Measurement of gastric acidity. Tests of gastric secretory function per se are of limited diagnostic value and are most useful in patients in whom a lesion has been demonstrated by x-ray or gastroscopy.

Various test meals were formerly used to stimulate gastric secretion. At present, drugs such as caffeine, histamine, or histalog, which are vigorous stimulants to gastric secretion, are used to determine the amount of acid produced.

GASTRIC ANALYSIS provides information on the rate of gastric emptying, the quantity of acid and pepsin secretion, and gastric cytology. Two methods are used: (1) intubation, in which a nasogastric tube is passed into the empty stomach and the contents are withdrawn for examination before a test "meal" and at specified intervals following the test "meal"; or (2) tubeless, which involves administration of a resin that exchanges a cation for hydrogen. The cation or dye is absorbed and excreted in the urine where its concentration indicates the amount of gastric acid exchanged.

The results of gastric analysis are usually described in terms of the total acid produced. The total amount of acid secreted varies from one individual to another. Some persons continually secrete

Table 32–1. Factors That Modify Acid Secretion and Gastrointestinal Motility and Tone

Increased Flow of Acid and Enzyme Production	Decreased Flow of Acid and Enzyme Production
1. Chemical stimulation—meat extractives, seasonings, certain spices, alcohol, acid foods	1. Large amounts of fat, especially as fried foods, pastries, nuts, etc.
2. Attractive, appetizing, well-liked foods	2. Large meals
3. State of happiness and contentment	3. Poor mastication of food
4. Pleasant surroundings for meals	4. Foods of poor appearance, flavor, or texture
	5. Foods acutely disliked
	6. Worry, anger, fear, pain*

Increased Tone and Motility	Decreased Tone and Motility
1. Warm foods	1. Cold foods
2. Liquid and soft foods	2. Dry, solid foods
3. Fibrous foods, as in certain fruits and vegetables	3. Low-fiber foods
4. High-carbohydrate low-fat intake	4. High-fat intake, especially as fried foods, pastries, etc.
5. Seasonings; concentrated sweets	5. Vitamin B complex deficiency, especially thiamin
6. Fear, anger, worry, nervous tension	6. Sedentary habits
	7. Fatigue
	8. Worry, anger, fear, pain

*In certain individuals these emotional disturbances may stimulate the flow of gastric juice.

Figure 32–1. Patient care conference. The physician points out site of gastric lesion to a dietitian, nurse, and student nurse. (Courtesy, Yale–New Haven Medical Center.)

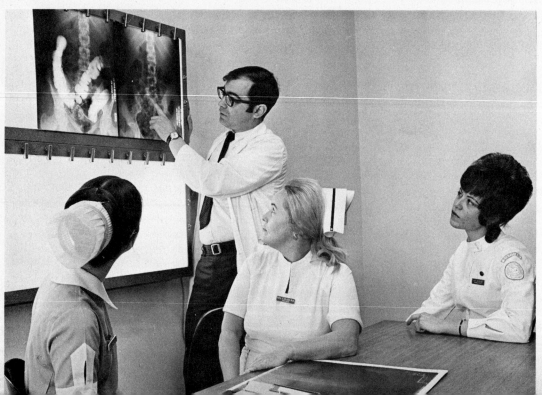

more gastric juice than normal without experiencing any discomfort. An excess secretion of acid is known as HYPERCHLORHYDRIA and is often accompanied by gastric distress. It may be associated with emotional or nervous upsets, or it may accompany organic disease such as peptic ulcer or cholecystitis.

HYPOCHLORHYDRIA denotes a diminished amount of free acid and may be present indefinitely in otherwise healthy persons. The cause should be determined, if possible, since hypochlorhydria also accompanies diseases such as pernicious anemia and is a common finding in sprue, chronic gastritis, and pellagra. It occurs occasionally in cancer, nephritis, cholecystitis, and diabetes. In ACHLORHYDRIA no free acid is present although there is some peptic activity; this finding suggests pernicious anemia and malignant gastric ulcer. ACHYLIA GASTRICA refers to the absence of both free and combined acid and of enzyme activity.

GENERAL DIETARY CONSIDERATIONS IN DISEASES OF THE GASTROINTESTINAL TRACT

Factors in dietary management. Many dietary recommendations have been made for the management of gastrointestinal diseases; yet actual knowledge of the specific effects of various foods on the digestive tract is rather limited. Any proposed dietary modifications should take into consideration the possible effects of ingested food upon (1) the secretory activity of the stomach, small intestine, pancreas, liver, and gallbladder; (2) motility of the tract; (3) the bacterial flora; (4) the comfort and ease of digestion; and (5) the maintenance and repair of the mucosal structures. In addition, some disorders interfere with the completeness of digestion or the absorption of one or more nutrients so that the nutrient intake must be modified in order to meet the net requirements of the body.

Influence of foods on gastric acidity. Most foods have a pH between 5 and 7, thus are considerably less acid than gastric juice. No food is sufficiently acid to have any adverse effect on a gastric lesion, although citrus juices and fruits might cause some discomfort to a lesion of the mouth, esophagus, or the achlorhydric stomach.[1]

Gastric secretion is initiated by the sight, smell, and taste of food. As food enters the stomach, the secretion continues and reaches its height sometime later. Protein foods stimulate more acid secretion than do carbohydrates and fats.

Protein foods initially have a temporary buffering effect; hence there is less free acid immediately available to erode the lesion when protein is fed. Milk has some buffering effect, although other protein foods appear to be more effective. Nevertheless, most patients with peptic ulcer have progressed well on diets in which milk feedings were used for their neutralizing effect. Regardless of buffering activity, the amount of free acid again is high within $\frac{1}{2}$ to 2 hours following a meal. No diet alone will maintain a 24-hour neutralization of gastric contents.

Fats inhibit gastric secretion. The entrance of fats into the duodenum stimulates the production of enterogastrone, a hormone, which in turn retards gastric secretion and likewise delays the emptying of the stomach. Dairy fats are not superior to other fats in this regard, but are useful as they are easily digested.

Meat extractives, tannins, caffeine, and alcohol are well known for their effect in stimulating the flow of acid. Spices are also commonly implicated in this respect, but experimental evidence on humans does not support this. Schneider and associates[2] tested the possible irritant effects of a number of spices and herbs on patients with active and healing ulcers. Subjective reactions by the patients, the rate of healing of the ulcer, and the gastroscopic appearance of the mucosa were not altered by allspice, caraway seeds, cinnamon, mace, paprika, thyme, or sage when given with foods. The elimination of these spices therefore is unnecessary. Slight reddening of the mucosa and some symptoms of gastric discomfort were noted with chili powder, cloves, mustard seeds, nutmeg, and black pepper. In gastric disorders these spices should be used with discretion, or not at all.

Influence of foods on motility. Recent evidence suggests that the rate of gastric emptying is related to the caloric density of the food given and is independent of the volume given; that is, isocaloric amounts of carbohydrate and triglyceride are equally effective in slowing gastric emptying.[3] This finding is consistent with the long-held belief that foods high in fiber increase peristaltic action, and low-fiber foods reduce such motility.

Fiber and residue defined. Tables of food composition list values for CRUDE FIBER. This is determined by subjecting a food sample to acid and then alkaline digestion according to standard laboratory procedures. It consists principally of cellulose and lignin. Other fibrous materials are partially or completely digested so that the resultant value is lower than the total fiber content of the sample.

DIETARY FIBER is the fiber that is resistant to hydrolysis by the digestive enzymes in the human intestinal tract. In addition to cellulose and lignin it includes variable amounts of hemicelluloses, pectins, gums, and mucilages. Some dietary fiber is disintegrated by intestinal bacteria. The data on the resistance of dietary fiber to digestion are extremely limited. Some earlier studies have indicated that the fiber in whole grains and in bran is almost completely resistant to hydrolysis. On the other hand, the fibers in vegetables and fruits are less resistant, but wide variations exist from one food to another.

RESIDUE refers to the volume of the materials remaining after the digestive processes have been completed and includes not only indigestible fiber but also the bacterial residues and desquamated cells from the mucosa. Whole-grain cereals and bran, for example, are considered to be high-residue foods because of their high fiber content. On the other hand, milk, a fiber-free food, is often cited as contributing to increased residue in the gastrointestinal tract.

The composition of the diet does not greatly influence the predominant type of intestinal organisms.[4,5]

Foods and their effect on lesions. Fibrous foods have often been omitted from diets for diseases of the gastrointestinal tract in the belief that they might mechanically injure or retard the healing of a lesion such as an ulcer. However, it is unlikely that fibrous foods, when sufficiently chewed, would be injurious to a peptic ulcer. Patients should be instructed to chew foods properly. Puréeing of foods is not necessary unless the teeth are poor or absent.[6] The individual can best determine tolerance for specific foods by trial and error.

Influence of foods upon digestive comfort. Ingestion of certain foods has long been associated with symptoms of belching, distention, epigastric distress, flatulence, constipation, or diarrhea in some persons with digestive disorders. Among these foods are baked beans, cabbage, fried foods, onions, and spicy foods. Tolerance to these and other foods is a highly individual matter.[6] Not all patients react to foods in the same way, nor does the same patient always react to a specific food in the same way. (See Figure 32–2.)

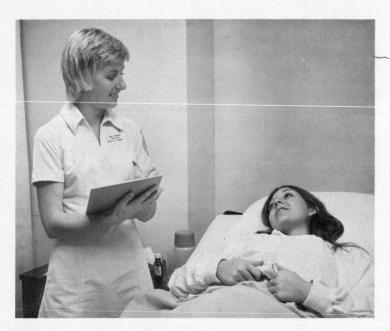

Figure 32–2. Tolerance for food is a highly individual matter. Patient is interviewed so that this can be taken into account in planning for her modified diet. (Courtesy, University of Minnesota Health Sciences Center, Minneapolis.)

Traditional diets. Clinicians who favor a conservative approach to the dietary management of gastrointestinal disease generally use diets based on recommendations made early in the century for treatment of peptic ulcer by Sippy (1915) and Meulengracht (1935).[7,8] Such diets are based on the principle that the presence of some food in the stomach at all times will dilute and neutralize excess acid and consequently lessen pain. In most of these, milk forms the basis of the diet with small feedings of "bland" foods being given at frequent intervals. Generally speaking, foods allowed are limited to those considered to be *chemically, mechanically,* and *thermally* nonirritating; other foods are rigidly excluded.

Foods believed to be *chemically* irritating because of their stimulatory effect on gastric secretion include meat extractives, caffeine, alcohol, citrus fruits and juices, and some spicy foods. (See page 432.) *Mechanically* irritating foods include those with indigestible carbohydrate, such as whole grains and most raw fruits and vegetables. Foods believed to be *thermally* irritating are those ordinarily served at extremes of temperature, such as very hot or iced liquids. In addition, certain foods traditionally forbidden include strongly flavored vegetables (Brussels sprouts, cabbage, cauliflower, onions, turnips, and others), baked beans, pork, and fried foods. Restriction of these foods is based on subjective evidence from patients who experienced distress following ingestion of these items.

Over the years, the practice of recommending or restricting certain foods in the management of ulcer disease has been carried over to treatment of other gastrointestinal disorders as well. Foods customarily allowed are described as bland, nonirritating, smooth, low fiber, or nonstimulating; those contraindicated are considered to be distending, gaseous, indigestible, stimulating, and so on. The soft diet, fiber-restricted diet, or stage 3 of the bland diet is appropriate for most gastrointestinal conditions; these diets are all very similar. The details of the soft diet are discussed in Chapter 27. The bland, fiber-restricted diet is on page 438.

Trend to more liberal diets. Current opinion among liberal clinicians is that strict diets are no longer appropriate for the majority of patients with gastrointestinal disease. Liberalization of foods used in diets for gastrointestinal disease has come about gradually as a result of (1) the realization that many of the dietary recommendations made in these diseases are not backed by scientific evidence; (2) evidence that traditional diets do not influence the rate of healing of ulcers; and (3) concern for the nutritional adequacy and patient acceptance of the diets.

DISORDERS OF THE ESOPHAGUS AND STOMACH

Esophagitis. This is an acute or chronic inflammation of the esophageal wall. *Acute* esophagitis is usually characterized by substernal pain brought on by swallowing. It may be a consequence of upper respiratory infections, extensive burns, prolonged gastric intubation, excessive vomiting, ingestion of poisonous substances such as lye, or diseases such as scarlet fever or diphtheria.

Most cases of *chronic* esophagitis are attributed to a sliding hernia that permits the reflux of gastric juice into the esophagus. Mucosal erosions and narrowing of the lumen occur. The disorder occurs most frequently in persons with high gastric acidity, many of whom have a history of duodenal ulcer.

Symptoms. Heartburn, intermittent at first, but becoming progressively worse, is often the chief complaint in esophagitis. Pain following ingestion of very hot or cold foods and spicy or acid foods and eventual dysphagia occur as the disease progresses.

Treatment. The objectives of therapy are to protect the esophagus, to reduce gastric acidity, and to reduce reflux of gastric contents into the esophagus. Antacid preparations are usually prescribed.

Dietary management consists of weight reduction (see Chapter 29) for obese individuals since excess abdominal fat is believed to increase gastric herniation and reflux. Large meals should be avoided in favor of more frequent small meals. A bland, fiber-restricted diet is desirable for most individuals (see page 438).

Hiatus hernia. A common disorder affecting the esophagus is the herniation of a portion of the stomach through the hiatus of the diaphragm. This disorder, known as HIATAL HERNIA, occurs most frequently in persons over 45 years of age. The incidence is greater in persons of stocky build and in overweight persons. Loss of muscle tone weakens muscles around the diaphragm and increased abdominal pressure helps push the stomach through the diaphragm. Symptoms occur when the herniated portion is irritated or injured or is large enough to affect other organs. Tight garments or belts appear to provoke symptoms and should be avoided. Substernal pain, belching, or hiccoughing occurs following meals or while lying down.

A bland, fiber-restricted diet with between-meal snacks is usually recommended (see page 438). Of equal importance are eating small amounts at any one time and omitting food for several hours before bedtime. Weight reduction is essential for obese individuals (see Chapter 29).

Esophageal reflux. The lower esophageal sphincter normally maintains a pressure barrier against reflux of gastric contents into the esophagus. Incompetence of the sphincter permits postural reflux of gastric contents and may cause esophagitis. Heartburn and dysphagia occur. Inadequate release of gastrin following a meal and other unknown factors are believed to cause the sphincter incompetence.[9] Esophageal reflux is not synonymous with hiatal hernia although both may occur together.[10]

Factors that decrease lower esophageal sphincter pressure include alcohol, caffeine, chocolate, fatty meals, and smoking, all of which should be avoided. Sphincter pressure is increased by proteins and antacids.[9] A bland diet with frequent small meals is used and antacids are prescribed. Weight reduction for overweight persons is encouraged.

Achalasia. This is a disorder of esophageal motility in which the lower esophageal sphincter fails to relax normally upon swallowing so that food can enter the stomach. Loss or absence of ganglion cells is believed to be involved. Long-continued intraesophageal pressure may lead to dilatation above the point of stricture. The primary symptom is dysphagia with possible vomiting and eventual weight loss.

Treatment consists of dilatation of the stricture. Dietary considerations include avoidance of excessively hot or iced beverages and any foods that may be irritating to the esophagus. If weight loss has been considerable, increased calories and protein are needed (see Chapter 30). Some individuals tolerate several small feedings better than larger ones.

Esophageal obstruction. This may result from a number of causes including pressure from adjacent organs, hiatal hernia, scar tissue formation, foreign bodies, diverticula, and neoplasms. Swallowed foods do not progress beyond the point of stricture owing to narrowing of the lumen, and if the condition is untreated, death from starvation follows. Measures to restore the normal passageway include dilatation, irradiation, or surgical intervention, depending on the nature of the obstruction.

Dietary management is the same for obstruction from any cause. Efforts are directed toward providing foods in suitable form and sufficient amounts to meet the patient's needs. In partial obstruction, liquids should be offered with progression to low-fiber foods (see page 438) as tolerated. Small amounts of food at frequent intervals are preferable. When it is not possible or desirable for food to pass through the esophagus, the patient is fed by means of a gastrostomy. Food is administered through a tube inserted directly into the stomach. (See Chapter 36 for characteristics of tube feedings.)

Indigestion. Indigestion, or dyspepsia, is a functional or organic disease manifested by symptoms of heartburn, acid regurgitation, epigastric pain, "fullness" or bloating especially after meals, flatulence, nausea, or vomiting.

The majority of cases of indigestion are of functional origin and are usually due to faulty dietary habits or emotional factors. The organic type is associated with diseases affecting the digestive organs; it may also be a symptom of generalized disease as in uremia. Treatment in organic types consists of treating the underlying disease.

Persons with functional dyspepsia need individualized dietary counseling in the essentials of a nutritionally adequate diet. Specific instructions should be given with emphasis on selection of foods from each of the Four Food Groups and the importance of regular mealtimes, sufficient time to eat in a relaxed atmosphere, rest after meals, and avoidance of emotional tension.

Gastritis. This is an inflammation of the mucosa of the stomach, occurring as an acute or chronic lesion with atrophy or hypertrophy in some persons. Causes are toxins of bacterial or metabolic origin (*Salmonella, Staphylococcus,* uremia, syphilis); irritation of the gastric mucosa by ingestion of ethyl alcohol, certain drugs (digitalis, glucogenic steroids, salicylates, and others), gastric irradiation, heavy metals, strong alkali or acid; or faulty dietary habits.

The latter may include excessive intake of fibrous, fried, or highly seasoned foods, very hot or very cold drinks, or rapid eating with poor mastication. Symptoms of indigestion usually occur.

Acute gastritis is characterized by a general inflammatory reaction of the mucosa with hyperemia, edema, and exudation; in more severe cases, erosion of localized areas and hemorrhages occur. Symptoms vary from anorexia, vague epigastric discomfort, or heartburn, to severe vomiting. The diagnosis of gastritis is based on biopsies of the gastric mucosa.

Since acute gastritis usually heals within three or four days, nutritional management is not the primary concern. Treatment is directed toward removal or neutralization of the offending agent by gastric lavage, antibiotics, withholding of food for 24 to 48 hours to allow the stomach to rest, and replacement of water and electrolyte losses due to severe vomiting. After one or two days small amounts of clear fluids (100 ml per hour) are administered with gradual progression to soft, easily digested foods (see page 394).

Chronic gastritis is characterized by recurrent inflammation of the gastric mucosa leading to glandular atrophy and changes in enzyme activities of the gastric mucosal cells. Complete atrophy results in the inability to absorb vitamin B_{12} and in pernicious anemia. Secretion of hydrochloric acid is impaired. Symptoms include epigastric distress, nausea, and vomiting. Chronic gastritis is often directly attributed to dietary indiscretion or indirectly to toxic substances; nevertheless, it may also occur in the absence of any known cause. Autoimmunologic factors, endocrine dysfunction, and nutritional deficiency, especially of iron, have been implicated.[1] Gastritis may be the cause of persistent symptoms in patients in whom peptic ulcer has seemingly healed.[12]

Dietary treatment of chronic gastritis consists in correcting faulty habits of eating or drinking, providing a relaxed atmosphere at mealtime, and emphasizing adequate caloric intake of soft or bland foods (see page 438). Arrangement of meals in four or six small feedings is sometimes preferred. Iron supplements may be desirable. Once symptoms have abated, progression to a normal diet may be made.

Carcinoma of the stomach. This usually occurs in persons over 50 years of age. Early diagnosis is essential for a complete cure. If the disease is not too far advanced a gastrectomy is done. Unfortunately, the disease is often well advanced before symptoms of anorexia, weight loss, fatigue, abdominal discomfort and pain, nausea, and vomiting appear. Since these symptoms are common to many disorders, positive evidence as shown by x-ray examination or cytologic studies is needed to establish the presence of malignancy. Iron-deficiency anemia, hypoalbuminemia, achlorhydria, or hypochlorhydria may also occur.

Following gastrectomy, the postoperative regimen is used (see page 483). Small, frequent meals are given. For those patients who develop the dumping syndrome, foods should be high in protein and fat and low in carbohydrate (see page 486).

When surgical intervention is not feasible, every effort is made to promote the patient's comfort. Frequent small feedings of soft, low-fiber foods are provided (see Chapter 27). It is most important that the meals be attractive to coax the patient's appetite, and that efforts be made to accommodate the patient's requests. Unnecessary dietary restrictions should be avoided.

Peptic Ulcer

The term *peptic ulcer* is used to describe any localized erosion of the mucosal lining of those portions of the alimentary tract that come in contact with gastric juice. The majority of ulcers are found in the duodenum, although they also occur in the esophagus, stomach, or jejunum. Similar symptoms are produced by the ulcer regardless of its location, and response to treatment is essentially the same. The same principles of dietary treatment apply to all regardless of etiology.

The incidence of peptic ulcer in the United States is approximately 10 per cent of the general population, occurring at any age, but particularly between the ages of 20 and 45. It occurs more frequently in males.

Etiology. In spite of extensive literature on the subject, the exact cause of peptic ulcer has not been determined. Multiple factors are probably involved. In duodenal ulcer, hypersecretion of acid is found, although tissue resistance is normal. In gastric ulcer, an abnormal pyloric sphincter is believed to permit reflux of bile salts from the duodenum into the stomach. Bile salts are capable of breaking the gastric mucosal barrier to hydrogen ions.[13]

Repeated irritation of the mucosa by dietary indiscretion or alcohol may lower the tissue resistance to acid, thereby making the individual more susceptible to ulcer formation. Likewise, certain drugs, such as the adrenal steroids and salicylates, may induce gastric ulceration either by their irritating effect on the mucosa or by a stimulating effect on acid secretion.

Personality type plays a role—highly nervous and emotional individuals seem to be more susceptible to the disease. Anxiety, worry, and strain may cause hypersecretion of acid and hypermotility. A positive family history of recurrent pain is not uncommon.

Symptoms and clinical findings. Epigastric pain occurring as deep hunger contractions one to three hours after meals is often the chief complaint. The pain may be described as dull, piercing, burning, or gnawing and is usually relieved by the taking of food or alkalies. The basis for the pain may be the action of unneutralized hydrochloric acid on exposed nerve fibers at the site of the ulcer. Pain is also associated with hypermotility of the stomach or gastric distention following ingestion of large amounts of food or liquids.

Low plasma protein levels are often present and delay rapid and complete healing of the ulcer. Weight loss and iron-deficiency anemia are common. The intake of iron, ascorbic acid, and the B-complex vitamins, particularly thiamin, may be less than desirable because of self-imposed limitation of leafy green vegetables and other food sources of these nutrients. (See Chapters 8, 11, and 12.)

In some instances, hemorrhage is the first indication of an ulcer and requires surgical intervention. Other complications such as intractability, obstruction, perforation, and carcinoma of gastric ulcer are treated surgically.

Rationale for treatment. Individualized attention to the whole person rather than to the ulcer per se is extremely important in the management of persons with ulcer disease. The patient must be taught to accept responsibility for his progress since medical and dietary therapies produce only symptomatic improvement. In general, treatment consists of drugs, rest, and diet therapy.

Drugs. Antacid preparations are prescribed to neutralize excess acid production. *Anticholinergic* drugs are used to inhibit acid secretion, and *antispasmodics* delay gastric emptying.

Rest. Good physical and mental hygiene is basic if the person is to learn to cope with his problems constructively. Mental and physical rest is important; modification of living and work habits is needed when overwork and physical stress cause exacerbations of the disease. Control of emotional stress is equally important.

Diet. Dietary management consists of providing a nutritionally adequate diet that includes frequent feedings. Such a diet is essential for persons with ulcers not only to promote rapid healing but to correct preexisting deficiencies. In some instances, intakes of nutrients in excess of the Recommended Dietary Allowances are desirable, with particular emphasis on high-quality protein, ascorbic acid, and iron. To help maintain neutrality of the gastric contents small feedings every two hours are often used initially with later progression to three meals plus snacks at midmorning, midafternoon, and bedtime. Establishing regularity of mealtimes is an important aspect of the diet. Some individuals experience fewer subjective symptoms if fiber is restricted (see below). Individualization of the diet to meet the patient's needs and preferences is essential.

BLAND FIBER-RESTRICTED DIET IN THREE STAGES

Characteristics and General Rules

The stages of diet are set up for gradual progression in quantity of food eaten at a meal, in fiber content, and in selection of foods.

The selection of foods includes those mild in flavor, and which infrequently bring forth complaints of intolerance. The lists should not be considered as restrictive, inasmuch as food tolerance is a highly individual matter. Additions or subtractions should be made according to individual need.

For patients with peptic ulcer, frequent feedings are essential. The six-meal sample menus listed below could be arranged for two-hourly feedings of smaller size, if the physician believes this to be necessary.

FOOD SELECTION FOR THREE STAGES OF DIET

Stages I and II

Beverages—milk and fruit juices

Breads—enriched white bread or toast; saltines; soda crackers; Melba toast; zwieback

Cereals—cornflakes, cornmeal, farina, hominy grits, oatmeal, Puffed Rice, rice flakes; macaroni, noodles, rice, spaghetti

Cheese—mild American in sauces; cream; cottage

Desserts—plain cake and cookies; custard; fruit whip; gelatin; plain ice cream; bread, cornstarch, rice, or tapioca puddings without raisins or nuts

Eggs—any way except fried

Fats—butter, cream, margarine, smooth peanut butter, cooking fat, vegetable oils

Fruits—fruit juices; avocado, banana, grapefruit and orange sections; baked apple without skin, applesauce; canned apricots, cherries, peaches, pears

Meat—tender or ground. Baked, broiled, creamed, roasted, stewed: beef, chicken, fish, lamb, liver, pork, sweetbreads, turkey, veal

Milk—in all forms

Seasonings—salt, sugar, flavoring extracts

Soups—cream

Vegetables—cooked; asparagus tips, green and wax beans, beets, carrots, white potato, winter squash, spinach, sweet potato

Stage III

All foods of stages I and II plus the following:

Beverages—decaffeinated coffee; 1 cup regular coffee with half milk, if desired; weak tea

Breads—rye without seeds; fine whole wheat

Cereals—all except coarse bran

Cheeses—all

Eggs—including fried

Fats—mayonnaise and salad dressings

Fruits—raw apple, cherries, peaches, pears, plums; stewed apricots and prunes

Seasonings—allspice, cinnamon, mace, paprika, sage, thyme

Soups—fish chowders

Vegetables—lettuce and other tender salad greens; celery; tomatoes; any others as tolerated

MEAL PATTERNS FOR STAGES I AND II

Stage I
(10–12 oz per meal)
ON AWAKING
Milk—8 oz
  BREAKFAST
Cereal—4 oz
Milk—4 oz
Sugar
Egg—1
White toast—1 slice
Butter

  MIDMORNING
Milk beverage—8 oz
Crackers, custard, plain pudding, gelatin—3 oz
  LUNCHEON
Cream soup—4 oz
Crackers—2

Stage II
(approximately 12–16 oz)

Milk—8 oz

Cooked or dry cereal
Milk
Sugar
Egg
Enriched toast
Butter
Fruit juice or fruit

Milk beverage—8 oz
Crackers, custard, plain pudding, gelatin

Cream soup
Crackers

Stage I (Cont.)
Egg—1; or mild cheese—1 oz; or tender meat—1 oz
White bread or toast—1 slice
Butter
Dessert—3 to 4 oz
Citrus juice—3 oz

MIDAFTERNOON
Milk beverage—8 oz
Crackers, custard, plain pudding, gelatin—3 oz
DINNER
Egg, soft cheese, or tender meat—1 oz
Potato or substitute—3 oz
Toast or bread—1 slice
Butter
Fruit—3 oz
Milk or cream soup—4 oz

EVENING
Milk beverage—8 oz
Crackers or dessert—3 oz

Stage II (Cont.)
Meat, fish, poultry, eggs, or cheese—2 to 3 oz
Potato or substitute
White bread or toast
Butter
Dessert
Fruit
Milk

Milk beverage or small meat sandwich
Plain dessert

Meat, fish, poultry, eggs, or cheese—3 oz
Potato or substitute
Cooked vegetable
Bread or roll
Butter
Fruit or dessert
Milk

Milk beverage or small meat sandwich
Crackers or plain dessert

A TYPICAL DAY'S MENU FOR STAGE III

BREAKFAST
Stewed apricots
Oatmeal with milk and sugar
Soft-cooked egg
Enriched toast with butter
Coffee with half milk—1 cup
MIDMORNING
Milk—8 oz
Saltines—4
LUNCHEON
Cream of asparagus soup
Baked rice with cheese
Buttered peas
Lettuce and sliced tomatoes with mayonnaise
Rye bread and butter

Vanilla ice cream
Milk
MIDAFTERNOON
Chicken sandwich
Jello
DINNER
Broiled lamb chop
Mashed potato
Diced buttered beets
Dinner roll with butter
Sliced peaches (fresh, frozen, or canned)
Milk

EVENING NOURISHMENT
Malted milk
Sugar cookies

Modification of diet in bleeding ulcer. The degree of dietary modification in bleeding ulcer depends on the peculiarities of the individual case. In severe hemorrhage, it is customary to give no food until the bleeding has been controlled and the patient's condition is stabilized. If hemorrhage is not severe, and if nausea and vomiting are not a problem, the patient may desire food and tolerate it well. Initial dietary treatment usually consists of milk alternated at two-hour intervals with small feedings of easily digested foods, such as egg, custards or simple puddings, toast, crackers, and tender cooked fruits and vegetables. Gradual progression in amounts and types of foods is made as the patient improves.

DIETARY COUNSELING

The patient with an ulcer needs careful counseling about his diet with emphasis on positive rather than negative aspects of the diet. He needs to know which foods are needed for a nutritionally adequate diet and the importance of including these daily. He should be taught to select an essentially normal diet from a wide variety of foods, omitting those foods which he knows to be distressing to him. Moderate use of seasonings is permitted and may greatly enhance the flavor of foods. The patient should be instructed to establish regularity of mealtimes, to include between-meal snacks—preferably of some protein foods, and to use moderation in amounts eaten. If the diet to be used at home is planned with the patient, giving consideration to his cultural pattern, he is more likely to follow recommendations made. Meals eaten in restaurants should pose no particular problems if the individual uses good judgment in food selection.

The dietitian or nurse should stress the importance of eating meals in a relaxed atmosphere with a happy frame of mind and advise the patient to try to forget personal or family problems while eating. A short rest before and after meals may be conducive to greater enjoyment of meals.

Ulcers frequently recur even after complete healing is believed to have taken place. To prevent recurrence of symptoms prompt treatment is advisable following great stress. The stomach tends to be empty of foods but full of highly acid gastric juice throughout the night and it is likely that this is the period when the greatest part of the injury to the gastric and duodenal mucosa occurs. In periods of great emotional strain, taking of food every few hours from dinnertime until 2 or 3 o'clock in the morning is recommended.

PROBLEMS AND REVIEW

1. List some of the nutritional disturbances which may develop when the stomach and intestinal tract are impaired.

2. Miss B. is a 28-year-old file clerk who is about 20 pounds overweight and has a hiatal hernia. Her physician has recommended a diet with small frequent feedings for her but she is afraid she will gain weight if she follows the diet. What suggestions could you offer to assist her in planning her diet?

3. Mrs. D. is a 33-year-old housewife who complains of indigestion. Name five dietary factors which could lead to development of this condition. What recommendations would you make concerning her diet?

4. Mrs. G. and Mrs. F. are discussing their husbands' recent hospitalizations for peptic ulcer. Mr. G.'s physician recommended a traditional bland diet; Mr. F. was advised to follow a liberal bland diet.
   a. In what respects would you expect their diets to be similar? How would you expect them to differ?
   b. Mr. G. will soon return to his teaching position and he plans to carry his lunch to school. Plan a day's menu for him.
   c. List five food combinations suitable for between-meal feedings for Mr. G.
   d. Mr. F. eats lunch in a restaurant. Plan a day's menu for him.

5. Mrs. G. does not understand the reasons for some of the recommendations made concerning her husband's diet. Explain the principle involved in each of the following:
   a. Milk.
   b. Those foods that depress acid secretion.
   c. Foods that are most effective in acid neutralization.
   d. Feedings at two-hour intervals.
   e. Omission of coffee and tea.

6. Mrs. F. has asked whether it makes any difference what foods her husband eats as long as he takes antacids. What would you tell her in regard to:
   a. Foods that are most likely to stimulate acid secretion.
   b. Those foods that depress acid secretion.
   c. Foods that are most effective in acid neutralization.
   d. Foods that increase motility of the gastrointestinal tract.

7. Mr. F. is concerned that his ulcer will recur when he returns to his job and his very demanding boss. What prophylactic measures can he take to prevent recurrence?

8. What possible role may diet play during the emotional stress to which some patients with peptic ulcer may be subjected?

CITED REFERENCES

1. Weinstein, L., *et al.:* "Diet as Related to Gastrointestinal Function," *J.A.M.A.,* **176:**935–41, 1961.
2. Schneider, M. A., *et al.:* "The Effect of Spice Ingestion upon the Stomach," *Am. J. Gastroenterol.,* **26:**722–32, 1956.
3. Hunt, J. N., and Stubbs, D. F.: "The Volume and Energy Content of Meals as Determinants of Gastric Emptying," *J. Physiol.,* **245:**209–25, 1975.
4. Haenel, H.: "Human Normal and Abnormal Gastrointestinal Flora," *Am. J. Clin. Nutr.,* **23:**1433–39, 1970.
5. Speck, R. S., *et al.:* "Human Fecal Flora under Controlled Diet Intake," *Am. J. Clin. Nutr.,* **23:**1488–94, 1970.
6. Shull, H. J.: "Diet in the Management of Peptic Ulcer," *J.A.M.A.,* **170:**1068–71, 1959.
7. Sippy, B. W.: "Gastric and Duodenal Ulcers. Medical Cure by an Efficient Removal of Gastric Juice Corrosion," *J.A.M.A.,* **64:**1625–30, 1915.
8. Meulengracht, E.: "Treatment of Haematemesis and Melaena with Food," *Lancet,* **2:**1220–22, 1935.
9. Castell, D. O.: "Diet and the Lower Esophageal Sphincter," *Am. J. Clin. Nutr.,* **28:**1296–98, 1975.
10. Cohen, S.: "Gastroesophageal Reflux," *Postgrad. Med.,* **57:**97–101, Jan. 1975.
11. Taylor, K. B.: "Gastritis," *N. Engl. J. Med.,* **280:**818–20, 1969.
12. Edwards, F. C., and Coghill, N. F.: "Clinical Manifestations in Patients with Chronic Atrophic Gastritis, Gastric Ulcer, and Duodenal Ulcer," *Q. J. Med.,* **37:**337–60, 1968.
13. Isenberg, J. I.: "Peptic Ulcer Disease," *Postgrad. Med.,* **57:**163–68, Jan. 1975.

ADDITIONAL REFERENCES

"The American Dietetic Association Position Paper on Bland Diet in the Treatment of Chronic Duodenal Ulcer Disease," *J. Am. Diet. Assoc.,* **59:**244–45, 1971.

Berman, P. M., and Kirsner, J. B.: "The Aging Gut: I. Diseases of the Esophagus, Small Intestine and Appendix," *Geriatrics,* **27:**84–89, March 1972.

Brooks, F. P.: "Clinical Usefulness of Gastric Acid Secretory Tests," *Postgrad. Med.,* **51:**188–93, Feb. 1972.

Cooke, A. R.: "Control of Gastric Emptying and Motility," *Gastroenterology,* **68:**804–16, 1975.

Cummings, J. H.: "Dietary Fibre," *Gut,* **14:**69–81, 1973.

Donaldson, R. M., Jr.: "The Muddle of Diets for Gastrointestinal Disorders," *J.A.M.A.,* **225:**1243, 1973.

Friedman, G. D.: "Cigarettes, Alcohol, Coffee, and Peptic Ulcer," *N. Engl. J. Med.,* **290:**469–73, 1974.

Hegedus, S., and Pelham, M.: "Dietetics in a Cancer Hospital," *J. Am. Diet. Assoc.,* **67:**235–40, 1975.

Jeffries, G. H.: "Gastritis," *DM:*3–32, 1973.

Katz, D., and Pitchumoni, C. S.: "Management of the Hiatal Hernia—Esophagitis Complex in the Elderly," *Geriatrics,* **28:**84–87, Oct. 1973.

Lipshutz, W. H., *et al.:* "Pathogenesis of Lower-Esophageal-Sphincter Incompetence," *N. Engl. J. Med.,* **289:**182–84, 1974.

Lowenfels, A. B.: "Etiological Aspects of Cancer of the Gastrointestinal Tract," *Surg. Gynecol. Obstet.,* **137:**291–99, 1973.

Roth, H. P., and Caron, H. S.: "Patients' Misconceptions About Their Peptic Ulcer Diets. Potential Obstacles to Cooperation," *J. Chronic Dis.,* **20:**5–11, 1967.

Sapp, O. L.: "Treatment of Duodenal Ulcer," *Am. Fam. Physician,* **7:**128–34, Feb. 1973.

Sheiner, H. J.: "Gastric Emptying Tests in Man," *Gut,* **16:**235–47, 1975.

Welch, C. E.: "Abdominal Surgery," *N. Engl. J. Med.,* **293:**858–63, 1975.

33 Diet in Disturbances of the Small Intestine and Colon

Very Low-Residue Diet; High-Fiber Diet

The functions of the small intestine may be unfavorably influenced by diseases affecting the tract itself or those organs closely related to the digestive process—the liver, gallbladder, and pancreas. In addition, many seemingly unrelated pathologic conditions to be discussed in chapters that follow have profound effects on the functioning of the gastrointestinal tract, for example, renal diseases. Depending upon the nature of the disease, there may be disturbances in motility, adequacy of enzyme production or release, hydrolytic activity, integrity of the mucosal surfaces, transport mechanisms, and so on. Any of these abnormalities interferes with the efficiency and completeness of absorption and hence the nutritional status of the individual. This chapter includes a discussion of alterations in bowel motility, inflammatory diseases

of the mucosa, and carcinoma of the bowel. The malabsorption syndrome will be discussed in the chapter that follows, and diseases of the liver, gallbladder, and pancreas in Chapter 35.

ALTERATIONS IN BOWEL MOTILITY

Diarrhea. Diarrhea is the passage of stools of liquid to semisolid consistency at frequent intervals. In diarrhea, a reduction in segmental activity of the sigmoid colon lowers intraluminal pressure and peripheral resistance, permitting more rapid passage of intestinal contents.[1] The number of stools varies from several per day to one every few minutes. Diarrhea is a symptom of underlying functional or organic disease and is acute or chronic in nature. Some causes of diarrhea are shown in Table 33–1.

Acute diarrhea is characterized by the sudden onset of frequent stools of watery consistency, abdominal pain, cramping, weakness, and sometimes fever and vomiting. Since the duration is usually 24 to 48 hours, nutritional losses are not a prime concern. Acute diarrhea may be the presenting symptom of systemic infection or chronic gastrointestinal disease such as regional enteritis or ulcerative colitis.

In chronic diarrhea, nutritional deficiencies eventually develop because the rapid passage of the intestinal contents does not allow sufficient time for absorption.

Nutritional considerations in diarrheas. Fluid, electrolyte, and tissue protein losses are usually severe if diarrhea is prolonged.

Fluids. Losses of fluids should be replaced by a liberal intake to prevent dehydration, especially in

Table 33–1. Some Causes of Diarrhea

Acute Types	Chronic Types
1. Chemical toxins, such as arsenic, lead, mercury, or cadmium	1. Malabsorptive lesions of anatomic, mucosal, or enzymatic origin
2. Bacterial toxins, such as *Salmonella* or staphylococcal food poisoning	2. Metabolic diseases, such as diabetic neuropathy, uremia, or Addison's disease
3. Bacterial infections, such as *Streptococcus, E. coli,* or *Shigella*	3. Alcoholism
4. Drugs, such as quinidine, colchicine, or neomycin	4. Carcinoma of small bowel or colon
5. Psychogenic factors, such as emotional instability	5. Postirradiation to small bowel or colon
6. Dietary factors, such as food sensitivity or allergy	6. Cirrhosis
	7. Laxative abuse

susceptible age groups such as the very young or elderly persons. Parenteral fluids are often administered to these individuals.

Electrolytes. Losses of sodium, potassium, and other electrolytes account for the profound weakness associated with severe diarrhea. Potassium loss, in particular, is detrimental as potassium is necessary for normal muscle tone of the gastrointestinal tract. Anorexia, vomiting, listlessness, and muscle weakness may occur unless losses are replaced by a liberal intake of fluids such as fruit juices that are high in potassium (see Chapter 42).

Nutrient malabsorption. Long-continued diarrhea may result in depletion of tissue proteins and decreased serum protein levels. Fat losses are considerable in certain disorders with consequent loss of calories and fat-soluble vitamins. Intake of calories must be great enough to replace losses and may need to be as high as 3000, with 100 to 150 gm protein, 100 to 120 gm fat, and the remainder as carbohydrate (see Chapter 30).

Vitamin deficiencies frequently seen in chronic diarrheas are related to the decreased intake of vitamins and the increased requirements because of losses in the stools. A temporary reduction of synthesis of some B-complex vitamins also occurs when antibiotic therapy is used. Vitamin B_{12}, folic acid, and niacin deficiencies have been observed in various diarrheas.

Iron deficiency is a prominent finding in patients with chronic diarrhea owing to the increased losses of iron in the feces, the occasional blood losses, and the reduced intake of iron-rich foods because of fear that some foods might aggravate an existing lesion. Patients often show remarkable improvement when given supplemental iron therapy.

Diet in diarrheal states. Any dietary modification in diarrheal states depends on the nature of the underlying defect. In acute diarrhea, clear liquids are usually tolerated best until the bowel has a chance to rest, usually 12 to 24 hours, after which progression to a soft (see Chapter 27) or regular diet is made.

Many patients with chronic diarrhea of functional or organic nature do not tolerate milk or foods high in fat or fiber content. Generally speaking, however, the need is for a diet high in protein (see Chapter 30) and calories, with adequate amounts of vitamins and minerals, and liberal amounts of fluids.

Constipation. In this condition, hypermotility of the sigmoid colon increases resistance to movement of intestinal contents; consequently, there is distention and infrequent or difficult evacuation of feces from the intestine. An accurate definition is related to personal habits since the frequency of bowel movements varies greatly among individuals. For some, daily elimination is normal; in other equally healthy persons, regular evacuation occurs every second or third day.

Infrequent or insufficient emptying of the bowel may lead to malaise, headache, coated tongue, foul breath, and lack of appetite. These symptoms usually disappear after satisfactory evacuation has taken place.

Temporary or chronic constipation can be due to any one of a number of factors such as: (1) failure to establish regular times for eating, adequate rest, and elimination; (2) faulty dietary habits, such as inadequate fluid intake or use of highly refined and concentrated foods that leave little residue in the colon; (3) interference with the urge to defecate brought on by poor personal hygiene or injury to the nervous mechanism; (4) changes in one's usual routine brought on by illness, nervous tension, or a trip away from home; (5) chronic use of laxatives and cathartics; (6) difficult or painful defecation due to hemorrhoids or fissures; (7) poor muscle tone of the intestine and stasis due to lack of exercise occurring especially in bedridden patients, invalids such as arthritics, the aged, and others; (8) organic disorders, such as diverticulosis or obstruction from adhesions or neoplasms; (9) ingestion of drugs, large amounts of sedatives, ganglionic blocking agents, or opiates; and (10) spasm of the intestine due to presence of irritating material, psychogenic influences, or others.

Determination of the cause is important so that proper treatment can be given. Correction of constipation depends in large measure on establishing regularity in habits—eating, rest, exercise, and elimination.

Dietary considerations. Attention to diet may be beneficial in *atonic* and *spastic* constipation (see Irritable Colon Syndrome, below). In the atonic type the diet should contain sufficient fiber to induce peristalsis and to contribute bulk to the intestine. A regular diet with an abundance of both raw and cooked fruits and vegetables is suitable for such patients. Whole-grain breads and cereals should be substituted for refined ones. Bran is useful for some patients but excesses are to be avoided since it may act as an irritant to sensitive intestinal tracts. Fat-containing foods such as bacon, butter, cream, and oils are useful for some because of the stimulating effect of the fatty acids on the mucous membranes. Excesses may cause diarrhea and should be avoided. Mineral oil if used should not be taken at mealtime because of its interference with the absorption of fat-soluble vitamins.

A fluid intake of 8 to 10 glasses a day aids in keeping the intestinal contents in a semisolid state for easier passage along the tract. Some individuals find that 1 or 2 glasses of hot or cold water, plain or with lemon, are helpful in initiating peristalsis when taken before breakfast.

Irritable colon syndrome. This condition, also known as *spastic colon,* is a functional disorder involving a disturbance in normal motor activity of the colon. This disorder probably accounts for 50 to 70 per cent of all gastrointestinal complaints. It is considered by some to be a forerunner of diverticular disease.

Etiology. Many factors contribute to this functional disorder. Included are excessive use of laxatives or cathartics; antibiotic therapy; food allergy; inadequate dietary fiber; poor hygiene in regard to rest, work, fluid intake, and elimination; and emotional upsets. Nervous, tense individuals are especially sensitive to gastrointestinal neurosis.

Symptoms. The most frequent symptom is pain, due to gaseous distention or to vigorous contractions of the colon. Pain is described as dull aching, cramping, or sharp and intermittent and may be accompanied by anorexia, nausea, and vomiting. Headache, palpitation, and heartburn sometimes occur. Constipation, or diarrhea, or both may occur in the same individual. Weight loss is uncommon.

Treatment. The underlying causes should be determined and corrected. Most patients need help in developing good personal and mental hygiene. Through counseling the individual will hopefully gain insight into the relationship between tension and his symptoms. Faulty eating habits must be corrected and the use of laxatives forbidden.

Dietary treatment for those patients with irritable colon syndrome who are constipated should consist of foods that increase intestinal residue enough to aid in evacuation.[2] Increased amounts of fruits, vegetables, and whole-grain cereals provide additional bulk. Some persons experience relief of symptoms when unprocessed bran is added to the diet.[3]

In recurrent diarrhea, a diet restricted in fiber and residue allows the colon the most rest (see page 446).

Intestinal obstruction. The movement of the intestinal contents is impaired or prevented by many causes such as tumors, impaction of material in the intestine, or paralytic ileus following surgery. As a rule, the obstruction must be removed by surgical intervention before an adequate diet can be administered. The postoperative diet should be fiber free (see page 446) for a period of time, following which a soft diet is usually ordered.

INFLAMMATORY DISEASE OF THE MUCOSA

Regional enteritis. (*Crohn's disease, granulomatous colitis*). This is a chronic, nonspecific inflammatory disease involving chiefly the terminal ileum, but which affects any part of the intestine. The cause is unknown, although genetic, environmental, and psychogenic factors have been implicated. The disease occurs most frequently in young adults and may have an acute or insidious onset.

The inflammatory reaction extends through the entire intestinal wall causing edema and fibrosis. It may be confined to one segment or involve multiple segments with normal areas in between.

Characteristic symptoms include abdominal pain, cramping, diarrhea, steatorrhea, weight loss, fever, and weakness. Systemic complications, malnutrition, and fistula formation are common.

Conservative management is used unless obstruction or other complications make surgical intervention (ileal resection) necessary.

Dietary considerations. The diet should provide at least 125 gm protein and 2500 kcal to overcome losses due to exudation and malabsorption (see Chapter 30). Medium-chain-triglyceride therapy (see Chapter 34) is effective in reducing steatorrhea and electrolyte losses in some patients. Foods high in potassium should be given in cases of prolonged diarrhea (see Chapter 42). During acute attacks, diets very low in residue (see below) are given initially in order to eliminate foods known to stimulate peristalsis and to prevent danger of obstruction.

Supplements of iron, folic acid, and vitamin B_{12} are needed to overcome deficiencies. Alternatively, synthetic low-residue diets (Chapter 34) or total parenteral nutrition (Chapter 36) is sometimes used to restore nutrition while permitting the bowel to rest. Progression to a regular diet is made, eliminating only those foods known by the patient to aggra-

vate symptoms.[4] For many persons some degree of fiber restriction is desirable.

Diverticulosis. In this condition, many small mucosal sacs, called DIVERTICULA, protrude through the intestinal wall. Most diverticula are found in the sigmoid colon, although they have been demon-

---

VERY LOW-RESIDUE DIET

Characteristics and General Rules

This diet is essentially fiber free and leaves a minimum of residue in the intestinal tract. See discussion on
  page 433.

If the diet is used for more than a few days, it should be supplemented with calcium, iron, and multivitamin
  concentrates.

As improvement takes place, the diet is liberalized by gradually adding tender cooked vegetables and fruits,
  and milk.

Foods Allowed

Beverages—coffee in limited amounts, tea

Breads—enriched bread or toast, crackers, plain rolls, Melba toast, zwieback

Cereals—cornmeal, farina, strained oatmeal; cornflakes, Puffed Rice, rice flakes; macaroni, noodles, rice, spaghetti

Cheese—cottage, cream, mild American in sauces

Desserts—plain cake, cookies, custard, gelatin, ice cream, puddings, rennet desserts

Eggs—cooked any way except fried

Fats—butter, cream, margarine, vegetable oils

Fruits—strained juices only. Occasionally applesauce is given to patients with diarrhea because of its pectin content.

Meats—tender or minced lean meat, fish, or poultry

Soups—clear: bouillon or broth without fat

Sweets—hard candy, honey, jelly, syrup, sugar in moderation

Vegetables—tomato juice; white potato

Miscellaneous—salt; spices in moderation

Foods to Avoid

Beverages—milk and milk drinks

Breads—whole-grain breads or crackers

Cereals—whole grain such as wheat flakes, wheat meal, granola type

Cheese—sharp

Desserts—with fruit or nuts; pies and pastries. Note: milk desserts are occasionally omitted.

Fruits—all except juices

Meats—tough; fried; fatty meats, fish, or poultry such as pork, mackerel, goose

Soups—fatty; cream; spicy

Sweets—with fruit or nuts; jam, marmalade

Vegetables—all except tomato juice and potato

Miscellaneous—nuts, popcorn, pickles, excessive seasonings

Meal Pattern

BREAKFAST
Strained fruit juice
Refined cereal with cream and sugar
Egg
White toast with butter
Coffee with cream and sugar

DINNER
Strained citrus juice
Tender meat, poultry, or fish

Potato or substitute
White bread with butter
Plain dessert
Coffee or tea
  LUNCHEON OR SUPPER
Broth
Tender meat, fowl, fish, or cheese
Potato, rice, macaroni, or noodles
White bread with butter
Plain dessert
Coffee or tea

strated throughout the length of the gastrointestinal tract. Diverticulosis is fairly common and the incidence increases with age.

The underlying defect is attributed to abnormal thickening of the muscle layers of the sigmoid colon resulting in narrowing of the lumen and increased intraluminal pressure.[5] Contraction of the colon further increases pressure within the lumen and leads to herniation of the mucosa through the intestinal wall at points where it is weakened by penetration of blood vessels. Intraluminal pressure is greater when the diet is low in residue. On the other hand, foods that leave a high residue increase the volume and weight of materials reaching the sigmoid colon, and, by distending the colon, may prevent development of high-pressure segments. For this reason, foods high in fiber (see below) have been recommended for use in diverticulosis.[6] Low-residue diets formerly used in this disorder are now considered to be contraindicated.[2]

DIVERTICULITIS occurs when one or more diverticula become inflamed and perforate. Inflammation usually results from accumulation of food particles or residues in the sacs and subsequent bacterial action. Symptoms include steady pain in the lower left abdomen, abdominal distention, changes in bowel habits—usually as constipation, colonic spasm, and occasionally fever. Steatorrhea and megaloblastic anemia, often associated with small bowel diverticula, are due to stasis.

The management of acute attacks of diverticulitis includes bed rest, antibiotics, and clear liquids with progression to a very low-residue diet (see page 446). In recurrent or persistent attacks, surgical resection of the involved portion of colon may be necessary. Complications, such as obstruction, perforation, or fistula formation, also necessitate surgical intervention.

DIETARY COUNSELING

Persons with diverticular disease who are placed on high-fiber diets need careful counseling in regard to the purpose of the diet. Those accustomed to restricting fiber intake may be especially apprehensive about such a drastic change in their diets and need frequent reassurance from the dietitian and the nurse. For most patients, increasing the fiber content of the diet should be made gradually. Whole-grain cereals should be used, and breads and other baked goods made with 100 per cent whole wheat or whole rye flour substituted for those made with white flour. Generous amounts of fruits and vegetables such as raw carrots, apples, oranges, and lettuce, stewed fruits, potatoes cooked in skins, and so on should be encouraged. Some physicians may recommend the use of bran, the amount depending on the fiber content of the rest of the diet. It is usually best to start with 1 tablespoon of bran per day in a liquid such as milk or juice, gradually increasing the amount of bran until one soft stool is produced daily or until symptoms are relieved. Some patients experience flatulence and distention at first but the diet should not be discontinued because of these. Bran can be mixed with foods such as cereals, soups, or puddings, or added to homemade breads, muffins, and cakes.

HIGH-FIBER DIET

Characteristics
This diet is essentially a regular diet with fiber content increased as follows:
  1. Substitute at least four servings whole-grain bread and cereals for refined breads and cereals.
  2. Emphasize raw fruits and vegetables that are high in fiber.
  3. Add 1 to 2 tablespoons bran each day.

The substitution of fibrous foods should be made gradually; for example, whole-grain breads and cereals are added first; then fibrous cooked fruits and vegetables followed by raw fruits and vegetables.

Foods Allowed
Beverages—all
Breads—breads, muffins, or rolls made from 100 per cent whole-wheat or whole-rye flour; graham, wheat, or rye crackers; Ry-Krisp
Cereals—whole grain such as oatmeal, rolled oats; bran flakes, granola; grapenuts; shredded wheat, wheat flakes; brown rice; bran, in moderation
Cheese—all
Desserts—all, with fruit and nuts, if tolerated
Eggs—all
Fats—all

Fruits—all, including dried; preferably raw
Meats—all
Soups—all, preferably vegetable
Sweets—jam, marmalade, preserves
Vegetables—all, especially raw; potatoes in skin
Miscellaneous—condiments and seasonings in moderation

Sample Menu
BREAKFAST
Orange sections
Oatmeal with milk and brown sugar
Poached egg
Bran muffins
Butter or margarine
Marmalade
Coffee
LUNCHEON OR SUPPER
Vegetable soup
Club sandwich:
Sliced turkey
Bacon
Whole-wheat bread
Lettuce and tomato
Mayonnaise
Baked apple with raisin stuffing
Milk
DINNER
Brown beef stew
Onions
Carrots
Oven-browned potato
Coleslaw with pineapple
Rye bread
Butter or margarine
Apricot fruit crisp
Tea with lemon and sugar
BEDTIME SNACK
Milk
Fresh pear
Graham crackers

Ulcerative colitis. This is a diffuse inflammatory and ulcerative disease of unknown etiology involving the mucosa and submucosa of the large intestine. No single etiologic factor has been identified, although genetic and autoimmune factors are thought to be involved. The role of psychologic factors in initiation of this disease is uncertain although such factors are probably involved in relapses.[7]

Symptoms and clinical findings. Ulcerative colitis may occur at any age but predominates in young adults. The onset is insidious in the majority of cases with mild abdominal discomfort, an urgent need to defecate several times a day, and diarrhea accompanied by rectal bleeding. Loss of water, electrolytes, blood, and protein from the colon produces systemic symptoms such as weight loss, dehydration, fever, anemia, and general debility. In early stages the mucosa is edematous and hyperemic. In more severe disease, necrosis and frank ulceration of the mucosa occur. The severity of the symptoms does not necessarily correlate with the extent of the disease. Patients with localized disease can be very seriously ill; on the other hand, persons with very troublesome symptoms may have mild disease.

Dietary considerations. One of the most important factors in the dietary management of this disorder is the individual attention given to the patient. Frequent visits by the dietitian and the nurse can do much toward convincing the patient of a sincere interest in his welfare. Many individuals with this disease are extremely apprehensive about what they can eat and seem to need constant reassurance. Mealtime visits provide an excellent opportunity to give encouragement and support.

Much patience and understanding are needed in helping ulcerative colitis patients with dietary problems. The diet must be highly individualized and yet be nutritionally adequate. Genuine efforts to meet the patient's requests must be made; he must never be made to feel that his numerous questions and frequent demands are troublesome. On the other hand, gentle, but firm guidance must be given in helping the patient select a nutritionally adequate diet. He must understand he is expected to eat his entire meal. Many patients have poor appetites, and it may be preferable to provide six or eight small feedings; for others, however, having less frequent meal intervals is a more satisfactory approach. (See Figure 33–1).

Liberal amounts of high-quality protein (up to 150 gm daily) are needed since nitrogen losses from the bowel may be considerable (see Chapter 30). Emphasis should be on tender meats, fish, poultry, and eggs for those patients who are allergic or intolerant to milk. Intakes of 3000 kcal, or more, are necessary to replace losses due to steatorrhea, and to promote weight gain. The very low-residue diet may be used at first; thereafter, some degree of fiber restriction is usually needed as many ulcerative colitis patients do not tolerate raw fruits or vegetables, and further damage to an already inflamed mucosa must be prevented. The bland, fiber-restricted diet (Chapter 32) is usually suitable. Supplementary vitamins and minerals are usually indicated to compensate for gastrointestinal losses and inadequate dietary intake. Especially important are iron salts when anemia is present, and calcium salts if milk is not tolerated.

CARCINOMA OF THE INTESTINE

Cancer of the colon is the second most frequent cause of death among all types of cancer in the United States.[8] This type of cancer progresses rapidly but is rarely symptomatic until the disease is well advanced. Pain, diarrhea or constipation, and weight loss are common symptoms.

The incidence of carcinoma of the bowel is higher in persons with long-standing Crohn's disease[9] or ulcerative colitis.[10]

The role of diet as an etiologic factor in cancer of the colon has been of considerable interest in recent years. Animal proteins, fats, and low-fiber intakes have all been implicated. [11-13] It is hypothesized that the typical Western diet favors the growth of bacteria that degrade sterols and bile acids to metabolites that are potentially carcinogenic. Moreover, the transit time through the intestinal tract is prolonged so that there is more time for potentially toxic materials to affect the mucosa.

Dietary treatment. When tumors can be excised, dietary management following operation is the same as that following any intestinal surgery (see Chapter 36). For inoperable tumors, the comfort of the patient is of prime concern. Most such patients are more comfortable if fiber is restricted and small, frequent meals are provided.

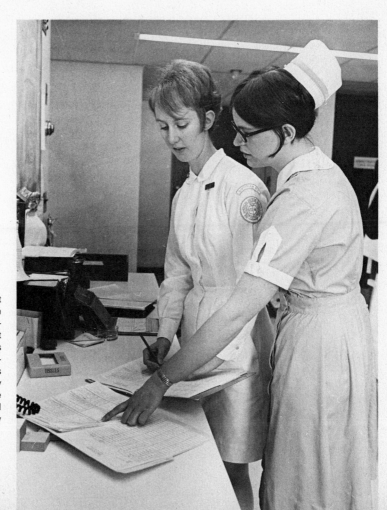

Figure 33–1. The patient's chart provides important information that must be considered in planning nutritional care. The chart should include progress notes concerning the patient's acceptance of his diet and any problems of nutritional adequacy that may be present. Sometime the intake of specific nutrients is calculated and charted. (Courtesy, Yale–New Haven Medical Center.)

PROBLEMS AND REVIEW

1. Discuss the role of diet in the incidence of diseases of the small intestine and colon.
2. What is the relationship of psychologic factors to the occurrence of gastrointestinal disorders? Cite examples.
3. What do the terms *fiber* and *residue* mean?
4. Mrs. K. is troubled with chronic diarrhea, although her physician has ruled out organic disease. What other factors might provoke diarrhea? In what ways would you expect her diet to be modified? What are the reasons for each modification?
5. Mrs. L. complains of constipation. List five possible causes.
   a. What type of person is likely to develop atonic constipation?
   b. What factors should be considered in treating constipation?
   c. What dietary recommendations would you make for Mrs. L.?
6. Mrs. R., now 75 years of age, has been troubled with diverticulosis for 20 years. For much of this time she has been on a low-residue diet. Her physician has recently recommended that she start eating whole-grain breads and cereals daily and that she add 2 tablespoons of bran to her diet daily.
   a. Mrs. R. is afraid to change her eating habits after all these years. How would you advise her in regard to the diet?
   b. What is the first change you would suggest Mrs. R. make in her diet?
   c. Mrs. R. states that she cannot afford to purchase the bran and fruits and vegetables. What suggestions would you make?
   d. Mrs. R. asks if a popular laxative, "nature's own," which is frequently advertised on TV, would serve the same purpose as the bran which her physician has recommended. What would you tell her?
   e. Show how you would modify Mrs. R.'s present very low-residue diet for a soft, low-fiber diet; for a diet with increased residue, but omitting raw fruits and vegetables; for a high-fiber diet.
7. List the recommendations you would make for a person with irritable colon.
8. Mr. P., a 16-year-old student, is hospitalized with ulcerative colitis. His doctor has ordered a 3500-kcal, 150-gm protein diet for him.
   a. Plan a day's menu for him. He has many food intolerances, does not eat raw fruits or vegetables, and dislikes milk. He is especially fond of pizza and carbonated beverages.
   b. Mr. P. will be going home soon but is somewhat apprehensive about this as he does not get along well with his parents. What advice would you give him concerning his diet?
   c. What suggestions could you offer Mr. P.'s mother to help her win her son's cooperation at mealtime?

CITED REFERENCES

1. Parks, T. G.: "Colonic Motility in Man," *Postgrad. Med. J.,* **49:**90–99, 1973.
2. Goldstein, F.: "Diet and Colonic Disease," *J. Am. Diet. Assoc.,* **60:**499–503, 1972.
3. Piepmeyer, J. L.: "Use of Unprocessed Bran in Treatment of Irritable Bowel Syndrome," *Am. J. Clin. Nutr.,* **27:**106–107, 1974.
4. Ament, M. E.: "Inflammatory Diseases of the Colon. Ulcerative Colitis and Crohn's Colitis," *J. Pediatr.,* **86:**322–24, 1975.
5. Morson, B. C.: "Pathology of Diverticular Disease of the Colon," *Clin. Gastroenterol.,* **4:**37–52, 1975.
6. Painter, N. S., *et al.:* "Unprocessed Bran in Treatment of Diverticular Disease of the Colon," *Br. Med. J.,* **2:**137–40, 1972.
7. Jackson, B.: "Ulcerative Colitis From An Etiological Perspective," *Am. J. Nurs.,* **73:**258–61, 1973.
8. Review: "Diet and Cancer of the Colon," *Nutr. Rev.,* **31:**110–11, 1973.
9. Weedon, D. D., *et al.:* "Crohn's Disease and Cancer," *N. Engl. J. Med.,* **289:**1099–1103, 1973.
10. Devroede, G. J., *et al.:* "Cancer Risk and Life Expectancy of Children with Ulcerative Colitis," *N. Engl. J. Med.,* **285:**17–21, 1971.
11. Howell, M. A.: "Diet as an Etiological Factor in the Development of Cancers of the Colon and Rectum," *J. Chronic Dis.,* **28:**67–80, 1975.

12. Wynder, E. E., and Reddy, B. S.: "Dietary Fat and Colon Cancer," *J. Nat. Cancer Inst.*, **54:**7–10, 1975.
13. Burkitt, D. P.: "Large Bowel Cancer: An Epidemiologic Jigsaw Puzzle," *J. Nat. Cancer Inst.*, **54:**3–6, 1975.

Additional References

Benson, J. A., Jr.: "Simple Chronic Constipation," *Postgrad. Med.*, **57:**55–60, Jan. 1975.
Burkitt, D. P., and Painter, N. S.: "Dietary Fiber and Disease," *J.A.M.A.*, **229:**1068–74, 1974.
Cummings, J. H.: "Dietary Fibre," *Gut*, **14:**69–81, 1973.
Eastwood, M. A.: "Medical and Dietary Management (Diverticular Disease)," *Clin. Gastroenterol.*, **4:**85–97, 1975.
————: "Idea Exchange: Fiber in the Diet," *J. Am. Diet. Assoc.*, **66:**50–53, 1975.
Kirwan, W. O., *et al.*: "Action of Different Bran Preparations on Colonic Function," *Br. Med. J.*, **2:**187–89, 1974.
Levitt, M. D.: "Intestinal Gas," *Postgrad. Med.*, **57:**77–80, Jan. 1975.
Painter, N. S.: "Diverticular Disease of the Colon and Constipation. 3. High Fibre Diet with Added Bran," *Nurs. Times*, **68:**620–21, 1972.
Phillips, S. F.: "Diarrhea. Pathogenesis and Diagnostic Techniques," *Postgrad. Med.*, **57:**65–71, Jan. 1975.
Plumley, P. F., and Francis, B.: "Dietary Management of Diverticular Disease," *J. Am. Diet. Assoc.*, **63:**527–30, 1973.
Reilly, R. W., and Kirsner, J. B.: "Fiber Deficiency and Colonic Disorders," *Am. J. Clin. Nutr.*, **28:**293–94, 1975.
Review: "Diet, Intestinal Flora, and Colon Cancer," *Nutr. Rev.*, **33:**136–37, 1975.
Sklar, M.: "Functional Bowel Distress and Constipation in the Aged," *Geriatrics*, **27:**79–85, Sept. 1972.

Instructional Material for the Patient

American Cancer Society (local chapters): *Nutrition for Patients Receiving Chemotherapy and Radiation Treatment.*

34 Malabsorption Syndrome

*Medium-Chain-Triglyceride Diet;
Lactose-Restricted Diet;
Sucrose-Restricted Diet;
Gluten-Restricted Diet*

GENERAL CHARACTERISTICS AND TREATMENT

The term *malabsorption syndrome* is used to describe a number of disorders that are characterized by steatorrhea and multiple abnormalities in absorption of nutrients. Malabsorption in these disorders may be due to defects in (1) the intestinal lumen, resulting in inadequate fat hydrolysis or altered bile salt metabolism; (2) the mucosal epithelial cells, affecting absorbing surfaces and interfering with transport functions; or (3) intestinal lymphatics. (See Table 34–1.)

Symptoms and laboratory findings. Symptoms present to a variable degree in most persons with this syndrome include (1) pale, bulky, frothy, and offensive stools due to abnormally high fat content; (2) muscle wasting and progressive weight loss due to steatorrhea, diarrhea, and anorexia; (3) abdominal distention in children, less marked in adults; (4) evidence of vitamin and mineral deficiencies, such as macrocytic anemia due to inadequate absorption of folic acid and vitamin B_{12}, iron-deficiency anemia, hypocalcemic tetany, glossitis, and so on.

Laboratory findings include decreases in serum concentrations of electrolytes, albumin, and carotene; impaired absorption of *d*-xylose, glucose, folic acid, and vitamin B_{12}; and increased fecal fat and nitrogen.

Diagnostic tests. The diagnosis of malabsorption syndrome is based upon findings from absorption tests, intestinal mucosal biopsy, and radiologic studies.

Direct tests of absorption involve measurement of *fecal fat*. The balance study method is widely used and involves the chemical analysis of a 72-hour stool collection. The patient is fed a diet containing a known amount of fat, usually 50 to 100 gm, for several days before and during the collection period. Stools are then analyzed for fat. Normal excretion is less than 5 gm per 24 hours. Stool collections are also used to measure fecal radioactivity following administration of a test dose of ^{131}I-labeled triolein. The triolein is mixed with a marker and stools are collected until the marker is no longer visible. Normal fecal radioactivity is less than 7 per cent of the test dose.

Table 34–1. Some Malabsorptive Disorders Responsive to Dietary Modification

Abnormalities in the Intestinal Lumen	Abnormalities in the Mucosa
Inadequate lipid hydrolysis*	Specific defects
1. Pancreatic insufficiency	1. Lactase insufficiency
2. Gastric resection	2. Sucrase-isomaltase deficiency
	3. Glucose-galactase deficiency
	4. A-beta-lipoproteinemia
Alteration of bile salt metabolism*	Nonspecific defects*
1. Hepatobiliary disease	1. Short-bowel syndrome
2. Intestinal resection	2. Gluten enteropathy
3. Bacterial overgrowth	3. Tropical sprue
	Intestinal lymphatic obstruction*
	Lymphangiectasia

*MCT therapy effective in disorders in this group.

The *serum carotene* level is a useful screening test, and malabsorption is suspected if levels of less than 60 micrograms per 100 ml are found.

Oral tolerance tests provide indirect evidence of malabsorption. Most commonly used are d-*xylose* and *lactose*. Urinary excretion of *d*-xylose following ingestion of a 25-gm load is used as an indication of carbohydrate absorption. Excretion of less than 4.5 gm in five hours in patients with normal renal function indicates decreased absorptive capacity. The *lactose tolerance test* is used in suspected lactase deficiency. Administration of 50 or 100 gm lactose is followed by determination of blood glucose levels for two hours. Lactase deficiency is indicated if the blood glucose fails to rise above the fasting level. Symptoms of abdominal distention, cramping, and diarrhea may occur following ingestion of the lactose in persons with malabsorption.

The *Schilling test* is frequently used as an index of vitamin B_{12} absorption; an oral dose of radioactive vitamin B_{12} is administered followed at two hours by an intramuscular injection of nonradioactive B_{12}. Urinary excretion of less than 5 to 8 per cent of the radioactive dose indicates malabsorption.

The *folic acid test* consists of assaying urine for 24 hours following injection of the vitamin and again after it is given orally 48 hours later. In malabsorption, excretion of folic acid is less after an oral dose than after injection.

Biopsy specimens of the jejunal mucosa showing villous atrophy provide nonspecific evidence of disturbances in absorptive function. Radiologic evidence of intestinal dilatation, altered motility, and bone demineralization may also be seen in malabsorption.

Treatment. Therapy is directed toward alleviation of symptoms by correction of the basic defect insofar as possible, dietary modification in accordance with the nature of the defect, vitamin and mineral supplements, and prevention or correction of complications by administration of appropriate agents.

Dietary modification. Generally speaking, the diet in malabsorption syndrome should be high in protein and calories (see Chapters 29 and 30). In a few of the disorders elimination of specific carbohydrates or proteins is necessary and the dietary management is outlined in the sections that follow. Modification of fat intake is often indicated. Vita-

min and mineral supplementation is usually needed. A soft or fiber-restricted diet is useful for patients with persistent diarrhea (see Chapter 27).

Fat absorption can be improved in some malabsorptive disorders by changing the type of fat ingested. Food fats are composed principally of fatty acids containing 12 to 18 carbon atoms (long-chain triglycerides). In contrast, fats composed almost entirely of fatty acids containing 8 and 10 carbon atoms (medium-chain triglycerides) have been synthesized. Substitution of medium-chain triglycerides (MCT) for longer-chain fats (LCT) is associated with reduced steatorrhea and decreased losses of calcium, sodium, and potassium in many of the disorders comprising the malabsorption syndrome. (See Table 34–1.)

The effectiveness of MCT over long-chain fats appears to be due to differences in the rate of hydrolysis, absorption, and route of transport. Medium-chain fats are hydrolyzed much more rapidly than long-chain fats in the intestinal lumen. The presence of pancreatic enzymes and bile salts is not required for absorption of the fats of medium-chain length. A mucosal enzyme system, specific for medium-chain-triglyceride hydrolysis, has been described. Medium-chain triglycerides are transported by way of the portal vein as free fatty acids bound to albumin whereas long-chain fats must undergo esterification and chylomicron formation and are transported by way of the lymph.[1]

Side effects of nausea, abdominal distention or cramps, and diarrhea have been noted in about 10 per cent of patients receiving MCT supplements. Symptoms are attributed to the hyperosmolar load produced by rapid hydrolysis of MCT and possible irritating effects of high levels of free fatty acids in the stomach and intestine. These symptoms can be overcome by slow ingestion of small amounts of the supplement.

Medium-chain triglycerides are available commercially as an oil preparation° or as a powdered formula.† A number of recipes have been developed

---

° MCT® from fractionated coconut oil, by Mead Johnson & Co., Evansville, Indiana. Provides 8.3 kcal per gram, or approximately 225 kcal per 30 ml.

† Portagen® by Mead Johnson & Co., Evansville, Indiana. An 8-ounce glass of the product reconstituted to 20 kcal per ounce provides 5.6 gm protein from sodium caseinate, 18.4 gm carbohydrate from corn syrup solids and sucrose, and 7.75 gm fat from MCT and corn oil.

for incorporating these products into the diet.° The oil provides a concentrated source of calories, and can be used in frying and in recipes such as salad dressings, hot breads, and desserts. It is a clear, odorless oil with a bland taste. The powder, on the other hand, is useful as a calorie-protein supplement to an otherwise very low-fat diet. A proprietary formula containing MCT is available for infants.†

Dietary management. From 50 to 70 per cent of the fat is supplied as MCT and the remainder as long-chain fats. To maintain this ratio, foods containing LCT are limited to

4 ounces meat, fish, or poultry
1 egg
3 teaspoons butter

This provides about 25 gm LCT daily.

The following diet is adapted from the plan described by Schizas et al.[2]

MEDIUM-CHAIN-TRIGLYCERIDE (MCT) DIET

Characteristics and General Rules
This diet provides for a reduction in long-chain triglycerides by substituting an oil containing medium-chain triglycerides as a source of fat. The diet is adjusted to provide 50 to 70 per cent of the fat calories as MCT.
The protein intake may be increased by adding nonfat dry milk to fluid skim milk, skim cottage cheese, egg whites, and cereal products.
The caloric level may be increased by adding high-carbohydrate foods such as fruits, sugar, jelly, and fat-free desserts.
Modifications in fiber and consistency may be made by applying restrictions concerning the soft diet (see Chapter 27) to the foods listed below.
Initially, small amounts of MCT should be taken with meals and gradually increased according to individual tolerance. Between-meal feedings may be desirable if large amounts of food are not tolerated.

Include These Foods Daily:
    2 or more cups skim milk
    4 ounces (cooked weight) lean meat, poultry, or fish
    1 egg
    3 or more fruits including
        1–2 servings citrus fruit or other good source of ascorbic acid
        1–2 other fruits
    3–4 servings vegetables including
        1 dark green or deep yellow
        1 potato
        1–2 other vegetables, raw or cooked, as tolerated
    5 servings bread and cereals
    3 teaspoons butter
MCT oil in amounts prescribed (usually 2 ounces)

Nutritive value: On the basis of specified amounts of foods above: protein, 75 gm (13 per cent of calories); fat, 35 gm (13 per cent of calories); carbohydrate, 315 gm (53 per cent of calories); MCT, 60 gm (21 per cent of calories); 2400 kcal.

Foods Allowed
Beverages—cereal beverages, coffee, tea, soft drinks
Breads and substitutes—hamburger rolls, hard rolls, white enriched, whole-wheat, pumpernickel, or rye bread.

Foods to Avoid

Commercial biscuits, coffeecake, cornbread, crackers, doughnuts, muffins, sweet rolls

° Available from Mead Johnson & Co., Evansville, Indiana.
† Pregestimil® by Mead Johnson & Co., Evansville, Indiana.

Bread products contain some LCT but are permitted to add palatability and variety to the diet.

Cooked or dry cereals, macaroni, noodles, rice, spaghetti

Cheese—skim cottage cheese

Desserts—angel cake, gelatin, meringues, any made from MCT special recipes

Egg—egg whites as desired; whole eggs and egg yolks only in prescribed amounts

Fats—butter in prescribed amounts, gravies made from clear soups and MCT oil

Fruits—all except avocado

Meats—lean meat, fish, and poultry only in prescribed amounts

Milk—skim milk

Soups—fat-free broth, bouillon, consommé

Sweets—jelly, syrups, sugars

Vegetables—all to which no fat is added except MCT

Miscellaneous—any special recipe in which MCT is substituted for long-chain fats

Cheese made from whole milk

Commercial cakes, pies, cookies, pastries, puddings and custards; mixes allowed only if they contain no LCT

Whole eggs and egg yolks except as prescribed

Oils and shortenings of all types, sauces and gravies except those made with MCT oil

Avocado

Fatty meats, fish, frankfurters, cold cuts, sausages

Buttermilk, partially skim milk, whole milk, light, heavy, or sour cream

Cream soups, others

Butter, chocolate, coconut, or cream candies

Creamed vegetables, or those with fats other than MCT added

Creamed dishes; commercial popcorn; frozen dinners; homemade products containing eggs, whole milk, and fats; mixes for biscuits, muffins, and cakes; olives

Sample Menu

BREAKFAST

Fresh grapefruit—1 half

MCT waffle—1

Butter—1 teaspoon

Maple syrup—2 tablespoons

Sugar—1 teaspoon

Coffee or tea

LUNCHEON OR SUPPER

Chicken sandwich

   Chicken—2 ounces

   MCT mayonnaise—1 tablespoon

   Whole-wheat bread—2 slices

   Lettuce and tomato

Fresh fruit cup—$\frac{1}{2}$ cup

MCT brownie—1

Skim milk—1 cup

DINNER

Veal chop—2 ounces

MCT scalloped potatoes—$\frac{1}{2}$ cup

Carrots—$\frac{1}{2}$ cup

   With lemon butter—2 teaspoons

Mixed green salad—1 serving

MCT Italian dressing—2 teaspoons

Angel cake—$\frac{1}{16}$ of 8 inch diameter

Fresh strawberries—1 cup

Coffee or tea

EVENING SNACK

Skim milk—1 cup

MCT sugar cookies—2

DIETARY COUNSELING

The patient must understand the importance of using the recommended amounts of MCT in the diet. He should be cautioned to take the oil slowly in small amounts; no more than 1 tablespoon of MCT should be taken at any given feeding. The diet to be used at home should be planned with consideration given to the individual's cultural background and usual meal pattern. He must be taught to use cuts of meat that are low in fat and to select only lean meats. Suggestions for incorporating the MCT oil into meals should be offered and suitable recipes supplied. Some persons prefer to take the oil mixed in fruit juice or as a "milkshake" composed of skim milk, fruit ice, and the oil. Others prefer to add the oil to solid foods such as cooked cereals, mashed potatoes, or sauces. The oil imparts a golden color to foods when used in frying; care should be taken to see that all the oil is removed from the frying pan, however, and actually consumed. Meals eaten away from home need not be a problem if the individual orders clear soups, lean meats trimmed of all visible fat, vegetables without cream sauces or other added fat, and so on. Desserts such as fruits, angel cake, and gelatin are suitable and usually available.

ABNORMALITIES IN THE INTESTINAL LUMEN

Inadequate digestion. Any condition that interferes with normal secretion or activity of pancreatic lipase causes inadequate hydrolysis of lipids in the intestinal lumen and results in malabsorption.

Pancreatic insufficiency. Inadequate production of lipase occurs in pancreatic insufficiency. This disorder may result from chronic pancreatitis, cystic fibrosis, carcinoma, pancreatectomy, or destruction of exocrine function by ligation of the duct. Steatorrhea and symptoms of generalized malabsorption occur due to poor utilization of fats and protein. Weight loss may be significant in spite of a good appetite.

The diet is designed to prevent further weight loss and to control gastrointestinal symptoms. From 2500 to 4000 kcal are required. The protein intake should be 80 to 150 gm. Carbohydrate (400 gm or more) is the chief source of calories since fat is poorly tolerated. Generally, long-chain fatty acids should be restricted to 40 to 60 gm daily. Pancreatic extract is given with meals to aid in fat absorption. MCT can be used to increase the calorie intake. (See page 453).

Gastric resection. Steatorrhea sometimes follows gastric resection because of inadequate mixing of food with pancreatic juice and bile or bacterial overgrowth in an afferent loop of intestine. In addition, anemia is frequently seen because of limited intake or impaired absorption of iron, vitamin B_{12}, and folic acid. Weight loss is common and persistent. Improved absorption of fats may be achieved by supplementing the diet with MCT. Other dietary considerations are described on page 483.

Altered bile salt metabolism. Steatorrhea occurs if adequate amounts of conjugated bile salts are not available for micelle formation and is frequently associated with the following conditions.

Hepatobiliary disease. Decreased amounts of bile salts in the lumen in hepatobiliary disease are due to impaired synthesis of bile acids or biliary stasis.

Ileal resection. Removal of the ileum reduces the bile salt pool thereby lowering the concentration of conjugated bile salts in the jejunum available for hydrolysis of fats. Unabsorbed fatty acids and bile salts may provoke diarrhea. Parenteral administration of vitamin B_{12} is indicated if the distal ileum is not functional.

Bacterial overgrowth (blind loop syndrome). Intestinal stasis is associated with changes in the bacterial flora. Deconjugation of bile salts by bacteria prevents adequate micelle formation. In some instances steatorrhea can be corrected by feeding conjugated bile salts. Bacteria also bind vitamin B_{12} so that it is unavailable for absorption, and replacement therapy is needed.

ABNORMALITIES IN MUCOSAL CELL TRANSPORT— SPECIFIC DISORDERS

Absence or deficiency of specific enzymes or failure of proper regulation of enzyme activity in the cell interferes with the absorption of certain nutrients and produces symptoms of malabsorption.

Lactase deficiency. Inability to utilize lactose may be due to lactase deficiency or may be secondary to conditions that produce alterations in absorptive surfaces. In the absence of lactase lactose is not hydrolyzed to glucose and galactose. The accumulation of lactose in the intestine causes fermentation, abdominal pain, cramping, and diarrhea. Failure to gain weight is an important symptom in infants.

Primary lactase deficiency occurs as a rare congenital abnormality in the intestinal mucosa. Symptoms occur following ingestion of milk by the infant. A strict lactose-free formula is used, several commercial products being available.° All products containing lactose in any form whatsoever are rigidly excluded.

Intestinal lactase activity is normally high during infancy but declines after weaning to low levels in adults. Throughout most of the world the majority of adults are unable to digest lactose, and they develop

° CHO-free Formula Base by Syntex Laboratories, Inc., Palo Alto, California. MBF (Meat-base formula) by Gerber Products Company, Fremont, Michigan, Mul-Soy® by Syntex Laboratories, Inc., Palo Alto, California. Nutramigen® and ProSobee® by Mead Johnson & Co., Evansville, Indiana.

symptoms of distention, cramping, and diarrhea following its ingestion. However, persons of northern European extraction and certain peoples of African descent generally are able to tolerate lactose. In general, populations in which dairying is traditional seem to tolerate lactose but peoples from nondairying parts of the world do not, and this inability to utilize lactose in the latter groups persists in successive generations in spite of migration. Some groups in dairying areas do not consume much milk as such, but process it into foods such as yogurt or cheese in which the lactose is converted to lactic acid. These groups are usually not able to digest lactose.

Several hypotheses have been proposed to explain the differences in ability to utilize lactose among various ethnic groups. One theory holds that a genetic mutation occurring as a result of some selective advantage may permit high levels of lactase to persist into the adult years in certain populations.[3]

Adults who have no history of gastrointestinal disease or childhood intolerance to milk, but who experience classical symptoms following excessive milk or lactose ingestion, can be kept asymptomatic by limiting their intake of milk products. A controlled lactose diet that restricts only obvious sources of lactose is used. The quantity of lactose allowed is a matter of individual tolerance. Some find that it is better tolerated if taken in small amounts several times daily, especially with meals, and at room temperature rather than cold. Many persons remain symptom free by limiting their intake of milk to one glass per day. If cheese, yoghurt, or other sources of calcium are not taken, supplements should be prescribed to replace the calcium ordinarily supplied by milk.

Secondary lactose intolerance is often observed following gastrectomy or extensive small bowel resection, and in celiac disease, sprue, colitis, enteritis, cystic fibrosis, kwashiorkor, and malnutrition. Drugs such as neomycin and colchicine may inhibit lactose absorption.[4]

DIETARY COUNSELING

Persons on lactose-free diets should be advised to carefully check labels on all commercial products. Foods containing milk in any form, butter, and margarine are to be avoided. Typical sources of lactose include breads, candies, cold cuts, mixes of all types, powdered soft drinks, preserves, soups, and so on. Fruit juices or water can be substituted for milk in many recipes. Meals eaten away from home should include foods prepared without breading, cream sauces, gravies, and so on. Broiled or roasted meats, baked potato, vegetables without added fat, salads, and desserts such as plain angel cake, fresh fruit, and gelatin are good choices. Kosher-style foods are suitable.

When patients with acquired lactose intolerance have responded well to a lactose-free diet, small amounts of lactose-containing foods are allowed. Milk or foods containing milk such as custards, puddings, cream soups, ice cream, and cottage cheese are tested, one at a time, in small amounts (for example, one-fourth cup milk at a meal) to determine levels that may be tolerated. Fermented dairy products such as yogurt, buttermilk, and many cheeses may be included if tolerated.

LACTOSE-FREE DIET

Characteristics and General Rules

This diet is designed to eliminate all sources of lactose.

All milk and milk products must be eliminated.

Lactose is used in the manufacture of many foods and medicines. It is essential to read labels of commercial products before use.

The diet is inadequate in calcium and riboflavin. Supplements of these nutrients should be prescribed.

The protein intake may be increased by adding meat, fish, poultry, or eggs, lactose-free milk substitutes, or breads and cereals from those allowed.

The caloric level may be increased by adding high-carbohydrate foods such as fruits, sugar, jelly, and desserts free of lactose.

Modifications in fiber and consistency may be made by applying restrictions concerning the soft diet (see Chapter 27) to the foods listed below.

Include the following foods daily:
  7 ounces meat, fish, or poultry
  1 egg
  3 or more fruits including
      1–2 servings citrus fruit or other good source of ascorbic acid
      1–2 other fruits
  3–4 servings vegetables including
      1 dark green or deep yellow
      1 potato
      1–2 other vegetables, raw or cooked, as tolerated
  6 servings enriched bread or cereals
  6 teaspoons fortified milk-free margarine
Other foods as needed to provide calories

Foods Allowed

Beverages—carbonated drinks, fruit drinks, coffee, tea

Breads and cereals—breads and rolls made without milk, cooked cereals, some prepared cereals (check labels), macaroni, spaghetti, soda crackers

Cheese—none

Desserts—angel cake, cakes made with vegetable oils, gelatin, puddings made with fruit juices, water, or allowed milk substitutes, water ices

Eggs—prepared any way except with milk or cheese

Fats—lard, peanut butter, pure mayonnaise, vegetable oils, margarines without milk or butter added, some cream substitutes (check labels)

Fruits—all except canned and frozen to which lactose is added

Milk—none

Meat, fish, or poultry—all kinds, cold cuts (check labels for added nonfat dry milk), kosher frankfurters

Vegetables—fresh, canned, or frozen—plain or with milk-free margarine (check labels of canned or frozen)

Soups—meat and vegetable only (check labels)

Miscellaneous—corn syrup, honey, nuts, nut butters, olives, pickles, pure seasonings and spices, pure jams and jellies, pure sugar candies, some cream substitutes, sugar

Foods to Avoid

Cereal beverages, cocoa, instant coffee

Bread with milk added, crackers made with butter or margarine, Cream of Rice or Cream of Wheat cereal, French toast, mixes of all types, pancakes, some dry cereals, waffles, zwieback.

All types

Cakes, cookies, pies, puddings or other desserts made with milk and butter or margarine, commercial fruit fillings, commercial sweet rolls, custards, custard and cream pies, ice cream, pie crust made with butter or margarine, sherbets

Any prepared with milk or cheese

Butter, cream substitutes, cream, sweet and sour, margarine with butter or milk added, salad dressings

Canned or frozen prepared with lactose

All types, infant food formulas, simulated mother's milk, yogurt

Brain, breaded or creamed dishes, cold cuts and frankfurters containing nonfat dry milk, liver, liver sausage, sweetbreads

Canned or frozen vegetables prepared with lactose, commercial French-fried potatoes, corn curls, creamed vegetables, instant or mashed potatoes, any seasoned with butter or margarine

All others

Ascorbic acid and citric acid mixtures, butterscotch, caramels, chewing gum, chocolate candy, cordials and liqueurs, cream sauces, cream soups, diabetic and dietetic preparations, dried soups, frozen cultures, frozen desserts, gravy, health and geriatric foods, molasses, monosodium glutamate extender, party dips, peppermints, powdered soft drinks, spice blends, starter cultures, sweetness reducers in candies, fruit pie fillings, icings, and preserves, toffee

Meal Pattern
  BREAKFAST
Fruit
Cereal with milk substitute and sugar
Egg
Bread or roll made without milk—2 slices
Margarine, milk free—2 teaspoons
Beverage with cream substitute and sugar
  LUNCHEON OR SUPPER
Lean meat, fish, or poultry—3 ounces
Potato or substitute
Cooked vegetable
Salad
Bread made without milk—2 slices
Margarine, milk free—2 teaspoons
Jelly
Fruit
Beverage
  DINNER
Lean meat, fish, or fowl—4 ounces
Potato
Vegetable
Bread or roll made without milk—2 slices
Margarine, milk free—2 teaspoons
Jelly
Fruit or dessert
Beverage

Sample Menu

Orange juice
Cornflakes with cream substitute and sugar
Soft-cooked egg
French bread, toasted enriched
Margarine—milk free
Coffee with cream substitute and sugar

Baked chicken breast
Parslied potato
Asparagus tips
Sliced tomato and lettuce
French or Italian bread, enriched
Margarine—milk free
Grape jelly
Canned peach halves
Tea with lemon and sugar

Roast beef sirloin
Baked potato
Diced carrots
French or Italian bread, enriched
Margarine—milk free
Apple jelly
Fresh fruit cup
Tea with lemon and sugar

Sucrase-isomaltase deficiency. Deficiencies of these enzymes lead to symptoms similar to those seen in lactase insufficiency following ingestion of significant amounts of sucrose and isomaltose. A sucrose tolerance test is used to confirm the diagnosis.

Sucrose is added to many foods during processing and preparation. In addition, naturally occurring sucrose is present in a number of foods, making a strict sucrose-free diet impractical. Nevertheless, elimination of foods containing relatively large amounts of sucrose should be made (see Table 34–2). Glucose is substituted as a sweetening agent. Products containing wheat and potato starches should be avoided as these yield more isomaltose upon hydrolysis than do other starches such as rice and corn.

Increased sucrase activity following fructose feeding has been reported in this disorder, thus

Table 34–2. Foods Containing More Then 5 gm Sucrose per 100 gm Edible Portion*

Apricots	Jams and jellies	Puddings
Bananas	Macadamia nuts	Syrups
Candy	Mangoes	Sorghum
Cane sugar	Milk chocolate	Soybeans
Cake	Molasses	Soybean flour or meal
Chestnuts, Va.	Oranges	Sugar beets
Chocolate, sweet	Pastries	Sweet breads and rolls
Condensed milk	Peaches	Sweet pickles
Cookies	Peanuts	Sweet potatoes
Dates	Peas	Tangerine
Honeydew melon	Pineapple	Watermelon
Ice cream	Prune plums, Italian	Wheat germ

*Adapted from Hardinge, M. G., *et al.*: "Carbohydrates in Foods," *J. Am. Diet. Assoc.*, **46**:197–204, 1965.

permitting ingestion of small amounts of sucrose without provoking symptoms. A sucrose-restricted diet containing 20 per cent of calories as fructose eliminated symptoms and permitted weight gain in a youngster with the disorder.[5]

Glucose-galactase deficiency. This rare disease is characterized by inability to absorb any carbohydrate that yields glucose or galactose upon hydrolysis. Substitution of fructose as the sole source of carbohydrate in the diet leads to improvement in symptoms. A special formula containing 4 to 8 per cent fructose has been devised for infants.[6] This formula is used almost exclusively for the first few months, after which it is gradually decreased and addition of foods low in starch is begun. Alternatively, a proprietary infant formula° containing no carbohydrate may be used as the basis for the diet. By the age of three, a regular diet for age is usually tolerated with limited amounts of milk and starch-containing foods. Some degree of dietary restriction is necessary throughout life in order to prevent recurrence of symptoms of diarrhea. If a galactose-free diet is ordered, the lactose-free diet (see page 457) is used with omission of sugar beets, peas, and Lima beans.

A-beta-lipoproteinemia. This is a rare congenital disorder which is believed to involve a defect in the release or synthesis of β-lipoprotein. As a result fat is not transported from the intestinal cells into the lacteals. Total β-lipoprotein deficiency is manifested by steatorrhea and failure to thrive among other symptoms in infants. The malabsorption of fats is associated with extremely low serum concentrations of β-lipoprotein, cholesterol, vitamin A, and phospholipids.

Substitution of medium-chain triglycerides for long-chain fats in the diet results in improved fat absorption since the shorter-chain fats are absorbed via the portal vein rather than by lymph.

ABNORMALITIES IN MUCOSAL CELL TRANSPORT—NONSPECIFIC DISORDERS

Reduction in the absorptive surface area by massive intestinal resection or by damage to the villi produced by disease may have profound effects on nutrient uptake and absorption.

° CHO-free Formula Base by Syntex Laboratories, Inc., Palo Alto, California.

Short-bowel syndrome. This term is used to describe those patients who are in metabolic imbalance as a consequence of massive resection of the small intestine. Removal of large portions of the bowel shortens the transit time of the contents through the intestine, thereby reducing the time for absorption. Attempts to increase absorption by delaying transit time include dietary modification, drug therapy, and surgical measures, such as small bowel reversal. In this syndrome, the length of the remaining bowel is generally less than 8 feet. The amount of bowel left intact and the site of resection have an important bearing on the patient's nutritional status.

Nutrients normally absorbed in the proximal intestine are shown in Figure 34–1. Following removal of the jejunum, some absorption of these nutrients may take place in the ileum by virtue of its ability to act as a functional intestinal reserve. On the other hand, the jejunum has a limited capacity to absorb water and electrolytes and cannot compensate for the massive losses that occur when the ileum is removed. Following ileal resection, steatorrhea occurs because of bile salt deficiency.

Typically, the patient goes through three stages after massive resection of the bowel. In the immediate postoperative period, diarrhea and fluid and electrolyte imbalance may be so severe as to be life threatening. Total parenteral nutrition is used as the sole source of nutrients for two or three months. The patient surviving this period enters the second stage when nutritional concerns are of prime importance. Steady weight loss occurs as a result of anorexia, diarrhea, and steatorrhea. Osteomalacia may develop. Oral intake during this period usually is not sufficient, and supplemental calories are provided by intravenous feedings. Carbohydrates low in fiber are the first foods added since they are well absorbed by the remaining intestine. From 50 to 100 gm per day are used initially. After the patient tolerates carbohydrates and proteins, small amounts of fat are gradually introduced. For many patients a maximum of 40 gm fat is tolerated. Amounts greater than this increase steatorrhea. Finally after three months or more, the patient's condition stabilizes, usually at a substantially lower weight. The fat intake can usually be increased to 50 to 60 gm daily.

The extreme losses of all nutrients in this syndrome require greatly increased intakes of calories, protein, vitamins, and minerals. Up to 5000 kcal and

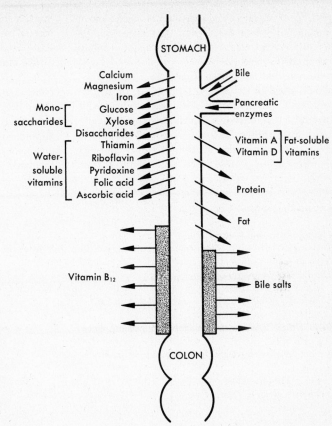

Figure 34–1. Sites of absorption in the small bowel. Most nutrients are absorbed from the proximal portion of the small intestine. (Adapted from Booth, C. C.: "Effect of Location Along Small Intestine on Absorption of Nutrients," Chapter 76 in *Handbook of Physiology. Alimentary Canal.* Vol. 1. American Physiological Society, Washington, D.C., 1967.)

175 gm of protein may be needed to prevent further weight loss. Substitution of medium-chain triglycerides for long-chain fats has led to decreased diarrhea and electrolyte losses and improvement in nutritional status.[7]

Synthetic low-residue diets have been useful in this and other malabsorptive disorders. These diets are designed to provide complete nutritional support for extended periods in patients in whom it is desirable to reduce gastrointestinal residue to a minimum. Synthetic low-residue diets, composed of purified amino acids, simple carbohydrates, fats, vitamins, and minerals, have no indigestible bulk, hence require minimum digestion, and are rapidly absorbed from the upper intestinal tract. Both frequency and volume of stools are decreased. Commercial powdered preparations, available in several flavors, when diluted with water may be used for tube feeding, beverages, or frozen as popsicles.

Gluten enteropathy. This is a disease of genetic origin characterized by intolerance to the gliadin fraction of gluten with consequent malabsorption. The disorder is known as *celiac disease* in childhood and as *adult celiac disease* or *nontropical sprue* in later life. The mechanism of the sensitivity to gluten is not understood.

The onset of this disease is insidious and is manifested by diarrhea, steatorrhea, weight loss, and other symptoms of the malabsorption syndrome. Stools are characteristically loose, pale, and frothy (due to fermentation of undigested carbohydrate) and contain excessive amounts of fat. Biopsy specimens of the mucosal surface have a flattened appearance; the villi become shorter and club shaped and appear to be fused. A marked decrease in the number of microvilli in the brush border drastically reduces the absorptive surface. Laboratory findings are consistent with those of the malabsorption syndrome (see page 452).

Exacerbations and remissions are common in this

disorder. Symptoms are provoked by ingestion of gluten from wheat, rye, barley, buckwheat, and, in some instances, oats. Gluten from rice and potato has no deleterious effect.

Elimination of gluten from the diet (below) should be given a trial of at least six weeks. Regeneration of villi and return of enzyme activity occur in most cases following strict adherence to a gluten-restricted diet. Lack of response to the diet in some cases may be due to failure to follow the diet or to secondary lactose intolerance resulting from mucosal damage. In this case, a gluten-restricted, lactose-free diet leads to improved fat and carbohydrate absorption.

The diet should provide 100 gm or more protein to replace wasted tissue. Some moderation in fiber content and fat intake may be needed initially as these are usually poorly tolerated. Improved fat absorption can be achieved through the use of MCT. Supplementary vitamins and minerals are needed to overcome nutritional deficiencies resulting from excessive losses in the stools.

GLUTEN-RESTRICTED DIET

Characteristics and General Rules
This diet excludes all products containing wheat, rye, oats, and barley. Read all labels carefully.
Aqueous multivitamins are usually prescribed in addition to the diet.
The diet may be progressed gradually; that is, small amounts of unsaturated fats may be used at first, adding harder fats later. Fiber may be reduced initially by using only cooked fruits and vegetables. Strongly flavored vegetables may be poorly tolerated at first.

Include these foods, or their nutritive equivalents, daily:
4 cups milk
6–8 ounces (cooked weight) lean meat, fish, or poultry
1 egg
4 vegetables including:
  1 dark green or deep yellow
  1 potato
  2 other vegetables
  Other to be served raw, if tolerated
3 fruits including:
  1–2 servings citrus fruit or other good source ascorbic acid
  1–2 other fruits
4 servings bread and cereals: corn, rice, soybean
  NO WHEAT, RYE, OATS, BARLEY
2 tablespoons fat
Additional calories are provided by using more of the foods listed, desserts, soups, sweets

Nutritive value of listed foods: Protein, 105 gm; fat, 110 gm; carbohydrate, 200 gm; 2200 kcal.
Minerals and vitamins in excess of recommended allowances.

Foods Allowed
Beverages—carbonated, cocoa, coffee, fruit juices, milk, tea

Breads—cornbread, muffins, and pone with no wheat flour; breads made with cornmeal, cornstarch, potato, rice, soybean, wheat starch flour

Cereals—cooked cornmeal, Cream of Rice, hominy or grits, rice; ready to eat: corn or rice cereals such as cornflakes, rice flakes, Puffed Rice

Foods to Avoid
Beverages—ale, beer, instant coffee containing cereal, malted milk, Postum, products containing cereal

Breads—all containing any wheat, rye, oats, or barley; bread crumbs, muffins, pancakes, rolls, rusks, waffles, zwieback; all commercial yeast and quick bread mixes; all crackers, pretzels, Ry-Krisp

Cereals—cooked or ready-to-eat breakfast cereals containing wheat, oats; barley, macaroni, noodles, pasta, spaghetti, wheat germ

Cheese—cottage; later, cream cheese

Desserts—custard, fruit ice, fruit whips, plain or fruit ice cream (homemade), plain or fruit gelatin, meringues; homemade puddings—cornstarch, rice, tapioca; rennet desserts; sherbet; cakes and cookies made with allowed flours

Eggs—as desired

Fats—oil: corn, cottonseed, olive, sesame, soybean; French dressing, pure mayonnaise, salad dressing with cornstarch thickening

Later addition: butter, cream, margarine, peanut oil, vegetable shortening

Flour—cornmeal, potato, rice, soybean

Fruits—all cooked, canned, and juices; fresh and frozen as tolerated, avoiding skin and seeds initially

Meat—all lean meats, poultry, fish: baked, broiled, roasted, stewed

Milk—all kinds

Soups—broth, bouillon, cream if thickened with cornstarch, vegetable

Sweets—candy, honey, jam, jelly, marmalade, marshmallows, molasses, syrup, sugar

Vegetables—cooked or canned: buttered; fresh as tolerated

Miscellaneous—gravy and sauces thickened with cornstarch; olives, peanut butter, pickles, popcorn, potato chips

Desserts—cake, cookies, doughnuts, pastries, pie; bisques, commercial ice cream, ice cream cones; prepared mixes containing wheat, rye, oats, or barley; puddings thickened with wheat flour

Fats—bacon, lard, suet, salad dressing with flour thickening

Flour—barley, oat, rye, wheat—bread, cake, entire wheat, graham, self-rising, whole wheat, wheat germ

Fruits—prunes, plums, and their juices; those with skins and seeds at first

Meat—breaded, creamed, croquettes, luncheon meats unless pure meat, meat loaf, stuffings with bread, scrapple, thickened stew

Fat meats such as corned beef, duck, frankfurters, goose, ham, luncheon meats, pork, sausage

Fatty fish such as herring, mackerel, sardines, swordfish, or canned in heavy oil

Soups—thickened with flour; containing barley, noodles, etc.

Sweets—candies with high fat content, nuts; candies containing wheat products

Vegetables—creamed if thickened with wheat, oat, rye, or barley products. Strongly flavored if they produce discomfort: baked beans, broccoli, Brussels sprouts, cabbage, cauliflower, corn, cucumber, lentils, onions, peppers, radishes, turnips

Miscellaneous—gravies and sauces thickened with flours not permitted

Meal Pattern

BREAKFAST

Fruit, preferably citrus or good source of ascorbic acid

Rice or corn cereal

Milk, sugar

Bread: rice or corn

Butter or margarine

Jelly, if desired

Eggs

Beverage

LUNCHEON OR SUPPER

Meat, poultry, or fish; or cheese; eggs (no thickened casserole dishes)

Potato, or substitute, or vegetable

Sample Menu

Tomato juice

Rice Krispies

Milk, sugar

Southern corn muffins

Butter or margarine

Currant jelly

Scrambled eggs

Coffee, with cream, sugar

Beef stew (not thickened)

Beef cubes

Potato

Carrots

Onions

Salad—vegetable or fruit, if tolerated

Bread: rice or corn
Butter or margarine
Milk
Dessert or fruit
  DINNER
Meat, poultry, or fish

Potato or rice
Cooked vegetable
Salad, if tolerated
Bread, corn or rice, if desired
Butter
Milk
Dessert or fruit
Tea or coffee

Tossed green salad
French dressing
Rice-flour bread
Butter or margarine
Milk
Vanilla cornstarch pudding with sliced frozen peaches

Broiled lamb patties (all meat)
Mint jelly
Rice with saffron seasoning
Buttered asparagus
Celery and olives

Milk
Lemon meringue pudding (thickened with cornstarch)
Coffee with cream, sugar

DIETARY COUNSELING

Proteins from lean meats, poultry, fish, cottage cheese, egg white, and skim milk are well utilized and should be encouraged. Individual tolerance for fibrous foods and strongly flavored vegetables should determine whether or not these foods are included. The patient should be advised to read labels on all commercial food products in order to avoid any foods containing wheat, rye, oats, or barley. Besides cereals and breads as obvious sources, many other foods contain wheat or other flour as a thickener. Canned soups, cheese spreads, cooked salad dressings, cold cuts, breaded meats, mixes of all kinds, catsup, ice cream, and pastries are but a few of the many foods that contain cereal products. Information on prepared and packaged foods known to be gluten free is available for patients.° Many standard cookbooks contain suitable recipes utilizing cornstarch, cornmeal, potato, rice, or tapioca instead of flour. Sources of special recipes utilizing arrowroot starch or wheat starch (from which the gluten is removed) should be supplied to the patient.° However, patients should be cautioned that mere substitu-

tion of other flours for wheat will not produce satisfactory results; other adjustments in mixing technique, baking time, and temperature are also needed. When meals are eaten away from home, plain foods, without breading, gravies, cream sauces, and so on, should be selected.

Tropical sprue. This disorder is a form of the malabsorption syndrome that occurs chiefly in the West Indies, Central America, and the Far East. In some respects it is similar to nontropical sprue, but the onset is more acute and it responds to different therapy. Both disorders are characterized by steatorrhea and secondary enzyme deficiencies in the intestinal mucosa. In tropical sprue there is also ileal involvement. Hypocalcemia with tetany and osteomalacia do not occur as commonly as in nontropical sprue; however, nutritional deficiencies of folic acid and vitamin B_{12} do occur and are manifested as macrocytic anemia. Dramatic improvement in symptoms is often shown following administration of folic acid and vitamin B_{12}.

The diet in tropical sprue should be high in protein and calories and restricted in fiber and in fat. The substitution of medium-chain triglycerides for some of the fat has resulted in weight gain and disappearance of steatorrhea. The restriction of gluten for patients with tropical sprue does not usually lead to further improvement.

° Available from Clinical Research Unit, University Hospital, Ann Arbor, Michigan.

ABNORMALITY OF INTESTINAL LYMPHATICS

Intestinal lymphangiectasia. This is a congenital defect in which obstruction of intestinal lymphatics is associated with leakage of chylomicron fat and plasma proteins into the intestinal lumen. In addition to decreased serum protein levels and associated edema and ascites formation, steatorrhea occurs. Protein losses are reduced considerably by use of medium-chain triglycerides or a fat-restricted diet (see page 474).

PROBLEMS AND REVIEW

1. What symptoms are characteristic of the malabsorption syndrome? In what ways is the diet modified?
2. What information is provided by each of the following tests:
   a. Serum carotene level
   b. Schilling test
   c. *d*-Xylose test
3. Plan a lactose-free diet for Mr. R., a single graduate student, who lives alone in an apartment with adequate cooking facilities. He enjoys Italian and Mexican foods. His caloric needs are estimated to be 2500 per day.
   a. List at least 10 foods that may contain lactose.
   b. Give suggestions for increasing calories in this diet.
   c. In which nutrients would this diet be inadequate?
   d. Which foods could be added if the diet is changed to controlled lactose?
   e. Mr. R. sometimes eats his lunch in a cafeteria. Give suggestions for suitable food choices.
4. Mrs. W. is a 45-year-old housewife and mother of four who was recently diagnosed as having adult celiac disease. The doctor prescribed a gluten-restricted diet for her.
   a. Explain what gluten is, and why it must be restricted in her diet.
   b. What are typical sources of gluten in the diet? Name some other less obvious foods that may contain gluten. What cereal grains can be substituted for those containing gluten?
   c. Mrs. W. is quite apprehensive about her diet. She states that she does not have time to bake special products for herself because her husband is a diabetic and one child has severe asthma. Give suggestions to help her in planning her diet. She wants to gain 10 pounds.
5. How could you change the diet you ate yesterday to make it free of gluten? To make it lactose free? To eliminate both lactose and gluten?
6. Mr. N. had a massive bowel resection. Which nutrients are likely to be poorly absorbed? Would MCT be useful in this disorder? Why?
7. Compare the dietary modifications used in nontropical and tropical sprue.

CITED REFERENCES

1. Isselbacher, K. J.: "Mechanisms of Absorption of Long and Medium Chain Triglycerides," in Senior, J. R., ed.: *Medium Chain Triglycerides*. University of Pennsylvania Press, Philadelphia, 1968, Chapter 3.
2. Schizas, A. A., *et al.*: "Medium-Chain Triglycerides—Use in Food Preparation," *J. Am. Diet. Assoc.*, **51**:228–32, 1967.
3. Johnson, J. D., *et al.*: "Lactose Malabsorption. Its Biology and History," *Adv. Pediatrics*, **21**:197–237, 1974.
4. Longstreth, G. F., and Newcomer, A. D.: "Drug-Induced Malabsorption," *Mayo Clin. Proc.*, **50**:284–93, 1975.
5. Greene, H. L., *et al.*: "Dietary Stimulation of Sucrase in a Patient with Sucrase-Isomaltase Deficiency," *Biochem. Med.*, **6**:409–18, 1972.
6. Lindquist, B., and Meeuwisse, G.: "Diets in Disaccharidase Deficiency and Defective Monosaccharide Absorption," *J. Am. Diet. Assoc.*, **48**:307–10, 1966.
7. Bayless, T. M., and Christopher, N. L.: "Disaccharide Deficiency," *Am. J. Clin. Nutr.*, **22**:181–90, 1969.

ADDITIONAL REFERENCES

Balacki, J. A., and Dobbins, W. O.: "Maldigestion and Malabsorption: Making Up for Lost Nutrients," *Geriatrics*, **29:**157–66, May 1974.

Dissanayake, A. S., *et al.:* "Lack of Harmful Effect of Oats on Small Intestinal Mucosa in Coeliac Disease," *Br. Med. J.*, **2:**189–91, 1974.

Evans, D. J., and Patey, A. L.: "Chemistry of Wheat Proteins and the Nature of the Damaging Substances," *Clin. Gastroenterology*, **3:**199–211, 1974.

Gallagher, C. R., *et al.:* "Lactose Intolerance and Fermented Dairy Products," *J. Am. Diet. Assoc.*, **65:**418–19, 1974.

"Lactase Deficiency," *Lancet*, **2:**910, 1975.

Review: "On the Pathogenesis of Gluten Sensitive Enteropathy," *Nutr. Rev.*, **32:**267–70, 1974.

Rosensweig, M. S.: "Diet and Intestinal Enzyme Adaptation: Implications for Gastrointestinal Disorders," *Am. J. Clin. Nutr.*, **28:**648–55, 1975.

Russell, R. I.: "Elemental Diets," *Gut*, **16:**68–79, 1975.

Stephenson, L. S., *et al.:* "Lactose Intolerance and Milk Consumption; the Relation of Tolerance to Symptoms," *Am. J. Clin. Nutr.*, **27:**296–303, 1974.

Wright, H. K., and Tilson, M. D.: "Short Gut Syndrome," *Current Prob. Surg.*, 3–51, June 1971.

SOURCES OF SPECIAL RECIPES

Medium-Chain-Triglyceride Diet

Mead Johnson Laboratories: *Recipes Using MCT Oil and Portagen.* Mead Johnson & Company, Evansville, Indiana.

Schizas, A. A., *et al.:* "Medium-Chain Triglycerides—Use in Food Preparation," *J. Am. Diet. Assoc.*, **51:**228–32, 1967.

Gluten-Restricted Diet

Allergy Recipes. American Dietetic Association, 430 North Michigan Ave., Chicago.

Celiac Disease Recipes. Hospital for Sick Children, Toronto, 1968.

French, A. B.: *Low Gluten Diet with Tested Recipes.* Clinical Research Unit, University Hospital, Ann Arbor, Michigan.

125 Great Recipes for Allergy Diets. Good Housekeeping Institute, 959 Eighth Ave., New York.

Sheedy, C. M., and Keifetz, N.: *Cooking for Your Celiac Child.* Dial Press, New York, 1969.

Lactose-Free Diet

Allergy Recipes: American Dietetic Association, Chicago.

Koch, R., *et al.:* "Nutrition in the Treatment of Galactosemia," *J. Am. Diet. Assoc.*, **43:**216–22, 1963.

125 Great Recipes for Allergy Diets. Good Housekeeping Institute, New York.

35 Diet in Disturbances of the Liver, Gallbladder, and Pancreas

*High-Protein,
High-Carbohydrate,
Moderate-Fat Diet;
Fat-Restricted Diet*

DISEASES OF THE LIVER—
GENERAL CONSIDERATIONS

The liver is the largest and most complex organ in the body. It performs many functions that have an important bearing on one's nutritional state. Diseases of this organ may therefore markedly affect health.

Functions. The role of the liver in intermediary metabolism with reference to proteins, fats, and carbohydrates has been described in Chapters 4, 5, and 6 and is briefly summarized as follows:

1. Protein metabolism (Chapter 4)—synthesis of plasma proteins; deaminization of amino acids; formation of urea.

2. Carbohydrate metabolism (Chapter 5)—synthesis, storage, and release of glycogen; synthesis of heparin.

3. Lipid metabolism (Chapter 6)—synthesis of lipoproteins, phospholipids, cholesterol; formation of bile; conjugation of bile salts; oxidation of fatty acids.

4. Mineral metabolism (Chapter 8)—storage of iron, copper, and other minerals.

5. Vitamin metabolism (Chapter 10)—storage of vitamins A and D; some conversion of carotene to vitamin A, and of vitamin K to prothrombin.

6. Detoxification of bacterial decomposition products, mineral poisons, and certain drugs and dyes.

Etiology. Liver diseases may have a number of causes: infectious agents, toxins, metabolic or nutritional factors, biliary obstruction, and carcinoma. The pathologic changes in the liver parenchymal cells are similar regardless of the etiology of the disease. Basic changes include atrophy, fatty infiltration, fibrosis, and necrosis.

Symptoms and clinical findings. *Jaundice* is a symptom common to many diseases of the liver and biliary tract and consists of a yellow pigmentation of the skin and body tissues because of the accumulation of bile pigments in the blood. *Obstructive jaundice* results from the interference of the flow of bile by stones, tumors, or inflammation of the mucosa of the ducts. *Hemolytic jaundice* results from an abnormally large destruction of blood cells such as occurs in yellow fever, pernicious anemia, and so forth. *Toxic jaundice* originates from poisons, drugs, or virus infections.

Other symptoms commonly seen in liver diseases include lassitude, weakness, fatigue, fever, anorexia, and weight loss; abdominal pain, flatulence, nausea, and vomiting; hepatomegaly; ascites and edema; and portal hypertension.

Nutritional considerations in liver disease. Protection of the parenchymal cells is the foremost consideration in all types of liver injury. Since the liver is so intimately involved in the metabolism of foodstuffs, a nutritious diet is an important part of therapy and should be designed to protect the liver from stress and to enable it to function as efficiently as possible. With the exception of hepatic coma, generous amounts of high-quality protein should be provided for tissue repair and for prevention of fatty infiltration and degeneration of liver cells. A high-carbohydrate intake ensures an adequate reserve of glycogen, which, together with adequate protein stores, has a protective effect. Moderate amounts of fat are indicated for many persons. Signs of nutritional deficiency such as glossitis, nutritional anemia, or peripheral neuropathy are not uncommon in patients with liver disease. Generous amounts of vitamins, especially of the B complex, must be provided to compensate for deficiencies. If edema and ascites are present, sodium restriction may be necessary.

HEPATITIS

Etiology and symptoms. This is an infectious disease characterized by inflammatory and degenerative changes of the liver. Two types are recognized, *viral* and *drug induced*. The viral type is more common and occurs as either *type A (infectious)* or *type B (serum)* hepatitis. Type A is due to an unidentified virus transmitted either by fecal contamination of water or food or parenterally. Epidemics occur from time to time in young people and are usually traced to a breakdown in sanitation. A specific antigen has been identified in type B viral hepatitis. This type is transmitted chiefly by the parenteral route in blood products containing the specific virus or through improperly sterilized needles. Drug-induced hepatitis may be due to alcohol, heroin, marihuana, or hashish, or to hypersensitivity to sulfa compounds or penicillin, or to a direct toxic effect on the liver by agents such as carbon tetrachloride.

Aside from mode of transmission and period of incubation, the two types of hepatitis are similar. Nonspecific symptoms such as anorexia, fatigue, nausea and vomiting, diarrhea, fever, weight loss, and abdominal discomfort usually precede the development of jaundice, which ordinarily subsides after one or two weeks. Complete recovery may take several months. Treatment consists of adequate rest, nutritious diet, and avoidance of further damage to the liver.

Dietary modification. The objectives of dietary treatment are to aid in the regeneration of liver tissue and to prevent further liver damage.

Energy. A high caloric intake, 3000 to 4000 daily,

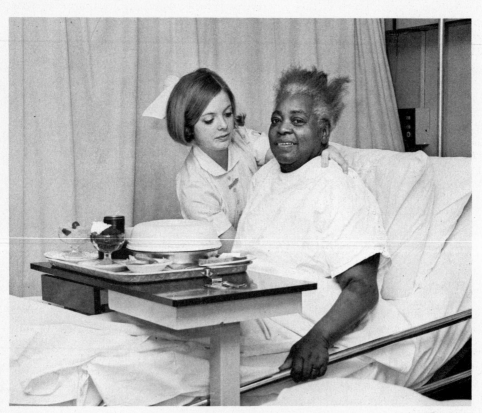

Figure 35-1. Many patients need some assistance at mealtime. The weak patient is better able to manage when shifted to a comfortable position. (Courtesy, School of Nursing, Thomas Jefferson University, Philadelphia.)

is needed to promote weight gain and to ensure maximum protein utilization.

Protein. An intake of 1½ to 2 gm protein per kilogram of body weight, or 100 to 150 gm protein daily, is needed to overcome negative nitrogen balance, to promote regeneration of parenchymal cells, and to prevent fatty infiltration of the liver.

Fat. Diets restricted in fats are not necessary in the majority of patients with hepatitis; in fact, their use may retard recovery if calories are thereby limited. Weight gain is more rapid and liver function tests revert to normal sooner when patients receive up to 150 gm fat daily.[1,2] Fats from dairy products, salad dressings, and cooking fats are easily utilized and add palatability to the diet without large amounts of bulk. If there is anorexia, fats may cause nausea and should be limited to amounts tolerated by the patient.

Carbohydrate. An intake of 300 to 400 gm carbohydrate ensures adequate glycogen reserves needed for the maintenance of liver function, for protection against further injury to the liver, and for its protein-sparing action.

Consistency. Foods of liquid to soft consistency (see Chapter 27) may be preferable if there is anorexia in the acute stages of the illness, progressing to a wider selection of foods with convalescence.

Dietary management. The patient must be convinced of the importance of the diet in promoting recovery and preventing relapses. Anorexia is frequently a problem; hence every effort must be made to encourage the patient to eat. Foods must be well prepared and attractively served with consideration given to the individual's food preferences. Judicious use of spices and condiments may help to stimulate the appetite. Small to moderate portions at mealtime with between-meal supplements of high-protein beverages are frequently more acceptable than larger meals. Some individuals need assistance in feeding themselves and should be allowed adequate time to eat at a leisurely pace. (See Figure 35–1.)

HIGH-PROTEIN, MODERATE-FAT, HIGH-CARBOHYDRATE DIET

Characteristics and General Rules

The caloric level may be increased by adding high-carbohydrate foods. Small amounts of cream and ice cream may be used when tolerated.

The protein intake may be increased by adding nonfat dry milk to liquid milk.

Modifications in fiber and consistency may be made by applying restrictions concerning the soft diet (Chapter 27) to the foods listed below.

Six or more small feedings may be preferred when there is lack of appetite.

When sodium restriction is ordered, all food must be prepared without salt. Low-sodium milk should replace part or all of the prescribed milk. See Sodium-Restricted Diets, Chapter 41.

Include These Foods Daily:

1 quart milk

8 ounces lean meat, poultry, or fish

1 egg

4 servings vegetables including:

    2 servings potato or substitute

    1 serving green leafy or yellow vegetable

    1–2 servings other vegetable

    One vegetable to be raw each day

3 servings fruit including:

    1 serving citrus fruit or other good source of ascorbic acid

    2 servings other fruit

1 serving enriched or whole-grain cereal

6 slices enriched or whole-grain bread

2 tablespoons butter or fortified margarine

4 tablespoons sugar, jelly, marmalade, or jam

Additional foods to further increase the carbohydrate as the patient is able to take them

Nutritive value of basic pattern on page 469: Protein, 135 gm; fat, 106 gm; carbohydrate, 236 gm; kcal, 2590; calcium, 2.53 gm; iron, 18.3 mg; vitamin A, 18,770 I.U.; thiamin, 2.11 mg; riboflavin, 3.39 mg; niacin, 27.6 mg; ascorbic acid, 159 mg.

Typical Food Selection
Beverages—carbonated beverages, milk and milk drinks, coffee, tea, fruit juices, cocoa flavoring
Breads and cereals—all kinds
Cheese—cottage, cream, mild Cheddar
Desserts—angel cake, plain cake and cookies, custard, plain or fruit gelatin, fruit whip, fruit pudding, Junket, milk and cereal desserts, sherbets, ices, plain ice cream
Eggs—any way
Fat—butter, fortified margarine, cream, cooking fat, vegetable oils
Fruits—all
Meat—lean beef, chicken, fish, lamb, liver, pork, turkey
Potato or substitute—hominy, macaroni, noodles, rice, spaghetti, sweet potato
Seasonings—salt, spices, vinegar (in moderation)
Soups—clear and cream
Sweets—honey, jam, jelly, sugar, sugar candy, syrups
Vegetables—all

Foods to Avoid
No foods are specifically contraindicated. Many patients complain of intolerance to the following groups of foods: strongly flavored vegetables; rich desserts; fried and fatty foods; chocolate; nuts; and highly seasoned foods. Although such complaints cannot always be explained on a physiologic basis, nothing is gained by giving the offending foods to the patient.

Meal Pattern	**Sample Menu**
BREAKFAST	
Fruit	Half grapefruit
Cereal with milk and sugar	Wheatena with milk and sugar
Egg	Scrambled egg
Whole-grain or enriched toast—2 slices	Whole-wheat toast
Butter or margarine—2 teaspoons	Butter
Marmalade—1 tablespoon	Orange marmalade
Beverage with cream and sugar	Coffee with cream and sugar
LUNCHEON OR SUPPER	
Lean meat, fish, or poultry—4 ounces	Broiled whitefish
Potato or substitute	Escalloped potatoes
Cooked vegetable	Buttered asparagus
Salad	Celery and carrot strips
Whole-grain or enriched bread—2 slices	Whole-wheat bread
Butter or margarine—2 teaspoons	Butter
Jelly—1 tablespoon	Grape jelly
Fruit	Sliced banana
Milk	Milk
MIDAFTERNOON	
Milk with nonfat dry milk	High-protein milk with strawberry flavor
DINNER	
Lean meat, fish, or fowl—4 ounces	Roast beef
Potato	Mashed potato
Vegetable	Baked acorn squash
Whole-grain or enriched bread—2 slices	Dinner rolls
Butter or margarine—2 teaspoons	Butter

Jelly—1 tablespoon
Fruit, or dessert
Milk—1 glass
Tea, if desired
  EVENING NOURISHMENT
Milk beverage

Apple jelly
Raspberry sherbet
Milk

High-protein milk flavored with caramel
Bread-and-jelly sandwich

CIRRHOSIS

Etiology. This chronic disease of the liver is characterized by diffuse degenerative changes, fibrosis, and nodular regeneration of the remaining cells. The causes include infectious hepatitis in a small percentage of patients, chronic alcoholism in association with malnutrition, underlying metabolic disturbances such as hemochromatosis or Wilson's disease, hepatotoxins derived from certain plants and fungi, and prolonged biliary stasis.

Laennec's cirrhosis. The most common type of cirrhosis in the United States is Laennec's (*alcoholic, portal*) cirrhosis. The exact etiology has not been established although alcohol and relative or absolute malnutrition are implicated in the majority of patients. Whether alcohol per se has a direct toxic effect on the liver is still controversial.[3,4] Pathologic changes include fatty infiltration, necrosis, and proliferation of fibrous tissue.

Symptoms and clinical findings. The onset of cirrhosis may be gradual with gastrointestinal disturbances such as anorexia, nausea, vomiting, pain, and distention. As the disease progresses, jaundice and other serious changes occur.

Ascites. Ascites is the accumulation of abnormal amounts of fluid in the abdomen. It may develop as a consequence of portal vein hypertension, obstruction of the hepatic vein, a fall in plasma colloid osmotic pressure due to impaired albumin synthesis, increased sodium retention, or impaired water excretion.

Esophageal varices (varicose veins). Varices in the esophagus and upper part of the stomach may develop as a complication of portal hypertension. Hemorrhage is then an ever-present danger and may be provoked by roughage of any kind. The hemorrhage itself may be fatal, or the blood may provide for the accumulation of ammonia and subsequent hepatic coma.

Modification of the diet. Regeneration of parenchymal cells occurs if appropriate diet therapy is initiated before the disease is well advanced. The high-protein, high-carbohydrate diet outlined for infectious hepatitis is satisfactory. In advanced cirrhosis, however, further dietary modification is needed.

Protein. Individual requirements for protein must be considered and intake must be adjusted as the disease progresses or improves. Most clinicians recommend an initial protein intake high enough to maintain nitrogen equilibrium, but low enough to prevent hepatic coma (approximately 35 to 50 gm per day).[5] Gradual increments to a maximal level of 1 gm protein per kilogram of body weight per day, or 65 to 85 gm daily, are associated with improved liver function and nutritional status. Intakes greater than this risk hepatic coma. Protein intake is restricted to less than 35 gm daily if signs of impending coma develop.

Fats. Malabsorption of fats occurs in many cirrhotics. For some patients the substitution of medium-chain triglycerides for part of the dietary fat is effective in reducing steatorrhea[6] (see Chapter 34).

Vitamins and minerals. Malabsorption of fat-soluble and B-complex vitamins occurs in alcoholic and biliary cirrhosis. Serum calcium, magnesium, and zinc are decreased. Potassium supplements are sometimes needed to correct deficiency resulting from nausea, vomiting, diarrhea, antibiotic therapy, or a reduced protein intake. Vitamin supplements may be advisable to replenish liver stores and repair tissue damage, especially if there is anorexia.

Sodium. Sodium restriction is prescribed if edema and ascites are present. Severe restriction of sodium for many months is often necessary for effective removal of excess fluid accumulation. Diets restricted to 250 mg sodium daily are not uncommon in this disorder. On such very low-sodium diets, all food used must be naturally low in sodium and prepared without sodium-containing compounds. Low-sodium milk is substituted for regular milk. Close attention to food selection is needed in order to provide an adequate protein intake without exceeding the sodium allowance (see Chapter 41).

Consistency. Reduction in fiber content of the diet is necessary in advanced cirrhosis when there is danger of hemorrhage from esophageal varices. A liquid or soft diet with small meals is used (see Chapter 27).

Hepatic Coma

Etiology. This is a complex syndrome characterized by neurologic disturbances which may develop as a complication of severe liver disease. It usually results from entrance of certain nitrogen-containing substances such as ammonia into the cerebral circulation without being metabolized by the liver. It may be a consequence of shunting of the portal blood into the systemic circulation in cirrhosis, or of severe damage to liver cells in hepatitis. Precipitating factors include gastrointestinal bleeding, severe infections, surgical procedures, excessive dietary protein, and sedatives.

Symptoms. Signs of impending coma include confusion, restlessness, irritability, inappropriate behavior, delirium, and drowsiness. There may also be incoordination and a flapping tremor of the arms and legs when extended. Electrolyte imbalance occurs. The patient may go into coma and may have convulsions. The breath has a fecal odor (*fetor hepaticus*). Prompt treatment is imperative or death occurs.

Dietary modification. The fundamental principle in the dietary management of hepatic coma is to reduce the protein intake to a minimum, thus decreasing the amount of ammonia produced. Catabolism of tissue proteins must also be avoided.

Calories. About 1500 to 2000 kcal are needed to prevent breakdown of tissue proteins for energy and are provided chiefly in the form of carbohydrates and fats. Although anorexia may occur, attempts should be made to keep the caloric intake as high as is practical to minimize tissue breakdown.

Protein. Some clinicians omit protein completely for two or three days and others permit 20 to 30 gm

daily. As the patient improves, the protein intake is gradually increased by 10 to 15 gm at a time until a maximum of 1 gm per kilogram of body weight is reached. The patient must be carefully watched following each increment lest signs of coma recur.

Levels of 40 to 50 gm protein daily may be used for long periods of time without detriment to nutritional status provided the diet is otherwise adequate. Nitrogen balance can be achieved on protein intakes as low as 35 gm daily[5] if high-quality protein is used and caloric intake is adequate.

Dietary management. These patients pose problems in feeding because of anorexia and behavioral patterns ranging from apathy, drowsiness, and confusion to irritability and hyperexcitability. The protein-free diet consisting of commercial sugar-fat emulsions, a butter-sugar mixture, or glucose in beverages or fruit juices may be used initially through oral or tube feeding. (See Chapter 42.) With improvements, the diets providing 20, 40, and 60 gm protein (see page 559) may be gradually introduced.

Diseases of the Gallbladder

Function of the gallbladder. The gallbladder concentrates bile formed in the liver and stores it until needed for digestion of fats. The entrance of fat into the duodenum stimulates secretion of the hormone *cholecystokinin* by the intestinal mucosa. The hormone is carried by way of the bloodstream to the gallbladder and forces it to contract, thus releasing bile into the common duct, and then into the small intestine where it is needed for the emulsification of fats. Interference with the flow of bile occurring in gallbladder disease may cause impaired fat digestion. From 5 to 10 per cent of the adult population have symptoms of gallbladder disease.

Inflammation of the gallbladder is known as CHOLECYSTITIS. Gallstone formation, or CHOLELITHIASIS, occurs when cholesterol, bile pigments, bile salts, calcium, and other substances precipitate out of the bile. An excess of cholesterol relative to other biliary lipids in bile favors gallstone formation. The etiology of gallstone growth is obscure although stasis, infection, and metabolic or chemical changes are all believed to play a role. In one study, autopsy data showed a higher incidence of gallstones in men who had consumed a diet high in polyunsaturated fats for some time. The authors speculated that alterations in bile salt metabolism (chenodeoxycholic acid) induced by the diet may have been responsible.[7] CHOLEDOCHOLITHIASIS refers to stones lodged in the common duct.

Symptoms and clinical findings. Mere presence of gallstones does not always produce symptoms; however, inflammation of the gallbladder or obstruction of the ducts by stones may cause severe pain whenever the gallbladder contracts. Ingestion of fatty foods may thus cause discomfort, and fat digestion may be impaired because of the diminished flow of bile. Intolerance to certain strongly flavored vegetables, legumes, melons, and berries occurs in many persons with gallbladder disease but the reason for this is not known.

Acute cholecystitis is usually associated with a gallstone lodged in the cystic duct and is accompanied by mild to severe pain, abdominal distention, nausea and vomiting, and fever.

Modification of the diet. The principal aim of dietary management in gallbladder disease is to reduce discomfort by providing a diet restricted in fat. Reduction of fibrous foods is sometimes desirable.

Energy. Many persons with gallbladder disease are overweight and should be given a calorie-restricted diet (see Chapter 29). Excessive calorie intake is associated with an increase in cholesterol gallstone formation.[8] With restriction of fats, carbohydrates are used more liberally to furnish the needed calories.

Fat. The patient receives no food initially during acute attacks of cholecystitis. Progression to a 20- to 30-gm fat diet is then made. If this is tolerated, the fat can then be increased to 50 to 60 gm daily, thus improving palatability of the diet. In chronic cholecystitis some degree of fat restriction is usually necessary.

Cholesterol. The chief component of most gallstones is cholesterol. High-cholesterol diets increase the biliary cholesterol level.[8] However, much more cholesterol is synthesized in the body from fragments of carbohydrates, amino acids, and fat metabolism. Dietary restriction of cholesterol, there-

Table 35–1. Food Allowances for Two Levels of Fat Restriction (Approximately 1500 kcal)

	20 gm Fat	50 gm Fat
Milk, skim	2 cups	2 cups
Meat, fish, poultry (lean	6 ounces*	6 ounces*
Eggs (3 per week)	$\frac{1}{2}$	$\frac{1}{2}$
Vegetables		
Dark green leafy or deep yellow	1 serving	1 serving
Potato	1 serving	1 serving
Other	1 or more servings	1 or more servings
Fruits		
Citrus	1 serving	1 serving
Other	3 servings	3 servings
Breads and cereals		
Cereals	1 serving	1 serving
Breads	6 slices	3 slices
Fats, vegetable	none	6 teaspoons
Sweets	3 tablespoons	2 tablespoons
Total fat, gm	20	50
Cholesterol, mg	270†	270†
Protein, gm	85	80
Kcal (approximate)	1500	1500

*Only lean cuts of meat, fish, poultry may be used. Each ounce is equivalent to 8 gm protein and 3 gm fat.

† Cholesterol level would be reduced to about half this level if eggs were not used. If butter is used instead of vegetable fat, the cholesterol level would be increased.

fore, is probably not very effective in prevention of gallstones. If a reduction in cholesterol content of the diet is ordered, egg yolks, liver, and other organ meats are omitted, and skim milk and margarine are substituted for whole milk and butter. See Table A–6 for cholesterol content of foods. Food allowances for two levels of fat restriction are shown in Table 35–1.

Fat-Restricted Diet

Foods Allowed

Beverages—whole milk, only 2 cups; skim milk as desired; coffee, coffee substitute, tea; fruit juices

Breads—all kinds except those with added fat

Cereals—all cooked or dry breakfast cereals, except possibly bran; macaroni, noodles, rice, spaghetti

Cheese—cottage only

Desserts—angel cake; fruit whip; fruit pudding; gelatin; ices and sherbets; milk and cereal puddings using part of milk allowance

Eggs—3 per week

Fats—vegetable oil or margarine

Fruits—all kinds when tolerated

Meats—broiled, baked, roasted, or stewed without fat: lean beef, chicken, lamb, pork, veal, fish

Seasonings—in moderation: salt, pepper, spices, herbs, flavoring extracts

Soups—clear

Sweets—all kinds: hard candy, jam, jelly, marmalade, sugars

Vegetables—all kinds when well tolerated; cooked without added butter, or cream

Foods to Avoid

Beverages—with cream; soda-fountain beverages with milk, cream, or ice cream

Breads—griddle cakes; sweet rolls with fat; French toast

Cheese—all whole-milk cheeses, both hard and soft

Desserts—any containing chocolate, cream, nuts, or fats: cookies, cake, doughnuts, ice cream, pastries, pies, rich puddings

Eggs—fried

Fats—cooking fats, cream, salad dressings

Fruits—avocado; raw apple, berries, melons may not be tolerated

Meats—fatty meats, poultry, or fish: bacon, corned beef, duck, goose, ham, fish canned in oil, mackerel, pork, sausage; organ meats
Smoked and spiced meats if they are poorly tolerated

Seasonings—sometimes not tolerated: pepper; curries; meat sauces; excessive spices; vinegar

Soups—cream, unless made with milk and fat allowance

Sweets—candy with chocolate and nuts

Vegetables—strongly flavored may be poorly tolerated: broccoli, Brussels sprouts, cabbage, cauliflower, cucumber, onion, peppers, radish, turnips; dried cooked peas and beans

Miscellaneous—fried foods; gravies; nuts; olives; peanut butter; pickles; popcorn; relishes

Meal Pattern (20 gm fat)

BREAKFAST

Fruit

Cereal with skim milk and sugar

Egg—1 only (3 per week)

Enriched or whole-grain toast

Jelly

Beverage with skim milk and sugar

LUNCHEON OR SUPPER

Lean meat, fish, poultry, or cottage cheese

Potato or substitute

Vegetable

Salad; no oil dressing

Sample Menu

Stewed apricots

Cornflakes with skim milk and sugar

Poached egg

Whole-wheat toast with jelly

Coffee with skim milk and sugar

Tomato bouillon

Fruit salad plate:
Cottage cheese
Sliced orange
Tokay grapes

Enriched or whole-grain bread
Dessert or fruit
Milk, skim—½ cup
   DINNER
Lean meat, poultry, or fish
Potato or substitute
Vegetable
Enriched or whole-grain bread
Jelly
Dessert or fruit
Milk, skim—1 glass

Diet following cholecystectomy. A fat-restricted diet may be used for some months following removal of the gallbladder. Thereafter, most individuals can tolerate a regular diet.

DIETARY COUNSELING

> Restriction of dietary fat influences the methods of food preparation permitted. The patient should be advised to prepare meats by baking, broiling, roasting, or stewing, and to use only lean meats trimmed of all visible fats. Meat drippings, cream sauces, and so on are not allowed, but spices and herbs in moderation can be used to enhance flavor of foods. Use of fortified skim milk and inclusion of green leafy or yellow vegetables is needed to help ensure adequate intake of vitamin A. The small amounts of fat permitted should be taken as butter or fortified margarine. Any foods known to cause distention should be omitted. Most individuals need guidance in selecting suitable substitutes for desserts that are high in fat.

PANCREATIC DISORDERS

Pancreatic disease may be due to congenital or inflammatory diseases, trauma, or tumors. Disorders of the pancreas usually involve inadequate production of enzymes needed for normal digestive processes. Interference with this process leads to impaired digestion and is manifested by the presence of excess fat and undigested protein in the stools.

Pear
Romaine
Sliced chicken sandwich
Vanilla blanc mange (using milk allowance)
Tea with milk, sugar

Roast lamb, trimmed of fat
Boiled new potatoes; no added fat
Zucchini squash
Parkerhouse roll
Jelly
Angel cake with sliced peaches
Milk, skim—1 glass

Some starch may also be present. Dietary treatment of pancreatic disorders depends on the nature and extent of digestive impairment rather than on the disease itself.

Acute pancreatitis. Acute inflammatory disease of the pancreas results from interference with the blood supply to the organ or from obstruction to the outflow of pancreatic juice. The usual causes are alcoholism and biliary tract disease; however, acute pancreatitis may also be due to trauma, virus infections, tumors, nutritional deficiency, certain vascular diseases, and a number of metabolic diseases. Acute pancreatitis and severe fat intolerance are also seen in types 1 and 5 hyperlipoproteinemias. (See Chapter 40.)

Acute pancreatitis may range from a mild inflammatory reaction to severe illness. The most predominant symptom is severe upper-abdominal pain radiating to the back and is aggravated by eating. Epigastric tenderness, distention, constipation, nausea, and vomiting occur.

Increased pressure in the ducts causes the activated pancreatic enzymes to escape into the interstitial tissues, thus leading to elevations in serum amylase and lipase. Other clinical findings include hyperlipemia and hypocalcemia. Alteration of structure or function of the pancreas or adjacent organs may be demonstrated radiographically. The islets of Langerhans are not necessarily involved.

Treatment. Conservative management is used. Aims are to alleviate pain, to keep pancreatic secretory activity at a minimum, and to replace fluids and electrolytes. Dietary management usually consists of giving the patient nothing by mouth during acute attacks. Progression from clear liquids to a soft (see Chapter 27) or bland (Chapter 32) diet is made as tolerated.

Chronic pancreatitis. This disease may be described as relapsing, recurrent, or continuous in nature. As in acute pancreatitis, alcoholism is the most common cause of attacks but the basic defect is not known. Alcohol indirectly stimulates pancreatic secretions, and one popular theory holds that it also obstructs pancreatic outflow.[9] Obstruction of the ducts leads to chronic changes including destruction of the islets of Langerhans in some patients, fibrosis, pseudocyst, and pancreatic calcification. Impaired digestion due to interference with enzyme activity leads to steatorrhea, creatorrhea, and deficiency of the B-complex and fat-soluble vitamins.

The chronic form is characterized by recurrent attacks of burning epigastric pain, especially after meals containing alcohol and fat. Other symptoms include flatulence, anorexia, weight loss, nausea, and vomiting.

Treatment. Conservative management is used unless the patient has unremitting pain or complications necessitating partial or complete pancreatectomy. Medications to alleviate pain and to inhibit pancreatic secretion are used.

The aim of dietary treatment is to minimize gastric secretion because of its stimulating effect on secretin output. Diet during attacks is the same as in acute pancreatitis. Thereafter, a soft diet, high in protein and calories, and low in fat, should be used. Some recommend 3000 to 6000 kcal, 100 to 150 gm protein, at least 400 gm carbohydrate, and 50 gm fat, gradually increasing fat according to the patient's tolerance.[10] Six small meals are better tolerated than large meals. Pancreatic extract is used to aid in fat absorption. Synthetic low-residue diets have been useful in the disease.[11]

Cystic fibrosis. This is a congenital disorder of unknown etiology in which there is generalized dysfunction of exocrine glands. The incidence is 1 per 2000 live births. About 10 million persons in the United States are carriers of the gene.[12]

Characteristics of the disease include abnormalities in mucus secretion and in sweat sodium and chloride levels. Secretion of abnormally thick mucus by exocrine glands obstructs ducts in the pancreas, lungs, and liver. Blockage of the ducts in the pancreas leads to fibrosis and cyst formation, and pancreatic enzymes are not released into the duodenum, interfering seriously with the utilization of proteins, fat, and carbohydrates. As much as 50 per cent of the protein and fat of the diet may be present in the feces. Impaired absorption of all nutrients occurs in many cases. Osteoporosis may be demonstrated radiologically. Chronic pulmonary disease and bronchial obstruction develop, and in some instances, obstruction of hepatic biliary ducts leads to portal hypertension and cirrhosis. Elevated levels of sodium and chloride—up to $2\frac{1}{2}$ times normal—are found in sweat. Massive salt loss in hot weather may cause heat stroke.

Symptoms. In the neonatal period, cystic fibrosis may present as meconium ileus, or there may be insidious onset of malnutrition in infants with good appetite but who nevertheless fail to grow and gain weight. Passage of foul-smelling, bulky, soft stools, haggard appearance, marked enlargement of the abdomen, and tissue wasting, especially about the buttocks, occur.

Treatment. General treatment consists of controlling pulmonary complications, maintaining good nutrition, and preventing abnormal salt loss. Measures designed to liquefy mucus, to minimize its formation, and to prevent obstruction are taken. Daily administration of pancreatic extract is prescribed.

Optimum nutrition should be maintained by careful attention to diet. A diet high in calories and protein with moderation in fat intake is needed in cases where fat is poorly tolerated. Calorie allowances must be sufficient to enable the individual to achieve desirable weight. The protein intake must be great enough to compensate for that lost in the stools. Protein hydrolysates may be useful in treating children who fail to grow. Medium-chain triglycerides are useful in this disorder and a proprietary formula containing these is available for infants.° Additional B-complex vitamins, ascorbic acid, and aqueous preparations of fat-soluble vitamins should be prescribed. Some recommend 2 to 4 gm of salt daily as a prophylactic measure.[13] Distribution of foods into six small feedings may be advisable for some persons, especially in the younger age groups.

° Pregestimil® by Mead Johnson & Co., Evansville, Indiana.

Problems and Review

1. Mr. T. is a 70-year-old retired bricklayer whose physician has recommended a soft, fat-restricted diet. Mr. T. lives alone since the recent death of his wife. He does some light cooking but usually eats his evening meal in a restaurant. He states that he does not have much of an appetite. Plan a day's menu for him. What recommendations would you make for foods eaten away from home?

2. Mr. J. is a 20-year-old unemployed laborer who has infectious hepatitis. Ordinarily, he eats all foods, but has lost 18 pounds due to marked anorexia. He still enjoys milkshakes, however.
   a. What type of diet would you expect his doctor to order for him?
   b. Plan two days' menus for him.
   c. He has a history of very irregular eating habits. Will this affect the course of his disease at present?

3. Mr. V. has cirrhosis of the liver and his physician has prescribed a 2500-kcal diet to help him regain some of the 22 pounds he has lost. The diet is to provide 75 gm protein, 80 gm fat, and 350 gm carbohydrate.
   a. Plan a day's menu for him.
   b. Show how you would modify this menu to reduce the sodium to 250 mg.
   c. Mr. and Mrs. V. depend on state aid for financial assistance. Because of their limited resources, they are accustomed to buying salt pork and other less expensive cuts of meat. How would you advise them in this regard?
   d. Mr. V.'s physician wants Mrs. V. to learn to adjust the protein intake at home so that she can adapt her husband's diet upon the physician's recommendation when signs of impending coma appear. How would you go about teaching her to do this?
   e. Mr. V. was later readmitted to the hospital in hepatic coma. The doctor has ordered a protein-free diet for him. Plan a day's menu that supplies 2000 kcal. Adjust this menu to provide 10, 20, 30, and 40 gm protein.

4. Mrs. M. is a 56-year-old woman with cholelithiasis whose physician has ordered a 1200-kcal fat restricted diet. What factors are important in the dietary management of this woman?
   a. What problems might she face in preparing meals if fat is limited to 25 gm per day?
   b. Plan a day's menu for her with 25 gm fat; adjust to provide 50 gm fat.

5. Mr. H. has chronic pancreatitis. What type of diet would you expect his doctor to order? Plan a day's menu. Should he take vitamin supplements?

Cited References

1. Sherlock, S.: "The Treatment of Hepatitis," *Bull. N.Y. Acad. Med.*, **45**:189–200, 1969.
2. Silverberg, M., *et al.*: "An Evaluation of Rest and Low Fat Diets in the Management of Acute Infectious Hepatitis," *J. Pediatr.*, **74**:260–64, 1969.
3. Rubin, E., and Lieber, C. S.: "Alcohol Induced Hepatic Injury in Non-Alcoholic Volunteers," *N. Engl. J. Med.*, **278**:869–76, 1968.
4. Davidson, C. S.: "Nutrition, Geography, and Liver Diseases," *Am. J. Clin. Nutr.*, **23**:427–36, 1970.
5. Gabuzda, G. J., and Shear, L.: "Metabolism of Dietary Protein in Hepatic Cirrhosis. Nutritional and Clinical Considerations," *Am. J. Clin. Nutr.*, **23**:479–87, 1970.
6. Linscheer, W. G.: "Malabsorption in Cirrhosis," *Am. J. Clin. Nutr.*, **23**:288–92, 1970.
7. Sturdevant, R. A., *et al.*: "Increased Prevalence of Cholelithiasis in Men Ingesting a Serum Cholesterol-Lowering Diet," *N. Engl. J. Med.*, **288**:24–27, 1973.
8. Sarles, H., *et al.*: "Diet, Cholesterol Gallstones, and Composition of the Bile," *Am. J. Dig. Dis.*, **15**:251–60, 1970.
9. Baum, R., and Iber, F. L.: "Alcohol, the Pancreas, Pancreatic Inflammation, and Pancreatic Insufficiency," *Am. J. Clin. Nutr.*, **26**:347–51, 1973.
10. Taubin, H. L., and Spiro, H. M.: "Nutritional Aspects of Chronic Pancreatitis," *Am. J. Clin. Nutr.*, **26**:369–73, 1973.
11. Voitk, A., *et al.*: "Use of an Elemental Diet in the Treatment of Complicated Pancreatitis," *Am. J. Surg.*, **125**:223–27, 1975.

12. Di Sant' Agnese, P. A.: "Cystic Fibrosis (Mucoviscidosis)," *Am. Fam. Physician,* **7:**102–11, Mar. 1973.
13. Crozier, D. N.: "Cystic Fibrosis. A Not-So-Fatal Disease," *Pediatr. Clin. North Am.,* **21:**935–50, 1974.

ADDITIONAL REFERENCES

Berry, H. K., *et al.:* "Dietary Supplement and Nutrition in Children with Cystic Fibrosis," *Am. J. Dis. Child.,* **129:**165–71, 1975.
Cooper, A. D., *et al.:* "Liver Disease in Nonparenteral Drug Abusers," *J.A.M.A.,* **233:**964–66, 1975.
Coyne, M. J., and Schoenfield, L. J.: "Gallstone Disease," *Postgrad. Med.,* **57:**153–58, Jan. 1975.
Davidson, C. S.: "Dietary Treatment of Hepatic Diseases," *J. Am. Diet. Assoc.,* **62:**515–19, 1973.
Kafka, E. C., and Kalser, M. H.: "Pancreatic Disease," *Postgrad. Med.,* **57:**140–45, Jan. 1975.
Leevy, C. M., *et al.:* "Vitamins and Liver Injury," *Am. J. Clin. Nutr.,* **23:**493–99, 1970.
Meyer, J. D., *et al.:* "Food-Borne Hepatitis A in a General Hospital," *J.A.M.A.,* **231:**1049–53, 1975.
Patek, A.: "Alcohol and Dietary Factors in Cirrhosis," *Arch. Intern. Med.,* **135:**1053–57, 1975.
Review: "Effects of Diet on Biliary Lipid Secretion and Bile Composition," *Nutr. Rev.,* **33:**72–74, 1975.
Rosenlund, M. L., and Lustig, H. S.: "Young Adults with Cystic Fibrosis: The Problems of a New Generation," *Ann. Intern. Med.,* **78:**959–61, 1973.
Schenker, S., *et al.:* "Hepatic Encephalopathy: Current Status," *Gastroenterology,* **66:**121–51, 1974.
Sherlock, S.: "Nutritional Complications of Biliary Cirrhosis," *Am. J. Clin. Nutr.,* **23:**640–44, 1970.
Simmons, S., and Given, B.: "Acute Pancreatitis," *Am. J. Nurs.,* **71:**934–39, 1971.
Wewalka, F.: "Clinical Course of Viral Hepatitis," *Clin. Gastroenterol.* **3:**355–76, 1974.

36 Nutrition in Surgical Conditions

*Tube Feedings;
High-Protein, High-Fat,
Low-Carbohydrate Diet*

Significant advances have been made in the area of surgical nutrition within the past decade. A better understanding of the effects of stress on metabolism, together with the development of numerous preparations suitable for oral, intravenous, or tube feeding, has made possible substantial improvement in the nutritional status of patients both before and after surgery.

Effects of surgery on the nutritive requirements. Good nutrition prior to and following surgery assures fewer postoperative complications, better wound healing, shorter convalescence, and lower mortality. The patient whose preoperative nutritional state is poor is at increased risk when he undergoes major surgery. Persons with chronic diseases are especially likely to have less than optimal nutriture. Hyperthyroidism or chronic infection as in bronchiectasis increases requirements. Serious malabsorption of nutrients may occur especially in liver diseases and those involving the gastrointestinal tract. Extensive losses of nutrients and fluids may have occurred through hemorrhage, vomiting, or diarrhea.

The extent of the deficiency is manifested by weight loss, poor wound healing, decreased intestinal motility, anemia, edema, or dehydration, and the presence of decubitus ulcers. The circulating blood volume and the concentration of the serum proteins, hemoglobin, and electrolytes may be reduced.

Following surgery or injury the need for nutrients is greatly increased as a result of loss of blood, plasma, or pus from the wound surface; hemorrhage from the gastrointestinal or pulmonary tract; vomiting; and fever. During immobilization, the loss of some nutrients such as protein is accelerated.

A fairly simple operation often involves moderate deficiency in food intake for a few days following the operation. Some nutrients may be supplied by parenteral fluids, but the full needs of the body usually are not met by that means alone. Provided that adequate oral intake is rapidly resumed, the metabolic losses are not of serious consequence. On the other hand, adequate oral intake is often delayed for a considerable period following cardiac or gastrointestinal surgery. Metabolic losses are great and alternative methods of nutritional support are needed.

Nutritional considerations. The objectives in the dietary management of surgical conditions are (1) to improve the preoperative nutrition whenever the operation is not of an emergency nature, (2) to maintain correct nutrition after operation or injury insofar as possible, and (3) to avoid harm from injudicious choice of foods.

Protein. A satisfactory state of protein nutrition ensures rapid wound healing by providing the correct assortment and quantity of essential amino acids, increases the resistance to infection, exerts a protective action upon the liver against the toxic effects of anesthesia, and reduces the possibility of edema at the site of the wound. The presence of edema is a hindrance to wound healing and, in operations on the gastrointestinal tract, may reduce motility thus leading to distention.

Concern for the protein nutritional status of surgical patients has been emphasized recently.[1,2] It is not always realistic to fully replace protein losses prior to surgery because the disease process itself may be such as to preclude a satisfactory intake of food. For selected patients, parenteral administration of amino acids and adequate calories is useful. The extent to which surgery should be delayed in order to improve the nutritional state is obviously a highly individual matter.

Protein catabolism is increased for several days immediately following surgery or injury; patients are characteristically in negative nitrogen balance even though the protein intake may be appreciable.

Well-nourished persons lose more nitrogen than poorly nourished persons whose labile protein stores are already depleted. The degree of negative balance can be reduced at higher intakes of protein and calories.

The level of protein to be used in preoperative and postoperative diets depends upon the previous state of nutrition, the nature of the operation, and the extent of the postoperative losses. Intakes of 100 gm protein, and frequently much more, are necessary as a rule.

Energy. The weight status is an important pre- and postoperative consideration, for it serves as a guide to the caloric level to be recommended. Without sufficient caloric intake, tissue proteins cannot be synthesized. Excessive metabolism of body fat may lead to acidosis, whereas depletion of the liver glycogen may increase the likelihood of damage to the liver.

In hyperthyroidism or fever, as much as 4000 kcal daily may be essential to bring about weight gain. Other patients will make satisfactory progress at 2500 to 3000 kcal.

Obesity constitutes a hazard in surgery. Whenever possible, it should be corrected, at least in part, by using one of the calorie-restricted diets (see page 410).

Minerals. Phosphorus and potassium are lost in proportion to the breakdown of body tissue. In addition, derangements of sodium and chloride metabolism may occur subsequent to vomiting, diarrhea, perspiration, drainage, anorexia, and diuresis or renal failure. The detection of electrolyte imbalance and appropriate parenteral fluid therapy requires careful study of clinical signs and biochemical evaluation.

Iron-deficiency anemia occurs in association with malabsorption or excessive blood loss. Diet alone is ineffective in correction of anemia, but a liberal intake of protein and ascorbic acid, together with administration of iron salts, is of value in convalescence. Transfusions are usually required to overcome severe reduction in hemoglobin level.

Fluids. The sources of water and the large amounts of fluids lost daily by the normal individual are outlined on page 127. The fluid balance may be upset prior to and following surgery owing to failure to ingest normal quantities of fluids and to increased losses from vomiting, exudates, hemorrhage, diuresis, and fever. A patient should not go to operation in a state of dehydration since the subsequent dangers of acidosis are great. When dehydration exists prior to operation, parenteral fluids are administered if the patient is unable to ingest sufficient liquid by mouth. Following major surgery the fluid balance is maintained by parenteral fluids until satisfactory oral intake can be established.

Vitamins. Ascorbic acid is especially important for wound healing and should be provided in increased amounts prior to and following surgery. Vitamin K is of concern to the surgeon since the failure to synthesize vitamin K in the small intestine, the inability to absorb it, or the defect in conversion to prothrombin is likely to result in bleeding. Hemorrhage is especially likely to occur in patients who have diseases of the liver.

Planning the preoperative diet. Patients who have lost much weight prior to surgery benefit considerably by ingesting a high-protein, high-calorie diet (see page 416) for even a week or two prior to surgery. The diet may be of liquid, soft, or regular consistency depending upon the nature of the pathologic condition. Certain patients may benefit from parenteral nutrition or use of synthetic low-residue diets.[3,4] In addition, the maintenance of metabolic equilibrium as in diabetes or other diseases must not be overlooked.

When surgery is delayed in order to improve the nutritional status, each day's intake should represent such improvement in nutrition that the delay is justified. This necessitates constant encouragement by the nurse and dietitian; it likewise requires imagination in varying the foods offered to the patient and ingenuity in getting the patient to eat. Foods which provide a maximum amount of nutrients in a minimum volume are essential. Small feedings at frequent intervals are likely to be better accepted than large meals which cannot be fully consumed.

For additional protein, milk beverages may be fortified with nonfat dry milk or commercial protein supplements. Strained meat in broth may be used when patients are unable to eat other meats. Fruit juices fortified with glucose, high-carbohydrate lemonade, jelly with crackers and bread, and hard candy may be used to increase the carbohydrate intake and to facilitate storage of glycogen. Butter incorporated into foods and light cream mixed with equal amounts of milk are also useful for increasing the caloric intake. The excessive use of sugars and fats may provoke nausea, however.

Food and fluids are generally allowed until midnight just preceding the day of operation, although a light breakfast may be given when the operation is scheduled for afternoon and local anesthesia is to be used. It is essential that the stomach be empty prior to administering the anesthesia so as to reduce the incidence of vomiting and the subsequent danger of aspiration of vomitus. When an operation is to be performed on the gastrointestinal tract, a diet very low in residue (page 446) may be ordered two to three days prior to operation. Synthetic low-residue diets (see Chapter 34) are useful for such cases.[5] In acute abdominal conditions such as appendicitis and cholecystitis, no food is allowed by mouth until nausea, vomiting, pain, and distention have passed in order to prevent the danger of peritonitis.

Planning the postoperative diet. Resumption of oral intake depends upon the nature of the surgery and the individual's progress. Following minor surgery, liquids are often tolerated within a few hours and rapid progression to a normal diet is made. After major surgery, however, oral intake may be delayed for days. Alternative methods for partial or complete nutritional support are provided by conventional intravenous feedings, total parenteral nutrition, tube feedings, or synthetic low-residue diets.

Parenteral feedings. During the interval when the patient is unable to ingest food or fluid by mouth, intravenous feedings are used for maintenance or restoration of fluid and electrolyte balance. These feedings furnish primarily fluids and salts. Some contain glucose, which serves to prevent ketosis and to minimize tissue catabolism. Amino acid solutions are sometimes used in place of glucose because of their nitrogen-sparing effects achieved through reduction of serum glucose and insulin levels and enhanced utilization of adipose stores.[6,7] None of these intravenous fluids can meet nutritional needs completely.

Total parenteral nutrition. For severely debilitated patients, TOTAL PARENTERAL NUTRITION is useful in providing complete nutritional support for extended periods. This method requires a careful consideration of the nature of the illness, physical examination to evaluate subjective changes, and laboratory analyses for blood glucose, electrolytes, pH, and proteins. The precise nutritional contributions made by such feedings and the details of management are beyond the scope of this text but have been reviewed elsewhere.[8] The method involves passage of an indwelling catheter into the superior vena cava with continuous infusion of a hypertonic solution of 20 to 25 per cent glucose, 3 to 5 per cent protein hydrolysate or amino acids, vitamins, and minerals. Essential fatty acid deficiency has been reported in adult patients who received no source of linoleic acid.[9] Balance studies using this method have shown that patients with moderate postoperative stress require at least 8 gm nitrogen and 1800 kcal daily for positive nitrogen balance. Most postoperative patients require 12 to 13 gm nitrogen and 2500 kcal.[10] Dudrick and coworkers have shown that up to 6000 kcal daily can be supplied using this technique.[11]

Intravenous fat emulsions make possible a substantial increase in caloric intake and promote positive nitrogen balance.[12] These emulsions, though widely used abroad, are approved for investigational use only in the United States.

Progression of oral feeding. Motility of the gastrointestinal tract is diminished following abdominal surgery. Small intestine motility recovers rapidly but return of gastric motility may take 24 hours or longer, and colonic motility three to five days.[13] Patients are given nothing by mouth for the first 24 hours following surgery. Oral feeding is begun after gastrointestinal secretions are being produced and peristalsis resumes. Feeding should not be delayed once such function has returned. The accumulation of gastrointestinal secretions may result in a feeling of fullness. Moreover, the wound strength is sufficient to permit digestion of food.

Progression from ice chips to sips of water, then clear liquids and full liquids is made in accordance with the patient's tolerance. Patients usually respond better once they are given solid foods. Initially, the feedings are small and may be restricted to a low-residue diet. (See also Chapter 32.) Foods which are high in protein and fat are believed to be less distending than those which are high in carbohydrate.[14] Perhaps of greater importance is the emphasis upon eating slowly and in small amounts to reduce the amount of air which is swallowed. As the patient improves, the selection of foods is that of a soft or regular diet, depending upon the nature of the surgery.

Tube Feedings

Feeding by tube may be required for a short period of time or indefinitely in a variety of circumstances: surgery of the head and neck; esophageal obstruction; gastrointestinal surgery; in severe burns; in anorexia nervosa; and in the comatose patient. For short-term use the feedings are ordinarily given by nasogastric tube, but for long-term use, the feeding is administered through a tube inserted into a new opening ("-*ostomy*") made in the stomach (GASTROSTOMY) or intestine.

Characteristics of tube feedings. A satisfactory tube feeding must be (1) nutritionally adequate; (2) well tolerated by the patient so that vomiting is not induced; (3) easily digested with no unfavorable reactions such as distention, diarrhea, or constipation; (4) easily prepared; and (5) inexpensive.

The concentration of the feeding may be adjusted from about $2/3$ to $1\frac{1}{3}$ kcal per milliliter. Lesser concentrations increase the volume which must be given to meet nutrient and energy needs, and greater concentrations are more likely to produce diarrhea and may be too thick to pass through a nasogastric tube. A concentration of about 1 kcal per milliliter is satisfactory. Two liters per 24 hours is a customary volume.

The proportion of protein, fat, and carbohydrate should approximate that of the normal diet. Adverse effects of excesses include azotemia, hypernatremia, dehydration, and death due to excessive protein intake,[15] and diarrhea as a result of high lactose content.[16] Adequate fluid intake is essential to prevent salt or protein overload.

Types of tube feedings. Three types of tube feedings are in common use: milk-base, blended, and synthetic formulas. Several commercial preparations are available for each of these types. Likewise, recipes are available for the preparation of milk-based and blended feedings within the hospital or home. Most of these recipes use whole or skim milk, eggs, and vitamin supplements together with some form of carbohydrate such as strained cooked cereals, sugar, or molasses. Vegetable oil or cream and nonfat dry milk are also incorporated to increase the calorie and protein levels, respectively.

Tube feedings prepared from the ordinary foods of a normal diet by using a high-speed blender are generally preferred to other types of formulas. Strained baby meats, fruits, and vegetables are used in addition to the foods listed above. Blenderized tube feedings are well tolerated and are only infrequently associated with diarrhea. They permit flexibility in meeting specific nutrient needs and are less expensive than commercial formulas. On the other hand, the commercial preparations possess the advantages of convenience, constant composition, presterilization, minimal preparation time, and ease of administration. The nutrient composition of several of these preparations is shown in Table 36–1.

Administration of tube feedings. Depending upon its nature, the feeding may be heated over hot water to body temperature, taking care that curdling does not occur with certain mixtures. Initially, small amounts of a dilute formula (50 ml) are given at hourly intervals. It is important that the feeding be given at a slow constant rate. A food pump is recommended for use with blenderized feedings.[17] In patients who do not have an adequate swallowing mechanism or who are comatose, special care must be taken to avoid vomiting and aspiration of the vomitus. The patient should be positioned to prevent aspiration, and suction should be readily available at the bedside if vomiting occurs. Close attention to individual water needs is essential.

When the small feedings are satisfactorily tolerated, the concentration and amount of the formula is gradually increased, with feedings not exceeding 12 ounces per three- to four-hour interval.

Synthetic low-residue diets. Mixtures of amino acids, sugars, vitamins, and minerals are used in both preoperative and postoperative patients in whom it is desirable to rest the bowel completely without compromising nutrition. (See Chapter 34.) They are given orally or by tube and have been used for extended periods. Palatability is a problem when the feedings are given orally. Frequent determinations of blood glucose and electrolytes and of urinary sugar and acetone are needed. The precautions needed in administration of tube feedings apply to use of these formulas as well.

Table 36–1. Composition of Some Products Suitable for Tube Feeding*

	Brand A Blenderized	Brand B Lactose free	Brand C Synthetic fiber free	Brand D Milk based
		per 100 ml		
Kcal	100	106	100	156
Protein, gm	4.00	3.71	2.00	6.00
Fat, gm	4.00	3.71	0.15	1.50
Carbohydrate, gm	12.00	14.45	22.60	17.00
Vitamin A, I.U.	313.00	265.00	278.00	440.00
Vitamin D, I.U.	25.00	21.00	22.00	35.00
Vitamin E, I.U.	2.00	3.20	1.70	0.90
Ascorbic acid, mg	4.00	16.00	4.00	26.50
Folic acid, mg	0.01	0.05	0.01	0.04
Thiamin, mg	0.10	0.17	0.07	0.90
Riboflavin, mg	0.10	0.18	0.07	0.90
Niacin, mg	0.60	2.12	0.74	8.80
Vitamin B_6, mg	0.10	0.20	0.11	0.44
Vitamin B_{12}, mcg	0.40	0.63	0.28	0.35
Calcium, mg	60.00	42.00	44.00	270.00
Phosphorus, mg	100.00	42.00	44.00	200.00
Iodine, mcg	8.00	3.50	0.01	15.00
Iron, mg	1.10	0.95	0.60	1.30
Magnesium, mg	21.00	21.00	19.40	40.00
Zinc, mg	0.90	1.59	0.69	2.00

*Brand A: Compleat B, Doyle Pharmaceutical Company, Minneapolis, Minnesota.
Brand B: Ensure, Ross Laboratories, Columbus, Ohio.
Brand C: Vivonex, Eaton Laboratories, Norwich, New York.
Brand D: Sustagen, Mead Johnson & Company, Evansville, Indiana.

DIET IN SPECIFIED SURGICAL CONDITIONS

Diet following operations on the mouth, throat, or esophagus. The period between full extraction of teeth and satisfactory adjustment to new dentures may take several weeks. For one or two days following the surgery, it may be necessary to restrict the diet to liquids taken through a drinking tube. Thereafter, any soft foods which require little if any chewing may be used for three weeks or longer.

Radical surgery of the mouth necessitates the use of full fluids or puréed foods, but immediately after surgery one of the regimens for tube feeding described in the previous section may be used. Following an operation on the esophagus, a gastrostomy tube feeding is used.

After tonsillectomy the patient is given cold fluids including milk, bland fruit juices, ginger ale, plain ice cream, and sherbets. Tart fruit juices and fibrous foods must be avoided. On the second day, soft foods such as custard, plain puddings, soft eggs, warm but not hot cereals, strained cream soups, mashed potatoes, and fruit and vegetable purées may be tolerated. As a rule, the regular diet is swallowed without difficulty within the week.

Diet following gastrectomy. A number of problems arise following gastrectomy, and their treatment should be anticipated. Weight loss is common, and studies undertaken up to 20 years following surgery indicate that most patients fail to regain weight to desirable levels.[18] The loss of a reservoir for food means that small feedings given at frequent intervals must be used if sufficient nutrients are to be ingested. Moreover, the absence of pepsin and hydrochloric acid entails the entire digestion of protein by the enzymes of the small intestine. Fat utilization is often impaired because of inadequate biliary and pancreatic secretions or defective mixing of food with the digestive juices. Intestinal motility is frequently increased.

Iron is less readily absorbed and hypochromic microcytic anemia is common. In the absence of gastric juice and its intrinsic factor vitamin B_{12} cannot be absorbed from the intestine, thereby eventually leading to macrocytic anemia unless injections of vitamin B_{12} are given.

Dietary progression. Oral feedings vary widely from one patient to another. The usual sequence consists of hourly feedings of 60 to 90 ml fluids for several days with progression from water to full liquids by the third day. Thereafter, the diet increases from day to day according to the individual's tolerance for food. By the fourth or fifth day, soft low-fiber foods are used. Eggs, custards, thickened soups, cereals, crackers, milk, and fruit purées are suitable. Tender meats, cottage cheese, and puréed vegetables are the next foods added. Meals are divided into five or six small feedings daily with emphasis on foods high in protein and fat; carbohydrate is kept relatively low. The selection of foods allowed for the first stage of the Bland Low-Fiber Diet (Chapter 32) or the Very Low-Residue Diet (Chapter 33) may be used initially. Many patients progress more satisfactorily if no liquids are taken with meals, and if the diet continues to be low in carbohydrate, especially the simple sugars. (See Figure 36–1.)

Diet following intestinal surgery. Obstruction, persistent ileitis or diverticulitis, perforation, and malignancy are among the reasons for removal of a section of the ileum (ILEECTOMY) or colon (COLECTOMY). A permanent opening is made in the abdominal wall for elimination of wastes. Following removal of part of the ileum and colon, the proximal end of the ileum is attached to the opening (ILEOSTOMY). Because the absorptive function of the colon

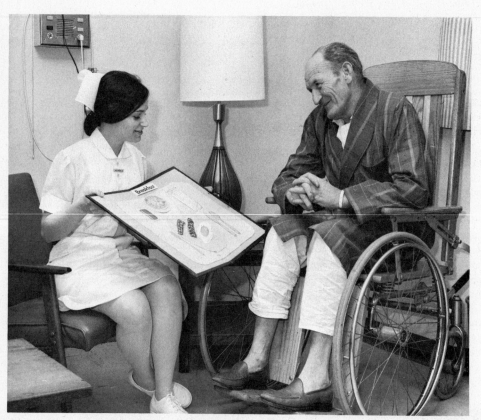

Figure 36–1. Convalescent patient receives some guidance for improving his diet when he goes home. (Courtesy, School of Nursing, Thomas Jefferson University, Philadelphia.)

has been eliminated by the surgery, the waste material is fluid and continuous. Fluid, sodium, and potassium losses may be considerable, fat absorption is often poor, and vitamin B_{12} absorption is reduced or absent.

A COLOSTOMY consists in attaching the proximal end of the resected colon to the opening in the abdominal wall. Some ability to absorb water is retained so that feces are more or less formed, and bowel regularity can be reestablished.

Following any operation upon the small intestine or colon, the initial oral intake is restricted to clear fluids and followed with a low-residue diet as a rule. Patients with an ileostomy are usually young and require a good deal of guidance and support from the nurse and dietitian. Gradually, they may add foods moderately low in fiber, but each food should be tested for tolerance before introducing a second. Weight loss may be considerable, and a high-protein, high-calorie diet is generally required. Vitamin B_{12} injections are required to prevent the occurrence of macrocytic anemia in later years.

Colostomy is performed more frequently on elderly persons. In time they may resume an essentially normal diet, but usually they require some counseling concerning the foods required for nutritive adequacy. They too require emotional support as well as assurance that foods will not be harmful.

Small intestinal bypass is used in treating selected persons with massive obesity. By means of a JEJUNOILEOSTOMY a short segment of the jejunum is joined to the terminal ileum, effectively bypassing about 90 per cent of the small bowel. Weight loss follows as a result of the shortened transit time and reduced surface area for absorption of nutrients. A number of serious metabolic consequences have been described, including diarrhea, electrolyte imbalance, anemia, calcium oxalate urinary calculi, hyperuricemia, osteoporosis, beriberi, fatty infiltration of the liver, cirrhosis, and death.[19-21] Some evidence suggests that the fatty changes in the liver can be reversed by amino acid infusions.[22] Average weight loss after one year is about 30 per cent; in some instances loss of an excessive amount of weight or failure to lose sufficiently has necessitated revision of the shunt.

Diarrhea and electrolyte imbalance are severe in the immediate postoperative period. Diarrhea is worsened by the ingestion of foods high in fat, fiber, or lactose, or by excessive fluids.[19] In severe diarrhea fluids are restricted to 1000 to 1200 ml per 24 hours, and are given between meals rather than at meals. A high-protein, low-fat, low-carbohydrate diet is given in six small feedings.[23] Multivitamins are usually recommended. Losses of potassium, calcium, and magnesium may be substantial and provision of good food sources of these minerals should be made.

Diet following other abdominal operations. The principles outlined on page 481 pertain to the planning of diet following appendectomy, cholecystectomy, and other abdominal operations. Adynamic ileus is present longer following cholecystectomy and hysterectomy than after removal of the appendix. Patients who have had the gallbladder removed may require a fat-restricted diet for several weeks after which a regular diet is used.

Following peritonitis and intestinal obstruction, nothing whatever is given by mouth until gastrointestinal function has been resumed. Drainage of the stomach and upper intestine is essential until there is reduction of distention and passage of gas. This may require several days, during which time nutrition is maintained by intravenous therapy. When the patient shows tolerance for water, broth, and weak tea, a very low-residue diet is introduced cautiously.

See Chapters 40 and 42 for nutritional considerations following coronary bypass surgery for advanced coronary artery disease and renal transplantation, respectively.

Diet following burns. Tremendous losses of protein, salts, and fluid take place when large areas of the body have been burned. Energy expenditure following major burns is increased 50 to 100 per cent above basal needs and the greatly increased nutritive requirements exist for weeks or months. Severe hypoproteinemia, edema at the site of injury, failure to obtain satisfactory skin growth, gastric atony, and weight loss are among the nutritional problems encountered. In patients with serious weight loss and inadequate oral intake, total parenteral nutrition or tube feeding, or both, may be needed to establish caloric equilibrium.[24] At least 150 gm protein, and often much more, are required daily together with 3500 to 5000 kcal. When oral feedings are tolerated, high-protein meals supplemented with high-protein beverages are used (see Chapter 30). The need for as much as 1.0 gm ascorbic acid has been definitely established, and additional B-complex vitamins are also considered essential.

Diet following fractures. Following fractures there is a tremendous catabolism of protein, which may not be reversed for several weeks. Nitrogen loss is accompanied by loss of phosphorus, potassium, and sulfur. Fever and infection may further accentuate such losses.

Calcium loss is also great but calcium therapy may lead to the formation of renal calculi and should not be attempted until the cast is removed and some mobilization is possible.

A liberal intake of protein is essential to permit restoration of the protein matrix of the bone so that calcium can be deposited. Sufficient calories to permit maximum use of the protein for synthesis should be provided.

DUMPING SYNDROME

Nature of the dumping syndrome. Following convalescence from gastric surgery a relatively high proportion of patients experience distressing symptoms about 10 to 15 minutes after eating. There is a sense of fullness in the epigastrium with weakness, nausea, pallor, sweating, and dizziness. The pulse rate increases and the patient seeks to obtain relief by lying down for a few minutes. Vomiting and diarrhea are infrequently present. Weight loss is common because of insufficient intake and malabsorption. About 16 per cent of patients who develop this syndrome continue to have severe symptoms as long as 12 years after the surgery.[25]

The exact etiology of the dumping has not been established, but may be partly explained as follows: Ingestion of large amounts of easily hydrolyzed carbohydrates following loss of the pylorus rapidly introduces a hyperosmolar mixture into the proximal intestine. Fluid withdrawn from the extracellular space to dilute this mixture leads to distention and the cardiovascular symptoms. Both the gastrointestinal[26] and the vasomotor[27] symptoms have been attributed to release of vasoactive hormones from the small intestine.

Modification of the diet. Dietary regimens developed to alleviate the symptoms of the dumping syndrome emphasize the following: (1) avoidance of sugar and concentrated forms of carbohydrate, (2) liberal protein, (3) small frequent feedings, and (4) dry meals with fluids taken only between meals.

Initially, calories from carbohydrates, proteins, and fats are supplied in a ratio of 1:1.5:5. The diet may have several stages, each providing for more liberalization in the foods allowed. The patient should be stabilized at a given stage before progressing to the next. Many persons who adhere to such dietary plans have achieved satisfactory weight status without marked nutritional deficiencies. Some are able to tolerate buttermilk, evaporated milk, nonfat dry milk, and heated milk in modest quantities when taken between meals. Although a few individuals eventually progress to a nearly regular diet, stage II below has been found to be the most satisfactory on a long-term basis.[28]

HIGH-PROTEIN, HIGH-FAT, LOW CARBOHYDRATE DIET[*]

Characteristics and General Rules

1. Three routines are employed, with progression from one to another as the patient's condition warrants. The composition of the three routines is approximately:

	ROUTINE I	ROUTINE II	ROUTINE III
Carbohydrate, gm	0	100	100
Protein, gm	115	150	150
Fat, gm	170	225	225
Energy, kcal	2000	3000	3000
Calorie ratio:			
Carbohydrate	0	1	1
Fat	5	5	5
Protein	1.5	1.5	1.5

[*]Adapted from Pittman, A. C., and Robinson, F. W.: "Dumping Syndrome—Control by Diet," *J. Am. Diet Assoc.*, 34:596–602, 1958.

2. Multiple vitamin supplements are prescribed; iron may be necessary.
3. Six small dry meals are given daily; meals must be eaten regularly without omissions.
4. Liquids are taken 30 to 45 minutes after meals.
5. Carbohydrate foods are severely restricted. Those allowed must be measured accurately.
6. Liberal portions of meat are used; 1 pat margarine or butter should be eaten with each ounce of meat.
7. Foods to avoid include: milk, ice cream and other frozen desserts; sugars, sweets, candy, syrup, chocolate; gravies and rich sauces.
8. Rest before meals, eating slowly and chewing well, and relaxation are essential.

Foods allowed for three routines

ROUTINE I

Meat, fish, poultry—all kinds: broiled, baked, poached, stewed, grilled. Luncheon meats without cereal filler

Eggs—2 to 3: poached, scrambled, coddled, shirred, hard cooked

Fats—1 pat margarine or butter per ounce meat; 2 to 3 strips crisp bacon

Beverages—never at meals, but 30 to 45 minutes *after* meals: small amounts of cool water, or coffee, tea, limeade or lemonade without sugar. Use artificial sweetener

Miscellaneous—salt; lemon or lime juice on fish, etc.

ROUTINE II. All foods of routine I plus

Bread—enriched day-old white toast, zwieback, soda crackers, Melba toast. Only 1 slice with each feeding

Bread substitutes—fresh Lima beans, sweet corn, cooked dried beans and peas, saltines, soda crackers, grits, noodles, macaroni, rice, spaghetti, parsnips, boiled potato, mashed potato, sweet potato. See Table A-4, Bread List, for equivalents

Cereals—thick, cooked. Only 1 serving

Fats—1 ounce whipping cream; cream cheese

Nuts, when tolerated—plain or salted; chew thoroughly

Vegetables—all kinds. Not more than one serving per meal

Miscellaneous—olives, pimiento

ROUTINE III. All foods of routines I and II plus

Fruits, fresh, canned, or frozen; *no sugar.* Drained of all liquid. Fruit juices may be taken only 30 to 40 minutes after meals.

SAMPLE MENU PLANS FOR PATIENTS WITH DUMPING SYNDROME

Routine I	Routine II	Routine III
MORNING		
2 eggs with	2 scrambled eggs with	2 scrambled eggs with
2–3 pats margarine or butter (or more)	3 pats margarine or butter	3 pats margarine or butter
2 or more strips crisp bacon	2 slices crisp bacon	2 strips crisp bacon
	1 average slice bread	½ slice bread
	1 pat margarine or butter	1 pat margarine or butter
		½ cup orange sections (no liquid)
MIDMORNING		
3 oz meat with	2 oz meat with	2 oz meat with
3 pats margarine or butter, if possible	1 pat margarine or butter	1 pat margarine or butter
	2 thin slices of bread for sandwich	2 thin slices bread for sandwich
NOON		
2 beef patties or hamburger, steak, chops, roast with	4 oz chicken with	4 oz chicken with
3 pats margarine or butter (or more)	2 pats margarine or butter	3 pats margarine or butter
	½ cup string beans with	½ cup string beans with
	1 pat margarine or butter	1 pat margarine or butter
	1 slice bread with	½ slice bread with
	2 pats margarine or butter	1 pat margarine or butter
		½ small banana
MIDAFTERNOON		
Meat or eggs with	2 oz meat or 4 tbsp peanut butter with	2 oz meat or 4 tbsp peanut butter
3 pats margarine or butter		

SAMPLE MENU PLANS FOR PATIENTS WITH DUMPLING SYNDROME (Cont.)

Routine I	Routine II	Routine III
	1 pat margarine or butter	1 pat margarine or butter
	2 thin slices bread for sandwich	2 thin slices bread for sandwich
EVENING		
Same as at noon	4 oz broiled fish with	4 oz broiled fish with
	2 pats margarine or butter	3 pats margarine or butter
	Asparagus tips with	Asparagus tips with
	1 pat margarine or butter	1 pat margarine or butter
	1 average slice bread	½ slice bread
	1 pat margarine or butter	½ cup applesauce
BEDTIME		
Same as midafternoon	Same as midafternoon	Same as midafternoon

PROBLEMS AND REVIEW

1. Mrs. N. needs to undergo major surgery but her physician has recommended that the surgery be delayed for two weeks in order to improve her nutritional status.
   a. List some symptoms and laboratory findings that indicate the need for specific attention to dietary management before surgery.
   b. Which nutrients will be especially important in Mrs. N.'s diet?
   c. Is a high-carbohydrate diet advantageous prior to surgery? Why?
   d. List several high-protein beverages which could be used to supplement Mrs. N.'s protein intake.
   e. Which fluids should be emphasized in the diet if a high potassium intake is ordered?
2. Study the charts of six postoperative patients and prepare a chart showing the following: nature of the surgery; orders for parenteral fluids; orders for diet. Indicate the length of time each diet was used, and explain the variations which were found.
3. Prepare a list of parenteral feedings, tube feedings, and synthetic low-residue diets used in your hospital and enumerate the chief nutritive contributions made by each.
4. Mr. E.'s physician ordered a tube feeding for him following surgery.
   a. Compare advantages and disadvantages of blenderized and commercial formula feedings.
   b. What adjustments might be made to correct diarrhea in patients receiving tube feedings?
   c. List several precautions that must be considered in administration of tube feedings.
5. List the factors important to consider in the dietary management of persons with a gastrostomy; an ileostomy; a colostomy.
6. Mrs. Q. recently underwent a subtotal gastrectomy.
   a. List some of the nutritional problems she may develop.
   b. What type of diet would you expect Mrs. Q.'s physician to order?
   c. Mrs. Q. has symptoms of the dumping syndrome; list some of these. What steps can she take to prevent occurrence of symptoms?
   d. What dietary modifications should be made for persons with this condition? Explain the rationale for each change. Plan a day's menu for Mrs. Q.

CITED REFERENCES

1. Bistrian, B. R., *et al.:* "Protein Status of General Surgical Patients," *J.A.M.A.*, **230:**858–60, 1974.
2. Butterworth, C. E., and Blackburn, G. L.: "Hospital Malnutrition," *Nutr. Today*, **10:**8–18, Mar.–Apr. 1975.

3. Rudman, D., *et al.:* "Elemental Balances During Intravenous Hyperalimentation of Underweight Adult Subjects," *J. Clin. Invest.,* **55:**94–104, 1975.

4. Nealon, T. F., *et al.:* "Use of Elemental Diets to Correct Catabolic States Prior to Surgery," *Ann. Surg.,* **180:**9–13, 1974.

5. Rosser, R. G.: "Dietary Preparation for Hemorrhoidectomy. Advantages of a Nutritionally Complete Chemically Defined Low Residue Diet," *Am. J. Surg.,* **130:**78–81, 1975.

6. Hoover, H. C., *et al.:* "Nitrogen-Sparing Intravenous Fluids in Postoperative Patients," *N. Engl. J. Med.,* **293:**172–75, 1975.

7. Flatt, J. P., and Blackburn, G. L.: "The Metabolic Fuel Regulatory System: Implications for Protein Sparing Therapies During Caloric Deprivation and Disease," *Am. J. Clin. Nutr.,* **27:**175–87, 1974.

8. Shils, M. E.: "Guidelines for Total Parenteral Nutrition," *J.A.M.A.,* **220:**1721–29, 1972.

9. Richardson, T. J., and Sgoutas, D.: "Essential Fatty Acid Deficiency in Four Adult Patients During Total Parenteral Nutrition," *Am. J. Clin. Nutr.,* **28:**258–63, 1975.

10. Van Way, C. W., *et al.:* "Nitrogen Balance in Postoperative Patients Receiving Parenteral Nutrition," *Arch. Surg.,* **110:**272–76, 1975.

11. Dudrick, S. J., and Rhoads, J. E.: "Total Intravenous Feeding," *Sci. Am.,* **226:**73–80, May 1972.

12. Gazzaniga, A. B. *et al,;* "Nitrogen Balance in Patients Receiving Either Fat or Carbohydrate for Total Intravenous Nutrition," *Ann. Surg.,* **182:**163–68, 1975.

13. Nachlas, M. M., *et al.:* "Gastrointestinal Motility Studies as a Guide to Postoperative Management," *Ann. Surg.,* **175:**510–22, 1972.

14. "Postoperative Distention and Fruit Juices," Questions and Answers. *J.A.M.A.,* **194:**476, 1965.

15. Gault, M. H., *et al.:* "Hypernatremia, Azotemia, and Dehydration Due to High-Protein Tube Feeding," *Ann. Intern. Med.,* **68:**778–91, 1968.

16. Walike, B. C., and Walike, J. W.: "Lactose Content of Tube Feeding Diets As a Cause of Diarrhea," *Laryngoscope,* **83:**1109–15, 1973.

17. Schuman, B. M.: "Tube Feeding Using a Food Pump," *Am. Fam. Physician,* **5:**85–88, Mar. 1972.

18. Glober, G. A., *et al.:* "Long Term Results of Gastrectomy with Respect to Blood Lipids, Blood Pressure, Weight, and Living Habits," *Ann. Surg.,* **179:**896–901, 1974.

19. Starkloff, G. B., *et al.:* "Metabolic Intestinal Surgery. Its Complications and Management," *Arch. Surg.,* **110:**652–57, 1975.

20. Spin, F. P., and Weismann, R. E.: "Death From Hepatic Failure After Jejunoileal Anastomosis," *Am. J. Surg.,* **130:**88–91, 1975.

21. Jewell, W. R., *et al.:* "Complications of Jejunoileal Bypass for Morbid Obesity," *Arch. Surg.,* **110:**1039–42, 1975.

22. Heimburger, S. L., *et al.:* "Reversal of Severe Fatty Hepatic Infiltration Following Intestinal Bypass for Morbid Obesity by Calorie-Free Amino Acid Infusion," *Am. J. Surg.,* **129:**229–35, 1975.

23. Swenson, S. A., and Oberst, B.: "Pre- and Postoperative Care of the Patient with Intestinal Bypass for Obesity," *Am. J. Surg.,* **129:**225–28, 1975.

24. Wilmore, D. W.: "Nutrition and Metabolism Following Thermal Injury," *Clin. Plast. Surg.,* **1:**603–19, 1974.

25. Chaimoff, C., and Dintsman, M.: "The Long-Term Fate of Patients with Dumping Syndrome," *Arch. Surg.,* **105:**554–56, 1972.

26. Toffolon, E. P., and Goldfinger, S. E.: "Malabsorption Following Gastrectomy and Ileal Resection," *Surg. Clin. North Am.,* **54:**647–53, 1974.

27. Wong, P. Y., *et al.:* "Kallikrein-Kinin System in Postgastrectomy Dumping Syndrome," *Ann. Intern. Med.,* **80:**577–81, 1974.

28. Pittman, A. C., and Robinson, F. W.: "Dietary Management of the Dumping Syndrome," *J. Am. Diet. Assoc.,* **40:**108–10, 1962.

ADDITIONAL REFERENCES

Chandler, J. G.: "Surgical Treatment of Massive Obesity," *Postgrad. Med.,* **56:**124–33, Aug. 1974.

Chen, W. J., *et al.:* "Amino Acid Metabolism in Parenteral Nutrition: With Special Reference to the Calorie:Nitrogen Ratio and the Blood Urea Nitrogen Level," *Metabolism,* **23:**1117–23, 1974.

Curreri, P. W., et al.: "Dietary Requirements of Patients With Major Burns," *J. Am. Diet. Assoc.*, **65:**415–17, 1974.

Cuthbertson, D. P., et al.: "Nutrition After Injury," *Proc. Nutr. Soc.*, **30:**150–90, 1971.

Gormican, A., et al.: "Nutritional Status of Patients After Extended Tube Feeding," *J. Am. Diet. Assoc.*, **63:**247–53, 1973.

Gutowski, F.: "Ostomy Procedure: Nursing Care Before and After," *Am. J. Nurs.*, **72:**262–67, 1972.

Holli, B. B., and Oates, J. B.: "Feeding the Burned Child," *J. Am. Diet. Assoc.*, **67:**240–42, 1975.

Jordon, G. L.: "Surgical Approach to Nutritional Problems," *Adv. Surg.*, **8:**85–128, 1974.

Lenneberg, E., and Mendelssohn, A. N.: "Colostomies: A Guide For the Patient," *Dis. Colon Rectum*, **12:**201–17, 1969.

Malt, R. A.: "Keep It Simple," *Nutr. Today*, **6:**30–33, May–June 1971.

Noone, R. B., and Graham, W. P.: "Nutritional Care After Head and Neck Surgery," *Postgrad. Med.*, **53:**80–86, June 1973.

Pryor, J. P.: "The Long-Term Metabolic Consequences of Partial Gastrectomy," *Am. J. Med.*, **51:**5–10, 1971.

Rivard, J. Y., and LaPointe, R.: "Clinical Experience in Using 'Elemental Diet' in the Management of Various Surgical Nutritional Problems," *Can. J. Surg.*, **18:**90–96, 1975.

Weber, B.: "Eating with a Trach," *Am. J. Nurs.*, **74:**1439, 1974.

37 Diabetes Mellitus

Diabetes mellitus is a chronic disease that has affected mankind throughout the world. The records of the ancient civilizations of Egypt, India, Japan, Greece, and Rome describe the symptoms of the disease and usually include recommendations for treatment. The wasting away of flesh, copious urination, and the sweet taste of the urine were frequently noted by the ancient medical writers. Aretaeus of Cappadocia, who lived between A.D. 30 and 90, not only named the disease *diabetes*, which means "to run through or to siphon," but also recommended milk, cereals, starch, autumn fruits, and sweet wines.[1] The term *mellitus*, which means honeylike, was added by a London physician, Willis, in 1675.

THE NATURE OF DIABETES

Insulin and metabolic defects. Diabetes mellitus is a genetic disease of metabolism in which there is a partial or total lack of functioning insulin; it is characterized by the lessened ability or complete inability of the tissues to utilize carbohydrate. The metabolism of fat and of protein is also altered. Hyperglycemia, glycosuria, and excessive urination are cardinal findings.

The insulin defect may be a failure in its formation, liberation, or action. Since insulin is produced by the beta cells of the islands of Langerhans, any reduction in the number of functioning cells will decrease the amount of insulin that can be synthesized. Many diabetics can produce sufficient insulin, but some stimulus to the islet tissue is needed in order that secretion can take place. Especially in the early stages of the disease the insulinlike activity (ILA) of the blood is often increased, but most of this insulin appears to be bound to protein and is not available for transport across the cell membrane and action within the cell.

The hormones of the anterior pituitary, adrenal cortex, thyroid, and alpha cells of the islands of Langerhans are glucogenic; that is, they increase the supply of glucose. Just how these hormones are involved in the etiology of diabetes is not fully understood. Possibly they could increase the demand, decrease the secretion, or antagonize and inhibit the action of insulin.

The role of glucagon, in particular, is of interest. Unger's research suggests that insulin deficiency alone does not account for the hyperglycemia seen in diabetes. An excess of glucagon is believed to be at least partly responsible for the high glucose levels seen in diabetic persons.[2]

Scope of the problem. Diabetes mellitus is a major public health problem for it affects about 4.4 million persons in the United States of whom about 1.6 million do not know that they have the disease.[3] Each year about 325,000 new cases are diagnosed, most of whom are over 40 years of age and who are also affected by one or more chronic conditions of the vascular system including heart disease, high blood pressure, neuropathy, nephropathy, and retinopathy. Diabetes ranks third as a cause of blindness with about 45,000 diabetics being blind.

About 35,000 deaths from diabetes are reported annually in the United States, placing diabetes eighth as a cause of death. In addition, an equal number of diabetics are estimated to die each year from the complications associated with the disease, principally ailments of the cardiovascular system.

The rate of diabetes among persons under 25 years is 2.3 per 1000; for persons over 45 years the rate is 62 per 1000, with the highest incidence occurring in the two decades 55 to 74 years.[3]

Diabetes is a major socioeconomic ill that costs more than two billion dollars annually in terms of loss of earnings and costs of hospitalization, physicians' fees, medication, and rehabilitation. The dis-

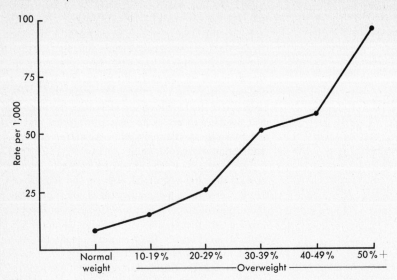

Figure 37-1. Diabetes rate increases as weight increases. (Data from diabetic screening of federal employees reported in *Diabetes Source Book,* U.S. Department of Health, Education, and Welfare, 1968, p. 31.)

ease is much more prevalent in lower economic groups, with the rate in families with annual incomes below $4000 being more than double that in families with incomes over $4000.

Factors influencing the incidence of diabetes. The high-risk individuals include: (1) Blood relatives of diabetics. The disease occurs with striking frequency among blood relatives. A number of genetic factors are probably involved but the mechanism is not fully understood. (2) Obese persons. The incidence of diabetes is 12 times more prevalent among those who are 50 per cent overweight than it is in persons of normal weight. (See Figure 37-1.) Although obesity and diabetes are highly associated, this does not mean that obesity is a cause of diabetes. It has been suggested by some that obesity may be a stress that uncovers the diabetic condition, and by others that obesity and diabetes are different manifestations of a common metabolic defect. (3) Persons over 40 years of age. Glucose tolerance decreases with age. (4) Women who have abnormal glucose tolerance curves during pregnancy. Some of these women become diabetic 10 or 20 years later. (5) Women who give birth to babies weighing 9 pounds or more. These heavy babies are also likely to become diabetic in later years.

Stages of diabetes. Diabetes is presumed to be present at birth, but detectable chemical and clinical manifestations of the disease may not be apparent for many years. The disease is often classified according to stages of development.

PREDIABETES is the period from birth until glucose intolerance is recognized. Studies on genetically predisposed persons have shown a delayed or decreased, or both, response to glucose. Vascular changes with thickening of the capillary basement membrane in muscle have been noted in some prediabetics.[4]

CHEMICAL DIABETES is characterized by an abnormal glucose tolerance test but no symptoms are yet evident. Sometimes the abnormality of glucose tolerance is evident only upon stimulation with cortisone (the CORTISONE GLUCOSE TOLERANCE TEST).

GESTATIONAL DIABETES is the abnormality of glucose tolerance seen particularly during the second and third trimesters of pregnancy, but disappearing within six weeks postpartum.

CLINICAL DIABETES is characterized by typical symptoms such as thirst, excessive urination, and increased appetite as well as an abnormal glucose tolerance curve.

Symptoms of juvenile and adult diabetes. Two types of diabetes are recognized, namely growth onset or juvenile diabetes, and maturity onset or adult diabetes.

GROWTH ONSET DIABETES occurs relatively infrequently and, as a rule, is seen prior to age 20 but occasionally it occurs up to age 40. The onset is usually acute, the abnormality of carbohydrate metabolism is severe, and insulin production is minimal or lacking. The patients are sensitive to insulin, unstable, difficult to manage, and fluctuate from diabetic coma on the one hand to hypoglycemia on the other. Most juvenile diabetics are of normal weight or have lost some weight. Most or all of the classic symptoms of diabetes are present in growth onset diabetes.

POLYURIA, or frequent urination and an abnormally large volume of urine
POLYDIPSIA, or excessive thirst
POLYPHAGIA, or increased appetite
Loss of weight
KETOSIS is sometimes the abnormality that brings the patient to the physician. It is a condition in which the accumulation of lower fatty acids in the blood leads to the excretion of ketones in the urine. The ketonuria is accompanied by loss of base, acidosis, dehydration, and eventually coma.

MATURITY ONSET DIABETES. The adult-type diabetes occurs primarily after age 30 years but has its highest incidence in the 50s and 60s. The onset is insidious and often does not present any of the classic symptoms. These patients may consult a physician because of a continued feeling of fatigue and because of symptoms associated with degenerative changes in the vascular system including high blood pressure, heart disease, retinitis, and peripheral neuritis. Sometimes they complain of increased thirst, more frequent urination, and itching. These patients are usually obese, have only a mild hyperglycemia, and seldom have ketosis except after a severe infection. They are not dependent upon insulin and can be controlled by diet alone or by diet and one of the oral hypoglycemic agents.

Laboratory studies. The diagnosis of diabetes is based upon the above-listed symptoms together with the results of several laboratory tests.

Glycosuria, or the presence of an abnormal amount of sugar in the urine, should be regarded as evidence of diabetes until proved otherwise. Sugar is present in the urine in many other conditions including pentosuria as a result of the body's failure to use the 5-carbon sugars; lactosuria in nursing mothers; alimentary glycosuria from excessive dietary loads of carbohydrate; fructosuria and galactosuria, resulting from enzyme deficiencies; and renal glycosuria because of a reduced ability of the tubules to reabsorb glucose.

Hyperglycemia, a high blood sugar, may be detected after a fast of 12 hours. A fasting blood sugar of more than 140 mg per 100 ml is suggestive of

diabetes. Many older persons have slightly elevated blood sugar levels without having diabetes.

The GLUCOSE TOLERANCE TEST is a measure of the ability of the body to utilize a known amount of glucose. At least three days prior to the test the patient is instructed to consume a diet containing at least 150 gm carbohydrate each day.[5] The test is performed 12 to 14 hours after the evening meal of the third day. A fasting blood sample is drawn and then a solution containing a weighed amount of glucose is given. Usually 100 gm glucose dissolved in 300 ml water and flavored with lemon juice is given to the adult. Blood samples are taken at $\frac{1}{2}$, 1, 2, and 3 hours after the ingestion of the glucose. The urine is also collected at each of these time intervals and tested for glucose. Under the conditions of the test, according to Public Health Service criteria,[6] diabetes is present if the fasting and three-hour sugar levels exceed the following levels, or if any three of the stated levels are exceeded:

	Whole Blood	Plasma
	(mg per 100 ml)	
Fasting	110	130
1 hour	170	195
2 hours	120	140
3 hours	110	130

(See Figure 37–2.)

Ketonuria, or excretion of ketones, occurs when fatty acids are incompletely oxidized in the body.

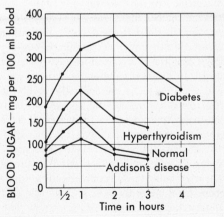

Figure 37–2. Glucose tolerance curves in various metabolic disorders.

Metabolism in diabetes. To understand the changes in metabolism that occur in diabetes, the student should first review the normal metabolism of proteins, carbohydrates, and fats (see Chapters 4, 5, and 6). A deficient supply of functioning insulin affects the metabolism of carbohydrates, fats, proteins, electrolytes, and water, and the consequences of the impairments are complex.

When insulin is not being produced or is ineffective, the formation of glycogen is decreased, and the utilization of glucose in the peripheral tissues is reduced. As a consequence the glucose that enters the circulation from various sources is removed more slowly and hyperglycemia follows. This is further accentuated by gluconeogenesis through which about 58 per cent of the protein molecule and 10 per cent of the fat molecule can yield glucose. When the blood glucose level exceeds the renal threshold (about 160 to 180 mg per 100 ml), glycosuria occurs. The loss of glucose in the urine represents a wastage of energy and entails an increased elimination of water and sodium. Ordinarily thirst and the increased ingestion of liquids compensate for the water loss, but interference with the intake such as occurs in nausea or through vomiting could lead to rapid dehydration.

With a deficiency of insulin lipogenesis decreases and lipolysis is greatly increased, these effects being of both immediate and long-range consequence. The fatty acids released from adipose tissue or available by absorption from the intestinal tract are oxidized by the liver to form "ketone bodies" including acetoacetic acid, β-hydroxybutyric acid, and acetone. The liver utilizes only limited quantities of the ketones and releases them to the circulation. Normally the peripheral tissues metabolize the ketones at a rate equal to their production by the liver so that the blood level at any given time is minimal. In diabetes mellitus the ketones are produced at a rate that far exceeds the ability of the tissues to utilize them and the concentration in the blood is greatly increased (KETONEMIA). Acetone is excreted by the lungs and gives the characteristic fruity odor to the breath. Acetoacetic acid and β-hydroxybutyric acid are excreted in the urine (ketonuria). Being fairly strong organic acids, these ketones combine with base so that the alkaline reserve is depleted, and acidosis results. The accompanying dehydration leads to circulatory failure, renal failure, and coma if not corrected. (See page 502.)

The rapid release of fatty acids into the blood circulation often results in a hyperlipemia and the blood serum may have a milky opalescent appearance. The blood levels of cholesterol are usually increased either because of increased synthesis or because of decreased destruction by the liver. The development of atherosclerosis in diabetic individuals occurs at an earlier age than in the nondiabetic and is more pronounced. (See page 526.)

The accelerated breakdown of protein tissues that occurs in uncontrolled diabetes not only adds to the glucose level of the blood, but increases the amount of nitrogen that must be excreted as a result of deaminization. The catabolism of protein tissues is accompanied by the release of cellular potassium and its excretion in the urine.

TREATMENT FOR DIABETES MELLITUS

Objectives for therapy. The goal of therapy in diabetes mellitus is to maintain and prolong a healthy, productive, satisfying life. This goal involves such specific aims as (1) optimum nutrition, (2) achieving normal weight, (3) a normal blood sugar level, (4) minimum glycosuria, (5) absence of ketoacidosis, and (6) minimum chronic degenerative complications. In planning the program of therapy the patient must always be considered with respect to his individual needs and desires; he must be fully involved in all aspects of the plans for his welfare. What constitutes a realistic goal for an 80-year-old with stable diabetes would be quite unsatisfactory for the adolescent diabetic who has his life ahead of him. For example, a level of control to reduce the degree of atherosclerosis may be important for the young diabetic, but is likely to be of limited value to the elderly person. On the other hand, the psychosocial problems of the adolescent may require primary consideration.

Dietary control is central to success. It is accompanied, when necessary, by insulin or oral hypoglycemic drugs. A regulated program of exercise and attention to personal hygiene are important to the total program. The many aspects of therapy require a continuing program of education for the patient together with periodic evaluation by the physician, nutritionist, and other specialists in health care.

Insulin. When the islands of Langerhans are unable to produce insulin, typically in growth onset diabetes, insulin must be supplied by injection. Insulin cannot be taken orally because the insulin molecule, being protein in nature, would be hydrolyzed in the digestive tract and thus inactivated.

Insulin is measured in units, 1 unit being the activity of 0.125 mg of the international standard. Insulin, formerly supplied in solutions of 40 or 80 units per milliliter (U-40 or U-80), is now available as U-100. A transition to use of U-100 exclusively was recommended by the American Diabetes Association in 1972 in order to lessen the possibility of error by patients in administering insulin.[7]

Specific circumstances vary the insulin requirement considerably. Exercise reduces the need and infections increase the need. Emotional upsets may also modify the utilization of insulin. The types of insulin and their action are listed in Table 37–1.

Oral hypoglycemic drugs. Two groups of oral compounds are now in use, namely, the sulfonylureas and the biguanides. These compounds do not have the same action as insulin and are of value only when the islands of Langerhans are able to produce some insulin.

Among the sulfonylurea compounds are tolbutamide (Orinase°), chlorpropamide (Diabinese†),

acetohexamide (Dymelor°), and tolazamide (Tolinase†). These drugs appear to stimulate the production or release of insulin by the beta cells of the islands of Langerhans.

Phenformin (DBI‡) is a phenethylbiguanide that has hypoglycemic activity. It appears to increase the uptake of glucose in the peripheral tissues but does not influence insulin production by the pancreas. Malabsorption of vitamin B_{12} has been reported in persons receiving this drug.[8]

The oral compounds are useful in the management of maturity onset diabetes which cannot be controlled by diet alone. Oral compounds may produce a hypoglycemia if food intake is delayed or inadequate. They should never be regarded as a substitute for a controlled diet, and they should not be used in complications of diabetes such as acidosis and coma. They are not satisfactory for the juvenile, unstable, severe diabetic.

Rationale for dietary management. The American Diabetes Association lists three goals for the dietary management of diabetes: (1) avoidance of detrimental metabolic derangements of diabetes; (2) reduction of risk factors associated with the development of atherosclerosis; and (3) lessening the risk of other complications of diabetes.[9] There are three points of view concerning the degree of dietary control needed.

° Dymelor®, Eli Lilly Company, Indianapolis, Indiana.

† Tolinase, The Upjohn Company, Kalamazoo, Michigan.

‡ DBI, U.S. Vitamin Pharmaceutical Corporation, New York, New York.

° Orinase, The Upjohn Company, Kalamazoo, Michigan.

† Diabinese, Chas. Pfizer & Co., Inc., New York, New York.

Table 37–1. Types of Insulin and Their Action°

Types	Onset Hours	Peak Action Hours	Duration Hours
Short acting Regular (crystalline) Semilente	1 or less	3–4	6–8
Intermediate acting Globin NPH (isophane) Lente	2	9	24
Long acting PZI (protamine zinc insulin) Ultralente	6	18	36–48

°Adapted from *Diabetes Guide for Nurses*. U.S. Public Health Service Pub. No. 861, U.S. Department of Health, Education, and Welfare, Washington, D.C., revised 1969, p. 20.

Chemical control. A measured diet and insulin dosage are carefully regulated so that the blood sugar is kept within normal limits and the urine is free or nearly free of sugar at all times. Such control is believed to reduce the incidence and severity of degenerative complications. One criticism sometimes leveled against it is that the treatment may tend to be directed to the diabetes and not to the person as a whole.

Clinical control. Hyperglycemia and glycosuria are disregarded, and insulin is used to control ketosis. The diet differs little if any from that of normal persons and is controlled only to the point of maintenance of normal weight. Some physicians use these so-called "free" diets in the most liberal sense, but others restrict concentrated carbohydrate foods, especially those from sources contributing no other nutrients. Those who favor clinical control believe that the patient has an increased sense of well-being and that the degenerative complications are not more frequent.

Intermediate control. The majority of physicians adopt a regimen that falls between the preceding two. The objectives are: (1) to treat the patient as an individual and not on the basis of his diabetes alone; (2) to provide adequate nutrition for the maintenance of normal weight, a sense of well-being, and a life of usefulness; (3) to keep the blood sugar almost at normal levels for a large part of the day by using insulin as needed and by avoiding hypoglycemia; (4) to keep the urine sugar free or with only traces of sugar for most of the day.

Nutritional needs. Dietary control is an integral part of management for the diabetic. The diet should always provide the essentials for good nutrition and adjustments must be made from time to time for changing metabolic needs, for example, during growth, pregnancy, or modified activity.

Energy. Control of calorie intake to achieve normal weight is a primary objective for all diabetics. The calorie allowance is essentially the same as that for normal individuals of the same activity, size, and sex. Obese individuals should be placed on a calorie-restricted diet until the desirable weight for height and age is attained. Such weight loss in middle-aged obese patients very often leads to return of normal glucose tolerance. From 30 to 40 per cent of diabetics do not need insulin if their diets are controlled.

One approach to planning the calorie level is to determine the patient's present food intake and to use it as a guide for the calculated diet. The patient's continuing weight status determines whether the diet, in fact, is satisfactory in its calorie level—assuming, of course, that the patient is adhering to it. A convenient guide for planning the energy level is as follows:

	Kcal per kg	Kcal per pound
	(Desirable Weight)	
For weight loss	20	9
For a bed patient	25	11
For light work	30	14
For medium work	35	16
For heavy work	40	18

Protein. The Recommended Dietary Allowance for protein for each age and sex category is satisfactory for the diabetic individual. Diets usually include 1 to $1\frac{1}{2}$ gm protein per kilogram ($\frac{1}{2}$ to $\frac{2}{3}$ gm per pound) of desirable body weight. The higher allowance is typical of American diets and lends satiety value to the diet.

Carbohydrate. A level of 100 gm carbohydrate will prevent ketosis. Several studies have shown that raising the carbohydrate intake does not adversely affect fasting blood glucose levels, glucose tolerance, or insulin requirements, provided that total calories are not increased. Insulin needs are more closely correlated with total calorie intake than with the carbohydrate level in the diet. Consequently, liberalization of the carbohydrate intake to more closely approximate that of the typical diet in the United States has been recommended. For the majority of diabetic persons, 45 per cent, or more, of calories as carbohydrate is considered appropriate.[9] Thus, the typical carbohydrate content of diets for adult diabetics might range from 135 gm at the 1200-kcal level to 340 gm or more at 3000 kcal.

Fat. After protein and carbohydrate levels have been established, the fat allowance makes up the remaining calories. For most diets, 30 to 35 per cent of the calories as fat is satisfactory.

Many clinicians now recommend that the type of fat in the diet be controlled, giving emphasis to fats rich in linoleic acid and sharply restricting those foods that are rich in saturated fatty acids. When such modification is prescribed, skim milk, low-fat meat, and polyunsaturated fats would be used for calculating the diet and planning the daily meals (See Table A–4.)

Fiber. Trowell has postulated that fiber-deficient diets may be involved in the etiology of diabetes mellitus.[10] Diets high in fiber tend to have a higher chromium content. Chromium is essential for synthesis of glucose tolerance factor, which facilitates the peripheral action of insulin. Improved glucose tolerance has been demonstrated in adult onset diabetes following dietary supplements of chromium. (See Chapter 8).

Regularity of meals. Establishing a regular meal pattern is desirable especially for persons taking insulin or oral hypoglycemic agents. Meals should be spaced to coincide with the availability of insulin. A delay in eating may produce hypoglycemia. On the other hand, hyperglycemia, brought on by eating an excess of rapidly hydrolyzed carbohydrate, is to be avoided. Physical activity influences insulin requirements and adjustments in the diet may be needed as well. Many patients are advised to have a snack before participating in vigorous physical exercise.

Calculation of the diabetic diet prescription. A number of procedures may be used to arrive at the diet prescription. This is the responsibility of the physician, but the nurse and dietitian should have an understanding of the basis for the calculation. One of the methods often used is described below.

Let us assume that a diet is to be planned for a secretary who is 25 years old and 170 cm (67 inches) tall. According to the table of heights and weights (Table A–10), her desirable weight is 60 kg (132 pounds) (medium frame).

1. Calories: 30 kcal per kilogram (14 per pound) of desirable body weight

$$60 \times 30 = 1800 \text{ kcal per day}$$

2. Protein: 1.0 to 1.5 gm per kilogram of desirable body weight

$$60 \times 1.25 = 75 \text{ gm protein per day}$$

3. Nonprotein calories: $1800 - 300 = 1500$ kcal to be divided between carbohydrate and fat.

4. Carbohydrate: allow 45 to 65 per cent of nonprotein calories

$$60 \text{ per cent of } 1500 \text{ kcal} = 900 \text{ kcal}$$

$$900 \div 4 = 225 \text{ gm carbohydrate per day}$$

5. Fat calories: total calories – calories from protein and carbohydrate

$$1800 - (300 + 900) = 600 \text{ kcal}$$

6. Fat: fat calories ÷ 9

$$600 \div 9 = 67 \text{ gm fat per day}$$

By rounding off the numbers, the prescription is: protein, 75 gm; carbohydrate, 225 gm; fat, 65 gm.

Distribution of carbohydrate. The meal distribu-

Table 37–2. Typical Meal Distribution of Carbohydrate*

Type of Insulin	Breakfast	Noon	Midafternoon	Evening	Bedtime*
None	1/3	1/3		1/3	Usually none
	1/5	2/5		2/5	
Short acting (before breakfast and dinner)	2/5	1/5		2/5	Usually none
Intermediate-acting					
NPH	1/7	2/7	1/7	2/7	1/7
Long acting	1/5	2/5		2/5	20–40 gm
With regular insulin at breakfast	1/3	1/3		1/3	20–40 gm

*When a bedtime feeding is prescribed, the carbohydrate is first subtracted from the day's total allowance. Then the meal fractions are applied to the remainder of the carbohydrate.

tion of carbohydrate is determined according to the type of insulin being used and is modified according to each patient's needs in order to achieve the best possible regulation of carbohydrate utilization. When moderate- or slow-acting insulins are used, a portion of the carbohydrate—usually 20 to 40 gm—is reserved for a midafternoon or bedtime feeding or both. This carbohydrate must be in slowly available form and should be accompanied by a portion of the day's protein. After the bedtime carbohydrate has been subtracted from the day's allowance, the remainder of the carbohydrate is distributed to correspond to the peak activity and the duration of the activity of the insulin that is being used (see Table 37-2).

Planning the meal pattern. The dietitian and the nurse must translate the prescription into terms of common foods, keeping the following points especially in mind.

1. The diet should be planned with the patient so that it can be adjusted to his pattern of living. This requires consideration of the patient's economic status, the availability and cost of food, national, religious, and social customs, personal idiosyncrasies, occupation, facilities for preparing or obtaining meals, and so on.

The diabetic diet need not be an expensive one, and, ideally, it should be so planned that it fits in with the menus of the rest of the family. However, if the family diet is a poor one, the entire family will benefit when the basic food groups become the center about which meals are planned. The diet for the diabetic person does not require many special foods; thus, the rest of the family should not be deprived.

2. The adequacy of the diet for minerals and vitamins is most easily assured if one includes minimum amounts of the Four Food Groups.

3. Including some of the protein and fat in each meal helps to provide satiety and balance of food selection.

4. The food exchange lists (Table A-4) permit reasonable dietary constancy from day to day and considerable flexibility in meal planning. The method for dietary calculation using these lists has been described in Chapter 28 and is illustrated in Table 28-2.

5. The meal distribution of the carbohydrate

can be adjusted to within 7 or 8 gm without using fractions of exchanges. The protein and fat should be adjusted within meals so that maximum flexibility is possible in meal planning. For example, the inclusion of milk at breakfast permits either cereal or bread to be selected from the bread exchanges; meat exchanges are wisely divided among the three meals with somewhat larger amounts being allocated to dinner. An example of the distribution of food exchanges into meal patterns is shown in Table 37-3 for the diet calculation illustrated on page 400.

DIETARY COUNSELING

Essential knowledge. The diabetic patient needs to know about (1) the nature of diabetes and the reasons for the measures that will be recommended, (2) the importance of weight control, (3) the details of his dietary program, (4) the amounts, time intervals, and method of administration of insulin or oral drugs, if needed, (5) skin care and personal hygiene, (6) procedures for testing the urine, (7) signs of hypoglycemia or acidosis and what steps to take in the event they occur, (8) emergency measures to take during infection and illness until medical help is available, and (9) the importance of periodic visits to his physician. (See Figure 37-3.)

Insofar as diet is concerned, the patient needs to be taught the amount of food exchanges he is to use at each meal, how to use the food exchange lists in daily meal planning, how to interpret labels when purchasing food, and how to prepare food for his meals. (See Figure 37-4.)

Responsibility for education. The physician, nurse, and dietitian share the responsibility for counseling the patient. The physician explains the nature of diabetes and the factors of importance in maintaining control. He also makes referrals to the dietitian and nurse for detailed aspects of education. In the hospital or outpatient clinic the dietitian usually initiates dietary instruction and arranges for a continuing program of education. The nurse instructs the patient regarding insulin administration, urine

Table 37–3. Meal Pattern and Sample Menu* Carbohydrate division: breakfast, 32 gm; luncheon, 64 gm; midafternoon, 32 gm; dinner, 64 gm; bedtime, 32 gm

		Carbohydrate		
Meal Pattern	**Exchanges**	**gm**	**Sample Menu**	**Measure**
Breakfast			*Breakfast*	
Fruit, list 3	1	10	Orange	1 small
Bread, list 4	1	15	Whole-wheat toast	1 slice
Milk, list 1	½	6	Skim milk	½ cup
Fat, list 6	1	—	Margarine	1 teaspoon
Coffee or tea			Coffee: no sugar	
		31		
Luncheon			*Luncheon*	
			Sandwich:	
Meat, list 5	2	—	Cold sliced chicken	2 ounces
Bread, list 4	3	45	White bread	2 slices
Fat, list 6	3	—	Mayonnaise	2 teaspoons
Vegetables, list 2	1	5	Sliced tomatoes on lettuce	
			French dressing	1 tablespoon
			Broth/saltines	6 squares
Fruit, list 3	2	20	Grapes	24
		70		
Midafternoon			*Midafternoon*	
Bread, list 4	1	15	Graham crackers	2 squares
Fat, list 6	1	—	Margarine	1 teaspoon
Milk, list 1	1	12	Skim milk	1 cup
		27		
Dinner			*Dinner*	
Meat, list 5	3	—	Chopped round steak	3 ounces
Bread, list 4	3	45	Parslied rice	1 cup
			Dinner roll	1, 2-in. diam.
Fat, list 6	3	—	Margarine	2 teaspoons
Vegetables, list 2	2	10	Wax beans with pimento	½ cup
			Sliced cucumber with oil and vinegar	2 teaspoons
Fruit, list 3	1	10	Cantaloupe	¼, small
Coffee or tea			Tea with lemon	
		65		
Bedtime			*Bedtime*	
Milk, list 1	½	6	Skim milk	½ cup
Bread, list 4	1	15	Popcorn	3 cups
Fruit, list 3	1	10	Apple	1 small
Fat, list 6	1	—	Margarine	1 teaspoon
		31		
Total carbohydrate		224		

*Calculation for food exchanges and day's total is shown on page 400.

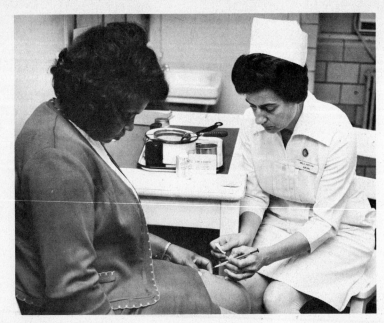

Figure 37–3. Nurse teaching patient how to administer insulin. (Courtesy, Medical College of Virginia, Health Sciences Division, Virginia Commonwealth University, Richmond.)

testing, and hygiene. She is a valuable assistant for dietary counseling and may be fully responsible for dietary instruction in some situations where no dietitian is available.

Experience has shown that the majority of diabetics fail to understand their diets. Some of the reasons for failure have been outlined recently, with suggestions for successful counseling.[11]

Satisfactory counseling of the patient includes individualized instruction which may be supplemented by group instruction. The patient must be involved throughout in order that he fully understand and adopt the program necessary for him. Frequent follow-up visits with the dietitian or public health nurse are essential to reinforce motivation, to answer questions, and to give added information.

Not only the patient but members of his family must be included in the counseling sessions. Each member of the family needs to understand that the diet for the diabetic patient is essentially a normal one, but that a regulated routine of meals and of the quantities of food is a vital aspect of the program. Members of the family also need to be aware of the complications that could arise and should know what to do in emergencies.

Teaching aids. Many books and pamphlets pertaining to diabetes have been prepared by health agencies, pharmaceutical firms, and physicians for the guidance of the patient. When these are selected at a reading level appropriate for the patient, these printed materials are useful for further study and reference. They should never be regarded as a substitute for personal counseling.

The patient's tray at each meal constitutes one of the best visual aids if the dietitian and nurse take the opportunity to so use it. If the patient has been introduced to the food exchange lists, the foods on the tray can be located in these lists and the amounts served identified in number of exchanges. Needless to say, careful checking of the tray before it is brought to the patient is important to emphasize dietary control. Measuring cups, measuring spoons, and various sizes of glasses and cups used for table service should be demonstrated during the instruction of the patient. Paper and plastic food models are useful in demonstrating menu planning and may be used by the patient for practice sessions in planning his own diet. In a relatively short time most patients can learn to estimate the portion sizes allowed on their diets. (See Figure 37–5.)

Programmed instruction, when available, can be an important teaching aid. Slides, filmstrips, and movies pertaining to the many aspects of diabetic care are especially useful for group instruction. Each patient should be encouraged to participate in some group events not only for their instructional value, but to afford him opportunity to share experiences with others.

Some problems in education of the diabetic patient. Lack of education, inability to read English, and failing vision are among the problems encountered in the use of printed materials. Sometimes a member of the family can assist in using printed materials. Posters, tapes, films, and food models may be used. The nurse and dietitian must expect to spend more time with patients who present these problems, but repeated verbal instruction can be successful.

About half the diabetic patients are from families with very limited incomes. Although the diabetic diet need not be more expensive than a normal diet, the daily meal pattern must be carefully planned to make the best use of inexpensive foods. Most patients and their families can profit by advice in the wise purchase of foods.

Patients often ask about the use of dietetic foods. Water-packed fruits are available in most supermarkets at costs only slightly above that of regular packs and are useful when fresh fruits are out of season. Many water-packed fruits are sweetened with artificial sweeteners.

Dietetic foods such as cookies, candies, ice cream, and gluten breads are not needed since most diabetic diets are sufficiently liberal to include a wide choice of foods. Some of the specialty products are expensive. Although low in carbohydrate, most of them contain protein and fat, thus contributing available glucose and calories. Products containing fructose or sorbitol should not be used freely as the calorie value of these sugars is equivalent to that of glucose. The patient who wishes to use such products should be advised about the specific changes he needs to make in his meal pattern.

Some patients ask about the use of alcoholic beverages. If the physician permits their use, the caloric content of the beverage is first subtracted from the day's allowance, and the balance of the diet is calculated accordingly.

Initially the patient should become thoroughly familiar with the kinds and amounts of foods allowed from the exchange lists. Once he has developed confidence in the use of these lists, he needs to be given some assistance in the use of food mixtures. A number of cookbooks have been prepared specifically for diabetic patients and include calculations of nutritive values. Some food processors have developed tables showing how their products can fit into the food exchanges. Patients usually need some assistance in the interpretation of these printed materials.

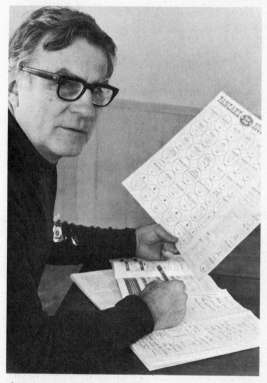

Figure 37–4. Ability to select appropriate foods for meals eaten away from home is an important part of the learning process for the diabetic. (Courtesy, Diabetes Education Center, Minneapolis.)

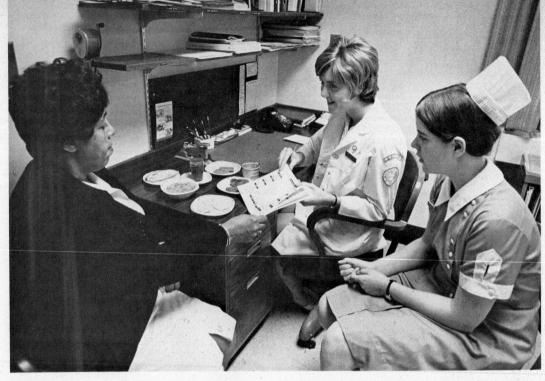

Figure 37–5. Use of food models helps the diabetic patient understand portion sizes for the exchange lists. (Courtesy, Yale–New Haven Medical Center.)

COMPLICATIONS OF DIABETES

Hypoglycemia. INSULIN SHOCK or hypoglycemia is caused by an overdose of insulin, a decrease in the available glucose because of delay in eating, omission of food, or loss of food by vomiting and diarrhea, or an increase in exercise without accompanying modification of the insulin dosage.

The patient going into insulin shock becomes uneasy, nervous, weak, and hungry. He is pale, his skin is moist, and he perspires excessively. He may complain of trembling, dizziness, faintness, headache, and double vision. His movements may be uncoordinated. Emotional instability may be indicated by crying, by hilarious behavior, or by belligerency. Occasionally, there may be nausea and vomiting or convulsions. Without treatment coma follows and death is impending. Laboratory studies show a blood sugar below 70 mg per 100 ml for mild symptoms and below 50 mg for coma.

Orange juice or other fruit juices, sugar, candy, syrup, honey, a carbonated beverage, or any readily available carbohydrate may be given. If absorption is normal, recovery follows in a few minutes. If there is stupor, intravenous glucose is necessary.

Most patients are now using one or another of the slowly acting insulins, in which case reactions may recur after a few hours. To avoid such subsequent reactions, it is necessary to follow the initial carbohydrate therapy in one or two hours and at later intervals with foods containing carbohydrate which is slowly absorbed—such as in milk and bread.

The patient must be impressed with the importance of balance between his diet and insulin dosage and the importance of close adherence to the physician's orders. He should always carry some sugar or hard candy to avert symptoms when they are still mild.

Diabetic acidosis and coma. A dreaded complication in diabetes is the state of coma which is brought about by acidosis. Diabetic coma often originates because the patient consumed additional foods for which his insulin did not provide, or because he failed to take the correct amount of insulin or omitted it entirely. The presence of diabetes is first detected in some persons who were not aware of the disease until coma occurred. Infection is an especially sinister influence since even a mild infection reduces the carbohydrate tolerance and severe acidosis may sometimes occur before the insulin dosage has been appropriately increased. Trauma of any kind, whether an injury or surgery, aggravates the diabetes so that acidosis is more likely.

Some of the signs of diabetic acidosis and coma are similar to those of insulin shock, and a differentiation cannot be made without information concerning the patient prior to the onset of the symptoms, together with blood and urine studies. The patient complains of feeling ill and weak; he may have a headache, anorexia, nausea and vomiting, abdominal pain, and aches and pains elsewhere. His skin is hot, flushed, and dry; his mouth is dry and he is thirsty. An acetone odor on the breath, painful, rapid breathing, and drowsiness are typical signs. Symptoms of shock, unconsciousness, and death follow unless prompt measures are taken. Sugar, acetone, and acetoacetic acid are present in the urine, the blood glucose is elevated to very high levels, and the blood carbon dioxide content is decreased.

When early signs of ketosis are present, small repeated doses of insulin are given together with small carbohydrate feedings. Diabetic coma, however, is a medical emergency best treated in a hospital where close nursing care can be given. The physician directs the therapy, which includes large doses of regular insulin with smaller doses repeated as needed every hour or so until the urine sugar is reduced and the blood sugar is lowered to less than 200 mg per 100 ml; saline infusions for the correction of dehydration; gastric lavage if the patient has been vomiting; and alkali therapy for the correction of the severe acidosis.

When the urine sugar decreases and the blood sugar begins to fall, glucose is given by infusion in order to avoid subsequent hypoglycemic reactions. As soon as fluids can be taken orally, the patient is given fruit juices, gruels, ginger ale, tea, and broth. All of these are useful for their fluid content; fruit juice, ginger ale, and gruels provide carbohydrate; broth and gruels contain sodium chloride; and fruit juices, broth and gruels contribute potassium. These fluids may be given in amounts of 100 ml, more or less, every hour or so during the first day. By the second day, the patient is usually able to take a soft diet which is calculated to contain 100 to 200 gm carbohydrate, and by the third day he may take the diet which meets his particular requirements.

Surgery. Ideally, the diabetic patient who is having surgery should have a normal blood sugar, no glycosuria, and no ketosis. A glycogen reserve is essential and can be assured only if sufficient carbohydrate is included up to 12 hours prior to the operation and if insulin is supplied in great enough amounts for the utilization of the carbohydrate. Fluids in abundance are indicated. When emergency surgery is needed, parenteral glucose is usually ordered.

Carbohydrate feedings should begin within three hours after operation, as a rule. Initially glucose may be given parenterally. When liquids can be taken by mouth, tea with sugar, orange juice, and ginger ale may be used. When a full fluid or soft diet can be tolerated, the diet can be calculated to provide the protein and fat as well as the carbohydrate allowances.

Infection. The guidance of a physician is important when a diabetic patient has an infection. An infection lowers the carbohydrate tolerance and increases the insulin requirement. A mild diabetic may become a severe case, and infections may precipitate coma. The physician sometimes orders insulin for patients who are not ordinarily required to use insulin.

Pregnancy. Diabetes increases the hazards of pregnancy because of the dangers of glycogen depletion, hypoglycemia, acidosis, and infection. Despite the increased hazards the diabetic woman can have an uneventful pregnancy and a healthy baby. She should have medical guidance throughout her pregnancy with emphasis on control of the rate of weight gain and the prevention of edema. The nutritional requirements are similar to those of the nondiabetic pregnant woman. The insulin requirements are usually increased. Most diabetic women are unable to produce enough milk for the baby and should not be encouraged to nurse their infants.

PROBLEMS AND REVIEW

1. Mr. White is an overweight 45-year-old factory worker who has just been diagnosed as a diabetic. Answer the following questions in relation to this patient.
   a. List the important predisposing factors in diabetes mellitus.

b. Explain how insulin deficiency affects the metabolism of carbohydrate; protein; fat; sodium; potassium; water.

c. Explain the typical symptoms of diabetes on the basis of the metabolic changes.

d. What advice might be appropriate for Mr. White's children in order to delay or avoid the onset of diabetes mellitus?

e. State the important objectives to be achieved in the therapy of this patient. What factors may influence the realization of these objectives?

f. What information do you need in order to plan a satisfactory dietary program for Mr. White?

2. The following diet prescription was ordered for Mr. White: protein, 85 gm; carbohydrate, 185 gm; fat, 65 gm. The carbohydrate should be distributed in thirds as Mr. White is taking tolbutamide. The fat allowance is to be chosen from foods low in saturated fat, and that are good sources of polyunsaturated fat. Mr. White carries his lunch to work.

a. Calculate the daily meal plan.

b. Plan one day's menu for Mr. White on a work day.

c. Explain the basis for the low saturated fat and increased polyunsaturated fat prescription.

3. Show how each of the following combinations could be used in the dinner pattern for Mr. White:

a. Tuna-noodle casserole

b. Beef stew with carrots, onion, potatoes, and celery

c. A picnic supper including ham and potato salad

4. Mr. White believes that he can eat as he pleases because the tolbutamide he takes will control his diabetes. Explain why this thinking is incorrect.

5. Mr. White is not feeling well and would prefer to have liquids at lunch. Calculate a full fluid diet to provide: protein, 28 gm; carbohydrate, 62 gm; fat, 22 gm.

6. Mr. Johnson, the patient in the next bed, is an insulin-dependent diabetic who has refused to eat the following foods on his tray: $\frac{1}{2}$ slice bread, $\frac{1}{2}$ cup carrots, $1\frac{1}{2}$ ounces meat, and 1 small potato. He has agreed to take a carbohydrate replacement as orange juice.

a. On the basis of the carbohydrate content of the foods refused, how much orange juice would be required?

b. If the amount of orange juice given was kept to $\frac{1}{2}$ cup, how much sugar would you need to add to the juice to cover the carbohydrate replacement?

c. List two other juices and the appropriate amounts of each that could be used if Mr. Johnson had not expressed a preference for orange juice.

d. If the replacement were based on the total glucose available from the foods refused, what changes would you need to make in items *a* and *b*?

CITED REFERENCES

1. Stowers, J. M.: "Nutrition in Diabetes," *Nutr. Abstr. Rev.*, **33**:1–15, 1963.

2. Unger, R. H.: "The Essential Role of Glucagon in the Pathogenesis of Diabetes Mellitus," *Lancet*, **1**:14–16, 1975.

3. Vavra, H. M.: *Diabetes Source Book*. Public Health Service Pub. 1168. U.S. Department of Health, Education, and Welfare, Washington, D.C., 1969.

4. Fajans, S. S.: "The Definition of Chemical Diabetes," *Metabolism*, **22**:211–17, 1973.

5. Siperstein, M. D.: "The Glucose Tolerance Test: A Pitfall in the Diagnosis of Diabetes Mellitus," *Adv. Intern. Med.*, **20**:297–323, 1975.

6. *Diabetes Control—A Public Health Program Guide*. Public Health Service Pub. 506, U.S. Department of Health, Education, and Welfare, Washington, D.C., 1969.

7. American Diabetes Association: "U-100 Insulin: A New Era in Diabetes Mellitus Therapy," *Diabetes*, **21**:832, 1972.

8. Jounela, A. J., *et al.*: "Drug Induced Malabsorption of Vitamin B_{12}. VI. Malabsorption of B_{12} During Treatment with Phenformin," *Acta Med. Scand.*, **196**:267–69, 1974.

9. Bierman, E. L., *et al.*: "Principles of Nutrition and Dietary Recommendations for Patients with Diabetes Mellitus: 1971," *Diabetes*, **20**:633–34, 1971.

10. Trowell, H.: "Dietary Fibre, Ischemic Heart Disease and Diabetes Mellitus," *Proc. Nutr. Soc.*, **32:**151–59, 1973.

11. West, K. M.: "Diet Therapy of Diabetes: An Analysis of Failure," *Ann. Intern. Med.*, **79:**425–34, 1973.

ADDITIONAL REFERENCES

Abiaka, M. H.: "Japanese-American Food Equivalents for Calculating Exchange Diets," *J. Am. Diet. Assoc.*, **62:**173–80, 1973.

Albrink, M. J.: "Dietary and Drug Treatment of Hyperlipidemia in Diabetes," *Diabetes*, **23:**913–18, 1974.

"Bingo Game Teaches Meal Planning to Diabetics," *Hospitals*, **49:**15, Mar. 1, 1975.

Cabot, E. E.: "The Exchange Lists, or How Diabetics Can Have Apple Pie and Ice Cream," *Mod. Hosp.*, **116:**147, April 1971.

Chalmers, T. C.: Editorial. "Settling the UGDP Controversy," *J.A.M.A.*, **231:**624–25, 1975.

Damron, J. J., and Olson, P. T.: "Tape-Recorded Instruction for Patients with Diabetes," *J. Am. Diet. Assoc.*, **62:**426–27, 1973.

Etzwiler, D. D.: "The Patient Is a Member of the Medical Team," *J. Am. Diet. Assoc.*, **61:**421–23, 1972.

Garcia, M. J.: "Morbidity and Mortality in Diabetics in the Framingham Population," *Diabetes*, **23:**105–11, 1974.

Grancio, S. D.: "Nursing Care of the Adult Diabetic Patient," *Nurs. Clin. North Am.*, **8:**605–15, 1973.

Guthrie, D. W., and Guthrie, R. A.: "Diabetes in Adolescence," *Am. J. Nurs.*, **75:**1740–44, 1975.

Hambidge, K. M.: "Chromium Nutrition in Man," *Am. J. Clin. Nutr.*, **27:**505–14, 1974.

Hassell, J., and Medved, E.: "Group/Audiovisual Instruction for Patients with Diabetes," *J. Am. Diet. Assoc.*, **66:**465–70, 1975.

Hillman, R. W.: "Sensible Eating for Older Diabetics," *Geriatrics*, **29:**123–26, May 1974.

Holland, W. M.: "The Diabetes Supplement of the National Health Survey. III. The Patient Reports on His Diet," *J. Am. Diet. Assoc.*, **52:**387–90, 1968.

LaBrenz, J. B.: "Planning Meals for the Backpacker with Diabetes—Nutritional Values of Freeze-Dried Foods," *J. Am. Diet. Assoc.*, **61:**42–48, 1972.

Levine, R., *et al.*: "The Diagnosis of Diabetes," (Programmed Instruction), *Am. Fam. Physician*, **1:**116–34, May; 111–25, June; 118–31, July; 119–33, Aug.; 99–115, Sept.; 113–27, Oct.; 151–63, Nov.; 109–25, Dec. 1970.

Mertz, W.: "Effects and Metabolism of Glucose Tolerance Factor," *Nutr. Rev.*, **33:**129–35, 1975.

Newmark, S. R., *et al.*: "Hyperglycemic and Hypoglycemic Crises," *J.A.M.A.*, **231:**185–87, 1975.

Power, L.: "New Approaches to the Old Problem of Diabetes Education," *J. Nutr. Educ.*, **5:**230–32, 1973.

Prater, B. M.: "The Diabetes Center: A Self-Care Living-In Program," *J. Am. Diet. Assoc.*, **64:**180–83, 1974.

Sharkey, T. P.: "Diabetes Mellitus—Present Problems and New Research," *J. Am. Diet. Assoc.*, **58:**201–209; 336–44; 442–44; 528–37, 1971.

Stuart, S.: "Day-to-Day Living with Diabetes," *Am. J. Nurs.*, **71:**1548–50, 1971.

Stulb, S. C.: "The Diabetes Supplement of the National Health Survey. IV. The Patient's Knowledge of the Food Exchanges," *J. Am. Diet. Assoc.*, **52:**391–93, 1968.

Tani, G. S., and Hankin, J. H.: "A Self-Learning Unit for Patients with Diabetes," *J. Am. Diet. Assoc.*, **58:**331–35, 1971.

Tokuhata, G. K., *et al.*: "Diabetes Mellitus: An Underestimated Public Health Problem," *J. Chronic Dis.*, **28:**23–35, 1975.

Weinsier, R. L., *et al.*: "Diet Therapy of Diabetes. Description of a Successful Methodologic Approach to Gaining Diet Adherence," *Diabetes*, **23:**669–73, 1974.

West, K. M.: "Prevention and Therapy of Diabetes Mellitus," *Nutr. Rev.*, **33:**193–98, 1975.

INSTRUCTIONAL MATERIALS FOR THE PATIENT

American Diabetes Association, New York
  Facts about Diabetes, 1966.
  Forecast (bimonthly magazine).

American Dietetic Association, Chicago
Exchange Lists for Meal Planning

Behrman, Sister M.: *A Cookbook for Diabetics*. American Diabetes Association, New York, 1959.

Bowen, A.: *The Diabetic Gourmet*. Harper & Row, New York, 1974.

Charleston District Dietetic Association: "Dining Delectables for the Diabetic," Medical Univ. Hosp., Dietary Dept., Charleston, S.C.

Duncan, G. G., and Duncan, T. G.: *A Modern Pilgrim's Progress with Further Revelations for Diabetics*, 2nd ed. W. B. Saunders Company, Philadelphia, 1967.

Jones, J.: *The Calculating Cook*. 101 Productions, San Francisco, 1974.

"Many People Have Diabetes Mellitus," Martland Hospital, Newark, New Jersey.

Middleton, K.: "Eats and Treats for the Young Diabetic," Diabetes Association of Greater Chicago, 620 No. Michigan Ave., Chicago.

Revell, D.: *Diabetes Control Cookery*. Berkley Publishing Corporation, New York, 1975.

Strachan, C. B.: *The Diabetic's Cookbook*. University of Texas Press, Austin, 1967.

U.S. Public Health Service
Answers to Questions That Are Often Asked About Diabetic Diets, Pub. 1847.
Diabetes and You, Pub. 567.

Weller, C.: *The New Way to Live with Diabetes*. Doubleday and Company, Inc., Garden City, N.Y., 1966.

38 Various Metabolic Disorders

Purine-Restricted Diet

Many diseases for which dietary modification is an effective part of treatment are deviations of normal metabolic pathways in the body. They occur because of abnormal production of one or more hormones, a deficiency of an enzyme, or a modification of excretion. Those which are discussed in this chapter fall into one or another of these categories but otherwise bear little, if any, relation to each other.

HYPOGLYCEMIA

Hypoglycemia refers to an abnormally low blood glucose level and may be of organic or functional origin. Organic causes include the following: (1) hyperinsulinism due to tumors or hyperplasia of islet cells; surgery rather than dietary management is essential; (2) hepatic diseases involving enzyme defects (see Chapter 46), alcoholism, or cirrhosis; and (3) endocrine disorders such as hypothyroidism and adrenocortical or pituitary insufficiency. Functional hypoglycemias are more common and may produce symptoms in the fasting state (spontaneous type) or, more frequently, in response to food intake (reactive type). An example of the latter is functional hyperinsulinism, in which there is oversecretion of insulin following carbohydrate ingestion, with the following effects on the blood glucose level: (1) a normal fasting blood sugar; (2) hypoglycemia two to four hours after meals, especially in the forenoon and late afternoon; (3) no hypoglycemia following fasting or the omission of meals; and (4) a glucose tolerance curve (see Figure 37–2) which shows a normal fasting sugar, initially elevated glucose level after taking the glucose, and a sharp fall to very low sugar levels.

Functional hypoglycemia may occur following gastrectomy or gastroenterostomy when nutrients are absorbed at an extremely rapid rate. In such situations the food reaches the small intestine much more rapidly than is normal, is very quickly absorbed, and the sudden elevation of the blood sugar serves as an extra stimulus to the islet cells and a subsequent hypoglycemia. See Chapter 36 for description of the dumping syndrome. Functional hypoglycemia may also be a manifestation of early adult onset diabetes or may be idiopathic in nature.

Symptoms. Rapid fall of the blood glucose level causes release of catecholamines and produces symptoms of weakness, nervousness, trembling, perspiring freely, rapid heartbeat, hunger, or nausea and vomiting. As a result of inadequate delivery of glucose to the brain, the person with chronic, severe hypoglycemia may experience headache, incoordination, irritability, confusion, emotional instability, and even coma.

Contrary to popular belief, occurrence of these symptoms does not necessarily indicate hypoglycemia. Diagnosis is based on laboratory evidence of low blood glucose levels, proof that the symptoms are due to hypoglycemia, relief of symptoms by food, and identification of the type of hypoglycemia.[1]

Modification of the diet. A diet prescription to meet each patient's needs is planned.

Carbohydrate. In hypoglycemias associated with some hepatic enzyme deficiencies or liver diseases, carbohydrate supplements are needed. In postprandial hypoglycemias the carbohydrate serves as a stimulus to further insulin secretion and is provocative of the hypoglycemic attack; thus, it is usually restricted to levels below 100 gm. The initial diet may be planned to contain 75 gm carbohydrate with further reduction to 50 gm if the patient shows no improvement.

Protein. A high-protein diet, 120 to 140 gm, is essential, since there is no appreciable increase in the blood sugar level following high-protein meals even though protein furnishes approximately 50 per cent of its weight in available glucose. This available glucose is released to the bloodstream so gradually that there is little stimulation to the islands of Langerhans.

Fat. When the levels of carbohydrate and protein have been established, the remaining calories are obtained from fat. Because the carbohydrate is so severely restricted, the fat level is, of necessity, high.

DIETARY COUNSELING

The exchange lists (see Table A–4) may be used for calculation of the diet prescription. Since carbohydrates are drastically restricted, it becomes apparent that the bread exchanges will usually be omitted. In order to include adequate amounts of fruits and vegetables, milk is limited to 2 or 3 cups; children should receive calcium supplements.

In order that absorption from the intestine will be gradual, the daily allowances of protein and fat, as well as carbohydrate, are divided into three approximately equal parts. Midmorning, midafternoon, and bedtime feedings are often desirable, in which case part of the food planned for the preceding meal can be used for the interval feeding. Carbohydrate-containing foods must be carefully measured.

ADRENOCORTICAL INSUFFICIENCY

Addison's disease is a comparatively rare condition resulting from an impairment of the functioning of the adrenal cortex because of atrophy of unknown origin, or, in some instances, because of tuberculosis. Sometimes adrenalectomy is necessary because of cancer, in which event the resultant metabolic effects are those of Addison's disease. Since the pituitary governs the activity of the adrenal cortex, hypophysectomy will also lead to characteristic symptoms of adrenal insufficiency.

Metabolic effects and related symptoms. The symptoms of insufficiency are directly related to the absence of hormones produced by the adrenal cortex.

Glucocorticoids. The principal action of these hormones, chiefly cortisol, is upon the regulation of the metabolism of carbohydrate, protein, and fat. Upon stimulation of cortisol, the liver forms glycogen from the amino acids supplied by the tissues. The hormone increases the rate of protein catabolism and decreases the permeability of the muscle cells to amino acids. On the other hand, the permeability of the liver cells is increased and the amino acids released as a result of protein catabolism are transported to the liver and may be used for synthesis of new protein. The glucocorticoids also influence the deposition of fatty tissue or the mobilization of fats.

In the absence of glucocorticoids rapid glycogen depletion occurs, followed by hypoglycemia a few hours after meals. Such hypoglycemia may be severe in a patient who has had no food for 10 or 12 hours. A glucose tolerance test shows a lower maximum blood sugar and a more rapid return to normal fasting levels than is obtained in normal individuals (see Figure 37–2.)

The production of glucocorticoids by the adrenal gland is governed by the adrenocorticotropic hormone (ACTH) of the pituitary. In the event hypophysectomy is performed, the adrenal cortex atrophies and glucocorticoids are not produced, just as they are not elaborated in Addison's disease.

Mineralocorticoids. Mineralocorticoids, of which aldosterone is of primary importance, are concerned with maintaining electrolyte homeostasis, especially for sodium and potassium. The production is regulated by the levels of sodium and potassium in the circulation. Aldosterone production leads to increased retention of sodium and greater excretion of potassium. Unlike the glucocorticoids, aldosterone production is not influenced by the pituitary. A deficiency of aldosterone, as seen in Addison's disease, leads to excessive excretion of sodium and increased retention of potassium. With the large salt loss much water is also excreted, thus leading to dehydration, hemoconcentration, reduced blood volume, and hypotension. In severe deficiency the patient experiences profound weakness and may have a craving for salt.

Androgenic hormones. These stimulate protein synthesis. In their absence tissue wasting, weight loss, reduction of muscle strength, and fatigue are present.

Patients with adrenal insufficiency frequently

experience anorexia, nausea, vomiting, abdominal discomfort, and diarrhea. Most of the patients have an increased pigmentation of the skin, often that of a deep tan or bronze. This results from the excessive production of *melanophore-stimulating hormone* by the pituitary when the adrenal steroids are lacking to exert an inhibitory effect.

Modification of the diet. Mild degrees of insufficiency are often satisfactorily treated by giving a higher salt intake, and by increasing the number of meals to five or six a day.[2] As the deficiency becomes more severe cortisone may be given to control the hypoglycemia, and, to some extent, to increase sodium retention. An increase in the salt intake is usually needed.[2]

Patients with severe insufficiency are treated with injections of deoxycorticosterone (DOCA) or by implantation of pellets of the synthetic hormone. The mineral metabolism is thereby controlled so that no change is usually required in the sodium and potassium levels of the diet.

DIETARY COUNSELING

A diet high in protein and relatively low in carbohydrate reduces the stimulation of insulin and helps to avoid the episodes of hypoglycemia. Meals should be given at frequent intervals—allowing between-meal feedings and a late bedtime feeding. Each of the feedings should include protein in order to reduce the rate of carbohydrate absorption. Simple carbohydrates—candy, sugar, and other sweets—are best avoided because of their rapid digestion and absorption and their stimulation of excessive insulin production.

METABOLIC EFFECTS OF ADRENOCORTICAL THERAPY

The adrenocorticotropic hormone of the anterior pituitary gland (ACTH) and the steroids of the adrenal cortex are used for the treatment of a wide variety of diseases such as arthritis, allergies, skin disturbances, adrenal insufficiency, many gastrointestinal diseases, and others. Although the various products used may vary somewhat in the degree of their effects on metabolism, it is important to be aware of possible nutritional implications of long-continued use of these hormones.

Water and electrolyte metabolism. Adrenocortical steroids in excess lead to retention of sodium and water and loss of potassium, as seen in Cushing's syndrome. Some sodium restriction is necessary for many patients. Usually, it is sufficient to avoid salty foods and to use no salt at the table, but a 1000-mg-sodium diet may occasionally be required (see Chapter 41). When the patient is eating well, the amounts of potassium in the diet are liberal. Foods especially high in potassium include broth, fruit juices, vegetables, whole-grain cereals, and meats.

Protein metabolism. A negative nitrogen balance may result when large doses of cortisone are used. This can be prevented when the diet is sufficiently liberal in carbohydrate to exert maximum protein-sparing effect and when high protein intakes are emphasized.

Carbohydrate metabolism. Cortisone therapy increases the storage of glycogen by increasing the amount of glycogen formation from protein. There also appears to be an insensitivity to insulin, as indicated by hyperglycemia and glycosuria. In diabetic patients who are also receiving cortisone, additional insulin may be required.

Gastrointestinal system. Hydrochloric acid secretion is increased following adrenocortical steroid therapy, and peptic ulceration may develop. In such a situation, the dietary modification described for peptic ulcer should be used (see Chapter 32.)

HYPERTHYROIDISM

Symptoms and clinical findings. Hyperthyroidism is a disturbance in which there is an excessive secretion of the thyroid gland with a consequent increase in the metabolic rate. The disease is also known as exophthalmic goiter, thyrotoxicosis, Graves' disease, or Basedow's disease. The chief symptoms are weight loss sometimes to the point of emaciation, excessive nervousness, prominence of the eyes, and a generally enlarged thyroid gland. The appetite is often increased, weakness may be marked, and signs of cardiac failure may be present.

Metabolism. All of the metabolic processes in the body are accelerated in hyperthyroidism. Serum protein-bound iodine values are elevated. The basal metabolic rate may be increased 50 per cent or more in severe cases. Moreover, the patient tends to be restless so that the total energy metabolism is further increased. When the level of calories is insufficient, the liver store of glycogen is rapidly depleted. This is especially serious just prior to surgery since postoperative shock is more likely.

The increased level of nitrogen metabolism leads to destruction of tissue proteins. Unless both protein and caloric levels are adequate, loss of weight may be rapid.

The excretion of calcium and phosphorus is greatly increased in hyperthyroidism. Osteoporosis and bone fractures are associated with severe losses. The increased level of energy metabolism increases the requirement for B-complex vitamins. For reasons not fully understood, the utilization of vitamin A and ascorbic acid is also speeded up.

Modification of the diet. Antithyroid compounds are now widely used to relieve the symptoms of hyperthyroidism, and in more severe instances to prepare the patient for surgery. These drugs reduce the basal metabolic rate to normal, but a liberal diet is still indicated because patients have usually experienced severe malnutrition prior to therapy.

DIETARY COUNSELING

Until normal nutrition is restored, approximately 4000 to 5000 kcal and 100 to 125 gm protein should be allowed (see High-Calorie Diet, Chapter 29). Calcium intakes of 2 to 3 gm daily are desirable together with supplements of vitamin D.[3] The calcium may be provided as calcium salts in addition to the liberal use of milk. The diet itself will include generous allowances of vitamin A, the B complex, and ascorbic acid, but supplements are often prescribed.

HYPOTHYROIDISM

Hypothyroidism, or decreased production of the thyroid hormone, is known as myxedema when severe in the adult, or cretinism when its symptoms become apparent shortly after birth (see Chapter 8). Myxedema is characterized by a lowered rate of energy metabolism—often 30 to 40 per cent below normal, muscular flabbiness, puffy face, eyelids, and hands, sensitivity to cold, marked fatigue with slight exertion, and a personality change including apathy and dullness. The patient frequently responds to therapy with desiccated thyroid.

Obesity is an occasional problem in patients with hypothyroidism since they may continue in their earlier patterns of eating even though the energy metabolism has been significantly reduced. In other patients, the appetite may be so poor that undernutrition results.

JOINT DISEASES

Incidence. Arthritis is the principal crippler in the United States. It affects about 20 million Americans, of whom some 3 million persons are limited in their usual activity. The incidence is higher in women, in people with low incomes, in the later years of life, and among residents of rural areas.

Eighty-three per cent of all cases of arthritis occur in persons over 45 years of age.[4]

Symptoms and clinical findings. The terms *arthritis* and *rheumatism* are applied to many joint diseases. Rheumatic fever is a special threat to the child or young adult because inadequate treatment may permanently damage the heart (see page 428). Gout, another of the joint diseases, is an error of uric acid metabolism and is discussed on page 512.

Osteoarthritis or *degenerative arthritis* is the most common form of arthritis and is usually associated with advancing age. Mechanical stress to a joint, for example, injury, overweight, or poor posture; aging factors; hereditary, metabolic, and endocrine factors are believed to be involved.[4] The joints of the fingers, knees, shoulders, and lumbar and cervical spines are most frequently affected. The onset is slow and noninflammatory. Gradual changes occur in the cartilages of the joints and new bone spurs grow at the edges. The joint stiffness is characteristic and pain is often severe.

Rheumatoid arthritis is a highly inflammatory and very painful condition having its onset in young adults, especially women. Autoimmunity and an infectious process have been proposed as etiologic factors.[4] Rheumatoid arthritis is characterized by fatigue, pain, stiffness, deformity which may be severe, and limited function. The disease is progressive but the symptoms may spontaneously disappear only to reappear again at a later time. With early diagnosis the disabling effects can be delayed but there is no known cure.

Treatment. Probably few diseases have had more theories offered concerning therapy. Arthritics spend over $435 million annually on phony diets and devices. None of the claims made by promoters have been supported by research. Over the years numerous diets have been tried by clinicians, but none has been effective in modifying the course of the disease. These trials have included diets high or low in protein, fat, and carbohydrate; modified for acid or alkaline ash; or supplemented with vitamins, especially ascorbic acid and vitamin D.

A number of drugs beginning with aspirin bring relief to the arthritic patient. Steroid therapy and gold salts have been effective for many. Since these drugs may bring about undesirable side effects, their use for each patient must be carefully evaluated.

Patients whose deformities limit their activities can be helped by physical and occupational therapy. The occupational therapist, home economist, dietitian, and nurse can help patients to greater independence by teaching them how to use many self-help devices that have been designed. (See Figure 38–1.) Homemakers need counseling on ways to accomplish their housekeeping activities with less effort. Sometimes a rearrangement of kitchen equipment is sufficient; in other instances some modification of the design of the kitchen itself is needed. (See also pages 385 to 387.)

DIETARY COUNSELING

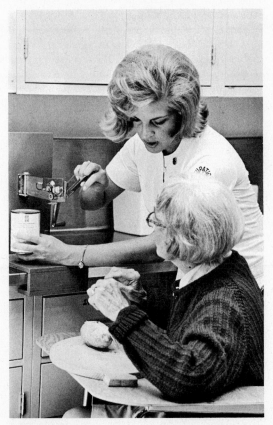

Figure 38–1. An occupational therapist shows a handicapped homemaker how to modify food preparation procedures for her physical limitations. (Courtesy, The Arthritis Foundation.)

Arthritic patients require the same foods for health that other persons need. When patients are of normal weight and in good nutritional status, the normal diet is suitable.

Obesity is a common problem in osteoarthritis, and weight loss should be brought about in order to reduce the added stress on weight-bearing joints. (See Chapter 29 for low-calorie diets.)

Many patients with rheumatoid arthritis have lost weight and are in poor nutritional status. For them a high-calorie high-protein diet is indicated until good nutritional status has been achieved. (See pages 416 and 422.)

Some individuals experience gastric irritation or even ulceration from aspirin or steroid therapy. These effects can be prevented by taking these medications with meals and with a bedtime snack containing protein foods for their buffering capacity. Steroid therapy also leads to sodium retention in some in which case mild sodium restriction is indicated. Usually it is sufficient to omit salty foods and the use of salt at the table; sometimes, a 1000-mg-sodium diet may be required. Continued steroid therapy adversely affects the calcium balance, leading to gradual bone demineralization. A liberal intake of milk, contrary to popular opinion, is desirable.

Gout

Incidence and etiology. Gout accounts for about 3 to 5 of every 100 persons afflicted with joint diseases. It is a hereditary disease occurring principally in males after 30 years of age. Women are more susceptible after the menopause. Hyperuricemia (high blood level of uric acid) is transmitted by a single dominant autosomal gene which is not sex linked. The cause for the hyperuricemia has not been fully established but various theories ascribe it to (1) decreased destruction of uric acid in the body, (2) increased production of uric acid in the body, or (3) decreased excretion of uric acid.

Overeating and excessive drinking of alcoholic beverages are not primary etiologic agents, but alcohol, high-fat diets, and obesity can aggravate an existing condition.

Nature and occurrence of uric acid. Cellular material of both plant and animal origin contains *nucleoproteins*. Glandular organs such as liver, pancreas, and kidney are among the richest sources; meats and the embryo or germ of grains and legumes, together with the growing parts of young plants, also furnish appreciable amounts. During digestion nucleoproteins are first split into proteins and nucleic acid. Further cleavage of nucleic acid leads to several products, one group of which are the purines. The latter in turn are oxidized to uric acid, probably by the liver.

In addition to the uric acid available from the metabolism of nucleic acid, the body can synthesize purines from the simplest carbon and nitrogen compounds such as carbon dioxide, acetic acid, and glycine. Thus any substances from which these materials originate, namely carbohydrate, fat, and protein, give rise to a considerable production of uric acid. Even in the fasting state there is a constant production of uric acid from cellular breakdown.

The liver and tissues store uric acid and its precursors for variable lengths of time and release them later. As a normal constituent of urine, uric acid represents a part of the daily nitrogenous excretion. Some uric acid is also excreted via the bile into the intestinal tract.

Symptoms and clinical findings. The range of plasma uric acid in normal individuals is 2 to 5 mg per cent, whereas in those with susceptibility to gout the concentration is above 7 mg per cent and may reach as high as 20 mg per cent. A large percentage of individuals with hyperuricemia sooner or later will have acute attacks of gout characterized by sudden inflammation and swelling accompanied by severe pain of the joints, especially the metatarsal, knee, and toe joints. The acute attack usually responds dramatically in 24 to 48 hours to treatment with colchicine.

Many patients have only occasional acute attacks of gout with moderate hyperuricemia and the disease does not progress. Others have attacks with greater and greater frequency, and deposits of sodium urate (tophi) in the tendon, cartilage, and kidneys lead to permanent damage of the joints and other tissues and increasing invalidism. Renal impairment is often present.

Treatment. A number of drugs are effective in the treatment of gout, and diet is considered to be an adjunct to drug therapy. Colchicine and a number of other drugs provide effective relief from the pain that accompanies the acute attack. In addition, these drugs reduce the frequency of attacks when they are also used as interval therapy.

Uricosuric drugs (probenecid and others) increase the excretion of uric acid, thereby bringing plasma levels within a normal range. With the lowering of the plasma uric acid levels, sodium urate deposits in the joints are gradually dissolved out. These drugs are not effective in reducing the pain of the acute attack and may exacerbate the symptoms during an attack. Therefore, they are used during the quiescent periods of the disease.

Allopurinol is a drug that inhibits the action of the enzyme *xanthine oxidase*, which is responsible for the formation of uric acid from xanthine and hypoxanthine. Therefore, the excretion of uric acid is diminished and that of xanthine is increased. Inasmuch as xanthine can precipitate out to form kidney stones, it is essential that the patient have a liberal fluid intake and excrete a urine that is neutral or slightly alkaline.

Modification of the diet. During the acute attacks a low-purine diet is often ordered in addition to drug therapy. Some physicians also recommend moderate restriction of purines as interval therapy for patients receiving uricosuric drugs.[5]

Dietary Counseling

Data on the purine content of foods are limited. Foods have been grouped in three categories in Table 38–1. As may be seen from this classification, all flesh foods and extractives from them such as gravies and soups must be eliminated for the low-purine diet. If purine restriction is also prescribed for interval therapy, the allowance of meat, poultry, and fish is limited to 2 to 3 ounces on each of three to five days.

Energy. Since obesity has adverse effects on general health as well as on gout, the overweight individual should gradually lose weight. Patients should not be placed on low-calorie diets during acute attacks of gout since the catabolism of adipose tissue reduces the excretion of uric acid. Rapid weight loss effected by starvation or by extremely low-calorie diets can precipitate an attack of gout. Usually, men can lose weight satisfactorily when their diets are restricted to 1200 to 1600 kcal. (See Chapter 29.)

Protein, fat, and carbohydrate. Because the nitrogen of the purine nucleus is supplied by protein, the intake is restricted to about 1 gm per kilogram. Fat is often restricted to about 60 gm daily. When the food intake is poor because of illness, it is essential that high-carbohydrate fluids be given so that adipose tissue is not excessively catabolized.

Fluid. The daily intake of fluids should be at least 3 liters. Coffee and tea may be used in moderate amounts. These beverages contain methylated purines, which are oxidized to

Table 38–1. Purine Content of Foods per 100 Grams*

Group I (0–15 mg)	Group II (50–150 mg)	Group III (150 mg and over)
Breads and cereals	Beans, dry	Anchovies
Butter and other fats*	Fish	Asparagus*
Caviar*	Lentils	Brains*
Cheese	Meats	Gravies*
Eggs	Oatmeal*	Kidney
Fish roe*	Peas, dry	Liver
Fruits	Poultry*	Meat extracts
Gelatin*	Seafood	Mincemeat*
Milk	Spinach	Mushrooms*
Nuts*		Sardines
Sugar, sweets*		Sweetbreads
Vegetables		

*Adapted from Turner, D.: *Handbook of Diet Therapy,* 5th ed. University of Chicago Press, Chicago, 1970, p. 117. Starred items are additions to Turner's list.

methyl uric acid. The latter is excreted in the urine and is not deposited in the tissues. Hence, the customary omission of coffee and tea may impose an unnecessary hardship. Alcohol is contraindicated.

To effect a neutral or slightly alkaline urine when allopurinol is prescribed, the diet should be liberal in its content of fruits and vegetables. In addition, the physician usually prescribes small amounts of sodium bicarbonate or sodium citrate.

Purine-Restricted Diet

General Rules

For a diet essentially free of exogenous purines, use foods only from group I, Table 38–1.

For a low-purine level, allow 3 to 5 small servings of lean meat, poultry, and fish from group II each week.

If a low-fat regimen is ordered, the butter is omitted, and skim milk is substituted for the whole milk.

Include These Foods Daily:

3–4 cups milk

  2 eggs

1–2 ounces cheese; allow 2 to 3 ounces lean beef, veal, lamb, poultry, or fish 3 to 5 times a week during interval therapy

3–4 servings vegetables including:
    1 medium potato
    1–2 servings green leafy or yellow vegetable
    1 serving other vegetable
2–3 servings fruit including:
    1 serving citrus fruit
    1–2 servings other fruits
1 serving enriched cereal
4–6 slices enriched bread
    2 tablespoons butter or fortified margarine
Additional calories are provided as needed by increasing the amount of potato, potato substitutes such as macaroni, rice, noodles, bread, sugars, sweets, fruits, and vegetables.

Nutritive value of basic foods above: Calories, 1850; protein, 68 gm; fat, 80 gm; carbohydrate, 220 gm; calcium, 1400 mg; iron, 11.3 mg; vitamin A, 11,350 I.U.; thiamin, 1.3 mg; riboflavin, 2.3 mg; niacin, 10 mg; ascorbic acid, 145 mg.

Foods to Avoid
All foods high in purines (see group III, Table 38–1)
Condiments and excessive seasoning
Alcohol
For low-fat diets:
    Pastries and rich desserts
    Cream and ice cream
    Fried foods
    Eggs not to exceed 2 daily; hard cheese not to exceed 1 ounce. Severe restriction may require the omission of eggs, whole milk, cheese, and butter. Skim milk and cottage cheese must then be used in ample amounts to provide the necessary protein.

Sample Menu
    BREAKFAST
Half grapefruit
Rice Krispies with milk and sugar
Buttered toast
Scrambled egg
Coffee with milk and sugar
    LUNCHEON OR SUPPER
Jelly omelet
Boiled rice
Broiled tomato
Half peach with cottage cheese on lettuce

Bread with 1 teaspoon butter
Milk—1 glass
    DINNER
Cheese soufflé
Baked potato
Beets
Green celery strips
Bread with 1 teaspoon butter
Apple snow
Milk—1 glass
    BEDTIME
Milk—1 glass

OSTEOPOROSIS

Osteoporosis is a bone disease of frequent occurrence in middle age, yet its etiology and its treatment are poorly understood. Various surveys of populations in homes for the aged and of other patients receiving ambulatory care have shown 15 to 50 per cent of the population over age 65 to be affected. A minimum of four million noninstitution-alized persons are believed to have severe osteoporosis. The disease occurs four times as frequently in women as in men.

Etiology. Osteoporosis is a deficiency disease, but it would be erroneous to assume that a deficit in dietary intake is primarily responsible. Rather, the aspects of deficiency are the result of many factors, among which are the following: gastrectomy; endocrine disorders such as hyperthyroidism, hyperparathyroidism, hyperadrenocorticism, and acromegaly; immobilization; rheumatoid arthritis; sickle-cell anemia; nutritional deficiencies such as of calcium, protein, ascorbic acid, and others.[6]

Some authorities consider osteoporosis to be a disease of the protein matrix and have associated this with the frequent occurrence of a low protein intake. Others have shown a close correlation between the degree of mineralization of the bone and the intake of calcium. Osteoporosis occurs far more frequently in women who have had a lifetime history of low calcium intake than it does in women who have always had a liberal calcium intake.

Metabolic changes and their effects. The principal symptoms of osteoporosis are low-back pain, sometimes severe, and often a history of vertebral fractures. Over a period of years the individual may have lost height—sometimes several inches. Roentgenographic changes are not diagnosed until as much as 30 per cent of the bone mass has been lost.

Osteoporosis is characterized by a reduction in the total bone mass, but with no known change in the structure or chemical composition of the bone. Because of the reduction in the number of cells, there is a decrease in the thickness of the cortex, a thinning of the trabeculae, and an increased porosity of the bone. As a result, fractures occur with greater frequency.

Blood levels of calcium, phosphorus, and alkaline phosphatase are normal, as are also the serum protein and lipoprotein levels. Calcium, phosphorus, and nitrogen balances are frequently negative. Inadequate dietary intake, defective absorption from the gastrointestinal tract, or excessive bone resorption could explain such negative balances. It is well to keep in mind that older individuals may require more calcium to achieve balance than those who are younger.

Treatment. The factors which may have initiated the osteoporosis must be determined before effective therapy can be instituted. Estrogens and androgens have been used advantageously in many patients, since the hormones exert an anabolic effect on proteins and also play a role in better retention of minerals in bone. Physiotherapy is required to relieve pain and to prevent immobilization.

DIETARY COUNSELING

A diet liberal in calcium is generally recommended. The inclusion of at least 1 quart of milk, some hard cheese, and a normal allowance of other foods would bring the daily intake of calcium to about 1.5 gm. A calcium supplement may also be used in the form of calcium gluconate or calcium lactate. In some instances a supplement of vitamin D has appeared to improve the absorption of calcium and the mineralization of bone. The resorption of bone is less in those areas where the water is fluoridated with 1 ppm of fluoride. A combined program of sodium fluoride, calcium, and vitamin D supplements has been recommended by some.[7] At best, the treatment of osteoporosis is likely to inhibit the progression of the disease; reversal of the disease is not likely.

The primary effort should be directed early in life to the prevention of bone loss. A diet adequate in calcium and protein is important for maintenance of bone structure; however, until more is known of the etiology of this disease the most effective prophylaxis as well as treatment cannot be prescribed.

PROBLEMS AND REVIEW

1. Mrs. H. is admitted to the hospital with the chief complaint of "hypoglycemia." She will undergo diagnostic tests to determine the cause of her symptoms.
   a. Differentiate between the hypoglycemia in functional hyperinsulinism, Addison's disease, and liver disease. What modification of carbohydrate level of the diet is required for each?
   b. What is the advantage of a high protein and high fat intake in hyperinsulinism?
   c. The tests revealed Mrs. H. has functional hyperinsulinism. Calculate a diet for her to provide: 2400 kcal, 130 gm protein, and 75 gm carbohydrate. Use the exchange lists for the calculation. Divide the day's allowance into three equal meals.

    d. Draw a typical glucose tolerance curve for a person who has functional hyperinsulinism, Addison's disease, hyperthyroidism, diabetes mellitus.

2. You are assigned to care for Mr. J., a 58-year-old patient with Addison's disease.
    a. What modifications of mineral and water metabolism are present in Addison's disease? In what way is this corrected by hormone therapy?
    b. Why is a sodium-restricted diet occasionally ordered for a patient receiving hormone therapy in Addison's disease? Under what circumstances would an increase in sodium intake be used?
    c. On the basis of your understanding of the metabolism in Addison's disease, what are some of the functions of the adrenal gland in the normal individual? What is the effect of the activity of the pituitary?
    d. What are the characteristic symptoms of hyperthyroidism?

3. A patient with hyperthyroidism was seen in the metabolism clinic and was asked to return in one month for surgery. The nutritionist instructed the patient on a diet to provide 5000 kcal and 125 gm protein.
    a. What are some of the characteristic symptoms of hyperthyroidism; of hypothyroidism?
    b. Compare the diet which might be used in a hyperthyroid patient who is well controlled with antithyroid drugs, and one who has an elevated metabolic rate.
    c. Suggest five ways in which the calories of a diet for a patient with hyperthyroidism might be increased.
    d. Why does a surgeon so frequently insist that a patient gain weight before an operation on the thyroid?
    e. What is myxedema? What is its chief cause? How can you explain the frequent occurrence of overweight?

4. Your grandmother shows you an ad for a booklet with a diet "guaranteed" to cure arthritis and aid in weight reduction.
    a. What would you tell her about the role of diet in arthritis?
    b. Outline briefly the dietary considerations in arthritis.
    c. What are the dietary implications of long-term use of cortisone in this disease or in other conditions?

5. You are asked to teach Mr. O. about gout. Consider the following questions in planning your remarks:
    a. What are the sources of uric acid to the body? In what ways is uric acid metabolism disturbed in gout?
    b. How can you explain the fact that a person who has gout may have an acute attack following surgery or during an acute infection?
    c. What is the basis for restricting the protein intake to 1 gm per kilogram in the dietary planning for a patient with gout?
    d. What problems are entailed when a purine-free diet is ordered for a patient, insofar as nutritional adequacy is concerned?
    e. Plan a menu for one day for a low-purine diet.

6. What is the role of each of these hormones on protein and mineral metabolism: thyroxine; parathormone; androgen; cortisone?

7. On the basis of current research related to osteoporosis, what dietary measures may be instrumental in preventing the disease?

8. What modifications of the normal diet may be helpful in the treatment of osteoporosis?

CITED REFERENCES

1. "Statement on Hypoglycemia," *J.A.M.A.*, **223**:682, 1973.
2. Greenblatt, R. B., and Metts, J. C., Jr.: "Addison's Disease," *Am. J. Nurs.*, **60**:1249–52, 1960.
3. Puppel, I. D., *et al.:* "Some Metabolic Factors in the Treatment of Hyperthyroidism," *Ann. Intern. Med.*, **48**:1300–1327, 1958.
4. *Arthritis, Prevention, Treatment, and Rehabilitation.* Hearing before the SubCommittee on Public Health and Environment. Committee on Interstate and Foreign Commerce. House of Representatives. 93rd Congress, 2nd Session, Nov. 25, 1974. Serial No. 93-109. U.S. Govt. Printing Office, Washington, D.C., 1975.
5. Zollner, N., and Griebach, A.: "Diet and Gout," *Adv. Exp. Med. Biol.*, **41**:435–42, 1974.
6. Ehtisham, M.: "Osteoporosis," *Nurs. Times*, **70**:1544–46, 1974.
7. Jowsey, J., *et al.:* "New Concepts in the Treatment of Osteoporosis," *Postgrad. Med.*, **52**:62–67, Oct. 1972.

ADDITIONAL REFERENCES

Berger, H.: "Hypoglycemia: A Perspective," *Postgrad. Med.*, **57:**81–85, Feb. 1975.
Blount, M., and Kinney, A. B.: "Chronic Steroid Therapy," *Am. J. Nurs.*, **74:**1626–31, 1974.
Boone, J. E.: "Juvenile Rheumatoid Arthritis," *Pediatr. Clin. North Am.*, **21:**885–915, 1974.
Eliott, D. D.: "Adrenocortical Insufficiency: A Self-Instruction Unit," *Am. J. Nurs.*, **74:**1115–30, 1974.
Evered, D. C., *et al.*: "Grades of Hypothyroidism," *Br. Med. J.*, **1:**657–62, 1973.
"Gout," *J.A.M.A.*, **224** (Suppl. 5): 757–66, 1973.
Hofeldt, F. D., *et al.*: "Diagnosis and Classification of Reactive Hypoglycemia Based on Hormonal Changes
    in Response to Oral and Intravenous Glucose Administration," *Am. J. Clin. Nutr.*, **25:**1193–1201, 1972.
Ibarra, J. D.: "Hypoglycemia," *Postgrad. Med.*, **51:**88–93, Feb. 1972.
Kogut, M. D.: "Hypoglycemia: Pathogenesis, Diagnosis and Treatment," *Curr. Probl. Pediatr.*, **4:**1–59, 1974.
Lutwak, L.: "Continuing Need for Dietary Calcium Throughout Life," *Geriatrics*, **29:**171–74, May 1974.
MacRae, I.: "Arthritis, Its Nature and Management," *Nurs. Clin. North Am.*, **8:**643–52, 1973.
Nerup, J.: "Addison's Disease. A Review of Some Clinical, Pathological and Immunological Features," *Dan.
    Med. Bull.*, **21:**201–17, 1974.
Newmark, S. R., *et al.*: "Hyperglycemic and Hypoglycemic Crises," *J.A.M.A.*, **231:**185–87, 1975.
Scott, C. W., ed.: "Hyperthyroidism," *South. Med. J.*, **65:**161–73, 1972.
Soika, C. V.: "Combatting Osteoporosis," *Am. J. Nurs.*, **73:**1193–97, 1973.
Yü, T. A.: "Milestones in the Treatment of Gout," *Am. J. Med.*, **56:**676–85, 1974.

INSTRUCTIONAL MATERIALS FOR THE PATIENT

Diet and Arthritis. Pub. 1857, Public Health Service, Diabetes and Arthritis Control Program, U.S.
    Department of Health, Education, and Welfare, Washington, D.C., 1969.
Hamilton, A.: "Good News about Gout," *Today's Health*, **45:**16, Dec. 1967.
Maddox, G.: *Food and Arthritis.* Taplinger Publishing Company, New York, 1969.

39 Nutrition in Neurologic Disturbances

Ketogenic Diet

Nutrition and the nervous system. The nervous tissues, like other tissues of the body, require energy for metabolic functions, protein for cell synthesis, vitamins as components of the enzyme systems, and mineral elements as activators of metabolic reactions and to maintain homeostasis of the fluid environment. The following discussion presents a brief summary of the principal effects of nutrient lack upon the functioning of the nervous system.

Energy. The brain normally utilizes glucose exclusively as its source of energy. To shut off the supply of glucose and oxygen from the brain for even a few minutes leads to irreversible damage. The body at rest utilizes up to 25 per cent of its total oxygen consumption for the brain alone.[1]

Protein. The influence of amino acid imbalances on mental development are dramatically illustrated by the severe mental retardation that accompanies inborn errors of metabolism. These are fully discussed in Chapter 46.

In recent years much research on experimental animals and on humans has shown that severe protein deficiency during pregnancy and during the first year of life especially can lead to profound alterations in brain development. Severe undernutrition is associated with deficits in physical, psychologic, and intellectual capacities and has long-lasting effects on behavior.[2] The retardation of development is accentuated when infection is also present. Although much evidence has been presented that implicates nutrition, it is exceedingly difficult to separate the effects of malnutrition from the economic, educational, emotional, and social deprivation that are simultaneously present. See also pages 345 to 349 for further discussion of protein-calorie malnutrition.

Vitamins. Deficiencies of the water-soluble vitamins bring about serious changes in functioning of the nervous system. (See Chapter 12.) Thiamin deficiency is characterized by reduced tendon reflexes, peripheral neuritis, incoordination of gait, muscle pains, irritability, inability to concentrate, lack of interest in affairs, and personality deterioration including hypochondriasis, depression and hysteria.[3]

Classic niacin deficiency, pellagra, is rarely seen in the United States. Its neurologic signs include poor memory, irritability, dizziness, hallucinations, delusions of persecution, and finally dementia.

Vitamin B_6 deficiency is characterized by weakness, ataxia, and convulsions. Pantothenic acid lack leads to mental depression, peripheral neuritis, sullenness, cramping pains in the arms and legs, and burning sensations of the feet. Irritability and forgetfulness are seen in folic acid deficiency. The inability to absorb vitamin B_{12} because of lack of intrinsic factor is the condition known as pernicious anemia and which presents such symptoms as unsteady gait, depression, and mental deterioration. (See Chapter 43.)

NUTRITION FOR THE MENTALLY ILL

Feeding older persons in nursing homes. Weiner[4] has described four categories of pathologic-psychologic reactions in aging persons in nursing homes: anxiety, depression, suspicion, and confusion. In some individuals all of these may be present to a varying degree or they may appear one after the other. Each type of reaction requires specific measures in feeding.

The anxious person requires assurance that everything is all right. He worries about the effects that foods may have on bowel function and often asks questions about which foods are constipating. Worry about his food may increase gastrointestinal motility so that he has cramps or may reduce motility so that he becomes distended. The anxious person needs to be comforted, to have someone around him, to be made to feel secure, and to be given special consideration by being served his favorite foods as often as possible.

The depressed individual feels that his situation is hopeless and has a conscious or unconscious desire to die. Reassurance only frightens him more and he will continue to demand more and more of it until there seems to be no end to his demands. He needs external control and should be told firmly exactly what he must do, that he must eat, that he will be taken care of, and that he will be helped to eat what he needs for his nourishment. Sometimes spoon feeding is needed to get him started. It is not advisable for him to choose his own menu.

The suspicious person is afraid that he will be hurt and often suspects that his food is poisoned. He feels that he must constantly be on watch lest something happens to his security. Efforts to reassure him to the contrary only increase his suspicions. Matter-of-factly he should be told that there is nothing wrong with his food, but it may be necessary for the attendant to taste the food in his presence to show that it is not poisoned. The suspicious person, unlike the depressed person, must not be forced to eat. He should be allowed to eat or not to eat what is presented to him.

The confused person has usually had some brain damage as in a stroke, from diabetic or hepatic coma, or from head injury. He does not know what is happening around him and he often becomes anxious, depressed, or suspicious. He may not know where he is, and regardless of what he is told he believes himself to be in his own home as an adult or in his childhood home. He needs help in understanding what is going on around him. With respect to feeding, he needs to be told that it is mealtime, what meal it is, and what foods are on his tray. When a favorite food is served, it is a good idea to specially identify it.

Diet for patients in the mental hospital. Diet is an important part of the total program of rehabilitation for the psychiatric patient. Aside from its nutritional necessity, food provides basic security and pleasurable satisfaction. The patient needs to feel that someone is genuinely concerned about his welfare and cares for him. The dietitian and nurse—through the care shown in meal planning, preparation, and service, and through their expressions of interest to the individual—are participants in the therapy.

Planning a nutritionally adequate diet is obviously not enough. The service of food that is attractive to the eye, tempting in aroma, and satisfying to the palate is just as important in the psychiatric hospital as in any other feeding situation. The mentally ill may express marked irritability when given foods they dislike. Food service in a cafeteria permits the patient to exercise some choice in his food selection, and thus helps to eliminate some of the irritations. On the other hand, staff-shared family-style meal service is favored by some and permits opportunity for closer rapport between staff and patients.[5]

Patients react favorably and are less destructive when an attractive dining environment is provided. A well-planned dining room with a cheerful color scheme, curtains or draperies at the windows, small attractive tables, and suitable background music is conducive to food acceptance and contributes to the therapy of the patient. Attention to birthdays, holidays, and other special events provides additional evidence that the patient is cared for.

Psychiatric patients frequently eat inadequate or excessive amounts of food. A regular schedule of weighing of patients—about once a month—will help to detect such changes, and correction can be started before marked weight change has occurred. Marked weight gain is not uncommon. It would seem easy to control this in a hospital by providing a diet designed for weight maintenance. However, the privileges of food purchases from a canteen and food gifts from relatives and friends must be taken into consideration. Patients are often known to eat food left by other patients.

Refusal to eat is a problem presented by other psychiatric patients. Hussar[6] recommends that the nurse or attendant should note any patient who refuses more than half of a meal. A four- or five-day simple checklist helps to identify whether the refusal follows a pattern with respect to a particular food or meal. Refusal of food sometimes denotes an underlying physical illness about which the patient who is withdrawn or mute does not complain. Those who need to gain weight may require close supervision in taking small, frequent feedings; some may be helped if butter is spread on the bread, milk and sugar are put on the cereal, the milk container is opened, the meat is cut, and so on; sincere words of encouragement should be offered when progress is made. Tube feeding (see Chapter 36) may be resorted to when all attempts to achieve satisfactory intake of food fail.

Feeding the mentally retarded presents many problems which may be especially acute in the child. The management of the diet for these patients is discussed in Chapter 45.

ANOREXIA NERVOSA

Anorexia nervosa is a psychiatric disorder seen primarily in females with onset usually occurring in early adolescence. It is characterized by extreme weight loss, even to the point of emaciation, as a consequence of refusal to eat. Mortality rates have ranged from 15 to 21 per cent in various series.[7] The individual often has a history of being "chubby" as a youngster. An overriding desire to lose weight leads to self-imposed starvation, bizarre food habits, self-induced vomiting, hyperactivity, laxative abuse, and so on as means of preventing weight gain. The individual usually is able to carry on normal school and social activities while denying hunger and fatigue. Amenorrhea, constipation, cold intolerance, hypotension, and bradycardia are characteristic findings. Anemia is not a common feature; serum iron and folate levels have been reported to be normal.[8,9] The clinical signs and symptoms are reversible with weight gain.

Treatment. Ultimately, individual and family psychotherapy is needed to resolve the basic conflict. For some individuals, short-term intervention is needed to prevent death by starvation. Various means have been used to induce the patient to eat. One approach uses behavior modification, in which privileges accorded the patient depend on achievement of a predetermined weight gain each day. Failure to gain the expected amount of weight results in suspension of privileges and use of supplemental feedings or tube feedings until the desired weight gain is reached.[10]

ALCOHOLISM

For about 9 million Americans chronic alcoholism severely affects health, job security, and family life.[11] Only about one fourth of these seek any kind of treatment. In the United States from 10 to 15 per cent of hospitalized patients have alcohol-related illnesses. Alcohol is a significant factor in approximately half of the highway fatalities each year in this country.[12] The American Academy of Pediatrics has expressed concern over the trend toward increased consumption of alcohol, and its related problems, in adolescents. Lowering of the drinking age and use of alcohol as an alternative to hard drugs have been cited as factors contributing to increased use.[13] Clearly, alcohol abuse is a major public health problem that must be considered in its physiologic, psychologic, economic, and social aspects.

Alcohol and metabolism. Alcohol is considered to be a food in that it yields 7 kcal per gram; however, it does not provide any nutrients to speak of. Alcohol is rapidly and almost completely absorbed. The presence of food in the stomach, as is well known, delays gastric absorption. However, from the small intestine absorption is rapid regardless of whether food is present or not.

Upon absorption alcohol is dispersed rapidly throughout the body water. The liver accounts for about 90 per cent of the total oxidation of alcohol. The first step in oxidation is to acetaldehyde, a reaction believed to be catalyzed by three enzyme systems: alcohol dehydrogenase, catalase, and a microsomal ethanol oxidizing system.[14] The reaction is limited in rate by the level of alcohol dehydrogenase that is present. Acetaldehyde is further oxidized to acetyl coenzyme A and enters the citric acid cycle where the oxidation is completed to yield energy, carbon dioxide, and water. (See page 69.)

Effects of alcohol upon nutrition. Alcohol reduces the appetite so that the heavy drinker eats poorly. Moreover, the chronic alcoholic often does not have the money to purchase an adequate diet inasmuch as he may be out of a job and he spends what money he has for alcohol. The incidence of malnutrition is not high according to Olson,[15] who claims that no more than 20 per cent of alcoholics show biochemical changes suggestive of mild deficiency and that only 3 per cent have frank deficiency symptoms. On the other hand, Iber[16] has emphasized the relationship of major illnesses to alcoholic malnutrition. Chronic alcoholics have a high incidence of hepatic, neurologic, gastrointestinal, and cardiac disorders.[17]

Formerly it was believed that alcohol was directly toxic to the liver; this view is now generally disputed. On the other hand, the liver is impaired because of the interfering effects of alcohol upon normal metabolic processes. Fatty infiltration of the liver results from one of several causes: increased synthesis of triglycerides; reduced synthesis of lipoproteins that are required for transport of fats; and possibly an increased mobilization of fat from adipose tissue during periods of starvation. In fatty infiltration there is little damage to the liver cells, but subsequently the hepatic cells are damaged, leading first to alcoholic hepatitis and then to cirrhosis. Even the early stages of cirrhosis can be reversed when a nutritious diet is given.

The urinary losses of amino acids, magnesium, potassium, and zinc are increased during periods of drinking. According to Flink, symptoms of *delirium tremens* have been associated with severe hypomagnesemia.[18]

Diet for alcoholics. A diet that meets normal nutritional requirements will restore the nutritional status of the alcoholic. When there is evidence of vitamin deficiencies, a supplement, especially of water-soluble factors, is indicated. It is a fallacy, however, that vitamin deficiencies are an etiologic factor in alcoholism, or that the correction of these deficiencies will cure the alcoholic.

When hepatitis or cirrhosis is present, the dietary modifications described on pages 468 to 471 should be considered. The possibility of hepatic coma and the need for drastic protein restriction when it occurs must always be kept in mind.

Nurses and dietitians can help the alcoholic return to better health by considering his food habits, by encouraging him to eat, and by providing dietary counseling. No useful purpose is served by assuming a critical, moralizing posture either by what one says or by one's attitude.

Wernicke's and Korsakoff's syndromes. Wernicke's syndrome and Korsakoff's psychoses are highly associated with alcoholism and appear to be different phases of the same disease. Wernicke's syndrome is characterized by ophthalmoplegia (paralysis of the eye muscles), ataxia (uncoordinated gait), and mental confusion. Nystagmus (rapid movement of the eyeballs) is a prominent feature.[19] The patient is often unable to stand or walk without support. The eye changes are dramatically corrected, often within hours, by the administration of thiamin.

Korsakoff's syndrome may not be apparent until several weeks after the changes in the eye and gait have become evident. The chief defect is the disturbance in memory and the inability to learn new things so that only the most routine tasks can be performed. Moreover, there is failure to associate past events in their proper sequence. Patients may be confused, anxious, fearful, and even delirious. Vitamin therapy has produced marked effects in restoring the patient to being responsive, alert, and attentive. However, when memory defects are present, they appear to persist despite therapy, suggesting that structural changes in the brain may be irreversible.

EPILEPSY

The nature of epilepsy. Epilepsy is a disease of the central nervous system characterized by loss of consciousness which may last for only a few seconds, as in petit mal attacks, or which may be accompanied by convulsions, as in grand mal attacks. It occurs more frequently in children than in adults. The disease in no way affects the individual's mental ability, but unthinking relatives and friends sometimes attach an entirely unwarranted stigma to the disease and thus may increase the tension states in the individual.

Treatment. Various drugs such as phenobarbital or phenytoin sodium or others have been employed with considerable success in the treatment of epilepsy and have largely replaced the ketogenic diet once so widely used. As a rule, a normal diet for the individual's age and activity is prescribed when drug therapy is used. Folate deficiency, anemia, and osteomalacia have been attributed to use of these drugs.[20]

Some individuals with minor motor seizures and petit mal epilepsy who do not respond to drug therapy have been successfully managed with a ketogenic diet. Preschool-age children seem to benefit most. The purpose of the diet, as described by Mike, is to produce ketosis by limiting very severely the amount of available glucose and increasing markedly the intake of fat so that complete combustion of fats cannot take place. The accumulation of acetone bodies (acetone, acetoacetic acid, and beta-hydroxybutyric acid) has a favorable effect on the irritability and restlessness of the child and does not dull the mental function as some drugs do.[21] The maintenance of a continuous state of acidosis is essential, for even small amounts of carbohydrate lead to seizures.

Some of the difficult features of the diet are that it permits selection from only a very limited list of foods, is severely restricted in carbohydrate, is unpalatable, lacks bulk, deviates sharply from customary food patterns, and requires great care in planning and preparation. A careful evaluation of the probable success of the diet for each patient and the ability of the parents to understand and adhere to the regulations is essential.

Modification of the diet. Sufficient calories for normal weight and for the maintenance of normal growth are necessary. The allowances recommended by Mike[21] are

Age (years)	kcal per kg
2–3	100 to 80
3–5	80 to 60
5–10	79 to 55

Protein. An allowance of 1 gm protein per kilogram of body weight is sufficient, but may be increased to 1.5 gm per kilogram for the older child.

Carbohydrate and fat. The nonprotein calories are so divided that a ketogenic to antiketogenic ratio of approximately 3 to 1 or 4 to 1 is maintained. Ketogenic factors (fatty acids) in the diet include 90 per cent of the fat, and about 50 per cent of the protein. The antiketogenic factors in the diet (available glucose) are derived from 100 per cent of the carbohydrate, plus approximately 50 per cent of the protein and 10 per cent of the fat. Obviously, to achieve a 3-to-1 or 4-to-1 ratio, the carbohydrate must be sharply restricted and the fat intake greatly increased. The level of carbohydrate usually needs to be less than 30 gm if ketosis is to be produced, but should never be less than 10 gm daily.

The diet for a five-year-old child weighing 25 kg illustrates the calculation of a diet prescription.

1. Kcal: $25 \times 70 = 1750$
2. Protein: $25 \times 1 = 25$ gm
3. Kcal from protein: $25 \times 4 = 100$
4. Kcal from carbohydrate and fat: $1750 - 100 = 1650$

If we allow 25 gm carbohydrate, the fat intake

would need to be 172 gm as noted in the following calculations:

5. Kcal from carbohydrate: $25 \times 4 = 100$
6. Kcal from fat: $1650 - 100 = 1550$
7. Grams of fat: $1550 \div 9 = 172$

The fatty acid to glucose ratio of this diet is as follows:

$$\frac{FA}{AG} = \frac{0.50\,(25) + 0.9\,(172)}{0.50\,(25) + 0.1\,(172) + 1.0\,(25)} = \frac{167}{55} = \frac{3}{1}$$

The maintenance of a constant acidosis requires that the protein, fat, and carbohydrate for the day be divided in three equal meals. The urine shows a positive test for acetoacetic acid when acidosis is being maintained.

Minerals and vitamins. Calcium gluconate or lactate is prescribed to furnish calcium. An iron supplement providing 7 to 10 mg elemental iron is also given. The vitamin needs are met by giving an aqueous multivitamin preparation.

Management of the diet. For the first 24 to 72 hours the child is given nothing but water, usually restricted to 500 to 1000 ml. Hunger disappears as ketosis increases. When ketosis is marked the diet is initiated, but is not forced until the transition has been accomplished. During this period nausea and vomiting may occur.

The diet may be calculated by using the values for individual foods as in Table A–1, or by using food groupings such as those developed by Mike[21] or Lasser.[22] The meal exchange lists are not satisfactory for the calculation. The predominant foods in the diet are carefully restricted amounts of meat, cheese, and eggs; cream, butter, bacon, mayonnaise; restricted amounts of low-carbohydrate vegetables and fruits. Other foods are avoided: sugar-containing beverages; breads and cereals; desserts such as cake, cookies, ice cream, pastries, pie, puddings; milk; all sweets including sugar, jellies, candy, preserves; vegetables and fruits high in carbohydrate.

The diet must be weighed on a gram scale and all food must be consumed at each meal. Foods may not be saved for later consumption. If no improvement occurs within six weeks, there is nothing to be gained by further continuance of the diet. If improvement does occur, the diet must be continued for a year or longer. Gradually the diet is liberalized with very small increases in the carbohydrate and corresponding caloric decreases in the fat. Table 39–1 illustrates a sample calculation for the ketogenic diet.

Signore[23] has described a ketogenic diet using medium-chain triglycerides. Inasmuch as medium-chain triglycerides are more ketogenic than conventional food fats, more carbohydrate is permitted on this diet. Foods need not be weighed.

Table 39–1. Sample Calculation for Ketogenic Diet*

Food	No. of Units	Household Measure	Weight gm	Protein gm	Fat gm	Carbohydrate gm
Breakfast						
Orange juice	4	⅙ cup	40	—	—	4.0
Canadian bacon	6	¾ slice	21	6.0	3.0	—
Whipping cream	2½	½ cup	115	2.5	42.5	3.8
Cellu wafers						
Butter	2	2¼ tsp	12	—	10.9	—
Apricot spread (Cellu)	½	1 teaspoon	5	—	—	0.5
				8.5	56.4	8.3
Luncheon or Supper						
Beef, lean	6	⅔ ounce	21	6.0	3.0	—
Tomato, raw	1	¼ small	25	0.2	—	1.0
Whipping cream	2½	½ cup	115	2.5	42.5	3.8
Peach, raw	3	⅓ small	30	—	—	3.0
Butter	2	2¼ tsp	12	—	10.9	—
Cellu wafers						
Blackberry jelly (Cellu)	½	1 teaspoon	5	—	—	0.5
				8.7	56.4	8.3
Dinner						
Cheddar cheese	5	⅔ ounce	20	5.0	5.0	—
Strawberries	4	4 large	40	—	—	4.0
Whipping cream	2½	½ cup	115	2.5	42.5	3.8
Butter	2	2¼ tsp	12	—	10.9	—
Cellu wafers						
Apricot spread (Cellu)	½	1 teaspoon	5	—	—	0.5
				7.5	58.4	8.3
Total for the day				(24.7)	(171.2)	(24.9)
(Prescribed order)				(25.0)	(172.0)	(25.0)

$$\frac{\text{Ketogenic factors}}{\text{Antiketogenic factors}} = \frac{166.4}{54.4} = 3.1$$

*Based on plan described by Lasser, J. L., and Brush, M. K.: "An Improved Ketogenic Diet for Treatment of Epilepsy," *J. Am. Diet. Assoc.*, **62**:281–85, 1973.

Problems and Review

1. Describe the development of the nervous system in relation to other factors in growth and development of the young child.
2. What is the principal source of energy for the brain? What proportion of oxygen consumption is required by the brain?
3. Why would you expect vitamin deficiencies to have an adverse effect on the functioning of the nervous system? Describe the changes that take place in deficiency of thiamin; of vitamin B_6.
4. What is the effect of alcoholism on the nutritional state of the individual? How can you explain some of the symptoms characteristic of Wernicke's syndrome?
5. What are some of the meanings of food that may have special relevance to the mentally ill? What recommendations could you make for the feeding of the mentally ill?
6. What is anorexia nervosa? What role does dietary therapy have in treatment?
7. What is epilepsy? What is the rationale for a ketogenic diet for the treatment of epilepsy? Why is the diet seldom used?
8. *Problem.* Modify the diet calculated in Table 39–1 so that it provides a ketogenic-antiketogenic ratio of 3.5 to 1.
9. *Problem.* List some ways in which the whipping cream and butter may be used in the ketogenic diet. What purpose is served by the Cellu wafers?

Cited References

1. Horwitt, M. K.: "Nutrition in Mental Health," *Nutr. Rev.*, **23**:289–91, 1965.
2. Coursin, D. B., *et al.:* "The Relationship of Nutrition to Brain Development and Behavior," *Nutr. Today*, **9**:12–17, July–Aug. 1974.
3. Brozek, J.: "Psychologic Effects of Thiamine Restriction and Deprivation in Normal Young Men," *Am. J. Clin. Nutr.*, **5**:109–18, 1957.
4. Weiner, M. F.: "A Practical Approach to Encouraging Geriatric Patients to Eat," *J. Am. Diet. Assoc.*, **55**:384–86, 1969.
5. Armstrong, R. G.: "Staff-Shared, Family Style Luncheon in a Mental Hospital—Therapeutic Advantages," *J. Am. Diet. Assoc.*, **60**:323–25, 1973.
6. Hussar, A. E., and Sturdevant, J. E.: "An Advisory Committee Considers Dietetic Problems in a Psychiatric Hospital," *J. Am. Diet. Assoc.*, **32**:1188–92, 1956.
7. Halmi, K., *et al.:* "Treatment of Anorexia Nervosa with Behavior Modification," *Arch. Gen. Psychiatry*, **32**:93–96, 1975.
8. Warren, M. P., and Vandewiele, R. L.: "Clinical and Metabolic Features of Anorexia Nervosa," *Am. J. Obstet. Gynecol.*, **117**:435–39, 1973.
9. Review: "The Hematology of Anorexia Nervosa," *Nutr. Rev.*, **31**:207–209, 1973.
10. Maxmen, J. S., *et al.:* "Anorexia Nervosa. Practical Initial Management in a General Hospital," *J.A.M.A.*, **229**:801–803, 1974.
11. Comprehensive Alcohol Abuse and Alcoholism Prevention, Treatment and Rehabilitation Act Amendments, 1973. Hearings before Subcommittee on Alcoholism and Narcotics. 93rd Congress. 1st Session. March 13–16, 1973.
12. "Alcohol: A Growing Danger," *WHO Chronicle*, **29**:102–105, 1975.
13. American Academy of Pediatrics: "Alcohol Consumption: An Adolescent Problem," *Pediatrics*, **55**:557–59, 1975.
14. Myerson, R. M.: "Metabolic Aspects of Alcohol and Their Biological Significance," *Med. Clin. North Am.*, **57**:925–40, 1973.
15. Olson, R. E.: "Nutrition and Alcoholism," in Goodhart, R. S., and Shils, M. E., eds.: *Modern Nutrition in Health and Disease*, 5th ed. Lea & Febiger, Philadelphia, 1973, Chap. 40.
16. Iber, F. L.: "In Alcoholism, the Liver Sets the Pace," *Nutr. Today*, **6**:2–9, Jan. 1971.

17. German, E.: "Medical Problems in Chronic Alcoholic Men," *J. Chronic Dis.*, **26**:661–68, 1973.
18. Flink, E. B.: "Mineral Metabolism," in Kissin, B., and Begleiter, H., eds.: *The Biology of Alcoholism*, Vol. 1. Plenum Press, New York, 1971, Chap. 12.
19. Victor, M.: "Deficiency Diseases of the Nervous System Secondary to Alcoholism," *Postgrad. Med.*, **50**:75–79, Sept. 1971.
20. Hooshmand, H.: "Toxic Effects of Anticonvulsants: General Principles," *Pediatrics*, **53**:551–56, 1974.
21. Mike, E. M.: "Practical Guide and Dietary Management of Children with Seizures Using the Ketogenic Diet," *Am. J. Clin. Nutr.*, **17**:399–405, 1965.
22. Lasser, J. L., and Brush, M. K.: "An Improved Ketogenic Diet for Treatment of Epilepsy," *J. Am. Diet. Assoc.*, **62**:281–85, 1973.
23. Signore, J. M.: "Ketogenic Diet Containing Medium-Chain Triglycerides," *J. Am. Diet. Assoc.*, **62**:285–90, 1973.

ADDITIONAL REFERENCES

Chappelle, M. L.: "The Language of Food," *Am. J. Nurs.*, **72**:1294–95, 1972.
Gabuzda, G. J.: "Nutrition and Liver Disease," *Med. Clin. North Am.*, **54**:1455–72, 1970.
Harkness, L.: "Bringing Epilepsy Out of the Closet," *Am. J. Nurs.*, **74**:875–76, 1974.
Livingston, S.: "Diagnosis and Treatment of Childhood Myoclonic Seizures," *Pediatrics*, **53**:542–48, 1974.
Martin, H. P.: "Nutrition: Its Relationship to Children's Physical, Mental, and Emotional Development," *Am. J. Clin. Nutr.*, **26**:766–75, 1973.
Mueller, J. F.: "Treatment for the Alcoholic: Cursing or Nursing?" *Am. J. Nurs.*, **74**:245–47, 1974.
Nicholson, R. E.: "Of Hooch and Hazards—Alcoholism and Accidents in Industry," *Occup. Health Nurs.*, **22**:10–12, May 1974.
Schmidt, M. P. W., and Duncan, B. A. B.: "Modifying Eating Behaviors in Anorexia Nervosa," *Am. J. Nurs.*, **74**:1646–68, 1974.
Shropshire, R. W.: "The Hidden Faces of Alcoholism," *Geriatrics*, **30**:99–102, Mar. 1975.
Southmayd, E. B.: "The Role of the Dietitian in Team Therapy for Chronic Alcoholism," *J. Am. Diet. Assoc.*, **64**:184–86, 1974.
Stunkard, A.: "New Therapies for the Eating Disorders. Behavior Modification of Obesity and Anorexia Nervosa," *Arch. Gen. Psychiatry*, **26**:391–98, 1972.
Weinberg, J.: "Psychologic Implications of the Nutritional Needs of the Elderly," *J. Am. Diet. Assoc.*, **60**:293–96, 1972.
Wiley, L.: "The Stigma of Epilepsy," *Nursing '74*, **4**:36–45, Jan. 1974.

40 Hyperlipidemia and Atherosclerosis

Fat-Controlled Diets;
Diets for Hyperlipoproteinemia

Cardiovascular disease, a major public health problem. The morbidity and mortality rates from cardiovascular diseases in the United States are among the highest in the world. Each year about a million persons in this country experience a heart attack or sudden death from coronary heart disease. More than 600,000 deaths each year are attributed to coronary heart disease and 200,000 more are due to atherosclerosis of other major vessels. About 165,000 of the coronary deaths occur in persons under 65 years of age. An adult male has about

1 chance in 5 of developing coronary heart disease before age 60, usually in the form of a heart attack. The probability of succumbing to heart disease within five years is 5 times greater in these men than in those with no history of coronary disease. In terms of economic losses, some 4.3 billion dollars were spent in 1967 for direct costs of illness from vascular and related diseases, and another billion dollars in wages were lost due to these diseases.[1]

Coronary heart disease may occur at any age, but it is not common until middle age at which time it assumes practically epidemic proportions. Males over 40 years of age are highly susceptible. Except for those who have hypertension or diabetes mellitus, coronary heart disease is not common in women until after the menopause.

Multiple risk factors in coronary disease. No single factor is an absolute cause either of atherosclerosis or of coronary disease. Many factors are interrelated and to the extent that they are present they increase the risk of disease. Major risk factors are elevated serum cholesterol, hypertension, and cigarette smoking. Presence of one of these factors doubles the risk of coronary disease. If all three are present, the risk of coronary disease is 10 times greater than if none is present. (See Figure 40–1.) Other risk factors include a family history of early heart disease, other lipid abnormalities, glucose intolerance, obesity, certain personality-behavior patterns, lack of physical activity, and stress.[1]

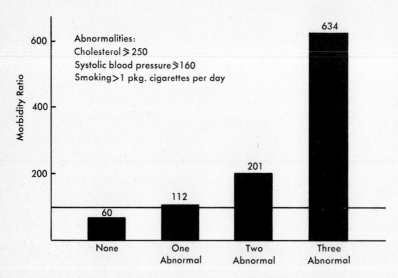

Abnormalities:
Cholesterol ≥ 250
Systolic blood pressure ≥ 160
Smoking > 1 pkg. cigarettes per day

Figure 40–1. The presence of a single risk factor doubles the risk of heart disease. If the three abnormalities listed in this chart are present, the risk is 10 times as high. (Courtesy, The Framingham Heart Study and National Heart and Lung Institute.)

Coronary Disease and the Role of Diet

The discussion in this chapter is concerned with (1) the rationale for dietary modification to reduce the incidence of atherosclerosis and coronary disease, (2) the fat-controlled diet, and (3) diets for five types of hyperlipoproteinemia. The dietary management of acute episodes of illness is discussed in the chapter that follows. The student should review normal fat and carbohydrate metabolism in order to understand the effects of altered physiology and biochemistry in coronary disease. (See Chapters 5 and 6.)

Coronary heart disease. Myocardial ischemia is a cardiac disability resulting from an inadequacy of the coronary arterial system to meet the needs of the heart muscle for oxygen and nutrients. It may be manifested as sudden death, myocardial infarction, or angina pectoris.

An *infarct* is a localized area of necrosis that results when the supply of blood to that area is inadequate for cellular survival. An infarct of the heart is known as myocardial infarction (heart attack), and one in the brain as a cerebrovascular accident (stroke). If the infarct is small, the remainder of the organ can function and healing takes place with the formation of scar tissue. The functional capacity of the organ is curtailed to the extent that tissue has been lost. Thus, repeated myocardial infarctions continue to reduce the functional capacity of the heart.

Angina pectoris refers to the tight, pressing, burning, and sometimes severe pain across the chest that follows exertion and that is a result of inadequate oxygen to the myocardium. As the coronary arteries become increasingly occluded, the pain develops with less and less exertion.

Atherosclerosis. This is a disease of the blood vessels resulting from the interaction of multiple factors such as heredity and the individual's environment (diet, activity, smoking, life style, etc.). Atheromatous plaques begin as soft, mushy accumulations of lipid material in the intima of the blood vessels. These plaques consist of a proliferation of the blood vessel wall of connective tissue into which lipids are deposited. The lipids include free cholesterol, cholesterol esters, and triglycerides in proportions that approximate those of the circulating blood lipids.

Atherosclerosis begins in the first decades of life and is almost universally present in people who live in affluent, highly developed countries. It develops gradually with increasing thickening of the arterial wall, loss of elasticity, and narrowing of the lumen. Finally, some event brings about occlusion of the vessel and ischemia of the affected part. (See Figure 40–2.)

Unquestionably, atherosclerosis sets the stage for coronary heart disease, but many people with atherosclerosis do not develop clinical disease. The conditions that bring about occlusion are not well understood. In some instances ulceration of the atheroma and hemorrhage into the lumen with clot formation occur. The anatomic location of the atheroma, the extent to which the lumen has been narrowed, the changes in the clearing of the blood lipids, and decrease in fibrinolytic activity are probably involved in the process.

Blood studies related to coronary disease. Measurements of various blood constituents can be used not only to determine the presence of abnormal concentrations but also to evaluate the effects of changes in diet and other therapy on the levels of these components. Hyperlipidemia is a general term that denotes an elevation of one or more lipids in the blood. Hypercholesterolemia refers to an elevation of serum cholesterol and hypertriglyceridemia to increased triglycerides. Although the specific levels separating normal from abnormal have not been determined, the National Heart and Lung Institute recommends treatment for all persons under 55 years of age whose serum cholesterol concentration is in excess of 220 mg per cent or whose fasting triglycerides are more than 150 mg per cent.[2] Hyperlipoproteinemia refers to elevation of any one of the classes of lipoproteins (see Chapter 6.) Hypertension, or elevated blood pressure, is generally considered to be present when the systolic pressure is 160 mm Hg or greater and the diastolic pressure is 95 mm Hg. Readings of 140/90 represent borderline hypertension.[3] (See Chapter 41.)

Determination of serum cholesterol is considered by some to be the best single measurement for estimating risk of atherosclerosis.[4] The hypothesis linking elevated serum cholesterol levels to athero-

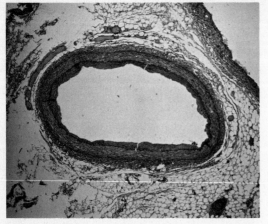

A. Normal artery

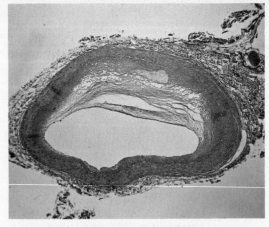

B. Deposits formed in inner lining of artery

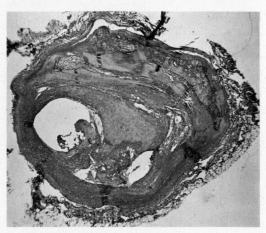

C. Deposits harden

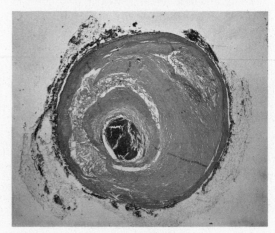

D. Channel is blocked by a blood clot

Figure 40–2. Gradual development of atherosclerosis in a coronary artery, leading to a heart attack. (Courtesy, American Heart Association.)

sclerosis and premature coronary heart disease may be summed up as follows. (1) Elevated serum cholesterol levels are associated with increased risk for coronary disease. This does not mean, however, that all persons with elevated serum cholesterol will develop coronary disease. (2) Serum cholesterol levels can be altered by dietary changes, particularly in cholesterol and fat intake. (3) There is insufficient evidence at present to state unequivocally that serum cholesterol is the direct cause of coronary disease. However, extensive epidemiologic data indicate that habitual consumption of a diet high in cholesterol and saturated fat is a key factor in the etiology.[4] (4) Further data are needed to confirm the assumption that lowering of serum cholesterol levels will reduce the risk of coronary disease.[5,6]

In some individuals hyperlipidemia is induced by carbohydrates, especially sucrose and fructose.[7] Serum triglyceride levels are increased in these persons.

Fredrickson and his associates have described five types of hyperlipoproteinemia.[8] The differentiation is based upon the appearance of the serum, the concentrations of cholesterol and triglyceride, and the classes of lipoproteins that serve as the vehicles for the lipids. The distinctions are important in determining whether the disorders are fat induced or carbohydrate induced so that appropriate diet therapy can be instituted. (See pages 530 to 532.)

Long-term studies on modified diets. Numerous studies have established that serum cholesterol can be lowered by dietary modification. Many investigators have sought to determine whether dietary modification could also lessen morbidity and mortality from coronary disease. In these studies, the ages and health characteristics of the subjects assigned to control and experimental groups were similar. The control groups ate their customary diets while the experimental groups consumed diets in which cholesterol was reduced and polyunsaturated fat was substituted for part of the saturated fats.

Well-known primary prevention studies include the Anti-coronary Club Project in New York,[9] the Los Angeles Veterans Study,[10] and the Helsinki study of patients in two mental hospitals.[11] A Norwegian study aimed at secondary prevention in subjects with established heart disease.[12] In all of these, sustained reduction of serum cholesterol by long-term dietary modification was associated with a decline in morbidity and mortality from coronary disease although the results were not statistically significant in all of the studies.

Dietary adjustments for hyperlipidemias. A joint statement by the Food and Nutrition Board and the Council on Foods and Nutrition has recommended that persons at increased risk because of elevated plasma lipids be given appropriate dietary advice with respect to a nutritionally adequate diet designed to maintain appropriate body weight, with reduction of saturated fat and cholesterol intake, and substitution of polyunsaturated fat for part of the saturated fat in the diet.[13]

Calorie balance. Obesity has long been recognized as one of the risk factors in cardiovascular disease. In the Framingham Heart Study overweight alone constituted only a slight risk; when obesity was associated with increased serum lipid levels, the risk was considerably greater.[14] When overweight is associated with diabetes mellitus, the serum cholesterol and triglyceride levels are customarily high. Reduction in body weight and blood lipids is ac-

complished by lowering calorie intake and substituting polyunsaturated fats for part of the saturated fats in the diet.

Increased body weight probably has its greatest effect by increasing the work load of the heart. A mild stenosis associated with obesity can be critical in a situation of added stress.

Normal weight is maintained only when energy intake and output are equal. Therefore, early in life it is important to develop a program of regular exercise that can be continued throughout the years. (See Chapter 29.)

Fat. Dietary fat is the single most important factor requiring adjustment in programs of prevention and control. (See also Figure 1–4.) The typical American diet furnishes about 40 per cent of the calories from fat. Moreover, the saturated fat in the diet is about four times as high as the polyunsaturated fat.

For the prevention of hyperlipidemia the total fat content should be kept below 40 per cent of the calories; a level of 30 to 35 per cent is preferable. The content of polyunsaturated fat should be increased and that of saturated fat strictly limited. Ratios of polyunsaturated fat to saturated fat (P-S ratio) range from 1 : 1 to 2 : 1.

Cholesterol. The cholesterol content of American diets ranges from 500 to 1000 mg daily, depending largely upon the number of eggs that are consumed. (See Table 6–2.) Increasing the dietary cholesterol from 0 to 400 mg daily without other dietary change results in a progressive increase in the blood cholesterol.[15] Thus, even the addition of one or two eggs a day can in part nullify the effects of a diet high in polyunsaturated fat. Most dietary regimens now restrict the cholesterol intake to 300 mg daily when hypercholesterolemia is present.

Carbohydrate. In the United States a marked decline has taken place in the consumption of breads and cereals, and the use of sugars and sugar-containing foods has increased considerably. Some investigators believe that the increase in sugars in the diet is as important in the elevation of blood lipids as is the increase in saturated fats.[16-18] A high-carbohydrate low-fat diet brings about an elevation in serum triglycerides even in normal individuals, although the effect is a temporary one.

For hyperglyceridemias that are carbohydrate induced the most important adjustment in diet is a reduction of the total carbohydrate and an elimination, insofar as possible, of sugars. This entails not only the elimination of sugar and sugar-containing foods, but control of the amounts of fruits and vegetables that are sources of fructose and sucrose. (See also pages 62 and 459.)

Other dietary factors. The mortality rate from cardiovascular diseases is significantly lower in areas where the drinking water is hard than in those areas where the water is soft. The higher levels of magnesium and calcium in the hard water may have a protective effect.[19,20] Pectins, gums, and hemicellulose as well as plant sterols interfere with the absorption of dietary cholesterol and therefore have a serum-cholesterol-lowering effect.[21] Ascorbic acid is needed for sulfation of intercellular substance in the arterial wall. Accumulation of nonsulfated substance in ascorbate deficiency is associated with increased binding of plasma lipids and fibrinogen in the arterial wall.[22]

FAT-CONTROLLED DIETS

Diet plans. The plans for fat-controlled meals at 1200 and 1800 kcal and for 2000 to 2600 kcal have been presented in two booklets prepared by a committee of dietitians and published by the American Heart Association.[23] The principal characteristics of these diets are summarized below.

1. About 30 to 35 per cent of the calories are supplied by fat.

2. Less than 10 per cent of the calories are furnished by saturated fat. Only skim milk and very lean meats, fish, and poultry may be used. Beef, lamb, and pork are restricted to three 3-ounce portions per week. Butter, cream, and whole-milk cheeses are not used.

3. Up to 10 per cent of the calories are supplied by polyunsaturated fats. The P/S ratio of the diets ranges from 1:1 to 2:1. The polyunsaturated fat content is increased principally by the use of safflower, corn, soy, or cottonseed oils. Limited amounts of special margarines may be included. (See Figure 40–3.)

4. Cholesterol is restricted to 300 mg daily or less. No more than 3 egg yolks per week may be used. Liver is used only as a substitute for egg yolk. Shellfish except shrimp are permitted as a substitute for meat.

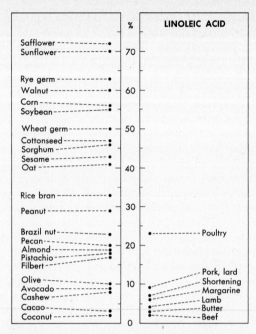

Figure 40–3. Percentage of linoleic acid in fats and oils of plant and animal origin. (Courtesy, Dr. Callie M. Coons and the *Journal of the American Dietetic Association.*)

5. Calorie adjustments may be made in the diet plans by including some sweets and desserts. These lists are not used when the hyperlipidemia is carbohydrate induced.

The dietary plans are adequate for men in all nutritional essentials, but for women the level of iron does not meet the recommended allowances.

Food lists. The food lists for fat-controlled diets are similar but not identical to the food exchange lists used for diabetic and other calculated diets. (See Table A–4.) The composition of food groups for fat-controlled diets is shown in Table 40–1, and the detailed listings of foods appear on page 534.

HYPERLIPOPROTEINEMIA

Types 1 to 5. Some hyperlipoproteinemias are induced by an excess of endogenous or exogenous fat, others by an intolerance to carbohydrates, especially sugars, and still others are influenced by dietary cholesterol.[3] These disorders of lipid metabolism may be hereditary or they may be caused by an intake of an abnormal diet. They are frequently associated with diabetes mellitus. Some types predispose to early atherosclerosis. Xanthomas are frequent, and in types 1 and 5 abdominal pain and acute pancreatitis may occur.

Type 1. An extremely high triglyceride concentration in the serum is characteristic of this type, with the serum cholesterol being normal to high. There is an inability to clear chylomicrons (dietary fat) from the blood, probably as a result of a genetic deficiency of lipoprotein lipase. The condition is rare, usually familial, and seen early in life. It may be associated with diabetes mellitus.

The diet must be very low in fat—25 to 35 gm daily for adults and about 15 gm for children. Cholesterol is not restricted. The carbohydrate is necessarily high in order to supply the needed calories. Alcohol is contraindicated because it increases the serum triglyceride levels when it is metabolized. The elimination of table spreads, cooking fats, and oils results in a dry diet. Medium-chain triglycerides are sometimes prescribed by the physician since they increase the calorie intake and may be used in food preparation. (See page 453.)

Type 2a and 2b. The beta-lipoprotein fraction and the serum cholesterol are increased, with triglycerides being normal in type 2a. This type is a common hereditary disorder, often detectable as early as the first year of life. It may also be associated with an excessive cholesterol intake or with nephrosis, myxedema, or liver disease. Xanthomas and vascular disease are often seen early in adult life. In type 2b cholesterol and triglycerides are both elevated.

Calories are not restricted in type 2a, but weight reduction is often indicated in type 2b. The cholesterol content of the diet is restricted to less than 300 mg daily. Protein is not restricted. Saturated fats are decreased and polyunsaturated fats increased so that a high P/S ratio is achieved. Carbohydrate may be limited in type 2b. Alcohol may be used with discretion.

Type 3. This relatively rare disorder is characterized by an abnormal form of beta-lipoproteins with an elevation of the serum cholesterol and triglycerides. The incidence of vascular diseases is increased. Lesions on the elbows, knees, and buttocks are common.

Overweight is frequent, and a calorie-restricted diet is indicated until the desirable weight is attained. The fat and carbohydrate are each limited to not more than 40 per cent of the calories. Concentrated sweets are eliminated and polyunsaturated fats are substituted for saturated fats. Cholesterol is restricted to 300 mg per day. Alcohol may be substituted for up to two servings bread or cereal.

Type 4. This is a very common pattern characterized by an increase in endogenous triglycerides. The pre-beta-lipoproteins and the triglycerides are elevated, but the serum cholesterol is often normal. Many patients in this group have an abnormal glucose tolerance and some have hyperuricemia. This disorder may be hereditary or associated with diabetes mellitus or another metabolic disorder. Obesity and the complications of atherosclerosis are frequent.

Initially the calories are restricted until desirable weight is achieved. Weight loss alone usually lowers the serum lipids, sometimes to normal. The maintenance diet provides not more than 45 per cent of the calories from carbohydrates and eliminates concentrated sweets. A P/S ratio of about 1 is maintained by substituting polyunsaturated fats for saturated fats. Cholesterol is restricted to 300 to 500 mg daily. Alcohol may be used at the physician's discretion.

Type 5. Chylomicrons and pre-beta-lipoproteins are elevated in this type, indicating intolerance to both endogenous and exogenous sources of fat. As with type 4, glucose tolerance and blood uric acid levels are often abnormal. This disorder is commonly associated with diabetic acidosis, nephrosis, alcoholism, and obesity. The liver and spleen may be enlarged, and abdominal pain is relatively common.

Calorie restriction is emphasized until the desired weight is achieved. The fat in the maintenance diet is kept as low as practical, but not more than 25 to 30 per cent of the calories. The P/S ratio, although not important, is somewhat higher than in typical diets because polyunsaturated fats are substituted for saturated fats. Cholesterol is restricted to 300 to 500 mg daily. The carbohydrate intake is not more than 50 per cent of the calories, thus necessitating a protein intake of 20 to 25 per cent of calories. Concentrated sweets and alcohol are contraindicated.

Dietary plans. A committee of the Heart and Lung Institute, National Institutes of Health, has

Table 40–1. Nutritive Composition of Food Groups for Fat-Controlled Diets*

Food	Measure	Energy kcal	Carbohydrate gm	Protein gm	Total Fat gm	Saturated Fat gm	Linoleic Acid gm	Cholesterol mg
Skim milk	8 ounces	80	12	8	tr	—	—	5†
Vegetables	½ cup	25	5	2	—	—	—	—
Fruit, unsweetened	Varies	40	10	—	—	—	—	—
Breads, cereals	Varies	70	15	2	—	—	—	—
Meat, fish, poultry (lean, weighted average)‡	1 ounce	50	—	8	2	0.6	0.1	21
Beef, lamb, pork, and ham, lean	1 ounce	65	—	9	3	1.3	—	21
Egg	1 whole	80	—	6	6	2.0	0.5	252†
Vegetable oils								
Corn	1 tablespoon	125	—	—	14	1.0	7.0	—
Cottonseed	1 tablespoon	125	—	—	14	4.0	7.0	—
Safflower	1 tablespoon	125	—	—	14	1.0	10.0	—
Soybean	1 tablespoon	125	—	—	14	2.0	7.0	—
Margarine, soft safflower	1 tablespoon	100	—	—	11	1.9	6.3	—
Other soft	1 tablespoon	100	—	—	11	2.5	3.7	—
Sugar	1 tablespoon	50	12	—	—	—	—	—

* Adapted from Zukel, M. C.: "Revising Booklets on Fat-controlled Meals," Tables 5 and 6. *J. Am. Diet. Assoc.*, 54: 23, 1969.

† Cholesterol values from Table A–6.

‡ Weighted average assumes weekly consumption to be: beef, lamb, pork, ham, three servings; poultry, four servings; veal, two servings; fish, five servings.

developed detailed dietary plans for the five types of hyperlipoproteinemia described above. These are available in separate booklets for the patient, including individualized dietary plans for the patient, food lists, guidelines for the purchase and preparation of food, and suggestions for eating out. The daily food allowances for the five diets are summarized in Table 40–2. Although the food lists for these diet plans differ in some details, the lists for the fat-controlled diet (page 534) may be used with complete confidence. The sample menus for diets for type 1, type 2, and type 4 hyperlipoproteinemia are shown in Table 40–3 to illustrate the variations that are applicable for a given menu.

DIETARY COUNSELING

The National Diet Heart Study established that dietary modification for the correction of hyperlipidemia is feasible for people living in a free-living society.[24] The diet is a palatable one that fits into family menus, the foods are selected from ordinary supplies in any food market, the cost is not greater than that of conventional diets, and the program can be followed indefinitely.

Food lists. The food lists must be meticulously followed with respect to the kinds and amounts of food that may be used and also those that must be avoided. Once the patient is familiar with the lists a great deal of flexibility is both possible and desirable. The food habits must be permanently changed and the connotation of a "special" diet should be avoided. Rather, it is a choice of foods for a more healthful way of living. The nurse and dietitian must recognize that even the most conscientious patient will break his diet once in a while, and he should not be made to feel guilty about an occasional indiscretion.

Motivation. Because the serum lipids generally respond within a few weeks following dietary modification, the lowering of lipid levels usually encourages dietary adherence. On the other hand, the patient needs to know that the full benefits of diet on the incidence of clinical disease may not become apparent for up to two or even three years.

Usually the patient who has had a heart attack is more highly motivated to adhere to a modified diet than is the coronary-prone individual. Periodic visits to the physician and the dietitian or nurse are helpful in giving support to the patient as well as in giving greater depth to the level of instruction. (Counseling continued page 536.)

Table 40–2. Food Allowances for Types 1 to 5 Hyperlipoproteinemia

Food	Type 1	Type 2	Type 3	Type 4	Type 5
Skim milk, cups	4	2	2	2	4
Lean meat, poultry, fish, ounces	5	6–9	6	6	6
Egg yolks as substitute for 1 ounce meat	3/week	None	None	3/week	3/week
Bread, cereals	6+	7+	7	8	9
Potato or other starchy vegetable	1+	1+	1	1	1
Vegetables	} 5	} 5	Ad lib.	Ad lib.	Ad lib.
Dark green or yellow, daily					
Fruit, servings			3	3	3
Citrus, daily					
Fat, teaspoons	None	6–9	12	Ad lib.	6
Sugars, sweets	Ad lib.	Ad lib.	None	None	None
Low-fat dessert	Ad lib.	Ad lib.	None	None	None
Alcohol	None	With discretion	Subst.*	Subst.*	None

*In these diets up to two servings of alcoholic beverage may be substituted for 2 slices bread. One slice of bread is equal to 1 ounce gin, rum, vodka, or whiskey; $1\frac{1}{2}$ ounces sweet or dessert wine; $2\frac{1}{2}$ ounces dry wine; or 5 ounces beer.

Food Lists for Fat-Controlled Diets*

Foods to Use

MILK LIST
Skim milk
Nonfat dry milk
Buttermilk

✴ **Foods to Avoid**

Whole milk, homogenized milk, canned milk; sweet cream, powdered cream; ice cream unless homemade with nonfat dry milk; sour cream; whole-milk buttermilk and whole-milk yogurt; cheese made from whole milk

VEGETABLES
See list 2, Table A–4

FRUITS
See list 3, Table A–4

Avocados
Olives

BREADS, CEREALS LIST
Breads: biscuits, cornbread, or muffins (all homemade); bread crumbs, bread sticks, rolls; griddlecakes (made with skim milk and fat from day's allowance), matso, melba toast, popcorn, pretzels, rye wafers; cereals: cooked or dry; barley, buckwheat groats, grits, hominy, rice; macaroni, noodles, spaghetti, cornmeal; flour; dried beans, peas, lentils, chickpeas; corn, kernel or cream style; potato, white or sweet

Commercial biscuits, muffins, cornbreads, waffles, griddle cakes, cookies, crackers; mixes for biscuits, muffins, and cakes; coffee cakes, cakes (except angel food), pies, sweet rolls, doughnuts, and pastries
Potato chips, French-fried potatoes

MEAT, FISH, AND POULTRY LIST
Make selections from this group for 11 of the 14 main meals
  Poultry without skin—chicken, Cornish hens, squab, turkey
  Fish—any kind except shrimp; veal—any lean cut; meat substitutes—cottage cheese (uncreamed), yogurt from partially skimmed milk; dried peas or beans, peanut butter, nuts (especially walnuts)
Make selections from this group for 3 of the 14 main meals
  Beef: hamburger—ground round or chuck; roasts, pot roasts, stew meats—sirloin tip, round, rump, chuck, arm; steaks—flank, sirloin, T bone, porterhouse, tenderloin, round, cube; soup meats—shank or shin; other—dried chipped beef; lamb: roast or steak—leg; chops, loin, rib, shoulder; pork: roast—loin, center cut ham; chops—loin; tenderloin; ham: baked, center cut steaks, picnic, butt, Canadian bacon

Skin of chicken or turkey; duck or goose; fish roe; caviar; fish canned in olive oil; shrimp
Coconut; macadamia nuts

Meats high in fat or marbled: beef, lamb, pork; bacon, salt port, spareribs; frankfurters, sausage, cold cuts; canned meats and meat mixtures: stew, hash; organ meats such as kidney, brain, sweetbread, liver (Note: 2 ounces liver, sweetbreads or heart may be substituted for 1 egg); any visible fat on meat; commercially fried meats, chicken, or fish; frozen or packaged casseroles or dinners

FAT LIST
Oils: corn, cottonseed, sesame, safflower, soybean, sunflower; mayonnaise, French dressing made with allowed oil, special margarine

Butter, ordinary margarines and solid shortenings, lard, salt pork, chicken fat, coconut oil, olive oil, chocolate

SUGARS AND SWEET LIST
Sugar: white, brown or maple; syrup—corn or maple; honey, molasses; jelly, jam, marmalade

* Adapted from food lists and text in *Planning Fat-Controlled Meals for 1200 and 1800 Calories*, revised 1966, and *Planning Fat-Controlled Meals for Approximately 2000–2600 Calories*, revised, 1967, American Heart Association, New York.

DESSERT LIST

Cakes made from allowed fat, skim milk, and eggs: chiffon, quick yellow or white, angel; candies: gum drops, marshmallows, hard fruit drops, mint patties (no chocolate); cookies: sugar; gelatin desserts; fruits, fruit whips; nut meringues; fruit pies; puddings made with fruit and fruit juice or with skim milk: cornstarch, tapioca; sherbet, preferably water ice

Cookies unless made with allowed fat or oil and egg; custards, puddings, and ice creams unless made with skim milk or nonfat dry milk; whipped cream desserts; candies made with butter, chocolate, cream, or coconut

MISCELLANEOUS

Cocoa (not chocolate) made with skim milk

Coffee, coffee substitutes, tea, carbonated beverages, artificial sweeteners, egg white, sugar, lemons and lemon juice, fat-free consommé and bouillon, pickles, relishes, catsup, vinegar, prepared mustard, herbs, spices

Sauces and gravies unless made with allowed fat or oil or made with skim milk; cream soups, creamed dishes unless made with skim milk and allowed oil; foods containing egg yolk except from day's allowance; commercial popcorn; substitutes for coffee cream

Table 40–3. Sample Menus for Three 1800-Kcal Diets*

	Fat-Controlled Diet (Type 2)	Very Low-Fat Diet (Type 1)	Carbohydrate-Restricted Diet (Type 4)
Breakfast			
Orange slices—$\frac{1}{2}$ cup		Same	Same
Whole-wheat cooked cereal—$\frac{1}{2}$ cup		Same	Same
Brown sugar—1 teaspoon		Same	None
Skim milk—1 cup		Same	Same
Homemade muffin—2		Toast—2 slices	Toast—2 slices
Special margarine—2 teaspoons		None; use jelly—2 teaspoons	Margarine—2 teaspoons
Coffee		Same	Same
Sugar for coffee—2 teaspoons		Same	None
Luncheon or Supper			
Broiled chicken—3 ounces brushed with oil—1 teaspoon		Roast chicken—2 ounces; no fat	Broiled chicken—3 ounces; brushed with 1 teaspoon oil
Mashed potato with 1 teaspoon special margarine		Mashed potato; no fat	Mashed potato—with 1 teaspoon margarine
Ripe tomato slices fried in 1 teaspoon oil		Tomato wedges; no fat	Tomato slices fried—1 teaspoon oil
Tossed green salad		Same	Same
French dressing—1 tablespoon		None	French dressing—1 tablespoon
Rye bread—1 slice		Same	Bread—2 slices
Special margarine—1 teaspoon		None; add jelly—1 teaspoon	Margarine—1 teaspoon
Skim milk—1 cup		Same	Same
Baked apple with 1 tablespoon sugar		Same	Fresh apple
Dinner			
Veal—3 ounces, baked in tomato sauce with oil—1 teaspoon		Same	Veal—3 ounces baked in sauce with oil—2 teaspoons
Rice—$\frac{1}{2}$ cup		Same	Same

*See Table 40–2 for food allowances.

Table 40–3. Sample Menus for Three 1800-Kcal Diets (Cont.)

Fat-Controlled Diet (Type 2)	Very-Low Fat Diet (Type 1)	Carbohydrate-Restricted Diet (Type 4)
Asparagus with pimento	Same	Same; add 1 teaspoon oil
Dinner roll	Hard roll	Dinner roll
Special margarine—1 teaspoon	None; use jelly—1 teaspoon	Margarine—2 teaspoons
Skim milk—1 cup	Same	Same
Fresh peach	Jello, ⅔ cup	Fresh peach
Angel cake—small slice	Same	None
Tea or coffee	Same	Same
Snack		
None	Skim milk—1 cup	None
	Fresh peach	
	Bread; jelly—1 teaspoon	

*See Table 40–2 for food allowances.

Some special problems. Some patients find it difficult for one reason or another to restrict beef, lamb, and pork to three meals a week. The market supply of fish and veal in some locations is limited, and some people dislike fish and poultry. When beef, lamb, and pork are used more often, the use of safflower oil in preference to other oils helps to counteract the effect of the higher saturated fatty acid content of these meats. (See Table 40–1.)

Food preparation. More food preparation "from scratch" is a key rule for these modified diets. Frozen dinners, casseroles, baked foods, and cake, bread, and pudding mixes usually contain more saturated fat than is permitted. Although home preparation implies that more time must be spent in the kitchen, the results can be rewarding in terms of creating numerous dishes that are delicious and lower in cost than the convenience foods of comparable quality. The person responsible for food preparation often needs some guidance in adapting recipes to the needs of the diet. Home economists for processors of fats and oils have developed many excellent recipes, and the dietitian or nurse should give the homemaker guidance in using those that are appropriate for the diet prescription. The following guidelines may be helpful:

1. Select only lean cuts of meat. Cut off any visible fat. Use only skim milk. (See Figure 40–4.)

2. Meat, fish, and poultry may be cooked in any way. If calories are restricted, frying should not be used. Part of the daily oil allowance may be used in meat preparation.

3. When including soups or stews prepare them a day before use. Chill them thoroughly and remove the fat when it is hardened.

4. The oil allowance may be used in these ways:

   a. Substitute oil for an equivalent amount of solid fat in recipes for muffins, griddle cakes, waffles, yeast breads. Special recipes are also available for pie crust, cake, and cookies made with oil.

   b. Brush meat, poultry, or fish with oil before broiling. Put drippings as a sauce over the food before serving.

   c. Make cream sauces by using oil instead of solid fat, flour, and skim milk; season with herbs.

   d. Marinate meat, poultry, or fish in a mixture of oil, lemon juice or vinegar, and herb seasonings. Use the marinade for basting meat when broiling.

   e. Cook vegetables in a tightly covered pan, using a minimum amount of water, and adding oil and seasonings for flavor. Remove the vegetables when cooked;

Figure 40–4. These cuts of meat show extremely lean portions and those that are lean with some marbling of fat. Some fat is easily separable from the meat. The individual who requires a fat-controlled diet would use the extremely lean portion of the meat. (Courtesy, National Live Stock and Meat Board.)

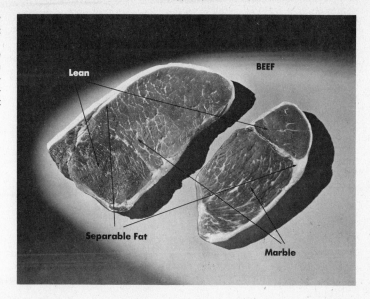

reduce the volume of liquid and pour over the vegetables as a sauce.

f. Oil may be blended with skim milk in a blender and flavored for a beverage. It should be consumed immediately after blending.

5. Special margarines may be substituted for part of the oil allowance.

Eating away from home. Adhering to a fat- or carbohydrate-controlled diet is more difficult in a restaurant, partly because the composition of foods is unknown and partly because the varied menu may be too tempting for the dieter. Nevertheless, an occasional meal away from home should be enjoyed. Those who must eat all their meals in a restaurant will need to determine which ones can best meet their dietary requirements. Some restaurants may be able to give a regular customer some special consideration if his needs are made known. The dieter can safely choose from these foods: fruit, fruit juice, or clear soup; roasted or broiled meat, fish or poultry without gravy; plain vegetables (many restaurants do not add much seasoning); tossed or fruit salad with or without dressing (no cheese dressing); hard rolls; fruit, plain gelatin, or fruit ice. Sauces, cream soups, butter, cream, ice cream, pastries, and puddings should be avoided.

Surgery for coronary artery disease. Surgical intervention is sometimes undertaken when severe atherosclerosis of the coronary arteries produces myocardial ischemia and disabling angina. The occluded vessels are bypassed by constructing new sources of blood supply to the heart by using portions of a vein or artery grafted from elsewhere in the body. In the immediate postoperative period fluids and sodium are restricted to prevent development of pulmonary edema or congestive heart failure (see Chapter 41). Thereafter, restriction of calories and a diet low in saturated fat and cholesterol are usually recommended to prevent recurrence or progression of the coronary artery disease.[25,26]

PROBLEMS AND REVIEW

1. List at least eight factors that have a bearing on the serum cholesterol level.
2. What relationship exists between the amount and nature of the dietary fat and the serum cholesterol level?

3. In what circumstances is a carbohydrate-restricted diet recommended?

4. *Problem.* Plan a normal diet for one day. Calculate the total fat, the saturated fat, and the linoleic acid content. Revise the diet so that the linoleic acid level is two times as high as the saturated fat. What measures can you suggest for making such a change acceptable to the patient?

5. Examine several pieces of advertising for food fats. Evaluate the statements made according to your understanding of the relationship of fat to the change in blood lipid levels.

6. *Problem.* Look up recipes for escalloped potatoes; fish chowder; waffles. How could you adjust these so that they are suitable for a fat-controlled diet?

7. What are some of the problems that the patient might encounter when restricted to a very low-fat diet for type 1 hyperlipoproteinemia?

8. Plan a week's lunches for a patient with type 2a hyperlipoproteinemia who carries his lunch to work.

CITED REFERENCES

1. "Primary Prevention of the Atherosclerotic Diseases," Report of Inter-Society Commission for Heart Disease Resources. *Circulation,* **42:**A55–A95, 1970. Revised 1972.

2. *Dietary Management of Hyperlipoproteinemia.* A Handbook for Physicians and Dietitians. National Heart and Lung Institute, Bethesda, Md., 1973.

3. Kannel, W. B.: "Role of Blood Pressure in Cardiovascular Disease: The Framingham Study," *Angiology,* **26:**1–14, 1975.

4. Stamler, J.: "Diet-Related Risk Factors for Human Atherosclerosis: Hyperlipidemia, Hypertension, Hyperglycemia—Current Status," *Adv. Exp. Med. Biol.,* **60:**125–58, 1975.

5. Podell, R. N.: "Current Status of the Cholesterol Hypothesis," *Am. Fam. Physician,* **9:**145–48, Jan. 1974.

6. Levy, R. I.: "The Meaning of Lipid Profiles," *Postgrad. Med.,* **57:**34–38, Apr. 1975.

7. MacDonald, I.: "Diet and Human Atherosclerosis—Carbohydrates," *Adv. Exp. Med. Biol.,* **60:**57–64, 1975.

8. Fredrickson, D. S., *et al.:* "Fat Transport in Lipoproteins—An Integrated Approach to Mechanisms and Disorders," *N. Engl. J. Med.,* **276:**34–44; 94–103; 148–56; 215–26; 273–81, 1967.

9. Christakis, G., *et al.:* "The Anti-coronary Club. A Dietary Approach to the Prevention of Coronary Heart Disease—A Seven-Year Report," *Am. J. Public Health,* **56:**299–314, 1966.

10. Review: "Los Angeles Veterans Administration Diet Study," *Nutr. Rev.,* **27:**311–16, 1969.

11. Turpeinen, O., *et al.:* "Dietary Prevention of Coronary Heart Disease: Long Term Experiment. I. Observations on Male Subjects," *Am. J. Clin. Nutr.,* **21:**255–76, 1968.

12. Leren, P.: "Effect of Plasma Cholesterol Lowering Diet in Male Survivors of Myocardial Infarction," *Bull. N.Y. Acad. Med.,* **44:**1012–20, 1968.

13. "Diet and Coronary Heart Disease," *J. Am. Diet. Assoc.,* **61:**379–80, 1972.

14. Dawber, T. R., and Kannel, W. B.: "Atherosclerosis and You: Pathogenetic Implications from Epidemiologic Observations," *J. Am. Geriatr. Soc.,* **10:**805–21, 1962.

15. Mattson, F. H., *et al.:* "Effect of Dietary Cholesterol on Serum Cholesterol in Man," *Am. J. Clin. Nutr.,* **25:**589–94, 1972.

16. Yudkin, J.: "Sugar Consumption and Myocardial Infarction," *Lancet,* **1:**296–97, 1971.

17. Albrink, M. J.: "Triglyceridemia," *J. Am. Diet. Assoc.,* **62:**626–30, 1973.

18. Ahrens, R. A.: "Sucrose, Hypertension and Heart Disease: An Historical Perspective," *Am. J. Clin. Nutr.,* **27:**403–22, 1974.

19. Seelig, M. S., and Heggtveit, H. A.: "Magnesium Interrelationships in Ischemic Heart Disease: A Review," *Am. J. Clin. Nutr.,* **27:**59–79, 1974.

20. Shaper, A. G.: "Soft Water, Heart Attacks, and Stroke," *J.A.M.A.,* **230:**130–31, 1974.

21. Hodges, R. E.: "Dietary and Other Factors Which Influence Serum Lipids," *J. Am. Diet. Assoc.,* **52:**198–201, 1968.

22. Krumdieck, C., and Butterworth, C. E.: "Ascorbate-Cholesterol-Lecithin Interactions: Factors of Potential Importance in the Pathogenesis of Atherosclerosis," *Am. J. Clin. Nutr.,* **27:**866–76, 1974.

23. Zukel, M. C.: "Revising Booklets on Fat-Controlled Meals," *J. Am. Diet. Assoc.,* **54:**20–24, 1969.

24. Remmell, P. S., *et al.:* "A Dietary Program to Lower Serum Cholesterol," *J. Am. Diet. Assoc.,* **54:**13–19, 1969.

25. Brener, E. R.: "Surgery for Coronary Artery Disease," *Am. J. Nurs.,* **72:**469–73, 1972.

26. Mundth, E. D., *et al.:* "Surgery in the Treatment of Coronary Artery Disease," *Postgrad. Med.,* **57:**68–72, Apr. 1975.

ADDITIONAL REFERENCES

Alfin-Slater, R. B.: "Fats, Essential Fatty Acids, and Ascorbic Acid," *J. Am. Diet. Assoc.,* **64:**168–70, 1974.

American Heart Association: "The National Diet-Heart Study. Final Report," Monograph No. 18, March, 1968, pp. 1–428.

Anderson, J. T., *et al.:* "Cholesterol-Lowering Diets," *J. Am. Diet. Assoc.,* **62:**133–42, 1973.

Aronow, W. S., *et al.:* "Response of Patients and Physicians to Mass Screening for Coronary Risk Factors," *Circulation,* **52:**586–88, 1975.

"Diet and Coronary Heart Disease," American Heart Association, New York, 1973.

Feeley, R. M., *et al.:* "Cholesterol Content of Foods," *J. Am. Diet. Assoc.,* **61:**134–49, 1972.

Freidman, G. M., *et al.:* "Alternate Approach to Low Fat-Low Saturated Fat-Low Cholesterol Diet," *J. Nutr. Educ.,* **6:**8–10, Jan.–Mar. 1974.

Gotto, A. M., and Scott, L.: "Dietary Aspects of Hyperlipidemia," *J. Am. Diet. Assoc.,* **62:**617–25, 1973.

Gotto, A. M., *et al.:* "Prudent Eating After 40," *Geriatrics,* **29:**109–18, May 1974.

Grande, F., *et al.:* "Sucrose and Various Carbohydrate-Containing Foods and Serum Lipids in Man," *Am. J. Clin. Nutr.,* **27:**1043–51, 1974.

Hodges, R. E.: "Vitamin E and Coronary Heart Disease," *J. Am. Diet. Assoc.,* **62:**638–42, 1973.

Jansen, C., *et al.:* "A Tool for Individualized Management of Fat-Controlled Diets," *J. Am. Diet. Assoc.,* **67:**28–35, 1975.

Marshall, M. W., *et al.:* "Composition of Diets Containing 25 and 35 Per Cent Calories from Fat," *J. Am. Diet. Assoc.,* **66:**470–81, 1975.

Moore, M. C., *et al.:* "Dietary-Atherosclerosis Study on Deceased Persons," *J. Am. Diet. Assoc.,* **67:**22–28, 1975.

Mueller, J. F.: "A Dietary Approach to Coronary Artery Disease," *J. Am. Diet. Assoc.,* **62:**613–16, 1973.

Perry, H. M.: "Minerals in Cardiovascular Disease," *J. Am. Diet. Assoc.,* **62:**631–37, 1973.

Posati, L. P., *et al.:* "Comprehensive Evaluation of Fatty Acids in Foods," *J. Am. Diet. Assoc.,* **66:**482–87, 1975.

Russek, H. I.: "Behavior Patterns, Stress, and Coronary Heart Disease," *Am. Fam. Physician,* **9:**117–22, Apr. 1974.

Shaefer, O.: "The Relative Roles of Diet and Physical Activity on Blood Lipids and Obesity," *Am. Heart J.,* **88:**673–74, 1974.

Sherwin, R.: "The Epidemiology of Atherosclerosis and Coronary Heart Disease," *Postgrad. Med.,* **56:**81–87, Nov. 1974.

Strong, J. P., *et al.:* "Pathology and Epidemiology of Atherosclerosis," *J. Am. Diet Assoc.,* **62:**262–68, 1973.

Wein, E. E., and Wilcox, E. B.: "Serum Cholesterol from Pre-adolescence Through Young Adulthood," *J. Am. Diet. Assoc.,* **61:**155–58, 1972.

INSTRUCTIONAL MATERIALS FOR THE PATIENT

American Heart Association, New York (or local chapters)
  Available Products for the Controlled Fat Diet, (revised), 1970.
  Eat Well But Eat Wisely, leaflet (revised), 1973.
  Heart Attack. How To Reduce Your Risk, 1970.
  The Heart and Blood Vessels, 1973.
  A Maximal Approach to the Dietary Treatment of the Hyperlipidemias. Booklets for Low Cholesterol,

Moderately Low Fat Diets, Low Cholesterol, High Polyunsaturated Fat Diet, and Extremely Low Fat Diet, 1973.

Planning Fat-Controlled Meals for 1200 and 1800 Calories (revised), 1966

Planning Fat-Controlled Meals for Approximately 2000–2600 Calories (revised), 1967.

Programmed Instruction for Fat-Controlled Diet, 1800 Calories, 1969.

Recipes for Fat-Controlled, Low Cholesterol Meals, leaflet, 1968.

Reduce Your Risk of Heart Attack, leaflet (revised), 1969.

The Way to a Man's Heart, 1968.

Blakeslee, A., and Stamler, J.: *Your Heart Has Nine Lives,* condensed ed. Corn Products Co., New York, 1966.

Bond, C-B. Y., *et al.: The Low Fat, Low Cholesterol Diet.* Doubleday & Co., Garden City, N.Y. 1971.

Cavaiani, M.: *The Low-Cholesterol Cookbook.* Henry Regnery Co., Cowles Book Company, Chicago, 1972.

Dietary Management of Hyperlipoproteinemia. Booklets for Type 1, Type 2, Type 3, Type 4, and Type 5. National Heart and Lung Institute, National Institutes of Health, Bethesda, Md., (revised), 1973.

Eshleman, R., and Winston, M.: *The American Heart Association Cookbook.* David McKay Company, Inc., New York, 1973.

Havenstein, N., and Richardson, E.: *The Anti-Coronary Cookbook,* rev. ed. Grosset & Dunlap, New York, 1971.

Jones, J.: *Diet for a Happy Heart.* 101 Productions, San Francisco, Calif., 1975.

Keys, A., and Keys, M.: *Eat Well and Stay Well,* 2nd ed. Doubleday & Co., Garden City, N.Y., 1963.

"Lipid Research Clinics Recipes, Moderately Low in Cholesterol, Fat-Controlled." Lipid Research Clinic, Johns Hopkins Hospital, Baltimore, Md.

125 Favorite Low-Fat, Low-Cholesterol Recipes. Good Housekeeping Institute, New York, 1968.

Payne, A. S., and Callahan, D.: *The Fat and Sodium Control Cookbook,* 4th ed. Little, Brown & Co., Boston, 1975.

Rosenthal, S.: *Live High on Low Fat.* J. B. Lippincott Co., Philadelphia, 1962.

Stead, E. S., and Warren, G. K.: *Low Fat Cookery.* McGraw-Hill Book Co., New York, 1959.

Stone, D. B., *et al.: A Low Cholesterol Diet Manual.* Dept. of Internal Medicine, College of Medicine, The University of Iowa, Iowa City, 1968.

41 Dietary Management of Acute and Chronic Diseases of the Heart

Sodium-Restricted Diet

Clinical findings related to dietary management. Heart disease affects people of all ages, but it is most frequent in those of middle age and is most often caused by atherosclerosis. (See Chapter 40.) Diseases of the heart may affect (1) the pericardium or outer covering of the organ, (2) the endocardium or membranes lining the heart, or (3) the myocardium or the heart muscle. In addition, the blood vessels within the heart or those leaving the heart or the heart valves may be diseased. Heart disease may be acute with no prior warning, as in a coronary occlusion, or chronic with progressively decreasing ability to maintain the circulation.

The heart may be only slightly damaged so that nearly normal circulation is maintained to all parts of the body; this is a period of *compensation.* The patient is able to continue normal activities with perhaps some restriction of vigorous activity. On the other hand, in severe damage, or *decompensation,* the heart is no longer able to maintain the normal circulation to supply nutrients and oxygen to the tissues, or to dispose of carbon dioxide and other wastes. Prompt measures including bed rest, oxygen, and drug therapy are essential to relieve the strain.

Impairment of the heart is manifested by dyspnea on exertion, weakness, and pain in the chest. In severe failure there is a marked dilation of the heart with enlargement of the liver. The circulation to the tissues and through the kidney is so impaired that sodium and water are held in the tissue spaces.

Edema fluid collects first in the extremities and, with increasing failure, in the abdominal and chest cavities. This is referred to as CONGESTIVE HEART FAILURE.

Infections, obesity, hypertension, and constipation complicate and make the treatment of diseases of the heart more difficult. Moreover, the heart is located close to several other organs, especially the stomach and intestines, and distention taking place in either of these organs is likely to press against and interfere with the functioning of the heart. Loss of appetite, nausea, vomiting, and other digestive disorders are common symptoms of heart disease.

Modification of the diet. Objectives in the dietary management of cardiac patients include (1) maximum rest for the heart, (2) prevention or elimination of edema, (3) maintenance of good nutrition, and (4) acceptability of the program by the patient. The following modifications of the diet are necessary to achieve these goals.

Energy. Loss of weight by the obese leads to considerable reduction in the work of the heart because the imbalance between body mass and strength of the heart muscle is corrected. There are a slowing of the heart rate, a drop in blood pressure, and thereby improved cardiac efficiency. Some physicians recommend a mild degree of weight loss even for the cardiac patient of normal weight. Usually a 1000- to 1200-kcal diet is suitable for an obese patient in bed; rarely is it necessary to reduce calories to a level below this.

Those patients whose weight is at a desirable level are permitted a maintenance level of calories during convalescence and their return to activity. Usually 1600 to 2000 kcal will suffice, with slight increases as the activity becomes greater.

Nutritive adequacy. Normal allowances of protein, minerals, and vitamins are recommended. The proportions and kinds of fat and carbohydrate may be modified so that polyunsaturated fatty acids and/or complex carbohydrates predominate (see Chapter 40). When sodium is restricted, other sources of iodine should be prescribed especially for pregnant women and children. A severe restriction of sodium also reduces the intake of vitamin A because carrots and some of the deep-green leafy vegetables that are high in sodium must be omitted.

Sodium. A sodium-restricted diet is indicated when there is retention of fluid and sodium. Usually a restriction of sodium to 500 mg is satisfactory in congestive heart failure, but occasionally sodium needs to be reduced further. Some patients who have associated renal disease are unable to reabsorb sodium in a normal fashion; these "salt wasters" become depleted of sodium on a severely restricted diet.

Once edema has disappeared, a moderately restricted sodium diet—about 1000 mg—is usually satisfactory. Many patients require only a mild restriction of sodium, or none at all.

Fluid. The restriction of fluid is not required so long as the sodium is restricted. Less work is required by the kidney when ample fluid is available for the excretion of wastes. Because of the homeostatic mechanisms afforded by adrenal and pituitary hormones, water is retained only when there is sufficient sodium to maintain physiologic concentrations. (See also page 136.) An intake of 2 liters of fluid daily is usually permitted.

In advanced congestive failure, especially with excessive use of diuretics, water may be retained even though the sodium intake is low. The hormonal controls are no longer balanced, and the sodium concentration of extracellular fluid is low even though the total body content of sodium is high. Such a circumstance necessitates the restriction of fluid as well as sodium.

Amount of food. Small amounts of food given in five or six meals are preferable to bulky, large meals that place an excessive burden upon the heart during digestion. Part of the food normally allowed at mealtime may be saved for between-meal feedings.

Consistency. When decompensation occurs, liquid or soft, easily digested foods that require little chewing should be used. During the early stages of illness, the patient may need to be fed. When his condition improves, he should be given foods that are easy to chew and to digest.

Choice of food. Abdominal distention must be avoided. Until the patient's food tolerances are known, it is best to omit vegetables of the cabbage family, onions, turnips, legumes, and melons. Occasionally a patient may complain that milk is distending to him. Because of its relaxing effect, the physician may prescribe small amounts of alcohol.

Constipation must be avoided by the judicious use of fruits and vegetables, prune juice, and a sufficient fluid intake.

Progression of the diet. During severe decompensation, as in coronary occlusion, rest is the primary consideration, and all attempts to feed the patient are avoided for the first few days. Liquids are then used for two or three days. All liquids are served at room temperature. Extremes of temperature such as very hot or iced beverages are contraindicated because they may induce arrhythmias. Beverages containing caffeine are omitted because of their stimulating effect on the heart rate.[1] When the acute phase has passed, more solid foods are permitted and small feedings of easily digested foods are given as tolerated. The foods may be selected from those permitted for the Soft Diet, page 394, giving only small amounts at each of five or six feedings. During this phase calories are usually limited to 1000 to 1200 daily, and cholesterol and saturated fat are restricted. In the rehabilitative stage, calories are adjusted as needed to bring about weight change if needed. The fat-controlled diet (see Chapter 40) is used with sodium restriction if needed. If decompensation is severe, sodium may be restricted to 500 mg or less daily.

SODIUM-RESTRICTED DIETS

Levels of sodium restriction. Sodium-restricted diets are used for the prevention, control, and elimination of edema in many pathologic conditions, and occasionally for the alleviation of hypertension. Since sodium is the ion of importance, it is incorrect to designate a diet as salt free, salt poor, or low salt. Moreover, to call a diet low sodium or sodium restricted is misleading, since any amount of sodium below the normal sodium intake would satisfy such a description, but would not necessarily be at therapeutic levels. Sodium-restricted diets should be prescribed in terms of milligrams of sodium, e.g., 500-mg-sodium diet.

The normal diet contains about 3 to 6 gm of sodium daily, although a liberal intake of salty food results in considerably higher sodium levels. The normal diet is modified for its sodium content as described in the following paragraphs.

250-mg-sodium diet (11 mEq°; severe sodium restriction). No salt used in cooking; careful selection of foods low in sodium; low-sodium milk substituted

_____
° 1 milliequivalent of sodium is 23 mg; thus, 250 ÷ 23 = 11 mEq.

for regular milk. This diet is used in conditions such as cirrhosis of the liver with ascites; very occasionally in hypertension; for congestive heart failure if the 500-mg level is ineffective.

500-mg-sodium diet (22 mEq; strict sodium restriction). No salt used in cooking; careful selection of foods in measured amounts; regular milk. This level is used for congestive heart failure; occasionally in renal diseases with edema, or cirrhosis with ascites.

1000-mg sodium diet (43 mEq; moderate sodium restriction). No salt in cooking; permits slightly higher protein level if needed, as in pregnancy; may include measured amount of salt, or salted bread and butter.

Mild sodium restriction. Some salt may be used in cooking, but no salty foods are permitted; no salt is used at the table. Sodium content varies from 2000 to 4500 mg. This level is used as a maintenance diet in cardiac and renal diseases.

Sources of sodium. The sodium-restricted diet must be planned with respect to the amount of naturally occurring sodium in foods and the sodium added in food preparation and processing. Sodium values for common foods are given in Table A–2. Most prepared foods show wide variations in sodium content, depending upon conditions of growth and processing of the food, sodium content of water used in preparation, and others.[2] The values listed in any table should not be considered absolute, but they do give reasonable approximations of foods which may be used and which should be avoided.

Naturally occurring sodium in foods. The natural sodium content of animal foods is relatively high and reasonably constant. Thus, meat, poultry, fish, eggs, milk, and cheese are the foods which, although nutritionally essential, must be used in measured amounts. Organ meats contain somewhat more sodium than muscle meats. Shellfish of all kinds are especially high in sodium, but other saltwater fish contain no more sodium than freshwater fish. A few plant foods, especially greens like spinach, chard, and kale, contain significant amounts of sodium and are omitted in the more severely restricted diets.

Fruits, cereals, and most vegetables are insignificant sources of sodium. Likewise, sugars, oils, shortenings, and unsalted butter and margarine are negligible sources of sodium.

The drinking water in many localities contains appreciable quantities of sodium, either naturally or through the use of water softeners. When the sodium content is in excess of 20 mg per liter, the daily intake from water alone may be appreciable.[3]

Sodium added to foods. Table salt is by far the most important source of sodium in the diet. Each gram of salt contains about 400 mg sodium; thus, a teaspoon of salt would furnish 2000 mg sodium. Salt is not only used in cooking and at the table but it also finds its way into many products through manufacturing processes: as in the preservation of ham, bacon, frozen and dried fish; in the brining of pickles, corned beef, and sauerkraut; in koshering of meat; as a rinse to prevent discoloration of fruits in canning; as a means of separating peas and Lima beans for quality before freezing or canning. Canned foods (except fruits), frozen casseroles, dinners, and baked foods, biscuit, bread, cookie, dessert, and sauce mixes contain high levels of salt.

Baking powder and baking soda are widely used in food preparation. Potassium bicarbonate may be used in place of sodium bicarbonate, and sodium-free baking powder may be substituted for regular baking powder.

Numerous sodium compounds other than sodium chloride, baking soda, and baking powder are used in food manufacture: sodium benzoate as a preservative in relishes, sauces, margarine; disodium phosphate to shorten the cooking time of cereals; sodium citrate to enhance the flavor of gelatin desserts and beverages; monosodium glutamate (MSG) as a widely used seasoning in restaurants and in food processing; sodium propionate in cheeses, breads, and cakes to retard mold growth; sodium alginate for smooth texture in chocolate milk and ice cream; and sodium sulfite as a bleach in the preparation of maraschino cherries and to prevent discoloration of dried fruits. (See Figure 41–1.)

Sodium in drugs. Many laxatives, antibiotics,

Figure 41–1. Watch for the words *salt* and *sodium* on labels when selecting foods for sodium-restricted diets. Leavenings and nonfat dry milk also contribute significant amounts of sodium.

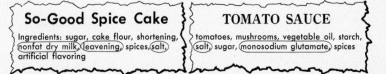

So-Good Spice Cake
Ingredients: sugar, cake flour, shortening, nonfat dry milk, leavening, spices, salt, artificial flavoring

TOMATO SAUCE
tomatoes, mushrooms, vegetable oil, starch, salt, sugar, monosodium glutamate, spices

alkalizers, cough medicines, and sedatives contain sodium, and the physician needs to determine whether the amount of a given drug will nullify the effects of a prescribed diet. Patients need to be especially warned against self-medication with sodium bicarbonate or antacids.

Unit lists for sodium-restricted diets. A joint committee of the American Dietetic Association, the American Heart Association, and the United States Public Health Service has grouped foods for sodium-restricted diets in *Unit Lists.* Each list corresponds closely to the meal exchange lists (Table A–4, Appendix), but foods which are not to be used are also listed. The group C vegetables of the unit lists are those included in the bread exchange lists. In addition, a "Free Choice" list providing 75 kcal per unit permits somewhat more flexibility in menu planning. (See Table 41–1.)

Table 41–1. Nutritive Values of Food Lists for Planning Sodium-Restricted Diets*

List	Amount	Energy kcal	Protein gm	Fat gm	Carbo-hydrate gm	Sodium mg
1. Milk, whole	1 cup, regular	170	8	10	12	120
	1 cup, low sodium	170	8	10	12	7
Milk, nonfat	1 cup, regular	85	8	—	12	120
	1 cup, low sodium	85	8	—	12	7
2. Vegetables						
List 2	½ cup	25	2	—	5	9
Starchy vegetables	Varies with choice	70	2	—	15	5
3. Fruits	Varies with choice	40	—	—	10	2
4. Low-sodium breads, cereals	Varies with choice	70	2	—	15	5
5. Meat, poultry, fish, eggs, or cheese	1 ounce meat or equivalent	75	7	5	—	25
6. Fats	1 teaspoon butter or equivalent	45	—	5	—	tr
7. Free choice	Varies with choice	75	See list; depends on selection made			10

*Arranged from *Your 500 Milligram Sodium Diet,* American Heart Association, New York, 1958.

Food Lists for Sodium-Restricted Diets

See Table A-4, page 660, for food groupings and portion sizes. For each list, note the items below that must be avoided.

Foods Allowed

List 1. Milk
Skim, whole, evaporated, low sodium

List 2. Vegetables
Fresh, frozen, or dietetic canned with no salt or other sodium compounds.

(See list 2, page 662)

Starchy vegetables (see Bread list, page 662)

Foods To Avoid

Commercial foods made with milk—chocolate milk, condensed milk, ice cream, malted milk, milk mixes, milk shakes, sherbet

Canned vegetables or juices except low-sodium dietetic

Artichoke, beet greens, celery, chard (Swiss), dandelion greens, kale, mustard greens, sauerkraut, spinach
Beets, carrots, frozen peas if processed with salt, white turnips
Frozen Lima beans if processed with salt, hominy, potato chips

List 3. Fruits
Fresh, frozen, canned, or dried
(See list 3, page 661)

Crystallized or glazed fruit, maraschino cherries, dried fruit with sodium sulfite added

List 4. Bread
Low-Sodium Breads, Cereals, and Cereal Products
Breads and rolls (yeast) made without salt; quick breads made with sodium-free baking powder or potassium bicarbonate and without salt, or made from low-sodium dietetic mix
Cereals, cooked, unsalted; dry cereals: puffed rice, puffed wheat, shredded wheat
Barley; cornmeal; cornstarch; crackers, low sodium; matzo, plain, unsalted; waffle, yeast

Yeast bread, rolls, or Melba toast made with salt or from commercial mixes; quick breads made with baking powder, baking soda, salt or MSG or made from commercial mixes
Quick-cooking and enriched cereals which contain a sodium compound. Read the label. Dry cereals except as listed
Graham crackers or any other except low-sodium dietetic; salted popcorn; self-rising cornmeal; pretzels; waffles containing salt, baking powder, baking soda, or egg white

List 5. Meat
Meat, Poultry, Fish, Eggs, and Low-Sodium Cheese and Peanut Butter
Meat or poultry: fresh, frozen, or canned low sodium
Liver (only once in 2 weeks)
Tongue, fresh

Fish or fish fillets, fresh only
Bass, bluefish, catfish, cod, eels, flounder, halibut, rockfish, salmon, sole, trout, tuna
Salmon, canned low-sodium dietetic
Tuna, canned low-sodium dietetic

Cheese, cottage, unsalted
Cheese, processed, low-sodium dietetic
Egg (limit, 1 per day)
Peanut butter, low-sodium dietetic

Brains or kidneys
Canned, salted, or smoked meat: bacon, bologna, chipped or corned beef, frankfurters, ham, kosher meats, luncheon meat, salt pork, sausage, smoked tongue, etc.
Frozen fish fillets
Canned, salted, or smoked fish: anchovies, caviar, salted and dried cod, herring, canned salmon (except dietetic low sodium), sardines, canned tuna (except low-sodium dietetic)
Shellfish: clams, crabs, lobsters, oysters, scallops, shrimp, etc.
Cheese, except low-sodium dietetic

Egg substitutes, frozen or powdered
Peanut butter unless low-sodium dietetic

List 6. Fat
Spreads, oils, cooking fats unsalted

Salted butter or margarine, bacon and bacon fat; salt pork; olives; commercial French or other dressing except low sodium; commercial mayonnaise, except low sodium; salted nuts

List 7. Free Choice
Bread list (1 unit)
Candy, homemade, salt free, or special low sodium (75 kcal)
Fat list (2 units)
Fruit list (2 units)
Sugar, white or brown (4 teaspoons)
Syrup, honey, jelly, jam, or marmalade (4 teaspoons)
Vegetable list, group C (1 unit)

Miscellaneous Foods
Beverages
Alcoholic with doctor's permission
Cocoa made with milk from diet
Coffee, instant, freeze dried, or regular; coffee substitutes
Lemonade; Postum; tea
Candy, homemade, salt free, or special low sodium
Gelatin, plain unflavored

Fountain beverages; instant cocoa mixes; prepared beverage mixes, including fruit-flavored powders

Commercial candies, cakes, cookies
Commercial sweetened gelatin desserts
Mixes of all types
Pastries

Leavening agents
Cream of tartar; sodium-free baking powder; potassium bicarbonate; yeast

Regular baking powder; baking soda (sodium bicarbonate)

Rennet dessert powder (not tablets)

Rennet tablets; pudding mixes; molasses

FLAVORING AIDS

		Avoid These Flavoring Aids
Allspice	Onion, fresh, juice or sliced	Barbecue sauce
Almond extract	Orange extract	Bouillon cube, regular
Anise seed	Oregano	Catsup
Basil	Paprika	Celery salt, seed, leaves
Bay leaf	Parsley	Chili sauce
Bouillon cube (low sodium)	Pepper	Cyclamates
Caraway seed	Peppermint extract	Garlic salt
Cardamom	Poppy seed	Horseradish prepared with salt
Chives	Poultry seasoning	Meat extracts, sauces, tenderizers
Cinnamon	Purslane	Monosodium glutamate
Cloves	Rosemary	Mustard, prepared
Cocoa (1–2 teaspoons)	Saccharin	Olives
Cumin	Saffron	Onion salt
Curry	Sage	Pickles
Dill	Salt substitutes (with physician's approval)	Relishes
Fennel		Salt
Garlic	Savory	Soy sauce
Ginger	Sesame seeds	Sugar substitutes containing sodium
Horseradish (prepared without salt)	Sorrel	Worcestershire sauce
Juniper	Sugar	
Lemon juice or extract	Tarragon	
Mace	Thyme	
Maple extract	Turmeric	
Marjoram	Vanilla extract	
Mint	Vinegar	
Mustard, dry	Wine, if allowed by physician	
Nutmeg	Walnut extract	

Meal planning with unit lists. The 500-gm sodium diet at three caloric levels is shown in Table 41–2.

Table 41–2. Food Allowances for 500-Milligram-Sodium Diet*

Food List	1200 Kcal units	1800 Kcal units	Unrestricted Calories units
Milk	2 (skim)	2 (whole)	2 (whole)
Vegetables, List 2	2	2	2 or more
Starchy vegetables	1	1	1 or more
Fruit	4	4	2 or more
Bread	5	7	4 or more
Meat	5	5	5 only
Fat	0	4	as desired
Free choice	1	2	as desired

Sample Menu for 500-mg Sodium Diet

1200 kcal | **1800 kcal**

1200 kcal	1800 kcal
BREAKFAST	
Honeydew melon, ⅛ medium	Same
Shredded wheat, 1 biscuit	Same
Low-sodium corn muffins, 2	Same
Unsalted margarine, 2 teaspoons	Same
Milk, 1 cup skim	1 cup whole
Coffee or tea, no sugar	Same
LUNCHEON OR SUPPER	
Toasted Sandwich:	
Low-sodium bread, 2 slices	Same
Low-sodium tuna fish, 2 ounces	Same
Low-sodium mayonnaise, none; use lemon juice	2 teaspoons
Lettuce	Same
Tomato	Same
Mixed green salad	Same
Low-sodium, low-calorie dressing, 1 tablespoon	Same
Fresh apple, medium	Baked apple with stuffing:
	Raisins, 2 tablespoons
	Brown sugar, 2 teaspoons
Milk, skim, 1 cup	1 cup whole
DINNER	
Broiled pork chop, 3 ounces	Same
Baked potato, small	Same
Baked acorn squash, ½ cup	Same
Low-sodium dinner roll, none	2
Low-sodium margarine, none	2 teaspoons
Fruit cup:	
Fresh pineapple, ½ cup	Same
Fresh strawberries, 1 cup	Same
Coffee or tea, no sugar	Same

Adjustments for sodium level. The 500-mg-sodium diet in Table 41–2 may be adjusted for lower or higher levels of sodium as follows:

250 mg sodium (11 mEq): substitute low-sodium milk for regular milk.

1000 mg sodium (43 mEq): substitute 2 slices ordinary salted bread (contains 400 mg sodium) and 2 teaspoons salted butter or margarine (contains 100 mg sodium) for 2 slices unsalted bread and 2 teaspoons unsalted butter; *or* put ¼ teaspoon salt in a shaker and use at the table.

Mild sodium restriction (2000 to 4500 mg): At 1200 kcal use lightly salted food and allow ordinary salted bread and regular milk. When 1800 kcal or more are allowed, it is possible to keep the sodium level around 2000–2500 kcal only by omitting salt in food preparation *or* by using unsalted bread and butter. Omit salting of food at the table. Omit salty foods such as potato chips, salted popcorn, and nuts, olives, pickles, relishes, meat sauces, smoked and salted meats.

Dangers of sodium restriction. Diets that are very low in sodium must be used with caution since there is occasional danger of depletion of body sodium. Hot weather may bring about great losses of sodium through the skin, and vomiting, diarrhea, surgery, renal damage, or the use of mercurial diuretics also increases the amounts of sodium lost from the body. Sodium depletion is characterized by weakness, abdominal cramps, lethargy, oliguria, azotemia, and disturbances in the acid-base balance. Patients must be instructed to recognize the symptoms of danger and to consult a physician immediately when they occur.

DIETARY COUNSELING

Perhaps no diet provides greater obstacles with respect to acceptance for taste appeal and understanding of the permissible food choices than does the sodium-restricted diet. Skilled counseling of the patient by dietitian, nurse, and physician is essential from the time the diet is first prescribed. Far too many patients have assumed that the omission of salt merely represented poor cookery and have eaten forbidden foods brought in by well-meaning but uninformed relatives and friends. (See Figure 41-2.)

When a sodium-restricted diet is to be continued in the home, the patient should be given some understanding of the purposes of the diet and some indication regarding the length of time he needs to use the diet. He needs information on the foods that are permitted on the diet, what foods are contraindicated, where foods may be purchased, and how to prepare palatable foods with flavoring aids. He should not expect foods to taste the same as those that are salted, but in time most patients learn to adjust to the change in flavors.

The individual responsible for meal preparation must be included in all phases of dietary counseling so that she understands the importance of the diet and learns what modifications in planning, purchasing, and preparation are required.

The American Heart Association has published detailed booklets concerning three levels of sodium restriction and low-calorie and maintenance energy allowances. For patients who find the details confusing, concise leaflets have also been prepared. Neither of these teaching aids should take the place of individualized instruction, nor should the patient be expected to comprehend all the information in one or two counseling sessions.

Cultural patterns must be considered, inasmuch as favorite dishes are often high in sodium. Usually, these dishes may be adapted within the sodium restriction rather than omitting them entirely.

Label information. The patient and the homemaker must be taught to read labels of food products, looking especially for the words *salt* and *sodium*. (See Figure 41-1.) Standards of

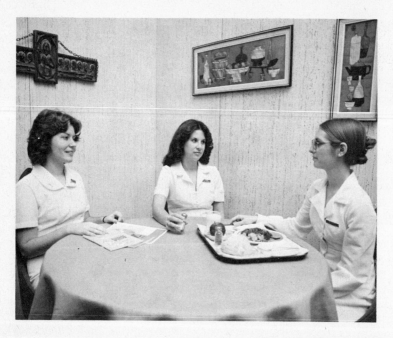

Figure 41–2. Students evaluate appearance and flavor of a sodium-restricted diet. They make comparisons with the essential characteristics outlined in the educational booklet prepared by the American Heart Association. (Courtesy, Department of Human Ecology, Marywood College, Scranton, Pennsylvania.)

identity have been established for many food products by the Food and Drug Administration. Such products do not need to carry a listing of ingredients. Thus, the fact that salt is not listed is no guarantee that it is a low-sodium product. Mayonnaise, catsup, and canned vegetables are examples of foods ordinarily prepared with salt but which belong in the category of foods for which a standard of identity has been set up.

Foods specially produced for sodium-restricted diets must be labeled according to regulations set up by the Food and Drug Administration. The label must indicate the sodium content in an average serving and also in 100 gm of the food. (See Figure 41–3.) Although foods may have been processed without added sodium compounds, some of them may exceed the limits allowed for a given category. For example, a vegetable that contains 50 mg sodium per serving is much higher than the average sodium content of vegetables. (See Table 41–1.)

Preparation of food. Ingenuity is required in the preparation of foods for sodium-restricted diets so that they will be accepted by the patient. A number of salt substitutes are available, but they should be used only upon the recommendation of the physician since some of them contain potassium, which may be contraindicated when there is renal damage.

Numerous flavoring aids are available (see page 546 for list) to provide taste appeal. Herbs and spices are especially useful, but they should be used with a light touch.

Delicious yeast breads, muffins, waffles, and doughnuts may be prepared using part of the milk and egg allowance of the diet. Low-sodium baking powder must be substituted for regular baking powder. When low-sodium milk is required in the diet, recipes may be successfully prepared by substituting low-sodium milk for regular milk. The calcium value of low-sodium milk is about 80 per cent of that of whole milk, the thiamin content is about half as great, and the potassium level is almost twice as high. In other nutrients low-sodium milk compares favorably with whole milk.[4]

The sodium content of kosher meats is too

DIETETIC PEACHES		
Nutritional Information per ½ cup serving		
Calories	40	
Protein	1	gm
Carbohydrate	14	gm
Fat	0	gm
Sodium	3.5	mg
(Less than 2.7 in 100 gm)		

Percentage of U.S. Recommended Daily Allowances (U.S.R.D.A.)	
Protein	*
Vitamin A	4
Vitamin C	2
Thiamin	*
Riboflavin	*
Niacin	4
Calcium	*
Iron	*

*Contains less than 2% of U.S.R.D.A. of these nutrients

Ingredients: Peaches, Pear, Apple, and
Grape Juices from Concentrates

Figure 41–3. Foods intended for use in therapeutic diets must be labeled with information concerning nutritive values. The sodium content per 100 gm and per average serving is included.

high for sodium-restricted diets. Orthodox Jewish patients should salt their meats lightly and allow them to stand for a minimum length of time to draw out the blood. Thoroughly washing with water will remove much of the salt. Then meats are simmered in a large volume of water, and the cooking liquid is discarded. The leaching is more effective if the meat is cut into pieces before cookery.[5]

HYPERTENSION

Hypertension, or elevation of the blood pressure above normal, is a symptom that accompanies many cardiovascular and renal diseases. In the Framingham study, hypertension was found to be the most important of the major risk factors that influence morbidity and mortality from cardiovascular disease. Fully three fourths of those who died of cardiovascular disease had some degree of hypertension.[6]

Hypertension occurs at any age but is found most frequently in persons over 40 years of age. It may be caused temporarily by emotional disturbances or by excessive smoking. Certain kidney disturbances or adrenal tumors are responsible for a small proportion of cases. However, about 85 to 90 per cent of patients belong to the group known as ESSENTIAL HYPERTENSION, for which the cause is unknown. Dahl[7] and others have suggested that a prolonged high salt intake increases the probability of high blood pressure.

Dietary modification. Hypertension is often reduced if weight loss is brought about in the obese patient. Sodium restriction has also been successfully used in lowering blood pressure, but the level of sodium used must be rigidly restricted for long periods of time.[8] Not only is it difficult to counsel patients regarding the rigid restrictions, but most patients find the diet to be monotonous and unpalatable. Today antihypertensive drugs have replaced the severely restricted sodium diets, but mild restriction of sodium is advocated by some clinicians.[9,10]

PROBLEMS AND REVIEW

1. For a patient with congestive heart failure, what are the dietary modifications with respect to calorie level; protein; fluid intake; frequency of feeding; selection of foods?
2. When is a 250-mg-sodium diet likely to be ordered? A 500-mg-sodium diet? A 1000-mg-sodium diet? A mildly-restricted-sodium diet? Outline the important differences in food allowances for each of these levels.
3. *Problem.* Plan a menu for one day that furnishes 500 mg sodium and 1800 kcal.
4. Suppose a 1000-mg-sodium diet has been ordered for a man who is going home. What are some of the questions that you should anticipate during the counseling?
5. Compare the sodium content of 1 slice (25 gm) regular bread and 1 slice low-sodium bread; 2 teaspoons (10 gm) regular butter and 2 teaspoons low-sodium butter; and ½ cup fresh peas and ½ cup canned peas.
6. Examine the labeling on five food products to find examples of different sodium compounds used in processing.
7. *Problem.* A 1000-mg-sodium-restricted diet has been ordered for a 60-year-old man. Neither he nor his wife has had much education and they read with difficulty. Their income is low. What steps would you take to provide guidance for them in the management of the diet at home?
8. *Problem.* Determine the sodium content of the local water supply. If a patient drinks 2 quarts of this water daily, how much sodium will be ingested? If the sodium content of the water is high, what recommendations would you make to a patient?
9. How does low-sodium milk compare with regular milk in nutritive value? Under what circumstances should it be used?
10. What foods may present problems in salt restrictions for the Jewish patient? The Chinese patient? The Puerto Rican? The Italian?

CITED REFERENCES

1. Christakis, G., and Winston, M.: "Nutritional Therapy in Acute Myocardial Infarction," *J. Am. Diet. Assoc.,* **63:**233–38, 1973.
2. Holinger, B. W., *et al.:* "Analyzed Sodium Values in Foods Ready to Serve," *J. Am. Diet. Assoc.,* **48:**501–504, 1966.
3. White, J. M., *et al.:* "Sodium Ion in Drinking Water," *J. Am. Diet. Assoc.,* **50:**32–36, 1967.
4. Council on Foods and Nutrition: "Low-Sodium Milk," *J.A.M.A.,* **163:**739, 1957.
5. Kaufman, M.: "Adapting Therapeutic Diets to Jewish Food Customs," *Am. J. Clin. Nutr.,* **5:**676–81, 1957.

6. Kannel, W. B.: "Role of Blood Pressure in Cardiovascular Disease: The Framingham Study," *Angiology*, **26**:1–14, 1975.
7. Dahl, L. K.: "Salt and Hypertension," *Am. J. Clin. Nutr.*, **25**:23–44, 1972.
8. Kempner, W.: "Treatment of Hypertensive Vascular Disease with Rice Diet," *Arch. Intern. Med.*, **133**:758–90, 1974. (Reprinted from *Am. J. Med.*, **4**:545–77, 1948.)
9. Dustan, H. R.: "Diuretic and Diet Treatment of Hypertension," *Arch. Intern. Med.*, **133**:1007–13, 1974.
10. Munro, A. B., and Woods, J. W.: "Present Day Management of Hypertension," *South. Med. J.*, **67**:847–52, 1974.

ADDITIONAL REFERENCES

Aagaard, G. N.: "Treatment of Hypertension," *Am. J. Nurs.*, **73**:621–23, 1973.

Feldschuh, J., and Yuceoglu, Y. Z.: "Study of Daily Caloric Intake of Patients in the Coronary Intensive Care Unit," *Angiology*, **26**:334–38, 1975.

Freis, E. D.: "Age, Race, Sex and Other Indices of Risk in Hypertension," *Am. J. Med.*, **55**:275–80, 1973.

Gordon, E. S.: "Dietary Problems in Hypertension," *Geriatrics*, **29**:139–41, May 1974.

King, J. F.: "Recent Advances in Therapy for Refractory Congestive Heart Failure," *Geriatrics*, **28**:94–102, Mar. 1973.

Parijs, J., *et al.*: "Moderate Sodium Restriction and Diuretics in the Treatment of Hypertension," *Am. Heart J.*, **85**:22–34, 1973.

Shank, L. F., and Ludewig, J.: "Hypertension," *Nurs. Clin. North Am.*, **9**:677–92, 1974.

Snively, W. D., *et al.*: "Sodium-Restricted Diet: Review and Current Status," *Nurs. Forum*, **13**:59–86, 1974.

Swaye, P. S., *et al.*: "Dietary Salt and Essential Hypertension," *Am. J. Cardiol.*, **29**:33-38, 1972.

INSTRUCTIONAL MATERIALS FOR THE PATIENT

American Heart Association (or local chapters):
    Your Sodium Restricted Diet: 500 mg, 1000 mg, Mild Restriction, 1958.
    Fold-out charts: *Sodium-Restricted Diet, 500 mg*, 1965.
                    Sodium-Restricted Diet, Mild Restriction, 1967.
                    Sodium-Restricted Diet, 1000 mg, 1966.

Payne, A. S., and Callahan, D.: *The Low-Sodium, Fat-Controlled Cookbook*, 4th ed. Little Brown & Co., Boston, 1975.

42 Diet in Diseases of the Kidney

Controlled Protein, Potassium, and Sodium Diet; Calcium- and Phosphorus-Restricted Diet

Renal function and disease. The important function of the kidneys is to maintain the normal composition and volume of the blood. They accomplish this by the excretion of nitrogenous and other metabolic wastes, by regulation of electrolyte and fluid excretion so that water balance is maintained, by making the final adjustment of acid-base balance, and by the synthesis of enzymes and other substances that influence metabolic activities. In view of the central role of the kidneys in maintaining the constant internal environment it is not surprising that renal disease and eventually renal failure affect every system and tissue in the body. A review of the functions of the normal kidney (see pages 132 to 135) is recommended before the student begins the study of dietary management in renal diseases (see Figure 42–1).

Disease may affect the glomeruli, the tubules, or both. NEPHRITIS means literally an inflammation of the nephrons. Although GLOMERULONEPHRITIS indicates that the glomeruli are particularly affected, the functioning of the tubules will also be disturbed. Renal disease may be acute, subacute or latent, or chronic. (See Figure 42–2.) The majority of patients with acute glomerulonephritis recover completely but a small group progress to chronic nephritis. In some patients disease may be in a latent stage for months or even years during which the individual is asymptomatic. Obviously, for each patient a careful evaluation must be made of the etiology, the presenting symptoms, and the level of renal function before any treatment including dietary control can be initiated.

ACUTE GLOMERULONEPHRITIS

Symptoms and clinical findings. Acute glomerulonephritis, also known as *hemorrhagic nephritis,* is primarily confined to the glomeruli. It occurs mostly in children and young adults as a frequent sequel to streptococcic infections such as scarlet fever, tonsillitis, pneumonia, and respiratory infections. In some patients the renal infection is so mild that there is no awareness of the disease until symptoms resulting from permanent damage appear much later. Others notice some swelling of the ankles and puffiness around the eyes and complain of headache, anorexia, nausea, and vomiting. Varying degrees of

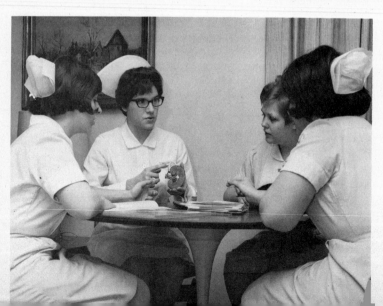

Figure 42–1. An understanding of the structure and function of the normal kidney is an essential foundation for developing the rationale for nutritional care in renal failure. (Courtesy, School of Nursing, Thomas Jefferson University, Philadelphia.)

Figure 42–2. Alternate courses for acute nephritis. (Courtesy, Duncan, G. G., *Diseases of Metabolism.* W. B. Saunders Company, Philadelphia, 1947.)

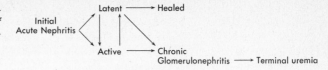

hypertension, dimness of vision, and even convulsions may occur. Usually there is a diminished urinary volume, hematuria, some albuminuria, and some nitrogen retention.

The acute phase of the illness lasts from several days to a week, but renal function returns to normal much more slowly. Full recovery is the rule, provided that treatment is prompt and appropriate. The recovery time varies from two or three weeks to several months, as determined by renal function tests.

Modification of the diet. During the acute phase of illness when nausea and vomiting are present it is unrealistic to provide a diet that fully meets nutritional requirements. An effort should be made to maintain fluid balance and to provide nonprotein calories, either orally or parenterally, to minimize the catabolism of tissue proteins. High-carbohydrate, low-electrolyte supplements,° fruit juices sweetened with glucose, sweetened tea, ginger ale, fruit ices, and hard candy contribute to the carbohydrate intake. Excessive amounts of sweet foods, however, may contribute to the nausea.

As the patient improves and the appetite returns, the following dietary modifications are appropriate:

Energy. The Recommended Dietary Allowances (page 31) provide a general guide to the caloric requirement for persons of various ages and body size. In the absence of fever and at bed rest, these allowances can be reduced somewhat if there is not a previous condition of malnutrition.

Protein. A low-protein diet, not exceeding 40 gm daily, is used initially.[1] The protein allowance for adults may be 0.5 gm per kilogram or less and 0.75 gm per kilogram for children. When there is marked albuminuria, the protein intake should be increased by the amount of protein lost in the urine.

Sodium. If there is edema or hypertension, sodium restriction to 500 or 1000 mg may be prescribed. Others recommend some sodium restriction

for all patients because of the dangers of hypertension, congestive failure, and pulmonary edema.[2]

Fluid. In the presence of oliguria, fluids are restricted to prevent further edema. The volume permitted depends on the previous day's output. Usually 500 to 1000 ml more fluid than the previous day's output is allowed. Larger amounts of fluid are given to replace losses by vomiting, diarrhea, or excessive perspiration.

Selection of foods. The food allowances for 20 gm-, 40 gm-, and 60-gm-protein diets listed in Table 42–2 (page 559) are used as the basis for meal planning. The emphasis is upon protein foods of high biologic value, especially eggs and milk; however, the amounts of each must be carefully controlled. Peas, Lima beans, dried beans and peas, nuts, peanut butter, and gelatin are high in protein of poor biologic value and they should be omitted.

Achieving a satisfactory caloric intake is doubly difficult; the limitations placed upon protein intake necessitate restriction of breads, cereals, potatoes, and similar foods that are good sources of calories, and poor appetite often interferes with food intake. The caloric intake can be increased by using appropriate supplements, low-protein desserts, sugars, jellies, hard candy, butter or margarine, vegetable oils, and carbonated beverages. Cream may be substituted for part of the milk allowance.

When sodium restriction is ordered, the food lists on pages 544 to 546 should be consulted. Regular milk can be used in the amounts listed, but all foods must be prepared without salt or other sodium-containing compounds for any restriction of 1000 mg or less.

CHRONIC GLOMERULONEPHRITIS

Clinical findings. Patients with chronic glomerulonephritis may be asymptomatic for months or even years. The nephritis may be detected only by laboratory studies. As the disease progresses there is gradually increasing involvement: proteinuria, he-

---

° Controlyte® by Doyle Pharmaceutical Co., Minneapolis, Minnesota.

maturia, hypertension, and vascular changes in the retina. The kidneys are unable to concentrate urine and there are both frequent urination and nocturia. Although the specific gravity of the urine is low, the large volume of urine makes possible the excretion of the metabolic wastes. In some patients the nephrotic syndrome (see below) characterized by massive edema and severe proteinuria develops. Hypoproteinemia and anemia are sometimes encountered. Eventually the symptoms of renal failure occur (see below).

Modification of the diet. The objectives of dietary management are (1) to maintain a state of good nutrition; (2) to control or correct protein deficiency; (3) to prevent edema; and (4) to provide palatable, easily digested meals adjusted to the individual patient's needs.

During the period when the kidneys are able to excrete wastes adequately the normal daily allowance of protein plus the amount of protein lost in the urine is allowed. With progression of the disease, elevated blood urea nitrogen levels may necessitate restriction of protein to 40 gm or less daily.

Sufficient carbohydrate and fat should be provided so that the energy needs of the body can be met without the breakdown of body protein. The daily caloric needs for the adult will usually range from 2000 to 3000 kcal.

Sodium restriction to 500 or 1000 mg is indicated only when edema is present. Some clinicians recommend a mild level of sodium restriction (see page 543) even when there is no edema. During the diuretic phase of nephritis increased amounts of sodium may be excreted because of the kidneys' inability to reabsorb the ion. Thus, a markedly restricted sodium diet could lead to body depletion with its attendant weakness, nausea, and symptoms of shock.

Nephrosis

Nephrosis is distinguished clinically from glomerulonephritis by the consistent absence of hypertension and hematuria and the usual absence of anemia and nitrogen retention. Like glomerulonephritis, it is characterized by proteinuria, but to an even more marked degree. The serum proteins are more seriously depleted than in glomerulonephritis, and this characteristic, which often results in massive edema, presents a primary problem in treatment. There is usually no associated cardiovascular disease.

The primary dietary factor requiring consideration is the replacement of protein, since urinary losses may be very large and plasma levels are low. Diets providing 100 gm protein daily are often prescribed. Because of the massive edema sodium is restricted, usually to less than 2 gm per day and even as low as 500 mg per day.

Nephrosclerosis

Nephrosclerosis, or hardening of the renal arteries, occurs in adults after 35 years of age, as a rule, and is associated with arteriosclerosis. The disease may run a benign course for many years. During late stages some albuminuria, nitrogen retention, and retinal changes develop. Death usually results from circulatory failure. In a small number of younger persons nephrosclerosis runs a stormy, rapid course leading to uremia and death. This is called *malignant hypertension.*

Modification of the diet. Weight reduction of the obese is desirable. A 200-mg-sodium diet has been used successfully in some instances. The protein intake is kept at a normal level until marked nitrogen retention indicates that the kidney is no longer able to eliminate wastes satisfactorily. The diet on page 559, Table 42–2, may be used with or without sodium restriction when a lower level of protein becomes necessary.

Renal Failure

Symptoms and biochemical findings. Chronic glomerulonephritis, nephrosclerosis, and chronic pyelonephritis are the principal diseases of the kidney leading to renal failure. This is a condition in which the kidneys are no longer able to maintain the normal composition of the blood. Uremia, a general term applied to the syndrome arising from the failing function of the kidney, refers to the retention of urea and other urinary constituents in the blood. AZOTEMIA, a more specific term, refers to the accumulation of nitrogenous constituents in the blood. OLIGURIA denotes a scanty output of urine (less than 500 ml), and ANURIA is the minimal production or absence of urine (less than 100 ml per day).

Renal failure may be acute or chronic. Acute renal failure occurs in severe acute glomerulonephritis or following inhalation or ingestion of poisons such as carbon tetrachloride or mercury, crushing injuries, or shock from surgery. The mortality rate is nearly 50 per cent. The patient is oliguric or even anuric. Dialysis is often employed until the kidney again resumes its function.

In chronic renal failure symptoms appear when the glomerular filtration rate (GFR) is inadequate to excrete nitrogenous wastes. When the GFR is less than 10 ml per minute (normal 120 ml per minute) and the blood urea nitrogen (BUN) is more than 80 mg per 100 ml (normal 8 to 18 mg per cent), dietary modifications usually bring about improvement in symptoms. Patients in whom the BUN is only mildly elevated usually do not experience symptoms and, therefore, dietary restrictions may not be needed. When the GFR falls to less than 3 ml per minute, dietary control alone is inadequate and dialysis is necessary.

Symptoms involving the gastrointestinal tract are often present in chronic renal failure and are especially trying because of the discomfort associated with them and the constant interference with food intake. The sight or smell of food may bring about nausea or vomiting. The breath has an ammoniacal odor that interferes with the taste of food. Ulcerations of the mouth and hiccups also interfere with food intake.

The nervous system is usually affected. Patients are irritable or drowsy and eventually sink into coma. Headache, dizziness, muscular twitchings, neuritis, and even failing vision occur, especially if there is also hypertension.

The functioning of the heart is seriously disturbed. Congestive failure occurs when the heart failure is associated with retention of sodium and water. Death results when HYPERKALEMIA (elevated serum potassium) blocks the contraction of the heart.

Patients with terminal uremia have a progressively worsening anemia. There is interference with the clotting mechanism, the capillaries are fragile, ulcerations in the gastrointestinal tract may lead to bleeding, the life-span of the red cells is reduced, hemolysis occurs readily, and hematopoiesis is reduced. Because the anemia reduces the effective exchange of oxygen and carbon dioxide at the tissues and in the lungs, fatigue and weakness are ever present.

When the GFR falls to 25 ml per minute, the serum phosphorus level is elevated and hypocalcemia occurs. The disturbed calcium and phosphorus metabolism leads to secondary hyperparathyroidism and RENAL OSTEODYSTROPHY, a term used to encompass osteomalacia, other bone deformities, and deposition of calcium in soft tissues. The kidney is unable to convert 25-hydroxy vitamin D_3 to its active form, 1,25-dihydroxy vitamin D_3, so that calcium absorption from the intestine is decreased.[4] (See Chapter 10 and Figure 10–6.) Excess fluoride may also play a role in the bone demineralization seen in uremia.[5] Glucose intolerance and elevated serum triglycerides are frequent and may increase the risk of premature cardiovascular disease.[6] As the function of the kidneys further deteriorates, hyperkalemia and acidosis become increasingly severe, and edema is marked. Progressive weakness, itching, and jaundice occur. Mental disorientation, severe gastrointestinal symptoms, bleeding, and coma are characteristic of the final stages.

DIALYSIS

In the management of end-stage renal disease, whether acute or chronic, dialysis is often used on a temporary or permanent basis. In *hemodialysis* the patient's blood circulates outside his body through coils or sheets of semipermeable membranes that are constantly bathed by a hypotonic dialyzing fluid so that the nitrogenous wastes are removed into the dialysate. The membranes do not permit bacteria to enter the blood nor can proteins escape from the blood. However, some amino acids are lost into the dialysate.

Although hemodialysis is a lifesaving measure, the patient does not return to a full normal life. He must be attached to a dialyzer for perhaps 24 hours each week. With dialysis for six to eight hours two or three times weekly, blood urea levels that range from 100 to 170 mg per 100 ml fall to 20 to 40 mg per 100 ml.[7] Dialysis does not eliminate the need for dietary control, however. Between dialyses nitrogenous end products, potassium, and sodium accumulate. If the diet is uncontrolled, dialysis will need to be more frequent. Since the artificial kidney does not correct the endocrine failure of the kidneys, most of the patients have severe anemia and hypertensive disease.

Dialysis and the associated diet require a great deal of the patient in terms of emotional stability, motivation, and intelligence. Those who are under 21 years especially resent the program, and those between 21 and 41 years seem to adapt best to the program. If home dialysis is used, the husband or wife, father or mother, or other relative or friend is trained to operate the dialyzer, and must also be able to provide moral support to the patient. Other considerations such as the scarcity of the equipment and the great cost limit the program to only a small number of those who could benefit.

Peritoneal dialysis. This is used when hemodialysis is not available. It consists in introducing 1 to 2 liters of dialysis fluid into the peritoneal cavity and 30 to 90 minutes later withdrawing the fluid. The process is repeated until the blood urea level drops to tolerable levels.

Some blood proteins (10 to 44 gm per dialysis period) as well as amino acids are lost through peritoneal dialysis and compensation must be made for this loss in order to avoid severe hypoproteinemia.

GENERAL DIETARY CONSIDERATIONS IN RENAL FAILURE

Present-day management of the diet in chronic renal disease is based on the principles outlined by Giordano[8] and Giovannetti[9] in the early 1960s. These investigators found that essential amino acid requirements could be met by providing diets containing limited amounts of high-biologic-value protein such as egg and milk. Other protein-containing foods were sharply restricted. Such a diet provides a minimum of nonessential amino acids, thereby enabling the patient to utilize his accumulated urea nitrogen for protein synthesis. Lowering of the blood urea nitrogen level and symptomatic improvement follow. Simultaneous provision of adequate nonprotein calories is essential to enhance protein utilization and to prevent endogenous protein catabolism. Sodium and potassium restriction is also employed.

A number of suitable diets have been developed utilizing the principles described above. In general, all of these aim for provision of adequate calories, regulation of protein, sodium, potassium, and fluid intake, restriction of phosphate, and supplements of calcium, iron, ascorbic acid, and the B vitamins.

Energy. The importance of adequate calories cannot be overemphasized, for without an adequate calorie intake body tissues will be rapidly catabolized, thus increasing the blood urea and potassium levels beyond the capacity of the kidney to excrete them. For adults, caloric needs range from 35 to 45 kcal per kilogram of ideal body weight,[1] or about 2000 to 3000 kcal per day. Carbohydrates are the main source of calories and should be ingested simultaneously with the protein so that the protein will not be utilized for energy. High-carbohydrate supplements that are protein free and low in electrolytes can greatly increase caloric intake if accepted by the patient.° In addition, a high-calorie supplement containing the essential amino acids plus histidine is available.† Many products made from low-protein wheat starch are suitable.‡ (See Figure 42–3.)

Protein. The optimal level of protein intake in advanced renal failure is not known, but is generally considered to be less than 0.5 gm per kilogram of body weight per day for patients who are not being dialyzed regularly. For those on maintenance dialysis the protein allowance is increased to 0.75 to 1.0 gm per kilogram, or about 70 gm per day, to compensate for losses of amino acids in the di-

° Controlyte® by Doyle Pharmaceutical Co., Minneapolis, Minnesota; Cal-Power by General Mills, Inc., Minneapolis, Minnesota; Hycal by Beecham Products, Inc., Clifton, New Jersey.

† Amin-aid by McGaw Laboratories, Santa Ana, California.

‡ Cellu Low Protein Baking Mix by Chicago Dietetic Supply Inc., La Grange, Illinois. Dietetic Paygel Baking Mix by General Mills, Inc., Minneapolis, Minnesota. Aproten Pasta by General Mills, Inc., Minneapolis, Minnesota.

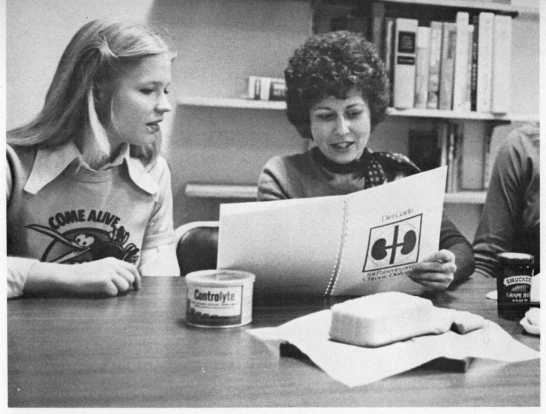

Figure 42–3. Instructor and student evaluate high-calorie, low-protein, low-electrolyte products used in diets for renal failure. (Courtesy, University of Minnesota, Coordinated Undergraduate Program in Dietetics, Minneapolis.)

alysate. Generally, the aim is to provide about three fourths of the protein allowance as high-biologic-value protein. Some recent evidence suggests that histidine may be an essential amino acid in uremia.[10]

Potassium. Excess or deficiency of potassium is detrimental to the patient, but in chronic renal failure hyperkalemia is the rule. Potassium intake is generally restricted to 2000 mg or less, depending somewhat on the protein allowance. Since potassium is so widely distributed in foods, even a level of 2000 mg places severe limitations upon food choices. Foods high in animal protein are usually high in potassium and many fruits and vegetables must be sharply limited or excluded from the diet because of their high potassium content.

Sodium. Sodium restriction is often needed because of edema, hypertension, and threat of congestive heart failure. The allowance may range from 500 to 2000 mg daily. Patients on dialysis are usually permitted intakes of 1500 to 2000 mg daily.

Other minerals. Blood levels of phosphorus gradually increase in the uremic patients, thus contributing to the acidosis and also to metastatic calcification. Aluminum hydroxide gel is often prescribed to bind some of the phosphate in the intestinal tract, thereby reducing the absorption. The diets are low in calcium and a supplement is usually prescribed. Diet alone cannot meet the iron requirements, and a supplement should be prescribed.

Vitamins. Losses of ascorbic acid and many of the B vitamins occur during dialysis. In addition, intake of these vitamins is likely to be low because raw fruits and vegetables are restricted and because foods may be cooked in large volumes of water to reduce the potassium content. Folic acid and pyridoxine requirements may be increased because of antagonistic effects of drug therapy. Impaired vitamin D metabolism occurs because the nonfunctioning kidney cannot convert the vitamin into its active form. Supplements of all of these vitamins are needed.

Fluids. Rigid control of fluid intake is necessary to prevent excess fluid retention between dialyses. The daily allowance is usually less than 1 liter.

CONTROLLED PROTEIN, POTASSIUM, AND SODIUM DIET

Food lists. A number of dietary regimens have been described for the control of protein, potassium, and sodium.[11-14] Each of these is based upon food groupings in which the foods within a given list are of approximately the same protein, potassium, and sodium value. Food choices for daily menus can therefore be made from a given group in the amounts specified. Generally speaking, the broad food groupings used in the various regimens are similar, but they differ in the specific foods included and the portion sizes, depending upon the criteria used in setting them up. For example, oranges are relatively high in potassium and are omitted from some lists; they are included in other lists in controlled amounts because of their popular appeal, their relatively low cost, and their content of ascorbic acid. Potatoes are excluded in some lists but included in others, provided that they are prepared by methods to minimize their potassium content. When the directions for the use of any of these regimens are explicitly followed any one of them will lead to satisfactory results.

Dietitians, nurses, and physicians must be aware of the many factors that modify the sodium and potassium content of foods. Actual diet contents may be higher or lower than published values. The methods of food preparation significantly modify the electrolyte levels. Those factors that enter into the sodium content of foods have been discussed in Chapter 41. With respect to potassium, considerable leaching out occurs when foods are cooked in large volumes of water. The amount lost to the water is greater if food is cut into small pieces.

One dietary regimen for these controlled diets is described in detail in the pages that follow. Table 42–1 lists the composition of the food groups that follow. Table 42–2 indicates the food allowances for four levels of protein. Each of these plans must be individualized according to the patient's caloric requirement, the nutritional status, and the level of biochemical control.

The 20-gm- and 40-gm-protein diets are used only for patients whose renal function has deteriorated so much that they are no longer able to avoid the gastrointestinal and other symptoms of renal failure, and who are not being dialyzed. These diets should be supplemented with B-complex vitamins, calcium, iron, and vitamin D.

DIETARY COUNSELING

Importance of adequate guidance. Dietary treatment in renal failure, with or without dialysis, is an integral part of therapy. Although the dietary modification cannot lead to improvement in kidney function, it can do much toward

Table 42–1. Protein, Sodium, and Potassium Values for Food Lists

Food List	Household Measure	Weight gm	Protein gm	Sodium* mg	Potassium mg
Milk, whole or skim	1 cup	240	8	120	335
Meat or substitute	1 ounce	30	7	25	65–100
Vegetables, Group 1	½ cup	100	1	9	110–190
Group 2	½ cup	100	2	9	160–245
Group 3	½ cup	100	3	9	210
Fruits, Group 1	½ cup	100	tr	2	85–145
Group 2	½ cup	100	1	2	135–200
Bread or substitute	Varies	Varies	2	5	30
Fats	Varies	Varies	—	—	—

*Except for milk, the values listed for sodium are those that apply when no salt is used in processing or preparation of the food. Also, certain high-sodium items in the meat and vegetable lists would be omitted for diets restricted in sodium.

Table 42–2. Food Selection for Controlled Protein, Sodium, and Potassium Diets

Food List	Measure	Protein			
		20 gm	40 gm	60 gm	70 gm
Milk, whole or skim	Cup	¾	1	1	1
Meat or substitute	Ounce	1	3	5	6
Vegetable, Group 1	½ cup	1	3	2	2
Group 2	½ cup	—	—	1	1
Fruit, Group 1	½ cup	2	2	2	2
Group 2	½ cup	—	1	2	2
Bread or substitute	Exchange	2	3	5	6
Low-protein bread	Slice	6	6	—	—
Fat	Exchange	Ad lib	Ad lib	Ad lib	Ad lib
Jelly, sweets	Varies	Ad lib	Ad lib	Ad lib	Ad lib
Low-protein dessert	Varies	Ad lib	Ad lib	Ad lib	Ad lib

alleviation of uncomfortable symptoms that interfere with adequate food intake. The rigid controls required make this diet as complex as any that can be prescribed. Particularly at 20- and 40-gm-protein levels, the diet lacks much in palatability, especially if sodium restriction is also severe, and the level of motivation of the patient and those who care for him must be high.

Many hours of dietary instruction are required for the patient and for those who will prepare the food for him at home. The counseling started in the hospital must be continued either in the out-patient clinic or by home visitation.

What the patient needs to know. Each patient needs to know why the diet is important, and what risks he encounters if he fails to follow the diet. He must understand that it is important to include the exact amounts of high-quality protein foods that have been prescribed. Likewise he needs to know the importance of eating sufficient quantities of low-protein low-electrolyte foods so that body weight is maintained and tissue catabolism does not take place.

High-calorie foods such as sugars, jams, honey, hard candies, butter or margarine, oils, and heavy cream should be used. Patients must be reminded frequently to make liberal use of these items. Growth failure is a common problem in children on dialysis whose calorie intake is inadequate.[15]

There must be a thorough familiarity with the food lists and the amounts of foods that may be used from each. Some practice in planning the daily meals from these lists is essential. If special products such as wheat starch are needed, the patient must be told where he can purchase them, and how much they will cost. Recipes for the use of these special products are needed together with precautions to take in food preparation.

Food preparation. The extraction of gluten from wheat flour yields a low-protein wheat starch that is also practically electrolyte free. Several sources of recipes using wheat starch are listed at the end of this chapter. With sodium and potassium restriction yeast must be used as a leavening agent; regular leavening agents are too high in sodium, and low-sodium leavening agents are too high in potassium. Breads and other products made from wheat starch do not have the same texture as those made from wheat flour because of the absence of the elastic gluten. Some patients find the bread more acceptable when toasted, or served with butter and jelly or jam, or prepared as cinnamon toast or French toast.

If potatoes are allowed they should be cut into small pieces and boiled in a large volume of water. Following this they may be pan fried with some of the fat or mashed with part of the milk and fat allowance. Meats that are simmered in a large volume of water also lose some of their potassium to the cooking liquid. Of course, these cooking procedures also result in greater losses of the water-soluble vitamins and of some other mineral elements.

Canned fruits are used, for the most part, instead of fresh raw fruits. Since part of the potassium has leached out into the syrup, only the solid fruit should be used.

Food Lists for Controlled Protein, Sodium, and Potassium Diets°

Milk List
1 cup equals 8 gm protein, 335 mg potassium

Buttermilk, unsalted
Evaporated milk, reconstituted
Low-sodium milk
Nonfat dry milk, reconstituted
Skim milk
Whole milk

Foods to Avoid
Commercial foods made of milk:
   Chocolate milk
   Condensed milk
   Ice cream
   Malted milk
   Milkshake
   Milk mixes
   Sherbet

Meat or Substitute List
1 ounce cooked equals 7 gm protein, 100 mg potassium

Beef, chicken, duck, lamb, liver, pork, tongue (unsalted), turkey, veal

Foods to Avoid
Brains, kidneys
Canned, salted, or smoked meats as: bacon, bologna, chipped beef, corned beef, frankfurters, ham, kosher meats, luncheon meats, salt pork, sausage, smoked tongue
Frozen fish fillets
Canned, salted, or smoked fish: anchovies, caviar, cod (dried and salted), herring, halibut, sardines, salmon, tuna

Cod, flatfish (flounder and sole), kingfish (whiting), haddock, perch; canned salmon and tuna (omit on sodium-restricted diet)
Clams, crab, lobster, oysters, scallops, shrimp (all omitted on sodium-restricted diet)
Egg (1 egg equals 7 gm protein, 65 mg potassium)
Cheese (1 ounce equals 7 gm protein, 25 mg potassium), Cheddar, cottage, American, Swiss

Omit on sodium-restricted diets

Vegetable List, Group I
1 gm protein, 110 mg potassium per serving

$\frac{1}{2}$ cup servings of raw cabbage, cucumber, lettuce, onion, tomato

1 gm protein, 125 mg potassium per serving

Foods to Avoid
All items marked (+) if diet is sodium restricted
Artichokes
Beans, baked
Beans, dried
Beans, Lima
Beet greens
Broccoli, fresh
Brussels sprouts

°Adapted from *Manual of Diets*, Departments of Dietetics, Hospital of St. Raphael, Veterans Administration Hospital, and Yale–New Haven Medical Center, New Haven, Conn., 1972. Diet revised by M.R.L., 1976.

½ cup servings of canned green or wax beans, carrots (+),
spinach (+); fresh cooked cabbage, eggplant, mustard
greens, onion, summer squash

Carrot, raw
Celery, raw
Chard
Endive, raw
Parsnips
Peas
Potato in skin, or frozen
Sauerkraut
Spinach, fresh or frozen
Squash, baked

The following may be used for diets with liberal potassium allowance:
1 gm protein, 190 mg potassium per serving

½ cup servings of canned beets (+), rutabagas, tomatoes;
fresh cooked carrots (+), turnips (+); frozen summer
squash, winter squash

Vegetable List, Group II
2 gm protein, 160 mg potassium per serving

½ cup servings of canned asparagus; fresh or frozen green
or wax beans, okra

The following may be used for diets with liberal potassium allowance:
2 gm protein, 245 mg potassium per serving

½ cup servings of fresh or frozen cauliflower; cooked
dandelion greens (+); potato, boiled (pared before
cooking), or mashed

Vegetable List, Group III
3 gm protein, 210 mg potassium per serving

½ cup servings of kale (+); frozen asparagus, broccoli,
collards (+), mixed vegetables (+), whole kernel corn

Fruit List, Group I
Less than 0.5 gm protein, 85 mg potassium per serving

Apple, raw   1 small
Grapes, European   12
½ cup servings of canned applesauce, pears, pineapple;
watermelon (diced)
½ cup of these juices: apple, grape, peach nectar, pear
nectar, orange-apricot, pineapple-grapefruit, pineap-
ple-orange

Foods to Avoid
All dried and frozen fruits with sodium sulfite added
Apricots, fresh
Avocado
Bananas
Glazed fruits
Maraschino cherries
Nectarines
Prunes
Raisins

The following may be used for diets with liberal potassium allowance:
Less than 0.5 gm protein, 145 mg potassium per serving

½ cup servings of apricot nectar, pineapple juice; canned
fruit cocktail, peaches, purple plums

Fruit List, Group II
1 gm protein, 135 mg potassium per serving

Pear, raw	1 small
Tangerine	1 small

½ cup servings of fresh or frozen blackberries, blueberries, boysenberries; canned cherries, figs; canned or fresh grapefruit; frozen red raspberries

The following may be used for diets with liberal potassium allowance:
1 gm protein, 200 mg potassium per serving

Orange	1 small
Peach, raw	1 small
Plums, fresh	2 medium
Strawberries, fresh	⅔ cup

½ cup servings of cantaloupe, honeydew, frozen melon balls, fresh or frozen rhubarb

½ cup of these juices: grapefruit, grapefruit-orange, orange, tomato

Avoid tomato juice if diet is sodium restricted

Breads and Substitutes
2 gm protein, 30 mg potassium per serving

Bread	1 slice
Cereals, dry	1 cup
Cornflakes, Puffed Rice, Puffed Wheat, shredded wheat	
Cereals, cooked	½ cup
cornmeal, farina, oatmeal, rice, rolled wheat	
Crackers, soda	3 squares
Flour	2 tablespoons
Grits	1 cup
Macaroni, noodles, or spaghetti	¼ cup
Rice	½ cup

Foods to Avoid

Yeast breads or rolls or melba toast made with salt or from commercial mixes

Quick breads made with baking powder, baking soda, or salt, or made from commercial mixes

Commercial baked products

Dry cereals except as listed

Self-rising cornmeal

Graham or other crackers except low-sodium dietetic

Self-rising flour

Salted popcorn

Potato chips

Pretzels

Waffles containing salt, baking powder, baking soda, or egg white

Fats
Negligible protein and potassium

Butter
Cream, light or heavy (1 ounce contains 35 mg potassium)
Fat or cooking oil
Margarine
Salad dressings: French or mayonnaise

Foods to Avoid

Salted fats on sodium-restricted diets

Avocado

Bacon, bacon fat

Olives

Nuts

Salt pork

Miscellaneous
Cornstarch
Flavoring extracts (see list, page 546)
Ginger ale
Hard candies
Herbs (see list, page 546)
Honey

Foods to Avoid

Antacids, laxatives

Bouillon, broth

Canned, dried, frozen soups

Chocolate

Cocoa, instant cocoa mixes

Jam or jelly
Jellybeans
Rice starch
Spices (see list, page 546)
Sugar, white, confectioners'
Syrup
Tapioca, granulated
Vinegar
Wheat starch

Coconut
Consommé
Fruit-flavored powders and prepared beverage mixes
Fountain beverages
Commercial candies except as listed
Commercial gelatin desserts
Regular baking powder and soda
Rennet tablets
Molasses
Pudding mixes
Peanut butter
Most carbonated beverages

Seasonings to Avoid
Catsup, celery leaves, celery salt, chili sauce, garlic salt,
prepared horseradish, meat extracts, meat sauces, meat
tenderizers, monosodium glutamate, prepared mustard,
onion salt, pickles, relishes, salt, and salt substitutes, soy
sauce, Worcestershire sauce

Diet following renal transplantation. Following successful renal transplantation most of the previous dietary restrictions are no longer needed. Mild sodium restriction (see Chapter 41) is usually necessary because prolonged administration of steroids favors fluid retention. Other side effects of long-term immunosuppressive therapy such as obesity, diabetes mellitus, and atherosclerosis[16] may make further dietary modifications necessary.

HYPOKALEMIA

Occurrence. Although the emphasis in the preceding discussion has been upon the problems of elevated levels of blood potassium, there are renal and extrarenal circumstances in which the plasma or serum level of potassium is below 3.3 mEq per liter. One situation in which this occurs is by dilution of the extracellular fluid volume. This results when the fluid intake exceeds the ability of the kidney to excrete it as in oliguria and anuria. The total amount of the ion in the extracellular fluid remains the same, but the concentration is lowered because of the expanded volume.

In the diuretic stage of nephritis, the kidneys do not conserve potassium as effectively as normal, and potassium depletion occurs, especially if the intake is low because of a poor appetite. Adrenocortical steroids and many diuretics are likely to accentuate the renal losses of potassium.

Hypokalemia also occurs when there is rapid uptake of potassium by the cells. Growth, cellular repair, cellular dehydration, glycogen formation, and administration of glucose and insulin in diabetic acidosis promote entrance of potassium into the cell. In dehydration and in the correction of diabetic acidosis emergency measures are required to replace the extracellular potassium.

Excessive losses of potassium occur with vomiting, diarrhea, and gastrointestinal drainage. Unless these losses are replaced the plasma levels are often lowered to dangerous levels.

Treatment. If hypokalemia is severe, the correction will require the parenteral administration of potassium-containing fluids. This is followed by emphasis on foods that are rich in potassium. When the appetite is good, any varied diet will supply a considerable amount of potassium. A few foods that are especially good sources of potassium include orange juice, tomato juice, milk, baked potato, and banana.

URINARY CALCULI

Nature of calculi. Urinary CALCULI (kidney stones) may be found in the kidney, ureter, bladder, or urethra. They consist of an organic matrix with interspersed crystals and vary in size from fine gravel to large stones.

About 90 per cent of all stones contain calcium as

the chief cation. More than half the stones are mixtures of calcium oxalate and magnesium ammonium phosphate. Uric acid stones occur rarely, and xanthine stones are extremely rare. Cystine stones are unique in that they are often pure and are a hereditary defect.

Incidence and etiology. About 1 person in every 1000 in the United States is admitted to a hospital each year for renal calculi.[17] In the southeastern United States the rate is 2 per 1000 persons, and in Wyoming and Missouri the rate is only one fourth as high.

In Thailand, India, and Turkey (known as stone belts) bladder stones are a common occurrence in children, especially small boys. Most of these are urate and oxalate stones and their cause is unknown. The incidence of bladder stones in adults is high in Syria, Bulgaria, India, China, Madagascar, and Turkey, but low in Africa. The reasons for these geographic variations are not known.

Renal calculi are more prevalent in sedentary people than in those who are active, with administrative workers being 20 times as susceptible as farmworkers.[17] No dietary relationship has been established, but kidney dehydration may be a factor and more fluid intake and exercise are urged as prophylaxis.

The formation of stones is more probable in the presence of urinary tract infections, during periods of high urinary excretion of calcium, and in disorders of cystine or uric acid metabolism. High urinary excretion of calcium occurs in hyperparathyroidism, following overdosage with vitamin D, in long periods of immobilization, in osteoporosis, or following excessive ingestion of calcium and of absorbable alkalies. Even though vitamin A deficiency has been cited as contributing to the formation of calculi, it is not believed to be an important factor in the United States.

Rationale of treatment. When the cause of urinary calculi is known, the physician can effectively direct treatment toward the correction of the disorder. For example, this might entail the treatment of an infection, or modification of the regimen for peptic ulcer, or avoidance of long immobilization. However, in a large percentage of urinary calculi, the cause is not known or the disorder is not easily corrected.

The solubility of salts may be increased and the tendency to stone formation minimized by means of acidifying or alkalinizing agents which increase or decrease the pH of the urine. Such treatment implies that the nature of the stones has been determined by laboratory analyses of the stones themselves or by appropriate urine and blood studies.

A liberal fluid intake is essential—3000 ml or more daily—to prevent the production of a urine at a concentration where the salts precipitate out. The patient should be impressed with the importance of taking fluids throughout the day, so that the urine dilution is maintained.

Binding agents are often used to reduce the absorption of calcium and phosphorus from the gastrointestinal tract. One study has shown that patients who form calcium oxalate stones and their relatives had significantly higher urinary calcium excretion than normal individuals and that this excretion was enhanced following the ingestion of glucose or sucrose.[18] The authors suggest that patients with a history of stone formation might avoid a large intake of carbohydrate-rich foods and beverages especially when the urine is more concentrated.

Modification of the diet. No diet of itself is effective in bringing about solution of stones already formed. However, for the predisposed individual it is thought that diet may be of some value in retarding the growth of stones or preventing their recurrence, although the effectiveness of such prophylaxis has not been fully established.

Calcium and phosphorus restriction. The diet on page 565 is planned to provide maintenance levels of calcium and phosphorus. Such a diet serves as the starting point for the prevention of calcium phosphate stones. Aluminum hydroxide gel is sometimes prescribed since it combines with phosphate to form an insoluble aluminum phosphate and thus diminishes the absorption of phosphorus and the subsequent formation of insoluble precipitates in the urinary tract. Sodium acid phosphate or sodium phytate similarly reduces the absorption of calcium.

Modification of urine pH. When stones are composed of calcium and magnesium phosphates and carbonates, therapy is directed toward maintaining an acid urine. On the other hand, if oxalate and uric acid stones are being formed, the urine should be kept alkaline. Acidifying or alkalinizing agents are more effective than dietary modification, although the diet should support the therapy by medications.

CALCIUM- AND PHOSPHORUS-RESTRICTED DIET*

Characteristics and General Rules

The diet provides maintenance levels of calcium and phosphorus. Milk constitutes the main source of calcium in the diet, and milk, eggs, and meat are the principal sources of phosphorus. (See Table 42–3.) When further restrictions of calcium and phosphorus are desired, the milk and egg may be eliminated. The calcium level is then reduced to 170 mg, the phosphorus level to 740 mg, and the protein level to 64 gm.

Table 42–3. Calcium- and Phosphorus-Restricted Diet

Include These Foods Daily*		Protein gm	Fat gm	Carbo- hydrate gm	Ca mg	P mg
Milk	1½ cups	12	14	18	430	340
Egg	1 whole	7	5	—	25	105
Meat, fish, or poultry	6 ounces	42	30	—	20	375
Vegetables:						
Potato	1 small	2	—	15	15	65
Leafy or yellow	½ cup	2	—	5	25	35
Other	½ cup	2	—	5	25	45
Fruits:						
Citrus	½ cup	—	—	10	30	20
Other	2 servings	—	—	20	25	40
Cereal, refined, without added calcium	2 servings	4	—	30	5	30
Bread, refined, without added calcium	6 slices	12	—	90	20	115
Fats	2 tablespoons	—	30	—	—	—
Sugars, sweets	2 tablespoons	—	—	30	—	—
		83	79	223	620	1170

*Protein, fat, and carbohydrate values on the basis of Meal Exchange Lists, Table A–4. Calcium and phosphorus values have been rounded off to the nearest 5 mg. Values for vegetables, fruits, cereals, and breads are averages of those permitted. Individual selections vary somewhat from these averages.

Foods Allowed

Beverages—milk in allowed amounts; coffee, tea

Breads—French or Italian without added milk; pretzels; saltines, matzoth; water rolls

Cereals—cornflakes, corn grits, farina, rice, rice flakes Puffed Rice; macaroni, noodles, spaghetti; cornmeal, cornstarch, tapioca, white flour

Cheese—½ ounce Cheddar or Swiss cheese may be used instead of ½ cup milk

Desserts—angel cake, white sugar cookies, gelatin, fruit pies, fruit tapioca, fruit whip, pudding with allowed milk and egg, shortbread, water ices

Foods to Avoid

Beverages—chocolate; cocoa; fountain beverages; proprietary beverages containing milk powder

Breads—biscuits; breads: brown, corn, cracked wheat, raisin, rye, white with nonfat dry milk, whole wheat; rye wafers; muffins; pancakes; waffles

Cereals—bran, bran flakes, corn and soy grits, oatmeal, wheat flakes, wheat germ, Puffed Wheat, Shredded Wheat; rye flour, soybean flour, self-rising flour, whole-wheat flour

Desserts—cakes and cake mixes, custard, doughnuts, ice cream, Junket, pies with cream filling or milk and eggs, milk puddings—except when daily allowance is used

* Modification of regimen described by Mary Alice White, unpublished report, Drexel Institute of Technology, 1958.

Eggs—1 whole. Whites as desired

Fats—butter, cooking oils and fats, lard, margarine, French dressing

Fruits—all, but restricting dried fruits to dates (3), prunes (2), raisins (1 tbsp.)

Meats—beef, ham, lamb, pork, veal; chicken, duck, turkey; bluefish, cod, haddock, halibut, scallops, shad, swordfish, tuna

Milk—1½ cups daily

Soups—broth of allowed meats; consommé; cream soups using allowed milk

Sweets—sugar, syrup, jam, jelly, preserves, hard candy, marshmallows, mints without chocolate

Vegetables—artichokes, asparagus, beans—green or wax, Brussels sprouts, cabbage, carrots, cauliflower, corn, cucumber, eggplant, escarole, lettuce, onions, peppers, potatoes—white and sweet, pumpkin, radishes, romaine, squash, tomatoes, turnips

Miscellaneous—pickles, mustard, salt, spices

Fats—mayonnaise, sweet and sour cream

Meats—clams, crab, herring, lobster, mackerel, oyster, fish roe, salmon, sardines, shrimp; brains, heart, kidney, liver, sweetbreads

Soups—cream in excess of milk allowance; bean, lentil, split pea

Sweets—caramels, fudge, milk chocolate, molasses, dark brown sugar

Vegetables—dry beans—kidney, Lima, navy, pea, soybean; beet greens, broccoli, chard, collards, chickpeas, dandelion greens, kale, okra, parsnips, peas—fresh and dried, rutabagas, soybeans, soybean sprouts, spinach, turnip greens, watercress

Miscellaneous—chocolate, cocoa, nuts, olives, brewers' yeast

Sample Menu

BREAKFAST

Fresh raspberries
Cornflakes
Milk—½ cup
Soft-cooked egg
Toasted Italian bread
Butter or margarine
Apple jelly
Coffee

LUNCH OR SUPPER

Cold sliced turkey
Potato salad (potato, diced cucumber, minced green pepper and onion, French dressing) on lettuce; tomato wedges

Italian bread
Butter or margarine
Angel cake with fresh strawberries
Milk—1 cup only

DINNER

Roast pork
Buttered noodles
Zucchini squash
Hard rolls, made without milk
Butter or margarine
Fruit gelatin
Tea with lemon

When an acid-ash diet is prescribed, acid-producing foods (see Table 42–4) are emphasized. Only 1 pint of milk, two servings of fruit, and two servings of vegetables are permitted.

On the other hand, for an alkaline-ash diet fruits and vegetables are used liberally, and the acid-producing foods are restricted to the amounts necessary for satisfactory nutrition.

Oxalate restriction. Some oxalate is produced in the body during the metabolism of foodstuffs. Dietary restriction of oxalates may be tried when calculi contain oxalate, but such restriction has not been shown conclusively to be of value. Oxalate-rich foods include green and wax beans, beets and beet greens, chard, endive, okra, spinach, sweet potatoes; currants, figs, gooseberries, Concord grapes, plums, rhubarb, raspberries; almonds, cashew nuts; chocolate, cocoa, tea.

Reduction of uric acid metabolism. The formation of uric acid stones may be minimized by using a Purine-Restricted Diet (see Chapter 38) and restricting the protein intake to 1 gm per kilogram body weight.

Cystine stones. A protein-restricted diet reduces the intake of sulfur-containing amino acids but has not been shown to be effective in the prevention of cystine stones.

Table 42–4. Acid-Producing, Alkali-Producing, and Neutral Foods

Acid Producing	Alkali Producing	Neutral
Bread, especially whole wheat	Milk	Butter
Cereals	Fruits	Candy, not chocolate
Cheese	Vegetables	Coffee
Corn		Cornstarch
Crackers	*Especially these*	Fats, cooking
Cranberries	Almonds	Honey
Eggs	Apricots, dried	Lard
Lentils	Beans, Lima, navy	Salad oils
Macaroni, spaghetti, noodles	Beet greens	Sugar
Meat, fish, poultry	Chard	Tapioca
Pastries	Dandelion greens	Tea
Peanuts	Dates	
Plums	Figs	
Prunes	Molasses	
Rice	Olives	
Walnuts	Parsnips	
	Peas, dried	
	Raisins	
	Spinach	
	Watercress	
	Foods prepared with baking powder or baking soda	

PROBLEMS AND REVIEW

1. What are the parts of the nephron? How do these parts function?
2. What are the chief wastes excreted by the kidney?
3. In addition to excreting wastes, what other functions are performed by the kidney?
4. What are the characteristic symptoms of acute glomerulonephritis? In what way do these symptoms affect dietary planning?
5. In what way do the abnormal excretion products in renal diseases affect dietary planning?
6. *Problem.* Outline the principles for a dietary regimen for a patient with acute glomerulonephritis, showing the progression of diet from time to time.
7. *Problem.* On the basis of the principles outlined in problem 6, write a menu for a patient for one day. Assume that the diet order restricts protein to 40 gm and sodium to 1000 mg.
8. What reasons can you give for using a protein-free, high-carbohydrate, high-fat diet in acute renal failure? Why are frequent small feedings preferable to three meals?
9. What is accomplished by dialysis with an artificial kidney? Why is a diet restricted in protein and potassium necessary?
10. What problems are you likely to encounter in planning a potassium-restricted diet?
11. *Problem.* Write a menu for one day for a 20-gm controlled protein, sodium, and potassium diet, using the plan in Table 42–2 and the food lists on pages 560 to 563. What foods can you suggest that would increase the caloric intake without increasing the protein and potassium levels?
12. What is meant by hypokalemia? Under what circumstances is it likely to occur? What foods could you suggest for increasing the potassium intake of a patient who has a poor appetite?
13. Why is a calcium-and-phosphorus-restricted diet often prescribed for certain patients with urinary calculi? What is the purpose of using a binding agent with such a diet?
14. Under what circumstances would an acid-ash diet be used? An alkaline-ash diet?

CITED REFERENCES

1. Burton, B. T.: "Current Concepts of Nutrition and Diet in Diseases of the Kidney. II. Dietary Regimen in Specific Kidney Disorders," *J. Am. Diet. Assoc.,* **65:**627–33, 1974.
2. Danowski, T. S.: "Low-Sodium Diets—Physiological Adaptation and Clinical Usefulness," *J.A.M.A.,* **168:**1886–90, 1958.
3. Burton, B. T.: "Current Concepts of Nutrition and Diet in Diseases of the Kidney. I. General Principles of Dietary Management," *J. Am. Diet. Assoc.,* **65:**623–26, 1974.
4. Schoolwerth, A. C., and Engle, J. E.: "Calcium and Phosphorus in Diet Therapy of Uremia," *J. Am. Diet. Assoc.,* **66:**460–64, 1975.
5. Rao, T. K. S., and Friedman, E. A.: "Fluoride and Bone Disease in Uremia," *Kidney Internatl.,* **7:**125–29, 1975.
6. Bagdade, J. D.: "Disorders of Carbohydrate and Lipid Metabolism in Uremia," *Nephron,* **14:**153–62, 1975.
7. Comty, C. M.: "Long Term Dietary Management of Dialysis Patients. I. Pathologic Problems and Dietary Requirements," *J. Am. Diet. Assoc.,* **53:**439–44, 1968.
8. Giordano, C.: "Use of Exogenous and Endogenous Urea for Protein Synthesis in Normal and Uremic Subjects," *J. Lab. Clin. Med.,* **62:**231–46, 1963.
9. Giovannetti, S., and Maggiore, Q.: "A Low Nitrogen Diet with Proteins of High Biological Value for Severe Chronic Uremia," *Lancet,* **1:**1000–1003, 1964.
10. Kopple, J. D., and Swendseid, M. E.: "Nitrogen Balance and Plasma Amino Acid Levels in Uremic Patients Fed an Essential Amino Acid Diet," *Am. J. Clin. Nutr.,* **27:**806–12, 1974.
11. de St. Jeor, S. T., *et al.:* "Planning Low-Protein Diets for Use in Chronic Renal Failure," *J. Am. Diet. Assoc.,* **54:**34–38, 1969.
12. Jordan, W. L., *et al.:* "Basic Pattern for a Controlled Protein, Sodium, and Potassium Diet," *J. Am. Diet. Assoc.,* **50:**137–41, 1967.
13. Bailey, G. L., and Sullivan, N. R.: "Selected-Protein Diet in Terminal Uremia," *J. Am. Diet. Assoc.,* **52:**125–29, 1968.
14. Mitchell, M. C., and Smith, E. J.: "Dietary Care of the Patient with Chronic Oliguria," *Am. J. Clin. Nutr.,* **19:**163–69, 1966.
15. Lewy, J. E., and New, M. I.: "Growth in Children with Renal Failure," *Am. J. Med.,* **58:**65–68, 1975.
16. Tilney, N. L.: "Treatment of Chronic Renal Failure by Transplantation and Dialysis: Two Decades of Cooperation," *Ann. Surg.,* **182:**108–15, 1975.
17. Lonsdale, K.: "Human Stones," *Science,* **159:**1199–1207, 1968.
18. Lemann, J., *et al.:* "Possible Role of Carbohydrate-Induced Calciuria in Calcium Oxalate Kidney-Stone Formation," *N. Engl. J. Med.,* **280:**232–37, 1969.

ADDITIONAL REFERENCES

Anderson, C. F., *et al.:* "Nutritional Therapy for Adults with Renal Disease," *J.A.M.A.,* **223:**68–72, 1973.
Calland, D. H.: "Iatrogenic Problems in End-Stage Renal Failure," *N. Engl. J. Med.,* **287:**334–36, 1972.
Chan, J. C. M., *et al.:* "1-α-Hydroxyvitamin D_3 in Chronic Renal Failure," *J.A.M.A.,* **234:**47–52, 1975.
Dyck, P. J., *et al.:* "Uremic Neuropathy. III. Controlled Study of Restricted Protein and Fluid Diet and Infrequent Hemodialysis versus Conventional Hemodialysis Treatment," *Mayo Clin. Proc.,* **50:**641–49, 1975.
Fiaschi, E., *et al.:* "Calcium and Phosphorus Metabolism in Chronic Uremia," *Nephron,* **14:**163–80, 1975.
Giovannetti, S., and Berlyne, G. M.: "An Outline of the Uremic Syndrome," *Nephron,* **14:**119–22, 1975.
Llach, F., *et al.:* "Dietary Management of Patients in Chronic Renal Failure," *Nephron,* **14:**401–12, 1975.
Loggie, J. M. H., *et al.:* "Renal Function and Diuretic Therapy in Infants and Children," Part 1. *J. Pediatr.,* **86:**485–96, 1975.

McCosh, E. J., *et al.:* "Hypertriglyceridemia in Patients with Chronic Renal Insufficiency," *Am. J. Clin. Nutr.,* **28:**1036–43, 1975.

Merrill, J. P., and Hampers, C. L.: "Uremia," *N. Engl. J. Med.,* **282:**953–61; 1014–21, 1970.

St. Jeor, S. T.: "First Annual Meeting of Council on Renal Nutrition," *J. Am. Diet. Assoc.,* **67:**135–36, 1975.

Stone, W. J., *et al.:* "Vitamin B_6 Deficiency in Uremia," *Am. J. Clin. Nutr.,* **28:**950–57, 1975.

Tsaltas, T. T.: "Dietetic Management of Uremic Patients. I. Extraction of Potassium from Foods for Uremic Patients," *Am. J. Clin. Nutr.,* **22:**490–93, 1969.

INSTRUCTIONAL MATERIALS FOR THE PATIENT

Cost, J. S.: *Dietary Management of Renal Disease.* Charles B. Slack, Inc., Thorofare, N.J., 1975.

de St. Jeor, S. T., *et al.: Low Protein Diets for the Treatment of Chronic Renal Failure.* University of Utah Press, Salt Lake City, 1970.

Diet Guide for Patients on Chronic Dialysis. National Institutes of Arthritis, Metabolism, and Digestive Diseases, Bethesda, Md., 1975.

Margie, J. D., *et al.: The Mayo Clinic Renal Diet Cookbook.* Golden Press, New York, 1975. (Distributed by the National Kidney Foundation.)

More Good Things Made with Dietetic Paygel-P Wheat Starch. Nutrition Services, General Mills, Inc., Minneapolis.

Recipes for Protein-Restricted Diets. The Doyle Pharmaceutical Company, Minneapolis.

Renal Failure Diet Manual. University of Alabama Hospitals and Clinics. Available from University of Alabama Book Store, Birmingham.

43 Anemias

Blood is a constantly changing, highly complex tissue which is concerned with the transport of cell nutrients, the elimination of wastes, and the maintenance of chemical equilibrium. Its intricate function and composition suggest the need for a considerable variety of nutrients, and these have been discussed especially in Part One. This chapter is concerned with some of the more common deficiencies that arise in the framework of the red blood cells and in the hemoglobin within these cells.

Synthesis of erythrocytes and hemoglobin. The red blood cells are synthesized in the bone marrow and proceed through a number of stages before they are released into the circulation as nonnucleated fully mature cells. For their synthesis many nutrients are required, including the amino acids. Vitamin B_{12} and folinic acid are required for the synthesis of DNA, which is essential for the growth and normal division of cells. When either or both of these vitamins are deficient, fewer cells can be produced, and they are released into the circulation as large, nucleated cells called megaloblasts. (See also Chapter 12, pages 185 and 188.)

Hemoglobin synthesis requires a constant source of iron for the formation of heme and of protein for the formation of globin. The rate of synthesis can be no more rapid than the supply of iron. The iron is made available to the erythroid marrow by the plasma, which in turn is supplied by the reserves held in the liver and by the absorption from the intestinal tract. (See page 112 for discussion of iron metabolism.)

The normal red cell count is about 5 million per cubic millimeter for males and 4.5 million for females. Normal hemoglobin levels for males range from 14 to 17 gm per 100 ml, and from 12 to 15 gm per 100 ml for females. The normal packed-cell volume (hematocrit) is about 45 per cent; for men the lower limit of normal is 42 per cent, for women, 36 per cent, and for pregnant women, 33 per cent.[1]

Anemia. ANEMIA is a condition in which there is a reduction in the total circulating hemoglobin. Anemias may be described biochemically in terms of lowered hemoglobin levels, number of red blood cells, and hematocrit. They are also differentiated on the basis of appearance of red cells: normocytic, macrocytic, or microcytic; nucleated or nonnucleated; normochromic, hyperchromic, or hypochromic. Other diagnostic aids include measurements of plasma iron levels, iron-binding capacity, and transferrin saturation.

Etiology. Anemias may be caused by several factors:

1. Blood loss.
2. Decreased production of blood. Failure to provide essential nutrients due to inadequate intake or defective utilization may lead to anemias. The anemias of nutritional origin may be microcytic or macrocytic, depending on the specific nutrient lacking. Exposure to x-ray or radium, bone tumors, cirrhosis of the liver, carcinoma, and leukemias are examples of conditions that may interfere with red cell formation within the bone marrow.
3. Increased destruction of blood. This may be the result of the action of intestinal parasites, hemolytic bacteria, chemical agents such as coal tar products and sulfonamide compounds, or abnormal red cell structure (sickle cells).

A number of drugs may interfere with vitamin B_{12} absorption and lead to anemia. Decreased serum vitamin B_{12} levels have been observed in women taking oral contraceptives although the significance of this is not yet known.[2] Impaired metabolism of folate polyglutamate has also been noted in some of these women. The mechanism involved is not clear, but is believed by some to occur only in women who have an underlying defect in absorption or whose diet is marginal in folate.[2,3]

Chronic diseases such as severe infections, malignancies, uremia, rheumatoid arthritis, liver disease, myxedema, and malabsorptive states following ileal resection or bypass are also associated with anemias.

Symptoms. Mild anemias diagnosed by laboratory studies are not closely associated with clinical symptoms or with changes in cardiorespiratory functions.[4] When anemias become more severe, however, the symptoms are more consistent and include skin pallor, weakness, easy fatigability, headaches, dizziness, sensitivity to cold, and paresthesia. Cheilosis, glossitis, loss of appetite, and loss of gastrointestinal tone with accompanying symptoms of distress are seen in severe anemias. Concave "spoon" fingernails (koilonychia) with longitudinal ridging of the nails is sometimes present. With increasing severity of anemia, the oxygenation of tissues is reduced—hence the feeling of fatigue. The heart rate increases, palpitation occurs, and there is shortness of breath.

Treatment. The treatment of anemias is dependent upon determination of the cause and eliminating it whenever possible. Nutritionally, specific supplements may be required to improve the formation of red cells and hemoglobin. A normal diet to restore good nutrition is usually emphasized to support the specific therapy.

IRON-DEFICIENCY ANEMIA

Incidence. Iron-deficiency anemias are widely prevalent throughout the world. Incidence in the various countries ranges from about 5 to 15 per cent in males, 10 to 50 per cent in women, and 15 to 92 per cent in children.[5] This type accounts for 30 per cent of the anemias in the United States.[6] Data from both the Ten-State Nutrition Survey and the Health and Nutrition Examination Survey (HANES) indicated widespread iron deficiency based on dietary intakes and biochemical data.[7,8] Generally, the incidence is high in preschool children, adolescents, and women in the childbearing years, and is higher among blacks and Spanish Americans than white individuals. It occurs more frequently among persons of low economic status, although it is by no means limited to this group. (See Figure 43–1.)

Iron deficiency follows a specific sequence.[9] First, the iron reserves drop to lower levels, the transferrin level of the blood increases slightly, and the hema-

tocrit and plasma iron levels remain normal. Then the iron reserves are used up, the transferrin level increases further, the hematocrit and plasma iron are reduced, and fewer red blood cells are produced. Finally, with no remaining iron reserves, the hematocrit and plasma iron continue to fall, and the cells are pale and reduced in size. Thus, the designation for the anemia is microcytic, hypochromic.

Etiology. Among the factors to be considered as initiating iron-deficiency anemia are these:

1. Blood loss (most common cause in adults)
   a. Accidental hemorrhage
   b. Chronic diseases, such as tuberculosis, ulcers or intestinal disorders, when accompanied by hemorrhage
   c. Excessive menstrual losses
   d. Excessive blood donation
   e. Parasites such as hookworm
2. Deficiency of iron in the diet during period of accelerated demand
   a. Infancy—rapidly expanding blood volume
   b. Adolescence—rapid growth, and onset of menses in girls
   c. Pregnancy and lactation
3. Inadequate absorption of iron
   a. Diarrhea, as in sprue, pellagra
   b. Lack of acid secretion by the stomach
4. Nutrition deficiencies such as severe protein depletion
   a. Protein-calorie malnutrition

Blood loss. Whenever hypochromic anemia occurs in adult males or in women past the menopause, blood loss, as from a bleeding ulcer or other cause, must always be suspected. Menstrual losses by some women may be sufficiently great to result in anemia, especially if the diet is poorly selected. Losses of iron in menses average about 0.5 mg per day, or about 15 mg per month.[1] The repeated donation of blood likewise could be a significant factor in anemia causation unless a liberal diet relatively rich in protein and iron is taken.

Whenever there is a loss of blood, fluid is quickly drawn in from the tissues to maintain the blood volume. The hemoglobin level and red cells are thus reduced in concentration, but the individual with adequate stores quickly replenishes the levels so

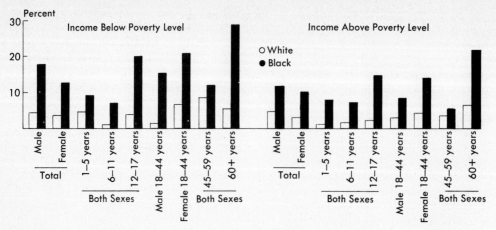

Figure 43–1. Percentage of persons with low hemoglobin values by age, sex, and race for income levels, United States, 1971–1972. (From Abraham, S., *et al.: Preliminary Findings of the First Health and Nutrition Examination Survey, United States, 1971–72: Dietary Intake and Biochemical Findings.* Pub. [HRA] 74-1219-1. U.S. Department of Health, Education and Welfare, Health Services Administration, Rockville, Md., 1974.)

that anemia is not evident unless hemorrhage is prolonged or repeated. From three weeks to three months may be required to replenish the losses from the donation of 1 pint of blood.

Infants and preschool children. The full-term infant born of a well-nourished mother has a sufficient hemoglobin supply for the first two or three months of life, after which iron-rich foods should be added to the milk diet. Many babies, however, are not born with this endowment of hemoglobin. Infants of low birth weight, those who are multiple births, and those whose mothers have had several previous pregnancies are least likely to have adequate reserves.

Iron-fortified cereals should be given to the infant as early as six weeks of life. When they are discontinued after six months of age, the foods substituted are likely to supply too little iron and thus an anemia follows. Many infants from low socioeconomic groups are anemic because mothers are unaware of the importance of using iron-fortified cereals or because they cannot afford to purchase them. Many pediatricians recommend that an iron-fortified formula be continued throughout the first year.

A cause of anemia in certain infants has been gastrointestinal bleeding resulting from the inges-

tion of homogenized milk. Heat-labile proteins in milk are believed to be responsible inasmuch as heat-processed cow's milk formulas do not produce the blood loss.[10]

Anemia in adolescent girls and women. Because of the lower calorie requirements of women the iron intake is likely to be no more than 10 to 12 mg per day, even though the other aspects of the diet may be fully adequate. With absorption at 5 to 10 per cent, these intakes are not adequate to cover fully the losses entailed by menstruation and to build up reserves. Adolescent girls, in addition, must have iron to meet their growth requirements; yet, during these years their diets are often of generally poor quality.

Pregnancy imposes substantial additional demands upon the iron supply. The woman who has had repeated pregnancies and the young girl who is still maturing are most likely to become anemic and to bear infants who have little or no reserves.

Treatment. For iron-deficiency anemia the primary emphasis in treatment is a supplement of iron salts such as ferrous sulfate, gluconate, or fumarate. Oral therapy is as effective as parenteral therapy except where there is severe interference with absorption as in ulcerative colitis or regional enteritis. Some individuals have an initial intolerance to iron salts, but usually become adjusted to the medication. It is helpful to take the salts after meals.

DIETARY COUNSELING

Although the specific therapy for iron-deficiency anemia is iron medication, the patient needs guidance in the selection of an adequate diet. The diet history will establish the previous pattern of food intake and will indicate the corrections that are to be recommended. Frequently, the choice of foods has been poor with respect to sources of iron. With special emphasis on the inclusion of liver every week, if possible, and on the liberal use of dried fruits, dark-green leafy vegetables, and enriched breads and cereals, the daily iron intake for women will be approximately 12 to 15 mg. Some animal foods at each meal help to improve the absorption of iron from the plant sources as well. Ascorbic-acid-rich juices also improve iron absorption and should be used generously. For many women, the importance of continuing to use a prophylactic supplement even after the anemia has been corrected may need to be emphasized.

In moderately severe anemias the regeneration of hemoglobin is improved if protein intakes are increased to 80 to 100 gm daily. The diets of many women and girls are low in protein, and suggestions for increasing the protein content of the diet should be given. When cost is an important factor, simple recipes for dishes that use non-fat dry milk, poultry, fish, and less expensive cuts of meat are useful if food is prepared in the home.

VITAMIN B_{12} DEFICIENCY

Pernicious anemia. This is caused by a lack of intrinsic factor in the gastric juice, and therefore vitamin B_{12} cannot be absorbed. With the absence of vitamin B_{12} the synthesis and maturation of the red blood cells are arrested. The anemia occurs chiefly in middle-aged to elderly persons and may be a genetic defect. Pernicious anemia also occurs following surgical removal of the portion of the stomach that produces the intrinsic factor, or the terminal ileum where absorption of vitamin B_{12} takes place. These effects of surgery do not become evident until three to five years postoperatively, depending upon the reserves of vitamin B_{12} ordinarily held in the body. The prolonged use of a strict vegetarian diet (vegan) has led to vitamin B_{12} deficiency anemia in a few cases. (See Chapter 15.)

In pernicious anemia the red cell count is often less than 2.5 million per cubic millimeter, with a large proportion of these cells being macrocytic. Patients have a lemon-yellow pallor, anorexia, glossitis, achlorhydria, abdominal discomfort, frequent diarrhea, weight loss, and general weakness. Numbness of the limbs, coldness of the extremities, and difficulty in walking are manifestations of neurologic changes in the untreated patient.

Treatment. Until Minot and Murphy introduced liver therapy in 1926, pernicious anemia was invariably fatal.[11] Their use of large amounts of liver started the search for the factor that was responsible for improvement. Liver extract replaced the liver diet and was in turn superseded by vitamin B_{12}.

When given parenterally, vitamin B_{12} produces marked hematopoietic response in dosages as small as 1 mcg daily. The vitamin is ineffective when given orally because of the absence of intrinsic factor.

Although folic acid brings about correction of the hematologic picture in pernicious anemia, it has no effect on the associated neurologic symptoms. Folic acid should never be used in place of vitamin B_{12} for the treatment of these patients, lest the neurologic symptoms become progressively worse. Because of this danger, multivitamin preparations may not contain more than 0.1 mg folic acid in a daily dosage.

DIETARY COUNSELING FOR PERNICIOUS ANEMIA

Poor appetite, sore mouth, and gastrointestinal discomfort seriously interfere with an adequate food intake so that patients often present a picture of general nutritional deficiency. Their diets must be corrected for adequate calories and for protein. Because of the achlorhydria in pernicious anemia the rate of digestion is retarded. Hence, the fat content of the diet should be kept to moderate levels, restricting especially fried foods that may further delay gastric emptying.

A soft, or even liquid, diet is preferable until the glossitis disappears. Tart and spicy foods should especially be avoided. (See Soft Diet, page 394, and Full-Fluid Diet, page 396.) Supplementation with ascorbic acid is essential if citrus fruits and other rich sources of the vitamin are not ingested. One practical way to supplement the usual diet is to use high-protein high-calorie beverages two or three times daily. They may be prepared from milk, nonfat dry milk, and flavorings, or one of several relatively inexpensive proprietary preparations may be used.

FOLIC ACID DEFICIENCY

A deficiency of folic acid leads to arrest of the synthesis and maturation of the red blood cells thus leading to megaloblastic anemia. Although the blood picture from folic acid lack resembles that occurring with vitamin B_{12} deficiency, it must be emphasized that one vitamin does not replace the other but that they are interrelated in function. Folic acid deficiency is observed in a variety of circumstances.

1. Elderly patients. A high incidence of folic acid deficiency has been noted in elderly patients, correlated with a poor intake of milk, fresh fruits, and vegetables.[12] The dietary fault results from lack of knowledge concerning the needs for foods in later life, insufficient income to purchase the essential foods, and organic diseases that interfere with food intake and further aggravate the deficiency. Malignancies, malabsorption, loss of blood, and certain drug therapies also reduce the serum folate levels. Additional folate therapy is recommended especially during acute stages of illness, but the blood levels of vitamin B_{12} should also be monitored.

2. Pregnancy. Megaloblastic anemia occurs with lesser frequency than iron-deficiency anemia. It is usually caused by inadequate diet and is corrected by folic acid therapy.

3. Infancy. Macrocytic anemia in babies is more frequent in those born to mothers who also have a folic acid deficiency. Anemia is present in infants who have scurvy, because lack of ascorbic acid reduces the conversion of folic acid to its active form folinic acid.

4. Disorders of absorption. Macrocytic anemia, often severe in tropical sprue, improves dramatically with folic acid therapy. Some improvement is often seen in the anemia of nontropical sprue and celiac disease with folic acid therapy. (See Chapter 34.)

SICKLE CELL ANEMIA

This is a hemolytic anemia of genetic origin occurring primarily in blacks. An abnormal hemoglobin causes the red cells to assume a crescent or sickle shape when deoxygenated. The distorted shape of the red cells prevents their passage through capillaries and leads to thrombosis and infarction. The sickle cells have a shortened life-span, and the individual becomes anemic because the red cells are destroyed more quickly than they can be replaced. In the United States, about 1 in 10 blacks are heterozygotes (carry one defective gene) for the sickle cell trait; these individuals usually do not have clinical manifestations.

In persons with the disease, symptoms usually develop after the age of one year and include decreased appetite, fatigue, pallor, bone pain, and so on. In older patients degenerative changes are seen in the retina, lungs, heart, kidneys, liver and spleen, bone, brain, and other tissues. Serious crises occur in young children following even minor infections; the frequency and severity of these crises decrease as the child grows older.

Dietary considerations. Children with sickle cell disease are frequently shorter in stature and weigh less than normal. Although nutritional requirements are the same as for any growing child, careful attention should be given to providing adequate calories and protein. Intakes of iron and folic acid may be less than desirable. The parents should be encouraged to have available foods enjoyed by the child which are good sources of these nutrients. Liquids may be preferred during crises. Recommendations made for older children and adults should include those considerations indicated in the sections on dietary counseling in iron and folic acid deficiencies.

Problems and Review

1. What nutrients are essential for the production of hemoglobin and red blood cells?
2. What are some of the etiologic agents that cause anemia? Which anemias originate because of a faulty diet? Which anemias may be classed as secondary nutritional deficiencies?
3. What are the laboratory findings and clinical symptoms of iron-deficiency anemia? Which groups are especially vulnerable?
4. What factors may interfere with the efficient use of iron in the body? Why is a so-called "high-iron" diet impractical in the treatment of iron-deficiency anemia?
5. What iron preparations are commonly provided for patients with iron-deficiency anemia? What dietary modification may be indicated?
6. List important steps that can be taken to prevent iron-deficiency anemia; folic-acid-deficiency anemia.
7. Why is vitamin B_{12} given parenterally to patients with pernicious anemia?
8. What problems may be encountered in the dietary intake by patients with pernicious anemia? How can these be controlled?
9. *Problem.* Plan a diet for a young woman who has iron-deficiency anemia to include 80 gm protein, 15 mg iron, and not more than 2000 kcal.

Cited References

1. Committee on Iron Deficiency, Council on Foods and Nutrition: "Iron Deficiency in the United States," *J.A.M.A.*, **203:**407–14, 1968.
2. Stebbins, R., *et al.:* "Drug-Induced Megaloblastic Anemias," *Semin. Hematol.,* **10:**235–51, 1973.
3. Shojania, A. M., and Hornady, G. J.: "Oral Contraceptives and Folate Absorption," *J. Lab. Clin. Med.,* **82:**869–75, 1973.
4. Elwood, P. C.: "Evaluation of the Clinical Importance of Anemia," *Am. J. Clin. Nutr.,* **26:**958–64, 1973.
5. FAO/WHO Expert Group: *Requirements of Ascorbic Acid, Vitamin D, Vitamin B_{12}, Folate and Iron. WHO Tech. Rep. Series* No. 452, Geneva, 1970.
6. Brunning, R. D.: "Differential Diagnosis of Anemia," *Geriatrics,* **29:**52–60, Feb. 1974.
7. "Highlights from the Ten-State Nutrition Survey," *Nutr. Today,* **7:**4–11, July–Aug. 1972.
8. Abraham, S., *et al.: Preliminary Findings of the First Health and Nutrition Examination Survey, United States, 1971–1972: Dietary Intake and Biochemical Findings.* Pub. (HRA) 74-1219-1. U.S. Public Health Service, Department of Health, Education, and Welfare, Health Services Administration, Rockville, Md., 1974.
9. Finch, C. A.: "Iron Metabolism," *Nutr. Today,* **4:**2–7, Summer 1969.
10. Wilson, J. F., *et al.:* "Studies on Iron Metabolism. V. Further Observations on Cow's Milk-Induced Gastrointestinal Bleeding in Infants with Iron-Deficiency Anemia," *J. Pediatr.,* **84:**335–44, 1974.
11. Minot, G. R., and Murphy, W. P.: "Treatment of Pernicious Anemia by a Special Diet," *J.A.M.A.,* **87:**470–76, 1926.
12. Meindok, H., and Dvorsky, R.: "Serum Folate and Vitamin B_{12} Levels in the Elderly," *J. Am. Geriatr. Soc.,* **18:**317–26, 1970.

Additional References

Camitta, B. M., and Nathan, D. G.: "Anemia in Adolescence. 1. Disturbances of Iron Balance," *Postgrad. Med.,* **57:**143–46, Feb. 1975.
Corn, M.: "What Is Nutritional Anemia?" *Postgrad. Med.,* **54:**105–107, Oct. 1973.
Markson, J. L.: "The Anemias. II. Pernicious Anemia," *Nurs. Times,* **67:**1562–64, 1971.
Owen, G. M., *et al.:* "A Study of the Nutritional Status of Pre-school Children in the United States, 1968–70," *Pediatrics,* **53** (Suppl.):597–646, 1974.

Pochedly, C.: "Sickle Cell Anemia: Recognition and Management," *Am. J. Nurs.*, **71**:1948–51, 1971.

Scott, D. E.: "Anemia in Pregnancy," *Obstet. Gynecol. Ann.*, **1**:219–44, 1972.

Streiff, R. R.: "Folate Deficiency and Oral Contraceptives," *J.A.M.A.*, **214**:105–108, 1970.

Trubowitz, S., *et al.:* "Survey of Vitamin B_{12} and Folate in the Serum and Marrow Tissue of Hospitalized Patients," *Am. J. Clin. Nutr.*, **27**:580–83, 1974.

Vaz, D. D. S.: "The Common Anemias: Nursing Approaches," *Nurs. Clin. North Am.*, **7**:711–25, 1972.

Wilson, P.: "Iron-Deficiency Anemia," *Am. J. Nurs.*, **72**:502–504, 1972.

44 Diet in Allergic and Skin Disturbances

Elimination Diets

Incidence. The National Institute of Allergy and Infectious Diseases estimates that, in 1971, nearly 32 million Americans (more than one in six persons) suffered from some form of allergy. Of these, 9 million had asthma, 14 million had hay fever, and 9 million had other related allergy problems. The high incidence of allergic diseases is an important health and economic problem. For example, time lost from work and school due to allergies totals 12 million days each year.[1] Food allergies account for a relatively small proportion of all allergies, but allergies to major food groups present serious problems in meal planning and in adequate nutrition. Moreover, many people who suffer from nonfood allergies find it difficult to ingest an adequate diet—the individual with severe asthma, for example.

The allergic reaction. A distinction must be made between food intolerance and food allergy. FOOD INTOLERANCE is characterized by a quantitative difference in the physiologic response to a substance whereas the response in ALLERGY is qualitatively different or abnormal. The substance that sets off the allergic reaction is an ALLERGEN. It is usually a protein, but it may be a polysaccharide or a complex of protein and polysaccharide. Simple substances such as aspirin that produce allergic reactions do not fit into these groups of compounds, but it is believed that they attach to body proteins and form a complex that becomes the active allergen.[2]

The ANTIBODY-ANTIGEN COMPLEX is the body's normal protective mechanism against foreign substances such as bacteria and viruses; thus antigens entering the body form complexes with antibodies to provide the immune mechanism. In allergic persons this mechanism is disturbed in some way; that is, the antibodies react with substances that are normally harmless and set off a chain of damaging reactions. The details of the mechanisms involved are beyond the scope of this text; however, theories concerning mechanisms were recently reviewed.[3]

Allergic reactions may be brought about by (1) ingestion of food or drugs; (2) contact with foods, pesticides, drugs, adhesive, fur, hair, feathers, molds, fungi, and so on; (3) inhalation of pollens, dust, molds, fungi, cosmetics, perfumes; and (4) injection of vaccines, serums, antibiotics, and hormones.

Allergic reactions may be immediate or delayed. *Immediate* reactions occur within a matter of minutes following exposure to the allergen and *delayed* reactions occur hours or days later. For example, individuals who are highly sensitive to eggs may experience immediate, violent symptoms due to a tiny amount of egg adhering to a poorly washed fork; on the other hand, mildly sensitive persons may be able to eat eggs for several days before characteristic symptoms develop. It is believed that the allergen involved is the whole food protein in the immediate type of reaction, and a breakdown product formed during digestion of the food in delayed reactions. The reaction time toward a given substance always remains the same in an individual; that is, if the reaction to eggs is immediate, it will always be so, and not delayed. An individual may have an immediate reaction toward one substance and a delayed response to another.

Heredity is important in the development of allergies. The incidence is increased in children whose parents have allergies, especially if both parents are affected. The child does not inherit a sensitivity to a specific substance or an identical manifestation of the allergy. The parent may be sensitive to wheat, for example, and the child to pollens. The parent may have eczema or a gastrointestinal disturbance whereas the child suffers from asthma.

Any kind of physical or emotional stress increases the severity of allergic reactions. However, the stress situation is not the cause of allergy, and too

577

often the genuinely allergic individual is regarded by his family and friends as well as professional health personnel as reacting because of his emotions. A number of other factors may influence the allergic reaction: for example, the frequency of eating the food, the amount eaten, the physical state of the food, and the season.

Food allergens. Any food may produce reactions, but the most frequent offenders are milk, eggs, wheat, citrus fruits, chocolate or cola, legumes, corn, fish, shellfish, and some spices. The incidence of allergy to these foods and the manifestations associated with each one have recently been reviewed.[4] The increasing incidence of food allergies due to use of soy products and food additives is of some concern.[5,6]

Foods unlike in flavor and structure but belonging to the same botanic group may result in allergic manifestations. For example, buckwheat is not of the cereal family but in a group which includes rhubarb. The sweet potato is not related to the white potato but is a member of the morning-glory family. Spinach, a frequent reactor, is in the same family with beets. The following botanic classification of a few common foods illustrates the relation of foods which at first appear to be dissimilar.

Cereal—wheat, rye, barley, rice, oats, malt, corn, sorghum, cane sugar
Lily—onion, garlic, asparagus, chives, leeks, shallots
Gourd—squash, pumpkin, cucumber, cantaloupe, watermelon
Cabbage and mustard—turnips, cabbage, collards, cauliflower, broccoli, kale, radish, horseradish, watercress, Brussels sprouts

Symptoms of food allergies. Manifestations of allergy may occur in any part of the body. The tissues of these systems are frequently involved: cutaneous, gastrointestinal, respiratory, and neurologic. The symptoms are consequently varied depending upon the parts affected.

1. Skin manifestations may include canker sores, dermatitis, edema, fever blisters, pruritus, and urticaria (hives).

2. Common gastrointestinal manifestations include cheilitis, stomatitis, colic in infants, abdominal distention, constipation, diarrhea, dyspepsia, and nausea and vomiting. The symptoms may be suggestive of appendicitis, colitis, gallbladder disease, or ulcers, and there may be confusion in diagnosis.

3. Respiratory symptoms include allergic rhinitis, asthma, bronchitis, and nasal polyps among others.

4. Neurologic symptoms such as migraine, neuralgias, and the tension-fatigue syndrome are sometimes due to food allergy. The latter syndrome is characterized by anxiety, fatigue, irritability, muscle and joint aching, restlessness, stomach pains, and so on.[4]

5. Miscellaneous symptoms such as anaphylactic reactions, arthralgias, arthritis, edema, and so on have been attributed to food allergy.

Diagnosis of food allergies. The procedures used include a careful diet history, skin testing, and testing with restricted diets.

History. A complete history is the single most important diagnostic tool. When a severe reaction occurs immediately, the patient is usually aware of the circumstances leading up to it. However, when reactions are delayed or when allergies are multiple in nature, the elucidation of the offending factors is often exceedingly difficult. The history must include a complete evaluation of the physical status and the conditions and events preceding the attack.

The patient is asked to keep a detailed diary of all foods ingested and of the occurrence of any symptoms. Individual likes and dislikes must be taken into consideration. One patient may like a food well enough to risk an allergic reaction by eating it while another may claim to be allergic to a food he dislikes.

Skin tests. Skin tests are sometimes used to confirm presence of allergies but their usefulness in the case of food allergy is limited.[7] A positive skin test does not necessarily mean that the patient is sensitive at the time to the material; it may represent a past or potential sensitivity. On the other hand, a negative skin reaction does not necessarily eliminate the possibility of food allergy, for symptoms may be manifested in other tissues. Verification of results from skin tests is made by recurrence of symptoms following ingestion of the food in a symptom-free patient.

Restricted diets. Many variants of restricted diets have been proposed as diagnostic aids. One approach is to restrict the patient to a list of foods to which no skin reactions were shown. The restricted diet may be tested for one to three weeks, after which new foods are added, one at a time, at three-day intervals. If symptoms develop following addition of a food, it is eliminated for a time and reintroduced later.

A number of *elimination diets* have been developed, based upon the principle that only those foods that are seldom responsible for allergy are included in the trial diet. Many elimination diets are modifications of the regimen advocated by Rowe (see diets below), who recommends its use for a minimum of three months in the diagnosis of food allergy.[8]

Rowe's patients are first placed on a cereal-free elimination diet. This diet eliminates all cereal grains, milk, egg, beef, pork (except bacon), fish, and a number of fruits and vegetables. Soybean oil is the only oil permitted; milk-free margarine made from soy oil is used. Bakery products are made from soy, Lima, or potato starch. Soymilk or meat-based formulas are used for infants. Calcium and vitamin supplements are needed. When the patient is free of allergic symptoms, fruits and vegetables are added, one at a time, every two to five days. Cereals are added in the following order; rice, oats, corn, rye, and wheat. Beef is added after one to two months. Tolerance for condiments and spices is determined by challenge testing. Subsequent additions of specified oils and other foods are made upon recommendation by the physician.

A fruit-free cereal-free elimination diet is used for patients who are allergic to fruits, spices, or condiments. On this diet careful planning is needed to ensure adequate calories, vitamins, and minerals, especially ascorbic acid, calcium, potassium, magnesium, iron, and iodine. A number of recipes suitable for use on cereal-free or fruit-free elimination diets are available.

Cereal-Free Elimination Diet*

Beverages—fruit juices: apricot, grapefruit, peach, pineapple, prune, or tomato; Neo-Mullsoy

Breads—Lima-potato, soy-potato; muffins made from allowed flours; pancakes or waffles made from soy-potato flours; soy crackers

*Adapted from Rowe, A. H.: *Food Allergy. Its Manifestations and Control and the Elimination Diets. A Compendium.* Charles C Thomas, Publisher, Springfield, Ill., 1972.

Desserts—cakes, cookies, cupcakes made from soy or potato flours; gelatin, plain; soy ice cream; puddings made from allowed flours; water ices made with allowed fruits

Flours and starches—Lima, potato, soy; pearl tapioca

Fruits—fresh, cooked, or canned apricots, grapefruit, peaches, pears, pineapple; lemon; prunes

Fats—sesame oil, soy oil, milk-free margarine made with soy oil

Gravy—thickened with potato starch

Meats—bacon; Canadian bacon; chicken (no hens); lamb; lamb liver

Soups—broth, chicken or lamb; Lima bean; split pea; tomato

Sweets—brown sugar, beet or cane sugar; jams, jellies, preserves made from allowed fruits; maple syrup; maple sugar candy, plain fondant

Vegetables—artichokes, asparagus, carrots, lettuce, Lima beans, peas, potatoes, spinach, squash, string beans, sweet potatoes, tomatoes, yams

Miscellaneous—baking powder (no cornstarch or tartaric acid); baking soda, cream of tartar, lemon extract, salt, vanilla extract, white vinegar

Sample Menu for Cereal-Free Elimination Diet

Breakfast

Half grapefruit with brown sugar
Canadian bacon
Hashed brown potatoes
Muffins, using soy-potato flour
Milk-free soy margarine
Peach preserves
Hot lemonade, pineapple, apricot, or prune juice

Luncheon or Supper

Tomato juice with lemon wedge
Fried chicken, using soy oil, potato flour
New potato, boiled
Peas
Mixed fruit cup with peach, pear, pineapple
Lemon gelatin salad with grated carrot and crushed pineapple
Soy-potato bread
Milk-free soy margarine
Jam or preserves from allowed fruits
Soy ice cream with caramel sauce
Soy cookies
Lemonade or apricot juice

Dinner

Broiled lamb chops
Baked potato
Mashed squash
Lettuce and tomato salad
Salad dressing, using soy oil, lemon juice, salt
Soy-potato bread

Milk-free soy margarine
Jam or preserves from allowed fruits
Pineapple upside-down cake, using soy-potato flour
Lemonade, apricot, or tomato juice

FRUIT-FREE CEREAL-FREE ELIMINATION DIET°

Beverages—Neo-Mullsoy; tea, if permitted by physician
Breads—Lima-potato, soy-potato; muffins made from allowed flours, pancakes or waffles from potato or soy flour
Desserts—cakes, cookies, cupcakes made from soy or potato flours; gelatin, plain; soy ice cream; puddings made from allowed flours
Fats—sesame oil; soy oil; milk-free soy margarine
Gravy—thickened with potato starch
Meats—bacon; Canadian bacon; chicken (no hens); lamb; lamb liver
Soups—broth, lamb or chicken; Lima bean, split pea
Flours and starches—Lima, potato, soy; pearl tapioca
Sweets—beet or cane sugar; brown sugar; syrup made with cane sugar
Vegetables—artichokes, carrots, Lima beans, peas, potatoes, string beans, squash, sweet potatoes, yams
Miscellaneous—corn-free tartaric acid baking powder; salt

Sample Menu for Fruit-Free Cereal-Free Elimination Diet

BREAKFAST

Waffles, using soy-potato flour
Bacon
Pearl tapioca cooked with water or Neo-Mullsoy and sugar
Milk-free soy margarine
Maple syrup
Tea, if permitted

LUNCHEON OR SUPPER

Split pea soup with bacon crumbs
Soy crackers
Sliced chicken sandwich on soy-potato bread
Milk-free soy margarine
Gelatin salad with shredded carrots
Frosted soy cupcake
Tea, if permitted

DINNER

Chicken broth with carrots, peas, Lima beans
Soy crackers
Roast lamb
String beans
Mashed potato, using Neo-Mullsoy and milk-free soy margarine, salt
Gravy, thickened with potato starch
Soy-potato muffin
Milk-free soy margarine

° Adapted from Rowe, A. H.: *Food Allergy. Its Manifestations and Control and the Elimination Diets. A Compendium.* Charles C Thomas, Publisher, Springfield, Ill., 1972.

Carrot marmalade
Soy ice cream
Butterscotch sauce, using Neo-Mullsoy and milk-free soy margarine
Tea, if permitted

Dietary treatment. If a single food such as strawberries or grapefruit is implicated, it is easy to omit this food from the diet. If allergy involves more than one food, the beginning diet is one that contains only those foods that produce no reactions. Thus, if improvement has occurred on an elimination diet, simple, not mixed, foods are added, one at a time, to the allowed list of foods. Several days to a week must elapse between the addition of each new food. Moreover, a given food should be tested on at least two, preferably three, occasions before it is permanently added to, or eliminated from, the diet. Because wheat, eggs, and milk are frequent allergens, these foods are added last.

Dietary adequacy becomes a matter of great concern when important foods are eliminated for a long period of time. This is especially true in infants and young children. For example, if milk cannot be used, additional amounts of meat should be included to provide the required allowance of protein, and vitamin D and calcium salts need to be prescribed.

Hyposensitization consists in decreasing the sensitivity to a given substance by giving minute doses of the allergen in gradually increasing amounts. It is a very tedious procedure and is seldom used in food allergy, and then only when a major food group is involved.

Dietary management for asthmatic patients. Those who have severe asthma often find it difficult to consume an adequate diet. The meals should be small and eaten slowly in an environment free from stress. Interval feedings are necessary to bolster the caloric intake. Fluid intake should be encouraged. Usually breakfast and lunch are the best meals of the day, and particular attention should be paid to their nutritional quality and attractiveness. A rest period after meals is helpful. Ordinarily, late-evening feedings are not advisable.[9] Some clinicians routinely eliminate highly allergenic foods such as chocolate, nuts, shellfish, and so on. Milk products are sometimes omitted because of their tendency to form mucus.[10]

Dietary Counseling

The importance of reading labels on food products every time purchases are made should be stressed to the patient. Formulations change from time to time and current ingredients are listed on the label. However, even conscientious checking of labels is not always adequate protection for the individual with food allergy. Foods for which a standard of identity has been established by the Food and Drug Administration need not be labeled with a complete listing of ingredients; only optional ingredients must be listed. For example, mayonnaise contains small amounts of egg, but this is not indicated on the label. A number of breads have been included under standards of identity, and thus the label would not indicate that milk is an ingredient.

Many patients may not be aware of the great number of food mixtures containing milk, eggs, cereal, or soy products. The patient should be provided with detailed lists showing typical uses of these foods and should be encouraged to ask specific questions concerning ingredients used in foods when in doubt. Examples of foods to be omitted for wheat, egg, milk, corn, or soy-free diets are given below.

Recipes and helpful hints on substitutions should be offered the patient. For example, water or fruit juices can usually be substituted in recipes using milk. Quick breads can be made from rice, potato, rye, or other flours, but adjustments in baking temperature and time must be made. The proportion of baking powder is increased because of the lack of gluten in these flours. The finished products differ in texture from those prepared from wheat. They should be stored in a freezer rather than in the refrigerator as they tend to dry out quickly. Sources of recipes are given at the end of this chapter.

Patients should be cautioned that improperly washed utensils or use of the same stirring or serving spoon in foods for allergic and nonallergic persons may be sources of prohibited foods for the food-sensitive individual.

Suggestions for ordering foods when eating away from home are useful for patients. Broiled meats, baked potato, plain vegetables without sauces, lettuce salads, and fruits for dessert are usually acceptable.

Diet Without Wheat—Foods to Avoid

Beverages—beer; Cocomalt; coffee substitutes; instant coffee unless 100 per cent coffee; gin; malted milk; whiskey

Breads, crackers, and rolls—all breads including pumpernickel, rye, oatmeal, and corn; baking powder biscuits; crackers; gluten bread; griddle cakes; hot breads and muffins; matzoth, pretzels; rusk; waffles; zwieback

Cereals—All-bran, bran flakes, Cheerios, Cream of Wheat, farina, Granola type, Grapenuts, Grape-nuts flakes, Kix, Krumbles, Maltex, Muffets, New oats, Pettijohn's, Puffed Wheat, Ralston cereals, Shredded Wheat, Special K, Total, Wheatena, Wheat flakes, wheat germ, Wheaties, Wheat Chex

Desserts—cake or cookies, homemade, from mixes, or bakery; doughnuts; ice cream, ice-cream cones; pies; popovers; puddings

Flour—all-purpose; graham, white, whole wheat

Gravies and sauces—thickened with flour

Meats—canned meat dishes such as stews; chili; frankfurters, luncheon meats, or sausage in which wheat has been used as a filler; prepared with bread, cracker crumbs or flour, such as croquettes and meatloaf; stews thickened with flour or made with dumplings; stuffings and commercial stuffing mixes

Pastas—macaroni, noodles, spaghetti, vermicelli, and so on

Salad dressings—thickened with flour

Soups—bouillon cubes; commercially canned

Diet Without Eggs—Foods to Avoid

Eggs—or commercial egg substitutes in any form

Beverages—Cocomalt; eggnog; malted beverages; Ovaltine; root beer; wine

Bread and rolls—containing eggs; crust glazed with egg; French toast; griddle cakes; muffins; pretzels; sweet rolls; waffles; zwieback

Desserts—cake; cream-filled pies, coconut, cream, custard, lemon, pumpkin; custard; doughnuts; ice cream; meringue; puddings; sherbet

Meat—breaded meats dipped in egg; meat loaf

Noodles

Salad dressings—cooked dressings; mayonnaise

Sauces—Hollandaise

Soups—bouillon; broth, consommé

Sweets—many cake icings; candies; chocolate, cream, fondant, marshmallow, nougat; whips

Miscellaneous—baking mixes; baking powder; cake flour; dessert powders; fondue; fritters; pastries; soufflé

Diet Without Milk—Foods to Avoid

Milk—all forms: buttermilk; evaporated; fresh whole or skim; malted; yogurt

Beverages—chocolate; cocoa; Cocomalt; Ovaltine

Breads and rolls—any made with milk (most breads contain milk); bread mixes; griddle cakes; soda crackers; waffles; zwieback

Cereals—Cream of Rice, Instant Cream of Wheat, Special K, Total

Cheese—all kinds; cheese dips and spreads

Desserts—cakes; cookies; custard; doughnuts; ice cream; mixes of all types; pie crust made with butter or margarine; pies with cream fillings such as chocolate, coconut, cream, custard, lemon, pumpkin; puddings with milk; sherbets

Fats—butter, cream, margarine

Meat—frankfurters, luncheon meats, meat loaf—unless 100 per cent meat

Sauces—any made with butter, margarine, milk, or cream

Soups—bisques; chowders; cream

Sweets—caramels; chocolate candy

Vegetables—au gratin; mashed potatoes; seasoned with butter or margarine; scalloped; with cream sauces

Diet Without Corn—Foods to Avoid

Beverages—ale; beer; carbonated; coffee lighteners; gin; grape juice; instant tea; milk substitutes; soy milks; whiskey

Breads, crackers, and rolls—corn breads or muffins; English muffins; graham crackers

Cereals—corn meal; hominy; ready-to-eat: cornflakes; Corn Chex; Grapenuts; Kix

Desserts—cakes; candied fruits; canned or frozen fruit or juices; cream pies; ice cream; pastries; pudding mixes; sherbet

Fats—corn oil; corn oil margarine; gravies, salad dressings thickened with cornstarch; mayonnaise, salad dressings, and shortenings unless source of oil is specified

Flours and thickeners—corn meal; cornstarch

Meats—bacon; hams (cured, tenderized); luncheon; sausage

Soups—all commercial; homemade thickened with cornstarch

Sweets—candy; cane sugar; corn syrups, corn sugars; imitation maple syrups; imitation vanilla; jams, jellies, preserves

Vegetables—beets, Harvard (thickened with cornstarch); corn; mixed vegetables containing corn; succotash

Miscellaneous—baking powders; batters for frying; catsup; chewing gum; cheese spreads; Chinese foods; commercial mixes of all types: baking, cake, pancake, pie crust, pudding; confectioner's sugar; distilled vinegar; monosodium glutamate; peanut butter; popcorn; sandwich spreads; sauces; toppings; vitamin capsules; yeast

Diet Without Soy—Foods to Avoid

Soy products are widely used in commercial food preparations. Omit all products for which labels state: soy, soybean oil, soy flour, soy milk, soy curd; vegetable protein; protein isolate; lecithin. Look for these terms especially on the following:

Beverages—beer, chocolate or cocoa mixes, coffee whiteners, soy milk, wine

Breads, crackers, or rolls—many commercial breads; frankfurter or hamburger rolls; dinner rolls; English muffins; biscuit/pancake mixes; bread or cereal stuffings

Cereals—natural or Granola type; flavored rice mixes; macaroni, spaghetti, noodle, or pizza mixes (canned or dry)

Desserts—cake and cake mixes; prepared frostings; chocolate pudding mixes

Fats—cooking oils, margarines, mayonnaise, salad oil, salad dressings, shortenings in which the type of oil is not specified

Flour—soy

Meat—meat extenders; frankfurters; luncheon meats; pork sausage; fish canned in oil

Soups—bouillon cubes; canned, dried, instant soups

Sweets—candy; chocolate chips; semisweet chocolate; caramels; some pancake syrups

Vegetables—frozen in sauces; au gratin potato mixes; instant mashed potatoes; prepared fried potatoes; potato chips

Miscellaneous—Baco's; pretzels; seasoned sauces: mushroom, soy, steak, tabasco, Worcestershire; dip mixes; powdered seasonings

Diseases of the Skin

The quality of the diet is a determining factor in skin health. Deficiencies of one or more nutrients are known to produce various cutaneous disorders. For example, there are the dermatitis associated with pellagra and resulting from lack of niacin (see page 180), the eruptions which accompany severe vitamin A deficiency (see page 153), the cheilosis of riboflavin lack (see page 177), and the eczema that occurs in infants with essential fatty acid deficiency (see page 80).

Some individuals may be allergic to certain substances and thus manifest skin disorders such as eczema or urticaria. Whenever allergy is suspected, it is essential to determine the offending agent as described in the preceding part of this chapter. No single food or food group predominates in producing allergic skin disorders.

Acne vulgaris is a particular problem during adolescence, and many boys and girls try bizarre diets in an effort to correct the situation. High-fat and concentrated carbohydrate diets have been considered to be undesirable. Chocolate, milk, nuts, cola, and iodized salt are among foods commonly implicated in exacerbation of symptoms. Nevertheless, a study on 65 persons with acne vulgaris who consumed large amounts of chocolate showed that the course of the acne was not adversely affected nor were the output and composition of sebum changed.[11] Controlled studies are needed to determine the influence of other foods in acne.

Dietary emphasis in skin disorders should be placed on nutritional adequacy; that is, the diet should contain sufficient milk, meat, eggs, fruits, vegetables, and whole-grain or enriched cereals and breads. Attention should be directed to improving the general hygiene, including skin cleanliness, regular meal hours, sufficient fluid intake, adequate rest, proper elimination, and psychologic support. There is no harm in excluding candies and sweets, fried foods, chocolate, and rich desserts, but such exclusion probably is most useful in that these foods are replaced by others that are more nutritionally satisfactory.

PROBLEMS AND REVIEW

1. What is the essential difference between food intolerance and food allergy?
2. List some of the characteristic symptoms of allergy.
3. List five foods that cause a great number of allergies. Name some foods that rarely cause sensitivity.
4. What is meant by skin test? Elimination diet?
5. What are the principles for the construction of elimination diets? What are some of the problems associated with using these diets?
6. *Problem.* Plan a day's menu for a patient who is sensitive to wheat, potatoes, and grapefruit.
7. What recommendation could you make to a 15-year-old girl who has acne vulgaris?
8. *Problem.* Prepare a table that shows the nature of skin disorders when a diet is markedly deficient in each of the following: protein, essential fatty acids, vitamin A, riboflavin, niacin, ascorbic acid. Under what circumstances would you expect these changes in the skin to become apparent? What is the incidence of these disorders in the United States?
9. List the considerations you would give to a patient who is severely asthmatic insofar as his nutrition is concerned.
10. What problems of dietary inadequacy should you anticipate if an individual is allergic to milk? To wheat? To many fruits?

CITED REFERENCES

1. Middleton, E.: "President's Address: Allergy, Allergists, and Accountability," *J. Allerg. Clin. Immunol.*, **51**:321–27, 1973.
2. Sanders, H. I.: "Allergy. A Protective Mechanism Out of Control," *Chem. Eng. News*, **48**:84–135, May 11, 1970.
3. Dolowitz, D. A.: "Theories of Allergy Brought Up-to-Date: Allergy as a Biologic Process," *Ann. Allerg.*, **32**:183–88, 1974.
4. Speer, F.: "Multiple Food Allergy," *Ann. Allerg.*, **34**:71–76, 1975.
5. Fries, J. H.: "Studies on the Allergenicity of Soybean," *Ann. Allerg.*, **29**:1–7, 1971.

6. Lockey, S. D.: "Sensitizing Properties of Food Additives and Other Commercial Products," *Ann. Allerg.*, **30:**638–41, 1972.

7. Slavin, R. G.: "Skin Tests in the Diagnosis of Allergies of the Immediate Type," *Med. Clin. North Amer.*, **58:**65–69, 1974.

8. Rowe, A. H.: *Food Allergy. Its Manifestations and Control and the Elimination Diets. A Compendium.* Charles C Thomas. Publisher, Springfield, Ill., 1972.

9. Fontana, V. J., and Strauss, M. B.: "Allergy and Diet," in Goodhart, R. S., and Shils, M. E., eds.: *Modern Nutrition in Health and Disease*, 5th ed. Lea & Febiger, Philadelphia, 1973, Chap. 33.

10. Fontana, V. J.: *Practical Management of the Allergic Child.* Appleton-Century-Crofts, New York, 1969.

11. Fulton, J. E., *et al.*: "Effects of Chocolate on Acne Vulgaris," *J.A.M.A.*, **210:**2071–74, 1969.

ADDITIONAL REFERENCES

Ament, M. E., and Rubin, C. E.: "Soy Protein—Another Cause of the Flat Intestinal Lesion," *Gastroenterology*, **62:**227–34, 1974.

American Academy of Pediatrics. Committee on Nutrition, "Should Milk Drinking by Children Be Discouraged?" *Nutr. Rev.*, **32:**363–69, 1974.

Cole, D.: "Feeding Allergic Patients," *Hospitals*, **45:**95–100, Feb. 16, 1971.

Draper, W. L.: "Food Testing in Allergy," *Arch. Otolaryngol.*, **95:**169–71, 1972.

Emerson, G. W., and Strauss, J. S.: "Acne and Acne Care," *Arch. Dermatol.*, **105:**407–11, 1972.

Food Allergy. Allergy Foundation of America, 801 Second Ave., New York, 10017.

Goldstein, G. B., and Heiner, D. C.: "Clinical and Immunological Perspectives in Food Sensitivity. A Review," *J. Allergy*, **46:**270–91, 1970.

Johnstone, D. E.: "Office Management of Food Allergy in Children," *Ann. Allergy*, **30:**173–80, 1972.

Kaufman, H. S.: "Diet and Heredity in Infantile Atopic Dermatitis," *Arch. Dermatol.*, **105:**400–404, 1972.

Mayer, J.: "Food Allergies," *Postgrad. Med.*, **47:**230–33, June 1970.

Noid, H. E., *et al:* "Diet Plan for Patients with Salicylate-Induced Urticaria," *Arch. Dermatol.*, **109:**866–69, 1974.

Randolph, T. G.: "Dynamics, Diagnosis, and Treatment of Food Allergy," *Otolaryngol. Clin. North Am.*, **7:**617–35, 1974.

Speer, F.: "The Allergic Child," *Am. Fam. Physician*, **11:**88–94, 1975.

INSTRUCTIONAL MATERIALS FOR THE PATIENT

Allergy Diets. Ralston Purina Company, Checkerboard Square, St. Louis.

Allergy Recipes. The American Dietetic Association, 430 North Michigan Ave., Chicago, 1969.

Baking for People with Food Allergies. HG 147, Government Printing Office, Washington, D.C., 1968.

"Food Allergy," (leaflet), National Institutes of Health, Bethesda, Md.

Frazier, C. A.: *Coping with Food Allergy.* Quadrangle/The New York Times Book Co., New York, 1974.

Good Recipes to Brighten the Allergy Diet. Best Foods, Division Corn Products Company, 717 Fifth Ave., New York, 1966.

Joseph, L.: *A Doctor Discusses Allergy: Facts and Fiction*, Budlong Press Co., Chicago.

125 Great Recipes for Allergy Diets. Good Housekeeping, 959 Fifth Ave., New York.

Shattuck, R. R.: *Creative Cooking Without Wheat, Milk and Eggs.* Barnes & Co., Inc., Cranbury, N.J., 1974.

Thomas, L. L.: *Caring and Cooking for the Allergic Child.* Drake Publishers Inc., New York, 1974.

45 Nutrition in Children's Diseases

Although the principles of normal and therapeutic nutrition that apply to the adult are also applicable to the sick child, additional factors that must be carefully considered for the child are (1) growth needs; (2) stage of physical, emotional, and social development; (3) the presence of physical handicaps in some; and (4) the more rapid nutritional deterioration which occurs.

The essentials of normal nutrition provide the base line for planning meals for the sick child (see Chapters 20 and 21). The factors affecting food acceptance must be considered (see Chapter 14), and the principles of nutritional care and counseling are similar to those for adults (see Chapters 25 and 26). The principles of dietary modification for many conditions are similar for adults and for children, and the preceding chapters pertaining to therapeutic nutrition should be consulted for specific regimens. The discussion that follows supplements the descriptive material set forth in the earlier chapters.

Feeding problems of the sick child. Like adults, children face many obstacles in illness. Eating a satisfactory diet may be difficult because of fatigue, nausea, lack of appetite occasioned by the illness and by drugs, and pain. Children often regress to an earlier stage of feeding; for example, the child who has learned to accept chopped foods may refuse them, or the child who can feed himself may refuse to eat unless someone feeds him. Older child- ren especially may experience a sense of failure and express it by excessive eating or refusal to eat. Illness produces emotional tensions in the child as well as in the adult. When the child must be placed in a hospital, he is also faced with the separation from his home and his parents. The principles of feeding the normal child apply in even greater degree to the child who is ill.

Insofar as possible the feeding program should establish a pattern of continuity with that to which the child is accustomed. A record of the child's feeding history is a first requisite so that the normal or therapeutic diet makes allowances for individual likes and dislikes. The period of a child's illness is no time in which to introduce new foods or to provide equipment that the child does not know how to handle. (See Figure 45–1.)

Even though careful menu planning takes into consideration the usual likes and dislikes of children and includes variations in both flavor and textures, foods may be refused. The illness itself and the strange environment are sufficient cause for such refusal; sometimes portions are a bit too large, or there may be a slight change in the flavoring or texture of a familiar food. Regardless of the reason for refusal, nothing can be gained by trying to force a child to eat.

Nurses and nutritionists must like children and must enjoy working with them if they expect to achieve good results in nutritional care. They must be observant of the child's behavior, of the acceptance or rejection of food, and of what the child says about his food. They have a special responsibility to communicate with the parents. From the parents they learn about the child's food habits at home, and about his attitudes toward food. In turn the parents are kept informed about the child's progress in food acceptance while in the hospital, and about changes that may be required after discharge.

Children often eat better when they are fed in groups. Family-style service in the pediatric ward to children who are well enough to sit up is more successful than individual tray service. Older children enjoy selecting their foods from a cafeteria arrangement whenever that is possible. Every advantage should be taken of birthdays and holidays to provide favorite foods and special treats. Many children are encouraged to eat when the mother can bring a favorite food, provided that it does not

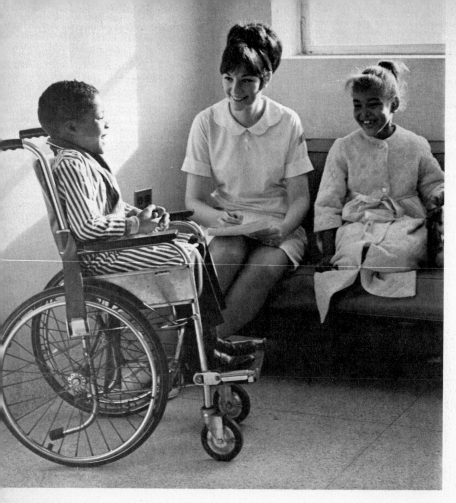

Figure 45–1. "Tell me what you like to eat." By learning something about the patient's food habits, the dietary technician can help to make his hospital stay more pleasant. Sometimes nutrition education can also be given on an informal basis. (Courtesy, Pittsburgh Dietetic Association and Pittsburgh Hospital Association.)

contradict the dietary regimen that has been ordered. Most hospitals now encourage parents to visit at any time they wish, and a young child fed by his mother may respond better than one who is fed by someone strange to him. (See Figure 45–2.)

DIETARY COUNSELING

Parents and children who are old enough to understand are jointly counseled regarding dietary modifications that will be required at home. Much less friction is likely to occur at home when the child is included in the interview. Parents assume the primary responsibility for nutritional care of the young child, but the child needs to know what is expected of him. As early as possible the child should begin to assume some responsibility for his care. Older children under

parental guidance gradually assume full responsibility for their own diets. In counseling it is important to direct the interview and the instructions to the child rather than to the parent.

One important aspect of counseling is to determine the attitudes of the parent toward the development of food habits, and likewise the child's attitudes not only toward his food but also toward his parents. Not infrequently the child uses food to achieve various ends.

If a modified diet will be required indefinitely as for diabetes mellitus, every effort must be made to plan this within the framework of the normal life pattern of the child; the diet must not become the dominating factor that interferes with the child's psychosocial development. Being like his peers is very important to the child, and for many reasons he may be reluctant to disclose that he is in any way different. Insofar as possible the diet should be planned so that it can include foods that are popular with other children. The child must be helped to understand that his condition does not make him abnormal in his relations with others of his group. Selecting foods from those offered by the school lunch would be better for the diabetic child, for example, than carrying a lunch.

Sometimes the hospital stay is sufficiently long that some nutrition education can be included in a group situation.[1] (See Figure 45–3.) Movies appropriate for young children are available from the National Dairy Council and other sources. Older children often view movies with interest in the hospital playroom that they might consider to be boring in the school situation. The teacher assigned to the hospital schoolroom may also be involved in the dietary instruction. For example, children can learn to keep records, to score their diets, and to learn about their needs for basic foods. The calculation of a diet with meal exchanges may be used as an arithmetic assignment. Eye-catching fliers on patient's trays have been used to introduce new ideas about foods such as a food custom of an ethnic group or a simple recipe.

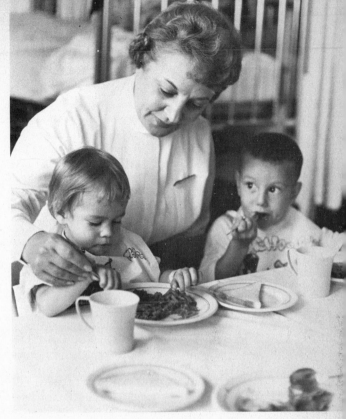

Figure 45–2. A guiding hand and a little encouragement will improve food intake greatly. Sick children away from home need the security of familiar foods and the understanding and affection of nurses, dietitians, and others. (Courtesy, Mrs. Elizabeth Wilcox and The Babies Hospital, New York City.)

Figure 45–3. Nurse demonstrates nutritive equivalents of fruits to three teen-agers. (Courtesy, Medical College of Virginia, Health Sciences Division, Virginia Commonwealth University, Richmond.)

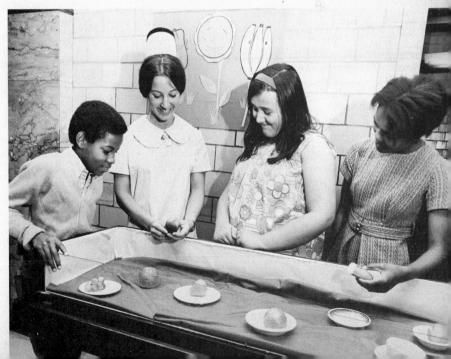

Weight Control

Obesity. The problem of obesity is not limited to adults. From 10 to 20 per cent of children and teen-agers are overweight and it is likely that many of these youngsters were overweight as infants. Excessive weight gain in the first year of life is highly correlated with development of obesity.[2] Juvenile-onset obesity is characterized by increased number and size of adipose cells. Once formed, the excess number of adipose cells cannot be altered by dieting; only the size can be reduced.[3] Since 80 per cent of youngsters who are obese remain so as adults, prevention, by regulation of food intake and activity patterns in childhood, has important implications for later years.[4]

Some children overeat because the pattern of overfeeding established in infancy is carried over into childhood. An abundance of rich, high-calorie foods is readily available and, together with relative inactivity, becomes part of the family pattern. Like adults, children may use food to cover up loneliness or lack of social relationships, or failure in everyday (school) activities. On the other hand, many obese children do not eat any more food than normal-weight children and, in fact, may eat less, but their energy expenditure is considerably less.[5] They avoid active sports, and when they do participate they manage to become involved as little as possible.

Because the energy requirements of children are relatively high, their diets are usually less restricted than those for adults. About 1200 to 1800 kcal may be included, depending upon the stature and activity of the child. Liberal protein, mineral, and vitamin allowances are essential so that tissue and stature development are not adversely affected. Equally important is a program of regular physical activity with emphasis on increasing energy expenditure. Some recommend reducing caloric intake by 200 per day and increasing energy expenditure by the same amount.[6] The low-calorie diets described on page 410 may be used as a basis for planning the child's diet. One cup of milk should be added to these diets daily so that the child receives his quota of 1 quart. Favorite foods need not be omitted entirely, but usually need to be limited. Learning to limit portion sizes and substituting low-calorie snacks are important concepts for the youngster to understand.

It is vital that the child (and his parents) realize what a loss of weight may mean to him. This may mean improved appearance, poise, and gracefulness; greater participation in sports, or winning the approval of fellow playmates and schoolmates. The physician, nurse, and dietitian who are guiding the child's weight-reduction program must show understanding of the child's problems and must maintain interest through a careful follow-up of the progress being made.

Underweight. Data from the Ten-State Nutrition Survey showed that a significant number of children are underweight and undersized.[7] Such children usually tire easily, are irritable and restless, and are more susceptible to infections. As in the correction of obesity, the cause for underweight must first be sought so that treatment may be properly directed. The diet is corrected with respect to its adequacy of the essential nutrients, after which increases in the level of kilocalories may be made gradually. A reasonable amount of outdoor exercise and regulated rest are important elements of the weight-gaining program. (For high-calorie diets, see Chapter 29.)

Growth failure. Infants sometimes fail to thrive when placed in institutions because they are deprived of the normal emotional environment of the home. Such growth failure also occurs in the home when parents reject their children, neglect them, or provide an otherwise hostile environment. Intellectual and neurologic development is impaired as well. Studies have shown that a disproportionately high number of children from such environments were low-birth-weight infants. Martin has suggested that the high incidence of brain damage in these children may be related to poor nutrition in utero. Postnatal undernutrition is also seen in many of these children. In a study of 42 abused and neglected children, 33 per cent were found to be undernourished. In children who were both undernourished and physically abused, the prognosis for normal intellectual development was much poorer.[8]

Gastrointestinal Disturbances in Infants and Children

Infant feeding problems. Many babies regurgitate small amounts of food, and this is no cause for concern. Usually it can be avoided by more frequent "burping" of the infant. Vomiting is more serious and should receive the attention of the physician.

Some babies cry loudly and for long intervals following feeding. Usually they have swallowed excessive amounts of air and have been inadequately "burped." However, some babies continue to cry even with "burping" and parents are likely to become quite distraught. These "colicky" babies usually grow well, and the parents need reassurance that they are progressing satisfactorily and will usually outgrow the colic within a few months. Colic sometimes occurs because the baby is overfed, is tired, or is cold.

Constipation. Formula-fed infants usually have but one bowel movement daily, whereas breast-fed infants have two or three. Only when the stools are hard and dry and eliminated with difficulty does constipation exist. Prune juice or strained prunes given daily usually suffice to correct the constipation.

In the young child, constipation is sometimes due to emotional upset arising out of conflict with his mother over toilet training. The child may learn to ignore the urge to defecate as a means of gaining attention. In time, delayed elimination weakens normal peristalsis and the stools become dry and hard and are difficult to evacuate.

The causes of constipation in older children are similar to those in adults. Corrective treatment includes emphasis upon regularity of habits, increased fluid intake, and a diet that includes raw and cooked vegetables and fruits and some whole-grain cereals and breads. (See Chapter 33.) Milk may need to be limited for some persons.

Diarrhea. Diarrhea occurring in infants and children may be functional or organic. It may be caused by the same factors as in adults or may be related to improper handling of the formula, or to its composition or concentration. Acute diarrhea can sometimes be traced to improper handling of foods or formulas. The incidence is several times higher in bottle-fed than in breast-fed infants and is greatly increased in the summer months when it is due to unsanitary preparation or inadequate refrigeration.

Serious consequences follow diarrhea in infants under one year of age if treatment is not prompt. The large loss of fluids and electrolytes quickly leads to dehydration, fever, loss of kidney function, and severe acidosis if electrolyte loss is chiefly through the intestinal tract. There may also be marked vomiting with loss of acid, in which case there may be no acidosis but a lowering of the total body anions and cations.

Modification of the diet. When mild diarrhea occurs in breast-fed infants, breast feeding may be continued but the baby is likely to take less milk for a few days. A 5 per cent glucose solution may also be offered at three- or four-hour intervals. Bottle-fed babies may be given a half-strength solution of skim milk or other fluids as directed by the physician. Both the volume of formula given and the concentration of the formula are increased gradually. Since it is important to maintain fluid balance, the formula may be supplemented with 5 per cent oral glucose solution.

In severe diarrhea, dehydration and acidosis are corrected by the intravenous administration of glucose and electrolyte solutions or through use of a synthetic low-residue diet by way of nasogastric tube. Many infants with moderate to severe diarrhea have a transient intolerance to lactose and sometimes to other carbohydrates as well.[9] For these infants soy-isolate or casein hydrolysate formulas are sometimes used.° Convalescence may be prolonged and the increases in concentration and in volume of the formula must be made cautiously.

The treatment of diarrhea in older children is similar to that for adults, namely, the omission of food during the first day or two, the gradual introduction of low-residue foods (Chapter 33), and progression to a soft diet.

Celiac disturbances. The celiac syndrome includes several disturbances in which the symptoms, the disorders of absorption, and the nutritional deficiencies are similar. They are gluten-induced enteropathy also known as primary idiopathic steatorrhea, celiac disease (in children), or nontropical sprue (in adults); cystic fibrosis of the pancreas; and kwashiorkor. The symptoms, metabolic alterations, and dietary management for gluten enteropathy have been discussed in Chapter 34, and for cystic fibrosis in Chapter 35. However, some adaptations of the diet will need to be made for the infant and toddler according to their food requirements for growth and development.

Modification of the diet. A high caloric intake is

° Isomil® by Ross Laboratories, Columbus, Ohio.

Mullsoy® and NeoMullsoy® by Syntex Laboratories, Inc., Palo Alto, California.

Nutramigen,® Pregestimil,® and ProSobee® by Mead Johnson & Company, Evansville, Indiana.

mandatory in these diseases because up to 50 per cent of the calories may be excreted in the stools. The intake should be increased by 50 to 75 per cent above normal levels. For infants during the acute phase of illness this necessitates 120 to 200 kcal per kilogram. A high protein intake is also recommended initially. As improvement occurs the protein intake is gradually reduced to normal levels. Supplements of the fat-soluble and water-soluble vitamins are always indicated, and iron supplementation may also be needed.

In celiac disease and in cystic fibrosis large amounts of fat are excreted. This may persist for a long time after subjective improvement occurs. Although fat restriction was formerly used, most pediatricians now allow a moderate fat intake. The increased intake of fat leads to greater quantities of fat in the stool, but the total amount of fat absorbed is also increased, thereby increasing the caloric intake. Pancreatin is prescribed for patients with cystic fibrosis of the pancreas and is taken with each meal. In hot weather the salt intake needs to be increased for patients with cystic fibrosis, but this is not necessary for celiac disease.

Children with cystic fibrosis vary widely in their tolerance to foods, and no single diet is appropriate for all patients. The levels of calories, protein, fat, and carbohydrate must be adjusted individually for each child. Some foods increase abdominal distention, pain, and steatorrhea in some children but not others.

For the young infant a high-protein formula such as *Probana*° supplies two thirds to three fourths of total caloric intake. The remaining calories are furnished by glucose and/or banana flakes or banana powder added to the formula. At two to four months these foods are gradually introduced: cottage cheese, egg yolk, strained beef or liver, apple juice, or applesauce, and banana or banana flakes.

With improvement, other foods are gradually added to include a wider variety of strained and then chopped meats, mild cheese, puréed and then chopped cooked vegetables and fruits, and plain gelatin. Wheat, oats, rye, and barley products must be rigorously excluded for the patient with gluten enteropathy, but these cereals may be gradually introduced into the diet of the patient with cystic fibrosis. (See also page 476.) The additions of food

° *Probana*® by Mead Johnson and Company, Evansville, Indiana.

are made much more gradually than for normal infants and children. Strained foods are used for a somewhat longer period of time, and raw fruits and vegetables are introduced at a later time.

Diabetes

The first patient treated with insulin prepared by Banting and Best in January 1922 was a 14-year-old diabetic boy. Approximately 1 in every 2000 children under 15 years is diabetic.

Comparison with adult diabetes. The disease in children differs in a number of important respects from that in adults. The onset of symptoms is usually more abrupt and the disease usually increases in severity during the period of growth. In contrast to the adult, obesity is uncommon; in fact, when first seen the diabetic child is likely to be underweight and not growing because he has not been metabolizing his food adequately.

All diabetic children need insulin, since there appear to be few if any functioning cells of the islands of Langerhans. The maintenance of control between acidosis on the one hand and hypoglycemia on the other is often difficult because of the greater frequency of infections and the erratic physical activity and emotional control.

Psychologic considerations. Too often the child and his parents feel that he is different from other children and that there is a certain stigma attached to the diabetic state. If the child experiences insulin reactions, he will be afraid to participate in the activities of other children, and he may become more dependent upon his parents. The diabetic adolescent is likely to be especially difficult to control. Like other adolescents he may rebel against authority, and may show his independence by failure to keep the disease in good control.

The guidance of the child in all aspects of his development, not only in the treatment of the diabetes, requires great patience, forbearance, and understanding on the part of the parent and physician. The child and the parent must recognize the interrelationship of diet, insulin, and activity and the importance of regulation. It is equally important that the child learn—and his parents understand— that he can take his place in the family and society just as does the nondiabetic child.

Modification of the diet. The principles of dietary

modification for the diabetic child are similar to those for the adult (see Chapter 37). The nutritive requirements are the same as those for the normal child of the same age, size, and activity (see Chapter 21). Briefly, these needs are as follows:

Calories: 75 to 90 kcal per kilogram (25 to 40 kcal per pound).

Protein: 3.3 gm per kilogram (1.5 gm per pound); 2.2 gm per kilogram for older children.

Carbohydrate and fat: About 45 per cent of the calories from carbohydrate with the remaining calories from fat. Some clinicians restrict carbohydrate to 225 or 250 gm per day, or even less, in which case the fat level is proportionately higher to ensure adequate caloric intake.

The additional calcium requirements are easily met when 3 to 4 cups of milk are included daily. Other minerals and vitamins are provided in satisfactory amounts when the exchange lists are used as the basis of meal planning. Children should receive vitamin D either in milk or as a supplement.

The diet prescription should be adjusted periodically to make allowances for satisfactory growth. A reasonable meal constancy from day to day is desirable. Between-meal snacks should be included. It is better that a child receive a snack before activity to forestall the possibility of insulin reaction.

Dietary control. Although the life-span of diabetic children has improved greatly, the incidence of degenerative diseases is unusually high after 10 to 20 years. The possibilities of diminished vision and even blindness, of coronary artery disease, and of kidney disease during the prime of life are serious, and as yet unsolved, problems.

The incidence of these complications in 73 persons with diabetes for more than 40 years was studied retrospectively at the Joslin Clinic.[10] (See Table 45–1.) The mean age in this group was 51 years (range 42 to 64 years). The onset of diabetes occurred before age 15 in all subjects. Retinopathy was seen in three fourths of the patients. Although visual changes were minor in 45 per cent, 12 per cent were legally blind. Almost half the patients were judged to be in good condition with only minor complications which did not interfere with their daily activities. One fourth were in poor condition with multiple serious complications in one of the categories shown in Table 45–1. Because of the nature of the study no correlation could be made between duration of the disease or degree of dia-

Table 45–1. Chronic Complications in 73 Persons with Diabetes of 40 Years' Duration*

Complications	Number	Per Cent
Retinopathy	55	75.2
Neuropathy	35	47.3
Nephropathy	30	41.0
Cardiac Involvement	15	20.5

*Adapted from Paz-Guevara, A. T., *et al.*: "Juvenile Diabetes Mellitus After Forty Years," *Diabetes,* **24:**559–65, 1975.

betic control and onset of complications. Jackson believes that the changes can be delayed many years if the diabetes is well controlled.[11] Under such control the blood sugar is kept as nearly normal as possible and glycosuria is avoided for the most part.

Some pediatricians use a so-called *free diet,* allowing the child to eat all family foods but usually restricting concentrated sweets and high-carbohydrate desserts. Enough insulin is given to metabolize food for normal growth and to avoid ketosis, but mild hyperglycemia and glycosuria are disregarded. At the other extreme are those pediatricians who maintain rigid chemical control and require weighed or carefully measured diets.

Insulin. In early stages of juvenile diabetes the pancreas sometimes produces small amounts of insulin, but this rapidly diminishes. As growth accelerates the insulin requirement increases greatly and control becomes much more difficult.

Jackson recommends at least two doses of intermediate-acting insulin for the desirable three-meal-plus-snack pattern. The morning dose is a mixture of regular and NPH insulin. A second dose of intermediate-acting insulin is given late in the afternoon (about 5:00 p.m.). With this program the blood sugar is maintained as nearly normal as possible throughout the 24-hour day. This regimen is intended to avoid glycosuria or insulin reactions.[11]

DIETARY COUNSELING

Whenever possible, initial hospitalization is desirable not only to stabilize the diabetes in the child but especially to set up an adequate program of education. The child and his parents must face the issue of diabetes squarely, but also

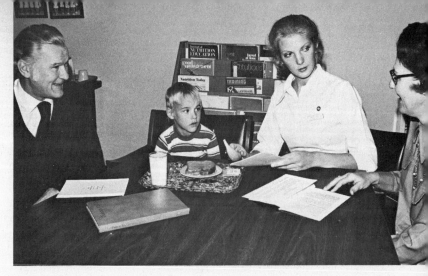

Figure 45-4. The child and his parents learn together about the important essentials of the diet through the use of food models and booklets. Although the parents assume responsibility for supervision of the dietary regimen, the child must be an active participant in making menu decisions. (Courtesy, St. Paul–Ramsey Hospital and Medical Center, St. Paul, Minnesota.)

recognize that the child can live a happy, useful life. Regardless of the opinions regarding chemical or clinical control, pediatricians agree that close adherence to the diet at the beginning provides security and guidance for the child and parent during the period of adjustment to the disease. The initial diet could be one that provides few substitutions until the patient is thoroughly accustomed to it; then gradually the diet is liberalized with respect to the food choices until the meal exchange lists are used with ease. (See Figure 45-4.)

Children, like adults, need to be taught the nature of the disease, how to administer insulin, how to select the daily diet from the plan set up, how to test the urine, and how to keep records. The importance of cleanliness and personal hygiene must be emphasized. The recognition of the signs of insulin reactions or of acidosis and what to do when these signs appear must be learned. See also pages 498 to 501 for further details on dietary counseling. (See Figures 45-5 and 45-6.)

Diabetic camps provide an unusual educational opportunity for children to learn more about the care of themselves and also to learn the important social adjustments with other children. Such camps are well staffed with recreational leaders, nurses, dietitians, physicians, and laboratory technicians.[12]

RENAL DISEASE

The causes of renal disease in children are similar to those in adults. The etiology, clinical manifestations, biochemical abnormalities, and principles of dietary modification are discussed in Chapter 42. These considerations hold for children as well, although quantitative differences must be taken into account. In this section nephrotic syndrome and chronic renal insufficiency in children are considered.

NEPHROTIC SYNDROME

Symptoms and clinical findings. The nephrotic syndrome includes so-called lipoid nephrosis and the nephrotic phase of glomerulonephritis. This rare syndrome occurs in young children at an average age of $2\frac{1}{2}$ years. Its onset is usually insidious and is characterized by marked edema, heavy proteinuria (more than 4 gm in 24 hours), serious depletion of plasma proteins, especially the albumin fraction, and hypercholesterolemia. The edema is often so marked that it seems as if the skin would burst. When diuresis occurs the severe depletion of tissue proteins and the accompanying undernutrition become fully apparent.

Excessive urinary wastage of ceruloplasmin, protein-bound iodine, iron-binding proteins, prothrombin, and complement also occur. Because of the loss

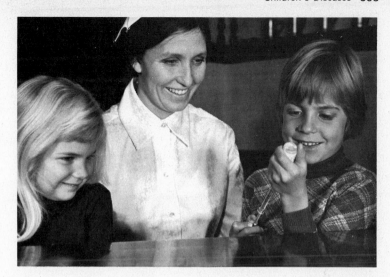

Figure 45–5. Success! Learning to measure his own insulin is an important first step toward independence for the young diabetic. (Courtesy, Diabetes Education Center, Minneapolis.)

of complement, the incidence of infections is high and is an important cause of death. Hematuria, hypertension, and azotemia are minimal or absent in lipoid nephrosis.

The aims of therapy include control of infections and edema and establishment of good nutrition. Corticosteroid therapy results in remission of clinical and biochemical aspects of the disease in over 95 per cent of patients.[13] Others may progress to terminal stages of nephritis or succumb to infections.

Modification of the diet. Patients with nephrosis have a particularly poor appetite, and the high-calorie high-protein diets that are often ordered are not necessarily consumed. Much attention must be given to the selection of foods that are acceptable to the child. With the loss of edema fluid the appetite usually improves.

The caloric intake should be based upon the child's desirable weight for his height and body build. Unless the caloric intake is adequate, effective tissue regeneration cannot take place. The protein intake is generally a little higher than normal; about 3 to 4 gm per kilogram is suitable for the preschool child and 2 to 3 gm per kilogram for school-age children.

Sodium restriction is prescribed in the presence of edema. Since unsalted foods are poorly accepted, prolonged restriction is undesirable. Diuretics may bring about such rapid diuresis that the blood levels of both sodium and potassium are reduced. In such

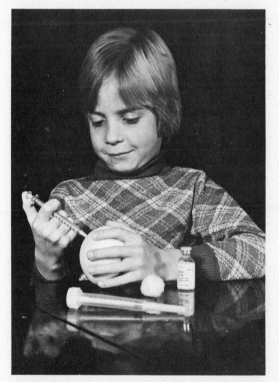

Figure 45–6. Young diabetic patient learns how to administer insulin. (Courtesy, Diabetes Education Center, Minneapolis.)

instances the sodium content of the diet should be increased, and juices rich in potassium offered. See Chapter 41 for planning of sodium-restricted diets.

CHRONIC RENAL INSUFFICIENCY

A major problem in most children on long-term dialysis for chronic renal disease is growth failure. The etiology is complex and inadequate caloric intake is just one of several factors involved. Poor appetite and multiple dietary restrictions make food less appealing. A major difficulty with the diet is providing adequate calories without exceeding the protein, mineral, and fluid allowances. The calorie intake needed for optimal growth is not known. Holliday has suggested that the needs for children on dialysis may be considerably more than 100 per cent of the Recommended Dietary Allowances for calories.[14] From 1.5 to 2.0 gm high-biologic-value protein per kilogram body weight daily has been recommended for children on dialysis.[15] Sodium usually is not restricted unless there is hypertension or edema. Hyperkalemia occurs and usually necessitates moderate potassium restriction. A number of suitable commercial products and recipes low in protein, sodium, and potassium are available, but monotony and lack of palatability limit their acceptance by many patients.

The active form of vitamin D, 1,25-dihydroxy-cholecalciferol, is synthesized in the kidney. As renal function deteriorates, osteodystrophy becomes a serious metabolic problem. Hyperparathyroidism, defective absorption of calcium, and altered metabolism of vitamin D are involved. Calcium supplements, 0.5 gm for younger children and 1.0 gm for older children, have been recommended.[15] Massive doses of vitamin D, 10,000 units or more, are used.

Because of the many nutritional problems in this disease, parents of these children require much guidance in meal planning in order that they can provide appropriate foods which are acceptable to the child.

ALLERGY

The designation of allergy has been used frequently for those conditions resulting from a sensitivity to a food. With the increased understanding of hereditary diseases, it is now apparent that many so-called allergies are, in fact, the failure to metabolize a given nutrient because of the congenital deficiency of one or more enzymes. There remain, however, many diseases which are not yet explained on any such basis and which are classified as allergies.

Foods are responsible for the majority of allergies in children under three years of age. The chief offending foods are milk, eggs, chocolate, cola, citrus fruits, legumes, corn products, tomato, wheat, and pork. When the child is young, it is relatively simple to determine which food is responsible by allowing only milk and crystalline vitamins. If a food other than milk is responsible, the symptoms, such as eczema, will be relieved in a few days; but if milk or nonfood allergy is responsible for the disturbance, no improvement will take place.

When the symptoms of allergy are mild, it is always necessary to consider the relative importance of the allergic disturbance in relation to the diet of the child. It is better management, for example, to treat a mild case of eczema locally than to subject the child to the dangers of an inadequate diet with its far more serious consequences.

For older children, the diagnosis of allergy is determined by the usual elimination diet, and noting reappearance of symptoms after the food is reintroduced into the diet. The treatment is planned as for adults (see Chapter 44).

Milk sensitivity. About 2 per cent of all children are sensitive to milk, according to various estimates.[16] In many instances this may be associated with infection and emotional stress; in others genetic factors may be a cause (see Galactose Disease, Chapter 46, and Lactose Intolerance, Chapter 34).

The response to the ingestion of milk is almost immediate in some and may lead to colic, spitting up of the feeding, irritability, diarrhea, and respiratory disorders. A delayed reaction may occur hours to days following the ingestion of milk, and thus it becomes difficult to determine the exact cause. The incidence of hypochromic anemia in some infants has been attributed to sensitivity to milk.[17] Following the ingestion of milk by these sensitive infants, some blood is lost from the gastrointestinal tract. This may average several milliliters per day and may go unnoticed until the anemia becomes appar-

ent months later. Some infants may have a sufficiently high intake of other iron-rich foods so that
the anemic tendency is counteracted.

Dietary treatment. Sometimes it is only necessary
to change the form of the milk to improve tolerance—that is, boiled, powdered, acidulated, or
evaporated milk may be satisfactory when fresh
cow's milk is not. Some children will tolerate no
milk whatsoever and it is necessary to substitute
formulas in which the protein is derived from meat°
or soybean (see page 456). The tolerance to milk
improves in many infants, but others need to continue a milk-free diet indefinitely.

FEEDING HANDICAPPED CHILDREN

Cerebral palsy. This is a disorder in which motor
control is disturbed due to brain damage. Feeding
problems are common.

Reverse swallowing wave. When the motor system of the tongue and throat is affected, food is not
pushed back to the throat, but the tongue motion
pushes the food forward. Initially such children
must be tube fed, but in time they learn to put food
at the back of the tongue and by tilting the head
backward learn to swallow. These children often
become severely undernourished because feeding is
such a prolonged process. Concentrated foods with
maximum protein and calorie value should be emphasized to keep the volume to a minimum. Vitamin and mineral supplements are usually required.

Athetoids are those who are constantly in motion
and who thus burn up a great deal of energy. Although they require a high-calorie high-protein diet,
the ingestion of the necessary amounts of food is
difficult because of the constant motion. Feeding is
quite time consuming and emphasis should be
placed upon concentrated foods of high caloric
value. Children should be encouraged to feed themselves by giving them foods that they can pick up
with their fingers such as pieces of fruit and sandwiches. Many devices have been developed as aids
in feeding. (See page 386.)

Spastics are very limited in their activity, and
they may also be indulged in eating by their par-

°MBF (Meat Base Formula) by Gerber Products Company,
Fremont, Michigan.

ents. Consequently they gain excessive amounts of
weight, and the obesity in turn further restricts their
ability to get around. These individuals require
marked restriction of caloric intake without jeopar-
dizing the intake of protein, minerals, and vitamins.

Cleft palate. Surgery for cleft palate is often not
completed for several years. In addition to the needs
for normal development, the infant and child must
build up reserves for surgery, the promotion of
healing, and the development of normal healthy
gums and teeth. Several considerations should be
borne in mind in feeding these children:

1. Infants may have difficulty in sucking, but
most of them learn to use chewing movements to
get the milk out of the nipple. An enlarged nipple
opening is helpful. Some babies may be fed with a
medicine dropper.

2. To counteract the tendency to choke, liquids
should be taken in small amounts and swallowed
slowly.

3. More frequent "burpings" are necessary because of the large amount of air which may be
swallowed.

4. Spicy and acid foods often irritate the mouth
and nose and should be avoided. If orange juice is
not well taken, ascorbic acid supplement should be
prescribed.

5. Among the foods which may get into the
opening of the palate are peanut butter, peelings of
raw fruit, nuts, leafy vegetables, and creamed
dishes. Some children have no difficulty with any
foods.

6. Puréed foods may be diluted with milk, fruit
juice, or broth and given from a bottle with a large
nipple opening. Some babies accept purées well if
they are thickened with vanilla wafer or graham-
cracker crumbs.

7. The time required for feeding may be long and
requires much patience on the part of parent and
nurse. For the older child, five or six small meals
may be better than three.[18]

When surgery has been performed, a liquid or
puréed diet is offered until healing is complete.

Mental retardation. Some 6 million persons in the
United States are estimated to be mentally retarded.
Of these, about 75 per cent have an I.Q. between 51
and 75 (educable) and are designated as "high
grade." Approximately 20 per cent of the mentally
retarded are "middle grade"; that is, they have an

I.Q. between 21 and 50 (trainable). The "low-grade" individual with an I.Q. below 20 is believed to account for 5 per cent of the mentally retarded and presents the problems in feeding; however, even the profoundly retarded can be trained to eat properly and to use good table manners.[19]

The nutritional requirements of the mentally retarded child and adult are like those of the individual of normal mental development. The nurse can help parents to understand the problems of feeding by giving encouragement and support.

The mentally retarded child may be kept on the bottle too long, thus increasing the difficulties of introducing other foods. The child may eat very slowly, and feeding may be messy. Hand sucking and vomiting are not uncommon. To obtain adequate food intake for growth may require frequent, small feedings, and certainly an abundance of patience and ingenuity. One must strike a balance between overprotectiveness and lack of caring.

The retarded individual, like the normal person, has an active emotional life. He feels the shunning of others and his failure to achieve, but will respond to loving attention. He resists new foods, has definite likes and dislikes, and finds it difficult to manage eating. He responds to the color of foods and like all children is fond of sweets.

When the individual is able to feed himself, he should be permitted to do so even though feeding may be messy. Food must be presented in a form that can be easily managed. Foods may be eaten with the fingers for a long time until simple utensils can be managed. The child unable to support himself should be held in a sitting position while he is being fed.

PROBLEMS AND REVIEW

1. What dietary problems may be anticipated in children who must be hospitalized? How can these problems be overcome?
2. How can a schoolchild be helped to adjust to a prolonged therapeutic diet?
3. *Problem.* List a number of ways in which you could encourage a boy with rheumatic fever to take an adequate diet.
4. What dietary considerations would apply for a seven-year-old child with scarlet fever?
5. *Problem.* Adjust a 1500-kcal diet of an adult so that it will be suitable for a 12-year-old boy. In what ways would you try to effect acceptance of this diet?
6. *Problem.* Plan six high-calorie after-school and bedtime snacks which could be added to the regular diet of a teen-age girl who is 20 pounds underweight.
7. What changes in diet might be indicated for an infant who is constipated? A four-year-old child?
8. *Problem.* Plan a day's meals for a three-year-old child with celiac disease for whom a gluten-restricted diet has been ordered. He is 34 inches tall and weighs 11 kg; he appears to be somewhat undernourished.
9. What are the similarities between celiac disease and cystic fibrosis? What differences are there?
10. A 10-year-old child has diabetes mellitus.
    a. List the differences between diabetes in children and in adults.
    b. What arguments can you give for, and against, chemical control in childhood diabetes?
    c. Enumerate the essential points in the instruction of the child and/or his parent with respect to diabetes.
    d. What is the effect of physical activity on the control of diabetes in the child?
    e. Prepare a plan for the organization of a diabetic club for children. Include suggestions for meetings for such a group.
    f. This child is invited to a birthday party. What plans can be made so that the child may eat at this party?
11. List several ways in which milk intolerance may be manifested. What substances in milk have been shown to produce such sensitivity? List three products that may be used satisfactorily in place of a milk formula.
12. *Problem.* For a two-year-old child with nephrosis plan a suitable diet containing 50 gm protein and 1200 kcal. How would you modify the diet for 500 mg sodium?

13. List some of the considerations to be kept in mind when planning the diet for a child undergoing chronic hemodialysis.

CITED REFERENCES

1. Rickard, K., and Farnum, S.: "Food for Fun and Thought: Nutrition Education in a Children's Hospital," *J. Am. Diet. Assoc.,* **65:**294–97, 1974.
2. Crawford, P. B., *et al.:* "An Obesity Index for Six-Month-Old Children," *Am. J. Clin. Nutr.,* **27:**706–11, 1974.
3. Winick, M.: "Childhood Obesity," *Nutr. Today,* **9:**6–12, May–June 1974.
4. Knittle, J. L.: "Obesity in Childhood: A Problem in Adipose Tissue Cellular Development," *J. Pediatr.,* **81:**1048–59, 1972.
5. Huenemann, R. L.: "Food Habits of Obese and Non-obese Adolescents," *Postgrad. Med.,* **51:**99–105, May 1972.
6. Dwyer, J. T., *et al.:* "Treating Obesity in Growing Children. 2. Specific Aspects. Activity and Diet," *Postgrad. Med.,* **51:**111–15, June 1972.
7. "Highlights from the Ten State Nutrition Survey," *Nutr. Today,* **7:**4–11, July–Aug. 1972.
8. Martin, H. P., *et al.:* "The Development of Abused Children," *Adv. Pediatr.,* **21:**25–73, 1974.
9. Fomon, S. J.: *Infant Nutrition,* 2nd ed. W. B. Saunders Company, Philadelphia, 1974, Chap. 19.
10. Paz-Guevara, A. T., *et al.:* "Juvenile Diabetes Mellitus After Forty Years," *Diabetes,* **24:**559–65, 1975.
11. Guthrie, R. A., and Jackson, R. L.: "Control of Diabetes in Children: Recent Concepts Concerning Vascular Complications and Growth Retardation," *Pediatr. Ann.,* **4:**48–58, June 1975.
12. Klam, W. P., and Silver, A. A.: "Camps for Diabetic Children," *Pediatr. Ann.,* **4:**80–87, June 1975.
13. Spitzer, A.: "Drug Therapy of Glomerular Disease," *Pediatr. Ann.,* **3:**43–57, April 1974.
14. Holliday, M. A.: "Calorie Deficiency in Children with Uremia: Effect Upon Growth," *Pediatrics,* **50:**590–97, 1972.
15. Cameron, J. S.: "The Treatment of Chronic Renal Failure in Children by Regular Dialysis and by Transplantation," *Nephron,* **11:**221–51, 1973.
16. American Academy of Pediatrics: "Should Milk Drinking by Children Be Discouraged?" *Pediatrics,* **53:**576–82, 1974.
17. Goldstein, G. B., and Heiner, D. C.: "Clinical and Immunological Perspectives in Food Sensitivity: A Review," *J. Allergy,* **46:**270–91, 1970.
18. Zickefoose, M.: "Feeding the Child with a Cleft Palate," *J. Am. Diet. Assoc.,* **36:**129–31, 1960.
19. Azrin, N. H., and Armstrong, P. M.: "The 'Mini-Meal'—A Method for Teaching Eating Skills to the Profoundly Retarded," *Ment. Retard.,* **11:**9–13, Feb. 1973.

ADDITIONAL REFERENCES

General References
Claxton, I.: "Nurses Explain Hospitals to Children," *Hospitals,* **49:**41–42, July 1, 1975.
Downey, T. J.: "All My Times in the Hospital—A Child Remembers," *Am. J. Nurs.,* **74:**2196–98, 1974.
Getty, G., and Hollensworth, M.: "Through a Child's Eye Seeing," *Nutr. Today,* **2:**17–20, 1967.
Jernigan, A. K.: "Suggestions for Feeding of Hospitalized Children," *Hospitals,* **44:**86–89, May 16, 1970.

Obesity
Heald, F. P., and Kahn, M. A.: "Teenage Obesity," *Pediatr. Clin. North Am.,* **20:**807–17, 1973.
Huenemann, R. L.: "Environmental Factors Associated with Preschool Obesity," *J. Am. Diet. Assoc.,* **64:**480–91, 1974.
Kaufmann, N. A., *et al.:* "Eating Habits and Opinions of Teenagers on Nutrition and Obesity," *J. Am. Diet. Assoc.,* **66:**264–68, 1975.
Kenna, A. P.: "Infant Feeding and Obesity," *Nurs. Times,* **70:**312–13, 1974.

Leveille, G. A., and Romsos, D. R.: "Meal Eating and Obesity," *Nutr. Today,* **9:**4–9, Nov.–Dec. 1974.

Matsumo, A. S., *et al.:* "Four Factors Affect Weight Control for Obese Children," *J. Nutr. Educ.,* **6:**104–107, 1974.

Ounsted, M., and Sleigh, G.: "The Infant's Self-Regulation of Food Intake and Weight Gain," *Lancet,* **1:**1393–97, 1975.

Thompson, R. J., and Palmer S.: "Treatment of Feeding Problems—A Behavioral Approach," *J. Nutr. Educ.,* **6:**63–66, 1974.

Celiac Disturbances

Ament, M. E.: "Malabsorption Syndrome in Infancy and Childhood," *J. Pediatr.,* **81:**685–97; 867–84, 1972.

Crozier, D. N.: "Cystic Fibrosis. A Not So Fatal Disease," *Pediatr. Clin. North Am.,* **21:**935–50, 1974.

Gall, D. G., and Hamilton, J. R.: "Chronic Diarrhea in Childhood," *Pediatr. Clin. North Am.,* **21:**1001–17, 1974.

Kuitunen, P., *et al.:* "Malabsorption Syndrome with Cow's Milk Intolerance," *Arch. Dis. Child.,* **50:**351–56, 1975.

Poley, J. R.: "Chronic Diarrhea in Infants and Children," *South. Med. J.,* **66:**1035–49; 1133–41, 1973.

Diabetes Mellitus

American Diabetes Association: "Principles of Nutrition and Dietary Recommendations for Patients with Diabetes Mellitus: 1971," *Diabetes,* **20:**633–34, 1971.

Collier, R. N., Jr., and Etzwiler, D. D.: "Comparative Study of Diabetes Knowledge Among Juvenile Diabetics and Their Parents," *Diabetes,* **20:**51–57, 1971.

Ehrlich, R. M.: "Diabetes in Childhood," *Pediatr. Clin. North Am.,* **21:**871–74, 1974.

Klam, W. P., *et al.:* "Care of the Diabetic Adolescent," *Pediatr. Ann.,* **4:**38–47, June 1975.

McFarlane, J.: "Children With Diabetes. Special Needs During Growth Years," *Am. J. Nurs.,* **73:**1360–63, 1973.

Prazar, G., and Felice, M.: "The Psychologic and Social Effects of Juvenile Diabetes," *Pediatr. Ann.,* **4:**59–70, June 1975.

Robinson, W.: "Learning to Live with Diabetes," *Nurs. Times,* **70:**383–84, 1974.

Renal Diseases

Barnett, H. L., *et al.:* "Classification of Glomerular Disease in Children," *Pediatr. Ann.,* **3:**22–42, April 1974.

Boichis, H., and Winterborn, M. H.: "Acute Renal Failure in Childhood," *Pediatr. Ann.,* **3:**58–68, April 1974.

Broyer, M., *et al.:* "Growth in Children Treated with Long Term Hemodialysis," *J. Pediatr.,* **84:**642–49, 1974.

Burton, B. T.: "Current Concepts of Nutrition and Diet in Diseases of the Kidney," *J. Am. Diet. Assoc.,* **65:**623–33, 1974.

Edelmann, C. M.: "Chronic Renal Insufficiency," *Pediatr. Ann.,* **3:**69–80, April 1974.

Makker, S. P., and Heymann, W.: "The Idiopathic Nephrotic Syndrome of Childhood," *Am. J. Dis. Child.,* **127:**830–37, 1974.

Potter, D. E., *et al.:* "Hyperparathyroid Bone Disease in Children Undergoing Long Term Hemodialysis; Treatment with Vitamin D," *J. Pediatr.,* **85:**60–66, 1974.

Other Childhood Diseases

Blair, J., and Fitzgerald, J. F.: "Treatment of Non Specific Diarrhea in Infants," *Clin. Pediatr.,* **13:**333–37, 1974.

Hanks, T. G.: "Milk as Obstipant," *J.A.M.A.,* **230:**538–39, 1974.

Laurance, B. M.: "The Underweight Child," *Practitioner,* **208:**220–26, 1972.

Sherman, J. O., *et al.:* "Use of an Oral Elemental Diet in Infants with Severe Intractable Diarrhea," *J. Pediatr.,* **86:**518–23, 1975.

Speer, F.: "The Allergic Child," *Am. Fam. Physician,* **11:**88–94, Feb. 1975.

Feeding the Handicapped

Feeding the Child with a Handicap. Children's Bureau, Pub. 2091, U.S. Department of Health, Education, and Welfare, Washington, D.C., 1967.

Wallace, H. M.: "Nutrition and Handicapped Children," *J. Am. Diet. Assoc.*, **61:**127–33, 1972.

Instructional Material for the Patient

"Nutrition and Feeding Techniques for Handicapped Children," California Department of Health, Sacramento.

46 Inborn Errors of Metabolism

Phenylalanine-Restricted Diet; Galactose-Free Diet

Many professional and lay groups have united in their efforts to understand the nature of the ever-growing number of inborn errors of metabolism and to seek methods of prevention and treatment. To the physician, the problems are those of diagnosis, of early detection before damage has occurred, and of effective treatment. To the biochemist falls the task of identifying the metabolic defect so that a possible rationale of therapy can be developed. To the nurse and dietitian fall the practical aspects of nursing care and of dietary planning and implementation. The problem of control through genetic counseling belongs to the geneticist. Most of all, to the parent of a child affected the problem is immediate and urgent; in some disorders treatment is effective, but in others no remedy is available.

Nature of inborn errors. The term INBORN ERROR was coined at the beginning of this century by Sir Archibald E. Garrod who wrote a book in which he described four diseases of a hereditary nature.[1] These were alkaptonuria, a defect of phenylalanine metabolism in which a metabolite excreted into the urine becomes dark upon standing; albinism, also a defect in phenylalanine metabolism characterized by a lack of pigmentation; cystinuria, or an excessive excretion of cystine because of a defect in the renal tubules which prevents the reabsorption of the amino acid cystine; and pentosuria, characterized by the presence of pentose in the urine owing to the lack of an enzyme in metabolism.

Inborn errors of metabolism include well over 100 disorders that originate in one or more mutations of the gene so that normal function is disrupted. These diseases are also referred to as *genetic diseases* or as *hereditary molecular diseases*. The effects of genetic mutation vary widely and may alter the metabolism of specific amino acids, carbohydrates, lipids, vitamins, or minerals. They may affect the synthesis of a body product; interfere with the transport of materials across a cell membrane; or produce toxic effects on tissues because of the accumulation of intermediate products.

Some errors of metabolism result in no serious limitations upon the individual; others lead to rapid changes in the central nervous system so that mental retardation is severe; still others may be lethal shortly after birth. Some become evident a few days after birth, whereas other hereditary diseases such as diabetes mellitus and gout may show no signs until adult life. Dietary management is effective in the control of many disorders but no known therapy is yet available for others.

Some of the inborn errors of metabolism are characterized by serious mental retardation if the condition is not treated promptly. During the first years of life the brain is developing so rapidly that any interference with its growth cannot be fully corrected at a later time. Thus, diagnosis at a very early age is important if effective treatment is to take place before serious damage has occurred. Inexpensive screening tests may be applied to some conditions during the first weeks of life. Several conditions for which dietary treatment has been successful are discussed in this chapter.

PHENYLKETONURIA

PHENYLKETONURIA (often abbreviated PKU) was first diagnosed by Asbjörn Fölling, a Norwegian biochemist, in 1934, and has been successfully treated with a phenylalanine-restricted diet since 1952. When the disorder is discovered early in infancy and is treated with the phenylalanine-restricted diet, mental development is normal.

Incidence. About 1 child in each 10,000 births has phenylketonuria, although 1 person in 50 is a carrier of the trait. About 1 per cent of all patients in mental institutions are estimated to be phenyl-ketonurics.

Phenylketonuria is transmitted by an autosomal recessive gene. Thus, each of the parents would have one defective gene and would be clinically normal. Each birth from the mating of two heterozygotes involves a one in four chance that the child will be phenylketonuric, two chances that he will be a heterozygote but clinically normal, and one chance that he will be entirely normal.

Biochemical defect. An enzyme, PHENYLALANINE HYDROXYLASE, is missing in the phenylketonuric individual. As a consequence the hydroxyl (OH) grouping cannot be incorporated into the phenylalanine molecule to form tyrosine. Tyrosine levels remain normal but phenylalanine and several metabolites accumulate in the blood circulation and are excreted in the urine. One of these, phenylpyruvic acid, is a ketone which accounts for the naming of the condition. It reacts with ferric chloride to give a vivid green color, thus forming the basis for the widely used "diaper" tests. Another intermediate product is phenylacetic acid, which accounts for the characteristic "wild," "gamey," or "mousy" odor from the skin and urine of these patients. (See Figure 46–1.)

Testing for phenylketonuria. Most states require the testing of newborn infants, using the "diaper" tests. To avoid false interpretations these should be followed by blood tests in four to six weeks. The acceptable range of phenylalanine in the blood serum is 3 to 7 mg per cent. In phenylketonuric infants the initial blood level is usually above 15 mg per cent and as high as 30 mg per cent by 10 days of age. In untreated persons with PKU, the serum level reaches as high as 75 mg per cent.[2]

In some children phenylalanine hydroxylase is not missing but is present in reduced amounts and there is consequent elevation of serum phenylalanine levels. Neurologic development in these youngsters is usually normal.[3] Occasionally infants have an initial elevation of serum phenylalanine that later returns to normal. Other infants, especially prematures, show a slight elevation of serum phenylalanine, and sometimes tyrosine, because of delayed maturation of the tyrosine-oxidizing system. Usually this is corrected by the administration of ascorbic acid. It is important to distinguish these conditions from true PKU so that children are not

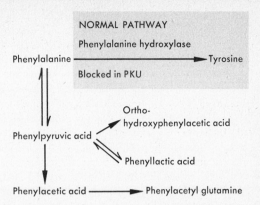

Figure 46–1. In the absence of phenylalanine hydroxylase, the normal pathway of phenylalanine to tyrosine is blocked, and a number of alternate by-products are excreted in the urine.

subjected to the phenylalanine-restricted diet unnecessarily.

Clinical changes. Mental retardation in untreated subjects is usually severe with most patients having an intelligence quotient below 50. The child appears to be normal at birth but within the first few days or weeks of life the various intermediate products of faulty phenylalanine metabolism accumulate and can be detected in the blood and urine. If treatment is not initiated promptly progressive irreversible brain damage occurs. Although the faulty phenylalanine metabolism is clearly understood as the cause of the brain damage, it is not yet known just how this change takes place.

Because of the block in tyrosine formation, the production of pigments is reduced. Consequently, these children are usually blond, blue eyed, and have a fair skin, even though their parents may be of darker skin, eye, and hair coloring. Eczema is a common finding.

The behavior of untreated children is considerably altered. They are hyperactive, wave their arms, rock back and forth, and grind their teeth. They show poor coordination, are irritable, immature, and overdependent. At times they may have seizures. Their behavior can be extremely trying even to the most loving parents.

Treatment. The successful treatment of PKU depends upon (1) early diagnosis; (2) restriction of phenylalanine intake to maintain an acceptable range of serum phenylalanine; (3) a nutritionally adequate diet adjusted from time to time to meet the requirements for normal growth and development; (4) continuing clinical and biochemical monitoring; and (5) a comprehensive program of education of the parents. Children for whom such treatment is begun within the first few weeks or months of life show apparently normal mental and physical development. The team approach is essential, including the physician, nurse, clinical chemist, social workers, dietitian, parents, and sometimes others. (See Figure 46-2.)

A delay in the initiation of the diet reduces the likelihood of satisfactory mental development. Once brain damage has occurred reversal does not take place. After three years of age, little improvement in mental development can be expected. However, even for the older child the phenylalanine-restricted diet is believed to be of some benefit in modifying the behavior characteristics.

Modification of the diet. The allowances for protein and for calories are essentially the same as those for normal children. Phenylalanine needs to be restricted but it cannot be totally eliminated from the diet since it is an essential amino acid. Proteins contain 4 to 6 per cent phenylalanine, which is excessive for the child with PKU. A commercial preparation (Lofenalac),° from which 95 per cent of the phenylalanine has been removed, is used as the source of protein. Some clinicians allow slightly more protein and calories initially since casein hydrolysate is used rather than natural protein. The allowances for protein, energy, and phenylalanine are summarized in Table 46-1.

Clinical experience has shown that a balance must be maintained between the amount of low-phenylalanine formula and the amount of natural foods that are fed.[4] The formula supplies most of the energy, protein, and other nutrients, and if inadequate amounts are fed, the amino acid and other nutritional requirements of the child will not be

° Lofenalac®, Mead Johnson & Company, Evansville, Indiana.

Figure 46-2. An important part of patient care involves adequate planning for the patient's discharge. Here the social worker shares information with the occupational therapist, nurse, physician, and dietitian. (Courtesy, University of Minnesota Health Sciences Center, Minneapolis.)

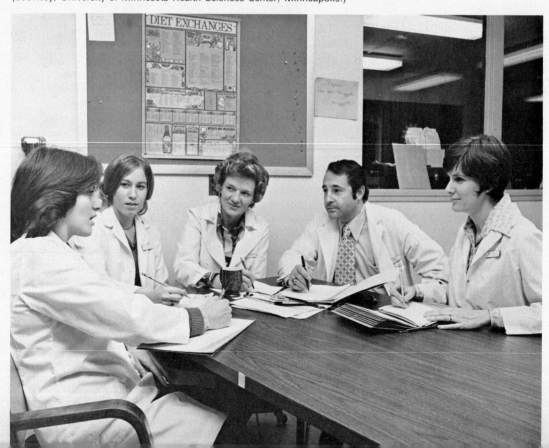

Table 46–1. Phenylalanine, Protein, and Calories Recommended for Various Age Groups of Phenylketonuric Patients*

Age	Phenylalanine mg per pound	Protein gm per pound	Kilocalories per pound
0–3 months	20–22	1.75–2.0	60–65
4–12 months	18–20	1.5	55–60
1–3 years	16–18	32 gm total	50–55
4–7 years	10–16	40 gm total	40–50

*Acosta, P. B.: "Nutritional Aspects of Phenylketonuria," in *The Clinical Team Looks at Phenylketonuria,* Revised. Children's Bureau, U.S. Department of Health, Education, and Welfare, Washington, D.C., 1964, p. 45.

met. On the other hand, if insufficient amounts of natural foods are given, the phenylalanine intake will be too low to meet growth requirements. Catabolism of tissue proteins then leads to a temporary increase in the serum phenylalanine level.

The signs of inadequate phenylalanine intake include anorexia, vomiting, listlessness, inconsistent growth or failure to grow, pallor, and skin rash.

Management of the diet. The diet is so unlike a normal diet that many problems are encountered in its administration. A skillful approach by physician, nurses, and nutritionist is required to achieve acceptance on the part of the parent as well as the child.

Considerations in planning the diet are as follows:

1. Estimate the daily protein, calorie, and phenylalanine requirements in accordance with the child's age and weight.

2. Calculate the amount of Lofenalac required to meet the protein and calorie allowances.

3. Determine amounts of other foods needed to meet the phenylalanine allowance.

Lofenalac provides the basis for this diet. Except for phenylalanine, this preparation is nutritionally complete, containing amino acids, unsaturated fat, carbohydrate, vitamins, and minerals. It is a satisfactory substitute for milk and other protein foods. Measured amounts are used to supply protein and calories for the young infant who is not yet receiving other foods, and to provide 85 per cent of the protein needs for the older child. To meet the phenylalanine requirement for the infant, from 1 to 2 ounces of milk are added to the Lofenalac formula. Milk contains about 55 mg per cent phenylalanine and should always be incorporated into the formula so that the infant does not develop a taste

for milk. The diet should be progressed as for a normal infant and child. (See Table 46–2.) Appropriate amounts of fruits, vegetables, and cereal foods are introduced as the child grows, and Lofenalac may be incorporated into these and other allowed foods. A variety of recipes have been developed for such use. Planning the diet is made easier by the use of special serving lists in which all foods within a given group provide the same amount of phenylalanine, protein, and calories when given in the specified amounts. (See Tables 46–3 and 46–4.)

The optimal age for discontinuing the diet is not known. For psychologic reasons it is usually discontinued about the time the child enters school. Follow-up studies have shown no significant deterioration in I.Q. after termination of the diet at age six.[5] Some recommend that the intake of high-biologic-value protein be limited after the diet is discontinued so that serum phenylalanine levels are not above 25 to 35 mg per cent.[6] Some phenylalanine restriction appears to be beneficial during pregnancy of the phenylketonuric woman.[7]

DIETARY COUNSELING

Eating problems are encountered frequently in the phenylketonuric children. These may be the result of great parental anxiety and feelings of guilt. The parent may overemphasize diet and allow it to dominate the relationships with the child. Initially, the acceptance of Lofenalac may be poor. If it is forced at first, or if the parent or brothers and sisters indicate dislike for the diet, the child may continue to refuse the formula. It

Table 46–2. Phenylalanine-Restricted Diets for Infants and Children*

Age	1 Month	8 Months	2 Years	4 Years
Weight, pounds	8	18	26	36
Diet prescription				
Phenylalanine, mg	160–176	324–360	416–468	360–576
Protein, gm	14–16	27	32	40
Energy, kcal	440	810	1300	1700
Lofenalac, measures†	10	18	19	23
Water to make	24 oz	32 oz	24 oz	24 oz
Milk as necessary	1½ oz	1 oz	—	—
Vegetables, servings	—	2	4	4
Fruits, servings	1	1	4	4
Breads, servings	—	3	5	4
Fats, servings	—	—	1	1
Desserts,‡ servings	—	—		1
Free foods§	—	—	As desired	As desired
Nutritive values				
Phenylalanine, mg	172	325	417	447
Protein, gm	16.8	30.4	33.1	40.6
Energy, kcal	540	944	1302	1724

*Acosta, P. B.: ''Nutritional Aspects of Phenylketonuria,'' in *The Clinical Team Looks at Phenylketonuria,* 1964. Children's Bureau, U.S. Department of Health, Education, and Welfare, Washington, D.C., p. 52.

†One measure = 1 tablespoon

‡Special recipes are required for desserts.

§If free foods are given in excessive amounts child may not consume proper amounts of other foods.

Table 46–3. Phenylalanine, Protein, and Caloric Content of Serving Lists Used on Phenylalanine-Restricted Diets*

	Phenylalanine mg	Protein gm	Kilocalories
Lofenalac, 1 measure (1 tablespoon)	7.5	1.5	43
Vegetables	15	0.3	5
Fruits	15	0.2	80
Breads	30	0.5	20
Fats	5	0.1	45
Desserts (special recipes required)	30	2.0	270
Free foods	0	0.0	varies
Milk (per ounce)	55	1.1	20

*Acosta, P. B.: ''Nutritional Aspects of Phenylketonuria,'' in *The Clinical Team Looks at Phenylketonuria,* revised. Children's Bureau, U.S. Department of Health, Education, and Welfare, 1964, p. 40.

Table 46–4. Serving Lists for Phenylalanine-Restricted Diet*

Food	Amount	Food	Amount
Vegetables—15 mg phenylalanine per serving		Cantaloupe, diced	½ cup†
Asparagus	1 stalk	Dates, dried	2
Beans, green, cooked	3 tbsp	Fruit cocktail, canned	2 tbsp
junior	2 tbsp	Grapefruit, sections or juice	⅓ cup
strained	2 tbsp	Grapes, green, seedless	20 medium
Beets, cooked	3 tbsp	Grape juice	⅓ cup
strained	2 tbsp	Guava, raw	⅓ medium
Cabbage, raw, shredded	4 tbsp	Lemon or lime juice	3 tbsp
Carrots, raw	½ large	frozen, diluted	½ cup
canned	4 tbsp	Mango	½ small
junior	3 tbsp	Orange	1 medium†
strained	3 tbsp	Papaya, cubed	¼ cup
Cauliflower	2 tbsp	juice	½ cup
Celery, raw, 5-in. stalks	2 stalks	Peach, raw	1 medium†
Cucumber, raw	⅓ medium	canned in syrup	1½ halves
Lettuce, head	2 leaves	junior	7 tbsp
Mushrooms, cooked	2 tbsp	strained	5 tbsp
Okra, pod, cooked	1 pod	Pear, raw	1⅓ medium†
Onion, green	2 medium	canned in syrup	3 halves
mature	¼ medium	junior	10 tbsp
Parsley	2 sprigs	strained	10 tbsp
Pumpkin, cooked	2 tbsp	Pear-pineapple, junior	
Radish	3 small	and strained	7 tbsp
Spinach, cooked	1 tbsp	Pineapple, raw	⅓ cup
creamed, junior and strained	2 tbsp	canned in syrup	1½ small slices
Squash, summer, cooked	4 tbsp	juice	½ cup
Squash, winter, cooked	2 tbsp	Plums, canned	1 medium
junior	6 tbsp	with tapioca, junior	7 tbsp
strained	3 tbsp	with tapioca, strained	5 tbsp
Tomato, raw	¼ small	Popsicle with fruit juice	2 medium
canned	2 tbsp	Prunes, dried	2 large†
juice	2 tbsp	juice	⅓ cup
Turnip	4 tbsp	strained	3 tbsp
Yam or sweet potato, strained	2 tbsp	Raisins, dried	2 tbsp†
		Strawberries	3 large
Fruits—15 mg phenylalanine per serving		Tangerine	⅔ small
Apple, raw	2 medium†	Watermelon	⅓ cup
Apricots, canned	2 halves		
dried, halves	4 large†	*Breads and Cereals*—30 mg phenylalanine per serving	
juice	¼ cup	Barley cereal, Gerber's dry	2 tbsp
Apricot-applesauce,		Biscuit‡	1 small
junior	10 tbsp	Cereal food, Gerber's dry	2 tbsp
strained	10 tbsp	Corn, cooked	2 tbsp
Avocado	2 tbsp	Cornflakes	⅓ cup
Banana, 6 in. long	½†	Crackers, Barnum animal	6

*Arranged from Acosta, P. B.: "Nutritional Aspects of Phenylketonuria," in *The Clinical Team Looks at Phenylketonuria,* revised 1964. Children's Bureau, U.S. Department of Health, Education, and Welfare, Washington, D.C., 1964, pp. 40–44.

†Miller, G. T., *et al.:* "Phenylalanine Content of Fruit," *J. Am. Diet. Assoc.,* **46**:43, 1965.

‡Special recipes required.

Table 46-4. (Cont.)

Food	Amount	Food
Crackers, graham	1	*Free Foods*—negligible phenylalanine; may be used
Crackers, soda	1	as desired
Crackers, saltines	2	Apple juice ⎱ Count as fruit if more than 1 cup
Cream of Rice, cooked	2 tbsp	Applesauce ⎰
Cream of Wheat, cooked	2 tbsp	Butter
Hominy	3 tbsp	Candy
Hominy grits, cooked	3 tbsp	butterscotch
Mixed cereal, Pablum, dry	3 tbsp	cream mints
Muffin, pineapple‡	2	fondant
Oatmeal, Gerber's, strained	2 tbsp	gum drops
Pablum, dry	2 tbsp	hard
Popcorn, popped	1/3 cup	jelly beans
Potato, white	2 tbsp	lollipops
Rice, cooked	2 tbsp	Cornstarch
Rice Flakes, Quaker	1/3 cup	Gingerbread‡
Rice Krispies, Kellogg's	1/3 cup	Guava butter
Rice Pablum	4 tbsp	Honey
Rice, Puffed, Quaker	1/3 cup	Jams, jellies, marmalades
Sugar Crisps	1/4 cup	Margarine
Wheat, Puffed, Quaker	1/3 cup	Molasses
Yam, sweet potato, cooked	2 tbsp	Oil
		Pepper
Fats—5 mg phenylalanine per serving		Popsicle (with fruit flavor only)
Cream, heavy	1 tsp	Rich's topping
Mayonnaise	2 tsp	Salt
Olives, ripe	1 large	Sauces: lemon‡, white‡
		Sugar, brown or white
Desserts—30 mg phenylalanine per serving		Syrups, corn, maple
Cake‡	1/2 of cake	Tapioca
Cookies—rice flour‡	2	*Foods to Avoid*—very high in phenylalanine
corn starch‡	2	Breads
Cookies, Arrowroot	1 1/2	Cheese, all kinds
Ice cream—chocolate‡	2/3 cup	Eggs
pineapple‡	2/3 cup	Flour, all kinds
strawberry‡	2/3 cup	Meat, poultry, fish
Jello	1/3 cup	Legumes (dried peas, beans and seeds)
Puddings‡	1/2 cup	Nuts; nut butters
Sauce, Hershey	2 tbsp	Milk (55 mg phenylalanine per ounce)
Wafers, sugar, Nabisco	6	except as calculated for formula

is best to offer the formula at the beginning of the feeding when the child is hungry, and to avoid any show of concern if it is not fully accepted. When parents begin to see the improvement in the child, encouragement is provided for the considerable effort needed to maintain careful vigilance in its preparation.

Both parents must receive detailed information concerning the amounts of phenylalanine permitted daily and the amounts of foods that will provide them. They should be asked to demonstrate the measurement and preparation of the formula and to plan a series of daily menus showing the phenylalanine, protein, and calorie content. The diet must be continually moni-tored. A record of the child's daily intake should be kept and brought along each time the child is seen in the PKU clinic so that the physician and nutritionist can assess the child's progress in relation to his diet. A program of home services is invaluable in assuring that the diet is being used as planned. (See Figure 46–3.) The public health nurse often supervises the home care and also consults with the dietitian or nutritionist in the planning and in problems of dietary manage-ment. Printed recipe materials should be care-fully explained to the parent.

Tyrosinosis

Hereditary TYROSINOSIS is transmitted as an auto-somal recessive gene. A deficiency of PARAHYDROXY-PHENYLPYRUVIC ACID OXIDASE places a block upon the conversion of tyrosine to homogentisic acid. Consequently, the tyrosine levels of the blood are elevated, and increased amounts of tyrosine, p-hydroxyphenylpyruvic acid, other amino acids, and phosphates are excreted in the urine.

Patients with this deficiency show extensive liver and renal damage. Abdominal distention is present because of the enlarged liver and spleen. Liver

disease may progress so rapidly that death results from liver failure. The reduced levels of blood phos-phate are associated with vitamin-D-resistant rick-ets. Mental retardation is present.

Dietary modification. A diet low in phenylala-nine and in tyrosine has been described, using a casein hydrolysate as the source of protein and calories. Limited amounts of other foods low in these two amino acids are permitted.[8]

Transient Tyrosinemia

Newborn infants sometimes have a transient form of tyrosinemia and tyrosyluria.[9] These abnormalities occur especially in premature infants and are di-rectly correlated with the level of protein intake. This appears to be a benign condition and is not associated with specific symptoms. The increased tyrosine levels in the blood and in the urine return to normal as the infant matures. The blood levels are reduced if adequate ascorbic acid is given early.

Maple Syrup Urine Disease

This inborn error of metabolism derives its name from the maple syrup odor of urine, a valuable clue in the diagnosis. The disease is also known as BRANCHED-CHAIN KETOACIDURIA, a term which

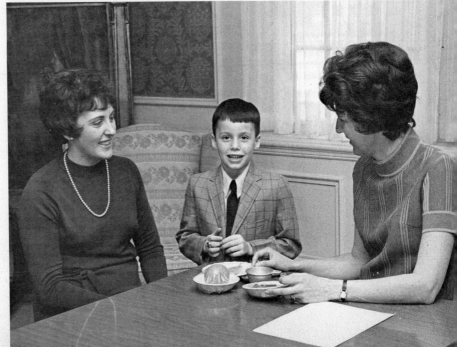

Figure 46–3. Nutritionist counsels boy with PKU and his mother about the kinds and amounts of foods that may be included in his diet. (Courtesy, Children's Reha-bilitation Center, Buffalo, New York.)

relates to the biochemical defect. It was first recognized in the United States in 1954 and since then has been described in several other countries. It is transmitted as an autosomal recessive trait. The incidence is not known.

Biochemical defect and clinical changes. Three branched-chain amino acids, namely, leucine, isoleucine, and valine, are normally metabolized to keto acids and then further degraded through decarboxylation to simple acids. In maple syrup urine disease an OXIDATIVE DECARBOXYLASE in the white blood cells is missing. Because the carboxyl group cannot be removed, the amino acids and their keto acids accumulate in the blood and are excreted in excessive amounts in the urine. A metabolite related to isoleucine is believed to be responsible for the odor of the urine and of the sweat.

Infants appear normal at birth but begin to show symptoms within the first few days. They are unable to suck and swallow satisfactorily, respiration is irregular, and there are intermittent periods of rigidity and flaccidity. Seizures of the grand mal type may occur. If the infants survive, mental retardation is severe. Hypoglycemia has been observed in several patients and may be related to leucine sensitivity. Frequent infections lead to increased tissue catabolism and thus to a further accumulation of the offending metabolites in the circulation.

Dietary treatment. A diet restricted in leucine, isoleucine, and valine has given some encouraging results.[10] After a synthetic formula has reduced the high blood levels of leucine, isoleucine, and valine together with their incompletely metabolized products, small amounts of milk are added to provide for the growth requirements of the infant. Fruits, vegetables, and cereals low in protein are added as the child grows. A gelatin base with added amino acids is used to provide nitrogen.[11] The dietary modifications are needed permanently.

HOMOCYSTINURIA

Biochemical and clinical findings. This is a disorder of methionine metabolism. The enzyme CYSTATHIONINE SYNTHETASE is essential for the conversion of homocysteine to cystathionine, both of which are intermediate products formed in the metabolism of methionine. When the enzyme is lacking, increased amounts of methionine and homocystine are found in the plasma, and large amounts of homocystine are excreted in the urine. Lack of the enzyme is an autosomal recessive trait.

HOMOCYSTINURIA occurs almost as frequently as phenylketonuria. Severe mental retardation is present in almost all patients. The optic lens is dislocated in all patients, and glaucoma and cataracts occur in some. There is a weakness of the muscles of the pelvic girdle and a shuffling gait. Skeletal abnormalities include long extremities, osteoporosis, and curvature of the spine. Pulmonary embolism, thrombosis, and cerebral accidents are common.

Dietary modification. Some patients respond to pyridoxine therapy. For these patients a normal, but not excessive, protein intake is recommended.[12] Low-methionine diets with adequate cysteine have been used for those patients who do not respond to pyridoxine therapy. Folic acid deficiency may occur in these patients.[12] Methionine exchange lists and recipes have been described.[12] Soy and gelatin are used as protein sources because of their low methionine content. Supplements of synthetic amino acids—leucine, isoleucine, phenylalanine, tryptophan, and valine—are needed to meet growth requirements. (See Table 4–2.)

LEUCINE-INDUCED HYPOGLYCEMIA

A relatively rare inborn error of metabolism, LEUCINE-INDUCED HYPOGLYCEMIA becomes apparent after about the fourth month of life. Convulsions may be the first indication of an abnormality. Infants with this disorder fail to thrive and show some evidence of delayed mental development. Signs typical of Cushing's syndrome—acne, hirsutism, obesity, and osteoporosis—are often present.

When L-leucine is given in a test dose to the infant, a profound lowering of the blood glucose occurs in the leucine-sensitive infant. The exact reason for the increased sensitivity is not known. Among the several theories suggested, the most likely one appears to be that leucine may act as a stimulus to insulin production or as an enhancement of insulin utilization.

Dietary management. A diet low in leucine is used,[13] but the minimum leucine requirement of 150 to 230 mg per kilogram must be included. Since all protein foods are sources of leucine, a restriction of this amino acid places restrictions upon the inclusion of protein-rich foods. The diet is planned to furnish the minimum requirements of protein for normal development. Fruits and vegetables are added to the diet according to the infant's normal feeding schedule. To counteract the hypoglycemic effects of the leucine, a carbohydrate feeding (equivalent to 10 gm) is given 30 to 40 minutes after each meal. By the age of five to six years the disease has run its course, and from that time on the child is able to tolerate a normal diet.

GALACTOSE DISEASE

Biochemical defect. Galactose disease is caused by the absence of an enzyme (GALACTOSE-1-PHOSPHATE URIDYL TRANSFERASE, sometimes abbreviated P-Gal-transferase) which is needed in the liver for the conversion of galactose to glucose. Galactose is derived from the hydrolysis of lactose in the intestine. It is absorbed normally in this inborn error, but in the absence of transferase, galactose, galactose-1-phosphate, and galactitol accumulate in the blood and tissues. Analysis of the red blood cells shows little or no transferase in those who have the disease, and only half the normal levels in carriers of the defect.[14] Urine tests show the presence of galactose, albumin, and amino acids. A galactose tolerance test helps to establish the diagnosis. Mothers of galactosemic infants have a diminished ability to metabolize galactose. If they drink unlimited amounts of milk during pregnancy, the possibility of damage to the fetus exists since galactose may pass the placenta.[14] The enzyme defect is inherited as an autosomal recessive trait.

Clinical changes. The disease becomes apparent within a few days after birth by such symptoms as anorexia, vomiting, occasional diarrhea, drowsiness, jaundice, puffiness of the face, edema of the lower extremities, and weight loss. The spleen and liver enlarge, and in some there may be evidences of liver failure within a short time leading to ascites, bleeding, and early death. Mental retardation becomes evident very early in the course of the disease, and cataracts develop within the first year.

Dietary treatment. Milk is the important dietary source of lactose which in turn yields galactose.

Human milk is especially high in galactose, and thus the breast-fed infant who lacks the necessary enzyme shows symptoms very early. The substitution of a nonmilk formula leads to rapid improvement as a rule. All of the symptoms disappear except that mental retardation which has already occurred is not reversible. Damage to the central nervous system is greatest during the first few weeks and months of life when growth is rapid. Therefore, the prompt initiation of therapy is essential.

A number of nonmilk formula products are available. These include Nutramigen,° ProSobee,° and Mul-Soy,† and a meat-base formula.‡ Some pediatricians do not use the soybean preparations since STACHYOSE, a tetrasaccharide in soybeans, is believed to be hydrolyzed to galactose. Others have used such formulas with success. The maintenance of a galactose-free diet is monitored by testing red blood cells for their content of galactose-1-phosphate transferase.

The formulas are supplemented with calcium gluconate or chloride, iron, and vitamins. Since milk is the only food which supplies lactose, other foods may be introduced into the infant's diet at the appropriate times. These include breads, crackers, and cereals made without milk, eggs, meat, poultry, fish, fruits, vegetables, and gelatin desserts. All foods that contain milk must be rigidly excluded: most commercial breads, cookies, cakes, puddings, pudding mixes, some ready-to-eat cereals, all cheeses, cream, ice cream, butter, margarine churned with milk, chocolate, cold cuts, and others. See the list of foods to avoid for lactose-free diets, page 458. Liver, brains, and pancreas store galactose and are usually avoided. The stachyose present in soybeans, beets, Lima beans, and peas is not hydrolyzed to free galactose; thus, limited amounts of these foods are permitted.[15]

As with phenylketonuria, dietary counseling is of paramount importance. Infants accept the substitute formulas quite well, but older children may refuse them for a time. Parents must avoid showing too much anxiety about refusal of food. They need to become thoroughly familiar with lists of foods

---

° Nutramigen® and ProSobee® by Mead Johnson & Co., Evansville, Indiana.

† Mul-Soy by the Syntex Laboratories, Palo Alto, California.

‡ Meat-base formula by Gerber Products Company, Fremont, Michigan.

that contain milk and must learn to read labels with care. The diet is successful only when repeated opportunities are available for follow-up, whether in the clinic or in the home. Such follow-up visits not only reinforce dietary instruction but provide encouragement to the parents.

Complete elimination of galactose is necessary for the very young child but breads and other prepared foods containing milk are usually permitted when the child enters school.[15] Milk must be permanently excluded from the diet, however.

FRUCTOSEMIA

Fructosemia is an inborn error in which the introduction of sucrose or fructose in the infant's diet before six months of age results in anorexia, vomiting, failure to thrive, hypoglycemic convulsions, and dysfunction of the liver and kidney.[16] Older children with the defect are often asymptomatic or they may have spontaneous hypoglycemia. When an oral dose of fructose is given, the blood fructose and magnesium levels rise, but the levels of glucose and phosphate fall. The hypoglycemia that occurs is believed to be caused by reduced glycogenolysis and gluconeogenesis.

Treatment. This condition is controlled by a diet that eliminates all sources of fructose from the diet. Most fruits contain some fructose,[17] and the intestinal hydrolysis of sucrose also yields fructose. Sorbitol is oxidized to fructose; thus, foods containing this sugar should be avoided. Glucose should be used in place of sucrose, and starches are utilized normally. For the infant a formula is calculated to meet normal requirements, using glucose as the source of carbohydrate. Unsweetened cereals, egg yolk, strained meats, and strained vegetables are added at intervals as in normal infant feeding. Sugar beets, sweet potatoes, and peas contain appreciable amounts of sucrose.[17] (See also Table 34-2.) Most patients learn to avoid sweets.

WILSON'S DISEASE

HEPATOLENTICULAR DEGENERATION, or Wilson's disease, is a hereditary disorder transmitted by an autosomal recessive gene. The characteristic defect includes low serum levels of copper and CERULO-PLASMIN, the latter a copper-containing protein of the blood. Radioisotope studies have shown that the increased deposits of copper in the brain, liver, and kidney are due to decreased biliary excretion.[18] Because of renal intoxication by the copper, there is a marked aminoaciduria and a negative phosphate balance.

Clinical findings. The onset of symptoms is correlated with the time required for sufficient copper to accumulate in the tissues to produce damage. They may appear as early as four or five years of age, or as late as the thirties. A characteristic sign is the Kayser-Fleischer ring, a greenish-brown discoloration seen in the eye. Other signs and symptoms include splenomegaly, jaundice, liver enlargement, easy bruisability, and neurologic involvement. The common neurologic signs include indistinct speech, a fixed unblinking stare, hypertonus or rigidity, tremor, seizures, and dementia.

Treatment. A chelating agent is used to increase the urinary excretion of copper. Patients are usually advised to avoid foods that are excessively high in copper such as organ meats, shellfish, mushrooms, legumes, whole-grain cereals, bran, chocolate, and nuts. The normal copper intake is about 2 to 3 mg. To establish negative copper balance, a more restricted intake is necessary, usually 1.5 mg or less.[19] For such diets, distilled water must be used if the water supply contains more than 1 ppm copper. Cooking utensils made of copper cannot be used. A paucity of data on the copper content of foods introduces difficulty in planning a diet that is reliably low in copper. Because of the presence of copper in most foods, it is difficult to maintain a sufficiently high caloric intake.

FAMILIAL HYPERCHOLESTEROLEMIA

Familial hypercholesterolemia is transmitted as an autosomal dominant trait and is said to occur in 1 of every 250 newborns. It is characterized by plasma cholesterol levels in excess of 230 mg per cent and elevated β-lipoproteins. Plasma triglyceride levels are normal. The risk of developing atherosclerotic heart disease is greatly increased in affected individuals. Attempts to delay the atherosclerotic changes by dietary intervention in young children have been reported by Tsang and colleagues.[20]

Diets containing less than 150 mg cholesterol daily and a P/S ratio of 0.9:1 are effective in lowering serum cholesterol to normal levels in hypercholesterolemic 2-to-4-year-olds.[21] See Chapter 40 for diets restricted in cholesterol.

See Chapter 34 for discussion of the following genetic errors characterized by malabsorption: lactose intolerance; invertase-isomaltase deficiency; glucose-galactose malabsorption.

Problems and Review

1. A one-month-old infant, weighing 4 kg, is diagnosed as having phenylketonuria.
   a. Why is prompt diet therapy essential for the treatment of this disorder and other errors of metabolism?
   b. What is phenylalanine? In what way is its function modified in phenylketonuria?
   c. What is Lofenalac? Why is it necessary to include some source of phenylalanine in the diet of the infant with phenylketonuria? What food source may be used?
   d. Plan a diet appropriate for this infant. Calculate the phenylalanine, protein, and calorie content of the diet.
   e. Outline the essential points to be covered in the counseling of the parents of this patient.
2. What is the principal defect in galactose disease?
   a. Examine the labels of a variety of packaged foods in a market, and prepare a list of those which contain milk.
   b. Plan a day's menu for a child with galactosemia.
   c. What points would you emphasize in counseling the parents of such a child?
3. Examine the labels of proprietary compounds such as Nutramigen, ProSobee, Mullsoy, and Lofenalac. What supplements, if any, to these formulas are needed? What is the cost of any of these formulas for one day for a three-month-old infant weighing 6 kg?
4. Why is carbohydrate given after meals to infants who are sensitive to leucine? What class of foods must be restricted when a leucine-restricted diet is used?
5. List some of the foods that would not be permitted for a patient who has Wilson's disease and who has been advised by his physician to omit foods high in copper.

Cited References

1. Garrod, A. E.: *Inborn Errors of Metabolism.* Frowde, Hodder & Stoughton, London, 1909.
2. *Phenylketonuria—Low-Phenylalanine Dietary Management with Lofenalac.*® Mead Johnson Laboratories, Evansville, Ind., 1969.
3. Patel, M. S., and Arinze, I. J.: "Phenylketonuria: Metabolic Alterations Induced by Phenylalanine and Phenylpyruvate," *Am. J. Clin. Nutr.,* **28:**183–88, 1975.
4. Sutherland, B. S., *et al.:* "Growth and Nutrition in Treated Phenylketonuric Patients," *J.A.M.A.,* **211:**270–76, 1970.
5. Johnson, C. F.: "What Is the Best Age to Discontinue the Low Phenylalanine Diet in Phenylketonuria?" *Clin. Pediatr.,* **11:**148–56, 1972.
6. Clayton, B. E.: "The Principles of Treatment by Dietary Restriction as Illustrated by Phenylketonuria," in Raine, D. N., ed.: *The Treatment of Inherited Metabolic Disease.* MTP, Medical and Technical Publishing Co. Ltd., Lancaster, Lancs, Great Britain, 1975, Chap. 1.
7. MacCready, R. A., and Levy, H. L.: "The Problem of Maternal Phenylketonuria," *Am. J. Obstet. Gynecol.,* **113:**121–27, 1972.
8. Hill, A., *et al.:* "Dietary Treatment of Tyrosinosis," *J. Am. Diet. Assoc.,* **56:**308–12, 1970.
9. Martin, H. P., *et al.:* "The Development of Children with Transient Neonatal Tyrosinemia," *J. Pediatr.,* **84:**212–16, 1974.
10. Smith, B. A., and Waisman, H. A.: "Leucine Equivalency System in Managing Branched Chain Ketoaciduria," *J. Am. Diet. Assoc.,* **59:**342–46, 1971.

11. Snyderman, S. E.: "Maple Sirup Urine Disease," in *The Treatment of Inherited Metabolic Disease,* Chap. 3. (See Reference 6.)

12. Carson, N. A. J.: "Homocystinuria," in *The Treatment of Inherited Metabolic Disease,* Chap. 2. (See Reference 6.)

13. Roth, H., and Segal, S.: "The Dietary Management of Leucine Sensitive Hypoglycemia with Report of a Case," *Pediatrics,* **34:**831–38, 1964.

14. Hansen, R. G.: "Hereditary Galactosemia," *J.A.M.A.,* **208:**2077–82, 1969.

15. Donnell, G. N., and Bergren, W. R.: "The Galactosaemias," in *The Treatment of Inherited Metabolic Disease,* Chap. 4. (See Reference 6.)

16. Froesch, E. R.: "Hereditary Fructose Intolerance and Fructose 1, 6-Diphosphatase Deficiency," in *The Treatment of Inherited Metabolic Disease,* Chap. 6. (See Reference 6.)

17. Hardinge, M. G., *et al.:* "Carbohydrates in Foods," *J. Am. Diet. Assoc.,* **46:**197–204, 1965.

18. Strickland, G. T., and Leu, M. L.: "Wilson's Disease. Clinical and Laboratory Manifestations in 40 Patients," *Medicine,* **54:**113–37, 1975.

19. Goldstein, N. P., and Owen, C. A.: "Introduction: Symposium on Copper Metabolism and Wilson's Disease," *Mayo Clin. Proc.,* **49:**363–67, 1974.

20. Tsang, R. C., *et al.:* "Neonatal Familial Hypercholesterolemia," *Am. J. Dis. Child.,* **129:**83–91, 1975.

21. Larsen, R., *et al.:* "Special Diet for Familial Type II Hyperlipoproteinemia," *Am. J. Dis. Child.,* **128:**67–72, 1974.

ADDITIONAL REFERENCES

General

Dancis, J.: "Nutritional Management of Hereditary Disorders," *Med. Clin. North Amer.,* **54:**1431–48, 1970.

Frimpter, G. W.: "Aminoacidurias Due to Inherited Disorders of Metabolism," *N. Engl. J. Med.,* **289:**835–41, 1973.

James, L. F.: "Diet-Related Birth Defects," *Nutr. Today,* **9:**4–11, July–Aug. 1974.

Scriver, C. R.: "Inborn Errors of Metabolism: A New Frontier of Nutrition," *Nutr. Today,* **9:**14–15, Sept.–Oct. 1974.

Galactosemia

Cook, J. G. H., *et al.:* "Hereditary Galactokinase Deficiency," *Arch. Dis. Child.,* **46:**465–69, 1971.

Koch, R., *et al.:* "Nutrition in the Treatment of Galactosemia," *J. Am. Diet. Assoc.,* **43:**216–22, 1963.

Monteleone, J. A., *et al.:* "Cataracts, Galactosuria, and Hypergalactosemia Due to Galactokinase Deficiency in a Child," *Am. J. Med.,* **50:**403–407, 1971.

Tedesco, T. A., *et al.:* "The Genetic Defect in Galactosemia," *N. Engl. J. Med.,* **292:**737–40, 1975.

Phenylketonuria

Ampola, M. G.: "PKU and Other Disorders of Amino Acid Metabolism," *Pediatr. Clin. North Am.,* **20:**507–36, 1973.

Berry, H. K., *et al.:* "Amino Acid Balance in the Treatment of Phenylketonuria," *J. Am. Diet. Assoc.,* **58:**210–14, 1971.

Children's Bureau: *The Clinical Team Looks at Phenylketonuria,* U.S. Department of Health, Education and Welfare, Washington, D.C., 1964.

Hunt, M. M., *et al.:* "Nutritional Management in Phenylketonuria," *Am. J. Dis. Child.,* **122:**1–6, 1971.

Koch, R., *et al.:* "Nutrition in the Treatment of Phenylketonuria," *J. Am. Diet. Assoc.,* **43:**212–15, 1963.

Other Metabolic Errors

Berry, W. R., *et al.:* "Effects of Penicillamine Therapy and Low Copper Diet in Dysarthria in Wilson's Disease (Hepatolenticular Degeneration)," *Mayo Clin. Proc.,* **49:**405–408, 1974.

Committee on Nutrition: "Childhood Diet and Coronary Heart Disease," *Pediatrics,* **49:**305–307, 1972.

Corey, J. E.: "Dietary Factors and Atherosclerosis: Prevention Should Begin Early," *J. School Health,* **44:**511–13, 1974.

Jagenburg, R., *et al.:* "Hereditary Tyrosinemia: Metabolic Studies in a Patient with Partial p-Hydroxy-phenylpyruvate Hydroxylase Activity," *J. Pediatr.,* **80:**994–1004, 1972.

Kannel, W. B., and Dawber, T. R.: "Atherosclerosis as a Pediatric Problem," *J. Pediatr.,* **80:**544–54, 1972.

Light, I. J., *et al.:* "Clinical Significance of Tyrosinemia of Prematurity," *Am. J. Dis. Child.,* **125:**243–47, 1973.

Lin-Fu, J. S.: *Maple Sirup Urine Disease.* Children's Bureau, U.S. Department of Health, Education, and Welfare, Washington, D.C., 1964.

Mellies, M., *et al.:* "Familial and Acquired Hyperlipoproteinemias in Children and Adolescents," *Postgrad. Med.,* **56:**94–100, Nov. 1974.

Menkes, H. H., *et al.:* "Relationship of Elevated Blood Tyrosine to the Ultimate Intellectual Performance of Premature Infants," *Pediatrics,* **49:**1218–24, 1972.

Perheentupa, J., *et al.:* "Hereditary Fructose Intolerance," *Acta Med. Scand. Suppl.,* **542:**65–75, 1972.

Snyder, R. D., and Robinson, A.: "Leucine-Induced Hypoglycemia," *Am. J. Dis. Child.,* **113:**566–70, 1967.

Snyderman, S. E.: "The Therapy of Maple Sirup Urine Disease," *Am. J. Dis. Child.,* **113:**68–73, 1967.

Strickland, G. T., *et al.:* "Metabolic Studies in Wilson's Disease," *Am. J. Med.,* **41:**31–40, 1971.

Appendixes

TABULAR MATERIALS

Foreword 616
Tables
A-1 Nutritive Values of the Edible Part of Foods 617
A-2 Mineral and Vitamin Content of Foods: Sodium, Potassium, Phosphorus, Magnesium, and Zinc; Folacin, Pantothenic Acid, Vitamin B_6, Vitamin B_{12}, and Vitamin E 641
A-3 Nutritive Values of Baby Foods 658
A-4 Exchange Lists for Meal Planning 660
A-5 Amino Acid Content of Selected Foods 665
A-6 Cholesterol Content of the Edible Portion of Food 670
A-7 Composition of Some Alcoholic Beverages 674
A-8 Growth Standards for Boys from Birth to Age 18 675
A-9 Growth Standards for Girls from Birth to Age 18 676
A-10 Suggested Weights for Heights for Men and Women 677
A-11 Normal Constituents of Human Blood 678
A-12 Normal Constituents of the Urine of the Adult 682
A-13 Conversions to and from Metric Measures 683
A-14 Recommended Daily Nutrient Intakes—Canada, Revised 1974 684

LIST OF AUDIOVISUAL MATERIALS 686
COMMON ABBREVIATIONS 694
GLOSSARY 695

Tabular Materials

Included in this section are seven tables of nutritive values of foods; three weight-height tables for age-sex categories; a table of Canadian Dietary Allowances; a table of conversion to and from metric measures; and two tables of blood and urine constituents.

The student should take time to review the arrangement and content of each of the tables so that he is able to refer to them rapidly and use them with skill. Probably more questions asked by the public pertain to the composition of foods than to any other aspect of nutrition. Tables of food values provide an invaluable reference source to answer such questions. Moreover, the quantitation of diets is possible only when nutritive values are known.

The uses of tables of food composition, as well as their limitations, have been described in Chapter 3. Tables A–1 and A–4 are for specific household measures of food. Other tables of nutritive values are stated for 100 gm of food. If a student, for example, wishes to determine the sodium content of 1 cup of milk, he will follow this procedure:

1 cup milk weighs 244 gm (see Table A–1)

100 gm milk contains 50 mg sodium (see Table A–2)

$$\frac{244}{100} \times 50 = 122 \text{ mg sodium in 1 cup milk}$$

TABLE A-1 EXPLANATION

Table A-1 is an alphabetic arrangement of items listed in the publication of the Consumer and Food Economics Research Division in 1970 *Nutritive Value of Foods*. A few additional items from Agriculture Handbook 8 *Composition of Foods—Raw, Processed, Prepared* are also included. The explanation provided in the bulletin for this table is reproduced here in part: °

Weight in grams—rounded to the nearest whole gram—is shown for an approximate measure of each food as it is described; if inedible parts are included in the description, both measure and weight include these parts.

The approximate measure shown for each food is in cups, ounces, pounds, some other well-known unit, or a piece of certain size. Usually, the measure shown can be calculated to larger or smaller amounts by multiplying or dividing. Because the measures are approximate (some are rounded for convenient use), calculated nutritive values for larger quantities of some food items may be less representative than those calculated for smaller quantities.

The cup measure refers to the standard measuring cup of 8 fluid ounces or ½ liquid pint. The ounce refers to ¹⁄₁₆ of a pound avoirdupois, unless fluid ounce is indicated. The weight of a fluid ounce varies according to the food measured. . . .

The values for food energy (calories) and nutrients

° Consumer and Food Economics Research Division, Agricultural Research Service: *Nutritive Value of Foods*. Home and Garden Bull. 72, U.S. Department of Agriculture, Washington, D.C., 1970.

shown in Table A-1 are the amounts present in the edible part of the item, that is, in only that portion of the weight of the item customarily eaten—corn without cob, meat without bone, potatoes without skin, European-type grapes without seeds. If additional parts are eaten—the skin of the potato, for example—amounts of some nutrients obtained will be somewhat greater than those shown.

For many of the prepared items, values have been calculated from the ingredients in typical recipes. Examples of such items are biscuits, corn muffins, oyster stew, macaroni and cheese, custard, and a number of other dessert-type items.

For toast and for vegetables, values are without fat added, either during preparation or at the table. Values for the thiamine content of toast are about 20 per cent lower than for fresh bread; it was impossible to show this loss adequately because of the small amount of thiamine present in a slice of bread. Some destruction of vitamins in vegetables, especially of ascorbic acid, may occur when foods are cut or shredded. Such losses are variable, and no deduction for these losses has been made.

For meat, values are for meat as cooked, drained, and without drippings. For many cuts, two sets of values are shown: Meat including the fat, and meat from which the fat has been trimmed off in the kitchen or on the plate.

A variety of manufactured items, such as some of the milk products, ready-to-eat breakfast cereals, imitation cream products, fruit drinks, and various mixes are included in Table A-1. Frequently these foods are fortified with one or more nutrients. If nutrients are added, this information is on the label. Values shown in this bulletin for these foods are usually based on products from several manufacturers and may differ somewhat from the values provided by any one source.

Table A–1. Nutritive Values of the Edible Part of Foods*

[Dashes in the columns for nutrients show that no suitable value could be found although there is reason to believe that a measurable amount of the nutrient may be present]

Milk, Cheese, Cream, Imitation Cream; Related Products

	Food, Approximate Measure, and Weight	(in grams) gm	Water per cent	Food Energy calories	Protein gm	Fat gm	Saturated (total) gm	Oleic gm	Linoleic gm	Carbohydrate gm	Calcium mg	Iron mg	Vitamin A Value I.U.	Thiamin mg	Riboflavin mg	Niacin mg	Ascorbic Acid mg
	Milk:																
	Fluid:																
1	Whole, 3.5% fat	1 cup	244	87	160	9	9	5	3	Trace	12	288	0.1	350	0.07	0.41	0.2	2
2	Nonfat (skim)	1 cup	245	90	90	9	Trace	—	—	—	12	296	0.1	10	0.09	0.44	0.2	2
3	Partly skimmed, 2% nonfat milk solids added	1 cup	246	87	145	10	5	3	2	Trace	15	352	0.1	200	0.10	0.52	0.2	2
	Canned, concentrated, undiluted:																
4	Evaporated, unsweetened	1 cup	252	74	345	18	20	11	7	1	24	635	0.3	810	0.10	0.86	0.5	3
5	Condensed, sweetened	1 cup	306	27	980	25	27	15	9	1	166	802	0.3	1,100	0.24	1.16	0.6	3
	Dry, nonfat instant:																
6	Low-density (1 1/3 cups needed for reconstitution to 1 qt)	1 cup	68	4	245	24	Trace	—	—	—	35	879	0.4	120	0.24	1.21	0.6	5
7	High-density (7/8 cup needed for reconstitution to 1 qt)	1 cup	104	4	375	37	1	—	—	—	54	1,345	0.6	130	0.36	1.85	0.9	7
	Buttermilk:																
8	Fluid, cultured, made from skim milk	1 cup	245	90	90	9	Trace	—	—	—	12	296	0.1	10	0.10	0.44	0.2	2
9	Dried, packaged	1 cup	120	3	465	41	6	3	2	Trace	60	1,498	0.7	260	0.31	2.06	1.1	—
	Cheese:																
	Natural:																
	Blue or Roquefort type:																
10	Ounce	1 oz.	28	40	105	6	9	5	3	Trace	1	89	0.1	350	0.01	0.17	0.3	0
11	Cubic inch	1 cu. in.	17	40	65	4	5	3	2	Trace	Trace	54	0.1	210	0.01	0.11	0.2	0
12	Camembert, packaged in 4-oz pkg. with 3 wedges per pkg.	1 wedge	38	52	115	7	9	5	3	Trace	1	40	0.2	380	0.02	0.29	0.3	0
	Cheddar:																
13	Ounce	1 oz	28	37	115	7	9	5	3	Trace	1	213	0.3	370	0.01	0.13	Trace	0
14	Cubic inch	1 cu in	17	37	70	4	6	3	2	Trace	Trace	129	0.2	230	0.01	0.08	Trace	0
	Cottage, large or small curd:																
	Creamed:																
15	Package of 12 oz, net wt.	1 pkg	340	78	360	46	14	8	5	Trace	10	320	1.0	580	0.10	0.85	0.3	0
16	Cup, curd pressed down	1 cup	245	78	260	33	10	6	3	Trace	7	230	0.7	420	0.07	0.61	0.2	0
	Uncreamed:																
17	Package of 12 oz net wt.	1 pkg	340	79	290	58	1	1	Trace	Trace	9	306	1.4	30	0.10	0.95	0.3	0
18	Cup, curd pressed down	1 cup	200	79	170	34	1	Trace	Trace	Trace	5	180	0.8	20	0.06	0.56	0.2	0

	Cream:																	
19	Package of 8 oz, net wt.	1 pkg	227	51	850	18	86	48	28	3	5	141	0.5	3,500	0.05	0.54	0.2	0
20	Package of 3 oz, net wt.	1 pkg	85	51	320	7	32	18	11	1	2	53	0.2	1,310	0.02	0.20	0.1	0
21	Cubic inch	1 cu in	16	51	60	1	6	3	2	Trace	Trace	10	Trace	250	Trace	0.04	Trace	0
	Parmesan, grated:																	
22	Cup, pressed down	1 cup	140	17	655	60	43	24	14	1	5	1,893	0.7	1,760	0.03	1.22	0.3	0
23	Tablespoon	1 tbsp	5	17	25	2	2	1	Trace	Trace	Trace	68	Trace	60	Trace	0.04	Trace	0
24	Ounce	1 oz	28	17	130	12	9	5	3	Trace	1	383	0.1	360	0.01	0.25	0.1	0
	Swiss:																	
25	Ounce	1 oz	28	39	105	8	8	4	3	Trace	1	262	0.3	320	Trace	0.11	Trace	0
26	Cubic inch	1 cu in	15	39	55	4	4	2	1	Trace	Trace	139	0.1	170	Trace	0.06	Trace	0
	Pasteurized processed cheese:																	
	American:																	
27	Ounce	1 oz	28	40	105	7	9	5	3	Trace	1	198	0.3	350	0.01	0.12	Trace	0
28	Cubic inch	1 cu in	18	40	65	4	5	3	2	Trace	Trace	122	0.2	210	Trace	0.07	Trace	0
	Swiss:																	
29	Ounce	1 oz	28	40	100	8	8	4	3	Trace	1	251	0.3	310	Trace	0.11	Trace	0
30	Cubic inch	1 cu in	18	40	65	5	5	3	2	Trace	Trace	159	0.2	200	Trace	0.07	Trace	0
	Pasteurized process cheese food, American:																	
31	Tablespoon	1 tbsp	14	43	45	3	3	2	1	Trace	1	80	0.1	140	Trace	0.08	Trace	0
32	Cubic inch	1 cu in	18	43	60	4	4	2	1	Trace	1	100	0.1	170	Trace	0.10	Trace	0
33	Pasteurized process cheese spread, American	1 oz	28	49	80	5	6	3	2	Trace	2	160	0.2	250	Trace	0.15	Trace	0
	Cream:																	
34	Half-and-half (cream and milk)	1 cup	242	80	325	8	28	15	9	1	11	261	0.1	1,160	0.07	0.39	0.1	2
35		1 tbsp	15	80	20	1	2	1	1	Trace	1	16	Trace	70	Trace	0.02	Trace	Trace
36	Light, coffee or table	1 cup	240	72	505	7	49	27	16	1	10	245	0.1	2,020	0.07	0.36	0.1	2
		1 tbsp	15	72	30	1	3	2	1	Trace	1	15	Trace	130	Trace	0.02	Trace	Trace
38	Sour	1 cup	230	72	485	7	47	26	16	1	10	235	0.1	1,930	0.07	0.35	0.1	2
		1 tbsp	12	72	25	Trace	2	1	1	Trace	1	12	Trace	100	Trace	0.02	Trace	Trace
40	Whipped topping (pressurized)	1 cup	60	62	155	2	14	8	5	Trace	6	67	—	570	—	0.04	—	—
		1 tbsp	3	62	10	Trace	1	Trace	Trace	Trace	Trace	3	—	30	—	Trace	—	—
	Whipping, unwhipped (volume about double when whipped):																	
42	Light	1 cup	239	62	715	6	75	41	25	2	9	203	0.1	3,060	0.05	0.29	0.1	2
43		1 tbsp	15	62	45	Trace	5	3	2	Trace	1	13	Trace	190	Trace	0.02	Trace	Trace
44	Heavy	1 cup	238	57	840	5	90	50	30	3	7	179	0.1	3,670	0.05	0.26	0.1	2
45		1 tbsp	15	57	55	Trace	6	3	2	Trace	1	11	Trace	230	Trace	0.02	Trace	Trace
	Imitation cream products (made with vegetable fat):																	
	Creamers:																	
46	Powdered	1 cup	94	2	505	4	33	31	1	0	52	21	0.6	[2]200	—	—	Trace	—
47		1 tsp	2	2	10	Trace	1	Trace	Trace	0	1	1	Trace	[2]Trace	—	—	—	—
48	Liquid (frozen)	1 cup	245	77	345	3	27	25	1	0	25	29	—	[2]100	0	0	—	—
49		1 tbsp	15	77	20	Trace	2	1	Trace	0	2	2	—	[2]10	0	0	—	—
50	Sour dressing (imitation sour cream) made with nonfat dry milk	1 cup	235	72	440	9	38	35	1	Trace	17	277	0.1	10	0.07	0.38	0.2	1
51		1 tbsp	12	72	20	Trace	2	2	Trace	Trace	1	14	Trace	Trace	Trace	Trace	Trace	Trace
	Whipped topping:																	
52	Pressurized	1 cup	70	61	190	1	17	15	1	0	9	5	—	[2]340	—	0	—	—
53		1 tbsp	4	61	10	Trace	1	1	Trace	0	Trace	Trace	—	[2]20	—	0	—	—

**Nutritive Value of Foods*, Home and Garden Bulletin No. 72. U.S. Department of Agriculture, Washington, D.C., 1970.

[1]Value applies to unfortified product; value for fortified low-density product would be 1500 I.U. and the fortified high-density product would be 2290 I.U.

[2]Contributed largely from beta-carotene used for coloring.

Table A–1. (Cont.)

	Food, Approximate Measure, and Weight (in grams)	Measure	Weight gm	Water per cent	Food Energy calories	Protein gm	Fat gm	Fatty Acids Saturated (total) gm	Unsaturated Oleic gm	Unsaturated Linoleic gm	Carbohydrate gm	Calcium mg	Iron mg	Vitamin A Value I.U.	Thiamin mg	Riboflavin mg	Niacin mg	Ascorbic Acid mg
	Whipped topping (cont.)																	
54	Frozen	1 cup	75	52	230	1	20	18	Trace	0	15	5	—	2560	—	0	—	—
55		1 tbsp	4	52	10	Trace	1	1	Trace	0	1	Trace	—	230	—	0	—	—
56	Powdered, made with whole milk	1 cup	75	58	175	3	12	10	1	Trace	15	62	Trace	2330	0.02	0.08	0.1	Trace
57		1 tbsp	4	58	10	Trace	1	1	Trace	Trace	1	3	Trace	220	Trace	Trace	Trace	Trace
	Milk beverages:																	
58	Cocoa, homemade	1 cup	250	79	245	10	12	7	4	Trace	27	295	1.0	400	0.10	0.45	0.5	3
59	Chocolate-flavored drink made with skim milk and 2% added butterfat	1 cup	250	83	190	8	6	3	2	Trace	27	270	0.5	210	0.10	0.40	0.3	3
	Malted milk:																	
60	Dry powder, approx. 3 heaping teaspoons per ounce	1 oz	28	3	115	4	2	—	—	—	20	82	0.6	290	0.09	0.15	0.1	0
61	Beverage	1 cup	235	78	245	11	10	—	—	—	28	317	0.7	590	0.14	0.49	0.2	2
	Milk desserts:																	
62	Custard	1 cup	265	77	305	14	15	7	5	1	29	297	1.1	930	0.11	0.50	0.3	1
	Ice cream:																	
63	Regular (approx. 10% fat)	1/2 gal	1,064	63	2,055	48	113	62	37	3	221	1,553	0.5	4,680	0.43	2.23	1.1	11
64		1 cup	133	63	255	6	14	8	5	Trace	28	194	0.1	590	0.05	0.28	0.1	1
65		3-fl-oz cup	50	63	95	2	5	3	2	Trace	10	73	Trace	220	0.02	0.11	0.1	1
66	Rich (approx. 16% fat)	1/2 gal	1,188	63	2,635	31	191	105	63	6	214	927	0.2	7,840	0.24	1.31	1.2	12
67		1 cup	148	63	330	4	24	13	8	1	27	115	Trace	980	0.03	0.16	0.1	1
	Ice milk:																	
68	Hardened	1/2 gal	1,048	67	1,595	50	53	29	17	2	235	1,635	1.0	2,200	0.52	2.31	1.0	10
69		1 cup	131	67	200	6	7	4	2	Trace	29	204	0.1	280	0.07	0.29	0.1	1
70	Soft-serve	1 cup	175	67	265	8	9	5	3	Trace	39	273	0.2	370	0.09	0.39	0.2	2
	Yoghurt:																	
71	Made from partially skimmed milk	1 cup	245	89	125	8	4	2	1	Trace	13	294	0.1	170	0.10	0.44	0.2	2
72	Made from whole milk	1 cup	245	88	150	7	8	5	3	Trace	12	272	0.1	340	0.07	0.39	0.2	2
	Eggs																	
	Eggs, large, 24 ounces per dozen: Raw or cooked in shell or with nothing added:																	
73	Whole, without shell	1 egg	50	74	80	6	6	2	3	Trace	Trace	27	1.1	590	0.05	0.15	Trace	0
74	White of egg	1 white	33	88	15	4	Trace	—	—	—	Trace	3	Trace	0	Trace	0.09	Trace	0
75	Yolk of egg	1 yolk	17	51	60	3	5	2	2	Trace	Trace	24	0.9	580	0.04	0.07	Trace	0
76	Scrambled with milk and fat	1 egg	64	72	110	7	8	3	3	Trace	1	51	1.1	690	0.05	0.18	Trace	0
	Meat, Poultry, Fish, Shellfish; Related Products																	
77	Bacon (20 slices per lb raw), broiled or fried crisp	2 slices	15	8	90	5	8	3	4	1	1	2	0.5	0	0.08	0.05	0.8	—
	Beef,[3] cooked: Cuts braised, simmered, or pot-roasted:																	
78	Lean and fat	3 ounces	85	53	245	23	16	8	7	Trace	0	10	2.9	30	0.04	0.18	3.5	—

No.	Item	Amount																
79	Lean only	2.5 ounces	72	62	140	22	5	2	2	Trace	0	10	2.7	10	0.04	0.16	3.3	—
	Hamburger (ground beef), broiled:																	
80	Lean	3 ounces	85	60	185	23	10	5	4	Trace	0	10	3.0	20	0.08	0.20	5.1	—
81	Regular	3 ounces	85	54	245	21	17	8	8	Trace	0	9	2.7	30	0.07	0.18	4.6	—
	Roast, oven-cooked, no liquid added:																	
	Relatively fat, such as rib:																	
82	Lean and fat	3 ounces	85	40	375	17	34	16	15	1	0	8	2.2	70	0.05	0.13	3.1	—
83	Lean only	1.8 ounces	51	57	125	14	7	3	3	Trace	0	6	1.8	10	0.04	0.11	2.6	—
	Relatively lean, such as heel of round:																	
84	Lean and fat	3 ounces	85	62	165	25	7	3	3	Trace	0	11	3.2	10	0.06	0.19	4.5	—
85	Lean only	2.7 ounces	78	65	125	24	3	1	1	Trace	0	10	3.0	Trace	0.06	0.18	4.3	—
	Steak, broiled:																	
	Relatively fat, such as sirloin:																	
86	Lean and fat	3 ounces	85	44	330	20	27	13	12	1	0	9	2.5	50	0.05	0.16	4.0	—
87	Lean only	2.0 ounces	56	59	115	18	4	2	2	Trace	0	7	2.2	10	0.05	0.14	3.6	—
	Relatively lean, such as round:																	
88	Lean and fat	3 ounces	85	55	220	24	13	6	6	Trace	0	10	3.0	20	0.07	0.19	4.8	—
89	Lean only	2.4 ounces	68	61	130	21	4	2	2	Trace	0	9	2.5	10	0.06	0.16	4.1	—
	Beef, canned:																	
90	Corned beef	3 ounces	85	59	185	22	10	5	4	Trace	0	17	3.7	20	0.01	0.20	2.9	—
91	Corned beef hash	3 ounces	85	67	155	7	10	5	4	Trace	9	11	1.7	—	0.01	0.08	1.8	—
92	Beef, dried or chipped	2 ounces	57	48	115	19	4	2	2	Trace	0	11	2.9	—	0.04	0.18	2.2	—
93	Beef and vegetable stew	1 cup	235	82	210	15	10	5	4	Trace	15	28	2.8	2,310	0.13	0.17	4.4	15
94	Beef potpie, baked, 4 1/4-inch diam., weight before baking about 8 ounces	1 pie	227	55	560	23	33	9	20	2	43	32	4.1	1,860	0.25	0.27	4.5	7
	Chicken, cooked:																	
95	Flesh only, broiled	3 ounces	85	71	115	20	3	1	1	1	0	8	1.4	80	0.05	0.16	7.4	—
	Breast, fried, 1/2 breast:																	
96	With bone	3.3 ounces	94	58	155	25	5	1	2	1	1	9	1.3	70	0.04	0.17	11.2	—
97	Flesh and skin only	2.7 ounces	76	58	155	25	5	1	2	1	1	9	1.3	70	0.04	0.17	11.2	—
	Drumstick, fried:																	
98	With bone	2.1 ounces	59	55	90	12	4	1	2	1	Trace	6	0.9	50	0.03	0.15	2.7	—
99	Flesh and skin only	1.3 ounces	38	55	90	12	4	1	2	1	Trace	6	0.9	50	0.03	0.15	2.7	—
100	Chicken, canned, boneless	3 ounces	85	65	170	18	10	3	4	3	0	18	1.3	200	0.03	0.11	3.7	3
101	Chicken potpie, baked 4 1/4-inch diam., weight before baking about 8 ounces	1 pie	227	57	535	23	31	10	15	3	42	68	3.0	3,020	0.25	0.26	4.1	5
	Chili con carne, canned:																	
102	With beans	1 cup	250	72	335	19	15	7	7	Trace	30	80	4.2	150	0.08	0.18	3.2	—
103	Without beans	1 cup	255	67	510	26	38	18	17	1	15	97	3.6	380	0.05	0.31	5.6	—
104	Heart, beef, lean, braised	3 ounces	85	61	160	27	5	—	—	—	1	5	5.0	20	0.21	1.04	6.5	1
	Lamb[3] cooked:																	
105	Chop, thick, with bone, broiled	1 chop 4.8 ounces	137	47	400	25	33	18	12	1	0	10	1.5	—	0.14	0.25	5.6	—
106	Lean and fat	4.0 ounces	112	47	400	25	33	18	12	1	0	10	1.5	—	0.14	0.25	5.6	—
107	Lean only	2.6 ounces	74	62	140	21	6	3	2	Trace	0	9	1.5	—	0.11	0.20	4.5	—
	Leg, roasted:																	
108	Lean and fat	3 ounces	85	54	235	22	16	9	6	Trace	0	9	1.4	—	0.13	0.23	4.7	—
109	Lean only	2.5 ounces	71	62	130	20	5	3	3	Trace	0	9	1.4	—	0.12	0.21	4.4	—
	Shoulder, roasted:																	
110	Lean and fat	3 ounces	85	50	285	18	23	13	8	Trace	0	9	1.0	—	0.11	0.20	4.0	—
111	Lean only	2.3 ounces	64	61	130	17	6	3	2	Trace	0	8	1.0	—	0.10	0.18	3.7	—
112	Liver, beef, fried	2 ounces	57	57	130	15	6	—	—	—	3	6	5.0	30,280	0.15	2.37	9.4	15

[2]Contributed largely from beta-carotene used for coloring.

[3]Outer layer of fat on the cut was removed to within approximately 1/2-inch of the lean. Deposits of fat within the cut were not removed.

Table A–1. (Cont.)

	Food, Approximate Measure, and Weight	Weight gm	Water per cent	Food Energy calories	Protein gm	Fat gm	Fatty Acids Saturated (total) gm	Unsaturated Oleic gm	Unsaturated Linoleic gm	Carbohydrate gm	Calcium mg	Iron mg	Vitamin A Value I.U.	Thiamin mg	Riboflavin mg	Niacin mg	Ascorbic Acid mg
	Pork, cured, cooked:																
113	Ham, light cure, lean and fat, roasted	3 ounces	85	54	245	18	19	7	8	2	0	8	2.2	0	0.40	0.16	3.1	—
	Luncheon meat:																
114	Boiled ham, sliced	2 ounces	57	59	135	11	10	4	4	1	0	6	1.6	0	0.25	0.09	1.5	—
115	Canned, spiced or unspiced	2 ounces	57	55	165	8	14	5	6	1	1	5	1.2	0	0.18	0.12	1.6	—
	Pork, fresh,[3] cooked:																
116	Chop, thick, with bone	1 chop, 3.5 ounces	98	42	260	16	21	8	9	2	0	8	2.2	0	0.63	0.18	3.8	—
117	Lean and fat	2.3 ounces	66	42	260	16	21	8	9	2	0	8	2.2	0	0.63	0.18	3.8	—
118	Lean only	1.7 ounces	48	53	130	15	7	2	3	1	0	7	1.9	0	0.54	0.16	3.3	—
	Roast, oven-cooked, no liquid added:																
119	Lean and fat	3 ounces	85	46	310	21	24	9	10	2	0	9	2.7	0	0.78	0.22	4.7	—
120	Lean only	2.4 ounces	68	55	175	20	10	3	4	1	0	9	2.6	0	0.73	0.21	4.4	—
	Cuts, simmered:																
121	Lean and fat	3 ounces	85	46	320	20	26	9	11	2	0	8	2.5	0	0.46	0.21	4.1	—
122	Lean only	2.2 ounces	63	60	135	18	6	2	3	1	0	8	2.3	0	0.42	0.19	3.7	—
	Sausage:																
123	Bologna, slice, 3-in diam. by 1/8 inch	2 slices	26	56	80	3	7	—	—	—	Trace	2	0.5	—	0.04	0.06	0.7	—
124	Braunschweiger, slice 2-in diam. by 1/4 inch	2 slices	20	53	65	3	5	—	—	—	Trace	2	1.2	1,310	0.03	0.29	1.6	—
125	Deviled ham, canned	1 tbsp	13	51	45	2	4	2	2	Trace	0	1	0.3	—	0.02	0.01	0.2	—
126	Frankfurter, heated (8 per lb purchased pkg)	1 frank	56	57	170	7	15	—	—	—	1	3	0.8	—	0.08	0.11	1.4	—
127	Pork links, cooked (16 links per lb raw)	2 links	26	35	125	5	11	4	5	1	Trace	2	0.6	0	0.21	0.09	1.0	—
128	Salami, dry type	1 oz	28	30	130	7	11	—	—	—	Trace	4	1.0	—	0.10	0.07	1.5	—
129	Salami, cooked	1 oz	28	51	90	5	7	—	—	—	Trace	3	0.7	—	0.07	0.07	1.2	—
130	Vienna, canned (7 sausages per 5-oz can)	1 sausage	16	63	40	2	3	—	—	—	Trace	1	0.3	—	0.01	0.02	0.4	—
	Veal, medium fat, cooked, bone removed:																
131	Cutlet	3 oz	85	60	185	23	9	5	4	Trace	0	9	2.7	—	0.06	0.21	4.6	—
132	Roast	3 oz	85	55	230	23	14	7	6	Trace	0	10	2.9	—	0.11	0.26	6.6	—
	Fish and shellfish:																
133	Bluefish, baked with table fat	3 oz	85	68	135	22	4	—	—	—	0	25	0.6	40	0.09	0.08	1.6	—
	Clams:																
134	Raw, meat only	3 oz	85	82	65	11	1	—	—	—	2	59	5.2	90	0.08	0.15	1.1	8
135	Canned, solids and liquid	3 oz	85	86	45	7	1	—	—	—	2	47	3.5	—	0.01	0.09	0.9	—
136	Crabmeat, canned	3 oz	85	77	85	15	2	—	—	—	1	38	0.7	—	0.07	0.07	1.6	—
137	Fish sticks, breaded, cooked, frozen; stick 3 3/4 by 1 by 1/2 inch	10 sticks or 8 oz pkg.	227	66	400	38	20	5	4	10	15	25	0.9	—	0.09	0.16	3.6	—
138	Haddock, breaded, fried	3 oz	85	66	140	17	5	1	3	Trace	5	34	1.0	—	0.03	0.06	2.7	2
139	Ocean perch, breaded, fried	3 oz	85	59	195	16	11	—	—	—	6	28	1.1	—	0.08	0.09	1.5	—
140	Oysters, raw, meat only (13–19 med. selects)	1 cup	240	85	160	20	4	—	—	—	8	226	13.2	740	0.33	0.43	6.0	—

Mature Dry Beans and Peas, Nuts, Peanuts; Related Products

Vegetables and Vegetable Products

No.	Food	Measure	Grams	Water (%)	Food energy (cal)	Protein (g)	Fat (g)	Saturated (g)	Oleic (g)	Linoleic (g)	Carbohydrate (g)	Calcium (mg)	Iron (mg)	Vitamin A (I.U.)	Thiamin (mg)	Riboflavin (mg)	Niacin (mg)	Ascorbic acid (mg)
141	Salmon, pink, canned	3 oz	85	71	120	17	5	1	1	Trace	0	[4]167	0.7	60	0.03	0.16	6.8	—
142	Sardines, Atlantic, canned in oil, drained solids	3 oz	85	62	175	20	9	—	—	—	0	372	2.5	190	0.02	0.17	4.6	—
143	Shad, baked with table fat and bacon	3 oz	85	64	170	20	10	—	—	—	0	20	0.5	20	0.11	0.22	7.3	—
144	Shrimp, canned, meat	3 oz	85	70	100	21	1	—	—	—	1	98	2.6	50	0.01	0.03	1.5	—
145	Swordfish, broiled with butter or margarine	3 oz	85	65	150	24	5	—	—	—	0	23	1.1	1,750	0.03	0.04	9.3	—
146	Tuna, canned in oil, drained solids	3 oz	85	61	170	24	7	2	1	1	0	7	1.6	70	0.04	0.10	10.1	—
147	Almonds, shelled, whole kernels	1 cup	142	5	850	26	77	6	52	15	28	332	6.7	0	0.34	1.31	5.0	Trace
	Beans, dry:																	
	Common varieties as Great Northern, navy and others:																	
	Cooked, drained:																	
148	Great Northern	1 cup	180	69	210	14	1	—	—	—	38	90	4.9	0	0.25	0.13	1.3	0
149	Navy (pea)	1 cup	190	69	225	15	1	—	—	—	40	95	5.1	0	0.27	0.13	1.3	0
	Canned, solids and liquid:																	
	White with—																	
150	Frankfurters (sliced)	1 cup	255	71	365	19	18	—	—	—	32	94	4.8	330	0.18	0.15	3.3	Trace
151	Pork and tomato sauce	1 cup	255	71	310	16	7	1	3	1	49	138	4.6	330	0.20	0.08	1.5	5
152	Pork and sweet sauce	1 cup	255	66	385	16	12	4	5	1	54	161	5.9	—	0.15	0.10	1.3	—
153	Red kidney	1 cup	255	76	230	15	1	—	1	1	42	74	4.6	10	0.13	0.10	1.5	—
154	Lima, cooked, drained	1 cup	190	64	260	16	1	—	1	—	49	55	5.9	—	0.25	0.11	1.3	—
155	Cashew nuts, roasted	1 cup	140	5	785	24	64	11	45	4	41	53	5.3	140	0.60	0.35	2.5	—
	Coconut, fresh, meat only:																	
156	Pieces, approx. 2 by 2 by 1/2 inch	1 piece	45	51	155	2	16	14	1	Trace	4	6	0.8	0	0.02	0.01	0.2	1
157	Shredded or grated, firmly packed	1 cup	130	51	450	5	46	39	3	Trace	12	17	2.2	0	0.07	0.03	0.7	4
158	Cowpeas or blackeye peas, dry, cooked	1 cup	248	80	190	13	1	—	—	—	34	42	3.2	20	0.41	0.11	1.1	Trace
159	Peanuts, roasted, salted, halves	1 cup	144	2	840	37	72	16	31	21	27	107	3.0	—	0.46	0.19	24.7	0
160	Peanut butter	1 tbsp	16	2	95	4	8	2	4	2	3	9	0.3	—	0.02	0.02	2.4	0
161	Peas, split, dry, cooked	1 cup	250	70	290	20	1	—	—	—	52	28	4.2	100	0.37	0.22	2.2	—
162	Pecans, halves	1 cup	108	3	740	10	77	5	48	15	16	79	2.6	140	0.93	0.14	1.0	2
163	Walnuts, black or native, chopped	1 cup	126	3	790	26	75	4	26	36	19	Trace	7.6	380	0.28	0.14	0.9	—
	Asparagus, green:																	
	Cooked, drained:																	
164	Spears, 1/2-in. diam. at base	4 spears	60	94	10	1	Trace	—	—	—	2	13	0.4	540	0.10	0.11	0.8	16
165	Pieces, 1 1/2 to 2-in. lengths	1 cup	145	94	30	3	Trace	—	—	—	5	30	0.9	1,310	0.23	0.26	2.0	38
166	Canned, solids and liquid	1 cup	244	94	45	5	1	—	—	—	7	44	4.1	1,240	0.15	0.22	2.0	37

[3] Outer layer of fat on the cut was removed to within approximately 1/2-inch of the lean. Deposits of fat within the cut were not removed.

[4] If bones are discarded, value will be greatly reduced.

Table A–1. (Cont.)

	Food, Approximate Measure, and Weight (in grams)		Water per cent	Food Energy calories	Protein gm	Fat gm	Fatty Acids Saturated (total) gm	Unsaturated Oleic gm	Unsaturated Linoleic gm	Carbohydrate gm	Calcium mg	Iron mg	Vitamin A Value I.U.	Thiamin mg	Riboflavin mg	Niacin mg	Ascorbic Acid mg
		gm															
	Beans:																
167	Lima, immature seeds, cooked, drained	1 cup	170	71	190	13	1	—	—	—	34	80	4.3	480	0.31	0.17	2.2	29
	Snap:																
	Green:																
168	Cooked, drained	1 cup	125	92	30	2	Trace	—	—	—	7	63	0.8	680	0.09	0.11	0.6	15
169	Canned, solids and liquid	1 cup	239	94	45	2	Trace	—	—	—	10	81	2.9	690	0.07	0.10	0.7	10
	Yellow or wax:																
170	Cooked, drained	1 cup	125	93	30	2	Trace	—	—	—	6	63	0.8	290	0.09	0.11	0.6	16
171	Canned, solids and liquid	1 cup	239	94	45	2	1	—	—	—	10	81	2.9	140	0.07	0.10	0.7	12
172	Sprouted mung beans, cooked, drained	1 cup	125	91	35	4	Trace	—	—	—	7	21	1.1	30	0.11	0.13	0.9	8
	Beets:																
	Cooked, drained, peeled:																
173	Whole beets, 2-in. diam.	2 beets	100	91	30	1	Trace	—	—	—	7	14	0.5	20	0.03	0.04	0.3	6
174	Diced or sliced	1 cup	170	91	55	2	Trace	—	—	—	12	24	0.9	30	0.05	0.07	0.5	10
175	Canned, solids and liquid	1 cup	246	90	85	2	Trace	—	—	—	19	34	1.5	20	0.02	0.05	0.2	7
176	Beet greens, leaves and stems, cooked, drained	1 cup	145	94	25	3	Trace	—	—	—	5	144	2.8	7,400	0.10	0.22	0.4	22
	Blackeye peas. See Cowpeas																
	Broccoli, cooked, drained:																
177	Whole stalks, medium size	1 stalk	180	91	45	6	1	—	—	—	8	158	1.4	4,500	0.16	0.36	1.4	162
178	Stalks cut into 1/2-in pieces	1 cup	155	91	40	5	1	—	—	—	7	136	1.2	3,880	0.14	0.31	1.2	140
179	Chopped, yield from 10-oz frozen pkg	1 3/8 cups	250	92	65	7	1	—	—	—	12	135	1.8	6,500	0.15	0.30	1.3	143
180	Brussels sprouts, 7–8 sprouts (1 1/4 to 1 1/2 in diam.) per cup, cooked	1 cup	155	88	55	7	1	—	—	—	10	50	1.7	810	0.12	0.22	1.2	135
	Cabbage:																
	Common varieties:																
	Raw:																
181	Coarsely shredded or sliced	1 cup	70	92	15	1	Trace	—	—	—	4	34	0.3	90	0.04	0.04	0.2	33
182	Finely shredded or chopped	1 cup	90	92	20	1	Trace	—	—	—	5	44	0.4	120	0.05	0.05	0.3	42
183	Cooked	1 cup	145	94	30	2	Trace	—	—	—	6	64	0.4	190	0.06	0.06	0.4	48
184	Red, raw, coarsely shredded	1 cup	70	90	20	1	Trace	—	—	—	5	29	0.6	30	0.06	0.04	0.3	43
185	Savoy, raw, coarsely shredded	1 cup	70	92	15	2	Trace	—	—	—	3	47	0.6	140	0.04	0.06	0.2	39
186	Cabbage, celery or Chinese raw, cut in 1-in pieces	1 cup	75	95	10	1	Trace	—	—	—	2	32	0.5	110	0.04	0.03	0.5	19
187	Cabbage, spoon (or pakchoy), cooked	1 cup	170	95	25	2	Trace	—	—	—	4	252	1.0	5,270	0.07	0.14	1.2	26
	Carrots:																
	Raw:																
188	Whole, 5 1/2 by 1 inch, (25 thin strips)	1 carrot	50	88	20	1	Trace	—	—	—	5	18	0.4	5,500	0.03	0.03	0.3	4

No.	Food, approximate measure	Measure	Grams	Water (%)	Food energy (cal.)	Protein (g)	Fat (g)	Saturated	Oleic	Linoleic	Carbohydrate (g)	Calcium (mg)	Iron (mg)	Vitamin A (I.U.)	Thiamin (mg)	Riboflavin (mg)	Niacin (mg)	Ascorbic acid (mg)
189	Grated	1 cup	110	88	45	1	Trace	—	—	—	11	41	0.8	12,100	0.06	0.06	0.7	9
190	Cooked, diced	1 cup	145	91	45	1	Trace	—	—	—	10	48	0.9	15,220	0.08	0.07	0.7	9
191	Canned, strained or chopped (baby food)	1 ounce	28	92	10	Trace	Trace	—	—	—	2	7	0.1	3,690	0.01	0.01	0.1	1
192	Cauliflower, cooked, flower-buds	1 cup	120	93	25	3	Trace	—	—	—	5	25	0.8	70	0.11	0.10	0.7	66
193	Celery, raw: Stalk, large outer, 8 by about 1 1/2 inches, at root end	1 stalk	40	94	5	Trace	Trace	—	—	—	2	16	0.1	100	0.01	0.01	0.1	4
194	Pieces, diced	1 cup	100	94	15	1	Trace	—	—	—	4	39	0.3	240	0.03	0.03	0.3	9
195	Collards, cooked	1 cup	190	91	55	5	1	—	—	—	9	289	1.1	10,260	0.27	0.37	2.4	87
196	Corn sweet: Cooked, ear 5 by 1 3/4 inches[5]	1 ear	140	74	70	3	1	—	—	—	16	2	0.5	[6]310	0.09	0.08	1.0	7
197	Canned, solids and liquid	1 cup	256	81	170	5	2	—	—	—	40	10	1.0	[6]690	0.07	0.12	2.3	13
198	Cowpeas, cooked immature seeds	1 cup	160	72	175	13	1	—	—	—	29	38	3.4	560	0.49	0.18	2.3	28
	Cucumbers, 10-ounce; 7 1/2 by about 2 inches:																	
199	Raw, pared	1 cucumber	207	96	30	1	Trace	—	—	—	7	35	0.6	Trace	0.07	0.09	0.4	23
200	Raw, pared, center slice 1/8-inch thick	6 slices	50	96	5	Trace	Trace	—	—	—	2	8	0.2	Trace	0.02	0.02	0.1	6
201	Dandelion greens, cooked	1 cup	180	90	60	4	1	—	—	—	12	252	3.2	21,060	0.24	0.29	—	32
202	Endive, curly (including escarole)	2 ounces	57	93	10	1	Trace	—	—	—	2	46	1.0	1,870	0.04	0.08	0.3	6
203	Kale, leaves including stems, cooked	1 cup	110	91	30	4	1	—	—	—	4	147	1.3	8,140	—	—	—	68
	Lettuce, raw:																	
204	Butterhead, as Boston types; head, 4-inch diameter	1 head	220	95	30	3	Trace	—	—	—	6	77	4.4	2,130	0.14	0.13	0.6	18
205	Crisphead, as Iceberg; head, 4 3/4 inch diameter	1 head	454	96	60	4	Trace	—	—	—	13	91	2.3	1,500	0.29	0.27	1.3	29
206	Looseleaf, or bunching varieties, leaves	2 large	50	94	10	1	Trace	—	—	—	2	34	0.7	950	0.03	0.04	0.2	9
207	Mushrooms, canned, solids and liquid	1 cup	244	93	40	5	Trace	—	—	—	6	15	1.2	Trace	0.04	0.60	4.8	4
208	Mustard greens, cooked	1 cup	140	93	35	3	1	—	—	—	6	193	2.5	8,120	0.11	0.19	0.9	68
209	Okra, cooked, pod 3 by 5/8 inch	8 pods	85	91	25	2	Trace	—	—	—	5	78	0.4	420	0.11	0.15	0.8	17
	Onions: Mature:																	
210	Raw, onion 2 1/2-inch diameter	1 onion	110	89	40	2	Trace	—	—	—	10	30	0.6	40	0.04	0.04	0.2	11
211	Cooked	1 cup	210	92	60	3	Trace	—	—	—	14	50	0.8	80	0.06	0.06	0.4	14
212	Young green, small, without tops	6 onions	50	88	20	1	Trace	—	—	—	5	20	0.3	Trace	0.02	0.02	0.2	12
213	Parsley, raw, chopped	1 tablespoon	4	85	Trace	Trace	Trace	—	—	—	Trace	8	0.2	340	Trace	0.01	Trace	7
214	Parsnips, cooked	1 cup	155	82	100	2	1	—	—	—	23	70	0.9	50	0.11	0.12	0.2	16
	Peas, green:																	
215	Cooked	1 cup	160	82	115	9	1	—	—	—	19	37	2.9	860	0.44	0.17	3.7	33
216	Canned, solids and liquid	1 cup	249	83	165	9	1	—	—	—	31	50	4.2	1,120	0.23	0.13	2.2	22
217	Canned, strained (baby food)	1 ounce	28	86	15	1	Trace	—	—	—	3	3	0.4	140	0.02	0.02	0.4	3

[5]Measure and weight apply to entire vegetable or fruit including parts not usually eaten.
[6]Based on yellow varieties; white varieties contain only a trace of cryptoxanthin and carotenes, the pigments in corn that have biologic activity.

Table A-1. (Cont.)

	Food, Approximate Measure, and Weight (in grams)	gm	Water per cent	Food Energy calories	Protein gm	Fat gm	Fatty Acids Saturated (total) gm	Unsaturated Oleic gm	Unsaturated Linoleic gm	Carbohydrate gm	Calcium mg	Iron mg	Vitamin A Value I.U.	Thiamin mg	Riboflavin mg	Niacin mg	Ascorbic Acid mg
218	Peppers, hot, red, without seeds, dried (ground chili powder, added seasonings)	1 tablespoon	15	8	50	2	2	—	—	—	8	40	2.3	9,750	0.03	0.17	1.3	2
	Peppers, sweet: Raw, about 5 per pound:																	
219	Green pod without stem and seeds	1 pod	74	93	15	1	Trace	—	—	—	4	7	0.5	310	0.06	0.06	0.4	94
220	Cooked, boiled, drained	1 pod	73	95	15	1	Trace	—	—	—	3	7	0.4	310	0.05	0.05	0.4	70
	Potatoes, medium (about 3 per pound raw):																	
221	Baked, peeled after baking	1 potato	99	75	90	3	Trace	—	—	—	21	9	0.7	Trace	0.10	0.04	1.7	20
	Boiled:																	
222	Peeled after boiling	1 potato	136	80	105	3	Trace	—	—	—	23	10	0.8	Trace	0.13	0.05	2.0	22
223	Peeled before boiling	1 potato	122	83	80	2	Trace	—	—	—	18	7	0.6	Trace	0.11	0.04	1.4	20
224	French-fried, piece 2 by 1/2 by 1/2 inch: Cooked in deep fat	10 pieces	57	45	155	2	7	2	2	4	20	9	0.7	Trace	0.07	0.04	1.8	12
225	Frozen, heated	10 pieces	57	53	125	2	5	1	1	2	19	5	1.0	Trace	0.08	0.01	1.5	12
	Mashed:																	
226	Milk added	1 cup	195	83	125	4	1	—	—	—	25	47	0.8	50	0.16	0.10	2.0	19
227	Milk and butter added	1 cup	195	80	185	4	8	4	3	Trace	24	47	0.8	330	0.16	0.10	1.9	18
228	Potato chips, medium, 2-inch diameter	10 chips	20	2	115	1	8	2	2	4	10	8	0.4	Trace	0.04	0.01	1.0	3
229	Pumpkin, canned	1 cup	228	90	75	2	1	—	—	—	18	57	0.9	14,590	0.07	0.12	1.3	12
230	Radishes, raw, small, without tops	4 radishes	40	94	5	Trace	Trace	—	—	—	1	12	0.4	Trace	0.01	0.01	0.1	10
231	Sauerkraut, canned, solids and liquid	1 cup	235	93	45	2	Trace	—	—	—	9	85	1.2	120	0.07	0.09	0.4	33
	Spinach:																	
232	Cooked	1 cup	180	92	40	5	1	—	—	—	6	167	4.0	14,580	0.13	0.25	1.0	50
233	Canned, drained solids	1 cup	180	91	45	5	1	—	—	—	6	212	4.7	14,400	0.03	0.21	0.6	24
	Squash: Cooked:																	
234	Summer, diced	1 cup	210	96	30	2	Trace	—	—	—	7	52	0.8	820	0.10	0.16	1.6	21
235	Winter, baked, mashed	1 cup	205	81	130	4	1	—	—	—	32	57	1.6	8,610	0.10	0.27	1.4	27
	Sweetpotatoes: Cooked, medium, 5 by 2 inches, weight raw about 6 ounces:																	
236	Baked, peeled after baking	1 sweetpotato	110	64	155	2	1	—	—	—	36	44	1.0	8,910	0.10	0.07	0.7	24
237	Boiled, peeled after boiling	1 sweetpotato	147	71	170	2	1	—	—	—	39	47	1.0	11,610	0.13	0.09	0.9	25
238	Candied, 3 1/2 by 2 1/4 inches	1 sweetpotato	175	60	295	2	6	2	3	1	60	65	1.6	11,030	0.10	0.08	0.8	17
239	Canned, vacuum or solid pack	1 cup	218	72	235	4	Trace	—	—	—	54	54	1.7	17,000	0.10	0.10	1.4	30
	Tomatoes:																	
240	Raw, approx. 3-in diam. 2 1/8 in high; wt. 7 oz	1 tomato	200	94	40	2	Trace	—	—	—	9	24	0.9	1,640	0.11	0.07	1.3	742
241	Canned, solids and liquid	1 cup	241	94	50	2	1	—	—	—	10	14	1.2	2,170	0.12	0.07	1.7	41

No.	Food, approximate measure	Measure	Grams	Water (%)	Food energy (cal.)	Protein (g)	Fat (g)	Saturated (total) (g)	Oleic (g)	Linoleic (g)	Carbohydrate (g)	Calcium (mg)	Iron (mg)	Vitamin A (I.U.)	Thiamine (mg)	Riboflavin (mg)	Niacin (mg)	Ascorbic acid (mg)
	Tomato catsup:																	
242	Cup	1 cup	273	69	290	6	1	—	—	—	69	60	2.2	3,820	0.25	0.19	4.4	41
243	Tablespoon	1 tbsp.	15	69	15	Trace	Trace	—	—	—	4	3	0.1	210	0.01	0.01	0.2	2
	Tomato juice, canned:																	
244	Cup	1 cup	243	94	45	2	Trace	—	—	—	10	17	2.2	1,940	0.12	0.07	1.9	39
245	Glass (6 fl oz)	1 glass	182	94	35	2	Trace	—	—	—	8	13	1.6	1,460	0.09	0.05	1.5	29
246	Turnips, cooked, diced	1 cup	155	94	35	1	Trace	—	—	—	8	54	0.6	Trace	0.06	0.08	0.5	34
247	Turnip greens, cooked	1 cup	145	94	30	3	Trace	—	—	—	5	252	1.5	8,270	0.15	0.33	0.7	68
	Fruits and Fruit Products																	
248	Apples, raw (about 3 per lb)[5]	1 apple	150	85	70	Trace	Trace	—	—	—	18	8	0.4	50	0.04	0.02	0.1	3
249	Apple juice, bottled or canned	1 cup	248	88	120	Trace	Trace	—	—	—	30	15	1.5	—	0.02	0.05	0.2	2
	Applesauce, canned:																	
250	Sweetened	1 cup	255	76	230	1	Trace	—	—	—	61	10	1.3	100	0.05	0.03	0.1	83
251	Unsweetened or artificially sweetened	1 cup	244	88	100	1	Trace	—	—	—	26	10	1.2	100	0.05	0.02	0.1	82
	Apricots:																	
252	Raw (about 12 per lb)[5]	3 apricots	114	85	55	1	Trace	—	—	—	14	18	0.5	2,890	0.03	0.04	0.7	10
253	Canned in heavy syrup	1 cup	259	77	220	2	Trace	—	—	—	57	28	0.8	4,510	0.05	0.06	0.9	10
254	Dried, uncooked (40 halves per cup)	1 cup	150	25	390	8	1	—	—	—	100	100	8.2	16,350	0.02	0.23	4.9	19
255	Cooked, unsweetened, fruit and liquid	1 cup	285	76	240	5	1	—	—	—	62	63	5.1	8,550	0.01	0.13	2.8	8
256	Apricot nectar, canned	1 cup	251	85	140	1	Trace	—	—	—	37	23	0.5	2,380	0.03	0.03	0.5	8[8]
257	Avocados, whole fruit, raw[5]: California (mid- and late-winter; diam. 3 1/8 in)	1 avocado	284	74	370	5	37	7	17	5	13	22	1.3	630	0.24	0.43	3.5	30
258	Florida (late summer, fall; diam. 3 5/8 in)	1 avocado	454	78	390	4	33	7	15	4	27	30	1.8	880	0.33	0.61	4.9	43
259	Bananas, raw, medium size[5]	1 banana	175	76	100	1	Trace	—	—	—	26	10	0.8	230	0.06	0.07	0.8	12
260	Banana flakes	1 cup	100	3	340	4	1	—	—	—	89	32	2.8	760	0.18	0.24	2.8	7
261	Blackberries, raw	1 cup	144	84	85	2	1	—	—	—	19	46	1.3	290	0.05	0.06	0.5	30
262	Blueberries, raw	1 cup	140	83	85	1	1	—	—	—	21	21	1.4	140	0.04	0.08	0.6	20
263	Cantaloups, raw; medium, 5-inch diameter about 1 2/3 pounds[5]	1/2 melon	385	91	60	1	Trace	—	—	—	14	27	0.8	6,540[9]	0.08	0.06	1.2	63
264	Cherries, canned, red, sour, pitted, water pack	1 cup	244	88	105	2	Trace	—	—	—	26	37	0.7	1,660	0.07	0.05	0.5	12
265	Cranberry juice cocktail, canned	1 cup	250	83	165	Trace	Trace	—	—	—	42	13	0.8	Trace	0.03	0.03	0.1	40[10]
266	Cranberry sauce, sweetened, canned, strained	1 cup	277	62	405	Trace	1	—	—	—	104	17	0.6	60	0.03	0.03	0.1	6
267	Dates, pitted, cut	1 cup	178	22	490	4	1	—	—	—	130	105	5.3	90	0.16	0.17	3.9	0
268	Figs, dried, large, 2 by 1 in	1 fig	21	23	60	1	Trace	—	—	—	15	26	0.6	20	0.02	0.02	0.1	0
269	Fruit cocktail, canned, in heavy syrup	1 cup	256	80	195	1	Trace	—	—	—	50	23	1.0	360	0.05	0.03	1.3	5
	Grapefruit: Raw, medium, 3 3/4-in diam.[5]																	
270	White	1/2 grapefruit	241	89	45	1	Trace	—	—	—	12	19	0.5	10	0.05	0.02	0.2	44
271	Pink or red	1/2 grapefruit	241	89	50	1	Trace	—	—	—	13	20	0.5	540	0.05	0.02	0.2	44
272	Canned, syrup pack	1 cup	254	80	180	2	Trace	—	—	—	45	33	0.8	30	0.08	0.05	0.5	76

[5] Measure and weight apply to entire vegetable or fruit including parts not usually eaten.

[7] Year-round average. Samples marketed from November through May, average 20 milligrams per 200-gram tomato; from June through October, around 52 milligrams.

[8] This is the amount from the fruit. Additional ascorbic acid may be added by the manufacturer. Refer to the label for this information.

[9] Value for varieties with orange-colored flesh; value for varieties with green flesh would be about 540 I.U.

[10] Value listed is based on products with label stating 30 mg per 6-fl-oz serving.

Table A–1. (Cont.)

	Food, Approximate Measure, and Weight (in grams)		Weight gm	Water per cent	Food Energy calories	Protein gm	Fat gm	Fatty Acids Saturated (total) gm	Unsaturated Oleic gm	Linoleic gm	Carbohydrate gm	Calcium mg	Iron mg	Vitamin A Value I.U.	Thiamin mg	Riboflavin mg	Niacin mg	Ascorbic Acid mg
	Grapefruit juice:																	
273	Fresh	1 cup	246	90	95	1	Trace	—	—	—	23	22	0.5	(11)	0.09	0.04	0.4	92
	Canned, white:																	
274	Unsweetened	1 cup	247	89	100	1	Trace	—	—	—	24	20	1.0	20	0.07	0.04	0.4	84
275	Sweetened	1 cup	250	86	130	1	Trace	—	—	—	32	20	1.0	20	0.07	0.04	0.4	78
	Frozen, concentrate, unsweetened:																	
276	Undiluted, can, 6 fluid ounces	1 can	207	62	300	4	1	—	—	—	72	70	0.8	60	0.29	0.12	1.4	286
277	Diluted with 3 parts water, by volume	1 cup	247	89	100	1	Trace	—	—	—	24	25	0.2	20	0.10	0.04	0.5	96
278	Dehydrated crystals	4 oz	113	1	410	6	1	—	—	—	102	100	1.2	80	0.40	0.20	2.0	396
279	Prepared with water (1 pound yields about 1 gallon)	1 cup	247	90	100	1	Trace	—	—	—	24	22	0.2	20	0.10	0.05	0.5	91
	Grapes, raw:[5]																	
280	American type (slip skin)	1 cup	153	82	65	1	1	—	—	—	15	15	0.4	100	0.05	0.03	0.2	3
281	European type (adherent skin)	1 cup	160	81	95	1	Trace	—	—	—	25	17	0.6	140	0.07	0.04	0.4	6
	Grapejuice:																	
282	Canned or bottled	1 cup	253	83	165	1	Trace	—	—	—	42	28	0.8	—	0.10	0.05	0.5	Trace
	Frozen concentrate, sweetened:																	
283	Undiluted, can, 6 fluid ounces	1 can	216	53	395	1	Trace	—	—	—	100	22	0.9	40	0.13	0.22	1.5	(12)
284	Diluted with 3 parts water, by volume	1 cup	250	86	135	1	Trace	—	—	—	33	8	0.3	10	0.05	0.08	0.5	(12)
285	Grapejuice drink, canned	1 cup	250	86	135	Trace	Trace	—	—	—	35	8	0.3	—	0.03	0.03	0.3	(12)
286	Lemons, raw, 2 1/8-in diam., size 165.[5] Used for juice	1 lemon	110	90	20	1	Trace	—	—	—	6	19	0.4	10	0.03	0.01	0.1	39
287	Lemon juice, raw	1 cup	244	91	60	1	Trace	—	—	—	20	17	0.5	50	0.07	0.02	0.2	112
	Lemonade concentrate:																	
288	Frozen, 6 fl oz per can	1 can	219	48	430	Trace	Trace	—	—	—	112	9	0.4	40	0.04	0.07	0.7	66
289	Diluted with 4 1/3 parts water, by volume	1 cup	248	88	110	Trace	Trace	—	—	—	28	2	Trace	Trace	Trace	0.02	0.2	17
	Lime juice:																	
290	Fresh	1 cup	246	90	65	1	Trace	—	—	—	22	22	0.5	20	0.05	0.02	0.2	79
291	Canned, unsweetened	1 cup	246	90	65	1	Trace	—	—	—	22	22	0.5	20	0.05	0.02	0.2	52
292	Limeade concentrate, frozen: Undiluted, can, 6 fluid ounces	1 can	218	50	410	Trace	Trace	—	—	—	108	11	0.2	Trace	0.02	0.02	0.2	26
293	Diluted with 4 1/3 parts water, by volume	1 cup	247	90	100	Trace	Trace	—	—	—	27	2	Trace	Trace	Trace	Trace	Trace	5
294	Oranges, raw, 2 5/8-in diam., all commercial varieties[5]	1 orange	180	86	65	1	Trace	—	—	—	16	54	0.5	260	0.13	0.05	0.5	66
295	Orange juice, fresh, all varieties	1 cup	248	88	110	2	1	—	—	—	26	27	0.5	500	0.22	0.07	1.0	124
296	Canned, unsweetened	1 cup	249	87	120	2	Trace	—	—	—	28	25	1.0	500	0.17	0.05	0.7	100
	Frozen concentrate:																	
297	Undiluted, can, 6 fluid ounces	1 can	213	55	360	5	Trace	—	—	—	87	75	0.9	1,620	0.68	0.11	2.8	360

Item No.	Food, approximate measure	Measure	Grams	Water (%)	Food energy (Cal.)	Protein (g)	Fat (g)	Saturated (g)	Oleic (g)	Linoleic (g)	Carbohydrate (g)	Calcium (mg)	Iron (mg)	Vitamin A (I.U.)	Thiamine (mg)	Riboflavin (mg)	Niacin (mg)	Ascorbic acid (mg)
298	Diluted with 3 parts water, by volume	1 cup	249	87	120	Trace	Trace	—	—	—	29	25	0.2	550	0.22	0.02	1.0	120
299	Dehydrated crystals	4 oz	113	1	430	6	2	—	—	—	100	95	1.9	1,900	0.76	0.24	3.3	408
300	Prepared with water (1 pound yields about 1 gallon)	1 cup	248	88	115	2	1	—	—	—	27	25	0.5	500	0.20	0.07	1.0	109
301	Orange-apricot juice drink	1 cup	249	87	125	1	Trace	—	—	—	32	12	0.2	1,440	0.05	0.02	0.5	[10]40
	Orange and grapefruit juice: Frozen concentrate:																	
302	Undiluted, can, 6 fluid ounces	1 can	210	59	330	4	1	—	—	—	78	61	0.8	800	0.48	0.06	2.3	302
303	Diluted with 3 parts water, by volume	1 cup	248	88	110	1	Trace	—	—	—	26	20	0.2	270	0.16	0.02	0.8	102
304	Papayas, raw, 1/2-inch cubes	1 cup	182	89	70	1	Trace	—	—	—	18	36	0.5	3,190	0.07	0.08	0.5	102
	Peaches: Raw:																	
305	Whole, medium, 2-inch diameter, about 4 per pound[5]	1 peach	114	89	35	1	Trace	—	—	—	10	9	0.5	[13]1,320	0.02	0.05	1.0	7
306	Sliced	1 cup	168	89	65	1	Trace	—	—	—	16	15	0.8	[13]2,230	0.03	0.08	1.6	12
	Canned, yellow-fleshed, solids and liquid: Syrup pack, heavy:																	
307	Halves or slices	1 cup	257	79	200	1	Trace	—	—	—	52	10	0.8	1,100	0.02	0.06	1.4	7
308	Water pack	1 cup	245	91	75	1	Trace	—	—	—	20	10	0.7	1,100	0.02	0.06	1.4	7
309	Dried, uncooked	1 cup	160	25	420	5	1	—	—	—	109	77	9.6	6,240	0.02	0.31	8.5	28
310	Cooked, unsweetened, 10–12 halves and juice	1 cup	270	77	220	3	1	—	—	—	58	41	5.1	3,290	0.01	0.15	4.2	6
	Frozen:																	
311	Carton, 12 ounces, not thawed	1 carton	340	76	300	1	Trace	—	—	—	77	14	1.7	2,210	0.03	0.14	2.4	[14]135
	Pears:																	
312	Raw, 3 by 2 1/2-inch diameter[5]	1 pear	182	83	100	1	1	—	—	—	25	13	0.5	30	0.04	0.07	0.2	7
	Canned, solids, and liquid: Syrup pack, heavy:																	
313	Halves or slices	1 cup	255	80	195	1	1	—	—	—	50	13	0.5	Trace	0.03	0.05	0.3	4
	Pineapple:																	
314	Raw, diced	1 cup	140	85	75	1	Trace	—	—	—	19	24	0.7	100	0.12	0.04	0.3	24
	Canned, heavy syrup pack, solids and liquids:																	
315	Crushed	1 cup	260	80	195	1	Trace	—	—	—	50	29	0.8	120	0.20	0.06	0.5	17
316	Sliced, slices and juice	2 small or 1 large	122	80	90	Trace	Trace	—	—	—	24	13	0.4	50	0.09	0.03	0.2	8
317	Pineapple juice, canned	1 cup	249	86	135	1	Trace	—	—	—	34	37	0.7	120	0.12	0.04	0.5	[8]22
	Plums, all except prunes:																	
318	Raw, 2-inch diameter, about 2 ounces[5]	1 plum	60	87	25	Trace	Trace	—	—	—	7	7	0.3	140	0.02	0.02	0.3	3
	Canned, syrup pack (Italian prunes):																	
319	Plums (with pits) and juice[5]	1 cup	256	77	205	1	Trace	—	—	—	53	22	2.2	2,970	0.05	0.05	0.9	4

[5]Measure and weight apply to entire vegetable or fruit including parts not usually eaten.
[8]This is the amount from the fruit. Additional ascorbic acid may be added by the manufacturer. Refer to the label for this information.
[10]Value listed is based on product with label stating 30 milligrams per 6-fl-oz serving.
[11]For white-fleshed varieties value is about 20 I.U. per cup; for red-fleshed varieties, 1,080 I.U. per cup.
[12]Present only if added by the manufacturer. Refer to the label for this information.
[13]Based on yellow-fleshed varieties; for white-fleshed varieties value is about 50 I.U. per 114-gm peach and 80 I.U. per cup of sliced peaches.
[14]This value includes ascorbic acid added by manufacturer.

Table A–1. (Cont.)

Food, Approximate Measure, and Weight (in grams)		Water per cent	Food Energy calories	Protein gm	Fat gm	Fatty Acids			Carbohydrate gm	Calcium mg	Iron mg	Vitamin A Value I.U.	Thiamin mg	Riboflavin mg	Niacin mg	Ascorbic Acid mg
						Saturated (total) gm	Unsaturated									
							Oleic gm	Linoleic gm								
	gm															
320 Prunes, dried, "softenized," medium: Uncooked[5]	4 prunes	32	28	70	1	Trace	—	—	—	18	14	1.1	440	0.02	0.04	0.4	1
321 Cooked, unsweetened, 17–18 prunes and 1/3 cup liquid[5]	1 cup	270	66	295	2	1	—	—	—	78	60	4.5	1,860	0.08	0.18	1.7	2
322 Prune juice, canned or bottled	1 cup	256	80	200	1	Trace	—	—	—	49	36	10.5	—	0.03	0.03	1.0	85
Raisins, seedless:																	
323 Packaged, 1/2 oz or 1 1/2 tbsp per pkg	1 pkg	14	18	40	Trace	Trace	—	—	—	11	9	0.5	Trace	0.02	0.01	0.1	Trace
324 Cup, pressed down	1 cup	165	18	480	4	Trace	—	—	—	128	102	5.8	30	0.18	0.13	0.8	2
Raspberries, red:																	
325 Raw	1 cup	123	84	70	1	1	—	—	—	17	27	1.1	160	0.04	0.11	1.1	31
326 Frozen, 10-ounce carton, not thawed	1 carton	284	74	275	2	1	—	—	—	70	37	1.7	200	0.06	0.17	1.7	59
327 Rhubarb, cooked, sugar added	1 cup	272	63	385	1	Trace	—	—	—	98	212	1.6	220	0.06	0.15	0.7	17
Strawberries:																	
328 Raw, capped	1 cup	149	90	55	1	1	—	—	—	13	31	1.5	90	0.04	0.10	1.0	88
329 Frozen, 10-ounce carton, not thawed	1 carton	284	71	310	1	1	—	—	—	79	40	2.0	90	0.06	0.17	1.5	150
330 Tangerines, raw, medium, 2 3/8-in diam., size 176[5]	1 tangerine	116	87	40	1	Trace	—	—	—	10	34	0.3	360	0.05	0.02	0.1	27
331 Tangerine juice, canned, sweetened	1 cup	249	87	125	1	1	—	—	—	30	45	0.5	1,050	0.15	0.05	0.2	55
332 Watermelon, raw, wedge, 4 by 8 inches (1/16 of 10 by 16-inch melon, about 2 pounds with rind)[5]	1 wedge	925	93	115	2	1	—	—	—	27	30	2.1	2,510	0.13	0.13	0.7	30
Grain Products																	
Bagel, 3-in diam.:																	
333 Egg	1 bagel	55	32	165	6	2	—	—	—	28	9	1.2	30	0.14	0.10	1.2	0
334 Water	1 bagel	55	29	165	6	2	—	—	—	30	8	1.2	0	0.15	0.11	1.4	0
335 Barley, pearled, light, uncooked	1 cup	200	11	700	16	2	Trace	1	1	158	32	4.0	0	0.24	0.10	6.2	0
336 Biscuits, baking powder from home recipe with enriched flour, 2-in diam.	1 biscuit	28	27	105	2	5	1	2	1	13	34	0.4	Trace	0.06	0.06	0.1	Trace
337 Biscuits, baking powder from mix, 2-in diam.	1 biscuit	28	28	90	2	3	1	1	1	15	19	0.6	Trace	0.08	0.07	0.6	Trace
338 Bran flakes (40% bran), added thiamin and iron	1 cup	35	3	105	4	1	—	—	—	28	25	12.3	0	0.14	0.06	2.2	0
339 Bran flakes with raisins, added thiamin and iron	1 cup	50	7	145	4	1	—	—	—	40	28	13.5	Trace	0.16	0.07	2.7	0
Breads:																	
340 Boston brown bread, slice 3 by 3/4 in	1 slice	48	45	100	3	1	—	—	—	22	43	0.9	0	0.05	0.03	0.6	0
Cracked-wheat bread:																	
341 Loaf, 1 lb	1 loaf	454	35	1,190	40	10	2	5	2	236	399	5.0	Trace	0.53	0.41	5.9	Trace
342 Slice, 18 slices per loaf	1 slice	25	35	65	2	1	—	—	—	13	22	0.3	Trace	0.03	0.02	0.3	Trace

No.	Food, approximate measure		Grams	Water (%)	Food energy (Cal.)	Protein (g)	Fat (g)	Saturated (g)	Oleic (g)	Linoleic (g)	Carbohydrate (g)	Calcium (mg)	Iron (mg)	Vitamin A (I.U.)	Thiamin (mg)	Riboflavin (mg)	Niacin (mg)	Ascorbic acid (mg)
	French or Vienna bread:																	
343	Enriched, 1-lb loaf	1 loaf	454	31	1,315	41	14	3	8	2	251	195	10.0	Trace	1.27	1.00	11.3	Trace
344	Unenriched, 1-lb loaf	1 loaf	454	31	1,315	41	14	3	8	2	251	195	3.2	Trace	0.36	0.36	3.6	Trace
	Italian bread:																	
345	Enriched, 1-lb loaf	1 loaf	454	32	1,250	41	4	Trace	1	2	256	77	10.0	0	1.32	0.91	11.8	0
346	Unenriched, 1-lb loaf	1 loaf	454	32	1,250	41	4	Trace	1	2	256	77	3.2	0	0.41	0.27	3.6	0
	Raisin bread:																	
347	Loaf, 1 lb	1 loaf	454	35	1,190	30	13	3	8	2	243	322	5.9	Trace	0.23	0.41	3.2	Trace
348	Slice, 18 slices per loaf	1 slice	25	35	65	2	1	—	—	—	13	18	0.3	Trace	0.01	0.02	0.2	Trace
	Rye bread:																	
	American, light (1/3 rye, 2/3 wheat):																	
349	Loaf, 1 lb	1 loaf	454	36	1,100	41	5	—	—	—	236	340	7.3	0	0.82	0.32	6.4	0
350	Slice, 18 slices per loaf	1 slice	25	36	60	2	Trace	—	—	—	13	19	0.4	0	0.05	0.02	0.4	0
351	Pumpernickel, loaf, 1 lb	1 loaf	454	34	1,115	41	5	—	—	—	241	381	10.9	0	1.04	0.64	5.4	0
	White bread, enriched:[15]																	
	Soft-crumb type:																	
352	Loaf, 1 lb	1 loaf	454	36	1,225	39	15	3	8	2	229	381	11.3	Trace	1.13	0.95	10.9	Trace
353	Slice, 18 slices per loaf	1 slice	25	36	70	2	1	—	—	—	13	21	0.6	Trace	0.06	0.05	0.6	Trace
354	Slice, toasted	1 slice	22	25	70	2	1	—	—	—	13	17	0.6	Trace	0.05	0.04	0.6	Trace
355	Slice, 22 slices per loaf	1 slice	20	25	55	2	1	—	—	—	10	17	0.5	Trace	0.05	0.04	0.5	Trace
356	Slice, toasted	1 slice	17	25	55	2	1	—	—	—	10	17	0.5	Trace	0.05	0.04	0.5	Trace
357	Loaf, 1 1/2 lb	1 loaf	680	36	1,835	59	22	5	12	3	343	571	17.0	Trace	1.70	1.43	16.3	Trace
358	Slice, 24 slices per loaf	1 slice	28	36	75	2	1	—	—	—	14	24	0.7	Trace	0.07	0.06	0.7	Trace
359	Slice, toasted	1 slice	24	25	75	2	1	—	—	—	14	24	0.7	Trace	0.06	0.06	0.7	Trace
360	Slice, 28 slices per loaf	1 slice	24	36	65	2	1	—	—	—	12	20	0.6	Trace	0.06	0.05	0.6	Trace
361	Slice, toasted	1 slice	21	25	65	2	1	—	—	—	12	20	0.6	Trace	0.06	0.05	0.6	Trace
	Firm-crumb type:																	
362	Loaf, 1 lb	1 loaf	454	35	1,245	41	17	4	10	2	228	435	11.3	Trace	1.22	0.91	10.9	Trace
363	Slice, 20 slices per loaf	1 slice	23	35	65	2	1	—	—	—	12	22	0.6	Trace	0.06	0.05	0.6	Trace
364	Slice, toasted	1 slice	20	24	65	2	1	—	—	—	12	22	0.6	Trace	0.06	0.05	0.6	Trace
365	Loaf, 2 lb	1 loaf	907	35	2,495	82	34	8	20	4	455	871	22.7	Trace	2.45	1.81	21.8	Trace
366	Slice, 34 slices per loaf	1 slice	27	35	75	2	1	—	—	—	14	26	0.7	Trace	0.07	0.05	0.6	Trace
367	Slice, toasted	1 slice	23	35	75	2	1	—	—	—	14	26	0.7	Trace	0.07	0.05	0.6	Trace
	Whole-wheat bread, soft-crumb type:																	
368	Loaf, 1 lb	1 loaf	454	36	1,095	41	12	2	6	2	224	381	13.6	Trace	1.36	0.45	12.7	Trace
369	Slice, 16 slices per loaf	1 slice	28	36	65	3	1	—	—	—	14	24	0.8	Trace	0.09	0.03	0.8	Trace
370	Slice, toasted	1 slice	24	24	65	3	1	—	—	—	14	24	0.8	Trace	0.09	0.03	0.8	Trace
	Whole-wheat bread, firm-crumb type:																	
371	Loaf, 1 lb	1 loaf	454	36	1,100	48	14	3	6	3	216	449	13.6	Trace	1.18	0.54	12.7	Trace
372	Slice, 18 slices per loaf	1 slice	25	36	60	3	1	—	—	—	12	25	0.8	Trace	0.06	0.03	0.7	Trace
373	Slice, toasted	1 slice	21	24	60	3	1	—	—	—	12	25	0.8	Trace	0.06	0.03	0.7	Trace
374	Breadcrumbs, dry, grated	1 cup	100	6	390	13	5	1	2	1	73	122	3.6	Trace	0.22	0.30	3.5	0
375	Buckwheat flour, light, sifted	1 cup	98	12	340	6	1	—	—	—	78	11	1.0	0	0.08	0.04	0.4	0
376	Bulgur, canned, seasoned	1 cup	135	56	245	8	4	—	—	—	44	27	1.9	0	0.08	0.05	4.1	0
	Cakes made from cake mixes:																	
	Angel food:																	
377	Whole cake	1 cake	635	34	1,645	36	1	—	—	—	377	603	1.9	0	0.03	0.70	0.6	0
378	Piece, 1/12 of 10-in diam. cake	1 piece	53	34	135	3	Trace	—	—	—	32	50	0.2	0	Trace	0.06	0.1	0

[5] Measure and weight apply to entire vegetable or fruit including parts not usually eaten.

[8] This is the amount from the fruit. Additional ascorbic acid may be added by the manufacturer. Refer to the label for this information.

[15] Values for iron, thiamin, riboflavin, and niacin per pound of unenriched white bread would be as follows:

	Iron mg	Thiamin mg	Riboflavin mg	Niacin mg
Soft crumb	3.2	.31	.39	5.0
Firm crumb	3.2	.32	.59	4.1

Table A-1. (Cont.)

	Food, Approximate Measure, and Weight (in grams)		Water per cent	Food Energy calories	Protein gm	Fat gm	Fatty Acids Saturated (total) gm	Unsaturated Oleic gm	Unsaturated Linoleic gm	Carbohydrate gm	Calcium mg	Iron mg	Vitamin A Value I.U.	Thiamin mg	Riboflavin mg	Niacin mg	Ascorbic Acid mg
		gm															
	Cakes made from cake mixes (cont.)																
	Cupcakes, small, 2 1/2 in diam.:																
379	Without icing	1 cupcake	25	26	90	1	3	1	1	1	14	40	0.1	40	0.01	0.03	0.1	Trace
380	With chocolate icing	1 cupcake	36	22	130	2	5	2	2	1	21	47	0.3	60	0.01	0.04	0.1	Trace
	Devil's food, 2-layer, with chocolate icing:																
381	Whole cake	1 cake	1,107	24	3,755	49	136	54	58	16	645	653	8.9	1,660	0.33	0.89	3.3	1
382	Piece, 1/16 of 9-in diam. cake	1 piece	69	24	235	3	9	3	4	1	40	41	0.6	100	0.02	0.06	0.2	Trace
383	Cupcake, small, 2 1/2-in diam	1 cupcake	35	24	120	2	4	1	2	Trace	20	21	0.3	50	0.01	0.03	0.1	Trace
	Gingerbread:																
384	Whole cake	1 cake	570	37	1,575	18	39	10	19	9	291	513	9.1	Trace	0.17	0.51	4.6	2
385	Piece, 1/9 of 8-in square cake	1 piece	63	37	175	2	4	1	2	1	32	57	1.0	Trace	0.02	0.06	0.5	Trace
	White, 2-layer, with chocolate icing:																
386	Whole cake	1 cake	1,140	21	4,000	45	122	45	54	17	716	1,129	5.7	680	0.23	0.91	2.3	2
387	Piece, 1/16 of 9-in diam. cake	1 piece	71	21	250	3	8	3	3	1	45	70	0.4	40	0.01	0.06	0.1	Trace
	Cakes made from home recipes:16																
388	Boston cream pie; piece 1/12 of 8-in diam.	1 piece	69	35	210	4	6	2	3	1	34	46	0.3	140	0.02	0.08	0.1	Trace
	Fruitcake, dark, made with enriched flour:																
389	Loaf, 1 lb	1 loaf	454	18	1,720	22	69	15	37	13	271	327	11.8	540	0.59	0.64	3.6	2
390	Slice, 1/30 of 8-in loaf	1 slice	15	18	55	1	2	Trace	1	Trace	9	11	0.4	20	0.02	0.02	0.1	Trace
	Plain sheet cake:																
	Without icing:																
391	Whole cake	1 cake	777	25	2,830	35	108	30	52	21	434	497	3.1	1,320	0.16	0.70	1.6	2
392	Piece, 1/9 of 9-in square cake	1 piece	86	25	315	4	12	3	6	2	48	55	0.3	150	0.02	0.08	0.2	Trace
393	With boiled white icing, piece, 1/9 of 9-in square cake	1 piece	114	23	400	4	12	3	6	2	71	56	0.3	150	0.02	0.08	0.2	Trace
	Pound:																
394	Loaf, 8 1/2 by 3 1/2 by 3 in	1 loaf	514	17	2,430	29	152	34	68	17	242	108	4.1	1,440	0.15	0.46	1.0	0
395	Slice, 1/2-in thick	1 slice	30	17	140	2	9	2	4	1	14	6	0.2	80	0.01	0.03	0.1	0
	Sponge:																
396	Whole cake	1 cake	790	32	2,345	60	45	14	20	4	427	237	9.5	3,560	0.40	1.11	1.6	Trace
397	Piece, 1/12 of 10-in diam. cake	1 piece	66	32	195	5	4	1	2	Trace	36	20	0.8	300	0.03	0.09	0.1	Trace
	Yellow, 2 layer, without icing:																
398	Whole cake	1 cake	870	24	3,160	39	111	31	53	22	506	618	3.5	1,310	0.17	0.70	1.7	2
399	Piece, 1/16 of 9-in diam. cake	1 piece	54	24	200	2	7	2	3	1	32	39	0.2	80	0.01	0.04	0.1	Trace
	Yellow, 2-layer, with chocolate icing:																
400	Whole cake	1 cake	1,203	21	4,390	51	156	55	69	23	727	818	7.2	1,920	0.24	0.96	2.4	Trace
401	Piece, 1/16 of 9-in diam. cake	1 piece	75	21	275	3	10	3	4	1	45	51	0.5	120	0.02	0.06	0.2	Trace

Cake icings. See Sugars, Sweets

No.	Food, approximate measure, and weight (in grams)		Grams	Water (%)	Food energy (Cal.)	Pro-tein (g)	Fat (g)	Saturated (total) (g)	Unsaturated Oleic (g)	Unsaturated Linoleic (g)	Carbo-hydrate (g)	Cal-cium (mg)	Iron (mg)	Vita-min A (IU)	Thia-min (mg)	Ribo-flavin (mg)	Nia-cin (mg)	Ascorbic acid (mg)
	Cookies:																	
	Brownies with nuts:																	
402	Made from home recipe with enriched flour	1 brownie	20	10	95	1	6	1	3	1	10	8	0.4	40	0.04	0.02	0.1	Trace
403	Made from mix	1 brownie	20	11	85	1	4	1	2	1	13	9	0.4	20	0.03	0.02	0.1	Trace
	Chocolate chip:																	
404	Made from home recipe with enriched flour	1 cookie	10	3	50	1	3	1	1	1	6	4	0.2	10	0.01	0.01	0.1	Trace
405	Commercial	1 cookie	10	3	50	1	2	1	1	Trace	7	4	0.2	10	Trace	0.01	Trace	Trace
406	Fig bars, commercial	1 cookie	14	14	50	1	1	—	—	—	11	11	0.2	20	Trace	0.01	0.1	Trace
407	Sandwich, chocolate or vanilla, commercial	1 cookie	10	2	50	1	2	1	1	Trace	7	2	0.1	0	Trace	Trace	0.1	0
	Corn flakes, added nutrients:																	
408	Plain	1 cup	25	4	100	2	Trace	—	—	—	21	4	0.4	0	0.11	0.02	0.5	0
409	Sugar-covered	1 cup	40	2	155	2	Trace	—	—	—	36	5	0.4	0	0.16	0.02	0.8	0
	Corn (hominy) grits, degermed, cooked:																	
410	Enriched	1 cup	245	87	125	3	Trace	—	—	—	27	2	0.7	[17]150	0.10	0.07	1.0	0
411	Unenriched	1 cup	245	87	125	3	Trace	—	—	—	27	2	0.2	[17]150	0.05	0.02	0.5	0
	Cornmeal:																	
412	Whole-ground, unbolted, dry	1 cup	122	12	435	11	5	1	2	2	90	24	2.9	[17]620	0.46	0.13	2.4	0
413	Bolted (nearly whole-grain) dry	1 cup	122	12	440	11	4	Trace	1	2	91	21	2.2	[17]590	0.37	0.10	2.3	0
	Degermed, enriched:																	
414	Dry form	1 cup	138	12	500	11	2	—	—	—	108	8	4.0	[17]610	0.61	0.36	4.8	0
415	Cooked	1 cup	240	88	120	3	1	—	—	—	26	2	1.0	[17]140	0.14	0.10	1.2	0
	Degermed, unenriched:																	
416	Dry form	1 cup	138	12	500	11	2	—	—	—	108	8	1.5	[17]610	0.19	0.07	1.4	0
417	Cooked	1 cup	240	88	120	3	1	—	—	—	26	2	0.5	[17]140	0.05	0.02	0.2	0
418	Corn muffins, made with enriched degermed cornmeal and enriched flour; muffin 2 3/8-in diam.	1 muffin	40	33	125	3	4	2	2	Trace	19	42	0.7	[17]120	0.08	0.09	0.6	Trace
419	Corn muffins, made with mix, egg, and milk; muffin 2 3/8-in diam.	1 muffin	40	30	130	3	4	1	2	1	20	96	0.6	100	0.07	0.08	0.6	Trace
420	Corn, puffed, presweetened, added nutrients	1 cup	30	2	115	1	Trace	—	—	—	27	3	0.5	0	0.13	0.05	0.6	0
421	Corn, shredded, added nutrients	1 cup	25	3	100	2	Trace	—	—	—	22	1	0.6	0	0.11	0.05	0.5	0
	Crackers:																	
422	Graham, 2 1/2-in square	4 crackers	28	6	110	2	3	—	—	—	21	11	0.4	0	0.01	0.06	0.4	0
423	Saltines	4 crackers	11	4	50	1	1	—	—	—	8	2	0.1	0	Trace	Trace	0.1	0
	Danish pastry, plain (without fruit or nuts):																	
424	Packaged ring, 12 ounces	1 ring	340	22	1,435	25	80	24	37	15	155	170	3.1	1,050	0.24	0.51	2.7	Trace
425	Round piece, approx. 4 1/4-in diam. by 1 in	1 pastry	65	22	275	5	15	5	7	3	30	33	0.6	200	0.05	0.10	0.5	Trace
426	Ounce	1 oz	28	22	120	2	7	2	3	2	13	14	0.3	90	0.02	0.04	0.2	Trace
427	Doughnuts, cake type	1 doughnut	32	24	125	1	6	1	4	1	16	13	[18]0.4	30	[18]0.05	[18]0.05	[18]0.4	Trace
428	Farina, quick-cooking, enriched, cooked	1 cup	245	89	105	3	Trace	—	—	—	22	147	[19]0.7	0	[19]0.12	[19]0.07	[19]1.0	0

[16] Unenriched cake flour used unless otherwise specified.

[17] This value is based on product made from yellow varieties of corn; white varieties contain only a trace.

[18] Based on product made with enriched flour. With unenriched flour, approximate values per doughnut are: iron, 0.2 mg; thiamin, 0.01 mg; riboflavin, 0.03 mg; niacin, 0.2 mg.

[19] Iron, thiamin, riboflavin, and niacin are based on the minimum levels of enrichment specified in standards of identity promulgated under the Federal Food, Drug, and Cosmetic Act.

Table A–1. (Cont.)

	Food, Approximate Measure, and Weight (in grams)	gm	Water per cent	Food Energy calories	Pro-tein gm	Fat gm	Fatty Acids Satu-rated (total) gm	Unsaturated Oleic gm	Lin-oleic gm	Carbo-hy-drate gm	Cal-cium mg	Iron mg	Vita-min A Value I.U.	Thia-min mg	Ribo-flavin mg	Niacin mg	Ascor-bic Acid mg
	Macaroni, cooked:																
	Enriched:																
429	Cooked, firm stage (undergoes additional cooking in a food mixture) 1 cup	130	64	190	6	1	—	—	—	39	14	1.4	0	0.23	0.14	1.8	0
430	Cooked until tender 1 cup	140	72	155	5	1	—	—	—	32	8	1.3	0	0.20	0.11	1.5	0
	Unenriched:																
431	Cooked, firm stage (undergoes additional cooking in a food mixture) 1 cup	130	64	190	6	1	—	—	—	39	14	0.7	0	0.03	0.03	0.5	0
432	Cooked until tender 1 cup	140	72	155	5	1	—	—	—	32	11	0.6	0	0.01	0.01	0.4	0
433	Macaroni (enriched) and cheese, baked 1 cup	200	58	430	17	22	10	9	2	40	362	1.8	860	0.20	0.40	1.8	Trace
434	Canned 1 cup	240	80	230	9	10	4	3	1	26	199	1.0	260	0.12	0.24	1.0	Trace
435	Muffins, with enriched white flour; muffin, 3-inch diam. 1 muffin	40	38	120	3	4	1	2	1	17	42	0.6	40	0.07	0.09	0.6	Trace
	Noodles (egg noodles), cooked:																
436	Enriched 1 cup	160	70	200	7	2	1	1	Trace	37	16	1.4	110	0.22	0.13	1.9	0
437	Unenriched 1 cup	160	70	200	7	2	1	1	Trace	37	16	1.0	110	0.05	0.03	0.6	0
438	Oats (with or without corn) puffed, added nutrients 1 cup	25	3	100	3	1	—	—	—	19	44	1.2	0	0.24	0.04	0.5	0
439	Oatmeal or rolled oats, cooked 1 cup	240	87	130	5	2	—	—	1	23	22	1.4	0	0.19	0.05	0.2	0
	Pancakes, 4-inch diam.:																
440	Wheat, enriched flour (home recipe) 1 cake	27	50	60	2	2	Trace	1	Trace	9	27	0.4	30	0.05	0.06	0.4	Trace
441	Buckwheat (made from mix with egg and milk) 1 cake	27	58	55	2	2	1	1	Trace	6	59	0.4	60	0.03	0.04	0.2	Trace
442	Plain or buttermilk (made from mix with egg and milk) 1 cake	27	51	60	2	2	1	1	Trace	9	58	0.3	70	0.04	0.06	0.2	Trace
	Pie (piecrust made with unenriched flour): Sector, 4-in, 1/7 of 9-in-diam. pie:																
443	Apple 1 sector	135	48	350	3	15	4	7	3	51	11	0.4	40	0.03	0.03	0.5	1
444	Butterscotch 1 sector	130	45	350	6	14	5	6	2	50	98	1.2	340	0.04	0.13	0.3	Trace
445	Cherry 1 sector	135	47	350	4	15	5	7	3	52	19	0.4	590	0.03	0.03	0.7	Trace
446	Custard 1 sector	130	58	285	8	14	5	6	2	30	125	0.8	300	0.07	0.21	0.4	0
447	Lemon meringue 1 sector	120	47	305	4	12	4	6	2	45	17	0.6	200	0.04	0.10	0.2	4
448	Mince 1 sector	135	43	365	3	16	4	8	3	56	38	1.4	Trace	0.09	0.05	0.5	1
449	Pecan 1 sector	118	20	490	6	27	4	16	5	60	55	3.3	190	0.19	0.08	0.4	Trace
450	Pineapple chiffon 1 sector	93	41	265	6	11	3	5	2	36	22	0.8	320	0.04	0.08	0.4	1
451	Pumpkin 1 sector	130	59	275	5	15	5	6	2	32	66	0.7	3,210	0.04	0.13	0.7	Trace
	Piecrust, baked shell for pie made with:																
452	Enriched flour 1 shell	180	15	900	11	60	16	28	12	79	25	3.1	0	0.36	0.25	3.2	0
453	Unenriched flour 1 shell	180	15	900	11	60	16	28	12	79	25	0.9	0	0.05	0.05	0.9	0

No.	Food, approximate measure	Grams	Water (%)	Food energy (Cal.)	Protein (g)	Fat (g)	Saturated fat (g)	Oleic (g)	Linoleic (g)	Carbohydrate (g)	Calcium (mg)	Iron (mg)	Vitamin A (I.U.)	Thiamin (mg)	Riboflavin (mg)	Niacin (mg)	Ascorbic acid (mg)
454	Piecrust mix including stick form: Package, 10 oz, for double crust — 1 pkg.	284	9	1,480	20	93	23	46	21	141	131	1.4	0	0.11	0.11	2.0	0
455	Pizza (cheese) 5 1/2-in sector; 1/8 of 14-in diam. pie — 1 sector	75	45	185	7	6	2	3	Trace	27	107	0.7	290	0.04	0.12	0.7	4
	Popcorn, popped:																
456	Plain, large kernel — 1 cup	6	4	25	1	Trace	—	—	—	5	1	0.2	—	—	0.01	0.1	0
457	With oil and salt — 1 cup	9	3	40	1	2	—	1	1	5	1	0.2	—	—	0.01	0.2	0
458	Sugar coated — 1 cup	35	4	135	2	1	—	—	—	30	2	0.5	0	—	0.02	0.4	0
	Pretzels:																
459	Dutch, twisted — 1 pretzel	16	5	60	2	1	—	—	—	12	4	0.2	0	Trace	Trace	0.1	0
460	Thin, twisted — 1 pretzel	6	5	25	1	Trace	—	—	—	5	1	0.1	0	Trace	Trace	Trace	0
461	Sticks, small 2 1/4 inches — 10 sticks	3	5	10	Trace	Trace	—	—	—	2	1	Trace	0	Trace	Trace	Trace	0
462	Stick, regular, 3 1/8 inches — 5 sticks	3	5	10	Trace	Trace	—	—	—	2	1	Trace	0	Trace	Trace	Trace	0
	Rice, white:																
	Enriched:																
463	Raw — 1 cup	185	12	670	12	1	—	—	—	149	44	[20]5.4	0	[20]0.81	[20]0.06	[20]6.5	0
464	Cooked — 1 cup	205	73	225	4	Trace	—	—	—	50	21	[20]1.8	0	[20]0.23	[20]0.02	[20]2.1	0
465	Instant, ready to serve — 1 cup	165	73	180	4	Trace	—	—	—	40	5	[20]1.3	0	[20]0.21	[20]—	[20]1.7	0
466	Unenriched, cooked — 1 cup	205	73	225	4	Trace	—	—	—	50	21	0.4	0	0.04	0.02	0.8	0
467	Parboiled, cooked — 1 cup	175	73	185	4	Trace	—	—	—	41	33	[20]1.4	0	[20]0.19	[20]0.02	[20]2.1	0
468	Rice, puffed, added nutrients — 1 cup	15	4	60	1	Trace	—	—	—	13	3	0.3	0	0.07	0.01	0.7	0
	Rolls, enriched:																
	Cloverleaf or pan:																
469	Home recipe — 1 roll	35	26	120	3	3	1	1	1	20	16	0.7	30	0.09	0.09	0.8	Trace
470	Commercial — 1 roll	28	31	85	2	2	Trace	1	Trace	15	21	0.5	Trace	0.08	0.05	0.6	Trace
471	Frankfurter or hamburger — 1 roll	40	31	120	3	2	Trace	1	Trace	21	30	0.8	Trace	0.11	0.07	0.9	Trace
472	Hard, round or rectangular — 1 roll	50	25	155	5	2	Trace	1	1	30	24	1.2	Trace	0.13	0.12	1.4	Trace
473	Rye wafers, whole-grain, 1 7/8 by 3 1/2 inches — 2 wafers	13	6	45	2	Trace	—	—	—	10	7	0.5	0	0.04	0.03	0.2	0
474	Spaghetti, cooked, tender stage, enriched — 1 cup	140	72	155	5	1	—	—	—	32	11	[19]1.3	0	[19]0.20	[19]0.11	[19]1.5	0
	Spaghetti with meat balls, and tomato sauce:																
475	Home recipe — 1 cup	248	70	330	19	12	4	6	1	39	124	3.7	1,590	0.25	0.30	4.0	22
476	Canned — 1 cup	250	78	260	12	10	2	3	2	28	53	3.3	1,000	0.15	0.18	2.3	5
	Spaghetti in tomato sauce with cheese:																
477	Home recipe — 1 cup	250	77	260	9	9	2	5	1	37	80	2.3	1,080	0.25	0.18	2.3	13
478	Canned — 1 cup	250	80	190	6	7	2	4	2	38	40	2.8	930	0.35	0.28	4.5	10
479	Waffles, with enriched flour, 7-in diam. — 1 waffle	75	41	210	7	7	2	4	1	28	85	1.3	250	0.13	0.19	1.0	Trace
480	Waffles, made from mix, enriched, egg and milk added, 7-in diam. — 1 waffle	75	42	205	7	8	3	3	1	27	179	1.0	170	0.11	0.17	0.7	Trace
481	Wheat, puffed, added nutrients — 1 cup	15	3	55	2	Trace	—	—	—	12	4	0.6	0	0.08	0.03	1.2	0
482	Wheat, shredded, plain — 1 biscuit	25	7	90	2	1	—	—	—	20	11	0.9	0	0.06	0.03	1.1	0
483	Wheat flakes, added nutrients — 1 cup	30	4	105	3	Trace	—	—	—	24	12	1.3	0	0.19	0.04	1.5	0
	Wheat flours:																
484	Whole wheat, from hard wheats, stirred — 1 cup	120	12	400	16	2	Trace	—	1	85	49	4.0	0	0.66	0.14	5.2	0

[19] Iron, thiamin, riboflavin, and niacin are based on the minimum levels of enrichment specified in standards of identity promulgated under the Federal Food, Drug, and Cosmetic Act.

[20] Iron, thiamin, and niacin are based on the minimum levels of enrichment specified in standards of identity promulgated under the Federal Food, Drug, and Cosmetic Act. Riboflavin is based on unenriched rice. When the minimum level of enrichment specified in the standards of identity becomes effective the value will be 0.12 mg per cup of parboiled rice and of white rice.

Table A–1. (Cont.)

No.	Food, Approximate Measure, and Weight	Weight (gm)	Water (per cent)	Food Energy (calories)	Protein (gm)	Fat (gm)	Saturated total (gm)	Oleic (gm)	Linoleic (gm)	Carbohydrate (gm)	Calcium (mg)	Iron (mg)	Vitamin A Value (I.U.)	Thiamin (mg)	Riboflavin (mg)	Niacin (mg)	Ascorbic Acid (mg)
	Wheat flours (cont.)																
	All-purpose or family flour, enriched:																
485	Sifted — 1 cup	115	12	420	12	1	—	—	—	88	18	[19]3.3	0	[19]0.51	[19]0.30	[19]4.0	0
486	Unsifted — 1 cup	125	12	455	13	1	—	—	—	95	20	[19]3.6	0	[19]0.55	[19]0.33	[19]4.4	0
487	Self-rising, enriched — 1 cup	125	12	440	12	1	—	—	—	93	331	[19]3.6	0	[19]0.55	[19]0.33	[19]4.4	0
488	Cake or pastry flour, sifted — 1 cup	96	12	350	7	1	—	—	—	76	16	0.5	0	0.03	0.03	0.7	0
	Fats, Oils																
	Butter:																
	Regular, 4 sticks per pound:																
489	Stick — 1/2 cup	113	16	810	1	92	51	30	3	1	23	0	[21]3,750	—	—	—	0
490	Tablespoon (approx. 1/8 stick) — 1 tbsp.	14	16	100	Trace	12	6	4	Trace	Trace	3	0	[21]470	—	—	—	0
491	Pat (1-in sq. 1/3-in high; 90 per lb) — 1 pat	5	16	35	Trace	4	2	1	Trace	Trace	1	0	[21]170	—	—	—	0
	Whipped, 6 sticks or 2, 8-oz containers per pound:																
492	Stick — 1/2 cup	76	16	540	1	61	34	20	2	Trace	15	0	[21]2,500	—	—	—	0
493	Tablespoon (approx. 1/8 stick) — 1 tbsp.	9	16	65	Trace	8	4	3	Trace	Trace	2	0	[21]310	—	—	—	0
494	Pat (1 1/4-in sq 1/3-in high; 120 per lb) — 1 pat	4	16	25	Trace	3	2	1	Trace	Trace	1	0	[21]130	—	—	—	0
	Fats, cooking:																
495	Lard — 1 cup	205	0	1,850	0	205	78	94	20	0	0	0	0	0	0	0	0
496	Lard — 1 tbsp.	13	0	115	0	13	5	6	1	0	0	0	0	0	0	0	0
497	Vegetable fats — 1 cup	200	0	1,770	0	200	50	100	44	0	0	0	—	0	0	0	0
498	Vegetable fats — 1 tbsp.	13	0	110	0	13	3	6	3	0	0	0	—	0	0	0	0
	Margarine:																
	Regular, 4 sticks per pound:																
499	Stick — 1/2 cup	113	16	815	1	92	17	46	25	1	23	0	[22]3,750	—	—	—	0
500	Tablespoon (approx. 1/8 stick) — 1 tbsp	14	16	100	Trace	12	2	6	3	Trace	3	0	[22]470	—	—	—	0
501	Pat (1-in sq 1/3-in high; 90 per lb) — 1 pat	5	16	35	Trace	4	1	2	1	Trace	1	0	[22]170	—	—	—	0
	Whipped, 6 sticks per pound:																
502	Stick — 1/2 cup	76	16	545	1	61	11	31	17	Trace	15	0	[22]2,500	—	—	—	0
	Soft, 2 8-oz tubs per pound:																
503	Tub — 1 tub	227	16	1,635	1	184	34	68	68	1	45	0	[22]7,500	—	—	—	0
504	Tub — 1 tbsp	14	16	100	Trace	11	2	4	4	Trace	3	0	[22]470	—	—	—	0
	Oils, salad or cooking:																
505	Corn — 1 cup	220	0	1,945	0	220	22	62	117	0	0	0	—	0	0	0	0
506	Corn — 1 tbsp	14	0	125	0	14	1	4	7	0	0	0	—	0	0	0	0
507	Cottonseed — 1 cup	220	0	1,945	0	220	55	46	110	0	0	0	—	0	0	0	0
508	Cottonseed — 1 tbsp	14	0	125	0	14	4	3	7	0	0	0	—	0	0	0	0
509	Olive — 1 cup	220	0	1,945	0	220	24	167	15	0	0	0	—	0	0	0	0
510	Olive — 1 tbsp	14	0	125	0	14	2	11	1	0	0	0	—	0	0	0	0
511	Peanut — 1 cup	220	0	1,945	0	220	40	103	64	0	0	0	—	0	0	0	0
512	Peanut — 1 tbsp	14	0	125	0	14	3	7	4	0	0	0	—	0	0	0	0

513	Safflower	1 cup	220	0	1,945	0	220	18	37	165	0	0	0	—	0	0	0	0
514		1 tbsp	14	0	125	0	14	1	2	10	0	0	0	—	0	0	0	0
515	Soybean	1 cup	220	0	1,945	0	220	33	44	114	0	0	0	—	0	0	0	0
516		1 tbsp	14	0	125	0	14	2	3	7	0	0	0	—	0	0	0	0
	Salad dressing:																	
517	Blue cheese	1 tbsp	15	32	75	1	8	2	2	4	1	12	Trace	30	Trace	0.02	Trace	Trace
	Commercial, mayonnaise type:																	
518	Regular	1 tbsp	15	41	65	Trace	6	1	1	3	2	2	Trace	30	Trace	Trace	Trace	—
519	Special dietary, low calorie	1 tbsp	16	81	20	Trace	2	Trace	Trace	1	1	3	Trace	40	Trace	Trace	Trace	—
	French:																	
520	Regular	1 tbsp	16	39	65	Trace	6	1	1	3	3	2	0.1	—	—	—	—	—
521	Special dietary, low fat with artificial sweeteners	1 tbsp	15	95	Trace	Trace	Trace	—	—	—	Trace	2	0.1	—	—	—	—	—
522	Home cooked, boiled	1 tbsp	16	68	25	1	2	1	1	Trace	2	14	0.1	80	0.01	0.03	Trace	Trace
523	Mayonnaise	1 tbsp	14	15	100	Trace	11	2	2	6	Trace	3	0.1	40	Trace	0.01	Trace	—
524	Thousand island	1 tbsp	16	32	80	Trace	8	1	2	4	3	2	0.1	50	Trace	Trace	Trace	Trace
	Sugars, Sweets																	
	Cake icings:																	
525	Chocolate made with milk and table fat	1 cup	275	14	1,035	9	38	21	14	1	185	165	3.3	580	0.06	0.28	0.6	1
526	Coconut (with boiled icing)	1 cup	166	15	605	3	13	11	1	Trace	124	10	0.8	0	0.02	0.07	0.3	0
527	Creamy fudge from mix with water only	1 cup	245	15	830	7	16	5	8	3	183	96	2.7	Trace	0.05	0.20	0.7	Trace
528	White, boiled	1 cup	94	18	300	1	0	—	—	—	76	2	Trace	0	Trace	0.03	Trace	0
	Candy:																	
529	Carmels, plain or chocolate	1 oz	28	8	115	1	3	2	1	Trace	22	42	0.4	Trace	0.01	0.05	0.1	Trace
530	Chocolate, milk, plain	1 oz	28	1	145	2	9	5	3	Trace	16	65	0.3	80	0.02	0.10	0.1	Trace
531	Chocolate-coated peanuts	1 oz	28	1	160	5	12	3	6	2	11	33	0.4	Trace	0.10	0.05	2.1	Trace
532	Fondant; mints, uncoated; candy corn	1 oz	28	8	105	Trace	1	—	—	—	25	4	0.3	0	Trace	Trace	Trace	0
533	Fudge, plain	1 oz	28	8	115	1	4	2	1	Trace	21	22	0.3	Trace	0.01	0.03	0.1	Trace
534	Gum drops	1 oz	28	12	100	Trace	Trace	—	—	—	25	2	0.1	0	0	Trace	Trace	0
535	Hard	1 oz	28	1	110	0	Trace	—	—	—	28	6	0.5	0	0	0	0	0
536	Marshmallows	1 oz	28	17	90	1	Trace	—	—	—	23	5	0.5	0	0	Trace	Trace	0
	Chocolate-flavored syrup or topping:																	
537	Thin type	1 fl oz	38	32	90	1	1	Trace	Trace	Trace	24	6	0.6	Trace	0.01	0.03	0.2	0
538	Fudge type	1 fl oz	38	25	125	2	5	3	2	Trace	20	48	0.5	60	0.02	0.08	0.2	Trace
	Chocolate-flavored beverage powder (approx. 4 heaping teaspoons per oz):																	
539	With nonfat dry milk	1 oz	28	2	100	5	1	Trace	Trace	Trace	20	167	0.5	10	0.04	0.21	0.2	1
540	Without nonfat dry milk	1 oz	28	1	100	1	1	Trace	Trace	Trace	25	9	0.6	—	0.01	0.03	0.1	0
541	Honey, strained or extracted	1 tbsp	21	17	65	Trace	0	—	—	—	17	1	0.1	0	Trace	0.01	0.1	Trace
542	Jams and preserves	1 tbsp	20	29	55	Trace	Trace	—	—	—	14	4	0.2	Trace	Trace	0.01	Trace	Trace
543	Jellies	1 tbsp	18	29	50	Trace	Trace	—	—	—	13	4	0.3	Trace	Trace	0.01	Trace	1
	Molasses, cane:																	
544	Light (first extraction)	1 tbsp	20	24	50	—	—	—	—	—	13	33	0.9	—	0.01	0.01	Trace	—
545	Blackstrap (third extraction)	1 tbsp	20	24	45	—	—	—	—	—	11	137	3.2	—	0.02	0.04	0.4	—
	Syrups:																	
546	Sorghum	1 tbsp	21	23	55	—	—	—	—	—	14	35	2.6	—	—	0.02	Trace	—

[19] Iron, thiamin, riboflavin, and niacin are based on the minimum levels of enrichment specified in standards of identity promulgated under the Federal Food, Drug, and Cosmetic Act.

[21] Year-round average.

[22] Based on the average vitamin A content of fortified margarine. Federal specifications for fortified margarine require a minimum of 15,000 I.U. of vitamin A per pound.

Table A–1. (Cont.)

	Food, Approximate Measure, and Weight (in grams)	Weight gm	Water per cent	Food Energy calories	Protein gm	Fat gm	Fatty Acids Saturated (total) gm	Unsaturated Oleic gm	Unsaturated Linoleic gm	Carbohydrate gm	Calcium mg	Iron mg	Vitamin A Value I.U.	Thiamin mg	Riboflavin mg	Niacin mg	Ascorbic Acid mg
	Syrups (cont.)																
547	Table blends, chiefly corn, light and dark	1 tbsp	21	24	60	0	0	—	—	—	15	9	0.8	0	0	0	0	0
	Sugars:																	
548	Brown, firm packed	1 cup	220	2	820	0	0	—	—	—	212	187	7.5	0	0.02	0.07	0.4	0
	White:																	
549	Granulated	1 cup	200	Trace	770	0	0	—	—	—	199	0	0.2	0	0	0	0	0
550		1 tbsp	11	Trace	40	0	0	—	—	—	11	0	Trace	0	0	0	0	0
551	Powdered, stirred before measuring	1 cup	120	Trace	460	0	0	—	—	—	119	0	0.1	0	0	0	0	0
	Miscellaneous Items																	
552	Barbecue sauce	1 cup	250	81	230	4	17	2	5	9	20	53	2.0	900	0.03	0.03	0.8	13
	Beverages, alcoholic:																	
553	Beer	12 fl oz	360	92	150	1	0	—	—	—	14	18	Trace	—	0.01	0.11	2.2	—
	Gin, rum, vodka, whiskey:																	
554	80 proof	1 1/2 fl oz jigger	42	67	100	—	—	—	—	—	Trace	—	—	—	—	—	—	—
555	86 proof	1 1/2 fl oz jigger	42	64	105	—	—	—	—	—	Trace	—	—	—	—	—	—	—
556	90 proof	1 1/2 fl oz jigger	42	62	110	—	—	—	—	—	Trace	—	—	—	—	—	—	—
557	94 proof	1 1/2 fl oz jigger	42	60	115	—	—	—	—	—	Trace	—	—	—	—	—	—	—
558	100 proof	1 1/2 fl oz jigger	42	58	125	—	—	—	—	—	Trace	—	—	—	—	—	—	—
	Wines:																	
559	Dessert	3 1/2 fl oz glass	103	77	140	Trace	0	—	—	—	8	8	—	—	0.01	0.02	0.2	—
560	Table	3 1/2 fl oz glass	102	86	85	Trace	0	—	—	—	4	9	0.4	—	Trace	0.01	0.1	—
	Beverages, carbonated, sweetened, nonalcoholic:																	
561	Carbonated water	12 fl oz	366	92	115	0	0	—	—	—	29	—	—	0	0	0	0	0
562	Cola type	12 fl oz	369	90	145	0	0	—	—	—	37	—	—	0	0	0	0	0
563	Fruit-flavored sodas and Tom Collins mixes	12 fl oz	372	88	170	0	0	—	—	—	45	—	—	0	0	0	0	0
564	Ginger ale	12 fl oz	366	92	115	0	0	—	—	—	29	—	—	0	0	0	0	0
565	Root beer	12 fl oz	370	90	150	0	0	—	—	—	39	—	—	0	0	0	0	0
566	Bouillon cubes, approx. 1/2 in	1 cube	4	4	5	1	Trace	—	—	—	Trace	—	—	—	—	—	—	—
	Chocolate:																	
567	Bitter or baking	1 oz	28	2	145	3	15	8	6	Trace	8	22	1.9	20	0.01	0.07	0.4	0
568	Semisweet, small pieces	1 cup	170	1	860	7	61	34	22	1	97	51	4.4	30	0.02	0.14	0.9	0
	Gelatin:																	
569	Plain, dry powder in envelope	1 envelope	7	13	25	6	Trace	—	—	—	0	—	—	—	—	—	—	—
570	Dessert powder, 3-oz package	1 pkg	85	2	315	8	0	—	—	—	75	—	—	—	—	—	—	—
571	Gelatin dessert, prepared with water	1 cup	240	84	140	4	0	—	—	—	34	—	—	—	—	—	—	—

No.	Food, approximate measure, and weight	Measure	Grams	Water (%)	Food energy (cal)	Protein (g)	Fat (g)	Saturated (g)	Oleic (g)	Linoleic (g)	Carbohydrate (g)	Calcium (mg)	Iron (mg)	Vitamin A (IU)	Thiamin (mg)	Riboflavin (mg)	Niacin (mg)	Ascorbic acid (mg)
572	Olives, pickled: Green	4 medium or 3 extra large or 2 giant	16	78	15	Trace	2	Trace	2	Trace	Trace	8	0.2	40	—	Trace	—	—
573	Ripe: Mission	3 small or 2 large	10	73	15	Trace	2	Trace	2	Trace	Trace	9	0.1	10	Trace	Trace	—	—
	Pickles, cucumber:																	
574	Dill, medium, whole, 3 3/4 in long, 1 1/4 in diam.	1 pickle	65	93	10	1	Trace	—	—	—	1	17	0.7	70	Trace	0.01	Trace	4
575	Fresh, sliced, 1 1/2 in diam., 1/4 in thick	2 slices	15	79	10	Trace	Trace	—	—	—	3	5	0.3	20	Trace	Trace	Trace	1
576	Sweet, gherkin, small, whole, approx. 2 1/2 in long, 3/4 in diam.	1 pickle	15	61	20	Trace	Trace	—	—	—	6	2	0.2	10	Trace	Trace	Trace	1
577	Relish, finely chopped, sweet	1 tbsp	15	63	20	Trace	Trace	—	—	—	5	3	0.1	—	—	—	—	—
	Popcorn. See Grain Products																	
578	Popsicle, 3-fl oz size	1 popsicle	95	80	70	0	0	0	0	0	18	0	Trace	0	0	0	0	0
	Pudding, home recipe with starch base:																	
579	Chocolate	1 cup	260	66	385	8	12	7	4	Trace	67	250	1.3	390	0.05	0.36	0.3	1
580	Vanilla (blanc mange)	1 cup	255	76	285	9	10	5	3	Trace	41	298	Trace	410	0.08	0.41	0.3	2
581	Pudding mix, dry form, 4-oz package	1 pkg	113	2	410	3	2	1	1	Trace	103	23	1.8	Trace	0.02	0.08	0.5	0
582	Sherbet	1 cup	193	67	260	2	2	—	—	—	59	31	Trace	120	0.02	0.06	Trace	4
	Soups:																	
	Canned, condensed, ready-to-serve:																	
	Prepared with an equal volume of milk:																	
583	Cream of chicken	1 cup	245	85	180	7	10	3	3	3	15	172	0.5	610	0.05	0.27	0.7	2
584	Cream of mushroom	1 cup	245	83	215	7	14	4	4	5	16	191	0.5	250	0.05	0.34	0.7	1
585	Tomato	1 cup	250	84	175	7	7	3	2	1	23	168	0.8	1,200	0.10	0.25	1.3	15
	Prepared with an equal volume of water:																	
586	Bean with pork	1 cup	250	84	170	8	6	2	2	1	22	63	2.3	650	0.13	0.08	1.0	3
587	Beef broth, bouillon consommé	1 cup	240	96	30	5	0	—	—	—	3	Trace	0.5	Trace	Trace	0.02	1.2	—
588	Beef noodle	1 cup	240	93	70	4	3	1	1	1	7	7	1.0	50	0.05	0.07	1.0	Trace
589	Clam chowder, Manhattan type (with tomatoes, without milk)	1 cup	245	92	80	2	3	—	—	—	12	34	1.0	880	0.02	0.02	1.0	—
590	Cream of chicken	1 cup	240	92	95	3	6	3	2	1	8	24	0.5	410	0.02	0.05	0.5	Trace
591	Cream of mushroom	1 cup	240	90	135	2	10	2	3	5	10	41	0.5	70	0.02	0.12	0.7	Trace
592	Minestrone	1 cup	245	90	105	5	3	1	1	Trace	14	37	1.0	2,350	0.07	0.05	1.0	—
593	Split pea	1 cup	245	85	145	9	3	1	1	1	21	29	1.5	440	0.25	0.15	1.5	1
594	Tomato	1 cup	245	90	90	2	3	1	1	Trace	16	15	0.7	1,000	0.05	0.05	1.2	12
595	Vegetable beef	1 cup	245	92	80	5	2	Trace	—	—	10	12	0.7	2,700	0.05	0.05	1.0	—
596	Vegetarian	1 cup	245	92	80	2	2	—	—	—	13	20	1.0	2,940	0.05	0.05	1.0	—
	Dehydrated, dry form:																	
597	Chicken noodle (2-oz package)	1 pkg	57	6	220	8	6	2	3	1	33	34	1.4	190	0.30	0.15	2.4	3
598	Onion mix (1 1/2-oz package)	1 pkg	43	3	150	6	5	1	2	1	23	42	0.6	30	0.05	0.03	0.3	6
599	Tomato vegetable with noodles (2 1/2-oz pkg)	1 pkg	71	4	245	6	6	2	3	1	45	33	1.4	1,700	0.21	0.13	1.8	18
	Frozen, condensed: Clam chowder, New England type (with milk, without tomatoes):																	
600	Prepared with equal volume of milk	1 cup	245	83	210	9	12	—	—	—	16	240	1.0	250	0.07	0.29	0.5	Trace

Table A–1. (Cont.)

Food, Approximate Measure, and Weight (in grams)		gm	Water per cent	Food Energy calories	Protein gm	Fat gm	Fatty Acids Saturated (total) gm	Unsaturated Oleic gm	Linoleic gm	Carbohydrate gm	Calcium mg	Iron mg	Vitamin A Value I.U.	Thiamin mg	Riboflavin mg	Niacin mg	Ascorbic Acid mg
Soups, frozen (cont.)																	
Clam chowder, New England type																	
601	Prepared with equal volume of water	1 cup	240	89	130	4	8	—	—	—	11	91	1.0	50	0.05	0.10	0.5	—
Cream of potato:																	
602	Prepared with equal volume of milk	1 cup	245	83	185	8	10	5	3	Trace	18	208	1.0	590	0.10	0.27	0.5	Trace
603	Prepared with equal volume of water	1 cup	240	90	105	3	5	3	2	Trace	12	58	1.0	410	0.05	0.05	0.5	—
Cream of shrimp:																	
604	Prepared with equal volume of milk	1 cup	245	82	245	9	16	—	—	—	15	189	0.5	290	0.07	0.27	0.5	Trace
605	Prepared with equal volume of water	1 cup	240	88	160	5	12	—	—	—	8	38	0.5	120	0.05	0.05	0.5	—
Oyster stew:																	
606	Prepared with equal volume of milk	1 cup	240	83	200	10	12	—	—	—	14	305	1.4	410	0.12	0.41	0.5	Trace
607	Prepared with equal volume of water	1 cup	240	90	120	6	8	—	—	—	8	158	1.4	240	0.07	0.19	0.5	—
608	Tapioca, dry, quick cooking	1 cup	152	13	535	1	Trace	—	—	—	131	15	0.6	0	0	0	0	0
Tapioca desserts:																	
609	Apple	1 cup	250	70	295	1	Trace	—	—	—	74	8	0.5	30	Trace	Trace	Trace	Trace
610	Cream pudding	1 cup	165	72	220	8	8	4	3	Trace	28	173	0.7	480	0.07	0.30	0.2	2
611	Tartar sauce	1 tbsp	14	34	75	Trace	8	1	1	4	1	3	0.1	30	Trace	Trace	Trace	Trace
612	Vinegar	1 tbsp	15	94	Trace	Trace	0	—	—	—	1	1	0.1	—	—	—	—	—
613	White sauce, medium	1 cup	250	73	405	10	31	10	10	1	22	288	0.5	1,150	0.10	0.43	0.5	2
Yeast:																	
614	Bakers', dry, active	1 pkg	7	5	20	3	Trace	—	—	—	3	3	1.1	Trace	0.16	0.38	2.6	Trace
615	Brewers', dry	1 tbsp	8	5	25	3	Trace	—	—	—	3	17	1.4	Trace	1.25	0.34	3.0	Trace
Yogurt. See Milk, Cheese, Cream, Imitation Cream																	

TABLE A-2. MINERAL AND VITAMIN CONTENT OF FOODS

Explanatory notes. The data in this table are intended to provide assistance in the planning of diets modified for sodium and potassium, and to give information on food composition for nutrients recently listed for the first time in the table of Recommended Dietary Allowances. The data are derived from a number of sources listed below. For these nutrients many of the values must be regarded as tentative inasmuch as only a few determinations have been made on many kinds of foods. No recent data are available for folacin, and there is a paucity of data for vitamin E.

In some instances, the sources do not indicate whether the product analyzed was raw or cooked; it has been assumed that the values are for the raw product unless specifically stated. Cooking procedures would reduce the values somewhat.

Sodium. The values for sodium apply to foods as they are purchased in the retail market. Further additions for salt and leavening agents are accounted for in home-prepared products for which recipes state an exact measure.

Foods to which salt and other sodium compounds have ordinarily been added include canned vegetables, regular pack, assuming 0.6 per cent salt concentration; canned meats, fish, poultry, soups; cured meats; cheeses; baked products including bread, quick breads, rolls, cakes, cookies, pies; ready-to-eat and cooked breakfast cereals; salad dressings; butter, margarine.

The amount of salt added to some foods is so highly variable that the values listed in this table pertain to the unsalted product. Included are cooked fresh and frozen vegetables; cooked fresh meats, fish, and poultry; cooked legumes; cooked macaroni, spaghetti, noodles.

SOURCES OF DATA

Bunnell, R. H., *et al.*: "Alpha-Tocopherol Content of Foods," *Am. J. Clin. Nutr.*, **17**:1–10, 1965.

Composition of Foods—Raw, Processed, Prepared, Handbook No. 8. U.S. Department of Agriculture, Washington, D.C., 1963. (All values for mineral elements)

Hardinge, M. G., and Crooks, H.: "Lesser Known Vitamins in Foods," *J. Am. Diet. Assoc.*, **38**:240–45, 1961. (Folacin)

Meyer, B. H., *et al.*: "Pantothenic Acid and Vitamin B_6 in Beef," *J. Am. Diet. Assoc.*, **54**:122–25, 1969.

Murphy, E. W., *et al.*: "Provisional Tables on the Zinc Content of Foods," *J. Am. Diet. Assoc.*, **66**:345–55, 1975.

Orr, M. L.: *Pantothenic Acid, Vitamin B_6, and Vitamin B_{12} in Foods*, Home Economics Research Report No. 36, Agricultural Research Service. U.S. Department of Agriculture, Washington, D.C., 1969.

Polansky, M. M.: "Vitamin B_6 Components in Fresh and Dried Vegetables," *J. Am. Diet. Assoc.*, **54**:118–21, 1969.

Toepfer, E. W., *et al.*: *Folic Acid Content of Foods*, Handbook No. 29. U.S. Department of Agriculture, Washington, D.C., 1951.

Table A-2. Mineral and Vitamin Content of Foods; Sodium, Potassium, Phosphorus, Magnesium, and Zinc; Folacin, Pantothenic Acid, Vitamin B$_6$, Vitamin B$_{12}$, and Vitamin E (*Values for 100 gm edible portion*)

Item No.	Food	Sodium mg	Potassium mg	Phosphorus mg	Magnesium mg	Zinc mg	Folacin mcg	Pantothenic Acid mcg	Vitamin B$_6$ mcg	Vitamin B$_{12}$ mcg	Vitamin E mg
1	Almonds, dried	4	773	504	270		45	470	100	0	
2	Roasted, salted	198	773	504	—[1]			250	95	0	
3	Apples, raw, not peeled	1	110	10	8	0.05	2	105	30	0	0.31
4	Apple brown Betty	153	100	22	—						
5	Apple juice, bottled	1	101	9	4		Trace		30	0	
6	Applesauce, sweetened	2	65	5	5			85	30	0	
7	Apricots, raw	1	281	23	12	0.1	3	240	70	0	
8	Canned	1	234	15	7		1	92	54	0	
9	Dried, sulfured, uncooked	26	979	108	62		5[2]	753[2]	169[2]	0	
10	Cooked, sweetened	7	278	31	20						
11	Apricot nectar	Trace	151	12	—						
12	Asparagus, green, cooked	1	183	50	20 (raw)		109				
13	Canned, regular pack	236	166	53	— (raw)		27	195	55	0	
14	Low sodium	3	166	53	—						
15	Frozen, spears, cooked	1	238	67	14		109	410	155	0	
16	Avocado	4	604	42	45		30	1070	420	0	
17	Bacon, cooked, drained	1021	236	224	25		—	330 (raw)	125 (raw)	0.70 (raw)	0.53
18	Canadian, cooked	2555	432	218	24						
19	Baking powder, home use: Sodium aluminum sulfate	10,953	150	2904							
20	Straight phosphate	8220	170	9438							
21	Tartrate	7300	3800	0							
22	Low sodium, commercial	6	10,948								
23	Low sodium, noncommercial formula		20,729								
24	Banana	1	370	26	33	0.2	10	260	510	0	0.22
25	Barley, pearled, light	3	160	189	37			503	224	0	
26	Bass, sea, raw	68	256	—	—			512			
27	Beans, common, mature: White, dry	19	1196	425	170	2.8	125	725	560	0	0.47
28	Cooked	7	416	148	—	1.0					
29	Canned with pork and tomato sauce	463	210	92	37			92			

No.	Food	1	2	3	4	5	6	7	8	9	10
30	Red, dry	10	984	406	163		180[1]	500	441	0	
31	Cooked	3	340	140	—						
	Beans, Lima, immature:										
32	Cooked	1	422	121	67 (raw)		34				
33	Canned, regular pack	236	222	70	—		13	130	90	0	
34	Low sodium	4	222	70	—						
35	Frozen, Fordhook, cooked	101	426	90	48 (raw)		34	240	150	0	
36	Mature seeds, dry	4	1529	385	180	2.8	103	975	580	0	
37	Cooked	2	612	154	—	0.9	128				
38	Beans, Mung, sprouts, cooked	4	156	48	—		145				
39	Beans, snap, green, cooked	4	151	37	32 (raw)	0.3	28	190 (raw)	80 (raw)	0	
40	Canned, regular pack	236	95	25	14	0.3	12	75	40	0	0.03
41	Low sodium	2	95	25	—						
42	Frozen, cooked	1	152	32	21 (raw)		28	135	70	0	0.11
43	Yellow, cooked	3	151	37	—		32	250 (raw)	— (raw)	0	
44	Canned, regular pack	236	95	25	—			—	42	0	
45	Low sodium	2	95	25	—						
	Beef:										
46	All cuts, lean, broiled or roasted, average	60	370	246	29	5.8	11	620 (raw)	435 (raw)	1.8 (raw)	0.13
47	Simmered, average	60	370	194	18	6.2				(raw)	
48	Hamburger, regular, cooked	47	450	194	21		7				0.37
49	Beef, canned, roast beef	—	259	116	—						
50	Beef, corned, cooked	1740	150	93	—					1.84 (canned)	
51	Hash, canned	540	200	67	—				75 (with potato)	—	
52	Beef, dried	4300	200	404	—					1.84	
53	Beef potpie, commercial	366	93	48	—						
54	Home recipe	284	159	71	—						
55	Beef and vegetable stew, canned	411	174	45	—					0.65	
56	Home recipe	37	250	75	—						

[1] Dashes denote lack of reliable data for a constituent believed to be present in measurable amounts.

[2] Source of data does not indicate whether raw or cooked; it is assumed that the values are for the raw food.

Table A–2. (Cont.)

Item No.	Food	Sodium mg	Potassium mg	Phosphorus mg	Magnesium mg	Zinc mg	Folacin mcg	Pantothenic Acid mcg	Vitamin B6 mcg	Vitamin B12 mcg	Vitamin E mg
57	Beets, cooked	43	208	23	25 (raw)		14	150 (raw)	55 (raw)	0	
58	Canned, regular pack	236	167	18	15 (raw)		3	100 (raw)	50 (raw)	0	
59	Low sodium	46	167	18	—						
60	Beet greens, cooked	76	332	25	106 (raw)		60	250 (raw)	100 (raw)	0	
	Beverages, alcoholic										
61	Beer	7	25	30				80	60	0	
62	Gin	1	2								
63	Wine, table	5	92	10	10			30	40	0	
	Biscuits, baking powder:										
64	Enriched	626	117	175	—						
65	Self-rising flour	660³	64	317³	—						
66	Biscuit dough, commercial in cans	868	65	497	—						
67	Blackberries, raw	1	170	19	30		14	240	50	0	
68	Blueberries, raw	1	81	13	6		8	156	67	0	
69	Frozen, sweetened	1	66	11	4		8	121	54	0	
70	Bluefish, baked or broiled, prepared with butter	104	—	287	—						
71	Bouillon cube	24,000	100	—	—						
72	Bran, with sugar and malt extract	1060	1070	1176	—						
73	Bran flakes (40 per cent bran)	925	—	495	—	3.6		875	384	0	
74	Bran flakes with raisins	800	—	396	—						
75	Brazil nuts	1	715	693	225		5	231	170	0	
	Breads:										
76	Boston brown	251	292	160							
77	Cracked wheat	529	134	128	35		25	607	92	0	
78	French or Vienna	580	90	85	22		9	378	53	0	
79	Italian	585	74	77	24		—				
80	Raisin	365	233	87							
81	Rye, American	557	145	147	42	1.6	16	450	100	0	
82	Pumpernickel	569	454	229	71	0.6		500	160	0	
83	White, 3–4 per cent nonfat milk solids	507	105	97	22		15	430	40	Trace	0.10
84	Whole-wheat bread, 2 per cent nonfat milk solids	527	273	228	78	1.8	30	760	180	0	0.45

No.	Food										
85	Broccoli spears, cooked	10	267	62	24 (raw)		54				1.00
86	Frozen, cooked	12	220	58	21		54	525	170	0	
87	Brownies with nuts	251	190	148	—				175 (frozen)	0	
88	Brussels sprouts, cooked	10	273	72	29 (raw)		49	420 (frozen)	175 (frozen)		
89	Butter, salted	987	23	16	2	0.1			3	Trace	
90	Unsalted	Under 10									
91	Buttermilk	130	140	95	14		—	307	36	0.22	
92	Cabbage, raw	20	233	29	13	0.4	11	205	160	0	
93	Cooked, small amount of water	14	163	20	—	0.4	32²				
94	Cabbage, celery or Chinese	23	253	40	14						
	Cakes (home recipe)[4]:										
95	Angel food	283	88	22	—			200 (commercial)	—	—	
96	Chocolate with icing	235	154	131	—						
97	Fruitcake, dark	158	496	113	—						
98	Gingerbread	237	454	65	—						
99	Plain with icing	229	114	104	—						
100	Plain without icing	300	79	102	—	0.2		—	40⁵	—	1.10
101	Poundcake, old fashioned	110	60	79	—						
102	Sponge	167	87	112	—						
	Candy:										
103	Caramels	226	192	122	—						
104	Chocolate, milk, plain	94	384	231	58	0.4					1.10
105	Fudge, plain	190	147	84	—	0.3					
106	Hard	32	4	7	Trace	0.3					
107	Marshmallows	39	6	6	—						
108	Peanut brittle	31	151	95	—						
109	Cantaloupe	12	251	16	16		7	250	86	0	0.14
110	Carrots, raw	47	341	36	23		8	280	150	0	0.11²
111	Cooked	33	222	31	—						
112	Canned, regular pack	236	120	22	—		3	130	30	0	0.11
113	Low sodium	39	120	22	—						
114	Cashew nuts, unsalted	15	464	373	267			1300	—	0	
115	Cauliflower, raw	13	295	56	24		22²	1000	210	0	
116	Cooked	9	206	42	—						
117	Frozen, cooked	10	207	38	13 (raw)			540	190	0	

[2]Source of data does not indicate whether raw or cooked; it is assumed that the values are for the raw food.
[3]Based on use of self-rising flour containing anhydrous monocalcium phosphate.
[4]Based on calculations using sodium aluminum sulfate powder with monocalcium phosphate monohydrate.
[5]Nature of samples not clearly defined.

Table A–2. (Cont.)

Item No.	Food	Sodium mg	Potassium mg	Phosphorus mg	Magnesium mg	Zinc mg	Folacin mcg	Pantothenic Acid mcg	Vitamin B6 mcg	Vitamin B12 mcg	Vitamin E mg
118	Celery, raw	126	341	28	22		7	429	60	0	0.38
119	Cooked	88	239	22							
120	Chard, Swiss, cooked	86	321	24	65 (raw)		42	172 (raw)		0	
	Cheese:										
121	Cheddar or American	700	82	478	45	4.0	16	500	80	1	
122	Cheddar, process	1136[6]	80	771[6]			11	400	80	0.80	
123	Cottage, creamed	229	85	152			31	220	40	1	
124	Uncreamed	290	72	175							
125	Cream	250	74	95				270	55	0.22	
126	Parmesan	734	149	781	48			530	96	—	
127	Swiss	710	104	563				370	75	1.80	
128	Cherries, raw, sweet	2	191	19	14		6	261	32	0	
129	Canned, syrup pack	1	124	12	9		3	—	30	0	
130	Frozen, sweetened	2	130	15	8			83	58	0	
	Chicken, broiled:										
131	Light without skin	64	411	265	19	0.9	3	800	683	0.45	0.37
132	Dark without skin	86	321	229		2.8	3	1000	325	0.40	
133	Chicken, canned, boneless		138	247				850	300	0.79	
134	Chicken potpie, frozen, commercial	411	153	50							
135	Chicory	7	182	21	13		28	—	45	0	
136	Chili con carne, canned with beans	531	233	126	169			140	103	—	
137	Chili powder with seasonings	1574	1000	204	292						
138	Chocolate, bitter	4	830	384	63	0.9		190	35	0	
139	Chocolate syrup, thin	52	282	92							
140	Clams, raw, soft, meat only	36	235	183		1.5		300	80	98	
141	Hard, round, meat only	205	311	151		1.5					
142	Canned		140	137		1.2	2	—	83	—	
143	Cocoa, breakfast, dry powder	6	1522	648	420	5.6					
144	Processed with alkali	717	651	648							
145	Coconut, fresh, shredded	23	256	95	46		28	200	44	0	
146	Dried, sweetened		353	112	77						
147	Coffee, instant, dry powder	72	3256	383	456	0.6		400	32	0	
148	Beverage	1	36	4		0.03		4	Trace	0	

No.	Food									
149	Collards, cooked	25	234	39	57 (raw)		102	450 (frozen)	195 (frozen)	0
150	Cookies, plain and assorted	365	67	163	15	0.3				
151	Fig bars	252	198	60	—	0.4				
152	Corn, sweet, cooked	Trace	165	89	48 (raw)	0.4	28[2]	540 (raw)	161 (raw)	0
153	Canned, whole kernel, regular pack	236	97	49	19	0.4	8	220	200	0.05
154	Low-sodium pack	2	97	49	—					
	Corn cereals, ready to eat:									
155	Cornflakes	1005	120	45	16	0.3	6	185	65	0.12
156	Cornflakes, sugar coated	775	—	24	—					
157	Corn, puffed	1060	—	90	—			288	—	0
158	Corn, shredded	988	—	39	—					
159	Corn, rice, and wheat flakes	950	120	120	20					
160	Corn grits, dry	1	80	73	3	0.4		—	147	0.31
161	Cooked	—	11	10	—					
162	Cornbread, southern style, degermed	591	157	156	—					
	Cornmeal, white or yellow, dry:									
163	Whole ground	(1)	(284)	256	106	1.8	7	580[5]	250[5]	0.64[5]
164	Degermed, dry	1	120	99	47	0.8	9			
165	Cooked	—	16	14	7	0.1	41			
166	Cowpeas, immature, cooked	1	379	146	55			95 (frozen)		0
167	Canned, regular pack	236	352	112	—		26	162	53	0
168	Cowpeas, dry seeds, cooked	8	229	95	230	1.2	439	1050	562	0
169	Crabmeat, canned	1000	110	182	34	1.1	Trace	600	300	10
170	Crackers, graham, plain	670	384	149	51					
171	Saltines	(1100)	(120)	90	—	0.5		—		
172	Soda	1100	120	89	29				68	0
173	Cranberry juice	1	10	3	3					
174	Cranberry sauce	1	30	4	2			—	22	0
175	Cream, half-and-half	46	129	85	—					
176	Light, coffee	43	122	80	11			321	33	0.25
177	Whipping, light	36	102	67	9			—	29	0.20

[2]Source of data does not indicate whether raw or cooked; it is assumed that the values are for the raw food.

[5]Nature of samples not clearly defined.

[6]Values for phosphorus and sodium are based on use of 1.5 per cent anhydrous disodium phosphate as the emulsifying agent. If the emulsifying agent does not contain either phosphorus or sodium, the content of these nutrients per 100 gm is sodium, 650 mg; phosphorus, 444 mg.

Table A-2. (Cont.)

Item No.	Food	Sodium mg	Potassium mg	Phosphorus mg	Magnesium mg	Zinc mg	Folacin mcg	Pantothenic Acid mcg	Vitamin B₆ mcg	Vitamin B₁₂ mcg	Vitamin E mg
178	Cream substitute (cream, skim milk, lactose)	575	—	—	—						
179	Cucumbers, not peeled	6	160	27	11			250⁵	42⁵	0	
180	Custard, baked	79	146	117	—						
181	Dandelion greens, cooked	44	232	42	36 (raw)						
182	Dates, domestic	1	648	63	58		25	780	153	0	
183	Doughnuts, cake type	501	90	190	—	0.5		387⁵	—	—	
184	Duck, flesh only, raw	74	285	(203)	—						
185	Eggplant, cooked	1	150	21	16 (raw)		10	220 (raw)	81 (raw)	0	
186	Eggs, whole	122	129	205	11	1.0	5	1600 (raw)	110 (raw)	2.0 (raw)	0.46 (cooked)
187	White	146	139	15	9	0.02	1	200 (raw)	2 (raw)	0.10 (raw)	
188	Yolk	52	98	569	16	3.0	13	4400	300	6	
189	Endive, curly	14	294	54	10		47	90 (canned)	20 (canned)	0	
190	Farina, regular, dry	2	83	107	25	0.5	13	515	67	0	
191	Cooked, salted	144	9	12	3	0.06					
192	Instant cooking, cooked	188	13	60	4						
193	Fats, vegetable	0	0	0	0						
194	Figs, raw	2	194	22	20		14	300	113	0	
195	Canned	2	149	13				69		0	
196	Dried, uncooked	34	640	77	71		32	435	175	0	
197	Flounder, raw	78	342	195	—	0.7		850	170	1.2	
198	Fruit cocktail	5	161	12	7			—	33	0	
199	Gelatin, dry	—	—	—	33			—	7	—	
200	Sweetened, ready to eat	51									
201	Goose, flesh only, raw	86	420	203	—						
202	Grapefruit, raw	1	135	16	12		3	283	34	0	
203	Canned, sweetened	1	135	14	11			120	20	0	
204	Grapefruit juice, canned	1	162	14	—		2	130	11	0	0.04
205	Frozen, diluted	1	170	17	9		1	162	14	0	
206	Grapes, American	3	158	12	13		5	75⁵	80⁵	0	
207	European	3	173	20	6						

No.	Food										
208	Grape juice, bottled	2	116	12	12						
209	Haddock, raw	61	304	197	24	0.7		130	180	1.3	0.60 (broiled)
210	Fried (dipped in egg, milk, bread crumbs)	177	348	247	24						
211	Heart, beef, lean, raw	86	193	195	18			2500	250	11	
212	Cooked, braised	104	232	181	—						
213	Herring, raw, Pacific	74	420	225	—					2	
214	Smoked, hard	6231	157	—	—			500	200	7	
215	Honey, strained	5	51	6	3		3	200	20	0	
216	Honeydew melon	12	251	16	—		5	207	56	0	
217	Ice cream, no added salt, approximately 12% fat	40	112	99	14	0.5		492	—	—	0.06
218	Ice milk, no added salt	68	195	124	—						
219	Jams and preserves	12	88	9	5			—	25	0	
220	Jellies	17	75	7	4					0	
221	Kale, cooked, leaves with stems	43	221	46	37 (raw)		70	376 (frozen)	185 (frozen)	0	
222	Lamb, average of lean cuts, cooked	70	290	223	21	4.3	3	550 (raw)	275	2.15 (raw)	0.16
223	Lard	0	0	0	0	0.2		20	20	0	
224	Lemon juice, fresh	1	141	10	8		1	103	46	0	
225	Lemonade, frozen, diluted	Trace	16	1	1			11	5	0	
226	Lettuce, butterhead	9	264	26	—		25				
227	Crisphead	9	175	22	11		21[5]	200[5]	55[5]	0	0.06
228	Looseleaf	9	264	25	—		44				
229	Lime juice, fresh or canned	1	104	11	—			314 (sweet)		0	
230	Limeade, frozen, diluted	Trace	13	1	—						
231	Liver, cooked, fried: Beef	184	380	476	18	5.1	294 (raw)	7700 (raw)	840 (raw)	80 (raw)	0.63 (broiled)
232	Calf	118	453	537	26	6.1		8000 (raw)	670 (raw)	60 (raw)	
233	Pork	111	395	539	24		221	6400 (raw)	650 (raw)	32 (raw)	
234	Lobster, canned or cooked	210	180	192	22 (raw)	2.2		1500 (raw)	—	0.5 (raw)	
235	Macaroni, dry	2	197	162	48	1.5		—		0	
236	Cooked, firm state	1	79	65	20	0.5			64		
237	Tender	1	61	50	18						

[5] Nature of samples not clearly defined.

Table A–2. (Cont.)

Item No.	Food	Sodium mg	Potassium mg	Phosphorus mg	Magnesium mg	Zinc mg	Folacin mcg	Pantothenic Acid mcg	Vitamin B6 mcg	Vitamin B12 mcg	Vitamin E mg
238	Macaroni and cheese, baked	543	120	161	—		—				
239	Margarine, salted	987	23	16	—	0.2	—				0.04
240	Unsalted	Under 10									
241	Milk, whole	50	144	93	13	0.4	1	340	40	0.4	
242	Skim	52	145	95	14	0.4	Trace	370	42	0.4	
243	Dry, nonfat, instant	526	1725	1005	143	4.5		3600	380	3.2	
244	Evaporated, undiluted	118	303	205	25	0.8	1	640	50	0.16	
245	Milk, goat's	34	180	106	17			320	45	0.08	
246	Milk, human	16	51	14	4			220	10	0.04	
	Milk beverages:										
247	Chocolate flavored, with skim milk	46	142	91	—						
248	Malted, with whole milk	91	200	122	—						
249	Molasses, light	15	917	45	46		10[5]	350[5]	200[5]	0[5]	
250	Blackstrap	96	2927	84	258						
251	Muffins, corn, enriched degermed cornmeal	481	135	169	—						
252	Plain	441	125	151	—						
253	Mushrooms, raw	15	414	116	—		24	2200	125	0	
254	Canned	400	197	68	8		4	1000	60	0	
255	Mustard, prepared, yellow	1252	130	73	48						1.75
256	Mustard greens, cooked	18	220	32	27		60	164	133	0	1.75 (raw)
257	Nectarine	6	294	24	13		20	(frozen)	(frozen)	(frozen)	
258	Noodles, enriched, dry	5	136	183	—			—	17	0	
259	Cooked	2	44	59	—			—	88	Trace	
260	Oatmeal, dry	2	352	405	144	3.4	30	1500	140	0	
261	Cooked, salted	218	61	57	21	0.5	33				
262	Oil, vegetable	0	0	0	0	0.2	—				36.0 (corn)[7]
263	Okra, cooked	2	174	41	41 (raw)		24	215 (frozen)	45 (frozen)	0 (frozen)	2.27[2]
264	Olives, green	2400	55	17	22		—	18	—	0	
265	Ripe	813	34	16	—		1	15	14	0	
266	Onions, mature, raw	10	157	36	12	0.3	11	130	130	0	
267	Cooked	7	110	29	—		10				

No.	Food										
268	Onions, young green	5	231	39	—	0.3	14	144	—	0	
269	Oranges, peeled	1	200	20	11	0.2	5	250	60	0	
270	Orange juice, fresh	1	200	17	11	0.02	2	190	40	0	0.04
271	Canned	1	199	18	10	0.07	2	150	35	0	
272	Frozen, diluted	1	186	16	10	0.02	2	164	28	0	
273	Oysters, eastern, raw	73	121	143	32	74.7	11	250	50	18	
274	Pancakes, buckwheat, from mix	464	245	337	—	(canned)				0	
275	Wheat, home recipe	425	123	139	—						
276	Papayas, raw	3	234	16				218	—	0	
277	Parsley	45	727	63	41		38	300	164	0	
278	Parsnips, cooked	8	379	62	32 (raw)		23	600[2]	90[2]	0[2]	
279	Peaches, raw	1	202	19	10	0.2	4	170	24	0	
280	Canned	2	130	12	6	0.1	1	50	19	0	
281	Dried, sulfured, uncooked	16	950	117	48		5	—	100[2]	0[2]	
282	Cooked with sugar	4	261	32	15						
283	Frozen	2	124	13	6		4	132	18	0	
284	Peach nectar	1	78	11	—						
285	Peanuts, roasted	5	701	407	175	3.0	57	2100	400	0	7.70 (dry)
286	Salted	418	674	401	175		57			0	
287	Peanut butter	607	670	407	173	2.9	2	70	330	0	
288	Pears, raw	2	130	11	7			22	17	0	
289	Canned	1	84	7	5				14	0	
290	Pear nectar	1	39	5	—						
291	Peas, green, cooked	1	196	99	35 (raw)	0.7	25			0	0.55
292	Canned, regular pack	236	96	76	20	0.8	10	150	50	0	0.02
293	Low-sodium pack	3	96	76							
294	Frozen, not thawed[8]	129[8]	150	90	24		25	315	130	0	0.25
295	Peas, dry, split, raw	40	895	268	180	3.2	51[2]	2000	130	0	
296	Cooked	13	296	89	—	1.1		220	20	0	
297	Pecans	Trace	603	289	142		27	1707 (canned)	183 (canned)	0 (canned)	
298	Peppers, sweet, green, raw	13	213	22	18		7	230	260	0	
299	Perch, ocean, Atlantic, raw	79	269	207	—						

[2] Source of data does not indicate whether raw or cooked; it is assumed that the values are for the raw food.

[5] Nature of samples not clearly defined.

[7] Vitamin E in other oils as follows: cottonseed, 60.5; olive, 67.0; peanut, 61.0; safflower, 90.0; and soybean, 21.0 mg per 100 gm.

[8] Average weighted in accordance with commercial practices in freezing vegetables.

651

Table A–2. (Cont.)

Item No.	Food	Sodium mg	Potassium mg	Phosphorus mg	Magnesium mg	Zinc mg	Folacin mcg	Pantothenic Acid mcg	Vitamin B6 mcg	Vitamin B12 mcg	Vitamin E mg
300	Persimmons, Japanese	6	174	26	8			—			
301	Pickles, dill	1428	200	21	12				7[5]	0[5]	
302	Relish, sweet	712	—	14	—						
	Pies, home recipe:										
303	Apple	301	80	22	—			110	—	0	2.50
304	Cherry	304	105	25	—						
305	Custard	287	137	113	—			946	—	0	
306	Lemon meringue	282	50	49	—						
307	Mince	448	178	38	—						
308	Pumpkin	214	160	69	—			519	—	—	
309	Piecrust, baked	611	50	50	—						
310	Pike, walleye, raw	51	319	214	—			—	115	—	
311	Pineapple, raw	1	146	8	13		6	160	88	0	
312	Canned	1	96	5	8		1	100	74	0	
313	Pineapple juice, canned	1	149	9	12		1	100	96	0	
314	Pizza, cheese, home recipe	702	130	195							
315	Plums, raw	2	299	17	9			186	52	0	
316	Canned, purple	1	142	10	5		1	72	27	0	
317	Popcorn, salted	1940	—	216	—	3.0	1		204	0	
	Pork, fresh:										
318	Ham, lean, roasted	65	390	308	29	3.1	2 (loin)	790 (raw)	450 (raw)	0.70 (raw)	0.16 (chops, fried)
	Pork cured:										
319	Picnic ham, lean, simmered	65	390	176	18	4.0					
320	Ham, light cure, lean, cooked	930	326	200	20	4.0	11	675 (raw)	400 (raw)	0.60 (raw)	0.28 (fried)
321	Canned, spiced or unspiced	(1100)	(340)	156	22 (raw)						
322	Potatoes, baked	4	503	65	—			360	233[5] (raw)		0.03
323	Boiled, unsalted	2	285	42	—	0.3		540 (frozen)	174	0	0.04
324	French fried	6	853	111	—		7		180 (frozen)		0.28
325	Mashed, with milk, table fat, salted	331	250	48	—						
326	Potato chips	Variable to 1000	1130	139	—			—	180	0	6.40
327	Pretzels	1680[9]	130	131				540	19	Trace	0.15

No.	Food										
328	Prunes, dried, uncooked	118	694	79	40		5	460[2]	240[2]	0[2]	
329	Cooked, without sugar	4	327	37	20						
330	Prune juice, canned	2	235	20	10						
	Pudding, home recipe:										
331	Bread with raisins	201	215	114	—						
332	Chocolate	56	171	98	—						
333	Cornstarch (blanc mange)	65	138	91	—						
334	Rennin, using mix	46	128	92	—						
335	Rice with raisins	71	177	94	—						
336	Tapioca cream	156	135	109							
337	Pumpkin, canned, unsalted	2	240	26	12 (raw)		8	400	56	0	
338	Radishes, raw	18	322	31	15		7	184	75	0	
339	Raisins, dried	27	763	101	35		10	45	240	0	
340	Raspberries, red, raw	1	168	22	20		5	240	60	0	
341	Frozen	1	100	17			5	270	38	0	
342	Rhubarb, cooked	2	203	15	13		4[5]	70	25	0	
343	Rice, white, dry	5	92	94	28	1.3		550 (frozen)	170 (frozen)	0	
344	Cooked, salted	374	28	28	8	0.4	16				0.18
	Rice cereals:										
345	Flakes	987	180	132	—	1.4	8	340	125	0	0.04
346	Puffed, without salt	2	100	92	—	1.4		378	75	0	
347	Rolls, commercial, plain	506	95	85	—	0.6		310	35	—	
348	Sweet	389	124	107	—						
349	Whole wheat	564	292	281							
350	Rutabagas, cooked	4	167	31	15 (raw)		5	160[2]	100[2]	0[2]	
351	Rye flour, light	1	156	185	73		16	720	90	0	
352	Rye wafers	882	600	388	—						
	Salad dressings:[10]										
353	Blue cheese	1094	37	74							
354	Commercial, mayonnaise type	586	9	26							
355	French	1370	79	14	10	0.2					
356	Home cooked	728	116	93							
357	Mayonnaise	597	34	28	2	0.2					
358	Thousand island	700	113	17							

[2] Source of data does not indicate whether raw or cooked; it is assumed that the values are for the raw food.

[5] Nature of samples not clearly defined.

[9] Sodium content is variable. For example, very thin pretzel sticks contain about twice the average amount listed.

[10] For salad dressings without salt, sodium content is low, ranging from less than 10 mg to 50 mg per 100 gm; the amount is usually indicated on the label.

Table A-2. (Cont.)

Item No.	Food	Sodium mg	Potassium mg	Phosphorus mg	Magnesium mg	Zinc mg	Folacin mcg	Pantothenic Acid mcg	Vitamin B6 mcg	Vitamin B12 mcg	Vitamin E mg
359	Salmon, pink, raw	64	306	—	—			300	700	4	1.35 (broiled)
360	Canned	387[11]	361	286	30	0.9	1	550	300	6.89	
361	Sardines, Pacific, canned in tomato sauce	400	320	478	24		1	700	160	10	
362	Sauerkraut	747[12]	140	18	—			93	130	0	0.06
	Sausage:										
363	Bologna	1300	230	128	—	1.8		—	100	—	
364	Frankfurters, raw	1100	220	133	—	2.0		430	140	1.30	
365	Pork links, cooked	958	269	162	16		12	682	165	0.54	0.16 (fried)
366	Scallops, bay steamed	265	476	338				132 (raw)	—	1.20 (raw)	0.60 (frozen, deep fried)
367	Shad, raw	54	330	260	—			608	—	—	
368	Baked, with butter or margarine	79	377	313	—						
369	Sherbet, orange	10	22	13	—						
370	Shrimp, raw	140	220	166	42	1.5		280	100	0.90	0.60 (fried)
371	Canned, dry pack	—	122	263	51	2.1	2	210	60	—	
	Soup, canned, diluted with equal part water:										
372	Bean with pork	403	158	51	—						
373	Beef bouillon	326	54	13	—						
374	Beef noodle	382	32	20	—						
375	Chicken noodle	408	23	15	—						
376	Clam chowder, Manhattan type	383	75	19	—						
377	Cream soup (mushroom), prepared with milk	424	114	69							
378	Minestrone	406	128	24							
379	Pea, green	367	80	46							
380	Tomato	396	94	14	9						
381	Vegetable with beef broth	345	98	16				140	—	0	
382	Spaghetti, dry	2	197	162				—	64	0	
383	Cooked, tender	1	61	50							

No.	Food									
384	Spaghetti with meatballs, canned	488	98	45	—	—					
385	Spaghetti in tomato sauce with cheese, home recipe	(382)	163	54	—	—					
386	Spinach, raw	71	470	51	88	0.8	77	300	280	0	
387	Cooked	50	324	38	—	0.7	75	75	130	0	
388	Canned, regular pack	236	250	26	63	0.8	49	65 (frozen)	70 (frozen)	0	0.02
389	Low sodium	32	250	26	—					0	
390	Squash, summer, cooked	1	141	25	16		11	173	63	0	
391	Winter, cooked	1	258	32	17 (raw)		12	282 (frozen)	91 (frozen)	0	
392	Strawberries, raw	1	164	21	12		9	340 (frozen)	55 (frozen)	0	0.13
393	Frozen	1	112	17	9		9	135	43	0	0.21
394	Sugar, brown	30	344	19							
395	Granulated	1	3	0	Trace	0.06	12[5]				
396	Sweet potatoes, baked	12	300	58	31 (raw)		12[5]	820 (raw)	218 (raw)	0	
397	Boiled	10	243	47							
398	Candied	42	190	43							
399	Syrup, table blend	68	4	16							
400	Tangerines, raw	2	126	18	—		7	200	67	0	
401	Tangerine juice, canned	1	178	14				—	32	0	
402	Tapioca, dry	3	18	18	3		6				
403	Tea, instant, dry powder	—	4530	—	395						
404	Beverage	—	25		22	0.02					
405	Tomatoes, raw	3	244	27	14	0.2	8	330	100	0	0.40
406	Canned, regular pack	130	217	19	12	0.2	4	230	90	0	
407	Low sodium	3	217	19							
408	Tomato catsup, regular pack	1042	363	50	21				107	0	
409	Tomato juice, canned, regular pack	200	227	18	10		7	250	192	0	0.22
410	Canned, low sodium	3	227	18							
411	Tongue, beef, braised	61	164	117	16 (raw)						
412	Tuna, canned, in oil, solids and liquid	800	301	294		1.0	2	320	425	2.20	
413	Turkey, light, roasted	82	411	(251)	28	2.1	8[5]	591	—	—	
414	Dark, roasted	99	398	(251)	—	4.4		1128	—	—	

[2] Source of data does not indicate whether raw or cooked; it is assumed that the values are for the raw food.

[5] Nature of samples not clearly defined.

[11] If canned without salt, the sodium value is about the same as for raw salmon.

[12] Based on salt content of 1.9 per cent; may vary significantly from this level.

Table A-2. (Cont.)

Item No.	Food	Sodium mg	Potassium mg	Phosphorus mg	Magnesium mg	Zinc mg	Folacin mcg	Pantothenic Acid mcg	Vitamin B6 mcg	Vitamin B12 mcg	Vitamin E mg
415	Turnips, cooked, diced	34	188	24	20 (raw)		4	200 (raw)	90 (raw)	0	
416	Turnip greens, canned, regular pack	236	243	30	58 (raw)		42	68	—	0	
417	Frozen, not thawed	23	188	41	—			140	100	0	
418	Veal, lean, stewed	80	500	140	—	4.2	5	1060 (raw)	400 (raw)	1.75 (raw)	
419	Roasted	80	500	235	19	4.1					0.05 (fried)
420	Vinegar, cider	1	100	9	1					0	
421	Waffles, home recipe	475	145	173	—			650	1 [5]	—	
422	Walnuts, black	3	460	570	190		77		—		
423	English	2	450	380	131			900	730	0	
424	Watermelon	1	100	10	8		1	300	68	0	
425	Wheat bran, crude	9	1121	1276	490	9.8	195				
	Wheat cereals, cooked:										
426	Wheat and malted barley, dry	1	—	350	168	3.6	33				
427	Cooked	72	Trace	59	31	0.5					0.61 [2]

No.		C1	C2	C3	C4	C5	C6	C7	C8	C9
428	Wheat, rolled, cooked	Trace	84	76	—		49			
	Wheat cereals, ready to eat:									
429	Wheat flakes	1032	—	309	—	2.3	47	469	292	0
430	Wheat, puffed, without salt	4	340	322	—	2.6		—	170	0
431	Wheat, shredded, plain	3	348	388	133	2.8	55	706	244	0
	Wheat flours:									
432	All purpose or family	2	95	87	25	0.7	8	465	60	0
433	Cake	2	95	73	—	0.3	5	320	45	0
434	Self-rising	1079	90[13]	466						
435	Whole wheat	3	370	372	113	2.4	38	1100	340	0
436	Wheat germ	3	827	1118	336	14.3	305	1200	1150	0
437	White sauce, medium	379	139	93	—					
	Yeast, bakers':									
438	Compressed	16	610	394	59			3500	600	0
439	Dry active	(52)	(1998)	(1291)	—			11,000	2000	0
440	Brewers', dry	121	1894	1753	231		2022	12,000	2500	0
441	Yogurt, made from partially skimmed milk	51	143	94	—			313	46	0.11

[2] Source of data does not indicate whether raw or cooked; it is assumed that the values are for the raw food.

[5] Nature of samples not clearly defined.

[13] Ninety milligrams potassium per 100 gm contributed by flour. Small quantities of additional potassium may be contributed by other ingredients.

Table A–3 Nutritive Values of Baby Foods*

(Per 100 gm Edible Portion—About 7 Tablespoons)

Food	Energy cal	Protein gm	Fat gm	Carbo-hydrate gm	Calcium mg	Iron mg	Vitamin A Value I.U.	Thiamin mg	Riboflavin mg	Niacin mg	Ascorbic Acid mg
Cereals, Precooked, Dry and Other											
Cereal Products											
Barley, added nutrients	348	13.4	1.2	73.6	736	53.2	(0)	3.71	1.20	32.2	(0)
High protein, added nutrients	357	35.2	3.7	48.1	815	63.1	—	3.67	1.15	24.0	(0)
Mixed, added nutrients	368	15.2	2.9	70.6	820	56.4	—	3.15	1.35	22.3	(0)
Oatmeal, added nutrients	375	16.5	5.5	66.0	757	48.2	(0)	2.58	1.05	21.3	(0)
Rice, added nutrients	371	6.6	1.6	80.0	858	50.2	(0)	2.56	1.24	19.7	(0)
Dinners, Canned											
Cereal, vegetable, meat mixtures (approx. 2%–4% protein):											
Beef noodle dinner	48	2.8	1.1	6.8	12	0.5	620	0.02	0.05	0.5	2
Cereal, egg yolk, and bacon	82	2.9	4.9	6.6	29	0.8	520	0.05	0.06	0.4	—
Chicken noodle dinner	49	2.1	1.3	7.2	27	0.3	800	0.03	0.06	0.4	1
Macaroni, tomatoes, meat, and cereal	67	2.6	2.0	9.6	21	0.5	500	0.14	0.12	1.0	1
Split peas, vegetables, meat, or bacon	80	4.0	2.1	11.2	29	0.7	600	0.08	0.05	0.5	1
Vegetables and bacon, with cereal	68	1.7	2.9	8.7	17	0.6	2200	0.07	0.05	0.6	1
Vegetables and beef, with cereal	56	2.7	1.6	7.6	17	0.8	2800	0.03	0.04	0.9	1
Vegetables and chicken, with cereal	52	2.1	1.4	7.7	33	0.4	1000	0.03	0.04	0.5	Trace
Vegetables and ham, with cereal	64	2.8	2.2	8.3	25	0.3	1000	0.08	0.05	0.5	3
Vegetables and lamb, with cereal	58	2.2	2.0	7.7	23	0.7	2200	0.03	0.05	0.7	1
Vegetables and liver, with cereal	47	3.1	.4	7.8	17	2.7	4700	0.04	0.37	1.6	3
Vegetables and liver, with bacon and cereal	57	2.4	1.9	7.5	11	2.6	4600	0.03	0.33	1.3	2
Vegetables and turkey, with cereal	44	2.1	0.8	7.2	22	0.3	400	0.01	0.03	0.4	1
Meat or poultry (approx. 6%–8% protein)											
Beef with vegetables	87	7.4	3.7	6.0	13	1.2	1100	0.07	0.17	1.6	2
Chicken with vegetables	100	7.4	4.6	7.2	22	0.9	1000	0.09	0.15	1.6	2
Turkey with vegetables	86	6.7	3.2	7.6	38	0.6	1000	0.13	0.13	1.8	2
Veal with vegetables	63	7.1	1.6	5.1	11	0.8	800	0.08	0.15	2.0	2
Fruits and Fruit Products with or Without Thickening, Canned											
Applesauce	72	0.2	0.2	18.6	4	0.4	40	0.01	0.02	0.1	Trace
Applesauce and apricots	86	0.3	0.1	22.6	4	0.3	600	0.01	0.02	0.1	2

Food											
Bananas (with tapioca or cornstarch, added ascorbic acid) strained	84	0.4	0.2	21.6	13	0.2	70	0.02	0.02	0.2	35
Bananas and pineapple (with tapioca or cornstarch)	80	0.4	0.1	20.7	20	0.2	30	0.01	0.01	0.1	2
Fruit dessert with tapioca (apricot, pineapple and/or orange)	84	0.3	0.3	21.5	15	0.4	450	0.02	0.01	0.2	4
Peaches	81	0.6	0.2	20.7	6	0.3	500	0.01	0.02	0.7	3
Pears	66	0.3	0.1	17.1	7	0.2	30	0.02	0.02	0.2	2
Pears and pineapple	69	0.4	0.2	17.6	7	0.2	20	0.03	0.02	0.2	2
Plums with tapioca, strained	94	0.4	0.2	24.3	5	0.4	250	0.01	0.02	0.2	2
Prunes with tapioca	86	0.3	0.2	22.4	7	0.9	400	0.02	0.06	0.4	4

Meats, Poultry, and Eggs; Canned

Food											
Beef:											
Strained	99	14.7	4.0	(0)	8	2.0	—	0.01	0.16	3.5	0
Junior	118	19.3	3.9	(0)	8	2.5	—	0.02	0.20	4.3	0
Chicken	127	13.7	7.6	(0)	—	1.9	—	0.02	0.16	3.5	Trace
Egg yolks, strained	210	10.0	18.4	.2	81	3.0	1900	0.12	0.12	Trace	
Lamb:											
Strained	107	14.6	4.9	(0)	9	2.1	—	0.02	0.17	3.3	—
Junior	121	17.5	5.1	(0)	13	2.7	—	0.02	0.21	4.1	—
Liver, strained	97	14.1	3.4	1.5	6	5.6	24,000	0.05	2.00	7.6	10
Liver and bacon, strained	123	13.7	6.6	1.3	6	4.2	22,000	0.05	1.99	7.8	7
Pork:											
Strained	118	15.4	5.8	(0)	8	1.5	—	0.19	0.20	2.7	—
Junior	134	18.6	6.0	(0)	8	1.2	—	0.23	0.23	2.8	—
Veal:											
Strained	91	15.5	2.7	(0)	10	1.7	—	0.03	0.20	4.3	—
Junior	107	18.8	3.0	(0)	8	1.6	—	0.03	0.22	6.0	—

Vegetables, Canned

Food											
Beans, green	22	1.4	0.1	5.1	33	1.1	400	0.02	0.06	0.3	3
Beets, strained	37	1.4	0.1	8.3	18	0.7	20	0.02	0.03	0.1	3
Carrots	29	0.7	0.1	6.8	23	0.5	13,000	0.02	0.03	0.4	3
Mixed vegetables, including vegetable soup	37	1.6	0.3	8.5	22	0.9	4700	0.05	0.04	0.6	2
Peas, strained	54	4.2	0.2	9.3	11	1.2	500	0.08	0.09	1.2	10
Spinach, creamed	43	2.3	0.7	7.5	64	0.6	5000	0.02	0.13	0.3	6
Squash	25	0.7	0.1	6.2	24	0.4	2400	0.02	0.04	0.3	8
Sweetpotatoes	67	1.0	0.2	15.5	16	0.4	4900	0.04	0.03	0.4	8
Tomato soup, strained	54	1.9	0.1	13.5	24	0.4	1000	0.05	0.12	0.7	3

*Items selected from Table 1 in *Composition of Foods—Raw, Processed, Prepared*, by B. K. Watt and A. L. Merrill, Handbook No. 8, Consumer and Food Economics Research Division, U.S. Department of Agriculture, Washington, D.C., 1963.

Table A-4. Exchange Lists for Meal Planning*

Food Exchange List	Measure	Carbohydrate gm	Protein gm	Fat gm	Energy kcal
Milk, nonfat, list 1	1 cup	12	8	tr	80
Milk, whole, list 1	1 cup	12	8	9	160
Vegetables, list 2	½ cup	5	2		25
Fruits, list 3	Varies	10			40
Breads, cereals, and starchy vegetables, list 4	Varies	15	2		70
Meat, low fat, list 5	1 ounce		7	2.5	50
Meat, medium fat, list 5	1 ounce		7	5	75
Meat, high fat, list 5	1 ounce		7	7.5	95
Fat, list 6	1 teaspoon			5	45

*The data from this table and the *exchange lists* in this book are based on materials in *Exchange Lists for Meal Planning* prepared by Committees of the American Diabetes Association, Inc., and The American Dietetic Association in cooperation with The National Institute of Arthritis, Metabolism and Digestive Diseases and the National Heart and Lung Institute, National Institutes of Health, Public Health Service, U.S. Department of Health, Education, and Welfare.

List 1. Milk, nonfat, fortified. Use only this list for diets restricted in saturated fat.

	Amount to Use
Skim or nonfat milk	1 cup
Powdered (nonfat dry)	⅓ cup
Canned, evaporated, skim	½ cup
Buttermilk made from skim milk	1 cup
Yogurt, made from skimmed milk, plain unflavored	1 cup

Milk, low fat, fortified

1 per cent fat, fortified (omit ½ fat exchange)	1 cup
2 per cent fat, fortified (omit 1 fat exchange)	1 cup
Yogurt made from 2 per cent fortified, plain, unflavored (omit 1 fat exchange)	1 cup

Milk, Whole

Whole milk	1 cup
Canned evaporated	½ cup
Buttermilk made from whole milk	1 cup
Yogurt made from whole milk (plain, unflavored)	1 cup

List 2 Vegetables. One-half cup equals one exchange.

Asparagus°
Bean sprouts
Beets
Broccoli°†
Brussels sprouts°
Cabbage°
Carrots†
Cauliflower°
Celery

Cucumbers
Eggplant
Greens°†
  Beet greens
  Chard
  Collards
  Dandelion greens
  Kale
  Mustard greens

Greens°† (cont.)
  Spinach
  Turnip greens
Mushrooms
Okra
Onions
Rhubarb
Rutabaga

Sauerkraut
String beans, green or yellow
Summer squash
Tomatoes°
Tomato juice°
Turnips
Vegetable juice cocktail
Zucchini

These vegetables can be used as desired: chicory, Chinese cabbage, endive, escarole, lettuce, parsley, radishes, and watercress. See List 4, Bread Exchanges, for starchy vegetables.

° Good sources of ascorbic acid.
† Good sources of vitamin A.

Table A–4. (Cont.)

List 3. Fruit Exchanges	Amount to Use
Apple	1 small
Apple juice	⅓ cup
Applesauce (unsweetened)	½ cup
Apricots, fresh†	2 medium
Apricots, dried†	4 halves
Berries	
Blackberries	½ cup
Blueberries	½ cup
Raspberries	½ cup
Strawberries°	¾ cup
Cherries	10 large
Cider	⅓ cup
Dates	2
Figs, fresh	1
Figs, dried	1
Grapefruit°	½
Grapefruit juice°	½ cup
Grapes	12
Grape juice	¼ cup
Mango°†	½ small
Melon	
Cantaloupe°	¼ small
Honeydew°	⅛ medium
Watermelon	1 cup
Nectarine	1 medium
Orange°	1 small
Orange juice°	½ cup
Papaya°†	¾ cup
Peach†	1 medium
Pear	1 small
Persimmon	1 medium
Pineapple	½ cup
Pineapple juice	⅓ cup
Plums	2 medium
Prunes	2 medium
Prune juice	¼ cup
Raisins	2 tablespoons
Tangerine°	1 large

Cranberries may be used as desired if no sugar is added.

List 4. Bread, Cereal, and Starchy Vegetable Exchanges

Bread	Amount to Use
White (including French and Italian)	1 slice
Whole wheat	1 slice
Rye or pumpernickel	1 slice
Raisin	1 slice
Bagel, small	½
English muffin, small	½
Frankfurt roll	½
Hamburger bun	½

Plain roll (bread)	1
Dry bread crumbs	3 tablespoons
Tortillas, 6 in.	1

Cereal

Bran flakes	½ cup
Other ready-to-eat unsweetened cereal	¾ cup
Puffed cereal, unfrosted	1 cup
Cereal, cooked	½ cup
Grits, cooked	½ cup
Rice or barley, cooked	½ cup
Pastas, cooked; macaroni, noodles, spaghetti	½ cup
Popcorn, popped	3 cups
Cornmeal, dry	2 tablespoons
Flour	2½ tablespoons
Wheat germ	¼ cup

Crackers

Arrowroot	3
Graham, 2 ½ in.	2
Matzoth, 4 × 6 in.	½
Oyster	20
Pretzels, 3 ⅛ in. × ⅛ in.	15
Rye wafers, 2 × 3 ½ in.	3
Saltines	6
Soda, 2 ½ in. square	4

Dried Beans, Peas, and Lentils

Dried beans, peas, and lentils, cooked	½ cup
Baked beans, no pork	¼ cup

Starchy Vegetables

Corn	⅓ cup
Corn on cob	1 small
Lima beans	½ cup
Parsnips	⅔ cup
Peas, green, fresh, canned, or frozen	½ cup
Potato, white	1 small
Potato, mashed	½ cup
Pumpkin	¾ cup
Winter squash, acorn or butternut	½ cup
Yam or sweet potato	¼ cup

Prepared Foods

Biscuit, 2 in. diam. (omit 1 fat exchange)	1
Cornbread, 2 × 2 × 1 in. (omit 1 fat exchange)	1
Corn muffin, 2 in. diam. (omit 1 fat exchange)	1
Crackers, round, butter type (omit 1 fat exchange)	5
Muffin, plain, small (omit 1 fat exchange)	1
Pancake, 5 × ½ in. (omit 1 fat exchange)	1
Potatoes, French fried, 2 in. to 3½ in. (omit 1 fat exchange)	8 pieces
Potato or corn chips (omit 2 fat exchanges)	15
Waffle, 5 × ½ in. (omit 1 fat exchange)	1

Table A–4. (Cont.)

List 5. Meat and Protein-Rich Exchanges
Lean Meat, Protein-Rich Exchanges. Use only this list for diets low in saturated fat and cholesterol.

	Amount to Use
Beef: baby beef (very lean), chipped beef, chuck, flank steak, tenderloin, plate ribs, plate skirt steak, round (bottom, top), all cuts rump, spare ribs, tripe	1 ounce
Lamb: leg, rib, sirloin, loin (roast and chops), shank, shoulder	1 ounce
Pork: leg (whole rump, center shank), smoked ham (center slices)	1 ounce
Veal: leg, loin, rib, shank, shoulder, cutlets	1 ounce
Poultry: without skin of chicken, turkey, Cornish hen, Guinea hen, pheasant	1 ounce
Fish; any fresh or frozen	1 ounce
canned crab, lobster, mackerel, salmon, tuna	¼ cup
clams, oysters, scallops, shrimp	5 or 1 ounce
sardines, drained	3
Cheeses; containing less than 5 per cent butterfat	1 ounce
Cottage cheese: dry or 2 per cent butter fat	¼ cup
Dried peas and beans (omit 1 bread exchange)	½ cup

Medium Fat Meat and Protein-Rich Exchanges

	Amount to Use
Beef: ground, 15 per cent fat; corned beef, canned; rib eye; round, ground (commercial)	1 ounce
Pork: loin, all cuts tenderloin; shoulder arm (picnic); shoulder blade; Boston Butt; Canadian bacon; boiled ham	1 ounce
Liver, heart, kidney, and sweetbreads (high in cholesterol)	1 ounce
Cottage cheese, creamed	¼ cup
Cheese: Mozzarella, ricotta, farmer's, Neufchatel, Parmesan	1 ounce
	3 tablespoons
Eggs (high in cholesterol)	1
Peanut butter (omit 2 fat exchanges)	2 tablespoons

High-Fat Meat and Protein-Rich Exchanges

	Amount to Use
Beef: brisket; corned beef brisket; ground beef (over 20 per cent fat); hamburger (commercial); chuck, ground (commercial); rib roast; club and rib steak	1 ounce
Lamb: breast	1 ounce
Pork; spare ribs; loin (back ribs); pork, ground; country style ham; deviled ham	1 ounce
Veal: breast	1 ounce
Poultry; capon, duck (domestic), goose	1 ounce
Cheese; cheddar type	1 ounce
Cold cuts, 4½ × ⅛ in.	1 slice
Frankfurter	1 small

Table A–4. (Cont.)

List 6 Fat Exchanges   **Amount to Use**
For a diet low in saturated fat and higher in polyunsaturated fat select only from this list.
Margarine: soft, tub, or stick (made with corn,
    cottonseed, safflower, soy, or sunflower
    oil)   1 teaspoon
Avocado, 4 in. diam. $\frac{1}{8}$
Nuts
    Almonds°   10 whole
    Peanuts°
      Spanish   20 whole
      Virginia   10 whole
    Pecans°   2 large, whole
    Walnuts   6 small
    Other nuts°   6 small
Oil, corn, cottonseed, safflower, soy, sunflower   1 teaspoon
Oil, olive or peanut°   1 teaspoon
Olives°   5 small
Salad dressings, if made with corn, cottonseed,
    safflower, or soy oil
    French dressing   1 tablespoon
    Italian dressing   1 tablespoon
    Mayonnaise   1 teaspoon
    Salad dressing, mayonnaise type   2 teaspoons

° Fat content is primarily monounsaturated.

The following fats should not be used on a diet low in saturated fat.
Margarine, regular stick   1 teaspoon
Butter   1 teaspoon
Bacon fat   1 teaspoon
Bacon, crisp   1 strip
Cream, light   2 tablespoons
Cream, sour   2 tablespoons
Cream, heavy   1 tablespoon
Cream cheese   1 tablespoon
Lard   1 teaspoon
Salad dressings (permitted on restricted diets only if
    made with allowed oils)
    French dressing   1 tablespoon
    Italian dressing   1 tablespoon
    Mayonnaise   1 teaspoon
    Salad dressing, mayonnaise type   2 teaspoons
Salt pork $\frac{3}{4}$ in. cube

Table A–5. Amino Acid Content of Selected Foods*

(per 100 gm food, edible portion)

Food	Protein gm	Trypto-phan gm	Threo-nine gm	Iso-leucine gm	Leucine gm	Lysine gm	Sulfur Containing Methi-onine gm	Sulfur Containing Cys-tine gm	Phenyl-alanine gm	Tyro-sine gm	Valine gm	Argi-nine gm	Histi-dine gm
Milk													
Cow:													
Fluid, whole and nonfat	3.5	0.049	0.161	0.223	0.344	0.272	0.086	0.031	0.170	0.178	0.240	0.128	0.092
Canned:													
unsweetened	7.0	0.099	0.323	0.447	0.688	0.545	0.171	0.063	0.340	0.357	0.481	0.256	0.185
Condensed, sweetened	8.1	0.114	0.374	0.518	0.796	0.631	0.198	0.072	0.393	0.413	0.557	0.296	0.214
Dried													
Whole	25.8	0.364	1.191	1.648	2.535	2.009	0.632	0.231	1.251	1.316	1.774	0.944	0.680
Nonfat	35.6	0.502	1.641	2.271	3.493	2.768	0.870	0.318	1.724	1.814	2.444	1.300	0.937
Goat	3.3	0.039	0.217	0.087	0.278	0.312	0.065	—	0.121	—	0.139	0.174	0.068
Human	1.4	0.023	0.062	0.075	0.124	0.090	0.028	0.027	0.060	0.071	0.086	0.055	0.030
Milk Products													
Buttermilk	3.5	0.038	0.165	0.219	0.348	0.291	0.082	0.032	0.186	0.137	0.262	0.168	0.099
Casein	100.0	1.335	4.227	6.550	10.048	8.013	3.084	0.382	5.389	5.819	7.393	4.070	3.021
Cheese													
Blue mold	21.5	0.293	0.799	1.449	2.096	1.577	0.559	0.121	1.153	1.028	1.543	0.785	0.701
Camembert	17.5	0.239	0.650	1.179	1.706	1.284	0.455	0.099	0.938	0.837	1.256	0.639	0.571
Cheddar	25.0	0.341	0.929	1.685	2.437	1.834	0.650	0.141	1.340	1.195	1.794	0.913	0.815
Cheddar processed	23.2	0.316	0.862	1.563	2.262	1.702	0.604	0.131	1.244	1.109	1.665	0.847	0.756
Cottage	17.0	0.179	0.794	0.989	1.826	1.428	0.469	0.147	0.917	0.917	0.978	0.802	0.549
Cream cheese	9.0	0.080	0.408	0.519	0.923	0.721	0.229	0.085	0.547	0.408	0.538	0.313	0.278
Swiss	27.5	0.375	1.021	1.853	2.681	2.017	0.715	0.155	1.474	1.315	1.974	1.004	0.896
Swiss processed	26.4	0.360	0.981	1.779	2.574	1.937	0.687	0.149	1.415	1.262	1.895	0.964	0.861
Eggs													
Whole	12.8	0.211	0.637	0.850	1.126	0.819	0.401	0.299	0.739	0.551	0.950	0.840	0.307
Whites	10.8	0.164	0.477	0.698	0.950	0.648	0.420	0.263	0.689	0.449	0.842	0.634	0.233
Yolks	16.3	0.235	0.827	0.996	1.372	1.074	0.417	0.274	0.717	0.756	1.121	1.132	0.368
Meat and Poultry													
Beef cuts, medium fat													
Chuck	18.6	0.217	0.821	0.973	1.524	1.625	0.461	0.235	0.765	0.631	1.033	1.199	0.646
Hamburger	16.0	0.187	0.707	0.837	1.311	1.398	0.397	0.202	0.658	0.543	0.888	1.032	0.556
Porterhouse	16.4	0.192	0.724	0.858	1.343	1.433	0.407	0.207	0.674	0.556	0.911	1.057	0.569
Rib roast	17.4	0.203	0.768	0.910	1.425	1.520	0.432	0.220	0.715	0.590	0.966	1.122	0.604
Round	19.5	0.228	0.861	1.020	1.597	1.704	0.484	0.246	0.802	0.661	1.083	1.257	0.677
Rump	16.2	0.189	0.715	0.848	1.327	1.415	0.402	0.205	0.666	0.550	0.899	1.045	0.562
Sirloin	17.3	0.202	0.764	0.905	1.417	1.511	0.429	0.219	0.711	0.587	0.960	1.116	0.601
Beef, dried or chipped	34.3	0.401	1.515	1.795	2.810	2.996	0.851	0.434	1.410	1.163	1.904	2.212	1.191
Lamb cuts, medium fat													
Leg	18.0	0.233	0.824	0.933	1.394	1.457	0.432	0.236	0.732	0.625	0.887	1.172	0.501

*Items selected from *Amino Acid Content of Foods*, by M. L. Orr and B. K. Watt, Home Economics Research Rep. No. 4, Agricultural Research Service, U.S. Department of Agriculture, Washington, 1957.

Table A–5. (Cont.)

Food	Protein gm	Tryptophan gm	Threonine gm	Isoleucine gm	Leucine gm	Lysine gm	Sulfur Containing		Phenylalanine gm	Tyrosine gm	Valine gm	Arginine gm	Histidine gm
							Methionine gm	Cystine gm					
Rib	14.9	0.193	0.682	0.772	1.154	1.206	0.358	0.195	0.606	0.517	0.734	0.970	0.415
Shoulder	15.6	0.202	0.714	0.809	1.208	1.263	0.374	0.205	0.634	0.542	0.769	1.016	0.434
Pork cuts, medium fat, fresh													
Ham	15.2	0.197	0.705	0.781	1.119	1.248	0.379	0.178	0.598	0.542	0.790	0.931	0.525
Loin	16.4	0.213	0.761	0.842	1.207	1.346	0.409	0.192	0.646	0.585	0.853	1.005	0.567
Miscellaneous lean cuts	14.5	0.188	0.673	0.745	1.067	1.190	0.362	0.169	0.571	0.517	0.754	0.889	0.501
Pork, cured													
Bacon, medium fat	9.1	0.095	0.306	0.399	0.728	0.587	0.141	0.106	0.434	0.234	0.434	0.622	0.246
Fat back or salt pork	3.9	0.006	0.141	0.110	0.367	0.317	0.055	0.043	0.157	0.052	0.168	0.379	0.035
Ham	16.9	0.162	0.692	0.841	1.306	1.420	0.411	0.273	0.646	0.652	0.879	1.068	0.544
Luncheon meat													
Boiled ham	22.8	0.219	0.934	1.135	1.762	1.915	0.554	0.368	0.872	0.879	1.186	1.441	0.733
Canned, spiced	14.9	0.143	0.610	0.741	1.151	1.252	0.362	0.241	0.570	0.575	0.775	0.942	0.479
Veal cuts, medium fat													
Round	19.5	0.256	0.846	1.030	1.429	1.629	0.446	0.231	0.792	0.702	1.008	1.270	0.627
Shoulder	19.4	0.255	0.841	1.024	1.422	1.620	0.444	0.230	0.788	0.698	1.003	1.263	0.624
Stew meat	18.3	0.240	0.793	0.966	1.341	1.528	0.419	0.217	0.744	0.659	0.946	1.192	0.589
Chicken, flesh only													
Broilers or fryers	20.6	0.250	0.877	1.088	1.490	1.810	0.537	0.277	0.811	0.725	1.012	1.302	0.593
Hens	21.3	0.259	0.907	1.125	1.540	1.871	0.556	0.286	0.838	0.750	1.046	1.346	0.613
Fish and Shellfish													
Blue fish	20.5	0.203	0.889	1.040	1.548	1.797	0.597	0.276	0.761	0.554	1.092	1.155	—
Cod, fresh	16.5	0.164	0.715	0.837	1.246	1.447	0.480	0.222	0.612	0.446	0.879	0.929	—
dried	81.8	0.811	3.547	4.149	6.178	7.172	2.382	1.099	3.036	2.212	4.358	4.607	—
Flounder	14.9	0.148	0.646	0.756	1.125	1.306	0.434	0.200	0.553	0.403	0.794	0.839	—
Haddock	18.2	0.181	0.789	0.923	1.374	1.596	0.530	0.245	0.676	0.492	0.970	1.025	—
Halibut	18.6	0.185	0.806	0.943	1.405	1.631	0.542	0.250	0.690	0.503	0.991	1.048	—
Herring, Atlantic	18.3	0.182	0.793	0.928	1.382	1.605	0.533	0.246	0.679	0.495	0.975	1.031	—
Mackerel, raw, common													
Atlantic	18.7	0.186	0.811	0.948	1.412	1.640	0.545	0.251	0.694	0.506	0.996	1.053	—
Salmon, raw, Pacific													
canned, red, solids and liquid	17.4	0.173	0.754	0.883	1.314	1.526	0.507	0.234	0.646	0.470	0.927	0.980	—
Sardines, canned, solids and liquid, Atlantic	20.2	0.200	0.876	1.025	1.526	1.771	0.588	0.271	0.750	0.546	1.076	1.138	—
Shrimp, canned, solids and liquid	21.1	0.209	0.915	1.070	1.593	1.850	0.614	0.284	0.783	0.571	1.124	1.188	—
	18.7	0.186	0.811	0.948	1.412	1.640	0.545	0.251	0.694	0.506	0.996	1.053	—
Products from Meat, Poultry, and Fish													
Fish flour	76.0	0.754	4.378	4.232	6.189	7.381	2.019	—	2.845	—	3.916	5.204	1.289
Gelatin	85.6	0.006	1.912	1.357	2.930	4.226	0.787	0.077	2.036	0.401	2.421	7.866	0.771
Liver, beef or pork	19.7	0.296	0.936	1.031	1.819	1.475	0.463	0.243	0.993	0.738	1.239	1.201	0.523

Sausage													
Bologna	14.8	0.126	0.606	0.718	1.061	1.191	0.313	0.185	0.540	0.481	0.744	1.028	0.398
Frankfurters	14.2	0.120	0.582	0.688	1.018	1.143	0.300	0.177	0.518	0.461	0.713	0.986	0.382
Liverwurst	16.7	0.187	0.724	0.818	1.400	1.301	0.347	0.203	0.759	0.510	1.037	1.034	0.497
Pork, links or bulk, raw	10.8	0.092	0.442	0.524	0.774	0.869	0.228	0.135	0.394	0.351	0.543	0.750	0.290
Pork, bulk, canned	15.4	0.131	0.631	0.747	1.104	1.239	0.325	0.192	0.562	0.500	0.774	1.069	0.414
Salami	23.9	0.203	0.979	1.159	1.713	1.923	0.505	0.298	0.872	0.776	1.201	1.660	0.642
Tongue, beef	16.4	0.197	0.708	0.792	1.286	1.364	0.357	0.207	0.661	0.548	0.840	1.065	0.412
Legumes													
Beans													
Red kidney													
raw	23.1	0.214	1.002	1.312	1.985	1.715	0.233	0.229	1.275	0.891	1.401	1.390	0.658
canned, solids and liquid	5.7	0.053	0.247	0.324	0.490	0.423	0.057	0.057	0.315	0.220	0.346	0.343	0.162
Other common beans including navy, pea-bean, white marrow:													
raw	21.4	0.199	0.928	1.216	1.839	1.589	0.216	0.212	1.181	0.825	1.298	1.287	0.609
baked with pork, canned	5.8	0.057	0.274	0.291	0.486	0.354	0.059	0.018	0.333	0.165	0.312	0.251	0.186
Chickpeas	20.8	0.170	0.739	1.195	1.538	1.434	0.276	0.296	1.012	0.692	1.025	1.551	0.559
Cowpeas	22.9	0.220	0.901	1.110	1.715	1.491	0.352	0.297	1.198	0.678	1.293	1.473	0.692
Lentils, whole	25.0	0.216	0.896	1.316	1.760	1.528	0.180	0.204	1.104	0.664	1.360	1.908	0.548
Lima beans	20.7	0.195	0.980	1.199	1.760	1.378	0.331	0.311	1.222	0.543	1.298	1.315	0.669
Peanuts	26.9	0.340	0.828	1.266	1.722	1.099	0.271	0.463	1.557	1.104	1.532	3.296	0.749
Peanut flour	51.2	0.647	1.575	2.410	3.563	2.091	0.516	0.881	2.963	2.100	2.916	6.273	1.425
Peanut butter	26.1	0.330	0.803	1.228	1.816	1.066	0.263	0.449	1.510	1.071	1.487	3.198	0.727
Peas, split	24.5	0.259	0.945	1.380	2.027	1.795	0.294	0.318	1.235	0.988	1.372	2.164	0.670
Soybeans, whole	34.9	0.526	1.504	2.504	2.946	2.414	0.513	0.678	1.889	1.216	2.005	2.763	0.911
Soybean flour, flakes and grits													
Low fat	44.7	0.673	1.926	2.630	3.773	3.092	0.658	0.869	2.419	1.558	2.568	3.538	1.166
Full fat	35.9	0.541	1.547	2.112	3.030	2.483	0.528	0.698	1.943	1.251	2.062	2.842	0.937
Soybean milk	3.4	0.051	0.176	0.175	0.305	0.269	0.054	0.071	0.195	0.193	0.186	0.302	0.121
Nuts													
Almonds	18.6	0.176	0.610	0.873	1.454	0.582	0.259	0.377	1.146	0.618	1.124	2.729	0.517
Brazil nuts	14.4	0.187	0.422	0.593	1.129	0.443	0.941	0.504	0.617	0.483	0.823	2.247	0.367
Cashews	18.5	0.471	0.737	1.222	1.522	0.792	0.353	0.527	0.946	0.712	1.592	2.098	0.415
Coconut	3.4	0.033	0.129	0.180	0.269	0.152	0.071	0.062	0.174	0.101	0.212	0.486	0.069
Pecans	9.4	0.138	0.389	0.553	0.773	0.435	0.153	0.216	0.564	0.316	0.525	1.185	0.273
Walnuts (English or Persian)	15.0	0.175	0.589	0.767	1.228	0.441	0.306	0.320	0.767	0.583	0.974	2.287	0.405
Other Seeds													
Cottonseed flour and meal	42.3	0.591	1.764	1.884	2.945	2.139	0.686	0.814	2.610	1.365	2.458	5.603	1.325
Safflower seed meal	42.1	0.675	1.462	1.914	2.740	1.525	0.731	—	2.605	—	2.446	4.623	0.985
Sesame seed	19.3	0.331	0.707	0.951	1.679	0.583	0.637	0.495	1.457	0.951	0.885	1.992	0.441
Meal	33.4	0.573	1.223	1.645	2.905	1.008	1.103	0.857	2.521	1.645	1.531	3.447	0.763
Sunflower meal	39.5	0.589	1.565	2.191	2.981	1.491	0.760	0.797	2.094	1.110	2.325	4.069	1.006
Grains and Their Products													
Barley	12.8	0.160	0.433	0.545	0.889	0.433	0.184	0.257	0.661	0.466	0.643	0.659	0.239
Bread, white (4% nonfat dry milk, flour basis)	8.5	0.091	0.282	0.429	0.668	0.225	0.142	0.200	0.465	0.243	0.435	0.340	0.192

Table A–5. (Cont.)

Food	Protein gm	Tryptophan gm	Threonine gm	Isoleucine gm	Leucine gm	Lysine gm	Sulfur Containing Methionine gm	Cystine gm	Phenylalanine gm	Tyrosine gm	Valine gm	Arginine gm	Histidine gm
Cereal combinations													
Corn and soy grits	18.0	0.161	0.792	0.841	1.656	0.772	0.271	0.311	0.832	0.562	1.054	0.982	0.472
Infant food, precooked, mixed cereals with nonfat dry milk and yeast	19.4	0.118	—	—	—	0.273	0.310	0.137	0.543	0.447	—	0.447	0.233
Oat-corn-rye mixture, puffed	14.5	0.172	0.545	0.841	1.368	0.343	0.388	0.234	0.933	0.622	0.900	0.776	0.326
Corn grits	8.7	0.053	0.347	0.402	1.128	0.251	0.161	0.113	0.395	0.532	0.444	0.306	0.180
Cornmeal, degermed	7.9	0.048	0.315	0.365	1.024	0.228	0.147	0.102	0.359	0.483	0.403	0.278	0.163
Corn flakes	8.1	0.052	0.275	0.306	1.057	0.154	0.135	0.152	0.354	0.283	0.386	0.231	0.226
Oatmeal	14.2	0.183	0.470	0.733	1.065	0.521	0.209	0.309	0.758	0.524	0.845	0.935	0.261
Rice flakes or puffed	5.9	0.046	—	—	—	0.056	—	0.044	0.286	0.124	—	0.137	0.137
Rice, white and converted	7.6	0.082	0.298	0.356	0.655	0.300	0.137	0.103	0.382	0.347	0.531	0.438	0.128
Rye flour, medium	11.4	0.129	0.422	0.485	0.766	0.465	0.180	0.227	0.538	0.368	0.594	0.557	0.260
Wheat flour													
Whole grain	13.3	0.164	0.383	0.577	0.892	0.365	0.203	0.292	0.657	0.497	0.616	0.636	0.271
White	10.5	0.129	0.302	0.483	0.809	0.239	0.138	0.210	0.577	0.359	0.453	0.466	0.210
Wheat products													
Bran	12.0	0.196	0.342	0.485	0.717	0.491	0.145	0.270	0.434	0.259	0.552	0.742	0.280
Burghul	12.4	0.070	—	—	—	0.430	0.300	0.319	—	0.447	—	—	—
Farina	10.9	0.124	—	—	—	0.199	0.143	0.184	0.579	—	—	0.424	0.268
Flakes	10.8	0.121	0.356	0.496	0.891	0.360	0.127	0.191	0.478	0.311	0.572	0.559	0.231
Germ	25.2	0.265	1.343	1.177	1.708	1.534	0.404	0.287	0.908	0.882	1.364	1.825	0.687
Macaroni or spaghetti	12.8	0.150	0.499	0.642	0.849	0.413	0.193	0.243	0.669	0.422	0.728	0.582	0.303
Noodles, containing egg solids	12.6	0.133	0.533	0.621	0.834	0.411	0.212	0.245	0.610	0.312	0.745	0.621	0.301
Shredded wheat	10.1	0.085	0.405	0.449	0.684	0.331	0.139	0.204	0.481	0.236	0.577	0.523	0.236
Whole wheat with added germ	12.8	0.136	—	—	—	0.466	—	0.246	0.755	0.481	—	0.742	0.371
Fruit													
Bananas, ripe	1.2	0.018	—	—	—	0.055	0.011	—	—	0.031	—	—	—
Dates	2.2	0.061	0.061	0.074	0.077	0.065	0.027	—	0.063	—	0.094	0.049	0.049
Grapefruit	0.5	0.001	—	—	—	0.006	0.000	—	—	—	—	—	—
Guavas, common	1.0	0.010	—	—	—	0.030	0.010	—	—	—	—	—	—
Limes	0.8	0.003	—	—	—	0.015	0.002	—	—	—	—	—	—
Mangos	0.7	0.014	—	—	—	0.093	0.008	—	—	—	—	—	—
Muskmelons	0.6	0.001	—	—	—	0.015	0.002	—	—	—	—	—	—
Oranges	0.9	0.003	—	—	—	0.024	0.003	—	—	—	—	—	—
Papayas	0.6	0.012	—	—	—	0.038	0.002	—	—	—	—	—	—
Pineapple	0.4	0.005	—	—	—	0.009	0.001	—	—	—	—	—	—

Vegetables													
Asparagus, raw	2.2	0.027	0.066	0.080	0.096	0.103	0.032	—	0.069	—	0.106	0.123	0.036
Beans, snap	2.4	0.033	0.091	0.109	0.139	0.126	0.035	0.024	0.057	0.050	0.115	0.101	0.045
Beat greens	2.0	0.024	0.076	0.084	0.129	0.108	0.034	—	0.116	—	0.101	0.083	0.026
Beets	1.6	0.014	0.034	0.051	0.055	0.086	0.006	—	0.027	—	0.049	0.028	0.022
Broccoli	3.3	0.037	0.122	0.126	0.163	0.147	0.050	—	0.119	—	0.170	0.192	0.063
Brussels sprouts	4.4	0.044	0.153	0.186	0.194	0.197	0.046	—	0.148	—	0.193	0.279	0.106
Cabbage	1.4	0.011	0.039	0.040	0.057	0.066	0.013	0.028	0.030	0.030	0.043	0.105	0.025
Carrots	1.2	0.010	0.043	0.046	0.065	0.052	0.010	0.029	0.042	0.020	0.056	0.041	0.017
Cauliflower	2.4	0.033	0.102	0.104	0.162	0.134	0.047	—	0.075	0.034	0.144	0.110	0.048
Celery	1.3	0.012	—	—	—	0.021	0.015	0.006	—	0.016	—	—	—
Chard	1.4	0.014	0.058	0.060	0.076	0.055	0.004	—	0.046	—	0.055	0.035	0.018
Chicory	1.6	0.024	—	—	—	0.052	0.016	0.006	—	0.040	—	—	0.024
Corn, sweet	3.7	0.023	0.151	0.137	0.407	0.137	0.072	0.062	0.207	0.124	0.231	0.174	0.095
Cowpeas	9.4	0.099	0.353	0.465	0.653	0.617	0.131	—	0.523	—	0.513	0.615	0.310
Cucumbers	0.7	0.005	0.019	0.022	0.030	0.031	0.007	—	0.016	—	0.024	0.053	0.001
Eggplant	1.1	0.010	0.038	0.056	0.068	0.030	0.006	—	0.048	—	0.065	0.037	0.019
Kale	3.9	0.042	0.139	0.133	0.252	0.121	0.035	0.036	0.158	—	0.184	0.202	0.062
Lettuce	1.2	0.012	—	—	—	0.070	0.004	—	—	—	—	—	—
Lima beans	7.5	0.097	0.338	0.460	0.605	0.474	0.080	0.083	0.389	0.259	0.485	0.454	0.247
Mustard greens	2.3	0.037	0.060	0.075	0.062	0.111	0.024	0.035	0.074	0.121	0.108	0.167	0.041
Onions, mature	1.4	0.021	0.022	0.021	0.037	0.064	0.013	—	0.039	0.046	0.031	0.180	0.014
Peas	6.7	0.056	0.245	0.308	0.418	0.316	0.054	0.073	0.257	0.163	0.274	0.595	0.109
Peppers	1.2	0.009	0.050	0.046	0.046	0.051	0.016	—	0.055	—	0.033	0.024	0.014
Potatoes, raw	2.0	0.021	0.079	0.088	0.100	0.107	0.025	0.019	0.088	0.036	0.107	0.099	0.029
Spinach	2.3	0.037	0.102	0.107	0.176	0.142	0.039	0.046	0.099	0.073	0.126	0.116	0.049
Squash, summer	0.6	0.005	0.014	0.019	0.027	0.023	0.008	—	0.016	—	0.022	0.027	0.009
Sweetpotatoes, raw	1.8	0.031	0.085	0.087	0.103	0.085	0.033	0.029	0.100	0.081	0.135	0.094	0.036
Tomatoes	1.0	0.009	0.033	0.029	0.041	0.042	0.007	—	0.028	0.014	0.028	0.029	0.015
Turnips	1.1	—	—	0.020	—	0.057	0.012	—	0.020	0.029	—	—	—
Turnip greens	2.9	0.045	0.125	0.107	0.207	0.129	0.052	0.045	0.146	0.105	0.149	0.167	0.051
Miscellaneous Food Items													
Yeast													
Bakers', compressed	10.6†	0.122	0.655	0.655	1.151	0.914	0.248	0.120	0.607	0.580	0.840	0.536	0.353
Brewers', dried	36.9†	0.710	2.353	2.398	3.226	3.300	0.836	0.548	1.902	1.902	2.723	2.250	1.251
Primary, dried													
Saccharomyces cerevisiae	36.9†	0.636	2.353	2.708	3.300	3.337	0.851	0.444	1.813	2.472	2.553	1.931	1.103
Torulopsis utilis	36.9†	0.636	2.331	3.323	3.707	3.648	0.710	0.422	2.361	2.464	2.901	3.337	1.251

† Assumes 4/5 of total nitrogen is protein.

Table A–6. Cholesterol Content of the Edible Portion of Food*

Food	Household Measure	Weight gm	Cholesterol mg
Beef, lean, trimmed of separable fat, cooked	3 ounces	85	(77)†
Beef-vegetable stew			
Home recipe	1 cup	245	63
Canned	1 cup	245	36
Beef potpie			
Home prepared, baked	⅓ 9-in pie	210	44
Commercial, frozen, unheated	1 pie	216	38
Brains, raw		100	>2000
Butter	1 tablespoon	14	35
Buttermilk, from nonfat milk	1 cup	245	5
Cakes, home recipes			
Chocolate, chocolate frosting	¹⁄₁₆ 9-in diam.	75	32
Fruitcake, dark	¹⁄₃₀ 8-in loaf	15	7
Sponge	¹⁄₁₂ 10-in diam.	66	162
Yellow, chocolate frosting	¹⁄₁₆ 9-in diam.	75	33
Baked from mixes			
Angel food	¹⁄₁₂ 10-in diam.	53	0
Chocolate, with eggs, chocolate frosting	¹⁄₁₆ 9-in diam.	69	33
	cupcake, small	36	17
Gingerbread	⅑ 8-in square	63	trace
White, 2 layer, chocolate frosting	¹⁄₁₆ 9-in diam.	71	1
Yellow, 2 layer, with eggs, chocolate frosting	¹⁄₁₆ 9-in diam.	75	36
Caviar, sturgeon, granular	1 tablespoon	16	>48
Cheeses, natural			
Blue	1 ounce	28	(24)
Camembert	triangular wedge	38	(35)
Cheddar, mild or sharp	1 ounce	28	28
Cottage, creamed, 1% fat	1 cup	267	23
4% fat	1 cup	245	48
Uncreamed	1 cup	200	13
Cream cheese	1 tablespoon	14	16
Edam	1 ounce	28	(29)
Mozzarella, part skim	1 ounce	28	18
Muenster	1 ounce	28	(25)
Parmesan, grated	1 cup	100	(113)
Provolone	1 ounce	28	(28)
Ricotta, part skim	1 ounce	28	(14)
Swiss	slice, rectangular	35	35
Pasteurized process, American	1 ounce	28	(25)
Swiss	1 ounce	28	(26)
Pasteurized process spread	1 tablespoon	14	(9)
Cheese soufflé, home recipe	¼ of 7-in diam.	110	184
Chicken, breast, cooked meat and skin	½ breast	92	74
meat only	½ breast	80	63
Drumstick, meat and skin	1 drumstick	52	47
meat only	1 drumstick	43	39

*Adapted from Feeley, R. M., *et al.*: "Cholesterol Content of Foods," *J. Am. Diet. Assoc.*, **61**:134–49, 1972.

†Numbers in parentheses indicate imputed values.

Food	Household Measure	Weight gm	Cholesterol mg
Chicken à la king, home recipe	1 cup	245	185
Chicken fricassee, home recipe	1 cup	240	96
Chicken potpie, home recipe	⅓ 9-in diam.	232	71
Commercial, frozen, unheated	1 pie	227	29
Chop suey with meat, home recipe	1 cup	250	64
Canned	3 ounces	85	10
Chow mein, without noodles, home recipe	1 cup	250	77
Clams,‡ raw, meat only	1 cup (19 large soft or 7 round chowders)	227	114
Cod, raw, flesh only	3½ ounces	100	50
Cookies			
Brownies with nuts, home recipe	1 brownie 1¾ in square	20	17
Ladyfingers	4 ladyfingers	44	157
Corn pudding	1 cup	245	102
Cornbread, home recipe	piece, 2½ square	83	58
Baked from mix	piece	55	38
	muffin	40	28
Crab, steamed, meat only	1 cup	125	100
Canned, meat only	1 cup	160	(161)
Cream, half and half	1 tablespoon	15	6
Light, coffee	1 tablespoon	15	10
Sour	1 tablespoon	12	8
Whipped topping (pressurized)	1 cup	60	51
Heavy whipping (unwhipped)	1 tablespoon	15	20
Cream puff, custard filling	1 cream puff	130	188
Custard, baked	½ cup	133	139
Egg, whole	1 large	50	252
White	one	33	0
Yolk	one	17	252
Flounder, raw, flesh only	3½ ounces	100	50
Frog legs, raw (refuse 35%)	3½ ounces	100	50
Gizzard, chicken, cooked	3 ounces	85	(166)
Turkey, cooked	3 ounces	85	196
Haddock, raw, flesh only	3½ ounces	100	60
Halibut, cooked, flesh only	piece, 6½ × 2½ × ⅝	125	(60)
Heart, beef, cooked	1 cup chopped	145	(398)
Herring, raw, flesh only	3½ ounces	100	85
Ice cream, 10% fat	1 cup	133	53
Frozen custard or French	1 cup	133	97
Ice milk, hardened	1 cup	131	26
Soft-serve	1 cup	175	36
Kidneys, all kinds, cooked	1 cup sliced	140	(1125)
Lamb, lean, trimmed, cooked	3 ounces	85	(85)
Lard	1 cup	205	195
Liver, including beef, calf, hog, lamb, cooked	3 ounces	85	(372)
Chicken, cooked	1 liver	25	(187)
Turkey, cooked	1 cup chopped	140	839
Lobster, cooked, meat only	1 cup cubed	145	123

‡Cholesterol accounts for about 40 per cent of the total sterol content of clams.

Food	Household Measure	Weight gm	Cholesterol mg
Lobster Newburg, with butter, egg yolks, sherry, cream	1 cup	250	456
Macaroni and cheese, home recipe	1 cup	200	42
Mackerel, broiled	piece 8½ × 2½ × ½	105	(106)
Margarine			
All vegetable fat			0
⅔ animal fat, ½ vegetable fat	1 tablespoon	14	7
Milk, whole	1 cup	244	34
Low fat, 1% with 1 to 2% nonfat milk solids	1 cup	246	14
2% fat with 1 to 2% nonfat milk solids	1 cup	246	22
Nonfat, skim	1 cup	245	5
Canned, undiluted evaporated	1 cup	252	79
Condensed sweetened	1 cup	306	105
Dry, to make 1 quart diluted	1⅓ cups	91	20
Chocolate beverage, commercial flavored milk			
drink with 2% added butterfat	1 cup	250	20
Flavored milk	1 cup	250	32
Cocoa, homemade	1 cup	250	35
Muffins, plain, home recipe	1 muffin	40	21
Noodles, whole egg, dry	8-ounce package	227	213
Cooked	1 cup	160	50
Chow mein, canned	1 cup	45	5
Oysters,§ meat only, raw	1 cup, 13–19 medium; 19–31 small; 4–6 Pacific medium	240	120
Canned, solids and liquid	3 ounces	85	(38)
Oyster stew, home prepared, 1 part oysters, 2 parts milk	1 cup	240	63
Pancakes, mix, with eggs, milk	cake 6-in diam.	73	54
Pepper, stuffed with beef and crumbs	pepper with 1⅛ cup stuffing	185	56
Pies, baked			
Apple			0
Custard	⅛ of 9-in diam.	114	120
Lemon chiffon	⅛ of 9-in diam.	81	137
Lemon meringue	⅛ of 9-in diam.	105	98
Peach			0
Pumpkin	⅛ of 9-in diam.	114	70
Popovers, home recipe	1 popover (from ¼ cup batter)	40	59
Pork, lean, trimmed, cooked	3 ounces	85	(75)
Potatoes, au gratin, milk, cheese	1 cup	245	36
Scalloped, milk	1 cup	245	14
Salad, mayonnaise, hard-cooked egg	1 cup	250	162
Pudding, chocolate, mix	1 cup	260	30
Vanilla, home recipe (blanc mange)	1 cup	255	35

§ Cholesterol accounts for about 40 per cent of the total sterol of oysters.

Food	Household Measure	Weight gm	Cholesterol mg
Rabbit, domesticated, cooked	1 cup diced	140	(127)
Rice pudding with raisins	1 cup	265	29
Roe, salmon, raw	1 ounce	28	101
Salad dressing			
Mayonnaise, commercial	1 tablespoon	14	10
Salad dressing, home recipe	1 tablespoon	16	12
Mayonnaise-type, commercial	1 tablespoon	15	8
Salmon, red, broiled steak (refuse: 12%)	$6\frac{3}{4} \times 2\frac{1}{2} \times 1$ in	145	(59)
Canned, solids and liquid	3 ounces	85	30
Sardines, drained solids	can—$3\frac{1}{4}$ ounces	92	129
Sausage, frankfurter, all meat	1 frank	56	(34)
Scallops,‖ muscle only, steamed	3 ounces	85	(45)
Shrimp, raw, flesh only	$3\frac{1}{2}$ ounces	100	150
Canned, drained solids	1 cup— 22 large or 76 small	128	192
Spaghetti with meatballs in tomato sauce			
Home recipe	1 cup	248	75
Canned	1 cup	250	39
Sweetbreads (thymus), cooked	3 ounces	85	(396)
Tapioca cream pudding	1 cup	165	159
Tartar sauce, regular	1 tablespoon	14	7
Trout, raw, flesh only	$3\frac{1}{2}$ ounces	100	55
Tuna, canned in oil, drained	can (No. $\frac{1}{2}$); $5\frac{1}{2}$ ounces	157	102
Canned in water, solids and liquid	can (No. $\frac{1}{2}$); $6\frac{1}{2}$ ounces	184	(116)
Turkey, cooked, light meat, without skin	3 ounces	85	65
Dark meat, without skin	3 ounces	85	86
Turkey potpie, home prepared	$\frac{1}{3}$ 9-in diam.	232	71
Commercial, frozen	1 pie	227	20
Veal, lean, cooked	3 ounces	85	(84)
Waffles, mix, egg, milk	1 waffle 9×9 in	200	119
Welsh rarebit	1 cup	232	71
White sauce, thin	1 cup	250	36
Medium	1 cup	250	33
Thick	1 cup	250	30
Yogurt, nonfat, plain or vanilla	carton; 8 ounces	227	17
Fruit flavored	carton; 8 ounces	227	15

‖ Cholesterol accounts for about 30 per cent of total sterol of scallops.

Table A–7. Composition of Some Alcoholic Beverages

Beverage	Approximate Measure	Weight gm	Energy calories*	Alcohol gm	Carbohydrate gm
Ale, American	1 glass	250	150	15	11
Beer	1 glass	250	110	10	10
Brandy	1 cordial glass	20	50	7	
Cocktails†					
Daiquiri (1 1/2 jiggers rum)	1 cocktail glass	90	180	22	5
Manhattan (1 1/2 jiggers whiskey)	1 cocktail glass	90	200	28	1
Martini (1 1/2 jiggers gin)	1 cocktail glass	90	220	31	1
Creme de menthe	1 cordial glass	20	75	7	6
Gin—90 proof	1 jigger	45	126	18	
Rum—80 proof	1 jigger	45	105	15	
Vermouth, dry	1 jigger	45	47	7	1
Vermouth, sweet	1 jigger	45	75	8	5
Vodka—100 proof	1 jigger	45	135	19	
Whiskey—86 proof	1 jigger	45	112	16	
Wine					
Champagne, dry	1 champagne glass	135	105	13	3
Champagne, sweet	1 champagne glass	135	160	13	17
California, red	1 claret glass	120	100	12	4
white	1 claret glass	120	95	11	4
Port	1 sherry glass	30	50	5	4
Sherry	1 sherry glass	30	45	5	2

*Alcohol yields 7 calories per gram. The percentage of alcohol varies widely in different preparations.

†Recipes from Rombauer's *Joy of Cooking* used in these calculations and based upon the proof of the liquor listed in the above table. Calories and alcohol content of cocktails will vary widely depending upon the recipes used.

Table A-8. Growth Standards for Boys from Birth to Age 18*

Age	Height (inches) Percentiles			Weight (pounds) Percentiles			Height (centimeters) Percentiles			Weight (kilograms) Percentiles		
	5th	50th	95th	5th	50th	95th	5th	50th	95th	5th	50th	95th
Birth	18.4	19.8	21.1	5.9	7.5	9.1	47	50	54	2.7	3.4	4.1
1 mo	19.9	21.4	22.9	7.3	9.4	11.1	51	54	58	3.3	4.3	5.0
3 mo.	22.6	24.0	25.4	9.8	13.4	16.0	57	61	65	4.4	6.1	7.3
6 mo.	25.1	26.7	28.3	14.7	18.0	21.3	63	68	72	6.7	8.2	9.7
9 mo.	27.2	28.7	30.2	16.8	21.4	25.1	69	73	77	7.6	9.7	11.4
1 yr.	28.4	30.2	32.0	18.7	23.3	27.8	72	77	81	8.5	10.6	12.4
2 yr.	32.1	34.6	37.1	23.3	28.3	33.3	82	88	94	10.6	12.8	15.1
3 yr.	35.3	37.8	40.3	27.1	32.5	37.9	90	95	102	12.3	14.8	17.1
4 yr.	38.3	40.8	43.3	30.0	36.1	42.2	97	104	110	13.6	16.4	19.2
5 yr.	40.3	43.4	46.4	33.0	40.3	47.6	102	110	118	15.0	18.3	21.6
6 yr.	42.8	45.9	49.0	36.0	44.7	53.4	109	117	124	16.3	20.3	24.2
7 yr.	44.8	48.1	51.4	40.3	50.9	61.5	114	122	131	18.3	23.1	27.9
8 yr.	46.9	50.5	54.1	44.4	57.4	70.4	119	129	137	20.2	26.1	32.0
9 yr.	48.8	52.8	56.8	48.0	64.4	80.4	124	134	144	21.8	29.2	36.5
10 yr.	50.6	54.9	59.2	51.4	71.4	91.4	129	139	150	23.3	32.4	41.5
11 yr.	51.9	56.4	60.9	53.3	78.9	102.5	132	143	155	24.2	35.8	46.5
12 yr.	53.5	58.6	63.7	60.0	86.0	113.5	136	149	162	27.2	39.0	51.5
13 yr.	55.2	61.3	67.4	65.3	98.6	131.9	140	156	171	29.6	44.8	59.9
14 yr.	57.5	64.1	70.7	75.5	111.8	148.1	146	163	180	34.3	50.8	67.2
15 yr.	61.0	66.9	72.8	88.0	124.3	160.6	155	170	185	40.0	56.4	72.9
16 yr.	63.8	68.9	74.0	97.8	133.8	169.8	162	175	188	44.4	60.7	77.1
17 yr.	65.2	69.8	74.4	106.5	139.8	174.0	166	177	189	48.3	63.5	79.0
18 yr.	65.9	70.2	74.5	110.3	144.8	179.3	167	178	189	50.0	65.7	81.4

*Height in inches and weight in pounds from: *Obesity and Health,* Pub. 1485, Public Health Service, U.S. Department of Health, Education, and Welfare, 1966; height in centimeters and weight in kilograms calculated from these data.

Table A–9. Growth Standards for Girls from Birth to Age 18*

Age	Height (inches) Percentiles			Weight (pounds) Percentiles			Height (centimeters) Percentiles			Weight (kilograms) Percentiles		
	5th	50th	95th	5th	50th	95th	5th	50th	95th	5th	50th	95th
Birth	18.3	19.5	20.7	5.3	7.3	8.8	47	50	53	2.4	3.3	4.0
1 mo.	19.5	21.0	22.5	6.6	8.3	9.8	50	53	57	3.0	3.8	4.4
3 mo.	22.2	23.6	25.0	10.2	12.4	14.4	56	60	64	4.6	5.6	6.5
6 mo.	24.6	26.1	27.6	13.4	16.7	19.8	63	66	70	6.1	7.6	9.0
9 mo.	26.3	27.9	29.5	15.3	19.8	24.1	67	71	77	6.9	9.0	10.9
1 yr.	27.6	29.4	31.2	17.4	21.7	26.0	70	75	79	7.9	9.9	11.8
2 yr.	31.6	33.8	36.0	22.3	27.1	31.9	80	86	91	10.1	12.3	14.5
3 yr.	35.3	37.5	39.7	26.3	32.3	38.3	90	95	101	11.9	14.7	17.4
4 yr.	38.1	40.7	43.3	28.8	36.1	43.4	97	103	110	13.1	16.4	19.7
5 yr.	40.6	43.4	46.2	32.2	40.9	49.6	103	110	117	14.6	18.6	22.5
6 yr.	42.8	45.9	49.0	35.5	45.7	55.9	109	117	124	16.1	20.7	25.4
7 yr.	44.5	47.8	51.1	38.3	51.0	63.7	113	121	130	17.4	23.2	28.9
8 yr.	46.4	50.0	53.6	42.0	57.2	72.4	118	127	136	19.1	26.0	32.9
9 yr.	48.2	52.2	56.2	45.1	63.6	82.1	122	133	143	20.5	28.9	37.3
10 yr.	49.9	54.5	59.1	48.2	71.0	95.0	128	138	150	21.9	32.2	43.1
11 yr.	51.9	57.0	62.1	55.4	82.0	108.6	132	145	158	25.1	37.2	49.3
12 yr.	54.1	59.5	64.9	63.9	94.4	124.9	137	151	165	29.0	42.9	56.7
13 yr.	57.1	62.2	66.8	72.8	105.5	138.2	145	158	170	33.1	47.9	62.7
14 yr.	58.5	63.1	67.7	83.0	113.0	144.0	149	160	172	37.7	51.3	65.4
15 yr.	59.5	63.8	68.1	89.5	120.0	150.5	151	162	173	40.6	54.5	68.3
16 yr.	59.8	64.1	68.4	95.1	123.0	150.1	152	163	174	43.2	55.9	68.1
17 yr.	60.1	64.2	68.3	97.9	125.8	153.7	153	163	174	44.4	57.1	69.8
18 yr.	60.1	64.4	68.7	96.0	126.2	156.4	153	164	174	43.6	57.3	71.0

*Height in inches and weight in pounds from: *Obesity and Health*, Pub. 1485, Public Health Service, U.S. Department of Health, Education, and Welfare, 1966; height in centimeters and weight in kilograms calculated from these data.

Table A–10. Suggested Weights for Heights for Men and Women*

Height (without shoes) inches	Weight (without clothing) Low	Median pounds	High	Height centimeters	Low	Weight Median kilograms	High
Men							
63	118	129	141	160	54	59	64
64	122	133	145	163	55	60	66
65	126	137	149	165	57	62	68
66	130	142	155	167	59	65	70
67	134	147	161	170	61	67	73
68	139	151	166	173	63	69	75
69	143	155	170	175	65	70	77
70	147	159	174	178	67	72	80
71	150	163	178	180	68	74	81
72	154	167	183	183	70	76	83
73	158	171	188	185	72	77	85
74	162	175	192	188	74	80	87
75	165	178	195	191	75	81	89
Women							
60	100	109	118	152	45	50	54
61	104	112	121	155	47	51	55
62	107	115	125	157	49	52	57
63	110	118	128	160	50	54	58
64	113	122	132	163	51	55	60
65	116	125	135	165	53	57	61
66	120	129	139	167	55	59	63
67	123	132	142	170	56	60	65
68	126	136	146	173	57	62	66
69	130	140	151	175	59	64	69
70	133	144	156	178	60	65	71
71	137	148	161	180	62	67	73
72	141	152	166	183	64	69	75

*Data for heights in inches and weights in pounds taken from: Hathaway, M. L., and Foard, E. D.: *Heights and Weights of Adults in the United States*. Home Economics Research Report No. 10, U.S. Department of Agriculture, Washington, D.C., Table 80, p. 111.

Conversions to centimeters and kilograms were rounded off to the nearest whole number.

Table A–11. Normal Constituents of Human Blood (*B = whole blood; P = plasma; S = serum*)

Constituent	Normal Range		Examples of Deviations
Physical Measurements			
Specific gravity (S)	1.025–1.029		
Bleeding time, capillary	1–3	min	
Prothrombin time (Quick, P)	10–20	sec	
Sedimentation rate (Wintrobe)			
Men	0–9	mm/hr	
Women	0–20	mm/hr	
Viscosity (water as unity) (B)	4.5–5.5		
Acid-Base Constituents			
Base, total fixed cations (Na + K + Ca + Mg) (S)	143–150	mEq/L	Low in alkali deficit; diabetic acidosis
Sodium (S)	320–335	mg/100 ml	Low in alkali deficit, diabetic acidosis, excessive fluid administration
	139–146	mEq/L	
Potassium (S)	16–22	mg/100 ml	High in acute infections, pneumonia, Addison's disease; low in diarrhea, vomiting, correction of diabetic acidosis
	4.1–5.6	mEq/L	
Calcium (S)	9–11	mg/100 ml	High with excessive vitamin D, hyperparathyroidism; low in infantile tetany, steatorrhea, severe nephritis, defective vitamin D absorption
	4.5–5.5	mEq/L	
Calcium, ionized (S)	50–60	per cent	
Magnesium (S)	2–3	mg/100 ml	High in chronic nephritis, liver disease; low in uremia, tetany, severe diarrhea
	1.65–2.5	mEq/L	
Chloride (S)	340–372	mg/100 ml	High in congestive heart failure, eclampsia, nephritis
	96–105	mEq/L	
As NaCl (S)	560–614	mg/100 ml	
	96–105	mEq/L	
Phosphorus, inorganic as P (S)			
Child	4.0–6.5	mg/100 ml	High in chronic nephritis, hypoparathyroidism; low during treatment of diabetic coma, hyperparathyroidism
Adult	2.5–4.5	mg/100 ml	
Sulfates as SO_4^{--} (S)	2.5–5.0	mg/100 ml	
	0.5–1.0	mEq/L	
Bicarbonate cation-binding power (S)	19–30	mEq/L	
Serum protein cation-binding power (S)	15.5–18.0	mEq/L	
Lactic acid (S)	10–20	mg/100 ml	
	1.1–2.2	mEq/L	
pH at 38°C (B, P, or S)	7.30–7.45		High in uncompensated alkalosis; low in uncompensated acidosis
Blood Gases			
CO_2 content (venous S)	45–70	vol %	Low in primary alkali deficit, diarrhea; high in hypoventilation
	20.3–31.5	mM/L	
CO_2 content (venous B)	40–60	vol %	
	18–27	mM/L	
CO_2 tension (pCO_2) arterial blood	35–45	mm Hg	pCO_2 in venous blood is about 6 mm higher than arterial or capillary blood

Constituent	Normal Range		Examples of Deviations
Oxygen content (arterial B)	15–22	vol %	High in polycythemia; low in emphysema
Oxygen content (venous B)	11–16	vol %	
Oxygen capacity (B)	16–24	vol %	
Oxygen tension (pO_2)	85–100	mm Hg	
Carbohydrates			
Glucose			
Reducing substances (B)	90–120	mg/100 ml	High in diabetes mellitus; low in hyperinsulinism
"True"	60–85	mg/100 ml	
Glucose tolerance			
Fasting sugar	90–120	mg/100 ml	
Highest value	130–140	mg/100 ml	
Highest value reached in	45–60	minutes	
Return to fasting in	1.5–2.5	hr	
Lactose tolerance			
Fasting blood glucose (B)	90–120	mg/100 ml	In lactase deficiency the rise in blood
Increase in blood glucose after test dose lactose	20	mg/100 ml	glucose after test dose of lactose is less than 20 mg in 1 hour
Citric acid (B)	1.3–2.3	mg/100 ml	
(P)	1.6–2.7	mg/100 ml	
Lactic acid (see acid-base constituents)			
Pyruvic acid, fasting (B)	0.7–1.2	mg/100 ml	
Enzymes			
Amylase (Somogyi) (S)	60–180	units/100 ml	High in acute pancreatitis, acute appendicitis
Lactic dehydrogenase (S)	25–100	units/ml	High in myocardial infarction
Lipase (S)	0.2–1.5	units/ml	High in pancreatitis
Leucine-aminopeptidase (S)	1–3.5	units/ml	High in hemolytic anemias
Phosphatase, alkaline			
(Bodansky) (S) Child	5–14	units/100 ml	High in rickets, bone cancer, Paget's
Adult	1–4		disease, hyperparathyroidism, vitamin D inadequacy; indicates rapid bone growth in young
Transaminases			
Glutamic-oxalacetic			
(SGOT) (Karmen) (S)	10–40	units/ml	Increased within 24 hours in myocardial infarction; normal after 6 to 7 days
Glutamic-pyruvic			
(SGPT) (Karmen) (S)	5–35	units/ml	High in hepatic disease, and trauma after surgery
Hematologic Studies			
Cell volume	39–50	per cent	High in polycythemia; low in anemia, prolonged iron deficiency
Red blood cells	4.25–5.25	million per cu mm	High in polycythemia, dehydration; low in anemia, hemorrhage
White blood cells	5000–9000	per cu mm	Increased in acute infections, leukemias

Table A–11. (Cont.)

Constituent	Normal Range		Examples of Deviations
Lymphocytes	25–30	per cent	
Neutrophils	60–65	per cent	
Monocytes	4–8	per cent	
Eosinophils	0.5–4	per cent	
Basophils	0–1.5	per cent	
Platelets	125,000–300,000	per cu mm	
Lipids			
Acetone (S)	0.3–2.0	mg/100 ml	High in uncontrolled diabetes and starvation
Cholesterol, total (S)	125–225	mg/100 ml	High in uncontrolled diabetes mellitus,
esters	50–67	per cent	nephrosis, hypothyroidism,
free	33–50	per cent	hyperlipidemias
Fatty acids, unesterified (P)	8–31	mg/100 ml	
17-Hydroxycorticosteroids (P)	10–13.5	mcg/100 ml	
Lipids, total (P)	570–820	mg/100 ml	
Phospholipid (S)	150–300	mg/100 ml	
Triglycerides (S)	30–140	mg/100 ml	Increased in hyperlipidemias
Nitrogenous Constituents			
Alpha-amino acid nitrogen (S)	3.5–5.5	mg/100 ml	High in severe liver disease; low in nephrosis
Ammonia (B)	40–70	mcg/100 ml	High in liver disease
Creatinine (S)	0.5–1.2	mg/100 ml	Increased in renal insufficiency
Creatinine clearance endogenous (B)	120±20	ml	Blood cleared per min by kidney; measure of glomerular filtration
Nonprotein N (NPN) (B)	25–35	mg/100 ml	High in acute glomerulonephritis, dehydration, metallic poisoning, intestinal obstruction, renal failure
Phenylalanine (S)	0.7–4	mg/100 ml	Increased in phenylketonuria
Urea nitrogen (BUN) (B)	8–18	mg/100 ml	High in renal failure, acute glomerulone-phritis, mercury poisoning, dehydration; low in hepatic failure
Urea clearance (B)	75	ml/min C_m	C_m = maximal clearance
	54	ml/min C_s	C_s = standard clearance
Uric acid (S)	2–6	mg/100 ml	High in gout, nephritis, arthritis
Proteins			
Total protein (S)	6.5–7.5	gm/100 ml	High in dehydration; low in liver disease, nephrosis
Albumin (S)	3.9–4.5	gm/100 ml	Low in starvation, cirrhosis, proteinuria
Globulin (S)	2.3–3.5	gm/100 ml	High in infections, liver disease, multiple myeloma
Albumin:globulin ratio	1.2–1.9		Low in liver disease, nephrosis
Fibrinogen (P)	0.2–0.5	gm/100 ml	High in infections; low in severe liver disease
Ceruloplasmin (S)	16–33	mg/100 ml	
Gamma globulin (S)	0.7–1.2	gm/100 ml	
Hemoglobin (B)			High in polycythemia; low in prolonged dietary deficiency of iron, anemia
Males	14–17	gm/100 ml	
Females	12–16	gm/100 ml	

Table A–11. (Cont.)

Constituent	Normal Range		Examples of Deviations
Vitamins			
Ascorbic acid (S)	0.3–1.4	mg/100 ml	
Folic acid (*L. casei*) (S)	6–10	mmcg/ml	
(*L. casei*) (B)	100–220	mmcg/ml	
Niacin (S)	30–150	mcg/100 ml	
Riboflavin (S)	2.3–3.7	mcg/100 ml	
Thiamin (B)	5.5–9.5	mcg/100 ml	
Tocopherol (S)	0.6–2.0	mg/100 ml	
Vitamin A (S)	25–90	mcg/100 ml	
Carotene (S)	40–125	mcg/100 ml	
Vitamin B_6 (B)	1–18	mcg/100 ml	
Vitamin B_{12} (S)	10–90	mcg/100 ml	
Miscellaneous			
Bilirubin (S)	0–1.5	mg/100 ml	High in red cell destruction, liver disease
Icterus index	4–6	units	High in jaundice
Copper (S)	80–240	mcg/100 ml	Low in anemia, Wilson's disease
Iron (S)			
Men	80–165	mcg/100 ml	High in hemochromatosis, liver disease,
Women	65–130	mcg/100 ml	transfusion hemosiderosis; low in iron-deficiency anemia
Iron-binding capacity (S)			
Men	250–430	mcg/100 ml	High in anemia
Women	220–415	mcg/100 ml	
Lead (S)	1–3	mcg/100 ml	
Manganese (S)	2–5	mcg/100 ml	
Protein-bound iodine (PBI) (S)	3–8	mcg/100 ml	High in hyperthyroidism; low in hypothyroidism
Zinc (S)	100–140	mcg/100 ml	

ml = milliliters   gm = grams
mg = milligrams   cu mm = cubic millimeters
mcg = micrograms
mEq = milliequivalents

$$\text{mEq per liter} = \frac{\text{mg per liter}}{\text{equivalent weight}} \qquad \text{mM (millimoles) per liter} = \frac{\text{mg per liter}}{\text{molecular weight}}$$

$$\text{equivalent weight} = \frac{\text{atomic weight}}{\text{valence of element}} \qquad \text{volumes per cent} = \text{mM per liter} \times 2.24$$

Sources of Data:
Oser, B. L., ed.: *Hawk's Physiological Chemistry*, 14th ed. McGraw-Hill Book Company, New York, 1965, pp. 977–79.
Robinson, H. W.: "Biochemistry," in *Rypins' Medical Licensure Examinations*, 11th ed., A. W. Wright, ed. J. B. Lippincott Company, Philadelphia, 1970, pp. 202–5.

Table A–12. Normal Constituents of the Urine of the Adult

Specific gravity		1.010–1.025
Reaction	pH	5.5–8.0
Volume	ml per 24 hr	800–1600
		gm per 24 hr
Total solids		*55–70*
Nitrogenous constituents		
Total nitrogen		10–17
Ammonia		0.5–1.0
Amino acid N		0.4–1
Creatine		None
Creatinine		1–1.5
Protein		None
Purine bases		0.016–0.060
Urea		20–35
Uric acid		0.5–0.7
Acetone bodies		0.003–0.015
Bile		None
Calcium		0.2–0.4
Chloride (as NaCl)		10–15
Glucose		None
Indican		0–0.030
Iron		0.001–0.005
Magnesium (as MgO)		0.15–0.30
Phosphate, total (as phosphoric acid)		2.5–3.5
Potassium (as K_2O)		2.0–3.0
Sodium (as Na_2O)		4.0–5.0
Sulfates, total (as sulfuric acid)		1.5–3.0

Table A–13. Conversions to and from Metric Measures

If measure is in	Multiply by	To find
Length		
inches	25.4	millimeters
inches	2.54	centimeters
feet	30.48	centimeters
feet	0.305	meters
centimeters	0.394	inches
meters	3.281	feet
Weight		
grains	64.799	milligrams
ounces (Av.)	28.35	grams
pounds (Av.)	454	grams
pounds	0.454	kilograms
grams	15.432	grains
grams	0.035	ounces (Av.)
grams	0.0022	pounds (Av.)
kilograms	2.205	pounds
Capacity (liquid)		
teaspoons	4.7	milliliters
tablespoons	14.1	milliliters
fluid ounces	29.573	milliliters
cups (8 ounces)	238	milliliters
pints	0.473	liters
quarts	0.946	liters
milliliters	0.034	fluid ounces
liters	1.057	quarts
Energy units		
kilocalories	4.184	kilojoules
kilojoules	0.239	kilocalories
Temperature		
Fahrenheit	subtract 32; then multiply by $\frac{5}{9}$	Celsius (Centigrade)
Celsius	multiply by $\frac{9}{5}$; then add 32	Fahrenheit

Metric equivalents
    1 kilogram (kg) = 1000 grams
    1 gram (gm) = 1000 milligrams
    1 milligram (mg) = 1000 micrograms
    1 microgram (mcg, μg, γ) = 1000 nanograms
    1 nanogram (ng) = 1000 picograms (pg)

Multiples
    deca- 10
    hecto- 10^2 (100)
    kilo- 10^3 (1000)
    mega- 10^6 (1,000,000)

Submultiples
    deci- = one tenth 10^{-1} (0.1)
    centi- = one hundredth 10^{-2} (0.01)
    milli- = one thousandth 10^{-3} (0.001)
    micro- = one millionth 10^{-6} (0.000,001)
    nano- = one billionth 10^{-9} (0.000,000,001)
    pico- = one trillionth 10^{-12} (0.000,000,000,001)

Table A–14. Recommended Daily Nutrient Intakes—Canada, Revised 1974 *Committee for Revision of the Canadian Dietary Standard, Bureau of Nutritional Sciences, Health and Welfare, Ottawa, Canada*

Age years	Sex	Weight kg	Height cm	Energy[a] kcal	Pro-tein gm	Thiamin mg	Niacin[e] mg	Ribo-flavin mg	Vita-min B_6[f] mg	Folate[g] mcg	Vita-min B_{12} mcg	Asco bic Aci mg
0–6 mos	both	6		kg × 117	kg × 2.2(2.0)[d]	0.3	5	0.4	0.3	40	0.3	20
1–11 mos	both	9		kg × 108	kg × 1.4	0.5	6	0.6	0.4	60	0.3	20
1–3	both	13	90	1400	22	0.7	9	0.8	0.8	100	0.9	20
4–6	both	19	110	1800	27	0.9	12	1.1	1.3	100	1.5	20
7–9	M	27	129	2200	33	1.1	14	1.3	1.6	100	1.5	30
	F	27	128	2000	33	1.0	13	1.2	1.4	100	1.5	30
10–12	M	36	144	2500	41	1.2	17	1.5	1.8	100	3.0	30
	F	38	145	2300	40	1.1	15	1.4	1.5	100	3.0	30
13–15	M	51	162	2800	52	1.4	19	1.7	2.0	200	3.0	30
	F	49	159	2200	43	1.1	15	1.4	1.5	200	3.0	30
16–18	M	64	172	3200	54	1.6	21	2.0	2.0	200	3.0	30
	F	54	161	2100	43	1.1	14	1.3	1.5	200	3.0	30
19–35	M	70	176	3000	56	1.5	20	1.8	2.0	200	3.0	30
	F	56	161	2100	41	1.1	14	1.3	1.5	200	3.0	30
36–50	M	70	176	2700	56	1.4	18	1.7	2.0	200	3.0	30
	F	56	161	1900	41	1.0	13	1.2	1.5	200	3.0	30
51+	M	70	176	2300[b]	56	1.4	18	1.7	2.0	200	3.0	30
	F	56	161	1800[b]	41	1.0	13	1.2	1.5	200	3.0	30
Pregnant				+300[c]	+20	+0.2	+2	+0.3	+0.5	+50	+1.0	+20
Lactating				+500	+24	+0.4	+7	+0.6	+0.6	+50	+0.5	+30

[a] Recommendations assume characteristic activity pattern for each age group.

[b] Recommended energy allowance for age 66+ years reduced to 2000 for men and 1500 for women.

[c] Increased energy allowance recommended during second and third trimesters. An increase of 100 kcal per day is recommended during the first trimester.

[d] Recommended protein allowance of 2.2 gm per kilogram body weight for infants aged 0 to 2 mos, and 2.0 gm per kilogram body weight for those aged 3 to 5 mos. Protein recommendation for infants, 0 to 11 mos, assumes consumption of breast milk or protein of equivalent quality.

[e] Approximately 1 mg of niacin is derived from each 60 mg of dietary tryptophan.

[f] Recommendations are based on the estimated average daily protein intake of Canadians.

[g] Recommendations given in terms of free folate.

[h] Considerably higher levels may be prudent for infants during the first week of life to guard against neonatal tyrosinemia.

Vitamin A[i] mcg RE	Vitamin D mcg cholecalciferol[j]	Vitamin E mg α-tocopherol	Calcium mg	Phosphorus mg	Magnesium mg	Iodine mcg	Iron mg	Zinc mg	Age years
			Fat-Soluble Vitamins		**Minerals**				
400	10	3	500[l]	250[l]	50[l]	35[l]	7[l]	4[l]	0–6 mos
400	10	3	500	400	50	50	7	5	7–11 mos
400	10	4	500	500	75	70	8	5	1–3
500	5	5	500	500	100	90	9	6	4–6
700	2.5[k]	6	700	700	150	110	10	7	7–9 M
700	2.5[k]	6	700	700	150	100	10	7	7–9 F
800	2.5[k]	7	900	900	175	130	11	8	10–12 M
800	2.5[k]	7	1000	1000	200	120	11	9	10–12 F
1000	2.5[k]	9	1200	1200	250	140	13	10	13–15 M
800	2.6[k]	7	800	800	250	110	14	10	13–15 F
1000	2.5[k]	10	1000	1000	300	160	14	12	16–18 M
800	2.5[k]	6	700	700	250	110	14	11	16–18 F
1000	2.5[k]	9	800	800	300	150	10	10	19–35 M
800	2.5[k]	6	700	700	250	110	14	9	19–35 F
1000	2.5[k]	8	800	800	300	140	10	10	36–50 M
800	2.5[k]	6	700	700	250	100	14	9	36–50 F
1000	2.5[k]	8	800	800	300	140	10	10	51+ M
800	2.5[k]	6	700	700	250	100	9	9	51+ F
+100	+2.5[k]	+1	+500	+500	+25	+15	+1[m]	+3[m]	Pregnant
+400	+2.5[k]	+2	+500	+500	+75	+25	+1[m]	+7	Lactating

[i] One microgram retinol equivalent (1 mcg RE) corresponds to a biologic activity in humans equal to 1 mcg retinol (3.33 IU) and 6 mcg carotene (10 IU).

[j] One microgram cholecalciferol is equivalent to 40 IU vitamin D activity.

[k] Most older children and adults receive enough vitamin D from irradiation but 2.5 mcg daily is recommended. This recommended allowance increases to 5.0 mcg daily for pregnant and lactating women and for those who are confined indoors or otherwise deprived of sunlight for extended periods.

[l] The intake of breast-fed infants may be less than the recommendation but is considered to be adequate.

[m] A recommended total intake of 15 mg daily during pregnancy and lactation assumes the presence of adequate stores of iron. If stores are suspected of being inadequate, additional iron as a supplement is recommended.

List of Audiovisual Materials

Representative audiovisual materials are listed below with suggested correlations with chapters of the text. When the title does not indicate the scope of the topics covered, a brief description of content is included. Approximate prices have been listed for purchase of some since many schools may wish to make gradual additions to their collections. Most movies are available for free loan or on a rental basis. The instructor should consult local groups for availability of films, filmstrips, and slides: the audiovisual department of local or state divisions of public education; departments of health; Dairy Council; district heart association; Modern Talking Picture Service, Associated Film Services, and other film services. Films should be ordered at least a month in advance of the expected showing.

FILMS (16 mm, color, sound, unless otherwise noted)

Chapter
Correlation

1. "Food, the Color of Life" (1965) 1
   Content: life continues through self-replacing cycle of which food is a part; motivational film toward better diet
   22½ minutes; National Dairy Council, Inc.
   free loan: Association-Sterling Films,
   866 Third Avenue, New York, NY 10022

Chapter
Correlation

2. "Food for a Modern World" 1, 24
   Content: development of U.S. food technology for past 50 years; compares our ability to produce food with that of other parts of the world
   22 minutes, California Dairy Council, rental from Perennial Education, Inc., 1825 Willow Road, Northfield, IL 60693
3. "Hunger in America" (1968) 1, 23
   Content: black sharecroppers, Navajo Indians, tenant farmers, Mexican-Americans; shows undernutrition
   CBS film, 54 minutes, black and white
   Rental fee: Audiovisual Services, Pennsylvania State University, University Park, PA 16802
4. "Hungry Angels" (1961) 1, 23, 24
   Content: nutritional problems related to poverty, ignorance; case studies shown; need for low-cost proteins
   20 minutes, rental: Association Films, Inc. 347 Madison Ave., New York, NY 10017
5. "The Human Body: Digestive System" 2
   Content: animation, x-rays, live action scenes; digestion of complex substances to simple; role and relationship of digestive organs
   13⅓ minutes, Coronet film, free loan, J. P. Lilley and Sons, Inc. Box 3035, 2009 N. Third St., Harrisburg, PA 17105
6. "How a Hamburger Turns into You" 2, 4
   Content: 12-year-old boy learns how protein is digested and resynthesized in cells according to DNA direction
   California Dairy Council, 22 minutes; rental from Perennial Education, Inc. (#2 above)
7. "The Big Dinner Table" 3
   Content: nutrition for people all over the world comes from the Four Food Groups; family mealtime in 35 world locations
   California Dairy Council, 11 minutes; rental from Perennial Education, Inc. (#2 above)
8. "Diet for a Small Planet" (1974) 4, 15, 24
   Content: foods to replace meat—grains and legumes, grains and dairy; concentrates on "no meat" rather than smaller amounts of meat; shows supplementary value of foods
   28 minutes; rental from Bullfrog Films, P.O. Box 114, Milford Square, PA 18935
9. "Food, Energy and You" (1972) 7
   Content: animated scenes showing process by which plants store energy; ATP-ADP system as control of energy in body
   California Dairy Council, 21 minutes; rental from Perennial Education, Inc. (# 2 above)

FILMS (16 mm, color, sound, unless otherwise noted)

10. "Calcium and Phosphorus Metabolism" (1964) 8
Content: sources of calcium and phosphorus; regulation of absorption, blood levels, excretion; diagnosis and treatment of metabolic disorders
Part I, 24 minutes; part 2, 23 minutes, black and white; loan, National Medical Audiovisual Center, Station "K", Atlanta, GA 30324

11. "Vitamins and Some Deficiency Diseases" (1955 revised) 11, 12
Content: laboratory scenes show deficiency in animals; clinical deficiency such as cheilosis, rickets, pellagra, scurvy, vitamin K
35 minutes, free loan: Lederle Laboratories, Division of American Cyanamid Co., Pearl River, NY 10965

12. "Vitamins from Food" 11, 12
Content: Dr. Lind cures scurvy; Dr. Eijkman cures beriberi; vitamins as coenzymes in animated scenes
California Dairy Council, 21 minutes: rental from Perennial Education, Inc. (#2)

13. "Eating on the Run" (1975) 13
Content: balanced meals need not require time-consuming preparation; breakfasts quickly prepared, lunches from fast-food service
$15\frac{1}{2}$ min, cost $215; Alfred Higgins Productions, Inc. 9100 Sunset Blvd., Los Angeles, CA 90069

14. "Eat, Drink and Be Wary" (1975) 14, 23
Content: emphasis on unprocessed and fresh foods; not overprocessed or fabricated; presents advertising emphasis on costs of processed foods; stimulates discussion on development of food habits
21 minutes, cost $265; Churchill Films, 662 N. Robertson Blvd., Los Angeles, CA 90069

15. "What You Eat, You Are" (1970) 15, 16
Content: situations in black families; planning, purchasing, preparing, serving food; protection against parasites
15 minutes, free loan; Audio Visual Aids, University of South Carolina, College of General Studies, Carolina Coliseum, Columbia, SC 29208

16. "The Vegetarian Gourmet" 15
Content: Alan Hooker, restaurateur, demonstrates preparation of vegetarian foods; also what foods can furnish adequate protein in vegetarian diet
Kikkoman International, Inc., $14\frac{1}{2}$ minutes, free loan: Association-Sterling Films (#1 above)

17. "Food: More for Your Money" 16
Content: comparing food items for quality and economy; shopping list, nutrition labeling, unit pricing, meat purchasing, convenience foods
14 minutes, cost $190: Alfred Higgins Productions, Inc. (#13 above)

18. "Mission Nutrition" (1971) 16
Content: tour through supermarket shows how to make wise food buys; nutritional values; reading labels; 1971 food prices date this film
15 min, cost $195, $15 preview: EPI/Evol Productions, Inc. 933 N. Kenmore St., Arlington, VA 22201

19. "That the Best Will Be Ours" 16, 18
Content: growth of meat and poultry inspection since 1906; inspection controls for processors; shopping, handling, preparation steps by consumer
18 min: loan, State Film Libraries, Agricultural Extension

20. "Read the Label, Set a Better Table" (1974) 18
Content: what is on the label; why; animated sequences of major nutrient classes, and functions of nutrients; narrated by Dick Van Dyke
Food and Drug Administration: free loan, regional FDA offices or Modern Talking Pictures, 2323 New Hyde Park Road, New Hyde Park, NY 11040

21. "Foods: Fads and Facts" (1974) 17, 18, 23
Content: nutritive value of health foods; organic and commercial growing methods; disadvantages of health food stores; some aspects of food processing and harvesting
17 minutes, cost $230: Alfred Higgins Productions, Inc., (#13 above)

22. "Prescription: Food" (1973) 19, 24
Content: problem of malnutrition in low-income area; home visits by nurse practitioners; classes for pregnant women; supervised play and meals
26 minutes, free loan: Director of Public Health Services, Ross Laboratories, Columbus, OH 43216

23. "Great Expectations" (1975) 19
Content: nutrition during pregnancy and lactation; variety of socioeconomic and ethnic backgrounds; meeting increased needs through food selection
22 minutes, cost $150: Society for Nutrition Education, 2140 Shattuck Ave., Berkeley, CA 94704; includes leader guides and 30 copies of "What Should I Eat?"

24. "Eating for Two" (1968) 19
Content: public health nurse helping young black mother learn nutritional needs; meal patterns for family, meal planning, economic shopping; food patterns typical of southeastern United States

FILMS (16 mm, color, sound, unless otherwise noted)

22 minutes: check local sources for loan; purchase, Bureau of Audio Visual Instruction, 1327 University Ave., Box 2093, Madison, WI 53701

25. "Nutrition: To Baby with Love" (1973) 20
Content: young parents with babies from different ethnic backgrounds; bottle feeding; supplementary foods
Gerber Products Company, 10 minutes: free loan, West Glen Films, 565 Fifth Ave., New York, NY 10017

26. "Jenny Is a Good Thing" (1969) 21
Content: Head Start centers: linking nutrition practices to play, learning, social experiences, language, development of self-concept
18 minutes, free loan: Modern Talking Pictures, (#20 above)

27. "Looking at Children" 21
Content: teachers and school nurses alerted to physical health problems of children; discusses anemia, obesity, malnutrition
24 minutes, free loan: Health and Welfare Division, Metropolitan Life Insurance Company, One Madison Ave., New York, NY 10010

28. "Big Problems for Little People" (1975) 21, 23
Content: lack of food and population pressures limit food available in mountain and seaside community in Philippines; infections further malnutrition
Helen A., and George M. Guthrie, rental $13.50: Audiovisual Services (#3 above)

29. "Food for Thought" (1974) 21
Content: explains and promotes school lunch programs; development, cost, type A lunch, nutrition education
Free loan: Illinois Office of Education, 100 N. First St., Springfield, IL 62777

30. "Lunch Bunch" (1973) 21
Content: needs for school lunch: working mother, children unable to go home; setting up a school lunch program
15½ minutes; rental $5 per day: Walter F. Colender, N.J. Department of Education, 225 W. State Street, Trenton, NJ 08625

31. "The Real Talking, Singing, Action Movie About Nutrition" (1972) 21
Content: teen-agers need to choose food wisely; white, middle-class values shown
Sunkist Growers, 14 minutes, rental $25: Oxford

Films, 1136 N. Las Palmas Ave., Los Angeles, CA 90036

32. "Food for Life" (1969) 21
Content: food selections by four teen-agers; two Americans choose poor diet even with abundant food supply; South American lacks variety; Asian lacks quantity, variety
California Dairy Council, 22 minutes; rental from Perennial Education, Inc. (#2 above)

33. "Don't Stop the Music" 22
Content: challenges myths and stereotypes of older persons; ways community can respond to needs of older persons
Department of Health, Education, and Welfare, 17½ minutes; free loan, Modern Talking Pictures, (#20 above)

34. "More than Food" (1965) 22
Content: filmed in nursing home; shows role of all personnel in meeting nutritional, physical, psychologic needs
23 minutes, check local source for loan: purchase, Colorado State Department of Public Health, Denver, CO 80203

35. "The Rights of Age" 22
Content: story of elderly widow, cut off from society, living alone, meager diet; film brings out various protective services
28 minutes: rental from International Film Bureau, Inc., 332 South Michigan Ave., Chicago, IL 60604

36. "Nutrition Quackery" (1973) 23
Content: food faddists giving TV lecture; film gives answers by showing scenes in food production; explains food safety, regulation
20 minutes, free loan: AIMS Instructional Media Services, Inc., P.O. Box 1010, Hollywood, CA 90028

37. "The Health Fraud Racket" (1967) 23
Content: traps of the quack; economic waste, risk to health of worthless products
Food and Drug Administration, 28 minutes; free loan, National Medical Audiovisual Center (#10 above)

38. "Three Times a Day" 24, 40
Content: one of every four Americans aged 55 to 62 has a coronary; diet a cause; should take steps to lower cholesterol
Best Foods, 25 minutes; free loan Association-Sterling Films (#1 above)

39. "Sorry, No Vacancy" (1973) 23, 24
Content: world food shortages, uncontrolled population growth, pollution; no simple solutions in film; raises questions for discussion

FILMS (16 mm, color, sound, unless otherwise noted)

J. Wilhite and P. Wilhite, cost $315: rental $35: Malibu Films, Inc., P.O. Box 428, Malibu, CA 90265

40. "Food or Famine" 24
Content: methods of using fertilizers, controlling pests, raising better cattle; Europe, southeast Asia, India, South America
28 minutes, free loan: Shell Film Library, 450 N. Meridian St., Indianapolis, IN 46204

41. "Feeding the Patient" (1959) 25
Content: appetite, digestion, feeding ambulatory and recumbent patients; physical, psychologic preparation for meals
15 minutes, black and white: rental, American Hospital Association, 840 N. Lake Shore Drive, Chicago, IL 60611

42. "The Missing Millions" (1968) 37
Content: young executive found to have typical symptoms of diabetes; nature of disease; effectiveness of treatment
14 minutes, free loan, National Medical Audiovisual Center (#10 above)

43. "Quiet Victory" (1967) 37
Content: nurse's responsibility to four persons with diabetes, teaching and guidance in detection, outpatient center, hospital, home
35 minutes, free loan: National Medical Audiovisual Center (#10 above)

44. "Understanding Diabetes" (1967) 37
Content: basic scientific concepts, epidemiology, management, prevention of acute problems. Live photography, animated drawings
35 minutes, free loan: National Medical Audiovisual Center (#10 above)

45. "Diabetes: Special Problems in the Older Patient" 37
22 minutes, loan, Upjohn Professional Film Library, 7000 Portage Road, Kalamazoo, MI 49001

45. "An Exchange for the Better" (1974) 37
Content: diabetic exchange system; simulated counseling session with portion sizes of food; useful review for established diabetic; use in small segments for new patient
S. Noyes and K. Noyes, rental $65 for 2 weeks, includes instructor's outline, self test, and 50 student supplements: Foodways System, 1615 Pandora Ave., Los Angeles, CA 90024

46. "Better Odds for a Longer Life" (1966) 40
Content: cartoon animation; functions of heart; atherosclerosis; ways to reduce risks
20 minutes, rental: American Heart Association Film Library, 267 W. 25th St., New York, NY 10001

47. "Eat to Your Heart's Content" 40
Content: case study of typical American family and dietary faults; some ways to correct diet
13 minutes, rental: American Heart Association Film Library (#46 above)

48. "A Pinch of Salt" (1974) 41
Content: sodium; history, role, individual or group counseling, modified diet
S. Noyes and K. Noyes, 16 minutes, rental $65 for 2 weeks, Foodways System (#45 above)

FILMSTRIPS, SLIDES (35 mm, color, record or script)

49. "Science of Nutrition" (1972) 1
Self-teaching unit—filmstrip, audiotape cassette, worksheet, post test
B. R. Rich, unit cost $16: Multi Media Office, San Jacinto College, 21400 Highway 79, Gilman Hot Springs, CA 92340

50. "How Food Affects You" (1969) 2, 3
Content: cartoon-type illustrations of functions of nutrition; names nutrients; examples of function; four food groups
Filmstrip, $5.50: Photo Lab, Inc., 3825 Georgia Ave., N.W., Washington, DC 20011
48 slides, $8.00; Office of Communications, Photography Division, U.S. Department of Agriculture, Washington, DC, 20250

51. "Gastric Function" (September 1971)° 2, 32
25 slides, 12 syllabi, $28.50: Nutrition Today, Educational Services, 101 Ridgely Ave., Annapolis, MD 21404

52. "Gastrointestinal Absorption" (March 1967) 2, 32
9 slides, 12 syllabi, $15.25: Nutrition Today, Educational Services (#51 above)

53. "The Esophagus" (January 1973) 2, 32
19 slides, 12 syllabi, $23.50; Nutrition Today, Educational Services (#51 above)

54. "Nutrition" (1969) 3
Content: how food is used by the body; nutrient functions and sources; Four Food Groups

° The dates for slides from *Nutrition Today* refer to articles appearing in the Journal. The articles, slides, and syllabi have been developed by internationally recognized authorities, and are highly recommended for dietetic and nursing programs.

FILMSTRIPS, SLIDES (35 mm, color, record or script)

20 multicolor transparencies for overhead projector, teacher supplement, $48.50: DCA Educational Products Inc., 4865 Stenton Ave., Philadelphia, PA 19144

55. "Food for Life: The Basic Four" (1975)   3,13
Bread and cereal group, 61 frames; meat group, 73 frames; milk group, 63 frames; vegetable-fruit group, 66 frames, $12.50: Tupperware Education Services, Orlando, FL 32802

56. "Proteins, the Building Blocks," (1972)   4
B. R. Rich, Nutrition Series (#49 above) ·

57. "Protein/Iron" (1973)   4, 8
Content: protein role, amino acids, protein synthesis, costs from various sources; iron, needs for high intake, iron absorption, role
35 slides, leader's guide, $6.00 per set: Visual Communications Office, 412 Roberts Hall, Cornell University, Ithaca, NY 14850

58. "Energy: Our Food and Our Needs" (1974)   4, 5, 6
Content: functions, digestion, food sources of protein, fat, carbohydrate; effects of imbalanced dietary regimens
65 slides, 25 page script, $10.00 per set: Visual Communications Office (#57 above)

59. "Energy and the Carbohydrates" (1972)   5, 7
B. R. Rich, Nutrition Series (#49 above)

60. "The Fats" (1972)   6
B. R. Rich, Nutrition Series (#49 above)

61. "Water and Minerals" (1972)   8, 9
B. R. Rich, Nutrition Series (#49 above)

62. "Iron Metabolism" (Summer 1969)   8
10 slides, 12 syllabi, $16.00: Nutrition Today, Educational Services (#51 above)

63. "How the Body Uses Water" (Spring 1970)   9
9 slides, 12 syllabi, $15.80: Nutrition Today, Educational Services (#51 above)

64. "Fat-Soluble Vitamins" (1972)   10
B. R. Rich, Nutrition Series (#49 above)

65. "Vitamin E" (July 1973)   10
14 slides, 12 syllabi, $24.50: Nutrition Today, Educational Services (#51 above)

66. "Vitamins and You"   10, 11, 12
Content: importance of vitamins for childhood
Filmstrip, $4.00: Vitamin Information Bureau, Inc., 575 Lexington, Ave., Dept. JN, New York, NY 10022

67. "Nutrition (Scope®) Manual"   10, 11, 12
Content: nutrition, deficiency diseases

49 slides, color, black and white, $20.00: The Upjohn Company, Unit 9435, Kalamazoo, MI 49001

68. "Water-Soluble Vitamins" (1972)   11, 12
B. R. Rich, Nutrition Series (#49 above)

69. "Vitamin C Makes the Difference" (1972)   11
Content: vitamin C sources, Four Food Groups, buying and storage of fruits and vegetables, meal planning, six citrus recipes
Filmstrip, 50 frames, narrative guide, $2.50; slides, $5.00: Sunkist Growers, Inc., Consumer Service, Box 7888, Valley Annex, Van Nuys, CA 91409

70. "Nutrition in the Home" (1972)   13
B. R. Rich, Nutrition Series (#49 above)

71. "Breakfast and the Bright Life"   13, 16
Content: social aspects of food; role of breakfast in weight control
Filmstrip, 96 frames, sound, teacher's guide: Educational Director, Cereal Institute, 135 S. La Salle St., Chicago, IL 60603

72. "Social Aspects of Nutrition" (1972)   14
B. R. Rich, Nutrition Series (#49 above)

73. "Puerto Rican Food Habits" (1971)   15
Content: culture, food habits, favorite foods, change within framework of culture
45 slides, script, $8.75: Visual Communications Office (#57 above)

74. "Spending Your Food Dollar"   16
77 frames, study guide, free loan: Money Management Institute, Household Finance Corporation, Prudential Plaza, Chicago, IL 60601

75. "The 130 Billion Dollar Food Assembly Line" (1972)   16
Content: movement of food from producer to consumer; emphasis on productivity, dollar value
Filmstrip, 47 frames, $5.50: Photo Lab, Inc. (#50 above)
Slides, $13.00: Office of Communications, Photography Division (#50 above)
Narrative cassette, $3.00; either source

76. "Our Incredible Shrinking Food Dollar" (1974)   16
Content: global reasons for rising food costs; buying economical protein sources; home cooking with economical dishes
Filmstrip, 104 frames, record, 20 booklets, free rental, $7.00 purchase: General Mills Consumer Center, P.O. Box 1113, Minneapolis, MN 55440

77. "What's Happening to Food Prices,"   16
Filmstrip, 153 frames, $15.00: Photo Lab, Inc. (#50 above)
Slides, $35.00: Office of Communications, Photography Division (#50 above)

FILMSTRIPS, SLIDES (35 mm, color, record or script)

**Chapter
Correlation**

78. "The Food Stamp Program and You" (1973) 16, 24
Filmstrip, 61 frames, cassette sound: Photo Lab.
(#50 above)
Slides, $18.50: Office of Communications, Photography Division (#50 above)

79. "It's Good Food, Keep It Safe" 17
Content: food contamination, maintaining sanitation
Filmstrip, 66 frames, cassette, $12.00: Our Baby's
First Seven Years, 5841 S. Maryland Ave.,
Chicago, IL 60637

80. "Food Additives" (July 1973) 17
14 slides, 12 syllabi, $19.95: Nutrition Today, Educational Services (#51 above)

81. "Ann's Additive Story (Its Meaning to Your Food and
Health)" 17
36 frames, filmstrip, $5.50: Photo Lab, Inc.
(#50 above)
36 slides, $11.00: Office of Communications, Photography Division (#50 above)

82. "Nutrition Labeling" (1973) 18
Content: FDA nutrition labeling regulations; need for
labeling; format; how to use information
J. Swanson, 29 slides, illustrated script, $4.75: Visual
Communications Office (#57 above)

83. "Diet and Birth Defects" (Nov. 1968 and
Sept. 1974) 19
18 slides, 12 syllabi, $18.50: Nutrition Today, Educational Services (#51 above)

84. "What Should a Pregnant Woman Eat" (Summer
1970) 19
16 slides, 12 syllabi, $20.90: Nutrition Today, Educational Services (#51 above)

85. "The Beginnings of Life" 19
Content: development of embryo, fetus; vitamins and
minerals
Filmstrip, wall chart, 25 student leaflets, $6.00: Vitamin Information Bureau, Inc. (#66 above)

86. "Prenatal Diet Counseling" 19
12 cards or slides, suggested narrative, $12.00: Creative Teaching Aids, 4161 Carmichael Ave.,
Suite 210, Jacksonville, FL 32207

87. "Straight Talk About Pregnancy and Prenatal Care"
(1972) 19
Content: wide range of income and ethnic groups;
parent education; food needs, shopping, weight
gain
Part 1, Straight Talk about Pregnancy, 80 slides;
part 2, What to Eat, 21 slides; part 3, Labor and
Delivery, 31 slides; teacher guide, scripts, record or

**Chapter
Correlation**

cassettes, $15.00: National Foundation, March of
Dimes, 1275 Mamaroneck Ave., White Plains, NY
10605

88. "Baby's First Year" (1972) 20
Content: development, feeding, nutrition advice; especially for new parent education
Filmstrip, 30 frames, cassette, narrative, $10.00;
slides, $15.00: Our Baby's First Seven Years
(#79 above)

89. "What Nutrients Do Our Infants Really Get?" (September 1973) 20
15 slides, 12 syllabi, $19.75: Nutrition Today, Educational Services (#51 above)

90. "Your Baby's Food" (1970) 20
Content: nutritional and psychologic adjustments
Filmstrip, record, $42.50; slides, $63.50: National
Medical Audiovisual (#10 above)

91. "Put Munch in Their Menu" 21
Content: how to introduce fresh vegetables
Filmstrip, 75 frames, $3.00 with printed script; $5.00
with cassette: Inter Harvest, P.O. Box 2115
Salinas, CA 93901

92. "Food for Teens, Snacks That Count" 21
34 frames, color, cassette, $10.00: Our Baby's First
Seven Years (#79 above)

93. "Children Can Cook" (1973) 21
Content: teacher uses social studies, math, science,
social awareness of food and cooking for preschool
and primary children
Filmstrip, 20 minutes, record, $14.00: Bank Street
Films, 470 Park Ave. South, New York, NY 10016

94. "Your Food—Chance or Choice" (1966) 21
Content: teen-agers' food choices; disc-jockey-type
narrative; rock music; awareness of food, principles
of nutrition, decision making
Filmstrip, 106 frames, teacher's guide, record, $5.00:
National Dairy Council, Inc. (#1 above)

95. "Where Old Age Begins" (1967) 22
11 slides, 12 syllabi, $17.25: Nutrition Today, Educational Services (#51 above)

96. "Natural Foods—Good, Bad, Different" (1973) 23
Content: good and bad aspects of buying and eating
"organically" grown foods
29 slides, cassette, 3 scripts, $12.00: Visual Communications Office (#57 above)

97. "Deficiency Disorders: How to Diagnose Nutritional Disorders in Daily Practice" (1969) 23
20 slides, 12 syllabi, $20.55: Nutrition Today, Educational Services (#51 above)

98. "World Food Situation" 24
Content: production of grains, corn, soybeans in less

FILMSTRIPS, SLIDES (35 mm, color, record or script)

Chapter
Correlation

developed and more developed countries; future world food production and trends

Filmstrip, 22 frames: Office of Communications, Photography Division (#50 above)

99. "Stress: On Just Being Sick" (1970)   25
13 slides, 12 syllabi, $19.25: Nutrition Today, Educational Services (#51 above)

100. "Nutrition in the Hospital" (1972)   25
B. R. Rich, Nutrition Series (#49 above)

101. "Liquid Diets"   27, 36
50 slides, cassette, script, 20 min: Mead Johnson Laboratories, Evansville, IN 47721

102. "Intestinal Malabsorption" (September 1968)   34
10 slides, 12 syllabi, $17.80: Nutrition Today, Educational Services (#51 above)

103. "Just One in a Crowd" (1965)   37
1. It's up to you (basic information, 10 minutes)
2. Watching what you eat (11 minutes)
3. Living with a diet (9 minutes)
4. Taking care of yourself (14 minutes)
5. Learning rules of health (9 minutes)
6. Joining the crowd (9 minutes)

Six filmstrips, tapes or record, $100: Creative Arts Studio, Inc., 814 H St. N.W., Washington, DC 20201

104. "Planning Diabetic Diets"   37
Content: food exchange lists, flexibility of meal planning; sample prescription, meals
Filmstrip, 16 minutes, guide, $47.50; slides, $85.00: National Medical Audiovisual Center (#10 above)

105. "Diabetes for Diabetics"   37
Content: the pancreas; identification insignia; measuring equipment; exchange lists; insulin; glucagon; urine testing
203 slides: Diabetes Press of America, Inc., 30 S.E. 8th St., Miami, FL 33131

Chapter
Correlation

106. "The Child with Diabetes" (1971)   37, 45
11 slides, 12 syllabi, $18.45: Nutrition Today, Educational Services (#51 above)

107. "Diet and Arthritis" (1967)   38
Content: susceptibility to faddism, basic food needs, equipment helpful to patient
Filmstrip, 26 frames, narrative guide, free loan:
Diabetes and Arthritis Control Program, Public Health Service, 4040 N. Fairfax Drive, Arlington, VA 22203

108. "Eat Heart-ily"   40
94 cartoon style slides regarding low-cholesterol, low-saturated fat, high-polyunsaturated fat diet, $30.00: Barbara Yee, Occupational Health Service, 222 N. Grand Ave., Los Angeles, CA 90012

109. "Planning Sodium Restricted Diets"   41
Content: basic information on sodium sources, food lists for planning diets; 500-mg diet and how to modify
Filmstrip, 19½ minutes, record, guide, $47.50; slides, $85.00: National Medical Audiovisual Center (#10 above)

110. "Inborn Errors of Metabolism" (1974)   46
17 slides, 12 syllabi, $23.25: Nutrition Today, Educational Services (#51 above)

111. "Phenylketonuria" (1964)   46
Content: biochemical, clinical, diagnostic, genetic, and diet aspects
Filmstrip, 116 frames, free loan: Audio Visual Division Mead Johnson and Company, 2404 Pennsylvania Ave., Evansville, IN 47721

112. "Treatment in Phenylketonuria" (1965)   46
Content: details of diet; role of physician, nurse, nutritionist
Filmstrip, 89 frames, free loan: Mead Johnson and Company (#111 above)

SOURCES OF NUTRITION EDUCATION MATERIALS

American Can Company. 730 Park Avenue, New York, NY 10017.
American Diabetes Association. 18 East 48th Street, New York, NY 10017.
American Dietetic Association. 430 North Michigan Avenue, Chicago, IL 60611.
American Heart Association. 44 East 23rd Street, New York, NY 10010.
American Home Economics Association. 1600 Twentieth Street, N.W., Washington, DC 20009.
American Institute of Baking. Consumer Service Department, 400 East Ontario Street, Chicago, IL 60611.
American Public Health Association. 1790 Broadway, New York, NY 10019.
American School Food Service Association. P.O. Box 10095, Denver, CO 80210.

The Borden Company. 350 Madison Avenue, New York, NY 10017.

Home Economics Department, The Campbell Soup Company. 385 Memorial Avenue, Camden, NJ 08101.

Cereal Institute, Inc., Educational Director. 135 South LaSalle Street, Chicago, IL 60603.

Chicago Dietetic Supply House, Inc. 1750 West Van Buren Street, Chicago, IL 60612.

Children's Bureau. Department of Health, Education, and Welfare. Washington, DC 20201.

Doyle Pharmaceutical Company, Minneapolis, MN 55416.

Evaporated Milk Association. 228 North LaSalle Street, Chicago, IL 60601.

Food and Drug Administration. Department of Health, Education, and Welfare, Washington, DC 20204.

Food and Nutrition Board, National Research Council. 2101 Constitution Avenue, Washington, DC 20418.

General Foods Corporation. 250 North Street, White Plains, NY 10602.

Public Relations Department. General Mills, Inc. 9200 Wayzata Boulevard, Minneapolis, MN 55426

Gerber Products. Department of Nutrition. Fremont, MI 49412.

John Hancock Life Insurance Company. 200 Berkeley Street, Boston, MA 02117.

Department of Home Economics Services. Kellogg Company. 215 Porter Street, Battle Creek, MI 49016.

Maternal and Child Health Service. Department of Health, Education, and Welfare, Rockville, MD 20852.

Mead Johnson and Company. 2404 Pennsylvania Avenue, Evansville, IN 47721.

Metropolitan Life Insurance Company. Health and Welfare Division. One Madison Avenue, New York, NY 10010.

National Dairy Council. 6300 N. River Rd., Rosemont, IL 60018.

National Live Stock and Meat Board, Home Economics Department. 36 South Wabash Avenue, Chicago, IL 60603.

The Nutrition Foundation, Inc. 99 Park Avenue, New York, NY 10016.

Poultry and Egg National Board. 250 West 57th Street, New York, NY 10019.

School Lunch Branch, Food Distribution Division, Agricultural Marketing Service, U.S. Department of Agriculture, Washington, DC 20250.

Sunkist Growers. Box 2706, Terminal Annex, Los Angeles, CA 90005.

Superintendent of Documents, U.S. Government Printing Office, Washington, DC 20402.

Office of Information, U.S. Department of Agriculture, Washington, DC 20250.

Common Abbreviations

AcCoA: acetyl coenzyme A
ACTH: adrenocorticotropic hormone
ADH: antidiuretic hormone
ADP: adenosine-5'-diphosphate
AMP: adenosine-5'-phosphate
ATP: adenosine-5'-triphosphate
ATPase: adenosine triphosphatase
BMR: basal metabolic rate
BUN: blood urea nitrogen
cal: calorie
cc: cubic centimeter
Co I: coenzyme I (NAD)
Co II: coenzyme II (NADP)
DNA: deoxyribonucleic acid
Dopa: dioxy-or dihydroxyphenylalanine
EAA: essential amino acid
EF: extrinsic factor
EFA: essential fatty acid
FAD: flavin adenine dinucleotide, oxidized form
FADH: flavin adenine dinucleotide, reduced form
FAO: Food and Agriculture Organization
FDA: Food and Drug Administration
FFA: free fatty acid
FMN: flavin mononucleotide
FSH: follicle-stimulating hormone
GFR: glomerular filtration rate
gm: gram(s)
GOT: glutamate oxalacetate transaminase
GTF: glucose tolerance factor
Hb: hemoglobin
HbO_2: oxyhemoglobin
HMP shunt: hexose monophosphate shunt
IF: intrinsic factor

INH: isonicotinic acid hydrazide
I.U.: international unit
J: joule
kcal: kilocalorie(s)
kg: kilogram
kJ: kilojoule
L: liter
lb: pound
LCT: long-chain triglyceride
LH: luteinizing hormone
mcg: microgram(s)
MCT: medium-chain triglyceride
mEq: milliequivalent(s)
mg: milligram(s)
ml: milliliter(s)
mm: millimeter(s)
mRNA: messenger ribonucleic acid
NAD: nicotinamide adenine dinucleotide
NADP: nicotinamide adenine dinucleotide phosphate
NEFA: nonesterified fatty acid
ng: nanogram(s)
NPN: nonprotein nitrogen
NRC: National Research Council
oz: ounce
PABA: para-amino benzoic acid
PBI: protein-bound iodine
PCBs: polychlorinated biphenyls
pg: picogram(s)
pH: hydrogen ion concentration
PKU: phenylketonuria
ppm: parts per million
PTH: parathyroid hormone
RDA: Recommended Dietary Allowances
RNA: ribonucleic acid
RNAse: ribonuclease
RQ: respiratory quotient
SH: sulfhydryl
TCA: tricarboxylic acid cycle
TPP: thiamin pyrophosphate
tRNA: transfer ribonucleic acid
TSH: thyroid-stimulating hormone
UNESCO: United Nations Educational, Scientific, and Cultural Organization
UNICEF: United Nations Children's Fund
USDA: United States Department of Agriculture
USP: United States Pharmacopeia
WHO: World Health Organization

Glossary

absorption (ab-sorp'shun): the transfer of nutrients across cell membranes; following digestion, nutrients are transferred from the intestinal lumen across the mucosa and into the blood and lymph circulation

acetoacetic acid (as'et-o-as-e'tik): a 4-carbon keto acid; one of the acetone bodies in diabetic urine

acetone (as'et-ōn): dimethyl ketone; accumulates in the blood and excretions when fats are incompletely oxidized as in diabetes mellitus; gives fruity odor to the breath

acetyl coenzyme A (as'et-il co-en'zīm): condensation product of acetic acid and coenzyme A; form by which 2-carbon fragment enters the tricarboxylic acid cycle

achlorhydria (a-klor-hi'drĭ-ah): absence of hydrochloric acid in gastric juice

acid: a substance that gives off or donates protons (H+ ions)

acidosis (as-ĭd-o'sis): condition caused by accumulation of an excess of acids (anions) in the body, or by excessive loss of base (mineral cations) from the body

acrolein (ak-ro'le-in): an irritating volatile decomposition product of glycerol that results from overheating fat

active transport: the movement of substances across cell membranes by pumping against a concentration gradient; requires source of energy

adenine (ad'en-in): one of the purines (bases) that are constituents of nucleic acid

adenosine triphosphate (ad-en'o-sin tri-fos'fāt): a compound consisting of 1 molecule each of adenine and ribose and 3 molecules of phosphoric acid; two of the phosphate groups are held by high-energy bonds; ATP

adipose (ad'ip-ōs): fat; fatty

aerobic (a-er-o'bik): growing in presence of air

agar (ah'gar): an indigestible polysaccharide prepared from moss and seaweed; has property of holding water and is often used to relieve constipation

alanine (al'an-in): a nonessential amino acid occurring widely in foods

albumin (al-bu'min): a protein in tissues and body fluids soluble in water and coagulated by heat; principal protein in blood regulating osmotic pressure; lactalbumin of milk

aldehyde (al'de-hīd): any of a large group of compounds containing the grouping -CHO

aldohexose (al-dō-hex'ōs): a 6-carbon sugar containing a -CHO grouping; glucose, galactose

aldosterone (al-dos'ter-ōn): a steroid hormone produced by the adrenal cortex; increases sodium retention and potassium loss

alkalosis (al-kah-lo'sis): increased alkali reserve (blood bicarbonate) of the blood and other body fluids; caused by excessive ingestion of sodium bicarbonate, persistent vomiting, or hyperventilation; pH of blood is usually increased

allergen (al'ler-jen): substance (usually protein) capable of producing altered response of cell, resulting in manifestation of allergy

amino acid (am'in-o as'id): an organic acid containing an amino (NH$_2$) group; the building blocks of protein molecules

amylase (am'ilās): salivary or pancreatic enzyme that hydrolyzes starch; ptyalin, amylopsin

amylopectin (am'il-o-pek'tin): polysaccharide found in starch consisting of branched chains of glucose

amylose (am'il-ōs): polysaccharide of starch consisting of unbranched chains of glucose

anabolism (an-ab'oh-lizm): processes for building complex substances from simple substances

anaerobic (an-aer-oh'bik): living in the absence of air

androgen (an'dro-jen): a substance such as testosterone that produces male sex characteristics

anemia (an-e'me-ah): deficiency in the circulating hemoglobin, red blood cells, or packed cell volume

anion (an'i-on): an ion that contains a negative charge of electricity and therefore goes to a positively charged anode

anorexia (an-o-rek'se-ah): loss of appetite

antagonist (an-tag'on-ist): a substance that opposes or neutralizes the action of another substance, e.g., a vitamin antagonist

anthropometry (an-thro-pom'et-re): branch of anthropology dealing with comparative measurements of the parts of the human body.

anti-: a prefix meaning against or opposing; e.g., antiscorbutic means preventing scurvy

antibiotic (an'ti-bi-ot'ik): a substance that inhibits the growth of bacteria

antibody (an'te-bod-e): a protein substance produced in an organism as a response to the presence of an antigen

antigen (an'ti-jen): any substance such as bacteria or foreign protein that, as a result of contact with tissues of the animal body, produces an immune response; an increased reaction such as hypersensitivity may result

antiketogenesis (an-ti-ke-tō-jen'es-is): the prevention of ketosis by stimulating the tricarboxylic acid cycle and thus bringing about oxidation of the ketone bodies

antioxidant (an-te-ok'sid-ant): a substance that prevents deterioration by hindering oxidation, e.g., tocopherols prevent oxidation and rancidity of fats

anuria (an-u're-ah): lack of urinary secretion

apathy (ap'ath-e): indifference; lack of interest or concern

apatite (ap'ah-tīt): complex calcium phosphate salt giving strength to bones

apoenzyme (ap-o-en'zīm): the protein part of an enzyme

arachidonic acid (ar-ak-id-on'ik): a 20-carbon fatty acid with four double bonds; the physiologically functioning essential fatty acid

arginase (ar'jin-ās): enzyme that splits arginine to urea and ornithine

arginine (ar'jin-in): a diamino acid; required for growth but not required by adults

arteriosclerosis (ar-te-re-o-skle-ro'sis): thickening and hardening of the inner walls of the arteries

ascites (a-si'tēz): accumulation of fluid in the abdominal cavity

ascorbic acid (a-skor'bik): water-soluble vitamin required for collagenous intercellular substance; prevents scurvy; also known as vitamin C

-ase: suffix that is used in naming an enzyme; for example, peptidase

aspartic acid (as-par'tik): a nonessential dibasic amino acid

asymptomatic (a-sim-tō-mat'ik): without symptoms

ataxia (a-tak'se-ah): loss of ability of muscular coordination

atherosclerosis (ath-er-o-skle-ro'sis): thickening of the walls of blood vessels by deposits of fatty materials, including cholesterol

atony (at'o-ne): lack of normal tone or strength

atrophy (at'ro-fe): a wasting away of cell, tissue, or organ

autosome (aw'tō-sōm): any chromosome other than a sex chromosome

avidin (av'id-in): protein substance in raw egg white which binds biotin and prevents its absorption from the digestive tract

azotemia (a-zo-te'me-ah): elevated levels of nitrogenous constituents in the blood; uremia

basal metabolism (ba'zal me-tab'o-lizm): energy expenditure of the body at rest in the postabsorptive state

base (bās): substance that combines with an acid to form a salt; any molecule or ion that will add on a hydrogen ion

benign (bi-nīn'): mild nature of an illness; with reference to a neoplasm, not malignant

beriberi (ber'ē-ber'ē): a deficiency disease caused by lack of thiamin and characterized by extreme weakness, polyneuritis, emaciation, edema, and cardiac failure

beta-hydroxybutyric acid (ba-tah-hi-drox'e-bu-tir'-ik): a 4-carbon intermediate in oxidation of fatty acids; one of the acetone bodies excreted in the urine in uncontrolled diabetes

bio- (bi-o-): prefix denoting life

bioassay (bi'-o-as-say): testing of activity or potency, as of a vitamin or hormone, on an animal or microorganism

biologic value: a measure of the effectiveness of a nutrient, such as protein, to the living organism

biopsy (bi'op-sē): examination of a piece of tissue removed from a living subject

biotin (bi'o-tin): a vitamin of the B complex; participates in fixation of carbon dioxide in fatty acid synthesis

Bitot's spots (be'tōz): gray, shiny spots on the conjunctiva resulting from malnutrition, especially vitamin A deficiency

botulism (bot'u-lizm): frequently fatal poisoning caused by toxin produced in inadequately sterilized canned food by the *Clostridium botulinum*

buffer (buf'er): a mixture of an acid and its conjugate base that is capable of neutralizing either an acid or a base without appreciably changing the original acidity or alkalinity, e.g., H_2CO_3/HCO_3-

calciferol (kal-sif'er-ol): vitamin D_2; fat-soluble vitamin of plant origin formed by irradiation of ergosterol; prevents rickets

calcification (kal-sif-ik-a'shun): hardening of tissue by a deposit of calcium and also magnesium salts

calcitonin (kal-sit-oh'-nin): hormone secreted by the thyroid gland; hypocalcemic effect; opposes action of parathormone

calculus (kal'ku-lus): an abnormal concretion occurring in any part of the body; usually consists of mineral salts around an organic nucleus

calorie (kal'o-rē): a unit of heat measurement; in nutrition, the kilocalorie is the amount of heat required to raise the temperature of 1 kg water 1° C

calorimetry (kal-or-im'et-rē): measurement of heat produced by the body, or from a food; *direct:* measure of heat produced by a subject in a closed chamber; *indirect:* measurement of heat by determining consumption of oxygen and sometimes carbon dioxide and calculating the amount of heat produced

carbonic acid (kar-bon'ik): the acid formed when carbon dioxide is dissolved in water; H_2CO_3

carboxylase (kar-bok'sil-ās): a thiamin-containing enzyme that catalyzes the removal of the carboxyl group of alpha keto acids, e.g., decarboxylation of pyruvic acid

carboxypeptidase (kar-box-e-pep'tid-ās): an intestinal enzyme which catalyzes the splitting of peptides

carotene (kar′o-tēn): precursor of vitamin A; yellow plant pigments occurring abundantly in dark-green leafy and deep-yellow vegetables

casein (ka′se-in): principal protein in milk; a phosphoprotein

catabolism (kat-ab′o-lizm): process for breaking down complex substances to simpler substances; usually yields energy

catalyst (kat′ah-list): a substance which in minute amounts initiates or modifies the speed of a chemical or physical change without itself being changed

cation (kat′i-on): an ion that carries a positive charge and migrates to the negatively charged pole

cellulose (sel′u-lōs): the structural fibers of plants; an indigestible polysaccharide

cephalin (sef′al-in): a phospholipid in brain and nervous tissue

ceruloplasmin (ser-ul′o-plaz-min): copper-containing protein in blood plasma

cheilosis (ki-lo′sis): lesions of the lips and the angles of the mouth; characteristic of riboflavin deficiency

chelation (ke-la′shun): formation of a bond between a metal ion and two or more polar groupings of a single molecule

cholecalciferol (ko-le-kal-sif′er-ol): vitamin D_3 formed from 7-dehydrocholesterol

cholecystitis (ko-le-sis-ti′tis): inflammation of the gallbladder

cholecystokinin (ko-le-sis-tō-kin′in): hormone produced in duodenum in presence of fat; stimulates contraction of gallbladder and release of bile

cholelithiasis (ko-le-lith-i′a-sis): gallstones in the gallbladder

cholesterol (ko-les′ter-ol): the commonest member of the sterol group; found in animal foods and made within the body; a constituent of gallstones and of atheroma

choline (ko′lēn): a nitrogenous base that donates methyl groups; a component of lecithin and acetylcholine; sometimes classed as a B complex vitamin

chondroitin sulfate (kon-droi′tin): a mucopolysaccharide widely distributed in skin and cartilage

chylomicrons (ki′lo-mi′krons): large molecules of fat occurring in lymph and plasma after a fat-rich meal; consist of triglycerides attached to a small amount of protein

chymotrypsin (ki-mo-trip′sin): enzyme produced in pancreas for the hydrolysis of protein

citric acid (sit′rik): an organic acid containing three carboxyl groups; one of compounds in the Krebs or citric acid cycle; a constituent of citrus fruits

citrovorum factor (sit-ro-vor′um): folinic acid, the active form of folic acid

citrulline (sit-rul′in): an amino acid formed from ornithine in the urea cycle

Clostridium (klos-trid′i-um): a genus of bacteria, chiefly anaerobic, found in soils and in the intestinal tract, e.g., *botulinum, perfringens*

coagulation (ko-ag-u-la′shun): process of changing into a clot, as in heating of an egg, curdling of milk

cobalamine (ko-bal′ah-min): compound containing cobalt grouping found in vitamin B_{12}

cocarboxylase (ko-kar-box′il-ās): thiamin-containing coenzyme of carboxylase

coenzyme (ko-en′zīm): the prosthetic group of an enzyme; a substance, for example, a vitamin, that conjugates with a protein molecule to form an active enzyme

coenzyme A: a complex nucleotide containing pantothenic acid; combines with acetyl groups to yield active acetate which can enter the Krebs cycle; involved in fatty acid oxidation and synthesis and cholesterol synthesis

coenzyme Q: involved in transfer of electrons in cytochrome chain

colitis (ko-li′tis): inflammation of the colon

collagen (kol′aj-in): widely distributed protein that makes up the matrix of bone, cartilage, and connective tissue

colloid (kol′oid): matter dispersed through another medium; particles are larger than crystalline molecules but not large enough to settle out; do not pass through an animal membrane

colostrum (ko-los′trum): milk secreted during the first few days after the birth of a baby

coma (ko′mah): state of unconsciousness

congenital (kon-jen′it-al): existing at or before birth with reference to certain physical or mental traits

coronary (kor′o-na-re): like a crown; related to blood vessels supplied to the heart muscle

cortex (kor′tex): outer layers of an organ, e.g., adrenal cortex

cortisone (kor′ti-sōn): hormone of the adrenal cortex; influences carbohydrate metabolism

creatine (kre′at-in): a nitrogenous constituent of muscle; phosphorylated form essential for muscle contraction

creatinine (kre-at′in-in): a nitrogen-containing substance derived from catabolism of creatine and present in the urine

crude fiber: plant fiber that remains after sample has been treated with sulfuric acid and sodium hydroxide; chiefly cellulose and lignin

cryptoxanthine (kript-o-zan′thin): a yellow pigment present in some foods; precursor of vitamin A

cystine (sis′tin): sulfur-containing nonessential amino acid

-cyte: suffix meaning cell; for example, adipocyte

cytochrome (si′tō-krom): a respiratory enzyme; consists of a number of hemochromogens; undergoes alternate reduction and oxidation

cytology (si-tol′oh-je): the anatomy, chemistry, physiology, and pathology of the cell

cytoplasm (si′to-plazm): substance within the cell exclusive of the nucleus

cytosine (si′tō-sin): one of the nitrogenous bases in nucleic acid

deamination, deaminization (de-am-in-a′shun): removal of the amino (NH_2) group from an amino acid

debility (de-bil′i-te): weakness

dehydrocholesterol, 7- (de-hi-dro-ko-les′ter-ol): cholesterol derivative in the skin that is converted to vitamin D

dehydrogenases (de-hi-dro′jen-ās-es): enzymes that catalyze oxidation by transferring hydrogen to a hydrogen acceptor

denaturation (de-na-tur-a′shun): to use chemical or physical means to alter the natural properties of a substance; e.g., heat coagulation of protein

deoxypyridoxine (de-ok′se-pir-id-oks′in): a compound similar in structure to pyridoxine that is antagonistic to the action of pyridoxine

deoxyribonucleic acid (DNA) (de-ok′se-ri-bo-nu-kla′ik): giant molecule in cell nucleus which determines hereditary traits; consists of four bases attached to ribose and phosphate

dermatitis (der-mat-i′tis): inflammation of the surface of the skin

dextrin (dex′trin): intermediate product in breakdown of starches; a polysaccharide

dicoumarin (di-koo′mah-rin): antiprothrombin; anticlotting factor first isolated from sweet clover

diffuse (dif-ūs′); not localized

digestion (di-jes′chun): the hydrolysis of foods in the digestive tract to simpler substances so they can be used by the body

diglyceride (di-glis′er-id): a fat containing 2 fatty acid molecules

disaccharidase (di-sak′ar-id-ās): enzyme which hydrolyzes disaccharides

disaccharide (di-sak′ar-id): a carbohydrate that yields two simple sugars upon hydrolysis; sucrose, maltose, lactose

distal (dis′tal): part of structure farthest from the point of attachment

diuresis (di-u-re′sis): increased secretion of urine

duodenum (du-o-de′num): first portion of the small intestine, extending from the pylorus to the jejunum

dys-: prefix meaning bad

dysgeusia (dis-goo′-se-ah): perverted sense of taste; "bad" taste

dysosmia (dis-ahs′-me-ah): impaired sense of smell; obnoxious odor

dyspepsia (dis-pep′se-ah): indigestion or upset stomach

dysphagia (dis-fa′je-ah): difficulty in swallowing

dyspnea (disp′ne-ah): difficulty or distress in breathing

eclampsia (ĕ-klamp′se-ah): convulsions occurring during pregnancy and associated with edema, hypertension, and proteinuria

edema (ĕ-de′mah): presence of abnormal amounts of fluid in intercellular spaces

elastin (ē-las′tin): insoluble yellow elastic protein in connective tissue

electrolyte (el-ek′tro-līt): any substance which dissociates into ions when dissolved and thus conducts an electric current

emaciation (e-ma-se-a′shun): wasting of the body; excessive leanness

-emia: suffix that denotes a condition of the blood; for example, hypoglycemia

emulsion (e-mul′shun): a system of two immiscible liquids in which one is finely divided and held in suspension by another

endemic (en-dem′ik): prevalence of a disease in a given region

endo-: prefix meaning inner or within

endocrine (en′do-krin): pertaining to glands that secrete substances into the blood for control of metabolic processes

endogenous (en-doj′en-us): originating in the cells or tissues of the body

endoplasmic reticulum (en′do-plaz-mik ret-ic′u-lum): the system of membranes within the cell that permits communication between cellular, nuclear, and extracellular environment

endosperm (en′do-sperm): reserve food material of the plant; the starchy center of the cereal grain

enter-: combining term denoting intestine

enteritis (en-ter-i′tis): inflammation of the intestine

enterocrinin (en-ter-o-krī′nin): hormone of small intestine that stimulates secretion of intestinal juice

enterogastrone (en-ter-o-gas′trōn): hormone secreted by duodenal mucosa upon stimulation by fat; inhibits secretion of gastric juice and reduces motility

enterokinase (en-ter-o-kīn′ās): enzyme of intestinal juice that converts trypsinogen to trypsin

enteropathy (en-ter-op′ath-e): any disease of the intestine

enzyme (en′zīm): an organic compound of protein nature produced by living tissue to accelerate metabolic reactions; hydrolases, oxidases, transferases, dehydrogenases, peptidases, and others

epinephrine (ep-in-ef′rin): secretion of the medulla of the adrenal gland that stimulates energy metabolism; adrenaline

epithelium (ep-ith-e′le-um): the covering layer of the skin and mucous membranes

ergosterol (er-gos′ter-ol): a sterol found chiefly in plants; when exposed to ultraviolet light becomes vitamin D

erythrocyte (er-ith′ro-sīt): mature red blood cell

erythropoieses (er-ith-ro-po-e′sis): formation of red blood cells

essential amino acid: an amino acid that must be supplied in the diet to provide the body's need for it

essential fatty acid: a fatty acid that must be present in the diet and that prevents certain deficiencies of the skin and blood capillaries; linoleic acid, arachidonic acid

estrogen (es'tro-jen): hormone secreted by the ovary

etiology (e-te-ol'o-je): cause of a disease

exacerbation (ex-as-er-ba'shun): increase in severity of symptoms

exogenous (ex-oj'en-us): originating or produced from the outside

extracellular (extra-sel'u-lar): situated or occurring outside the cells

extrinsic factor (ex-trin'sik): vitamin B_{12}; term used by Castle prior to identification of the nature of the compound

exudate (ex'u-dāt): a fluid discharged into the tissues or any cavity

familial (fam-il'e-al): common to a family

fatty acids (fat'e): open-chain monocarboxylic acids containing only carbon, hydrogen, and oxygen

favism (fa'vism): condition caused by eating certain species of beans, e.g., *Vicia faba*; symptoms include fever, abdominal pain, headache, anemia, coma

febrile (feb'ril): feverish; having a fever

ferritin (fer'it-in): an iron-protein complex containing up to 23 per cent iron and formed by combining iron with apoferritin

fetor hepaticus (fe'tor hep-at'ik-us): offensive odor to the breath present in persons with severe liver disease

fibrosis (fi-bro'sis): formation of fibrous tissue in repair processes

fistula (fis'tu-lah): a tubelike ulcer leading from an abscess cavity or organ to the surface, or from one abscess cavity to another

flatulence (flat'u-lens): distention of stomach or intestines with gases

flavin adenine dinucleotide, FAD (fla'vin ad'en-in di-nu'kle-o-tīd): a coenzyme consisting of riboflavin and adenosine diphosphate required for the action of various dehydrogenases

flavin mononucleotide, FMN (fla'vin mon-o-nu'kle-o-tīd): a riboflavin-containing coenzyme involved in the action of dehydrogenases

flavoprotein (fla-vo-pro'te-in): a conjugated protein that contains a flavin and is involved in tissue respiration

fluoridation (floo-or-id-a'shun): the use of fluorine, as in water, to reduce the incidence of tooth decay

folacin (fo'lah-sin): folic acid, a vitamin of the B complex

folic acid (fo'lik): a vitamin of the B complex necessary for the maturation of red blood cells and synthesis of nucleoproteins; also known as folacin and pteroylglutamic acid

folinic acid (fo-lin'ik): the active form of folacin; citrovorum factor

follicle (fol'ikl): small excretory sac or gland, e.g., hair follicle, ovarian follicle

fortification (for-ti-fik-a'shun): the addition of one or more nutrients to a food to make it richer than the unprocessed food, e.g., vitamin D milk

fructose (fruk'tōs): a 6-carbon sugar found in fruits and honey; also obtained from the hydrolysis of sucrose; fruit sugar, levulose

galactose (gal-ak'tōs): a single sugar resulting from the hydrolysis of lactose

galactosemia (gal-ak'tō-se'me-ah): accumulation of galactose in the blood owing to a hereditary lack of an enzyme to convert galactose to glucose; accompanied by severe mental retardation

gastrectomy (gas-trek'tō-me): surgical removal of part or all of the stomach

gastrin (gas'trin): hormone secreted by pyloric mucosa that stimulates secretion of hydrochloric acid by parietal cells

genetic (jen-et'ik): congenital or inherited

-genic: suffix meaning to produce or give rise to; for example, ketogenic

gingivitis (jin-jī-vi'tis): inflammation of the gums

gliadin (gli'ad-in): a protein fraction of wheat gluten

globulin (glob'u-lin): a class of proteins insoluble in water and alcohol; serum globulin, lactoglobulin, myosin

glomerulus (glom-er'u-lus): the tuft of capillaries at the beginning of each tubule in the kidney

glossitis (glos-i'tis): inflammation of the tongue

glucagon (gloo'kag-on): hormone produced by the alpha cells of the islands of Langerhans; raises blood sugar by increasing glycogen breakdown

glucocorticoid (glu'ko-kor-tī-koid): hormone produced by the adrenal cortex that influences glucose metabolism

glucogenic (glu-ko-jen'ik): glucose forming

gluconeogenesis (glu'ko-ne-o-jen'e-sis): formation of glucose from noncarbohydrate sources, namely certain amino acids and the glycerol fraction of fats

glucose (glu'kōs): a single sugar occurring in fruits and honey; also obtained by the hydrolysis of starch, sucrose, maltose, and lactose; the sugar found in the blood; dextrose, grape sugar

glutamic acid (glu-tam'ik): a dibasic nonessential amino acid widely distributed in proteins

glutathione (glu-ta-thi'ōn): a tripeptide of glycine, glutamic acid, and cystine; can act as hydrogen acceptor and hydrogen donor

gluten (glu'ten): protein in wheat and other cereals that gives elastic quality to a dough

glyceride (glis'er-id): organic ester of glycerol; fats are esters of fatty acids and glycerol

glycerol (glis'er-ol): a 3-carbon alcohol derived from the hydrolysis of fats

glycine (gli′sin): aminoacetic acid; a nonessential amino acid

glycogen (gli′ko-jen): polysaccharide produced from glucose by the liver or the muscle; "animal" starch

glycogenesis (gli′ko-jen′ĭ-sis): formation of glycogen from glucose by the liver or muscle

glycogenolysis (gli-ko-jen-ol′ĭ-sis): enzymatic breakdown of glycogen to glucose

glycolysis (gli-kol′ĭ-sis): the anaerobic conversion of glucose to lactose, an energy-yielding process

glycosuria (gli-ko-su′re-ah): presence of sugar in the urine

goiter (goi′ter): enlargement of the thyroid gland

goitrogen (goi′tro-jen): a substance that leads to goiter

guanine (gwan′in): one of the nitrogenous bases in nucleic acids

hem-, hema-, hemo-: prefixes referring to blood

hematocrit (he-mat′o-krit): separation of red cells from the plasma

hematuria (he-mat-u′re-ah): condition in which urine contains blood

heme (hēm): deep red pigment consisting of ferrous iron linked to protoporphyrin

hemicellulose (hem-i-sel′u-lōs): a class of indigestible polysaccharides that form the cell wall of plants

hemochromatosis (hem-o-kro-ma-to′sis): a condition in which excessive iron absorption leads to skin pigmentation and deposits of hemosiderin in the liver and other organs

hemoglobin (he-mo-glo′bin): the iron-protein pigment in the red blood cells; carries oxygen to the tissues

hemolytic (he-mo-lit′ik): causing separation of hemoglobin from the red blood cells

hemopoietic, hematopoietic (he-mo-poi-et′ik): concerned with the formation of blood

hemorrhage (hem′or-ej): loss of blood from the vessels; bleeding

hemosiderin (he′mo-sid′er-in): iron-containing pigment in liver and other organs in disorders of iron metabolism, including excessive iron absorption or excessive blood destruction

heparin (hep′ar-in): a mucopolysaccharide that prevents clotting of blood

hepatic (hep-at′ik): pertaining to the liver

hepatomegaly (hep-at-o-meg′ah-le): enlargement of the liver

heterozygous (het-er-o-zi′gus): possessing dissimilar pairs of genes for any hereditary trait

hexose (heks′ōs): a 6-carbon sugar; glucose, fructose, galactose

histidine (his′tid-in): an essential amino acid

homeostasis (ho-me-o-sta′sis): tendency to maintain equilibrium in normal body states

homogenize (ho-moj′en-īz): to make of uniform quality throughout

homozygous (ho-mo-zi′gus): having identical pairs of genes for any given pair of hereditary traits

hormone (hor′mōn): substance produced by an organ to produce a specific effect in another organ

hydrogenation (hi′dro-jen-a′shun): the addition of hydrogen to a compound, such as an unsaturated fatty acid to produce a solid fat

hydrolysate (hi-drol′is-āt): the product of hydrolysis; e.g., protein hydrolysate is a mixture of the constituent amino acids when the protein molecule is split by acids, alkalies, or enzymes

hydrolysis (hi-drol′is-is): the splitting up of a product by the addition of water

hydroxyproline (hi′drok-se-pro′lin): a nonessential amino acid occurring abundantly in collagen

hyper-: a prefix meaning above, beyond, or excessive

hypercalcemia (hi-per-kal-se′me-ah): abnormally high calcium level in the blood

hypercalciuria (hi-per-kal-se-u′re-ah): abnormal calcium excretion in the urine

hyperchlorhydria (hi-per-klor-hi′dre-ah): increased hydrochloric acid secretion by stomach cells

hyperchromic (hi-per-krōm′ik): abnormally high color

hyperemia (hi-per-e′me-ah): excess of blood in any part of the body

hyperesthesia (hi-per-es-the′zĭ-ah): increased sensitivity to touch or pain

hyperglycemia (hi-per-glī-se′me-ah): an excess of sugar in the blood

hyperkalemia (hi-per-kah-le′me-ah): an increased level of potassium in the blood

hyperlipoproteinemia: increased concentration of lipoproteins in the blood

hyperplasia (hi-per-pla′se-ah): abnormal multiplication of normal cells

hypertriglyceridemia: increased levels of triglycerides in the blood

hypertrophic (hi-per-tro′fik): pertaining to enlargement of an organ due to increase in size of its constituent cells

hyperuricemia (hi-per-u-ris-e′me-ah): excess of uric acid in the blood; one of the characteristics of gout

hypervitaminosis (hi-per-vi-tah-min-o′sis): condition produced by excessive ingestion of vitamins, especially vitamins A and D

hypo-: prefix meaning lack or deficiency

hypoalbuminemia (hi-po-al-bu-min-e′me-ah): low albumin level of the blood

hypochlorhydria (hi-po-klor-hid′re-ah): decreased secretion of hydrochloric acid by the cells of the stomach

hypochromic (hi-po-krom′ik): below normal color; e.g., pale red blood cells lacking hemoglobin

hypogeusia: diminished sense of taste

hypoglycemia (hi-po-gli-se′me-ah): a lower than normal level of glucose in the blood

hypokalemia (hi-po-kal-e′me-ah): decreased potassium level in the blood

hyposmia: diminished sense of smell

hypothalamus (hi-po-thal′am-us): a group of nuclei at the base of the brain; includes centers of appetite control, cells that produce antidiuretic hormone

idiopathic (id-e-o-path′ik): pertaining to a disease of unknown origin

idiosyncrasy (id-e-o-sin′kra-se): a susceptibility to action of food or drugs that is characteristic or peculiar to an individual person

ileum (il′e-um): lower portion of the small intestine extending from the jejunum to the cecum

ileus (il′e-us): obstruction of the bowel

infarction (in-fark′shun): the formation of an area of dead tissue resulting from obstruction of blood vessels supplying the part

ingest (in-jest′): to take food into the body

inositol (in-os′it-ol): a 6-carbon alcohol found especially in cereal grains; combines with phosphate to form phytic acid

insidious (in-sid′e-us): pertaining to the progress of a disease with few if any symptoms to indicate its seriousness

insulin (in′su-lin): hormone secreted by beta cells of the islands of Langerhans of the pancreas; promotes utilization of glucose and lowers blood sugar

interstitial (in-ter-stish′al): situated in spaces between tissues

intra-: prefix meaning within

intracellular (in-trah-sel′u-lar): within the cell

intravenous (in-trah-ve′nus): into or from within a vein

intrinsic factor (in-trin′sik): mucoprotein in gastric juice which facilitates absorption of vitamin B_{12}; deficient in patients with pernicious anemia

iodopsin (i-o-dop′sin): pigment found in cones of the retina; visual violet

ion (i′on): an atom or group of atoms carrying a charge of electricity; e.g., cations, anions

ionize (i′on-īz): to separate molecules into electrically charged atoms or group of atoms; the number of negative charges exactly equals the number of positive charges

ischemia (is-ke′me-ah): a local deficiency of blood, chiefly from narrowing of the arteries

isocaloric (i-sō-kal-or′ik): containing an equal number of calories

isoleucine (i-sō-lu′sin): an essential amino acid

isotopes (i′so-tōps): atoms of the same element having the same atomic numbers and chemical properties but differing in the nuclear masses

-itis: suffix denoting inflammation; for example, colitis

jaundice (jon′dis): condition characterized by elevated bilirubin level of the blood and deposit of bile pigments in skin and mucous membranes

jejunum (je-joo′num): middle portion of small intestine; extends from duodenum to ileum

joule (jool): the unit of energy in the metric system; 1 calorie equals 4.184 joules (J)

keratin (ker′at-in): an insoluble sulfur-containing protein found in the skin, nails, hair

keratomalacia (ker′at-o-mal-a′shah): dryness and ulceration of the cornea resulting from vitamin A deficiency

keto-: a prefix denoting the presence of the carbonyl (CO) group

ketogenesis (ke-to-jen′es-is): formation of ketones from fatty acids and some amino acids

α-ketoglutaric acid (ke-tō-gloo-tar′ik): one of the intermediates in the tricarboxylic acid cycle; also the product of oxidative deamination of glutamic acid

ketone (ke′tōn): any compound containing a ketone (CO) grouping; ketone bodies include acetone, beta-hydroxybutyric acid, and acetoacetic acid

ketosis (ke-tō′sis): condition resulting from incomplete oxidation of fatty acids, and the consequent accumulation of ketone bodies

kilocalorie (kil′o-ka′lo-re): the unit of heat used in nutrition; the amount of heat required to raise 1000 gm water 1° C (from 15.5 to 16.5° C); also known as the large calorie

kwashiorkor (kwash-e-or′kor): deficiency disease related principally to protein lack and seen in severely malnourished children; characterized by growth failure, edema, pigment changes in the skin

labile (la′bil): chemically unstable

lactalbumin (lak-tal-bu′min): a protein in milk

lactic acid (lak′tik): 3-carbon acid produced in milk by bacterial fermentation of lactose; also produced during muscle contraction by anaerobic glycolysis

lactose (lak′tōs): a disaccharide composed of glucose and galactose; the form of carbohydrate in milk

lamina propria (lam′in-ah pro′pre-ah): connective-tissue structure that supports the epithelial cells of the intestinal mucosa

lecithin (les′ith-in): a phospholipid occurring in nervous and organ tissues, and in egg yolk; effective emulsifier

leucine (lu′sin): an essential amino acid

linoleic acid (lin-o-le′ic): an 18-carbon fatty acid with two double bonds; essential for growth and skin health

linolenic acid (lin-o-len′ik): an 18-carbon fatty acid with three double bonds; not an essential fatty acid

lipase (lip′ās): an enzyme that hydrolyzes fat

lipid (lip′id): a term for fats including neutral fats, oils, fatty acids, phospholipids, cholesterol

lipogenesis (lip-o-jen′es-is): formation of fat

lipoic acid (lip-o′ik): thioctic acid; protogen; a factor that functions with thiamin pyrophosphate in removing the carboxyl group from alpha keto acids such as pyruvic acid

lipolysis (lip-ol′is-is): the splitting up of fat

lipoprotein (li-po-pro′te-in): a conjugated protein that incorporates lipids to facilitate transportation of the lipids in an aqueous medium

lipotropic (lip-o-trop′ik): pertaining to substances that prevent accumulation of fat in the liver

lithiasis (li-thi′a-sis): the formation of calculi of any kind

lysine (li′sēn): a diamino essential amino acid

lysosomes (li′so-sōms): structures of cell cytoplasm that contain digestive enzymes

macrocyte (mak′ro-sīt): an abnormally large red blood cell

malaise (mal-āz′): discomfort, distress, or uneasiness

malignant (mal-ig′nant): occurring in severe form, frequently fatal; in tumors refers to uncontrollable growth as in cancer

maltose (mawl′tōs): a disaccharide resulting from starch hydrolysis; yields 2 molecules glucose on further hydrolysis

marasmus (mar-az′mus): extreme protein-calorie malnutrition marked by emaciation, especially severe in young children who receive insufficient amounts of food

matrix (ma′trix): the groundwork in which something is cast; for example, protein is the bone matrix into which mineral salts are deposited

megaloblast (meg′al-o-blast): primitive red blood cell of large size with large nucleus; present in blood when there is deficiency of vitamin B_{12} and/or folic acid

menadione (men-a-di′on): synthetic compound with vitamin K activity

metabolic pool (met-ah-bol′ik): the assortment of nutrients available at any given moment of time for the metabolic activities of the body, e.g., amino acid pool, calcium pool

metabolism (me-tab′o-lism): physical and chemical changes occurring within the organism; includes synthesis of biologic materials and breakdown of substances to yield energy

metabolite: any substance that results from physical and chemical changes within the organism

methionine (meth-i′o-nin): an essential sulfur-containing amino acid; supplies labile methyl groups

micelle (mis-el′): a microscopic particle of lipids and bile salts

microcyte (mi′kro-sīt): small red blood cell

microvilli (mi′kro-vil′li): minute structures visible by electron microscope, present on surface of mucosal epithelium; the "brush border"

milliequivalent, mEq (mil′li-e-kwiv′ah-lent): concentration of a substance per liter of solution; obtained by dividing the milligrams per liter by the equivalent weight

mitochondria (mit-o-kon′dre-ah): rod-shaped or round structures in cell that trap energy-rich ATP

monoglyceride (mono-glis′er-id): an ester of glycerol with one fatty acid

monosaccharide (mon-o-sak′ar-id): a single sugar not affected by hydrolysis; includes glucose, fructose, galactose

monounsaturated (mon-o-un-sat′u-ra-ted): having a single double bond as in a fatty acid, e.g., oleic acid

morbidity (mor-bid′it-e): the proportion of disease to health in a community

motility (mo-til′it-e): ability to move spontaneously

mucin (mu′sin): a substance containing mucopolysaccharides secreted by goblet cells of the intestine and other glandular cells; has a protective and lubricating action

mucopolysaccharide (mu′ko-pol-e-sak′er-id): any of a group of polysaccharides combined with other groups such as protein

mucoprotein (mu′ko-pro′te-in): a conjugated protein containing a carbohydrate group such as chondroitin sulfuric acid

mucosa (mu-ko′sah): membrane lining the gastrointestinal, respiratory, and genitourinary tracts

myo-: prefix meaning muscle

myocardium (mi-o-kar′de-um): the heart muscle

myoglobin (mi-o-glo′bin): an iron-protein complex in muscle that transports oxygen; somewhat similar to hemoglobin

myosin (mi′o-sin): a soluble protein in muscle; combines with actin to form actomyosin, an enzyme that catalyzes the dephosphorylation of ATP during muscle contraction

nausea (naw′se-ah): sickness at the stomach; inclination to vomit

necrosis (ne-kro′sis): death of a cell or cells or of a portion of tissue

neonatal (ne-o-na′tal): pertaining to the newborn

neoplasm (ne′o-plazm): new or abnormal, uncontrolled growth, such as a tumor

nephron (nef′ron): the functional unit of the kidney consisting of a tuft of capillaries known as the glomerulus attached to the renal tubule

neuritic (nu-rit′ik): pertaining to inflammation of a nerve

neuropathy (nu-rop′ath-e): disease of the nervous system

niacin (ni′ah-sin): one of the water-soluble B complex vitamins which functions as a coenzyme in cell respiration; antipellagra factor

niacin equivalent: the total niacin available from the diet including preformed niacin plus that derived from the metabolism of tryptophan; 60 mg tryptophan = 1 mg niacin

niacinamide (ni′ah-sin-am′id): biologically active form of niacin occurring in the tissues

nicotinamide adenine dinucleotide, NAD (nik′o-tin-am′id

ad'en-in di-nu'kle-o-tid): coenzyme for a number of enzymes, chiefly dehydrogenases

nicotinic acid (nik-o-tin'ik): niacin

nocturia (nok-tu're-ah): excessive urination at night

nucleic acid (nu-kle'ik): complex organic acid containing four bases—adenine, guanine, cytosine, and thymine—attached to ribose and phosphate

nucleoprotein (nu-kle-o-pro'te-in): conjugated protein found in the nuclei of cells; yields a protein fraction and nucleic acid

nucleotide (nu'kle-o-tid): a hydrolytic product of nucleic acid; contains one purine or pyrimidine base and a sugar phosphate

nutrient (nu'tre-ent): chemical substance in foods which nourishes, e.g., amino acid, fat, calcium

nyctalopia (nik-tal-o'pe-ah): night blindness

nystagmus (nis-tag'mus): rhythmic rapid movement of the eyeball

oleic acid (o-le'ik): an 18-carbon fatty acid containing one double bond; widely distributed in foods

oliguria (ol-ig-u're-ah): scanty secretion of urine

-ology: suffix meaning science of, study of

ophthalmia (of-thal'me-ah): severe inflammation of the eye

organelles (or-gan-elz'): the various structures of the cell such as lysosomes, mitochondria

ornithine (or'nith-in): an amino acid formed from arginine when urea is split off

osmosis (oz-mo'sis): passage of a solvent from the lesser to the greater concentration when two solutions are separated by a membrane

ossification (os-if-ik-a'shun): formation of bone

osteo-: prefix meaning bone

osteomalacia (os-te-o-mal-a'se-ah): softening of the bone, chiefly in adults

osteoporosis (os-te-o-po-ro'sis): reduction of the quantity of bone, occurring principally in women after middle age; the remaining bone is normally mineralized

oxalic acid (oks-al'ik): a dicarboxylic acid present in foods such as spinach, chard, rhubarb; forms insoluble salts with calcium

oxaloacetic acid (oks-al-o-as-e'tik): a 3-carbon ketodicarboxylic acid; an intermediate in the tricarboxylic acid cycle

oxidation (oks-id-a'shun): increase in positive charges on an atom or loss of negative charges

palmitic acid (pal-mit'ik): a 16-carbon saturated fatty acid widespread in foods

pancreozymin (pan'kre-o-zi'min): hormone produced in duodenal mucosa that stimulates secretion of pancreatic enzymes

pantothenic acid (pan-to-then'ik): one of the B complex vitamins; a constituent of coenzyme A

parathormone: secretion of parathyroid gland that regulates calcium and phosphorus metabolism

parenchyma (par-en'ki-mah): functional tissue of an organ or gland as distinct from its supporting framework

parenteral (par-en'ter-al): by other means than through the gastrointestinal tract; introduction of nutrients by vein or into subcutaneous tissues

paresthesia (par-es-the'zi-ah): abnormal sensation such as numbness, burning, pricking

parturition (par-tu-rish'un): giving birth to a child

path-, patho-, -pathy: combining forms meaning disease, e.g., *patho*genic, nephro*pathy*

pathology (path-ol'o-je): science dealing with disease; structural and functional changes caused by disease

pectin (pek'tin): a polysaccharide found in many fruits and having gelling properties

pellagra (pel-lah'gra): a deficiency disease of the skin, gastrointestinal tract, and nervous system caused by lack of niacin and associated with other nutritional deficiencies

pentose (pen'tōs): a simple sugar containing 5 carbon atoms; ribose, arabinose, xylose

peptide linkage (pep'tid): the CO-NH linkage of two amino acids by condensation of the amino group of one amino acid with the carboxyl group of another amino acid

peptone (pep'tone): an intermediate product of protein digestion

perinatal (per-ī-na'tal): pertaining to before, during, or after the time of birth

peristalsis (per-is-tal'sis): the rhythmic, wavelike movement produced by muscles of the small intestine to move food forward

phagocyte (fag'o-sīt): a cell capable of ingesting bacteria or other foreign material

phenylalanine (fen-il-al'ah-nin): an essential amino acid; consists of a phenyl group attached to alanine

phenylketonuria (fe-nil-ke-to-nu're-ah): excretion of phenylpyruvic acid and other phenyl compounds in urine because of congenital lack of an enzyme required for conversion of phenylalanine to tyrosine; characterized by mental retardation

phospholipid (fos'fo-lip'id): a fatlike compound that contains a phosphate and another group such as a nitrogen base in addition to glycerol and fatty acids, e.g., lecithin, cephalin

phosphoprotein (fos-fo-pro'te-in): a conjugated protein that contains phosphorus, e.g., nucleoprotein, casein

phosphorylate (fos-fo'ril-ate): to introduce a phosphate grouping into an organic compound, e.g., glucose monophosphate produced by action of enzyme *phosphorylase*

photosynthesis (fo-to-sin'the-sis): the process whereby the chlorophyll in green plants utilizes the energy from the sun to synthesize carbohydrate from carbon dioxide and water

phylloquinone (fil'o-kwin-ōn): vitamin K

phytic acid (fi'tik): a phosphoric acid ester of inositol found in seeds; interferes with absorption of calcium, magnesium, iron, zinc

pica (pi'kah): a hunger for substances not fit for food

pinocytosis (pin-o-si-to'sis): the taking up of droplets (for example, fat) by a cell by surrounding the liquid with part of the membrane

plaque (plak): any patch or flat area; atherosclerotic plaque in a deposit of lipid material in the blood vessel

plasma (plaz'mah): fluid portion of the blood before clotting has taken place

poly-: prefix meaning much or many

polyneuritis (pol-e-nu-ri'tis): inflammation of a number of nerves

polypeptide (pol-e-pep'tid): a compound consisting of more than three amino acids; an intermediate stage in protein digestion

polyphagia (pol-e-fa'je-ah): excessive eating

polysaccharide (pol-e-sak'ar-id): a class of carbohydrates containing many single sugars; includes starch, glycogen, dextrins, pectins, cellulose, and others

polyunsaturated fatty acid: fatty acids containing two or more double bonds; linoleic, linolenic, and arachidonic acids

porphyrin (por'fir-in): a pigmented compound containing four pyrrole nuclei joined in a ring structure; combines with iron in hemoglobin

precursor: anything that precedes another or from which another is derived; for example, carotene is a precursor to vitamin A

prenatal (prē-na'tal): preceding birth

proenzyme (pro-en'zīm): inactive form of an enzyme, e.g., pepsinogen

progesterone (prō-jes'ter-ōn): hormone of corpus luteum which prepares endometrium for reception and development of the fertilized ovum

prognosis (prog-no'sis): forecast of probable result from attack of disease

proline (pro'lēn): a nonessential amino acid

prophylaxis (pro-fil-ak'sis): prevention of disease

prosthetic group (pros-thet'ik): chemical group attached to a molecule such as protein; nonprotein part of an enzyme

protease (pro'te-ās): an enzyme that digests protein

proteinuria (pro'te-in-u'ri-ah): excretion of protein in the urine

proteolytic (pro'te-o-lit'ik): effecting the hydrolysis of protein

proteose (pro'te-ōs): a derivative of protein formed during digestion

prothrombin (pro-throm'bin): factor in blood plasma for blood clotting; precursor of thrombin

protoplasm (pro'to-plazm): form of living matter in all cells

protoporphyrin (pro'tō-por'fir-in): a porphyrin combined with iron and globin forming hemoglobin

provitamin (pro-vi'tah-min): precursor of a vitamin

proximal (prok'sim-al): nearest to the head or point of attachment

pteroylglutamic acid (ter'o-il-glu-tam'ik): folic acid

puerperium (pur-pe'ri-um): the period after labor until involution of the uterus

purine (pu'rin): organic compounds containing heterocyclic nitrogen structures that are catabolized to uric acid; supplied especially by flesh foods and synthesized in the body

pyridoxal phosphate (pir-ī-dok'sal fos'fate): a coenzyme that contains vitamin B_6

pyridoxine (pi-ri-dox'in): one of the forms of vitamin B_6

pyruvic acid (pi-ru'vik): a 3-carbon keto acid; an intermediate in glucose metabolism

rancid (ran'sid): term that describes rank taste or smell that results from decomposition of fatty acids

regurgitation (re-gur-jit-a'shun): the backward flow of food; casting up of undigested food

relapsing (re-laps'ing): return of symptoms

remission (re-mish'un): a lessening of the severity or temporary abatement of symptoms

renal (re'nal): pertaining to the kidney

renal threshold: the level of concentration of a substance in the blood beyond which it is excreted in the urine

renin: enzyme produced by the kidney; pressor substance

rennin (ren'in): enzyme in gastric juice that coagulates milk protein

repletion (rep-le'shun): to fill up; to restore

resection (re-sek'shun): removal of part of an organ

residue (rez'i-du): remainder; the contents remaining in the intestinal tract after digestion of food; includes fiber and other unabsorbed products

resorption (re-sorp'shun): a loss of substance, e.g., loss of mineral salts from bone

reticulocyte (re-tik'u-lo-sīt): a young red blood cell occurring during active blood regeneration

reticuloendothelium (re-tik'u-lo-en-dō-the'le-um): a system of macrophages concerned with phagocytosis; present in spleen, liver, bone marrow, connective tissues, and lymph nodes

retinene (ret'in-ēn): vitamin A aldehyde; intermediate step in bleaching of visual purple

retinol (ret'in-ol): vitamin A alcohol

retinopathy (ret-in-op'ath-e): degenerative disease of the retina

rhodopsin (ro-dop'sin): visual purple; pigment of the rods of the retina bleached by light; vitamin A required for regeneration

riboflavin (ri'bo-fla'vin): heat-stable B complex vitamin and a constituent of flavin enzymes; vitamin B_{12}

ribonucleic acid, RNA (ri-bo-nu-kle'ik): molecules in cytoplasm which serve for transfer of amino acid code from nucleus and the synthesis of protein

ribose (ri′bōs): 5-carbon sugar; a constituent of nucleic acid

ribosomes (ri′bo-sōms): dense particles in cell cytoplasm that are the site of protein synthesis

rickets (rik′ets): a deficiency disease of the skeletal system caused by a lack of vitamin D or calcium or both, and often resulting in bone deformities

saccharin (sak′ah-rin): a sweetening agent that is 300 to 500 times as sweet as sugar; yields no calories

Salmonella (sal-mo-nel′ah): group of bacteria causing intestinal infection; frequently contaminates foods

saponification (sap-on′if-ik-a′shun): the action of alkali on a fat to form a soap

satiety (sat-i′et-e): feeling of satisfaction following meals

saturated (sat′u-ra-ted): a state in which a substance holds the most of another substance that it can

scurvy (skur′vē): a deficiency disease caused by lack of ascorbic acid and leading to swollen bleeding gums, hemorrhages of the skin and mucous membranes, and anemia

secretin (se-kre′tin): a hormone secreted by the epithelium of the duodenum upon stimulation by the acid chyme; stimulates secretion of pancreatic juice and bile

serine (se′rin): one of the amino acids occurring in protein; nonessential

serosa (ser-o′sah): the membranes lining the peritoneal, pericardial, and pleural cavities and covering their contents

serum (se′rum): the fluid portion of the blood that separates from the blood cells after clotting

siderophilin (sid′er-o-fil′in): an iron-transferring protein

sorbitol (sor′bit-ol): a 6-carbon sugar alcohol with a sweet taste; used commercially to maintain moisture and inhibit crystal formation

sphincter (sfink′ter): a muscle surrounding and closing an orifice

sphingomyelin (sfing-go-mi′el-in): a phospholipid found in the brain, spinal cord, and kidney

stasis (sta′sis): retardation or cessation of flow of blood in the vessels; congestion

steapsin (ste-ap′sin): a hormone in pancreatic juice that hydrolyzes fat; lipase

stearic acid (ste′rik): a saturated fatty acid containing 18 carbon atoms

steatorrhea (ste-at-o-re′ah): excessive amount of fat in the feces

stenosis (sten-o′sis): narrowing of a passage

steroid (ste′roid): a group of compounds similar in structure to cholesterol; includes bile acids, sterols, sex hormones

sterol (ste′rol): an alcohol of high molecular weight; cholesterol, ergosterol

stomatitis (sto-ma-ti′tis): inflammation of the mucous membranes of the mouth

sub-: prefix denoting beneath, or less than normal

substrate (sub′strāt): substance upon which an enzyme acts

succinic acid (suk-sen′ik): a 3-carbon dicarboxylic acid that is an intermediate in the tricarboxylic acid cycle

sucrose (su′krōs): cane or beet sugar; a disaccharide that yields glucose and fructose when hydrolyzed

syn-: prefix meaning with, together

syndrome (sin′drōm): a set of symptoms occurring together

synergism (sin′er-jizm): the joint action of agents which when taken together increases each other's effectiveness

synthesis (sin′thes-is): process of building up a compound

systemic (sis-tem′ik): pertaining to the body as a whole

tachycardia (tak-e-kar′de-ah): rapid beating of the heart

testosterone (tes-tos′ter-ōn): testicular hormone responsible for male secondary sex characteristics

tetany (tet′an-e): a condition marked by intermittent muscular contraction accompanied by fibrillar tremors and muscular pains; seen in hypocalcemia, alkalosis.

thiamin (thi′am-in): a B-complex vitamin; with phosphate forms coenzymes of decarboxylases; essential for carbohydrate metabolism

thio-: prefix meaning sulfur containing

threonine (thre′o-nin): an essential amino acid

thrombus (throm′bus): a clot in a blood vessel formed by coagulation of blood

thymine (thi′min): one of the four nitrogenous bases in nucleic acid

thyroxine (thī-rok′sin): iodine-containing hormone produced by the thyroid gland; regulates the rate of energy metabolism

tocopherol (tok-of′er-ōl): vitamin E; antioxidant alcohol occurring in vegetable germ oils; alpha-, beta-, gamma-, delta-tocopherol

-tomy: suffix meaning to cut into, e.g., gastrectomy

tophi (to′fi): sodium urate deposits in fibrous tissues near the joints; present in gout

tox-: prefix meaning poison

toxemia of pregnancy (tok-se′me-ah): a disorder of pregnancy characterized by hypertension, edema, albuminuria

transamination (trans′am-in-a′shun): transfer of an amino group to another molecule, e.g., transfer to a keto acid, thus forming another amino acid

transferase (trans′fer-ās): an enzyme that transfers a chemical grouping from one compound to another, for example, transaminase, transphosphorylase

transferrin (trans-fer′in): iron-binding protein for transport of iron in blood; siderophilin

trauma (traw-mah): wound or injury usually inflicted suddenly

trichinosis (trik-in-o′sis): illness caused by eating raw pork that is infested by *Trichinella spiralis,* a worm

triglyceride (tri-glis′er-id): an ester of glycerol and three fatty acids

trypsin (trip′sin): a protein-digesting enzyme secreted by the pancreas and released into the small intestine

trypsinogen (trip-sin′o-jen): inactive form of trypsin

tryptophan (trip′tō-fan): an essential amino acid that contains the indole ring; a precursor of niacin

tyramine (tir′am-en): a pressor amine that has an action similar to epinephrine; produced by decarboxylation of tyrosine; found especially in cheeses and some wines

tyrosine (ti′ro-sin): semiessential amino acid; spares phenylalanine; the amino acid in thyroxine

urea (u-re′ah): chief nitrogenous constituent of the urine; formed by the liver when amino acids are deaminized

uremia (u-re′me-ah): presence of urinary constituents in the blood resulting from deficient secretion of urine

uric acid (u-rik): a nitrogenous constituent formed in the metabolism of purines; excreted in the urine; blood levels increased in gout

valine (va′lin): an essential amino acid

vegan: one who excludes all animal foods from his diet

vegetarian: one who excludes one or more classes of animal foods from his diet; thus, vegans, lactovegetarian, lacto-ovo-vegetarian

villus (vil′us): fingerlike projection of the intestinal mucosa

viosterol (vi-os′ter-ol): vitamin D formed by irradiation of ergosterol

visual purple: photosensitive pigment found in the rods of the retina; rhodopsin

vitamin (vi′tah-min): organic compound occurring in minute amounts in foods and essential for numerous metabolic reactions; fat-soluble A, D, E, and K; water-soluble ascorbic acid and B complex including thiamin, riboflavin, niacin, pantothenic acid, biotin, vitamin B_6, vitamin B_{12}, folacin, and others

xanthine (zan′thin): an intermediate in the metabolism of purines; related to uric acid

xanthomatosis (zan-thō-mat-o′sis): accumulation of lipids in the form of tumors in various parts of the body

xerophthalmia (zer-of-thal′me-ah): dry infected eye condition caused by lack of vitamin A

xerosis (ze-ro′sis): abnormal dryness of skin and eye

xylose (zi′lōs): a 5-carbon aldehyde sugar that is not metabolized by the body

zein (za′in): a protein of low biologic value present in corn

zymogen (zi′mo-jen): the inactive form of an enzyme

Index

Information in tables is indicated by the letter *t*; illustrations are indicated by numbers in **boldface** type.

Abbreviations, list, 694
A-beta-lipoproteinemia, 460
Absorption, 23, 26
  amino acids, 46–47
  calcium, 104–105
  carbohydrates, 65
  fats, 82–83
  mechanisms, 23–26
  nature, 23
  sites, 23
  sodium pump, 65
  surface, 23
  vitamin A, 150
Acerola, 230
Acetoacetic acid, 86, 494, 521
Acetohexamide, 495
Acetone, 86, 494
Acetylcholine, 103, 183, 188
Acetyl coenzyme A, **69,** 70, 85, 86, 92, 183
Acetylsalicylic acid, 374*t*
Achalasia, 436
Achlorhydria, 112, 176, 330, 433
Achylia gastrica, 433
Acid, metabolism, 138
Acid-ash diet, 566
Acid-base balance, 138–41
  blood constituents, 678*t*
  chloride shift, 131–32
  measurement, 138
  reaction of foods, 138–39, 567
  regulation, 139–40
Acidity, gastric, factors affecting, 432*t*, 433
Acidosis, 140–41, **140**
  diabetic, 138, 141, 502–503
  ketogenic diet, 521–22
  metabolic, **140,** 141
  renal failure, 583
  respiratory, 140, **140**
Acid-producing foods, 138, 567
Acne vulgaris, 583

Acrolein, 80
ACTH (adrenocorticotropic hormone), 373*t*, 508, 509
Active acetate, 70
Active transport, 26, 46, 65, 104, 133
Activity, caloric expenditure, 96, **96,** 97*t*, 99, 407, 412, **412**
Addison's disease, 508–509
  glucose tolerance curve, **493**
Additives, 264–67
  amendment, federal, 272
  GRAS list, 272–73
  incidental, 266
  intentional, 264–66, 265*t*
  misinformation, 266–67
Adenine, 50
Adenosine triphosphate (ATP), 17, 68, 91, 103
ADH (antidiuretic hormone), 136
Adipose tissue, 80, 97, 406
  food intake, regulation, 216
  metabolism, 84, **84,** 167
Adolescence, anorexia nervosa, 520
  diet patterns, 321
  dietary allowances, 31*t*, 315–17
  growth rate, 315
  obesity, 321
  pregnancy, 287, 289, 292*t*
ADP (adenosine diphosphate), 68, 91
Adrenals, ascorbic acid, 167
  hormones, 49, 67, 137
  insufficiency, 131, 507
Adrenocortical insufficiency, 508–509
  diet, 509
  dietary counseling, 509
  hormones, 508–509
  symptoms, 508
Adrenocortical steroids, 373*t*
Adrenocorticotropic hormone (ACTH), 49, 67, 81, 84, 130, 131
  therapy and diet, 509
Adulterated food, 276
Adults, dietary allowances, 31*t*, 33*t*
  food plans, cost, 249*t*, 250*t*
  height-weight table, 677
  later maturity, 328–36
  nutrient intake, **9**
Adynamic ileus, 485
Aflatoxins, 257
Agar, 63
Aged (aging), anemia, 574
  biochemical changes, 329–30
  cellular changes, 329
  characteristics, 328
  community services, 334–35
  counseling, diet, **329, 331,** 333–34, **334**
  dietary allowances, 31*t*, 332
  dietary deficiencies, 331–32
  dietary management, 332–33
  feeding, 518–19
  food habits, 332
  gastrointestinal function, 330
  health problems, 188, 330–31, 574
  meal plans, 333
  metabolism, 99, 330
  nutrition, 331–32
  physiologic changes, 329–31
  socioeconomic factors, 328–29
  theories, 329–30

Agencies, community nutrition, 352–53t
Agency for International Development, 362
Alanine, 44t
Albinism, 600
Albumin, plasma, 135–36, 680t
  urine, 554
Alcaptonuria, 600
Alcohol, 373t
  beverages, 205, 674t
  calories, 92, 99, 674t
  modified diets, 501, 531, 533, 542
Alcoholism, 520–21
  cirrhosis, 471–72
  diet, 521
  Korsakoff's syndrome, 521
  metabolism, 520
  nutrient deficiencies, 111, 131, 175, 184, 419
  Wernicke's syndrome, 521
Aldohexose, 62
Aldosterone, 130, 136, 137, **137,** 508
Alginate, 63
Alkali-producing foods, 138, 567
Alkaline-ash diet, 138, 566
Alkaline phosphatase, 117, 515
Alkaline reserve, 134, 139
Alkaloids, poisonous, 256
Alkalosis, metabolic, **140,** 141
  respiratory, 140, **140**
Allergens, common, 577, 578
Allergy, 577–84
  asthma, 580
  children, 594
  diagnosis, 578–79
    cereal-free elimination diet, 579
    fruit-free cereal-free elimination diet, 580
    restricted diet, 578–79
  diet lists, without corn, 582
    without eggs, 581
    without milk, 582
    without soy, 582
    without wheat, 581
  dietary counseling, 581
  food preparation, 581
  hyposensitization, 580
  incidence, 577
  infants, 594
  milk sensitivity, 594
  reactions, 577
  skin tests, 578
  symptoms, 578
Alpha-glycerophosphate, 85
Alpha-ketoglutaric acid, 51, 92, 174
Alpha-lipoprotein, 83
Alphatocopherol, 159
Aluminum, 103
  cooking utensils, safety, 259
Aluminum hydroxide, 373t, 557, 564
Amanita, 257
Amebic dysentery, 255
American Diabetes Association, 495, 660–64t
American Dietetic Association, 278, 351
  exchange lists, meal planning, 660–64t
American Heart Association, 360
  fat in diet, recommended, 86
  fat-controlled diets, 530
  sodium-restricted diets, 544
American Home Economics Association, 278

American Institute of Nutrition, 278, 351
American Medical Association, 277, 360
American Nurses Association, 353
Amin-aid, 556
Amino acids, 41–60
  absorption, 46–47
  classification, 43, 44t
  conversion to glucose, fat, 51
  deamination, 47, 48, 51
  energy from, 51, **52**
  essential, 43, 53
  in foods, 665–69t
  functions, 45
  glucogenic, 51
  imbalance, 46, 363
  ketogenic, 51
  limiting, 49, 56
  metabolism, 47–52, **47**
  peptide linkage, 42, **43**
  pool, 49
  requirements, 53, 53t
  structure, 42
  supplementation of proteins, **44**
  synthesis, 51
  transamination, 51, 182
  transport, 49
  transulfuration, 182
  turnover, rate, 49
Aminoaciduria, 111, 600, 608
Aminopeptidase, 25t, 46t, 117
Aminopterin, 374t
Aminosalicylic acid, 374t
Ammonia, disposal, 51–52, **52,** 135
  intoxication, 472
  production, 51, 134, 140
Amphetamine, 413
Ampicillin, 373t
Amylase, 24t, 65
Amylopectin, 63, **63**
Amylose, 63, **63**
Anabolism, 26, 49–51
Androgenic hormone, 49, 508, 515
Anemia, 115, 570–76
  children, 10, 11, 314, 572
  etiology, 570–71
  elderly, 574
  folic acid deficiency, 188, 294, 574
  following gastrectomy, 484
  hemolytic, 115, 257
  incidence, 10, 571, **572**
  infants, 188, 572, 574
  iron deficiency, 115, 571–73
    dietary counseling, 573
    etiology, 571
    treatment, 572–73
  macrocytic, 187, 188, 573
  megaloblastic, 187–88, 574
  pernicious, 185, 187, 573
    diet, 573–74
    dietary counseling, 573–74
  pregnancy, 286, 294, 574
  renal disease, 554, 555
  sickle cell, 574
    diet, 574
  symptoms, 571
  vitamins, deficiencies, 168, 182, 185, 187, 573
  women, 572

Angina pectoris, 527
Angiotensin, 137, **137**
Angiotensinogen, 137, **137**
Anion, 127, 128*t*, 138
Annatto, 230, 265*t*
Anorexia nervosa, 131, 415, 520
Antacid, 373*t*
Antagonist, vitamin, 182, 183, 184
Anthropometric measurements, 405–406
Antibiotics, 373*t*
    foods, 263
    vitamin synthesis, 161, 427
Antibody-antigen complex, 577
Antibody formation, 45, 577
Anticoagulants, 374*t*
Anticonvulsants, 374*t*
Antidepressants, 374*t*
Antidiuretic hormone, 136
Antihypertensives, 374*t*
Antiketogenic factors, 522
Antimetabolites, 374*t*
Antioxidants, 80, 120, 159, 167, 265*t*
Antipyretics, 374*t*
Antituberculars, 374*t*
Anuria, 555
Apatite, 105
Apoenzyme, 18
Appendectomy, diet following, 485
Appetite, 217
    alcoholism, 520
    drug depressants, 413
    illness, 372
    older persons, 330
    thiamin, 175
Aproten pasta, 556
Arabinose, 62
Arachidic acid, 79*t*
Arachidonic acid, 77, 79*t*, 80, 182
Arginase, 51, 119
Arginine, 44*t*, **52**, 665–69*t*
    urea cycle, 52
Ariboflavinosis, 177
Armenian dietary patterns, 233
Arroz, 230
Arroz con pollo, 230
Arthritis, 510–11
    diet, role, 511
    faddism, 511
    incidence, 510
    rehabilitation, 385–87, **511**
    symptoms, 510
    treatment, 511, **511**
Ascites, 471
Ascorbic acid, 166–71
    absorption, 167
    blood, 167
    body distribution, 167
    chemistry, characteristics, 166, **166**
    deficiency, 10, 166, 168–69, **169**
    in diet, basic, **168**, 206*t*, 208
        infant, 301, 308
        United States, **9**, 167, 168, 196, 197*t*
    dietary allowances, 31*t*, 33*t*, 167
        Canada, 33*t*, 684*t*
        U.S. RDA, 279*t*
    discovery, 166
    excretion, 167

food sources, 167–68, 202, 618–40*t*, 658–59*t*
    retention, 168, 245
    functions, 167
    measurement, 166
    megadoses, 169–70
    metabolism, 166–67
    summary, 190
    synthesis, 166
    wound healing, 167, 168, 480
Aspartic acid, 44*t*, 51, 52
Aspergillus flavus, 257
Aspirin, 511
Asthma, 577, 578, 580
Atheroma, 527, **528**
Atherosclerosis, 526–40, **528**
    coronary heart disease, 527–29
    diet, 529–37
    dietary studies, 529
    risk factors, 526, **526**
Athetoids, 595
Athletes, diet, 322
Atole, 231
Atomic Energy Commission, 259
Atonic constipation, 444
ATP (adenosine triphosphate), 17, 68, 70, 85, 91
ATPase (adenine triphosphatase), 103
Atropine, 256, 374*t*
Atwater factors, 93
Audiovisual materials, 686–93
Aureomycin, 263
Avidin, 184
Azotemia, 555

Baby foods, composition, 658–59*t*
Bacalao, 230
Bacteria, action in digestive tract, 22
    growth, 260, **261**
    infections, food, 254
    intoxication, food, 255
Bacterial overgrowth, intestine, 456
Bagel, 228
Bal Ahar, 364
Bantu, hemosiderosis, 115
Barbiturates, 374*t*
Basal metabolism, 94–95
Base, 138
Basedow's disease, 509
Batata, 230
Beans, dry, nutritive value, 243, 623*t*, 667*t*
Beef, characteristics, 242
    consumption, United States, 199, **200**
    cost, protein, **243**
    grades, 242*t*
    nutritive values, 620–23*t*, 665–67*t*
Behavior and food intake. *See also* Food habits
    mentally ill, 519–20
    older persons, 328, 518–19
    preschool child, 317–20
    school child, 320
    teen-ager, 321–22
Behavior modification, weight loss, 409
Behemic acid, 79*t*
Benzoic acid, 202
Beriberi, 172, 175
Berzelius, 41
Beta-carotene, 149
Beta-hydroxybutyric acid, 86, 494, 521

Beta-lipoprotein, 83–84
Beta-oxidation, fatty acids, 85
Betaine, 85
Beverages, 205, 247
   alcoholic, composition, 674t
   nonalcoholic, composition, 638t
BHA (butylated hydroxyanisole), 265t
BHT (butylated hydroxytoluene), 265t
Bible, Jewish dietary pattern, 227–29
   reference to cereals, 203
Bicarbonate, acid-base balance, 139, 140, 141
Biguanides, 375t
Bile, cholesterol, 81
   composition, 24
   enterohepatic circulation, 83, 161
   fat-soluble vitamins, 150, 156, 159, 161
   functions, 24t, 81
   gallbladder, role, 472
   inadequacy, 456
   liver secretion, 135
Bioassay, 36
Biologic half-life, 259
Biologic value of protein, 43, 56
Biotin, **173**, 184
   dietary allowances, 184
      U.S. RDA, 279t
   summary, 191
Bisacodyl, 375t
Bishop, 159
Bitot's spots, 10, 153
Black Americans, food patterns, 229
Blacktongue, dogs, 178
Bland fiber-restricted diet, 435, 438–40
Blenderized feedings, 482
Blind loop syndrome, 456
Blindness, diabetes, 491
   vitamin A deficiency, 153
Blintzes, 228
Blood, cells, 112, 187, 188, 570
   circulation, pregnancy, 288
   clotting, 64, 103, 161
   constituents, normal, 678–81t
   glucose, 66–68, **67**
   lipids, 73, 83–84
   loss and anemia, 570, 571
   pH, 138
   regeneration, 570
   urea nitrogen, 555
Blood pressure, coronary risk, 526
   hypertension, 549
Body, anthropometric measurements, 405–406
   build, types, 408, **408**
   carbohydrate, 63
   chemical elements, 16, 103t
   composition, 16, 405–406
   electrolytes, 128t
   fluid compartments, 16, 125, **126**
   neutrality regulation, 135–37
   skinfold thickness, 405, **405**
   temperature maintenance, 97
Bomb calorimeter, 92
Bone, composition, 105, 129
   development, 105
   minerals, 105, 108, 109, 117, 129
   osteomalacia, 108, 159
   osteoporosis, 108, 119, 514–15
   protein, 105

   resorption, 105, 108
   rickets, 158
   trabeculae, 105
   vitamins in formation, 105, 152, 155, 156, 167, 169
Boron, 103t
Borsch, 228
Bottle feeding, 303–306, **305**
Botulism, 255
Bourglour, 233
Bowel, motility alterations, 443–44
   short bowel syndrome, 460
Bowman's capsule, 132
Boys, dietary allowances, 31t, 321t
      Canadian, 684–85t
   food habits, 321
   growth, 315, 675t
Brain, development, 286–87, 299
   glucose need, 518
Branched-chain ketoaciduria, 607–608
Bread, 202–205
   basic diet, 206t, **208**
   carbohydrate, 71
   dough conditioners, 116
   enriched, 278t
   kinds, 245
   list, controlled protein, potassium, and sodium diet, 562
      exchanges, meal planning, 400, 661–62t
      fat-controlled diet, 534
      sodium-restricted diet, 544–46
   lysine enriched, 363
   nutritive values, 203–205, **204**, 630–35t
   proteins, 54t, **55**, 204
   vitamins, 174, **174**, 177, **177**
Breakfast, 208–10, 218
   calculation, nutritive value, 37, 38t
   efficiency, 208–209
   habits, 315
   meal plans, 209, 210, **210**
   school, 324
Breast feeding, 301–303, **302**
Bromine, 103t
Brush border, intestinal mucosa, 23, 65, 82
Buddhist, vegetarianism, 221
Budget, food, 237–40
Buffer systems, acid-base balance, 139
Bulgur, 246, 364
Bulk, diet, *See* Fiber
Bulke, 228
Burns, 485–86
   fluid loss, 137
   potassium loss, 131
Butter, 87, 177, 205, 636t, 670t

Cacciatore, chicken, 232
Cadmium, 103, 258
Cafe con leche, 230
Caffeine, 205
Calabaza, 230
Calciferol, 155
Calcification, vitamin D, 155–56
Calcitonin, 105
Calcium, 103–108
   absorption, 104–105
   blood clotting, 64, 103
   body tissues, 103, 105–106
   calculi, renal, 563–67

carbonate, 373t
deficiency, 106, 108, 158–59, 515
diet, basic, **107**, 206t, **208**
  osteoporosis, 515
  restricted, 565–66
  United States, **9**, 196, 197t
dietary allowances, 31t, 33t, 106
  aging, 332
  Canadian, 33t, 684–85t
  childhood, 315–17
  infants, 299t, 300
  pregnancy, 289–91, 291t
  U.S. RDA, 279t
diffusible, 105
excretion, 106
food sources, 106, 107t, 197t, 199, 618–40t
functions, 103
metabolism, **104**, 105–106, 156
  immobilization, 385, 515
  lactose effect, 104
  magnesium, 109
  oxalic acid, 104, 202
  phosphorus ratio, 104, 105
  phytic acid, 104
  protein, 106
  steroid therapy, 511
  vitamin D, 104, 155–56
milk-alkali syndrome, 108
rickets, 158–59
salts, supplementation, 522, 580
stones, renal, 564–65
storage, body, 105
summary, 142t
teeth, 104
Calcium-phosphorus-restricted diet, 565–66
Calculation methods, daily diet, 37–39
  diabetic diet, 399, 497
  exchange lists, 399–403
  ketogenic diet, 522
  phenylalanine-restricted diet, 602–603
  purposes, 37
Calculi, diet, 563–67
  following fracture, 486
  renal, 563–67
Calories, from carbohydrate, 61, 64
  definition, 92
  diet, basic, **100**, 206t, **208**
    high-calorie, 415–16
    low-calorie, 410–11
    United States, 91, 196, 197t
  dietary allowances, 31t, 33t, 98
    activity, 96, **96**, 97t, 99
    age, 99, 332
    atherosclerosis, 529
    based on body size, 98t
    burns, 485
    Canadian, 33t, 106, 684–85t
    cardiovascular disease, 529, 541
    celiac syndrome, 589
    children, 315–17
    climate, 97, 99
    diabetes mellitus, 496, 591
    factors influencing, 95–98
    fevers, 426, 427
    gallbladder disease, 473
    gout, 513
    growth, 98

hepatic coma, 472
hepatitis, 468
hyperlipoproteinemia, 531
hyperthyroidism, 510
infants, 299, **300**
ketogenic diet, 522
lactation, 291t, 294
nephritis, 553, 554
obesity, 410–11
phenylketonuria, 603t
pregnancy, 289–90, 291t
protein deficiency, 421
reference standard, 98
renal failure, 556
short-bowel syndrome, 460
surgical conditions, 480
tube feeding, 482
underweight, 415–16
vitamin allowances, 174, 176, 179
fat, 76, 80, 87
foods, 99, **100**, 618–40t, 658–59t
intake, United States, 196, 197t
joule, relation, 92
measurement, food, 92
nutrition education, 100
protein, 45, 49
Calorigenic effect, food, 97
Calorimetry, bomb, 92, **93**
  respiration, 93–95, **94**
Canada, dietary standards, 32, 33t, 684–85t
Cancer, colon, 449
  stomach, 437
Candy, nutritive values, 637t
  school lunch policies, 324
Cannelloni, 232
Canning of food, 216–62
Cannoli, 232
Capric acid, 79t
Carbohydrate, 61–75
  absorption, 65
  amino acids, 67
  antiketogenic effect, 522
  atherosclerosis, 529
  available, 65, 522
  baby foods, 308
  blood, 66–68, **67**, 679t
  body, 16, 63–64
  classification, 61–63
  complex, 71t
  composition, 61
  consumption, United States, **7**, 8, 61, 70, 72, **72**, 196, 197t
  dental caries, 72
  derivatives, 63
  diet, 70–73
    basic, 206t
    high in, 469–71
    low in, dumping syndrome, 486–88
    significance, 61
  dietary allowances, 70
    Addison's disease, 508
    diabetes mellitus, 496, 497t
    dumping syndrome, 486
    fevers, 427
    hepatic coma, 472
    hepatitis, 469
    hyperlipidemia, 531

Carbohydrate, dietary allowances [*Cont.*]
    hypoglycemia, 507
    ketogenic diet, 522
    obesity, 410
    renal failure, 556
    surgical conditions, 481
  digestion, 24–25*t*, 64–65
  energy from, 61, 64
  excess, effect, 72–73
  excretion, urine, 66
  fats, conversion to, 68
  food sources, 71*t*, 71, 72, **72**, 202, 618–40*t*, 658–59*t*
  functions, 63–64
  hydrolysis, 25*t*, 64
  lysine linkage, 46
  metabolism, 66–70, **66, 69**
    citric acid cycle, 68, **69**, 70
    diabetes mellitus, 494
    glycolysis, 68, **69**
    hormonal control, 67, 68, 509
    interrelation, nutrients, 27, 65–66
    older persons, 330
    oxidation, glucose, 68, 70
    pentose shunt, 70
    role of insulin, 68
    role of liver, 66, **66**
    role of minerals, 66, 109, 130
    role of vitamins, 66, 68, 70, 173, 179, 182
  nutrition education, 73
  problems, consumption, 72–73
  protein-sparing action, 64, 421
  renal threshold, 66
  requirement, minimum, 70
  storage, liver, 66
  sweetness, 62
  synthesis, 61
  triglycerides, serum, 73, 531
  water of oxidation, 126
Carbonic acid, 138
Carbonic acid–bicarbonate buffer system, 139
Carbonic anhydrase, 117, 134
Carboxylase, 173
Carboxylation, 184
Carboxypeptidase, 25*t*, 46*t*, 117
Carcinogens, 257
Carcinoma, intestine, 449
  stomach, 437
Cardiac failure, 131, 541
Cardiovascular disease, 526–40, 541–51
  beriberi, 175
  blood studies, 527–29
  diet, adjustments, 541–42
    fat-controlled, 530–37
    sodium-restricted, 542–47
  dietary counseling, 533, 536–37
  public health problem, 526
  risk factors, 88, 526
CARE, 362
Carotene, absorption, 150
  blood, 151, 453
  conversion to vitamin A, 149
  foods, 149
Carrageen, 63
Carriers, absorption, 23, 26
Cascara, 375*t*
Casein, 198, 304
Cassava, 257

Castle, 185
Catabolism, 26, 49, 51–52, 426
Catalyst, enzyme, 18
Cataracts, genetic disease, 609
Catecholamines, 507
Cathartics, 444
Cations, 127, 128*t*, 138
Celiac disease, 461, 589–90
  diet, 462–63
  gluten-induced, 461–62
Cells, aging, change, 329
  functioning units, 16–18
  glycolysis, 68
  membranes, 17, 80, 103
  metabolism, 26–27
  mucosal abnormalities, 452*t*, 456–64
  nutrient absorption, 23, 26
  protein synthesis, 50
  role of minerals, 103, 109, 129, 130
  structure, 16–18, **17**
Cellu low-protein baking mix, 556
Cellulose, 63, 65
Cement substance, intercellular, 167, 168
Cephalin, 77
Cereal foods, 202–205, 245–46
  amino acids, 668*t*
  bread, 204, 245
  breakfast, 246
  carbohydrate, 71, 203
  diet, basic, 206*t*, 207*t*, **208**
    United States, 8
    world, 363
  economy, 246
  enrichment, 277
  in food plans, 249*t*, 250*t*
  grain, cross section, **203**
  infant diet, 309
  milk, as supplement, 204
  milling, effect, 203
  minerals in, 109, 110, 115, 117, 118, 120
  nutritive values, 54, **55**, 196, 203, **203**, 205
  phytic acid, 63, 104
  protein, 54*t*, **55**, 56, 204
  supplementation, protein, 204
  vitamins in, 174, **174**, 177, **177**, 204
Cereal-free elimination diet, 579
Cereal-free fruit-free elimination diet, 580
Cerebral palsy, 595
Cerebrosides, 77
Cerebrovascular accident, 527
Ceruloplasmin, 118, 610
Cesium-137, 259
Cestodes, 256
Challah, 228
Chappatties, **219**
Chayotes, 231
Cheese, 199, 241–42
  nutritive value, 199, 618*t*
  process, 241
  purchase, 242
  types, 199, 241–42
  tyramine, 258
Cheilosis, 177, **178**
Chemical diabetes, 492
Chemicals, combining power, 128
  foods, additives, 264–67
  plants, 256–58

poisoning, 258–59
preservation of foods, 263
Chicos, 231
Children, 313–27. *See also* Infant(s); Teen-agers
  amino acid requirements, 53
  anemia, 10, 314, 572, 574
  basal metabolism, 95, 316
  counseling, diet, 586–87
  day care centers, 359
  diabetes mellitus, 590–92
  diet(s), preschool, 317–20
    school, 320–21, 321*t*
    teen-age, 321–22, 321*t*
  dietary allowances, 31*t*, 315–17
    Canadian, 684–85*t*
  dietary errors, 315
  diseases, 585–96, 600–613. *See also* individual diseases
  energy requirement, 99, 221
  food habits, 221
    preschool child, **314**, 317–20
    school, 320
    sick, 585, **586**
    teen-age, 321–22
  food plans, cost, 249*t*, 250*t*
  food supplements, program, 360
  growth and development, 313, 315
  growth failure, 314, 588
  handicapped, feeding, 595–96
  hospitalized, 585
  inborn errors of metabolism, 600–611
  lead poisoning, 258
  malnutrition, 57, 314–15, 339, 340, 345–49, **362**
  mental retardation, 595–96
  milk sensitivity, 594–95
  nutrient intake, **9**
  nutrition programs, 322–25
  nutritional status, 10, 314–15
  obesity, 588
  renal insufficiency, 594
  school feeding, 322–25, **323, 324**
  snacks in diet, 211, 315, 318, 322
  sugar in diet, 72
  underweight, 588
  weight control, 588
  weight-height tables, 675–76*t*
Chili con carne, 231
Chinese dietary patterns, 234
  folklore, 218
Chloramphenicol, 373*t*
Chloride, 131–32
  summary, 143
Chlorophyll, 61
Chlorothiazide, 374*t*
Chlorpropamide, 495
Chlortetracycline, 263
Cholecalciferol, 155
Cholecystectomy, 475, 485
Cholecystitis, 472
Cholecystokinin, 21*t*, 81, 472
Cholelithiasis, 472
Cholent, 228
Cholesterol, absorption, 82
  ascorbic acid, 167
  atherosclerosis, 527, 528
  bile, 24*t*, 86
  blood, 83, 86, 531
  body distribution, 81

chemical formula, **77**
diet, restricted, 529, 530–37
excretion, 86
food sources, 87, 88*t*, 532*t*, 670–73*t*
functions, 80–81
gallstones, 473
metabolism, 86, 167
  lipoproteins, 83–84
  liver function, 85
  plant sterols, role, 530
  vitamin A, role, 152, 183
synthesis, 86
transport in blood, 86
Cholestyramine, 375*t*
Choline, 85, 186, 188–89, 191
Chondroitin sulfate, 64, 105, 111
Chow mein, 234
Christian, 176
Chromium, 120–21
  summary, 145
Chromoprotein, 43
Chylomicron, 83, 531
Chyme, 21*t*, 22
Chymotrypsin, 25*t*, 46*t*
Chymotrypsinogen, 25*t*, 46*t*
Cirrhosis of liver, 471–72
  diet, 471
  etiology, 471
  magnesium deficiency, 111
  symptoms, 471
  zinc need, 118
Citric acid cycle, 68, **69**, 70
Citrovorum factor, 187
Citrulline, 42, **52**
Clear-fluid diet, 396
Cleft palate, feeding, 595
Climate, energy need, 99
Clinical diabetes, 492
Clofibrate, 375*t*
Clostridium, botulinum, 255, 264
  perfringens, 253, 254
Cobalamin, 185
Cobalt, 121, 185, **186**
Cocarboxylase, 173
Coconut oil, 78
Cod-liver oil, 155
Coefficient digestibility, 23, 93
Coenzymes, 18, 111, 173, 176, 179, 182, 184
  I, II, 179
  A, **69**, 70, 183
  Q, 160
Cofactor, 18
Coffee, 205
Coffee whitener, 247, 619*t*
Colchicine, 375*t*, 457, 512
Cold, common, ascorbic acid, 169
Colic, infantile, 589
Colitis, granulomatous, 445
  spastic, 445
  ulcerative, 448–49
Collagen, 105, 118, 167, 329
Colloid osmotic pressure, 135–36
Colon, cancer, 449
  diseases, 443–51
  surgery, 484–85
Color Additive Amendment, 272
Colostomy, diet, 485

Colostrum, 302
Coma, diabetic, 502–503
  hepatic, 472
Committee on Maternal Nutrition, 284, 285, 288
Community nutrition, 337, 351–66
  agencies, 352–53*t*
  education, 353–56
  facilities, 351–53
  focus, 337
  food supply, increase, 362
  international agencies, 361–62
  low-income groups, helps for, 356–57
  older persons, 334–35
  programs, 358–61
  services, 351
  state programs, 358
Compleat B, 483*t*
Comprehensive care, concepts, 380, 383
  services, 384–87
Concepts, basic, nutrition, 354
Congestive heart failure, 541–42
Connective tissue, 64
Constipation, 444–45
  causes, 444
  diet, 444–45
  infants, 589
  physical handicaps, effect, 385
  pregnancy, 294
  spastic, 444, 445
Consumer and Food Economics Institute, U.S.D.A.,
    249–50
Consumerism, 272
Contraceptives, 183, 188, 375*t*
Controlled-fat diet, 530–37
Controlled protein, potassium, sodium diet, 558–63
Controlyte, 553, **557**
Convenience foods, 240
Cookery, food preservation, 261
Cooking utensils, safety, 259
Cool storage, food, 262
Cooperative Extension Service, 357
Coppa, 232
Copper, 118
  diet restricted, 610
  dietary allowance, 118
    U.S. RDA, 279*t*
  iron utilization, 113
  molybdenum, role, 118, 256
  summary, 144
  Wilson's disease, defect, 118, 610
Corn, in diet, 56, 245
  diet without, 582
  opaque-2, 363
Corneal vascularization, 177
Coronary heart disease, 526–29
  blood studies, 527–29
  diet, 529–36
  dietary counseling, 533, 536–37
  risk factors, 526
  surgery, 537
Coronary occlusion, 541
Corpus luteum, 288
Corticoids, 508
Cortisol, 428, 508, 509
Cottonseed, toxic pigment, 363
Counseling (dietary), 380–83. *See also* Education
    (nutrition)

adrenocortical insufficiency, 509
allergy, 581
anemia, 573
arthritis, 511
calorie-restricted diet, 413–15
children, 586–87, **587**
continuity, 383
controlled protein, potassium, sodium diet, 558–60
diabetes mellitus, 498–501, **500, 501, 502**
  children, 591–92, **592**
diet history, 381–82
diverticulitis, 447
family, 354–56
fat-controlled diet, 533, 536–37
fat-restricted diet, 475
gluten-restricted diet, 464
group, 383
high-protein diet, 421–22
hyperthyroidism, 510
hypoglycemia, 508
lactose-free diet, 457
low-purine diet, 513
medium-chain triglyceride diet, 455–56
older persons, **329, 331,** 333–34, **334**
osteoporosis, 515
patient's needs, 382–83
peptic ulcer, 440–41
phenylalanine-restricted diet, 603, 606–607
pregnancy, 291–93, **293**
protein deficiency, 421–22
rapport, 381
responsibility, 380–81
sodium-restricted diets, 548–49
techniques, 380–83
timing, 381
Cretinism, 116, 510
Crohn's disease, 445–46·
Cryptoxanthin, 149
C.S.M. (corn-soy-milk blend), 364
Culture, food acceptance, 224–34
  malnutrition, 341–42
Cushing's syndrome, 509, 608
Cyanocobalamin, 185
Cystathionine synthetase, 608
Cysteine, 44*t*, 182
Cystic fibrosis of pancreas, 476, 590
  diet, 476
  symptoms, 476
Cystine, 43, 44*t*
  calculi, 564, 566
  food sources, 665–69*t*
Cystinuria, 111, 600
Cytochrome system, 92, 118
Cytoplasm, cell, 17
Cytosine, 50

Daily Food Guide, **34-35,** 35*t*, 205–208
Davis, 149, 172
Day care, children, 359
DBI (phenformin), 495
DDT, 273
Deamination, 48, 51, 184
Decarboxylation, 70, 182, 184
  deficiency, maple syrup urine disease, 608
Deficiency diseases. *See also* individual nutrients
  economic cost, 339–40
  environmental factors, 340–43

incidence, 10
malabsorption, 452
primary, 338
protein, 57, 345–50
secondary, 338
signs, 339
summary, 338*t*
susceptibility, 340
Degenerative arthritis, 510
Dehydration, body, 136
diarrhea, 137, 443, 589
fevers, 137
food preservation, 263
hemorrhage, 137
hyperkalemia, 131
hypothalamus, 136
surgery, 137, 480
Dehydroascorbic acid, 166, **166**
7-Dehydrocholesterol, 155, 157
Dehydrofreezing, 263
Dehydrogenase, 92, 176
Delaney clause, food additives, 272
Delirium tremens, 521
Dental caries, 10
dietary factors, 72, 159
fluorine, 119
selenium, 120
Dental fluorosis, 119
Deoxycorticosterone, 509
Deoxypyridoxine, 182
Deoxyribonucleic acid, 17, 50, **50**, 64
Deoxyribose, 50
Depression, mental, 519
Dermatitis, biotin deficiency, 184–85
fatty acid deficiency, 80, **81**
niacin deficiency, 178, 180, **181**
protein deficiency, 57
riboflavin deficiency, 177, **178**
vitamin A deficiency, 153
vitamin B₆ deficiency, 183
Detoxification, 467
Dextrins, 63, 65
Dextrose, 62
Diabetes mellitus, 491–506, 590–91
acidosis, 86, 141, 502–503
adult, 493
atherosclerosis, 526, 531
camps, 592
chemical, 492
childhood, 491, 492, 590–91
chromium, 121
clinical, 492
coma, 502–503
complications, 502–503, 591, 591*t*
control levels, 492
diet, 494–98
calculation, 401–402, 497, 499
carbohydrate distribution, 497*t*
children, 590–91
exchange lists, 399–403, 660–64
"free," 496, 591
meal patterns, 498, 499
nutritional needs, 496–97
rationale, 495–96
dietary counseling, 498, 500–541, **501**, 502
children, 591–92, **592, 593**
essential knowledge, 498

problems, 501
responsibility, 498, 500
teaching aids, 500
dietetic foods, 501
electrolyte imbalance, 111, 131
glucose, blood, 493, **493**
growth-onset, 492
heredity, 492
hormones, 491
hyperlipoproteinemia, 531
hypoglycemia, 502
incidence, 491–92
infections, 503
insulin, 495, 495*t*, 591
insulin shock, 502
juvenile, 492–93
ketosis, 86, 503
laboratory studies, 493
maturity onset, 493
metabolism, 86, 491, 494
nature, 491–94
obesity, 492, **492, 500**
oral drugs, 495
potassium, role, 131
prediabetes, 492
pregnancy, 503
risk factors, 492
stages, 492
surgery, 503
symptoms, 492–93
treatment, 494–98
types, 492–93
Diabinese, 495
Dial-a-dietitian, **352**
Dialysis, 555
diet, 556–63
peritoneal, 556
Diaper test, PKU, 601
Diarrhea, 443
acidosis, 141
causes, 443*t*
diet, 444
electrolyte losses, 130, 131, 132
food-borne, 284–86
irritable colon, 445
malabsorption, 444
nutritional considerations, 443–44
regional enteritis, 445–46
ulcerative colitis, 448–49
water loss, 137
Dicoumarol, 161
Diet. *See also* individual nutrients and specific diseases
adults, 196, 208–12, 332–35
basic, 36, 205–208, 206*t*, 207*t*
calories, **100**
minerals, **107, 110, 114**
protein, **55**
vitamins, **152, 168, 174, 177, 180**
calculation, diabetes mellitus, 496–98
using exchange lists, 399–402
using long method, 37–39
children, 317–22
cost, two levels, plans, 249*t*, 250*t*
counseling, 380–83. *See also* Counseling (dietary)
cultural patterns, 224–36
economy, 237–48, **238, 239**
errors, children, 315

Diet [*Cont.*]
  evaluation, 37–39
  family, 196–213
  fat, 86–87
  guides, 29–36
  history, 381–83
  infant, 303–306, 307–10
  lactation, 294–95
  liquid, 396–97
  low cost, 249*t*
  macrobiotic, 56
  manuals, 392
  meal patterns, 208–11
  moderate cost, 250*t*
  modified, rationale, 390
  nomenclature, 392
  normal, 389–90, 391*t*
  pregnancy, 291–93, **293**
  regional, United States, 225
  routine hospital, 389–90, 391*t*, 393–97
  texture modification, 389–97
  therapeutic, 369–78
  therapy, purposes, 361
  trends, United States, 6–8, 87, 196
  vegetarian, 56, 225
Diet-drug interrelations, 372, 373–75*t*
Diet manuals, 392
Dietary allowances, 31*t*, 33*t*
  Canadian, 33*t*, 684–85*t*
  FAO/WHO, 33*t*
  United Kingdom, 33*t*
  U.S. RDA, 279*t*
Dietary counseling, 380–83. *See also* Counseling
  (dietary); Education (nutrition)
Dietary guides and uses, 29–40
Dietary surveys, 6–8, **7**, **9**
  children, 314–15
  HANES, 406*t*, 571, 572*t*
  older persons, 331
  pregnancy, 285–86
  ten-state, 10, 168
  U.S.D.A., 7–8, **9**
Dietetic foods, 281, 501, 549, **549**
Dietitian, goals, nutrition study, 12–13
  role, 351, 370
Diffusion, nutrient absorption, 23
Digestibility coefficient, 23, 93
Digestion, 19–23
  carbohydrate, 64–65
  chemical, 22
  comfort, 434
  controls, 19–20
  disturbances, deficiency disease, 175, 180
    gastrointestinal disease 431–42, 443–51, 452–65
  enzymes, 24–25*t*
  factors affecting, 432*t*, 433–34
  fat, 81–83
  fluid exchange, 135
  hormones regulating, 20, 21*t*
  infants, 298
  intestines, 20, 22
  juices, 22, 24–25*t*
  later years, 330
  mechanical, 20–22
  motility, 22, 81, 432*t*, 433–34
  mouth, 20, 24*t*
  organs, 19, **20**
  pancreas, 25*t*
  protein, 45–46, 46*t*
  purposes, 19
  secretions, 22, 24–25*t*
  stomach, 21
  water, role, 125, 135
Digitalis, 375*t*
Diglyceride, 76
1,25-Dihydroxycholecalciferol, 156
1,25-Dihydroxyvitamin D$_3$, 156, 159, 555
Diiodotyrosine, 116
Dinner, pattern, 211, **212**
Diphosphopyridine nucleotide, 179
Disaccharidase deficiency, 452, 456–60
Disaccharides, 62
Disaster feeding, 267–68
Disease, food-borne, 253–59
Diverticulosis, 446–47
  diet, 447–48
  dietary counseling, 447
DNA, 50, **50**, 108, 117, 186, 188, 329
Donath, 172
Drugs, 372–75
  anorexigenic, 413
  diuretic, 374
  interrelation, nutrition, 372, 373–75*t*
  oral hypoglycemic, 495
  peptic ulcer, 438
  uricosuric, 512
Dumping syndrome, 486–88
  diet, 486–88
  nature, 486
Duodenum, absorption, 23
  diseases, diet, 437–41
  hormones, 21*t*
Dwarfism, zinc, 117
Dymelor (acetohexamide), 495
Dynamic equilibrium, 26, 48–49, 102
Dysentery, amebic, 255
  bacillary, 254
Dysgeusia, 117
Dysosmia, 118
Dyspepsia, 436

Eating devices, handicapped, 386–87
Eclampsia, 286, 294
Ecology, food supply, 9, 226
  pesticides, 266
Economy of diet, 237–48, **238**, **239**
  plans, two cost levels, 249*t*, 250*t*
  ways of effecting, 238, 240
Ecosystem, children, 313
Ectomorph, 408
Eczema, 80, **81**
Edema, 137
  beriberi, 175
  heart disease, 137, 541
  kidney disease, 137, 552, 554, 555
  kwashiorkor, 347
  liver disease, 471
  nutritional, 137, 419, 420
  pregnancy, 294
  sodium imbalance, 130
Education (nutrition), 353–56. *See also* Counseling
  (dietary)
  basic concepts, 354
  children, 353–54

counseling, therapeutic diets, 380–83
family, guidelines, 354–56
knowledge, essential, 354
  lack and malnutrition, 341
nurse, 12–13
points for emphasis, carbohydrate, 73
  energy, 100
  fat, 88–89
  minerals, 141
  proteins, 57–58
  vitamins, 189–92
poor people, 357
program aides, 357, **358**
scope of program, 353–54
Egg(s), allergy, foods to avoid, 581
avidin, biotin, 184
basic diet, **55, 107, 110, 114, 152, 177**
cholesterol, 87, 88*t*
diet, 199, 200
  infants, 309
fats, 87, 88*t*
nutritive values, 54*t*, 56, 200, 201, 620*t*
quality, 242, 243
Egg foo young, 234
Egg rolls, 234
Egg white injury, 184
Eijkman, 172
Elastin, 43, 118
Elderly persons, malnutrition, 340
nursing homes, feeding, 518–19
nutrition, 328–36
Electrolytes, 127–29
acid-base balance, 138–41
balance, 125–41
  factors influencing, 134–35
  hormonal control, 136–37, 508
blood, 679*t*
composition, body fluids, 128*t*
definition, 127
extracellular fluid, 129
intracellular fluid, 129
losses, diarrhea, 444
low-, supplement, 553
measurement, 127–28
regulation, 136–37
role of kidney, 132–33
role of lungs, 139
Electron, acceptors, donors, 127
transport, 92, 118
Elementary school, nutrition education, 354
Elimination diets, cereal-free, 579
fruit-free cereal-free, 580
Elvehjem, 118, 178
Embden-Meyerhof glycolytic pathway, 68, **69,** 85
Emergency feeding, 267–68
Emotions, anorexia nervosa, 520
diabetes mellitus, children, 590
digestion, 432*t*
food, outlet for, 221–22
nutrient utilization, 321
obesity, 404
Emphysema, 429
Enchiladas, 231
Endamoeba histolytica, 255
Endemic goiter, 116
Endocrine glands, energy metabolism, 95
Endometrium, 288

Endomorph, 408
Endoplasmic reticulum, 18
Endosperm, cereal, 204
Energy. *See also* Calories
body stores, 91
calorimetry, 92–95, **93, 94**
catabolism, amino acids, 51
conservation, law, 91
definition, 91
diet, American, 91, 196*t*, 197*t*
  basic, **100**
dietary allowances, 31*t*, 33*t*, 95–99, 97*t*, 98*t*
  Canadian, 684*t*
  children, 31*t*, 98*t*, 316
  diabetes, 496
  infants, 98*t*, 299
  lactation, 291*t*, 295
  older persons, 98*t*, 330
  pregnancy, 98*t*, 289–90, 291*t*
forms, 91
fuel factors, 92–93
imbalance, obesity, 406–409
  thyroid disorders, 509–10
  underweight, 404, 415
measurement, 92
metabolism, 91–101
  basal, 94–95
  coenzymes, 176, 179, 183
  factors influencing, 95–98
  infants, 299
  measurement, body, 93–94
  nutritional priority, 91
  total energy, 95–98
nutrition education, emphasis, 100
protein, 45
requirement, 31*t*, 95–99
transformation, 91–92
  ATP, 91
  oxidative phosphorylation, 92
  TCA cycle, 92
value of foods, 99, **100,** 618–40*t*
Enfamil, 306
Enrichment of breads and cerals, 278, 278*t*
rice, 175
Ensure, 483*t*
Enteritis, food-borne, 254
regional, 445–46
  diet, 446
Enterocrinin, 21*t*
Enterogastrone, 21*t*
Enterohepatic circulation, 83, 185
Enterokinase, 46*t*
Enzymes, 18. *See also* specific names
action, factors influencing, 18
activation, 103
blood, 679*t*
cytochrome, 92
digestive, 24–25*t*, 46*t*, 64, 65, 81, 432
inhibitors, 46, 257, 258
minerals, role, 102, 103, 109, 112, 117, 118, 119, 130
nature, 18, 45
proenzyme, 18
vitamins as coenzymes, 173, 176, 179, 182, 183, 184, 185, 188
Epilepsy, 521–23
diet, 522, 523*t*
treatment, 521

Epinephrine, 67, 84, 95, 167
Epithelium, vitamin A, 151
Equilibrium, dynamic, 26, 48–49, 102
Equivalent weight, 128, 681
Ergocalciferol, 155
Ergosterol, 155
Erythrocyte transketolase, 175
Erythropoiesis, 112
Esophageal obstruction, 436
Esophageal reflux, 436
Esophagitis, 435
Esophagus, diet following surgery, 483
   diseases, 435–36
   varices, 471
Estrogens, 375t
   osteoporosis, 515
   pregnancy, 288
   protein metabolism, 49
Ethacrynic acid, 374t
Ethnic groups and diet, 224–34
Evans, 159
Exchange lists, 660–64t
   fat-controlled diet, 534–35
   phenylalanine-restricted diet, 605–606
   protein, sodium, potassium controlled diet, 560–63
   sodium-restricted diet, 544–46
Exercise, energy metabolism, 96, 97t, 407, 409, 412,
   412
Exophthalmic goiter, 509
Extracellular fluid, 16, 125, **126,** 129, 130, 131
Extrinsic factor, 185
Eye, cataracts in galactosemia, 609
   riboflavin deficiency, 177
   vitamin A deficiency, 153

Fabricated foods, 247
Factor U, 187
FAD (flavin adenine dinucleotide), 69, 92, 176
Faddism, combatting, 345
   identifying quack, 344–45
   obesity, 404
   older persons, 332–33
   pregnancy, 284–85
   types, 343–44
Fair Packaging and Labeling Act, 273–74
Fallout, radioactive, 259, **259**
Families, changes, life style, 6–7
   counseling, 354–56
   food allowances, two cost levels, 249–50t
   food habits, 218
   meal planning, 196, 205–11
FAO, 11, 361
Farfalleti dolci, 233
Farfel, 229
Fasting, religious, 221
   weight loss, 412
Fat(s), 77–90
   absorption, 82–83
   blood, 83, 680t
   body, 16
   calcium utilization, 105
   characteristics, 78, 80
   chemical structure, **76, 77**
   cholesterol, 81, 86, 672t, 673t
   cis and *trans* forms, 77
   classification, 78
   composition, 77

diet, 77
   basic, 88, 206t
   concerns, health, 76
   fat-controlled, 530–36
   high-fat, dumping syndrome, 486–88
   high-fat, epilepsy, 522, 523t
   restricted, 474–75
   United States, 87, 196, 197t
dietary allowances, 86–87
   atherosclerosis, 529
   cirrhosis, 471
   cystic fibrosis, 476
   diabetes mellitus, 496
   dumping syndrome, 486
   epilepsy, 522
   gallbladder disease, 473
   gout, 513
   hepatitis, 469
   hyperlipidemia, 531, 532t
   hypoglycemia, 508
   infants, 299–300
   malabsorption, 453
   obesity, 410
   pancreatic deficiency, 476
digestibility, 82–83
digestion, 81–82, 83, 432t, 433
emulsification, 78
energy value, 80
essential fatty acids, 80
excesses, diet, 10
exchanges, meal planning, 400, 664
food plans, 249–50t
food sources, 87, 88t, 205, 618–40t
functions, 80–81
hardness, 78
heating, effect, 80
hydrogenated, 78
ketogenesis, 86
lipoproteins, 83, 84
metabolism, **82,** 83–86, **84**
   adipose tissue, 84, **84**
   ascorbic acid, role, 167
   carbohydrate, 64
   diabetes mellitus, 494
   insulin, 84
   hormones, 84
   lipotropic factors, 85
   older persons, 330
   role of liver, 85, 467
nutrition education, emphasis, 88–89
nutrition labeling, 87
nutritive values, 205, 636–37t
oxidation, 85–86, 126
phospholipids, 80
problems, fat intake, 87–88
P/S ratio, 86, 529, 531
purchase, food, 246
rancidity, 80, 153
saponification, 78
saturated, 77, 78, **78,** 79t
synthesis, **84,** 85
test, feces, 452
transport, circulation, 83–84
unsaturated, 77, 78, **78,** 79t
Fat-controlled diet, 532–37
Fat exchanges, 664
Fat-restricted diet, 473–75

Fat-soluble vitamins, 148–65
Fatty acids, 77–78
  blood, 84
  essential, 80
    infant needs, 299
  foods, 79*t*, 87, 198, 618–40*t*
  glucose ratio, 522
  metabolism, 83–86
    kidney, role, 133
    lipoproteins, 83, 84
    oxidation, **84,** 85–86
    vitamin E need, 160
  milk, 198
  monounsaturated, 77
  saturated, 77, **78,** 79*t*
  structure, 77–78, **78**
  unsaturated, 77, **78,** 79*t*
Favism, 257
FDA (Food and Drug Administration), 274–77
Federal Radiation Council, 259
Federal Trade Commission, 281
Feedback mechanism, food intake, 215
Feeding, bottle, 303–306
  breast, 301–303
  children, handicapped, 595–96
    sick, 585–86
  emergency, 267–68
  frequency, 392–93
  handicapped, 385–87
  intravenous, 397, 480, 481
  mentally ill, 519–20
  patient, 376–77
  premature infants, 306–307
  problems, infant, 588–89
    psychiatric, 518–20
  tube, 482, 483*t*
Ferric chloride test, 601
Ferritin, 112
Ferrous iron, 112
Ferrous sulfate, 375*t*
Fertilizers, 36
Fetal development, 287–88
Fevers and infections, 426–30
  classification, 426
  diets, 426–29
  dietary counseling, 429
  metabolism, 95, 419, 426
Fiber, cancer, relation to, 70
  definition, 65, 434
  dietary allowances, 70
  digestion, 65
  diverticulosis, 70, 446–47
  gastrointestinal diseases, 435
  high-fiber diet, 447–48
  low-residue diet, 446
  -restricted diet, 438–40
  sources, 72
Filtration, glomerular, 132, 555
Filtration pressure, 132, **133**
Fish, cholesterol, 671–73*t*
  consumption, 199
  mercury pollution, 258
  nutritive values, 200, 622–23*t*, 666*t*
  place in diet, 199, 363
  protein concentrate, 363
Flavin adenine dinucleotide (FAD), 92, 176
Flavins, 176

Flavoproteins, 43
Flavoring agents, sodium-restricted diet, 546
Flour, 245, 278*t*
Fluids. *See also* Water
  anions, 128, 128*t*
  balance, 127*t*, 137
    burns, 485
    dumping syndrome, 486
    heart disease, 541, 542
    kidney, role, 126–27
    potassium, 130, 555
    protein, 135–36
    regulation, 135–38, **136**
    sodium, 135
    surgical conditions, 480
  body, 16, 125
  cations, 128, 128*t*
    compartments, 125, **126**
  diets, 396–97
    blenderized, 482
    parenteral, 480, 481
    tube, 482, 483*t*
  digestive secretions, 135
  exchange, 135
  excretion, obligatory, 126
  losses, 126
  requirements, 127
  sources to body, 126
Fluorine, 118–19
  osteoporosis, 119, 515
  poisoning, 259
  summary, 145
  water supply, 119
Fluorosis, dental, 119
Fluorouracil, 374*t*
FMN (flavin mononucleotide), 176
Folacin, 187–88
  absorption test, 453
  ascorbic acid, 167, 188
  characteristics, 186, 187–88
  deficiency, 188, 452
  diet, basic, 207*t*
  dietary allowances, 31*t*, 188
    Canadian, 684*t*
    pregnancy 291
    U.S. RDA, 279*t*
  discovery, 187
  food sources, 188, 642–57*t*
  functions, 188
  metabolism, 188
  relation to vitamin B_{12}, 188
  summary, 191
Folic acid, 187–88
Folinic acid, 167
Folklore, food, 217–18
Follicular hyperkeratosis, 153
Food(s), acceptance, 215–22, 317–18, 320, 321–22
  acid-producing, 138–39, 567
  additives, 264–67
  adulterated, 276
  alkali-producing, 138–39, 567
  allergens, 578
  baby, 307–10, 658–59*t*
  basic diet, 35, 206*t*, 207*t*, **208**
  breakfast, 246
  budget, 237–40, **239**
  chemicals in, 256–58

Food(s) [*Cont.*]
  composition, factors affecting, 36
    tables, 37, 617–73
  consumption, United States, 7–8, 197, **200**
  convenience, 240
  cookery, effect on enzymes, 261
    vitamin losses, 168, 174–75
  cost, plans, two levels, 249–50*t*
  cultural patterns, 224–36
  dietetic, 281, 414, 501, 549, **549**
  digestion, 19–23, 434
  economy, 237–48
  enrichment, 277–78
  fabricated, 247
  faddism, 332–33, 343–45, 404
  flavoring aids, 546
  fortification, 277–78
  Four Food Groups, **34–35**, 35
  functions, 19
  gastrointestinal function, effect, 432*t*, 433–35
  habits, 215–23
  health, relation to, 3–13
  illness from, 253–59
  industry, 271
  labeling, 278–81, **280**
  laws, 271–74
    enforcement, 274–77
  marketing systems, 237
  misbranded, 276
  mixtures, protein, 364
  nutrients, 33, 617–73*t*
  plans, two cost levels, 249–50*t*
  political significance, 218–19
  preservation, 259–64
  radioactivity, 259
  safety, legal controls, 271–81
  satiety value, 22, 76
  selection, 237–48
  service, mentally ill, 518–20
    patients, 376–77
  spoilage, 259–61
  standards, FDA, 276–77
  strongly flavored, 435
  supply, national, 9, 196
    world, 362–64
  water, 126
Food Additives Amendment, 272
Food and Agriculture Organization, 361
Food and Drug Administration, 274–77
  inspections, 274, **275**
  regulations, additives, 272–73
    enrichment, 278, 278*t*
    labeling, 279–80, **280**
    packaging, 273
    pesticides control, 273, 344
    standards, identity, 245, 276–77
Food, Drug, and Cosmetic Act, 272
Food for Freedom Program, 362
Food habits, 215–23
  age, influence, 221
  appetite, 217
  changes, 224–25
  children, 313
  communications media, influence, 218
  cultural influences, 217–22, 341–42
  development, 313
    infants, 307
    preschool children, 318–20
    school children, 320
    teen-agers, 321–22
  emotional outlets, 221–22
  family influence, 6–7, 218
  folklore, 217–18, 284–85
  hunger, 217
  illness, children, 585
    effect, 222, 371–72
  meal patterns, 218
  meanings of food, 3, 220–21
  modified diets, 372
  movements affecting, 219
  older persons, 332–33
  pattern of living, 6
  physiologic bases, 215–16, **216**
  political significance, 218–19
  psychologic influence, 518–19
  religious influence, 221
  sex, role, 221
  social value, 220–21
  taboos, 217–18
Food and Nutrition Board, 29, 31*t*, 86, 278
Food patterns, Black Americans, 229
  Chinese, 234
  Italian, 232–33
  Japanese, 224
  Jewish, Orthodox, 227–29
  Mexican-American, 230–32
  Near East, 233–34
  Puerto Rican, 229–30
  regional, U.S., 225
  vegetarian, 225–27
Food preservation, 259–64
Food programs, 359–60
  stamps, 357
  women, infants, children, 359–60
Food Protection Committee, 281
Formula diet, obesity, 411
Formulas for infants, 304–305
Four Food Groups, 34–35, **35**, 205–208
Fractures, diet following, 486
  osteoporosis, 515
Freezing of food, 262–63
Frijoles refritos, 231
Frittata, 232
Frölich, 166
Fructose, 61, 62, **62**, 65
  diabetic diets, 501
Fructosemia, 610
Fructosuria, 492
Fruit(s), 20, 201–202, 243–45
  acid-base balance, 139
  carbohydrates, 71, 72, 202
  diet, basic, 35, **100**, 201–202, 206*t*, 207*t*, **208**
  lists, controlled protein, potassium, and sodium diet,
    561–62
    exchanges for meal planning, 400, 661
    phenylalanine-restricted diet, 605
  minerals, **107**, **110**, **114**, 131, 202
  nutritive value, 100, 196, 197*t*, 201–202, 627–30*t*, 668*t*
  protein, 54*t*, **55**, 202
  purchase, 245
  vitamins, 152, **152**, 167, **168**, **174**, **177**, 202
Fruit-free cereal-free elimination diet, 580
Fruitarians, 225
Fuel factors, 92–93
Full-fluid diet, 396–97
Funk, 172

Galactase deficiency, 460
Galactolipins, 64
Galactose, 61, 62, **62**, 65
Galactose disease, 609–10
Galactose-free diet, 460, 609–10
Galactose-1-phosphate uridyl transferase, 609
Galactosuria, 493
Gallbladder, cholesterol, 473
    disease, 472–75
    fat-restricted diet, 473–75
    function, 81, 472
Ganglionic blockers, 374t
Ganglionic stimulators, 375t
Gastrectomy, anemia, 187
    diet following, 483
    dumping syndrome, diet, 486–88
    iron absorption, 484
Gastric analysis, 431
Gastric atony, 431
Gastric juice, 24t, 135, 431, 432t
Gastric resection, 456
Gastric surgery, 483–85
Gastrin, 21t
Gastritis, 436–37
Gastroesophageal sphincter, 19
Gastrointestinal function, acidity, 432t, 433
    adrenocortical therapy, 509
    carbohydrate, 64, 73
    children, 314, 318
    dehydration, effect, 137
    digestive comfort, 434
    electrolytes, 129, 131, 132
    fats, 82–83
    fiber, 65
    indigestible polysaccharides, 63, 64
    motility, influence of food, 432t, 433–34
    older persons, 330
    pregnancy, changes, 288
    protein deficiency, 419
    steroid therapy, influence, 509
    tests, 431–33
    tone, 432t
    vitamin deficiencies, 175, 180
Gastrointestinal system diseases, 431–65
    allergic manifestations, 578
    bowel motility, alterations, 443–45
    diagnostic tests, 431–33
    dietary considerations, 433–34
    diets, liberal, 435
        traditional, 435
    diverticulitis, 446–47
    esophagus, 435–36
    food-borne, 253–56
    gallbladder disease, 472–75
    gluten-induced enteropathy, 452–64
    lactase deficiency, 456–60
    lesions, effect of food, 434
    liver, 467–72
    lumen, abnormalities, 456
    malabsorption, 452–66
    mucosa, inflammatory disease, 445–49
    mucosal cell transport, 456–64
    pancreatitis, 475–76
    peptic ulcer, 437–41
    small intestine, problems, 443–49
    stomach, 436–37
    surgery, 483–85, 486–88
    ulcerative colitis, 448

Gastrostomy, 482
Gefillte fish, 228
Gelatin, 45
Genetic code, 50
Genetic diseases, allergy, 577
    diabetes, 491–505
    favism, 257
    fructosemia, 610
    galactose disease, 609–10
    homocystinuria, 608
    hypercholesterolemia, 610–11
    hypoglycemia, leucine-induced, 608–609
    maple syrup urine disease, 607–608
    phenylketonuria, 600–607
    tyrosinemia, 607
    tyrosinosis, 607
    Wilson's disease, 610
Geriatrics, 328
Gerontology, 328
Giordano-Giovanetti diet, 556
Girls, adolescent, anemia, 572
    dietary needs, 321–22
    food habits, 321, 322
    growth rate, 315
    height-weight table, 676
    nutritional requirements, 31t, 321t
    pregnancy, 287, 289, 291, 292t
Gliadin, 43, 461
Globin, 43, 113
Glomerular filtration rate, 132, 555
Glomerulonephritis, acute, 552–53
    chronic, 553–54
Glomerulus, **132**
Glossitis, 177, 180, 187
Glucagon, 67, 84, 491
Glucocorticoids, 373t, 508
Glucogenesis, 51, 491
Glucokinase, 68
Gluconeogenesis, 67, **67**, 494
Glucose, 61, 62, **62**
    absorption, 65
    available, 522
    blood, 66–68, **67**
    chemical structure, **62**
    malabsorption, 460
    metabolism, 65–70, **69**
        chromium, role, 120
        conversion to fat, 68
        diabetes, 494
        energy yield, 92
        glycogen formation, 68, **69**, 70, 508
        hormones, 67, 216, 508
        hydrolysis, 62, 64
        oxidation, 68, **69**, 70
        phosphorylation, 68
        sodium pump, 65
        synthesis, 67
        transport, 65
        vitamins, 68, 70, 173, 176, 179, 182, 183, 185, 188
    sources, 62
    tolerance, 492, 493, **493**
        diabetes, 492
        hyperlipidemia, 531
        older persons, 330, 492
Glucose-galactase deficiency, 460
Glucose tolerance factor, 120
Glucose-1-phosphate, **69**
Glucose-6-phosphate, 68, **69**

Glucostatic theory, 215–16
Glucosuria, 66
Glucuronic acid, 64
Glutamic acid, 44t, 187
  transamination, 51
Glutathione, 111, 257
Glutathione oxidase, 120
Gluten, 245
Gluten-induced enteropathy, 461–64
Gluten-restricted diet, 462–64
Glutenin, 43
Glyceraldehyde, 69
Glycerokinase, 85
Glycerol, 63, 76, **82**, 83, 85
Glycine, 42, 44t
Glycogen, 63, 72
  metabolism, 66, **66**, **67**, 68, **68**, **69**, 70
    conversion to glucose, 64, 67, 182
    diabetes mellitus, 494
    hormones, 67, 508
    phosphorylation, 182
    synthesis, 63, **66**, **67**, 68, **69**, 130, 131
  storage, body, 66, **67**, 68
Glycogenesis, **67**, 68
Glycogenolysis, 67, **67**, 130
Glycolipids, 77
Glycolysis, 68, 133
Glycosides, 64, 257
Glycosuria, 66, 493, 494, 496
Goiter, endemic, 116
  exophthalmic, 509
Goitrogens, 116, 257, 258
Goldberger, 178, 181
Golgi complex, 18
Gonadotropins, pregnancy, 288
Gossypol, 257
Gout, 512–14
  dietary counseling, 513
  purine-restricted diet, 513–14
Granos, 230
GRAS list, 272
Graves' disease, 509
Greece, dietary patterns, 233–34
Green revolution, 363
Grijns, 172
Griseofulvin, 375t
Group feeding, elderly, 334, **335**
Growth, development, infant, 298–99, 313
  energy metabolism, 95, 98
  failure, 10, 588
  hormone, 49
  rate, boys and girls, 315
    infants, 298
Growth retardation, 314–15
Guanethidine, 374t
Guanine, 50

Half-life, radioisotope, 259
Handicapped, 385–87
  children, feeding, 595–96
  food preparation aids, 386–87
  nutrition, 385
  self-help devices, 386
HANES survey, 406t, 571, 572t
Harosseth, 228
Health, agencies, 352t, 353t
  carbohydrate, role, 10, 72–73

defined, 3
  fat, role, 10, 87–88
  food, relationship, 3–14
  goals, 12–13
  problems, elderly, 330–31
  professionals, role, 351
Health aide, home, 384, **384**
"Health" foods, 343–44
Heart diseases, 541–51
  atherosclerosis, 526–37
  clinical findings, 541
  control programs, 360
  diet, 541–42
    fat-controlled, 530–37
    sodium-restricted, 542–47
  dietary counseling, 548–49
  vegetarian benefits, 226
Heat, effect on protein, 46
Heat regulation, body, 97, 126
Height, nutritional status, 286
  -weight tables, children, 657t, 676t
    men and women, 677t
Helminths, 256
Hematologic studies, 679–80t
Hematopoiesis, 187
Heme, 113
Hemicellulose, 63, 64, 65
Hemodialysis, 555
Hemoglobin, 45, 112, 118, 570
  acid-base balance, 139
  formation, 112, 113, 182
  infants, 298, 300
  -oxyhemoglobin system, 139
  pregnancy, 288
Hemolysis, vitamin E lack, 160
Hemorrhage, anemia, 571
  ascorbic acid deficiency, 169
  cirrhosis, 471
  infants, vitamin K deficiency, 161
  ulcer, 440
Hemorrhagic nephritis, 552
Hemosiderosis, 115
Henle, loop, tubule, 132
Heparin, 64, 111, 374t
Hepatic coma, 472
Hepatitis, 468–71
  diet, 468–71
  etiology, 468
  symptoms, 468
  zinc need, 118
Hepatolenticular degeneration, 118, 610
Herbs, low-sodium diets, 546
Heredity. *See* Genetic diseases
Hernia, hiatal, 435–36
Hess, 155
Hexose monophosphate shunt, 70
Hexoses, 61–62, 62
High-calorie diet, 416
High-energy phosphate compounds, 68
High-fiber diet, 447–48
High-protein diet, 422–23
  fluid, 423–24
  high-fat, low-carbohydrate, 486–88
  moderate-fat, high-carbohydrate, 469–71
Hindus, food prohibitions, 221
Histidine, 43, 44t, 53t, 665–69t
Holst, 166

Home-delivered meals, 384
Home health aides, 383
Homemaker, services, 384
Homeostatic mechanisms, 26, 27
    calcium, 104, 105
    ionic balance, 136–37
    nitrogen balance, 48
    parathyroid hormone, 105
    renal function, 132–34, **133, 134**
    water balance, 136, **136**
Homocystinuria, 608
Hookworm infestation, 256
Hormones, adrenal, 136
    aldosterone, 130, 136, 137, 508
    androgenic, 49, 508, 515
    antidiuretic, 136
    carbohydrate metabolism, 67, 68
    digestion, regulation, 21t
    elderly, imbalance, 330
    fat metabolism, 84
    food intake, regulation, 216
    glucogenic, 491
    hypothalamus, 136
    mineralocorticoid, 508
    obesity, 408, 412
    osteoporosis, 514, 515
    pregnancy, 288
    protein metabolism, 49
    protein nature, 45
    sex, 81
    sodium metabolism, 136
    thyroid, 95, 115
    thyroid-stimulating hormone (TSH), 116
    vitamin D, 156
    water balance, **136, 137**
"Hot dog" syndrome, 266
Hunger, 217
Hyaluronic acid, 64
Hydralazine, 374t
Hydrochloric acid, 24t
    absorption, minerals, 104, 109, 112
Hydrogen ion concentration, 138–40
Hydrogen transport, 92
Hydrogenation, fats, 78
Hydrostatic pressure, 133
Hydroxyapatite, 105
25-Hydroxycholecalciferol, 156
Hydroxylysine, 44t
Hydroxyproline, 44t
25-Hydroxyvitamin D_3, 156, 159
Hyperalimentation. *See* Parenteral nutrition
Hypercalcemia, 108
Hyperchlorhydria, 433
Hypercholesterolemia, 527, 610
Hyperglycemia, 66, 493, **493,** 496
Hyperinsulinism, 507
Hyperkalemia, 131, 555
Hyperlipidemia, 526–37
    definition, 527
    diabetes, 494
    dietary adjustments, 529
    dietary counseling, 533, 536–37
    dietary studies, long term, 529
    fat-controlled diet, 530
    five types, diet, 530–36
    types, 530–31
Hyperlipoproteinemia, 84, 527

Hypermagnesemia, 111
Hyperparathyroidism, 555, 564
Hyperperistalsis, 431
Hyperpotassemia, 131
Hypertension, 527, 549–50
    malignant, 554
    pregnancy, 294
    renal disease, 553, 554
    role of sodium, 130
    sodium restriction, 550
Hyperthyroidism, 95, 176, 479, 509–10
    diet, 510
    dietary counseling, 510
Hypertriglyceridemia, 527
Hyperuricemia, 512
Hyperventilation, 140, **140**
Hypervitaminosis, A, 155
    D, 158
Hypoalbuminemia, 420
Hypocalcemic tetany, 108
Hypochloremic alkalosis, **140,** 141
Hypochlorhydria, 433
Hypocholesteremic agents, 375t
Hypogeusia, 117
Hypoglycemia, 67
    Addison's disease, 508–509
    causes, 507
    fructosemia, 610
    hyperinsulinism, 507
        diet, 507
        dietary counseling, 508
        treatment, 502
    insulin shock, 502
    leucine-induced, 608–609
    oral drugs, 495
    types, 507
Hypoglycemic drugs, 375t, 495
Hypokalemia, 131, 563
Hypoproteinemia, 57, 420, 485, 554
Hyposensitization, allergy, 580
Hyposmia, 117
Hypothalamus, fluid regulation, 136
    hunger regulation, 215–16
Hypothyroidism, 95, 510
Hypoventilation, 140
Hysterectomy, diet following, 485

Ileal bypass surgery, 485
Ileostomy, 485
Ileum, absorption, 23
    disease, 445–46
    resection, 456, 484–85
Illness, caused by food, 253–59
    comprehensive care, 380
    food acceptance, during, 371–72
    food problems, children, 585
        older persons, 518–19
    nutritional stress, 371
Immobilization, nutrition following, 371, 385, 419
    urinary calculi, 564
Immunopolysaccharides, 64
Inborn errors of metabolism, 26, 600–611
Incaparina, 56, 364
Income, diet of older persons, 328
    food cost, 237, **238**
    poor people, aids to nutrition, 357
    restriction on diet, 340–41

Indigestion, 436
Indomethacin, 374t
Infant(s), amino acid requirements, 53t
　anemia, 188, 572, 574
　beriberi, 175
　bone development, 105, 298
　bottle feeding, 303–306
　　home preparation, 304–305
　　proprietary, 304
　　technique, 305–306
　brain development, 299, 518
　breast feeding, 301–303, **302**
　　adequacy, 303
　　advantages, 301
　　contraindications, 301
　　technique, 302–303
　celiac disease, 589–90
　colic, 589
　condition at birth, mother's diet, 285–87
　constipation, 589
　diarrhea, 589
　diet, 307–10
　dietary allowances, 31t, 299t
　　Canadian, 684–85t
　digestion, 298
　eczema, 80, **81,** 594
　energy, 299
　feeding, intervals, 303
　　problems, 588–89
　　self-demand, 303
　food habits, 307
　food plans, cost, 249t, 250t
　food programs, 359–60
　foods, 307–10, 658–59t
　　home-prepared vs. proprietary, 307–308
　　introducing new, 307, 308, **308**
　glucose-galactase deficiency, 460
　growth and development, 298–99
　growth failure, 588
　height-weight tables, 675–76
　hemorrhagic disease, 161
　hypercalcemia, 108
　hypocalcemia, 300
　inborn errors of metabolism, 600–611
　kidney function, 298
　lactase deficiency, 456
　linoleic acid, 87
　malnutrition, 57, 340, 342, 345–49
　mineral needs, 114t, 115, 300–301
　mortality, neonatal, 284
　neonatal tetany, 304
　nutrition, 298–312
　nutritional requirements, 31t, 299–301, 299t
　overnutrition, 310
　phenylketonuria, 600–607
　premature, development, 306
　　feeding technique, 306–307
　　formula, 306
　　nutritional needs, 306
　　schedule, 307
　protein, 299
　rickets, 158, **158**
　salt excesses, 310
　scurvy, 169, **169**
　supplementary foods, vitamins, 307–10
　vitamin B₆ deficiency, 182
　vitamin needs, 161, 301

　water balance, 127, 300
　weaning, 303
　weight gain, 298
Infections, common cold, 169
　diabetes, 503
　diet, 426–30
　food-borne, 254
　nutrition, 151, 169
Infectious hepatitis, 468
Inositol, 63, 85, 189, 191
Insalata, 232
Insecticides, 266
Insensible perspiration, 127
Instruction, patient. *See* Counseling (dietary); Education
　(nutrition)
Insulin, 68, 111
　administration, **500**
　carbohydrate, action, **67,** 68
　carbohydrate distribution, 497t
　chromium, 120
　defect, diabetes mellitus, 491, 494
　fat metabolism, 68, 84, 85
　juvenile diabetes, 591
　-like activity, 491
　shock, 502
　tissue synthesis, 49
　types, 495t
　unitage, 495
Interagency Committee on Nutrition Education, 354
Intercellular cement substance, 167, 168
International unit, vitamin A, 149, 150
　vitamin D, 155
　vitamin E, 159
Interstitial fluid, 125, 136
Intestinal juice, 25t, 135
Intestinal lymphangiectasia, 465
Intestines, **21,** 22
　absorption sites, 23, **461**
　digestion, 20–22
　diseases, 443–51
　　carcinoma, 449
　　colon, 443–45, 448–49
　　ileum, 445–46
　　inflammatory, 445–50
　　lumen, 456
　　motility, alterations, 443–44
　　mucosal transport, 456–65
　enzymes, 24, 25t
　large, functions, 22
　mucosa, structure, **21**
　obstruction, 445, 485
　small, functions, 22
　surgery, 456, 483–88
Intoxication, bacterial food, 255
Intracellular fluid, 16, 125, **126,** 129, 130
Intravenous feedings, 307, 397, 481, 485
Intrinsic factor, 185, 187, 484
Iodine, 115–16
　diet, children, 316
　　pregnancy, 290, 291t
　dietary allowances, 31t, 116
　　Canadian, 685t
　　U.S. RDA, 279t
　food sources, 116
　functions, 115
　goitrogens, 116
　protein bound, 95, 115, 510, 681t

summary, 143
Iodine-131, 116, 259
Iodized salt, 116
Iodopsin, 151
Ion, 127
Iron, 112–15
 absorption, 112, **113**
 ascorbic acid, 167
 blood, 112, 681*t*
 cytochromes, 92
 deficiency, 115, 571–73, **572**
 diet, basic, **114**, 206*t*
  United States, **9**, 197*t*
 dietary allowances, 31*t*, 33*t*, 113–14, 114*t*
  Canadian, 33*t*, 685*t*
  infants, 114*t*, 300
  pregnancy, 114*t*, 290, 291*t*
  U.S. RDA, 279*t*
 distribution, body, 103, 112
 enrichment, 278*t*
 excess, 115
 excretion, 113
 food sources, 114–15, **204**, 206*t*, **208**, 618–40*t*
  availability to body, 115
  effect of cookery, 115
 functions, 112, 113
 metabolism, 112–13, **113**
 storage, body, 112
 summary, 144
 supplements, anemia, 572
 transport, blood, 112–13
 turnover, 113
Irradiation of foods, 264
Irritable colon syndrome, 445
Ischemia, 527
Islamites, 221
Islands of Langerhans, 68, 491
Isohydric transport, 139
Isoleucine, 44*t*, 46
 content of foods, 665–69*t*
 maple syrup urine disease, 607–608
 requirements, 53*t*
Isomaltase deficiency, 459
Isoniazid therapy, 374*t*
 vitamin B₆, 183, 429
Italians, food habits, 232–33

Japanese, dietary changes, 224–25
Jaundice, 467
Jejunoileostomy, 485
Jejunum, absorption, **461**
 resection, 460
Jewish food habits, 227–29, **228**
Joints, diseases, 510–12
Joule, 92

Kasha, 229
Kashruth, 227
Keratin, 43
Keratinization, vitamin A lack, 153
Keto acid, 51
Ketogenesis, 51, 86, 522
Ketogenic diet, 522, 523*t*
 obesity, 412
α-Ketoglutaric acid, 51, **69**, 70
Ketohexose, 62

Ketone bodies, 86, 494, 522
Ketonemia, 494
Ketonuria, 86, 493, 522
 maple syrup urine disease, 607–608
 phenylketonuria, 600–607
Ketosis, 64, 493, 521
Kidneys, acid-base balance, 139–40
 acid secretion, 139–40
 ammonia production, 140
 calculi, 563–67
 dialysis, 555–56
 diseases, 552–69
  diet, 553, 554, 556–63
  dietary counseling, 558–60
 electrolyte balance, 132, 136, 137, **137**
 energy requirement, 133
 failure, 554–63
 functions, 132–34
 infants, 298, 306
 glomerular filtration, 132, **133**
 glucose threshold, 66, **67**
 secretory activity, 134
 transplants, 563
 tubules, 133–34, **134**
 urine, composition, 134, 682*t*
 water balance, 132, 136, **136**
 water loss, 126
Kilocalorie, 92
Kilojoule, 92
King, 166
Kishke, 228
Kloese, 229
Knishes, 228
Korsakoff's syndrome, 521
Krebs cycle, **69**, 70
Krebs-Henseleit cycle, 51–52, **52**
Kreplach, 228
Kuchen, 229
Kuhn, 176
Kwashiorkor, 10, 57, **57**, 345–49, **346**
 biochemical changes, 347
 etiology, 345
 mineral deficiencies, 111, 117
 prevention, 348
 symptoms, 57, 347
 treatment, 348

Labeling, 33, 277, 278–81, **280**
 diets for allergy, 581
 Fair Packaging and, Act, 273–74
 fats, 87
 sodium-restricted diet, **543**, 548–49, **549**
Lactalbumin, 43, 198, 303
Lactase, 25*t*
Lactase deficiency, 73, 456–57
 diet, 457–59
  counseling, 457
 test, 453
Lactation, diet, 292*t*, 294
 dietary allowances, 31*t*, 291*t*
  Canadian, 684–85*t*
 food plans, two cost levels, 249–50*t*
Lactic acid, 68, **69**, 70, 241
Lactic dehydrogenase, 117
Lactoflavin, 176
Lactoglobulin, 43, 198
Lacto-ovovegetarian diets, 56, 225

Lactose, 25t, 62
  intolerance, 73, 456–57
  milk, 198, 457
  tolerance test, 453
Lactose-controlled diet, 457
Lactose-free diet, 457–59
Lactosuria, 493
Lactovegetarian diets, 56, 225
Laennec's cirrhosis, 471
Lamb, 199, **200,** 242t
Lasagne, 232
Lathyrism, 257
Latkes, 229
Lauric acid, 78
L-casei factor, 187
LCT (long-chain triglycerides), 453, 454
Lead poisoning, 258
Leche Alim, 364
Lecithin, 77, **77,** 265t
Lecithinase, 25t
Leckach, 229
Legislation, 271–74
Legumes, 200, 243, 363
  nutrients, 56, 118, 119, 120, 184, 200, 623t
  toxicants, 257
Legumin, 43
Lenticular degeneration, 118
Leucine, 44t, 46
  content in foods, 665–69t
  diet low in, 608
  hypoglycemia induced by, 608–609
  maple syrup urine disease, 607–608
  requirements, 53t
Leukemia, 188
Levodopa, 375t
Levulose, 62
Lincomycin, 373t
Lind, 166
Line test, 155, **156**
Linmarin, 257
Linoleic acid, 77, 85
  chemical formula, **78**
  conversion to arachidonic acid, 80, 182
  deficiency, 80, **81**
  dietary allowances, 87
  food sources, 78, 79t, 87, **88, 530,** 532t, 618–40t
  function, 80
  vitamin needs, 160
Linolenic acid, 77, **78,** 79t, 80
Lipase, 24–25t
Lipids, 76–90. *See also* Cholesterol; Fat(s); Fatty acids
  absorption, 82–83
  atherosclerosis, 527–30
  blood, 83–84, 680t
  characteristics, **76, 77,** 78, 80
  classification, 76–77
  composition, 76
  dietary significance, 76
  digestion, 25t, 81–82
  food sources, 87, 618–40t
  functions, 80–81
  metabolism, 83–86
  peroxidation, 330
  role in health, 87–88
Lipogenesis, 67, 68, 83, 84, 494
Lipoic acid, 70, 189
Lipolysis, 83, 494

Lipoprotein(s), 43, 77, 83–84
  disease risks, 84, 527
  synthesis, 85
Lipoprotein lipase, 83, 531
Lipoproteinemia, α-beta, 460
Lipotropic factors, 85, 186, 188
Liquid diets, 396–97
Liver, diseases, 467–76
  alcoholism, 520
  cirrhosis, 471–72
  hepatic coma, 472
  hepatitis, 468–71
  functions, 24t, 467
  alcohol metabolism, 520
  bile production, 24t
  carbohydrate metabolism, 63, 66, 67, 68, 72
  fat metabolism, **84,** 85, 86
  protein metabolism, 49, 51, 420
  urea synthesis, 51
Lofenalac, 602, 604t
Long-chain triglycerides, 453, 454
Low-calorie diet, 410–11
Low-residue diet, 446
Lunch, patterns, 210
  poor habits, 315
  school, 322–24, **323**
Lungs, acid-base balance, 139, 140
  water losses, 126, 127
Lymph, 23, 83
Lymphangiectasia, 452t, 465
Lysine, **42,** 44t, 56, 204
  food sources, 665–69t
  heat, carbohydrate linkage, 46
  hydroxylation, ascorbic acid, 167
  opaque-2 corn, 363
  requirement, 53t
  supplementation, **44,** 56, 198
Lysosomes, 17

McCollum, 149, 172
Macrobiotic diet, 56
Macronutrients, 102
Magnesium, 109–11
  absorption, 109–10
  deficiency, 110–11
  diet, basic, **110,** 207t
    United States, 110, 196, 197t
  dietary allowances, 31t, 110
    Canadian, 685t
    U.S. RDA, 279t
  food sources, 110, **110,** 641–57t
  functions, 109
  metabolism, 68, 109–10
  summary, 142
Magnesium hydroxide, 373t
Malabsorption, 23, 452–65. *See also* Gastrointestinal
    system diseases
  deficiencies, 111, 419, 452, 460
  diagnostic tests, 452–53
  diarrhea, 444
  diet, medium-chain-triglyceride, 453
  dietary counseling, 455–56, 457, 464
  disorders, 452t
  inborn errors of metabolism, 600–611
  laboratory findings, 452
  symptoms, 452
  treatment, 453

vitamin lack, 176
Malnutrition, 5, 11. *See also* Anemia; Deficiency
    diseases; Protein-calorie malnutrition;
    Underweight
  diseases, summary, 338t
  economic cost, 339
  factors contributing, 340–43
  infection, 346, **347**
  programs against, 351–64
  United States, 8–10
  vulnerable groups, 340
Maltase, 25t, 64
Maltose, 25t, 62
Manganese, 119, 681t
Manicotti, 232
Mannose, 61, 62, **62**
MAO inhibitors, 374t
Maple syrup urine disease, 607–608
Marasmus, 10, 57, 347, **348**
Margarine, 78, 87
Masa, 231
Maternal-child health, 284
Maternal mortality, 284
Matsoth, 227, 229
Maturity, later, 328–36
MCT (medium-chain triglycerides), 453, 476
Meal planning, 208–12
  basic pattern, 35–36
  economy, 237–50
  factors in, 209t
  food plans, two cost levels, 249t, 250t
  meal patterns, 208–11, **210, 212**
  snacks, 211, **212**
Meal service, patients, 376–77
Meals on Wheels, 335
Meat, 199–201, 242–43
  analogs, 247
  characteristics, 242
  cholesterol, 87, 88t, 201, 670–73t
  cookery, vitamin retention, 175, 177
  cost, 242, **243**
  diet, basic, 54, 206t, 207t
    United States, 19, **55**, 199, 200
  extractives, 201
  fat content, 87, **88**, 201
  fatty acids, 78, 79t
  inspection, 274, **275**
  lists, exchanges, meal planning, 400, 663
    fat-controlled diet, 534
    protein-controlled diet, 560
    sodium-restricted diet, 545
  minerals, **106, 107**, 109, 110, **110, 114**, 115, 117, 118,
    120, 201
  nitrite/nitrates, 264–65
  nutritive value, 196, 197t, 200–201, 620–22t, 659t,
    665–66t, 667t
  protein, 54t, **55**, 200, 201
  selection, 242
  trichinella, 256, 264
  vitamins, **152**, 174, **174**, 177, **177**, 179, **180**, 184, 188,
    201
Meat-base formula, 609
Meat Inspection Act, 274
Mechanical soft diet, 393
Medium-chain-triglyceride diet, 454–55
  dietary counseling, 455–56
Megadoses, vitamins, 69, 183

Megaloblastic anemia, 187, 188
Melanin, 118
Melanophore-stimulating hormone, 509
Mellanby, 155
Men, dietary allowances, 31t
    Canadian, 684–85t
  height-weight table, 677t
Menadione, 161
Menaquinone, 161
Mendel, 43, 149
Menstruation, iron loss, 571
Mental development, malnutrition, 57, 347–48
  nutritional factors, 518
Mental effort, caloric need, 96
Mental illness, diet, 518–20
  nutritional deficiencies, 175, 180, 187, 518
Mental retardation, 595–96
  inborn errors, 601, 607, 608, 609
  iodine lack, 116
  role of nutrition, 347–48
Mercury poisoning, fish, 258
Mesomorph, 408
Metabolic acidosis, 141
Metabolic alkalosis, 141
Metabolic pool, 26
Metabolic rate, 94–95
Metabolism, 18–19
  alcohol, 520
  basal, 94–95
  calcium, 105–106
  carbohydrate, 65–70, **66, 69**
  common pathways, 27, **27, 52**
  defined, 18
  dynamic equilibrium, 26
  energy, 91–101
  errors of, 600–611
  fat, **82, 83**–86, **84**
  intermediary, 26–27, **27**
  iron, 112–13
  magnesium, 109
  phosphorus, 109
  potassium, 130–31
  pregnancy, 95
  protein, 47–52, **47, 50, 52**
  purine, 512
  sodium, 129
  water from, 126
Metalloproteins, 43
Metformin, 375t
Methionine, **42**, 43, 44t, 46, 46t, 56
  foods, 665–69t
  function, 45, 85
  homocystinuria, 608
  requirements, 53t
  sulfur, 111, 112
Methotrexate, 374t
Methyl groups, 45, 85, 186, 188
Methyldopa, 374t
Metric system, conversion to, 683t
Meulengracht diet, 435
Mexicans, food patterns, 225, 230–32
Micelles, 82
Micronutrients, 102, 112–21
Microvilli, 23
Middle West, foods, 225
Milk, 196, 198–99, 240–42
  calcium, 106, 107t, 107, 198, 199

Milk [*Cont.*]
  carbohydrate, 62, 72, 198
  Daily Food Guide, 35*t*
  diet, basic, **198**, 206*t*, 207*t*
  economy, 242
  fat, 78, 79*t*, 87, 198
  filled, 241
  fortified, 157, 199
  human, compared with cow's, 303–304, 304*t*
  imitation, 247
  infant formulas, 304–305
  intolerance, 594
    allergy, diet without, 582
    anemia, infants, 572
    galactose disease, 609–10
    lactase deficiency, 456–59
  lists, exchanges for meal planning, 400, 660
    fat-controlled diet, 534
    protein-controlled diet, 560
    sodium-restricted diet, 544
  market forms, 240–41
  nutritive values, 196, 198–99, 206*t*, 207*t*, 618*t*, 665*t*
  overuse, 315
  pasteurization, 261
  protein, 54*t*, **55**
  school lunch, 324, 325
  symbolic meaning, 221
  vitamins, **152**, 174, **174**, 176, **177**
Milk-alkali syndrome, 108
Milk sensitivity, 594
Milliequivalents, 127, 128, 681
Mineral elements, 102–21. *See also* specific minerals
  acid-base balance, 138–39
  body distribution, 102, 103*t*
  deficiency, 106–107, 108, 115, 116, 117
  dietary allowances, 31*t*
    Canadian, 33*t*, 684–85*t*
    FAO/WHO, 33*t*
    United Kingdom, 33*t*
    U.S. RDA, 279*t*
  dynamic equilibrium, 102–103
  food sources, 102–103, 618–40*t*, 641–57*t*
  functions, 102
  nutrition education, 141
  summary, 142–45
  trace, 112–21
  urine, 682*t*
Mineral oil, 83, 150, 375*t*
Mineralocorticoids, 508
Minestrone soup, 232
Minimum daily requirements, 279
Misbranding food, 276
Mitochondria, 17, **17**, 68, 70
Modified diets, 390–93
Modified food starches, 308
Molds, toxins, 257
Molybdenum, 120
  copper metabolism, 120, 256
  summary, 145
Monkshood, 257
Monoamine oxidase inhibitor, 258, 374*t*
Monoglycerides, 76
Monosaccharides, 61–62, **62**
Monosodium glutamate, 543
Mortadella, 232
Motility, gastrointestinal tract, 22, 81–82, 431, 432*t*, 433
Mouth, digestion, 20, 24*t*

surgery, 483
Mozzarella cheese, 232
Mucin, 22, 24*t*
Mucopolysaccharides, 105, 111, 151
Mucoproteins, 43, 151
Mucosa, **21**, 23, 151
Mucosal cell transport, abnormalities, 460–64
Mulder, 41
Mul-Soy, 609
Muscle, activity, metabolism, 96
  contraction, 103
    fat oxidation, 84
    glycogen, 64, **67, 69**
Muscular dystrophy, 160
Mushroom poisoning, 257
Mycotoxins, 120, 257
Myocardial infarction, 527
Myoglobin, 112
Myristic acid, 79*t*
Myxedema, 510

NAD, 68, 92, 179
NADP, 68, 109, 179
NADPH, 70, 85, 109
Name, 230
National Communicable Disease Center, 253, 254
National Dairy Council, 353*t*
National Livestock and Meat Board, 353*t*
National nutrition policy, 351
National Nutrition Survey, 10, 168
National Research Council, 29, 31*t*
National School Lunch Act, 322
"Natural" foods, 266, 344
Nausea, pregnancy, 293–94
Near East, dietary patterns, 233–34
Nematodes, 256
Neomycin, 373*t*, 457
Neonatal tetany, 304
Nephritis, 552–54
Nephron, 132, **132**, 134
Nephrosclerosis, 554
Nephrosis, 554, 592–94
  diet, 593
Nervous system, allergic reaction, 578
  disturbances, 518–25
  mineral elements, role, 80, 102, 103, 109, 129
  nutrition, 518
  transmission, impulse, 103
  vitamin deficiencies, 175, 180, 187, 518
Neuropathy, alcoholism, 521
  liver disease, 472
  pernicious anemia, 573
New England, foods, 225
Niacin, 177–80
  chemistry and characteristics, **173**, 178
  deficiency, 180, **181**, 518
  diet, basic, **180**, 206*t*, **208**
    United States, 196, 197*t*
  dietary allowances, 31*t*, 33*t*, 179
    Canadian, 33*t*, 684*t*
    U.S. RDA, 279*t*
  early studies, 177–78
  enrichment, 278
  excretion products, 179
  food sources, 179, 197*t*, 618–40*t*
  function, 179
  hyperlipoproteinemia, 179

measurement, 179
NADPH, 85
physiology, 179
retention in food, 180
storage, body, 179
summary, 190
tryptophan, 45, 179, 182
Niacinamide, 177, 180
Nickel, 103*t*
Nicotinamide adenine dinucleotide (NAD), 68, 92, 179
Nicotinamide adenine dinucleotide phosphate (NADP), 68, 179
Nicotine, 375*t*
Nicotinic acid, 177, 178, 375*t*
Night blindness, 153, **154**
Nitrates/nitrites, 264–65
Nitrogen, balance, 47–48
  constituents, blood, 680*t*
    urine, 682*t*
  excretion, 48
  retention, renal disease, 555
Nitrosamines, 265
Nomenclature, diets, 392
Nontropical sprue, 461
Nopalitos, 231
Norepinephrine, 84
Normal diet, 389–90, 391*t*
  modifications, 390–93
Nuclear attack, food safety, 259
Nucleic acid, 25*t*, 160
Nucleoproteins, 43, 138, 512
Nucleus, cell, 17
Nurse, goals, nutrition study, 11–13
  role, nutrition education, 12
    patient care, 12, 370–71
    public health, 12
Nursing homes, feeding, 518–19
Nutramigen, 609
Nutrients, 4
  absorption, 23–24
  carbohydrate, 64–70, **66**
  common pathways, 27, **27**
  digestion, 19–22, 24–25
  fats, 81–86, **82, 84**
  minerals, 102–24, 127–32
  proteins, 45–52
  vitamins, 148–65, 166–71, 172–95
Nutrition, aides, 357, **358**
  balance, 10
  children, 313–25
  community, 351–66
  disciplines, related, 5, **6**
  education, 12, 57, 73, 88, 100, 141, 189, 192, 353–56.
    See also Counseling (dietary)
  excesses, 10
  infants, 298–310
  infections, 426
  labeling, 278–81, **280**
  later maturity, 328–36
  needs of sick, 369
  objectives for study, 11–13
  policy, national, 351
  pregnancy, lactation, 284–95
  preventive, primary, 10
  problems, international, 11, 337–50
    United States, 8–10, 337–45
  professional opportunities, 12

rehabilitation, 385–87, **386, 387**
relation to sciences, **6**
services, 351
surgical conditions, 479–88
surveys, 8, **9,** 10, 168, 286
therapeutic, 369–77
Nutrition agencies, 352*t*, 353*t*
Nutritional care, 5, 380
  counseling, 380–83
  illness, 371–72
  patient, 369–71
  rehabilitation, 385–87
  team, 369–70, **369, 370**
Nutritional deficiencies, 337–40, 338*t. See also* specific deficiencies
Nutritional status, 4
  children, 314–15
  elderly, 329–31
  pregnancy, 284–86
Nyctalopia, 153

Obesity, 404–13
  adipose cell development, 84, 406
  atherosclerosis, 526
  body composition, 405–406, 408, **408**
  causes, 406–409, **407**
  childhood, 588
  diabetes mellitus, 492, **492, 502**
  diet, 410–12, 410*t*
  dietary counseling, 413–15
  exercise, 412
  faddism, 404
  food habits, 407
  genetic factors, 408
  hazards, 10, 404
  incidence, 406
  infant, 310
  maintenance of weight loss, 415
  measurement, skinfold, 405, **405**
  metabolism, 408–409
  older persons, 330
  pregnancy, 294
  prevention, 409
  psychologic aspects, 408
  treatment, 409–15
    assessment of patient, 409–10
    drugs, 412–13
    group therapy, 413
    hormones, 412
    surgical, 413
  types, 406, 408, **408**
  water retention, 406
  weight loss, rate, 406
Obstruction, esophagus, 436
  intestine, 445, 485
Occupational therapy, 386
Oils, 205
  coconut, 78
  fatty acids, 78, 79*t*, 87, **88**
  food preparation with, 536
  nutritive values, 197*t*, 205
  vitamin E, 160
Older Americans Act, 334
Older persons, diet, 328–36
Oleic acid, 77, 78, **78,** 79*t*, 85, 88*t*, 618–40*t*
Oliguria, 555
Opsin, 151

Oral contraceptives, 375*t*
Oral hypoglycemic drugs, 495
Organelle, 17
"Organic" foods, 266, 344
Orinase, 495
Ornithine, 42, 51, **52**
Osborne, 43, 149
Osmoreceptor system, 136
Osmosis, **133**, 135
Osmotic balance, 128, 130
Osmotic pressure, 128, 131, 132, **133**, 135, 136
Ossification, 105
Osteoarthritis, 510
Osteodystrophy, renal, 555
Osteomalacia, 108, 159
Osteoporosis, 108, 330, 514–15
    dietary counseling, 515
    etiology, 514
    fluoride, 119, 515
    metabolism, 515
    treatment, 515
Overnutrition, 5
    infants, 310
Overweight, 404–15
    pregnancy, 294
Oxalacetic acid, 69, 70
Oxalate-restricted diet, 566
Oxalic acid, 104, 109
    foods, 104, 202, 257, 566
    urinary calculi, 564, 566
Oxidase, 176
Oxidation, fatty acids, 85
    glucose, 68
    water, 126
Oxidative phosphorylation, 92, 109
Oxidative shunt, **69**, 70
Oxytetracycline, 263

Paklava, 234
Palatability, sensations affecting, 216–17
Palmitic acid, 78, 79*t*
Panapen, 230
Pancreas, cystic fibrosis, 476
    disease, diet, 475–76
    enzymes, 25*t*
    secretions, 25*t*, 135
Pancreatic extract, 476
Pancreatic insufficiency, 456
Pancreozymin, 21*t*
Pantothenic acid, 70, **173**, 183–84, 518
    deficiency, 184, 518
    diet, basic, 207*t*
    discovery, 183
    summary, 191
Para-aminobenzoic acid, 187
Para-aminosalicylic acid, 429
Parahydroxyphenylpyruvic acid oxidase, 607
Parasitic infestation of food, 255–56
Parathormone, 104, 105, 156
Paratyphoid fever, 254
Parenteral nutrition, 397, 480, 481
Parotid gland, 24*t*
Passive transport, 23, 24
Passover, 227
Pastafasiole soup, 232
Pastas, 232, 246
Pastasciutta, 232

Pasteurization, irradiation, 264
    milk, 177, 261
Patient, comprehensive care, 383–85
    factors influencing, 369–79
    counseling, diet, 380–83
    diet history, 381–82
    feeding, 376–77
        devices, self-help, 386–87
        mentally ill, 518–20
        older persons, 332
    food acceptance, illness, 371–72
    handicaps, 385
    home-delivered meals, 384
    homemaker services, 384
    interpersonal relationships, 372–76
    modified diets, 372
    needs for nursing, 370–71
    team approach, care, 369–70, **369, 370**
    tray service, 377
Paygel, Dietetic Baking Mix, 556
PBI (protein-bound iodine), 115
PCBs, 266
P-CM (protein-calorie malnutrition), 41, 57, 345–49
Pectin, 63, 65
Pellagra, 177–78, 180, **181**
Penicillamine, 183
Penicillin, 373
Pennsylvania Dutch, foods, 225
Pentoses, 62
    shunt, 68, **69**, 70, 174, 179
Pentosuria, 493, 600
Pepsin, 24*t*, 45, 46*t*
Pepsinogen, 24*t*, 46*t*
Peptic ulcer, 437–41
    bleeding, 440
    diagnostic tests, 431–33
    diet, bland, 438–40
        considerations, 433–34
        liberal/traditional, 435
    dietary counseling, 440–41
    etiology, 437
    symptoms, 438
    treatment, 438
Peptidase, 25*t*, 119
Peptide(s), 24*t*
Peptide linkage, 42, **43**
Perfringens poisoning, 254
Perinatal nutrition, 285–86
Periodontal disease, 10, 108
Peristalsis, 22, 431
Peritoneal dialysis, 556
Peritonitis, 485
Pernicious anemia, 185, 187, 573–74
Pernicious vomiting of pregnancy, 294
Peroxidation, lipid, 160, 330
Perspiration, losses in, 48, 127, 129, 137
Pesticides, 266, 344
    amendment, federal law, 272, 273
pH, 138, **140**
    chloride shift, 131
    gastric juice, 433
    variations in urine, diet, 564, 566
Phenethylbiguanide, 495
Phenformin, 375*t*, 495
Phenobarbital, 374*t*, 521
Phenolphthalein, 375*t*
Phenylacetic acid, 601

Phenylalanine, 43, 44t, 46t
  content in foods, 604t, 605–606t, 665–69t
  requirements, 53t, 603t
  tyrosine, conversion, 179, 183, 601, **601**
Phenylalanine hydroxylase, 601
Phenylalanine-restricted diet, 602–606
Phenylbutazone, 374t
Phenylketonuria, 600–607
  biochemical defect, 601, **601**
  clinical changes, 601
  diet, 602–606
  dietary counseling, 603, 606–607, **607**
  incidence, 600
  screening, 601
  treatment, 601
Phenylpyruvic acid, 601
Phenytoin, 374t, 521
Phosphatase, 109
Phosphate, high-energy compounds, 68, 91, 109
Phospholipids, 77, 80, 109, 118
Phosphoproteins, 43
Phosphorus, 108–109
  absorption, 109
  acid-base balance, 109
  body distribution, 103, 108, 128t, 129, 678t
  carbohydrate metabolism, 68, 109
  diet, basic, 207t
    calcium-phosphorus restricted, 565–66
  dietary allowances, 31t, 109
    Canadian, 685t
    U.S. RDA, 279t
  excess, calcium absorption, 300, 304
  foods, 109, 196, 197, 641–57t
  functions, 108, 109
  high-energy compounds, 68, 91, 109
  metabolism, 109
  protein synthesis, 50
  renal excretion, 140
  summary, 142
  urinary calculi, 564
  vitamin D, 155
Phosphorus-restricted diet, 565–66
Phosphorylation, 68, 92, 109
Photosynthesis, 61, 91
Phytic acid, 63, 104, 108, 110
Phytylmenaquinone, 161
Pica, 288
Pilavi, 233
Pinocytosis, 26, 82
Pituitary hormone, 136, 508, 509
PKU (phenylketonuria), 600–607
Placenta, development, 287–88
Plasma, electrolytes, 128t
  lipids, 83, 84
Pneumonia, 426
Poisoning, bacterial, 254–55
  chemical food, 258–59
  mushroom, 257
  natural food toxicants, 256–57
Polenta, 232, 233
Polychlorinated biphenyls (PCB), 266
Polysaccharides, 62–63
Polyunsaturated fatty acids, 77, **78**, 529
Poor people, characteristics, 356
  counseling, 354–56
  diet, 357
  malnutrition, 339, 340

nutrition, education, 357
  programs, nutrition, 358–61
Population and food, 11, 340–41, **341**
Pork, consumption, per capita, 199, **200**
  Trichinella, 256
Porphyrin, 182
Portagen, 453
Posole, 231
Postoperative diet, 481–82
Potassium, 130–31
  absorption, 130
  body distribution, 103t, 129
  deficiency, 131, 563
  diet, basic, 207t
    controlled, 558–63
  excess, 131, 557
  excretion, 131, 137, **137**
  foods, 131, 641–57t
  functions, 130
  metabolism, 130–31
    Addison's disease, 508
    fevers, 426, 427
    heart failure, 131
    renal failure, 555, 557
    surgery, 480
  requirement, 131
  summary, 143
Potassium, protein, and sodium controlled diet, 558–63
Potassium chloride, 375t
Poultry, consumption, 199
  inspection, 274
  nutritive values, 200, 621t, 670t
Poultry Inspection Act, 274
Poverty, 356–57
  undernutrition, 340
Pre-beta lipoproteins, 531
Precursor, niacin, 79
  vitamin A, 149
  vitamin D, 155
Prediabetes, 492
Prednisone, 373t
Preeclampsia, 286, 294
Pregestimil, 476, 589
Pregnancy, 284–97
  anemia, 294, 572, 574
  biochemical changes, 288
  complications, 293–94
  concept of care, WHO, 284
  constipation, 294
  diabetes, 492, 503
  diet, 291–93, 292t
    folklore, 284–85
  dietary allowances, 31t, 291t
    Canadian, 684–85t
  dietary counseling, 291–93
  fetal development, 105, 209t
  food plans, two cost levels, 249t, 250t
  gastrointestinal changes, 288
  hormones, 288
  malnutrition, vulnerability, 340
  metabolism, 95, 289
  mortality, 284
  nausea, 293–94
  nitrogen balance, 48
  nutrition before, 285
  nutrition during, 286, 289–91
  outcome, factors, 285, **285**

Pregnancy [*Cont.*]
  physiologic changes, 287–89, 290*t*
  stages, 287–89
  supplements, 293
  teen-age, 287, 291, 292*t*, 321
  toxemias, 294
  vomiting, 294
  weight status, 285–86
Premateral nutrition, 285
Premature infants, formula, 306–307
  nutrition of mother, 286
Prenatal nutrition, 286
Preoperative diet, 479–81
Preschool children, 317–20
Preservation, food, 259–64
Probana, 590
Probenecid, 375*t*, 512
Proenzyme, 18
Progesterone, 288, 375*t*
Program aides, nutrition, 357, **358**
Proline, 44*t*
Prosciutto, 232
ProSobee, 589, 609
Prostaglandins, 80
Protease, 45
Protein(s), 41–60
  absorption, amino acids, 46–47
  acid-base balance, 18, 128*t*, 139, 433
  amino acids, 42, 43, 53, 53*t*
  ammonia from, 51–52
  anabolism, 49–51
  biologic value, 43, 56
  blood, 45, 680*t*
  body, 16, 128*t*, 129
  brain development, 518
  calcium requirement, 106
  catabolism, 49, 51–52
  classification, 42–43
  complete, 43
  composition, 41
  deficiency, 11, 57, **57**, 347–49, 419–24
  diet, basic, 54, **55**, 206*t*, **208**
    for dumping syndrome, 486–88
    high-protein, 422–23
    high-protein, fluid, 423–24
    high-protein, moderate-fat, high-carbohydrate, 469–471
    high-protein, obesity, 410*t*, 411
    protein, sodium, potassium controlled, 558–63
    restricted protein, 559
    United States, 7, **7**, **9**, 54, 196, 197*t*
  dietary allowances, 31*t*, 33*t*, 53
    burns, 485
    Canadian, 33*t*, 684*t*
    celiac disturbances, 590
    children, 31*t*, 55, 316
    cirrhosis of the liver, 471
    colitis, 448
    diabetes mellitus, 496, 591
    fevers, 427
    gout, 513
    hepatic coma, 472
    hepatitis, 469
    hypoglycemia, 507
    infants, 31*t*, 299, 299*t*
    ketogenic diet, 522
    lactation, 31*t*, 55

    nephritis, 553
    nephrosis, 554, 593
    phenylketonuria, 603*t*, 604*t*
    pregnancy, 31*t*, 55, 290, 291*t*
    premature infant, 306
    protein deficiency, 421
    renal failure, 556
    short-bowel syndrome, 461
    surgical conditions, 479
    tuberculosis, 428
    U.S. RDA, 279*t*
  digestion, 24–25*t*, 45
  energy value, 45
  fluid balance, 135
  foods, cost, from meat and alternates, **243**
    mixtures, 56, 364
    sources, 54*t*, 54–57, **55**, 198, 200, 204, 206*t*, 618–40*t*
    textured vegetable protein, 247
  functions, 41, 45
  glucose formation, 51, 522
  hydrolysates, 602
  incomplete, 43
  intracellular fluids, 128
  lipoproteins, 43, 530–31
  malnutrition, 10, 57, 419–21
  metabolism, 47–52, **47**, **52**
    all-or-none law, 49
    carbohydrate, relationship, 66
    dynamic equilibrium, 48–49
    hormones affecting, 49, 508
    immobilization, effect, 385, 419
    liver, role, 48–49, 51
    nervous system, 518
    study methods, 47–48
  nitrogen balance, 47–48
  nutrition education, 57–58
  osmotic pressure, 135
  peptide linkage, 42, **43**
  plant, 56, 226, 363
  potassium, relationship, 130
  quality, 43, **44**, 56, 200–201
  reference, 200
  requirement, factors affecting, 52–53
    minimum, 48
  reserves, body, 49
  sparing action, carbohydrate, 64
  specific dynamic action, 97
  specificity, 42
  structure, 42
  supplementary value, 56
  synthesis, 50–51, **50**
  textured vegetable, 247
  urea from, 51–52
  vegetarianism, 56–57
Protein-bound iodine, 95, 115, 510
Protein-calorie malnutrition, 41, 345–49
  etiology, 345
  kwashiorkor, 57, **57**, 347
  marasmus, 57, 347, **348**
  mental development, 347–48
  synergism with infection, 346, **347**
  treatment, 348–49
Protein-free wheat starch, 556
Protein-restricted diet, 558–63
  phenylketonuria, 603–607
  protein, sodium, potassium controlled diet, 558–63
Proteose, 24*t*

Prothrombin, 161
Protogen, 189
Protoporphyrin, 113
Protozoa, food, 255
Provitamin, 149
Proximal tubule, nephron, 132
P/S ratio, fat, 86, 529, 530, 531
Psychiatric patients, feeding, 519–20
  nutritional deficiencies, 518
Psychology, diabetes, children, 590
  food habits, 215
  obesity, 404, 408, 413
Psychrophils, 260, **261**
Pteroylglutamic acid, 187
Ptyalin, 24*t*
Public health, illness from food, 253–59
  and the nurse, 12, 351
  nutrition, 337
Puerto Rican food habits, 229–30
Puma, 364
Pump, sodium, 65, 129
Purchase of foods, 237–50
Purine(s), metabolism, 184, 512
  sources, 201, 513*t*
  uric acid stones, 564, 566
Purine-restricted diet, 513–14
Pyloric valve, 19
Pyridoxal, **173,** 181
  phosphate, 51, 182
Pyridoxamine, **173,** 181
Pyridoxic acid, 182
Pyridoxine, **173,** 181. *See also* Vitamin B₆
Pyrimidine, 160
Pyruvic acid, 51, 68, **69,** 70, 92
  decarboxylation, 70, 173

Quackery, 343–45
Quail poisoning, 253

Radiation preservation of food, 264
Radioactive fallout, 259, **259**
Radioisotopes, 259
Rancidity, fats, 80, 153
Ravioli, 232
Recommended Dietary Allowances, 29–33, 31*t*
  comparison, other countries, 32–33, 33*t*
  interpretation, 29–30
  uses, 29
  U.S. RDA, 33, 279*t*
Red blood cells, formation, 112, 117, 188, 570
  hemolysis, 160
  iron, 112
  pernicious anemia, 187
  zinc, 117
Reference man, woman, 98
Reflux esophagitis, 436
Refrigeration of food, 262
Regional enteritis, 445–46
Regional food patterns, 225
Regular diet, 389–90
Rehabilitation, 385–87, **386**
Religion, regulations, Jewish diet, 227–29
  values attributed to food, 221
Renal calculi, 563–67
Renal failure, 554–63

acidosis, 141
biochemical findings, 554–63
calcium deficiency, 108, 555
children, 594
dialysis, 555–56
dietary considerations, 556–58
dietary counseling, 558–60
potassium retention, 131
symptoms, 554–55
Renal osteodystrophy, 555
Renal threshold, glucose, 66, 494
Renal transplants, 563
Renin, 136, **137**
Rennin, 24*t*
Reserpine, 374
Residue, diet low, 446
  definition, 434
Residue-free diet, synthetic, 461, 482
Residue-restricted diet, 446
Respiration, acid-base regulation, 139, 140
Respiratory acidosis, 140
Respiratory alkalosis, 140
Respiratory chain, 92
Respirometer, 94, **94**
Retina, 151, **151**
Retinal, 149
Retinaldehyde, 149
Retinene, 149
Retinoic acid, 149
Retinol, 149, **150**
  equivalents, 150
Retinopathy, diabetic, 491
Retinyl esters, 149
Rheumatic fever, diet, 428
Rheumatoid arthritis, 510
Rhodopsin, 151, **151**
Riboflavin, 175–77
  absorption, 176
  chemistry and characteristics, **173,** 176
  deficiency, 177, **178**
  diet, basic, **177,** 206*t*, **208**
    United States, **9,** 176, 196, 197*t*
  dietary allowances, 31*t*, 33*t*, 176
    Canadian, 684*t*
  discovery, 175–76
  foods, 176–77, 196, 199, 618–40*t*
  functions, 176
  measurement, 176
  physiology, 176
  retention in foods, 177
  storage in body, 176
  summary, 190
Ribonucleic acid, 50, 51, 62
Ribose, 50, 62, 70
Ribosomes, 18, 51
Rice, 174, 175, 204, 246
Rickets, 158, **158**
  adult, 159
  resistant, 158
Ricotta cheese, 232
Risotto alla Milanese, 232
RNA, 80, 81, 108, 117
Romano, 232
Rose, W. C., 43, 53
Rowe elimination diets, 579–80
Roughage. *See* Fiber
Rye, diet without, 462

Saccharin, 265t
Saci, 364
Safflower oil, **530**, 532t
Salicylates, 438
Salmonellosis, 243, 254
Salt, 129, 130
    excess, 10, 310
    iodized, 116
Saponification of fats, 78
Satiety value, foods, 22, 76, 215, 216
Schilling test, vitamin B$_{12}$, 453
School feeding, 322–25, **323**, **324**
    breakfast, 324
    legislation, 322
    type A lunch, 323, **323**
Scopalamine, 256
Scurvy, 166, 168–69, **169**
Seasonings, sodium-restricted diet, 546
Secretin, 21t
Secretion, renal, 134
Seder, 227, **228**
Selenium, 120
    summary, 145
    toxicity, 120, 258
Serine, 44t, 188
Serotonin, 167, 182
Serum hepatitis, 468
Seventh Day Adventists, vegetarianism, 221, 226
Sex factors, diabetes mellitus, 492
    heart disease, 526
    hormones, 81, 159, 160, 288
    obesity, 406t
    osteoporosis, 514
Shashlik, 233
Shigellosis, 254
Shock, insulin, 502
Short-bowel syndrome, 460–61
Sickle cell anemia, 574
Siderophilin, 112
Silicon, 103t
Similac, 306
Sippy diet, 435
Skin, allergic reactions, 578
    diseases, 582–83
    sodium losses, 129
    tests, allergy, 578
    vitamin deficiencies, 153, 177, **178**, 180, 181, 183
    water losses, 126, 127
Skinfold thickness, 405, **405**
Small intestine, **21**, 22–23, 25t, 26
    diseases, 443–49
    surgery, 484–85
Smoking, coronary risk, 526
Snacks, 211, 315, 318, **319**, 322
Social worker, 351
Sodium, 129–31
    absorption, 129
    acid-base balance, 138–39, 141
    active transport, 26
    alginate, 265t
    allowances, adrenocortical therapy, 509
        cardiac disease, 542
        cirrhosis, 471
        hypertension, 550
        nephritis, 553, 554
        pregnancy, 290
        renal failure, 557

balance, regulation, 129
    body, 103t, 129
    deficiency, 129, 130, 547
    diet, basic, 207t
    diet restriction, 542–47
        indications for, 542, 543
        nomenclature, 542
        protein, sodium, potassium controlled, 558–63
    dietary counseling, 548–49
    drugs, 543
    excretion, 126, 129, 135, 136–37
    extracellular fluid, 128t, 129, 137, **137**
    foods, 130, 543, 641–57t
        compounds added, 130, 543
        labeling, **543**, 548–49, **549**
        unit lists, 544–46
    functions, 129
    losses from body, 130
        adrenal insufficiency, 508
        cystic fibrosis, 476
        fevers, 426
        surgery, 480
    metabolism, 129
    osmotic pressure, 135
    pump, 65, 129
    requirements, 129–30
    retention, 130
    summary, 143
Sodium benzoate, 263
Sodium bicarbonate, 373t
Sodium chloride, 129, 130
Sodium-restricted diet, 542–47
Sofrito, 230
Soft diet, 394–95
    mechanical soft diet, 393–94
Soil, effect on nutrients, 36
Solanine, 257
Sopaipillas, 231
Sorbic acid, 265
Sorbitol, 63
Soul food, 229
South, food patterns, 225, 229
Southwestern states, food patterns, 225
Soy-free diet, allergy, 582
Soybeans, 56
    oil, **530**, 532
    textured protein, 247
    toxicants, 257
Spastic colitis, 445
Spastics, cerebral palsy, 595
Specific dynamic action, 97
Spices, flavoring effects, 546
    irritants, 433
Spies, 178, 187
Sprue, 108, 461–62
    anemia, 187, 188
    diet, 462–64
    dietary counseling, 464
    tropical, 464
Stachyose, 609
Standards, food, FDA, 276–77
Staphylococcic food poisoning, 255
Starch, 63
    digestion, 64–65
    modified, infant foods, 308
Starvation, acidosis, 141
    energy metabolism, 95

treatment, obesity, 412
Status foods, 221
Stearic acid, 78, **78**, 79t
Steatorrhea, 456, 460, 476
    test, 452
Steenbock, 149, 155
Sterilization, food, 261
    infant formulas, 305
    irradiation, 264
Steroid hormones, 67, 81
    adrenal insufficiency, 508
    pregnancy, 288
    vitamin role, 156, 167
Sterols, 77, 155
Stomach, acid, 431, 432t, 433
    atony, 431
    cancer, 437
    digestive function, 21, 24t
    diseases, diet, 431–42
    emptying time, 22, 433–34
    enzymes, 24t
    food influence, 433
    gastrectomy, diet, 483
    gastritis, 436–37
    link to hunger, 215
Stress and nutrition, 176, 371–72
Stroke, 527
Strontium-90, 259
Strudel, 229
Strychnine, 256
Succinic acid, **69**
Succus entericus, 25t
Sucrase, 25t
Sucrase-isomaltase deficiency, 459
Sucrose, 25t, 62, 459t
Sucrose-restricted diet, 459–60
Sugar, consumption, 72, **72**
    diet, excess, 10, 72–73
        restricted, 459–60
    sources, 205, 459t
Sugar alcohols, 63
Sulfolipids, 111
Sulfonamides, 373t
Sulfonylurea, 375t, 495
Sulfur, 103, 111–12
    dioxide, food preservation, 265t
    molybdenum, relationship, 120
    summary, 143
    thiamin component, 172
Sunlight, energy, 61, 91
    riboflavin loss, 177
    vitamin D, 157
Surgery, 479–90
    colostomy, 485
    coronary artery disease, 537
    diet, following, 481–82
        preceding, 480–81
    gallbladder, 485
    ileostomy, 485
    jejunoileostomy, 485
    mouth, throat, esophagus, 483
    nutrition, effect, 479
    obesity, 413
    resection, gastric, 483
        small intestine, 484
Surveys, children, 314–15
    diet, 6–8, **7, 9**

HANES, 406t, 571, 572t
    National Nutrition, 10, 168
    older persons, 331
    pregnancy, 285–86
Sustagen, 483t
Sweets, 247, 249t, 250t
Synergism, nutrition/infection, 346–47, **347**
Synthetic low-residue diet, 461, 482
Syria, dietary patterns, 233

Taco, 231
Takaki, 172
Tamales, 231
Tanier, 230
Tapeworms, 256
Taste, sensations, 117, 216–17, **216**
    zinc, role, 117
TCA cycle, 92
Technology, food, 271
Teen-agers, athletes, diet, 322
    dietary allowances, 31t, 316–17
        Canadian, 684–85t
    dietary problems, 321
    food selection, 321t, 322
    growth, 315
    nutritional status, 321
    obesity, 321
    pregnancy, 287, 289, 292t
    snacks, 322
Teeth, calcium turnover, 106
    carbohydrate, 72
    decay, 10, 72, 106
    extraction, diet following, 483
    fluorine, effect, 119
    missing, food choices, 334, 393
    nutrient needs, 105, 119, 152, 167
    selenium, role, 120
Teiglach, 229
Temperature, maintenance in body, 97, 126, 127
    role in food intake, 216
Ten-State Nutrition Survey, 10
Terramycin, 263
Tetany, hypocalcemic, 108, 158–59, 304, 452
Tetracycline, 263, 373t
Tetrahydrofolic acid, 188
Texture, dietary modification, 389–97
Theobromine, 205
Theophylline, 205
Therapeutic nutrition, 389–93
Thermophils, 260, 261
Thiamin, 172–75
    antagonist, 258
    chemistry and characteristics, 172, 173
    deficiency, 175, 518
    diet, basic, **174**, 206t, **208**
        United States, 174, 196, 197t
    dietary allowances, 31t, 33t, 174
        Canadian, 684t
        U.S. RDA, 279t
    discovery, 172
    excretion, 173
    foods, 174, 196, 199, 201, 618–40t
    functions, 70, 173–74
    measurement, 172
    physiology, 172
    pyrophosphate, 109, 172, 173
    retention, foods, 174–75

Thiamin [*Cont.*]
  storage, body, 172
  sulfur, 172
  summary, 190
Thiaminase, 173, 258
Thioctic acid, 189
Thirst, mechanisms, 136, **136**
Threonine, 44*t*, 46, 53*t*, 56
  content in foods, 204, 665–69*t*
Thrombin, 103
Thymine, 50
Thyroglobulin, 115, 116
Thyroid gland, carbohydrate metabolism, 67
  deficiency, 510
  hormones, 67, 115
  iodine, 115
  overactivity, 176, 479, 509–10
  pregnancy, 288
  radioactive iodine, 115
Thyroid-stimulating hormone, 116
Thyrotoxicosis, 509
Thyroxine, 49, 115, 116
Tin, 259
Tocopherol, 159, 160
Tofu, 234
Tolazamide, 495
Tolbutamide, 375*t*, 495
Tolinase, 495
Tonsillectomy, diet following, 483
Topopo, 231
Torta, 233
Tortellin, 232
Tortillas, 232
Toxemia of pregnancy, 286, 287, 294
Toxicity, 256
Toxin, bacterial, food, 255
TPN (triphosphopyridine nucleotide), 179
TPP (thiamin pyrophosphate), 109, 173
Trabeculae, 105
Trace elements, 112–21
Transamination, 51, 182
Transcobalamin, 185
Transferase, 609
Transferrin, 112
Transketolase, 174
Transmagnin, 119
Transmethylation, 186
Transport, active, 26
Transulfuration, 182
Trappists, vegetarians, 226
Tray service, standards, 377
Trematodes, 256
Tricarboxylic acid cycle, 68, **69**, 92
Trichinella, 256, 264
Trichinosis, 256
Triglycerides, 76, **76**, 83
  adipose tissue, 84, **84**
  carbohydrate, effect, 529, 531
  chylomicrons, 83
  hydrolysis, 81
  lipoproteins, 83, 84
  medium-chain, 476
  serum, coronary disease, 527, 531
  synthesis, 85
Triiodothyronine, 115, 116
Trioses, glycolysis, 68
Triparenol, 375*t*

Triphosphopyridine nucleotide (TPN), 179
Triticale, 363
Tropical sprue, 464
Trypsin, 18, 25*t*, 46*t*
  inhibitor, 46, 257
Trypsinogen, 18, 25*t*, 46*t*
Tryptamine, 182
Tryptophan, **42,** 44*t*, 45, 46*t*, 56
  decarboxylation, 182
  foods, 198, 204, 665–69*t*
  load test, 182
  niacin, relationship, 45, 179, 182
  requirement, 53*t*
  serotonin, 167
  vitamin B$_6$ lack, effect, 178
  vitamin C, role, 167
TSH (thyroid-stimulating hormone), 116
Tube feeding, 482–83
  blenderized, 482
  formulas, commercial, 483*t*
  hazards, 482
Tuberculosis, diet, 428–29
  dietary counseling, 429
  vitamin B$_6$ deficiency, 429
Tubule of kidney, 132–33, **133**
Turkey, dietary patterns, 233–34
Typhoid fever, 254
  diet, 427–28
Tyramine, foods high in, 258
Tyrosinase, 118
Tyrosine, 43, 44*t*, 46*t*, 115
  conversion from phenylalanine, 601, **601**
  diet restricted, 607
  foods, 665–69*t*
  thyroxine synthesis, 115
  tyramine, 258
Tyrosinemia, 301, 607
Tyrosinosis, 607
Tyrosyluria, 301, 607

Ulcer, bleeding, diet, 440
  diagnostic tests, 431–33
  dietary considerations, 433–35
  peptic, 437–41. *See also* Peptic ulcer
Ulcerative colitis, 448–49
Undernutrition, 5
  basal metabolism, 95
  factors contributing, 340–43
Underweight, 404, 405, 415–16
  causes, 415
  children, 588
  diet, 415–16
  pregnancy, 286
  problems, 404
  protein deficiency, 420
UNESCO, 11
UNICEF, 361
United Nations, Children's Fund, 361
  Educational, Scientific, and Cultural Organization, 11
  Food and Agriculture Organization, 361
  World Health Organization, 11, 284, 361
United States, cultural food patterns, 224–34
  Department of Agriculture, child nutrition programs, 322–25
    food consumption surveys, 6, **7**
    food safety, 259, **260**
    food stamp program, 357

meat inspection, 274
WIC program, 359
Department of Health, Education and Welfare, Food
and Drug Administration, 274
HANES survey, 406*t*, 571, 572*t*
Public Health Service, 279
Federal Trade Commission, 281
nutrition problems, 8–10
world nutrition, role, 362
Unsaturated fat, 77, 78, **78**, 79*t*
Uracil, 50
Urbanization, influence, nutrition, 342
Urea, 48
cycle, 51, **52**
excretion, 126, 133, 134
formation, 51, **52**, 138
nitrogen source, renal failure, 556
Uremia, 554
Uric acid, 135, 512, 513
stones, 564, 566
Uricase, 118
Urinary calculi, 563–67
diet, acid-ash, 566–67
alkaline-ash, 566–67
calcium-phosphorus restricted, 565–66
oxalate-restricted, 566
etiology, 564
incidence, 564
nature, 563
treatment, 564
Urine, composition, 134–35, 682*t*
obligatory excretion, 126
pH, 139, 564
production, 133–35
testing, diabetes, 493
phenylketonuria, 601
U.S. RDA, 279*t*

Valine, **42**, 44*t*, 46
content of foods, 665–69*t*
maple syrup urine disease, 607–608
requirements, 53*t*
Vanadium, 103*t*
Varicose veins, esophagus, 471
Veal, 242*t*
Vegans, 225
Vegetables, 201, 202, 243–45
amino acids, 669*t*
canned, 244–45
botulism, 255
carbohydrate, 71, 71*t*, 72, 202
Daily Food Guide, **34**, 35
diet, basic, 201, 206*t*, 207
infants, 309
exchanges, 660
food plans, two cost levels, 249–50*t*
frozen, 245
lists, exchanges, meal planning, 400, 660–61, 662
phenylalanine-restricted diet, 605
sodium-restricted diet, 544
minerals, 106, **107**, 110, **110**, **114**, 115, 130, 131
nutrient retention, 175
nutritive values, 196, 197*t*, 201–202, 618–40*t*, 641–57*t*
protein, 54, **55**, 202
purchase, 245
vitamins, 152, **152**, 167, **168**, 177, **177**, 179, **180**, 188,
202

Vegetarians, 56–57, 225–27, 344
definition, 225
health benefits, 226
nutrition, 226–27
phytic acid, 105
protein, 56–57
reasons for, 226
typical foods, 227
vitamin B$_{12}$ deficiency, 187
world prevalence, 225–26
Viandas, 230
Villi, **21**, 23
Viosterol, 155
Vision, vitamin A, 151, **151**
Visual aids, 686–93
Visual purple, 151
Visual violet, 151
Vitamin(s). *See also* individual vitamins
antagonists, 182, 183, 184, 258
classification, 148
dietary allowances, 31*t*
aging, 332
Canadian, 684–85*t*
children, 316–17
infants, 299*t*, 301
pregnancy, 291*t*
U.S. RDA, 279*t*
fat-soluble, 148–65
food sources, selection, 148–49
tables, 618–40, 641–57, 658–59
measurement, 148
megadoses, 169, 183
nomenclature, 148
nutrition education, 189, 192
study, introduction, 148–49
supplementation of diet, 149, 169
synthetic vs. natural, 166
toxicity, 149, 151
water-soluble, 166–71, 172–95
Vitamin A, 149–55
absorption, 150
carotenes, 149–51
chemistry and characteristics, 149, **150**
deficiency, 10, 152, 153–55, **154**
diet, basic, **152**, 206*t*
United States, **9**, 196, 197*t*
dietary allowances, 31*t*, 33*t*
Canadian, 33*t*, 685*t*
U.S. RDA, 279*t*
discovery, 149
food sources, 152, **152**, 618–40*t*
retention, 153
fortification, margarine, 278
functions, 151–52
measurement, 149
precursors, 149
rancidity, 149
storage, 151
summary, 162
transport, 150
vision, 151, **151**, **154**
vitamin-E sparing action, 150, 160
zinc, role, 117
Vitamin-B complex, 172–95
Vitamin B$_1$. *See* Thiamin
Vitamin B$_c$, 187
Vitamin B$_2$, 176. *See also* Riboflavin

Vitamin B$_6$, 181–83
  chemistry and characteristics, **173,** 181
  contraceptives, effect, 183
  deficiency, 182–83, 518
  diet, basic, 207*t*
    United States, 182, 196, 197*t*
  dietary allowances, 31*t*, 182
    Canadian, 684*t*
    pregnancy, 291
    U.S. RDA, 279*t*
  discovery, 181
  foods, 182, 641–57*t*
  functions, 182
  isoniazid, effect, 183, 429
  measurement, 181
  megadoses, 183
  physiology, 181–82
  stores, body, 182
  summary, 190
  transamination, 51, 182
Vitamin B$_{12}$, 85, 185–87
  absorption, 103, 185
  characteristics, 185, **186**
  deficiency, 187, 464, 484, 518, 555, 573
  diet, basic, 207*t*
    United States, 187, 196, 197*t*
  dietary allowances, 31*t*, 186–87
    Canadian, 684*t*
    U.S. RDA, 279*t*
  discovery, 185
  foods, 185–86, 641–57*t*
  functions, 185–86
  malabsorption, phenformin, 495
  metabolism, 185
  Schilling test, 453
  storage, 185
  summary, 191
  vegetarian diet, 227
Vitamin C, 166–71. *See also* Ascorbic acid
Vitamin D, 155–59
  absorption, 156
  calcium utilization, 104, 105, 155–56
  chemistry and characteristics, **150,** 155
  deficiency, 10, 158–59, **158**
  dietary allowances, 31*t*, 156
    Canadian, 685*t*
    U.S. RDA, 279*t*
  discovery, 155
  fortification, milk, 157, 199, 278
  function, 155
  hormone nature, 156
  hypercalcemia, 108
  hypervitaminosis, 158
  measurement, 155
  nomenclature, 155
  precursors, 155
  sources, 156–58
  storage, body, 156
  summary, 162
  synthesis, body, 157
Vitamin E, 150, 159–60
  absorption, 159
  antioxidant effect, 80, 150, 167
  body distribution, 159
  chemistry and characteristics, **150,** 159
  diet, basic, 207*t*
    United States, 160

dietary allowances, 31*t*, 160
  Canadian, 685*t*
  U.S. RDA, 279*t*
  exaggerated claims, 160
  functions, 159–60
  measurement, 159
  physiology, 159
  selenium, influence, 120
  sources, 160, 641–57*t*
  summary, 162
Vitamin G. *See* Riboflavin
Vitamin K, **150,** 160–61
  chemistry and characteristics, **150,** 160–61
  deficiency, 161
  dietary allowances, 161
  functions, 161
  measurement, 161
  newborn, 161, 301
  physiology, 161
  sources, 161
  summary, 162
Vitamin M, 187
Vitasoy, 364
Vivonex, 483*t*
Vomiting, alkalosis, 141
  pregnancy, 293–94

Warburg, 176
Water, 125–27. *See also* Fluids
  balance, 127, 127*t*, 135–36, **136**
    mechanisms, 133, 135–36
  body distribution, 16, 125, 298
    exchange, 135
  edema, 137, 175, 294, 419, 541, 552
  fluoridation, 119
  foods, 126, 618–40*t*
  functions, 125–26
  loss from body, 126–27
  oxidation, 126
  proteins, role, 45
  requirements, 127
    infant, 300
    older persons, 332
  sources to body, 126
Water-soluble vitamins, 166–71, 172–95
Weaning, 303
Weight, body composition, 405–406
  children, gain, 315
  control, 404–405
  desirable, 405
  exercise, 412
  gain and loss, 406
  infants, gain, 298
  pregnancy, 288, **289**
Weight-height tables, boys, 675*t*
  girls, 676*t*
  men and women, 677*t*
Wernicke's syndrome, 521
Wheat, bread, 204
  bulgur, 246
  diet without, for allergy, 581
    for gluten enteropathy, 462–64
  flour, 245
  grain, structure, **203**
  lysine deficiency, 204
  whole-, bread, 246
WHO, 11, 361

WIC program, 359
Wiley, H., 272
Williams, R. J., 183
Williams, R. R., 172, 175
Wilson's disease, 118, 610
    cirrhosis, 471
Women, basic diet, 206*t*
    dietary allowances, 31*t*
        Canadian, 684–85*t*
    height-weight table, 677*t*
    nutrition program, WIC, 359
World, food supply, 11, 362–64
    nutrition problems, 11
World Health Organization, 3, 153, 284, 361
Worm infestation, food, 255–56
Wound healing, nutrition, 479–80

Xanthine, gout, 512
    oxidase, 112, 120, 176, 512
    stones, 564
Xanthomas, hyperlipoproteinemia, 532
Xanthurenic acid, 182
Xerophthalmia, 153
Xerosis, 153
Xylose, 62
    absorption test, 453

Yellow enzyme, 176
Yogurt, 233, 241
Yom Kippur, 227
Yuca, 230

Zabaglione, 233
Zein, 45
Zen macrobiotic diet, 56
Zinc, 117–18
    absorption, 117
    blood, 117, 681*t*
    deficiency, 117, 257
    diet, basic, 207*t*
    dietary allowances, 31*t*, 117
        Canadian, 685*t*
        U.S. RDA, 279*t*
    distribution, body, 117
    food sources, 117, 641–57*t*
    functions, 117
    metabolism, 117
    toxicity, 118
    summary, 145
Zymogen, 18